Diagnosis of Genitourinary Disease

Diagnosis of Genitourinary Disease
Second Edition

Edited by

Martin I. Resnick, M.D.
Lester Persky Professor of Urology
Chairman, Department of Urology
Case Western Reserve University School of Medicine
University Hospitals of Cleveland
Cleveland, Ohio

Robert A. Older, M.D.
Associate Professor of Radiology
Head of Uroradiology
Department of Radiology
University of Virginia Health Sciences Center
Charlottesville, Virginia

*with 768 illustrations
including a color insert*

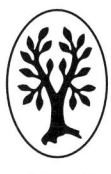

1997
Thieme
New York • Stuttgart

Thieme Medical Publishers, Inc.
381 Park Avenue South
New York, NY 10016

Diagnosis of Genitourinary Disease—Second edition
Martin I. Resnick, M.D.
Robert A. Older, M.D.

Library of Congress Cataloging-in-Publication Data

Diagnosis of genitourinary disease / edited by Martin I. Resnick,
  Robert A. Older.—2nd ed.
    p. cm.
  Includes bibliographical references and index.
  ISBN 0-86577-573-7 (hard). — ISBN 3-13-616902-6 (hard)
  1. Genitourinary organs—Diseases—Diagnosis. I. Resnick, Martin
I. II. Older, Robert A.
  [DNLM: 1. Urogenital Diseases—diagnosis, WJ 141 D5355 1997]
RC874.D47 1997
616.6'075—dc20
DNLM/DLC
for Library of Congress   96-26584
                                                                                             CIP

Copyright © 1997 by Thieme Medical Publishers, Inc. This book, including all parts thereof, is legally protected by copyright. Any use, exploitation or commercialization outside the narrow limits sets by copyright legislation, without the publisher's consent, is illegal and liable to prosecution. This applies in particular to photostat reproduction, copying, mimeographing or duplication of any kind, translating, preparation of microfilms, and electronic data processing and storage.

Important note: Medical knowledge is ever-changing. As new research and clinical experience broaden our knowledge, changes in treatment and drug therapy may be required. The authors and editors of the material herein have consulted sources believed to be reliable in their efforts to provide information that is complete and in accord with the standards accepted at the time of publication. However, in view of the possibility of human error by the authors, editors, or publisher of the work herein, or changes in medical knowledge, neither the authors, editors, publisher, nor any other party who has been involved in the preparation of this work, warrants that the information contained herein is in every respect accurate or complete, and they are not responsible for any errors or omissions or for the results obtained from use of such information. Readers are encouraged to confirm the information contained herein with other sources. For example, readers are advised to check the product information sheet included in the package of each drug they plan to administer to be certain that the information contained in this publication is accurate and that changes have not been made in the recommended dose or in the contraindications for administration. This recommendation is of particular importance in connection with new or infrequently used drugs.

Some of the product names, patents, and registered designs referred to in this book are in fact registered trademarks or proprietary names even though specific reference to this fact is not always made in the text. Therefore, the appearance of a name without designation as proprietary is not to be construed as a representation by the publisher that it is in the public domain.

Printed in the United States of America

5 4 3 2 1

TMP ISBN 0-86577-573-7
GTV ISBN 3-13-616902-6

Contents

Contents v

Contributors vii

Preface xi

1. History and Physical Examination of the Urologic Patient 1
   Mark D. Stovsky, M.D., Martin I. Resnick, M.D.

2. Laboratory Evaluation of the Urologic Patient 13
   Lee Anne Matthews, M.D., Martin I. Resnick, M.D.

3. Urodynamic Studies 21
   Stephen D. Mark, M.B., Ch.B., FRACS, George D. Webster, M.B., FRCS

4. The Abdominal Radiograph 35
   Robert A. Older, M.D.

5. Basic Radiologic Techniques for Imaging the Urinary Tract 45
   Robert A. Older, M.D.

6. Ultrasound of the Genitourinary Tract 79
   William Horstman, M.D., Laurence Watson, M.D.

7. Practical Use of Radionuclides in the Evaluation of Urinary Tract Disease 131
   David Teates, M.D., Jayashree S. Parekh, M.D.

8. Computed Tomography in Urologic Disease: A Practical Guide to the Uses
   and Limitations of CT Scanning 161
   Durba Dutta, M.D., John R. Haaga, M.D.

9. Magnetic Resonance Imaging of the Urinary Tract 179
   Elizabeth D. Brown, M.D., Richard C. Semelka, M.D.

10. *Section 1:* Endourology 205
    Alan D. Jenkins, M.D.

    Section 2: Renal Angiography 220
       John F. Angle, M.D., Charles J. Tegtmeyer, M.D.,
       Alan H. Matsumoto, M.D.

11. Pediatric Uroradiology 231
    Thomas E. Sumner, M.D., Sam T. Auringer, M.D.

12. Urinary Tract Infections 257
    Michael P. Donovan, M.D., Culley C. Carson, III, M.D.

13. Tuberculosis, Fungal Diseases, and Parasitic Diseases of the Urinary Tract 285
    Durwood E. Neal, Jr., M.D. Eric Walser, M.D.

14. Urinary Stone Disease 303
    Bruce I. Carlin, M.D., Martin I. Resnick, M.D.

15. *Section 1:* Urinary Tract Obstruction and Dilatation: Upper Urinary Tract 315
    Robert L. Waterhouse, Jr., M.D.

    Section 2: Bladder Outlet Obstruction 323
    David R. Couillard, M.D., Steve W. Waxman, M.D.,
    George D. Webster, M.B., FRCS

16. Cystic Disease of the Kidney 343
    Kenneth A. Kropp, M.D., Steven Arrowsmith, M.D.

17. The Complex Cystic Mass 349
    Robert A. Older, M.D., Marguerite C. Lippert, M.D.

18. Benign and Malignant Tumors of the Upper Urinary Tract 361
    Marguerite C. Lippert, M.D., Robert A. Older, M.D.

19. Benign and Malignant Tumors of the Lower Urinary Tract 395
    Gabriel P. Haas, M.D., David J. Grignon, M.D., James E. Montie, M.D.

20. Renal Tumors in Children 411
    Sandip P. Vasavada, M.D., Juan G. Corrales, M.D., Jack S. Elder, M.D.

21. *Section 1:* Upper Urinary Tract Trauma 425
    Hunter Wessells, M.D., Jack W. McAninch, M.D.

    Section 2: Lower Urinary Tract Trauma 438
    J. Patrick Spirnak, M.D., FACS

22. Diseases and Imaging of the Prostate 445
    David S. Sandock, M.D., Martin I. Resnick, M.D.

23. Disorders of the Scrotum and Its Contents 465
    David S. Sandock, M.D., Thomas E. Herbener, M.D., Martin I. Resnick, M.D.

24. New Tests for the Diagnosis of Erectile Dysfunction 485
    Mark D. Stovsky, M.D., Allen D. Seftel, M.D., and Thomas E. Herbener, M.D.

25. Neurogenic Bladder 501
    Stephen D. Mark, M.B., Ch.B., FRCSA, George D. Webster, M.B., FRCS

26. Urinary Incontinence 517
    William D. Steers, M.D., Burkhardt H. Zorn, M.D.

27. Diagnosis of Adrenal Disorders 529
    Robert A. Older, M.D., Alexander D. Zwart, M.D., Helmy M. Siragy, M.D.

28. Renal Transplantation 551
    Bashir R. Sankari, M.D., Andrew C. Novick, M.D.

29. Genitourinary Manifestations of HIV Infection 567
    Carole A. Sable, M.D., Brian Wispelwey, M.D.

    Index 577

Contributors

John F. Angle, M.D.
Assistant Professor
Division of Angiography and Interventional Radiology
University of Virginia Health Sciences Center
Charlottesville, VA

Steven Arrowsmith, M.D.
Resident
Department of Urology
Medical College of Ohio
Toledo, OH

Sam T. Auringer, M.D.
Associated Professor of Radiology
Department of Radiology
The Bowman Gray School of Medicine
Wake Forest University
Winston-Salem, NC

Elizabeth D. Brown, M.D.
Research Fellow
Department of Radiology
University of North Carolina Hospitals
Chapel Hill, NC

Bruce I. Carlin, M.D.
Resident in Neurosurgery
Case Western Reserve University
University Hospitals of Cleveland
Cleveland, OH

Culley C. Carson, III, M.D.
Professor and Chief
Department of Surgery
Division of Urology
University of North Carolina Hospitals
Chapel Hill, NC

Juan G. Corrales, M.D.
Assistant Professor of Urology
Department of Urology
San Marcos University School of Medicine
Instituto de Salud del Nino
Lima, Peru

David R. Couillard, M.D.
Fellow, Reconstructive Urology and Urodynamics
Duke University
Division of Urology
Department of Surgery
Duke University Medical Center
Durham, NC

Michael P. Donovan, M.D.
Resident
Department of Surgery
Division of Urology
University of North Carolina Hospitals
Chapel Hill, NC

Durba Dutta, M.D.
Department of Radiology
University Hospitals of Cleveland
Cleveland, OH

Jack S. Elder, M.D.
Director of Pediatric Urology
Rainbow Babies and Children's Hospital
Professor of Urology and Pediatrics
Case Western Reserve University School of Medicine
Cleveland, OH

David J. Grignon, M.D.
Department of Pathology
Wayne State University School of Medicine
Detroit, MI

John R. Haaga, M.D.
Department of Radiology
University Hospitals of Cleveland
Cleveland, OH

Gabriel P. Haas, M.D.
Professor and Chairman
Department of Urology
State University of New York Health Sciences Center
Syracuse, NY

Thomas E. Herbener, M.D.
Section Head, Ultrasound
Department of Radiology
Case Western Reserve University
University Hospitals of Cleveland
Cleveland, OH

William Horstman, M.D.
Assistant Professor of Radiology
Director of Ultrasound of Genitourinary Radiology
Co-director of the Radiology Residency Program
Eastern Virginia Medical School
Norfolk, VA

Alan D. Jenkins, M.D.
Associate Professor of Urology
Department of Urology
University of Virginia Health Sciences Center
Charlottesville, VA

Kenneth A. Kropp, M.D.
Professor of Urology and Pediatrics
Chairman, Department of Urology
Medical College of Ohio
Toledo, OH

Marguerite C. Lippert, M.D.
Associate Professor of Urology
Department of Urology
University of Virginia Health Sciences Center
Charlottesville, VA

Stephen D. Mark, M.B., Ch.B., FRACS
Fellow, Reconstructive Urology and Urodynamics
Division of Urologic Surgery
Duke University Medical Center
Durham, NC

Alan H. Matsumoto, M.D.
Associate Professor
Division of Angiography and Interventional
  Radiology
University of Virginia Health Sciences Center
Charlottesville, VA

Lee Anne Matthews, M.D.
Resident in Urology
Case Western Reserve University School of Medicine
Cleveland, OH

Jack W. McAninch, M.D.
Professor and Vice Chairman
Department of Urology
University of California, San Francisco

Chief of Urology
San Francisco General Hospital
San Francisco, CA

James E. Montie, M.D.
Professor of Urology
University of Michigan
Ann Arbor, MI

Durwood E. Neal, Jr., M.D.
Associate Professor of Surgery/Urology,
  Microbiology, and Internal Medicine
University of Texas Medical Branch at Galveston
Galveston, Texas

Andrew C. Novick, M.D.
Chairman, Department of Urology
Cleveland Clinic Foundation
Cleveland, OH

Robert A. Older, M.D.
Associate Professor of Radiology
Head of Uroradiology
Department of Radiology
University of Virginia Health Sciences Center
Charlottesville, VA

Jayashree S. Parekh, M.D.
Assistant Professor of Radiology
Department of Radiology
University of Virginia Health Sciences Center
Charlottesville, VA

Martin I. Resnick, M.D.
Lester Persky Professor of Urology
Chairman, Department of Urology
Case Western Reserve University School of Medicine
University Hospitals of Cleveland
Cleveland, OH

Carole A. Sable, M.D.
Assistant Professor of Medicine
University of Virginia Health Sciences Center
Department of Internal Medicine
Division of Infectious Disease
Charlottesville, VA

David S. Sandock, M.D.
Resident in Neurology
Department of Urology
Case Western Reserve University
School of Medicine
Cleveland, OH

Bashir R. Sankari, M.D.
Department of Urology
Cleveland Clinic Foundation
Cleveland, OH

Director of Renal Transplantation
Charleston Area Medical Center
Charleston, WV

Allen D. Seftel, M.D.
Assistant Professor of Urology and Reproductive
  Biology
Department of Urology
Case Western Reserve University
Cleveland, OH

Richard C. Semelka, M.D.
Associated Professor of Radiology and Director, MRI
  Division
Department of Radiology
University of North Carolina School of Medicine
Chapel Hill, NC

Helmy M. Siragy, M.D.
Associate Professor
Department of Medicine
Division of Endocrinology and Metabolism
University of Virginia Health Sciences Center
Charlottesville, VA

J. Patrick Spirnak, M.D., FACS
Associate Professor of Urology
Case Western Reserve University School of Medicine

Director of Urology
MetroHealth Medical Center
Cleveland, OH

William D. Steers, M.D.
Associate Professor of Urology
Department of Urology
University of Virginia Health Sciences Center
Charlottesville, VA

Mark D. Stovsky, M.D.
Department of Urology
Case Western Reserve University
University Hospitals of Cleveland
Cleveland, OH

Thomas E. Sumner, M.D.
Professor of Radiology and Pediatrics
Department of Radiology
The Bowman Gray School of Medicine
Wake Forest University
Winston-Salem, NC

David Teates, M.D.
Department of Radiology
University of Virginia Health Sciences Center
Charlottesville, VA

Charles J. Tegtmeyer, M.D.
Professor of Radiology and Anatomy
Chief, Division of Angiography and Interventional
  Radiology
University of Virginia Health Sciences Center
Charlottesville, VA

Sandip P. Vasavada, M.D.
Chief Resident
Department of Urology
Cleveland Clinic Foundation
Cleveland, OH

Eric Walser, M.D.
Assistant Professor of Radiology
Department of Radiology
University of Texas Medical Branch
Galveston, TX

Robert Waterhouse, M.D.
Associate Professor
Department of Urology
Mount Sinai Medical Center
New York, NY

Laurence Watson, M.D.
Director of Ultrasound and Computing
Department of Urology
University of Virginia Health Sciences Center
Charlottesville, NC

Steve W. Waxman, M.D.
Fellow, Reconstructive Urology and Urodynamics
Duke University
Division of Urology, Department of Surgery
Duke University Medical Center
Durham, NC

George D. Webster, M.B., FRCS
Professor of Urologic Surgery
Division of Urologic Surgery
Duke University Medical Center
Durham, NC

Hunter Wessells, M.D.
Clinical Instructor
Department of Urology
University of California, San Francisco
San Francisco, CA

Brian Wispelwey, M.D.
Associate Professor of Medicine
University of Virginia Medical Center
Department of Internal Medicine
Division of Infectious Disease
Charlottesville, VA

Burkhardt H. Zorn, M.D.
Department of Urology
University of Virginia Health Sciences Center
Charlottesville, VA

Alexander D. Zwart, M.D.
Fellow, Division of Endocrinology and Metabolism
Department of Medicine
University of Virginia Health Sciences Center
Charlottesville, VA

Preface

Much has transpired in clinical medicine since the publication of the first edition of this text in 1982. At that time, real time ultrasonography was becoming standard and CT scanning was being widely applied to the evaluation of many organ systems. Such used modalities as magnetic resonance imaging, color flow Doppler, positron emission tomography and radioimmunodetection were only in their developmental stages. Obviously, these latter studies have been and continue to be developed and are becoming commonplace in clinical practice today.

Additionally, many changes have occurred in laboratory technology as well. A most notable example is the development of prostate specific antigen whose widespread clinical use has not only been of value in the diagnosis of patients with carcinoma of the prostate but it is also being increasingly utilized not only for staging purposes but for follow-up purposes as well. New molecular techniques are being developed to more specifically identify cells of various origins that also are of value in the assessment of the specific disease processes. These studies, which were known to be experimental and investigational a decade ago, are in routine application in many hospital and commercial laboratories.

Associated with these new developments has been a decreased utilization of some studies as well. For instance, arteriography that had been routine in many clinical situations has limited used today. Other techniques such as percutaneous aspiration procedures may not be as useful as had been thought or have been replaced by less invasive imaging techniques. In many respects the replacement of invasive studies by more accurate and less invasive ones has been of significant value.

With these technological developments in both imaging departments and clinical laboratories there has been an increasing need to utilize these new studies in an efficacious and cost effective manner. All too often, repetitive examinations are carried out that may provide clinical information in a new format but oftentimes have little impact on the care of the patient. Additionally, some studies are carried out that will not help answer the questions being asked, and more prudent use of the most appropriate study would be a wiser choice. Changes in healthcare economics have in some respects forced these changes but in many respects have resulted in improved and more efficient patient care. The combined editorship of this text by a urologist and a radiologist has ensured that these issues are emphasized.

Further developments will continue. Though the solution of imaging techniques will probably improve it is unlikely that they will be able to determine the presence of microscopic disease. New molecular testing and laboratory studies will probably become of increasing value in patient assessment in the future. However, it is important for clinicians of various backgrounds to continue to interact and cooperate so that the most appropriate studies will be performed.

Martin I. Resnick, M.D.
Robert A. Older, M.D.

1 History and Physical Examination of the Urologic Patient

Mark D. Stovsky, Martin I. Resnick

The history and physical examination are central to the competent management of a patient with a urologic problem. A complete initial evaluation is essential not only for urologists but for primary care physicians, since a large proportion of patients seen by internists, family practitioners, and pediatricians present with complaints concerning the genitourinary system. The skillfully executed preliminary survey should establish a working diagnosis that identifies and guides the need for appropriate confirmatory radiologic and laboratory tests. In addition, a thorough history and physical examination must define the overall medical condition of the patient and identify pertinent findings that might influence the decision to pursue a surgical or medical course of treatment.

THE UROLOGIC HISTORY

Performing an efficient and proficient history is an art that requires substantial medical knowledge and sound clinical judgment. During the patient interview, the clinician must take a subjective complaint and, through directed questioning, elicit a clear impression of the patient's specific problem. The practitioner then extracts additional historical information that either facilitates the diagnosis, promotes the development of an appropriate treatment plan, or assists in general patient management.

The urologic history can be divided into eight broad sections. At the outset, a brief description of the patient's chief complaint is recorded. The chief complaint should be a concise interpretation of the patient's own subjective impression of the problem (e.g., "blood in the urine" or "pain in the side," as opposed to "gross hematuria" or "costovertebral angle tenderness"). The history of present illness should expand upon this short statement to illustrate the details of the current disorder by succinctly describing the period of time over which the problem developed and the pertinent signs and symptoms. Moreover, the history of present illness should outline those aspects of a patient's medical history that are relevant to the current problem (e.g., diabetes mellitus in an individual whose signs and symptoms are consistent with organic impotence).

Other essential components of the urologic history include a medication summary and a list of drug allergies. Many drugs—including a range of antihypertensives, analgesics, neuroleptics, antidepressants, anticholinergics, and endocrine agents—can directly affect the function of the genitourinary system and can be the source of urologic dysfunction. Moreover, an understanding of the patient's current pharmacologic regimen and any known allergic responses to medications is critical in the perioperative management of the patient.

The past medical history is meaningful since many urologic disorders demonstrate either a tendency toward recurrence or chronicity. Renal parenchymal and urothelial tumors, upper and lower tract calculi, and urinary tract infections are examples of common complaints that demonstrate a marked rate of recurrence. Benign prostatic hyperplasia, adenocarcinoma of the prostate, interstitial cystitis, neurogenic bladder dysfunction, and renal artery stenosis are among the myriad processes that may require treatment on a chronic basis. An appreciation of the chronic or recurring nature of urologic disease can, when indicated by the current signs and symptoms, allow the physician to concentrate and focus the investigative effort. Further, information concerning related medical conditions—including diabetes mellitus, hypertension, metabolic disorders, sickle cell anemia, tuberculosis, spinal cord injury, coronary artery and peripheral vascular disease, chronic pulmonary dysfunction, and tobacco/ethanol/illicit drug use—may add diagnostic insight or may significantly alter the management of the patient's urologic disease.

The past surgical history is consequential for two reasons. First, a prior history of abdominal or pelvic procedures makes surgical management technically demanding and compels the clinician to scrutinize and reexamine any planned open, endoscopic, or laparoscopic approach to a particular genitourinary problem. Second, the patient may present with either an early or a late complication of an antecedent operation. The past surgical history should be recorded chronologically and should include any instances of blood product transfusion.

The male sexual function history should document the specific nature of the problem. Many patients regard the term impotence as a catchall for the broad spectrum of disorders of male sexual function. A detailed inquiry must be made that distinguishes between true erectile dysfunction, the loss of sexual desire, the absence of seminal emission, difficulties achieving orgasm, and premature ejaculation. Once the disorder is outlined, a precise clinical investigation may be initiated, including hormonal studies (e.g., LH, FSH, prolactin, and testosterone), an evaluation of penile tumescence, a seminal fluid analysis, and psychological counseling.

Finally, since urologic disorders can have genetic or environmental determinants, comprehensive family and birth histories should be obtained. The family history should emphasize those processes that have established genetic (i.e., prostate adenocarcinoma) or environmental (i.e., bladder transitional cell carcinoma) aggregation patterns.[1] The birth history—including the notation of specific congenital genitourinary defects such as hypospadias, urethral valves, vesicoureteral reflux, duplicated collecting systems, hydronephrosis, and spina bifida/myelomeningocele—is a necessity because many of these anomalies require close follow-up and their long-term urologic sequelae may continue into adulthood.

Urologic Symptoms

PAIN

Urologic disease is typically manifested as a distinct set of symptoms. A comprehensive summary of these clinical indicators is central to a complete history of present illness and serves to direct the investigator to the source of the pathology. An accurate evaluation of pain is of primary importance in distinguishing urologic and nonurologic processes. In general, pain of any origin can be reliably characterized by recording the precipitating or palliating factors, the quality of the discomfort, the severity index, the radiation pattern, and the timing of episodes of discomfort.[2]

A knowledge of factors that induce or alleviate a patient's discomfort can be instrumental in localizing the problem and differentiating pain of urologic origin from abnormalities in other organ systems. For example, severe abdominal tenderness that is relieved by lying completely still is consistent with an intra-abdominal source of peritoneal irritation. Conversely, urologic pain, typically caused by either obstruction or inflammation of the upper or lower urinary tract in the retroperitoneum or pelvis, is commonly distinguished by the inability of the patient to find a comfortable position on the examining table. Similarly, pain of biliary or gastrointestinal etiology, often present in the right or left upper quadrants and frequently indistinguishable from flank pain of urologic origin, is commonly preceded by the consumption of specific substances (e.g., fatty food, alcohol, caffeine) that cause the secretion of either bile or gastric acid. In contrast, upper and lower urinary tract discomfort is not, in general, temporally related to controllable precipitating factors.

The concept of the quality of the discomfort refers to the characterization of pain in abstract terms. Adjectives such as sharp, dull, burning, squeezing, colicky, superficial, and deep are all used to describe the pain of urinary tract dysfunction caused by different pathologic mechanisms. Moreover, information concerning the severity of the pain on a scale from 0 to 10 along with an indication of whether the pain has progressed or improved is valuable in determining the need for further surgical or medical intervention.

The radiation pattern of pain is integral in discriminating urologic from nonurologic processes. Referred pain describes a phenomenon whereby sensory nerves innervating organs that have a similar embryonic origin but have been separated in the developmentally mature individual are stimulated by the same pathologic process. Genitourinary afferent pain fibers travel to the spinal cord with the sympathetic autonomic nerves that comprise the thoracolumbar plexus (spinal cord level T10 to L2) and with the parasympathetic autonomic nerves that form the pelvic plexus (spinal cord level S2 to S4).[3]

Pain of urologic origin, therefore, may be referred to areas that have a somatic sensory innervation that coincides, at the spinal cord level, with the sympathetic distribution of the urinary tract. Additionally, irritation of the subcostal, iliohypogastric, ilioinguinal, or genitofemoral nerves may result in a comparable radiating pattern of discomfort.[4] In comparison, intra-abdominal disorders such as peptic ulcer disease, pancreatitis, and cholelithiasis typically cause pain that radiates to the back and shoulder secondary to stimulation of sensory fibers of the phrenic nerve on the inferior margin of the diaphragm. This information can be used to differentiate these common disorders from upper and lower genitourinary problems that have differing patterns of radiation.

Finally, an accurate illustration of a patient's pain should include the timing of the episodes of discomfort. A painful stimulus caused by obstruction of the collecting system is typically intermittent and colicky, whereas discomfort from inflammation and infection is classically either continuous or occurs consistently after an act such as micturition.

Upper Urinary Tract

The genitourinary system is typically characterized as comprising an upper urinary tract, a lower urinary tract, and the external genitalia. The principal symptoms of upper urinary tract dysfunction include pain, fever, chills, nausea and vomiting, and hypertension. Pain in the upper urinary tract originates in either the kidney or the ureter and is transmitted to the spinal cord via sensory fibers that, as stated earlier, follow the sympathetic autonomic nerves. Painful stimuli that arise in the renal parenchyma are primarily the result of capsular distention from either obstruction of the collecting system, inflammation, or renal ischemia. The direct stimulation of receptors in the mucosa by noxious stimuli has also been postulated.[5]

Discomfort of renal origin during, for example, acute pyelonephritis, is commonly manifested as flank tenderness, which is often present at rest and can be precipitated by abdominal palpation. This tenderness cannot usually be palliated without significant narcotic analgesia and is generally described as a continuous ache of high intensity. Disorders of the kidney generally result in pain that radiates to the costovertebral angle.[6]

Ureteral pain is usually caused by distention of the collecting system from an intra- or extraluminal obstructive process. The most common etiology for a ureteral obstruction is urolithiasis. Other causes include ureteropelvic junction obstruction, blood clot, tumor, stricture disease, and retroperitoneal fibrosis. Tenderness from ureteral or renal pelvic distention typically has no precipitating factors and, depending on the level of pain, can be palliated with a range of medications, from nonsteroidal anti-inflammatory agents to intravenous narcotics.

The pain of renal colic is ordinarily intermittent and is produced by the intrinsic peristalsis of the ureter and renal pelvis that carries urine to the level of obstruction. The resultant increase in intraluminal pressure causes discomfort in direct proportion to the degree of distention of the collecting system.[7] Ureteral discomfort may, however, become steady and continuous after the acute obstructive period. This phenomenon occurs because, in high-grade obstruction, ureteral peristalsis tends to diminish in frequency and magnitude over time. Intraluminal hydrostatic pressure remains high until the obstruction is relieved.[8] During acute obstruction of the collecting system, patients commonly describe a sharp, squeezing pain with variable amplitude.

Ureteral discomfort may be felt in the flank, lower abdomen, groin, or scrotum/labium, depending on the site of the disorder. Upper ureteral obstruction causes pain referred to the flank. Mid-ureteral distention results in discomfort that radiates to the inguinal region. Lower ureteral dilation elicits tenderness in the suprapubic area.[6] It is important to note that distention at any point along the collecting system can produce, in the male, ipsilateral testicular tenderness, which must be differentiated from a primary process of the scrotum, testes, spermatic cord, or, in the female, the external genitalia.

With respect to upper tract pain, two significant caveats must be noted. First, many disease processes can mimic renal or ureteral discomfort. Notably, pathologic processes involving the costovertebral angle regions and the retroperitoneum such as musculoskeletal radiculitis, cholecystitis/cholelithiasis, pancreatitis, and splenomegaly can manifest tenderness very similar to that of upper urinary tract derangements. Conversely, renal and ureteral pain can radiate to the lower abdomen and simulate intra-abdominal disorders such as appendicitis and diverticulitis. Second, many urologic diseases arise insidiously (e.g., chronic pyelonephritis, chronic hydronephrosis, polycystic kidney disease, renal cell carcinoma) and never exhibit overt physical symptoms.[9] Thus, a high index of suspicion and judicious use of appropriate diagnostic tests are necessary when approaching the patient with a presumed urologic difficulty.

Fever and chills can be symptoms of upper urinary tract disorders, including pyelonephritis and perinephric abscess. A history of fever or chills, flank pain, and associated pyuria or bacteriuria is indicative of a severe upper tract infection that may require intravenous antimicrobial treatment. Evidence of urinary infection in combination with upper tract obstruction is particularly alarming and, in general, represents a urologic emergency requiring intervention (e.g., ureteral stent or nephrostomy) to prevent sepsis. Other noninfectious processes, including renal cell carcinoma, may also induce a febrile response by, presumably, a cytokine-mediated pathway utilizing an endogenous pyrogen.[10]

Nausea and vomiting can also comprise part of the symptom complex of upper urinary tract disease. The gastrointestinal and urinary systems have common autonomic and sensory spinal cord pathways. Stimulation of upper urinary tract afferent fibers may, therefore, result in a spinal reflex that activates the stomach or intestinal smooth muscle leading to spasm and, consequently, gastrointestinal (GI) upset.

Hypertension can be a manifestation of underlying renal or adrenal disease. Typically, high blood pressure associated with urologic pathology is uncontrolled and requires a multiple drug regimen for management. Conditions involving the adrenal gland that produce malignant hypertension include aldosterone-secreting tumors and pheochromocytoma. Renal artery stenosis, caused by either atherosclerosis or fibromuscular dysplasia, is the prototypic mechanism for high blood pressure originating in the kidney.

Lower Urinary Tract and External Genitalia

The cardinal indicators of lower urinary tract and external genital disease include pain, irritative voiding symptoms, obstructive voiding symptoms, incontinence/enuresis, male sexual dysfunction, and external genital dermatologic disorders. Pain in the lower urinary tract can arise from the bladder/urethra, penis, prostate, scrotum, or labia/vulva. Discomfort originating in the bladder is generally caused by inflammation or vesical overdistention. The sensory innervation of the urinary bladder is complex. The detrusor is primarily innervated by parasympathetic fibers from the pelvic plexus. Sensory afferent nerves coursing with these parasympathetics are responsible for the perception of stretch and fullness. The bladder outlet receives autonomic innervation predominantly from sympathetic nerves emanating from the thoracolumbar plexus. Sensory fibers carried with this autonomic innervation transmit the sensations of pain, touch, and temperature.[11] This differential innervation gives rise to the unique pattern of referred pain seen in pathologic conditions of the bladder.

Specifically, the discomfort associated with overdistention of the bladder during, for example, acute urinary retention from infravesical obstruction is typically described as a constant, excruciating sensation of pressure. This tenderness is heightened on palpation of the lower abdomen and can only be palliated by decompression of the bladder. The discomfort of vesical overdistention is referred to the suprapubic region. Of note, chronic processes resulting in vesical overdistention (e.g., urinary retention associated with diabetes mellitus and a flaccid neurogenic bladder) do not produce this level of pain, probably owing to a sensory deficit in combination with a mechanism of accommodation to large residual volumes.[12]

In contrast, inflammatory processes involving the bladder/urethra produce intermittent pain, occurring primarily during the act of voiding. These processes generally cause burning on urination (dysuria) that is mild or moderate in intensity. This sensation (seen, for instance, in episodes of acute bacterial cystitis, with bacterial and nonspecific urethritis, or in conjunction with transitional cell carcinoma of the bladder) can only be definitively palliated with treatment of the underlying disorder and commonly radiates to the distal urethra. Inflammatory and infectious diseases of the bladder do not routinely give rise to febrile illness.

Painful stimuli within the penis either are the product of a primary process within the organ or are referred from another segment of the urinary tract. Primary disorders that produce penile discomfort include urethritis, paraphimosis, urethral foreign bodies, priapism, Peyronie's disease, and external dermatologic conditions such as balanitis. Discomfort felt in the penis that is radiated from another area of the urinary tract is usually caused by cystitis with inflammation in the region of the trigone and bladder neck. Penile discomfort may be constant or intermittent, depending on the etiology, and is generally described as a burning/stinging sensation. This discomfort is routinely mild. Severe pain may accompany paraphimosis, urethral foreign bodies, priapism, and balanitis. Penile pain typically does not display a radiation pattern.

Prostatic pain is indicative of an underlying inflammatory process. In most instances, inflammation of the prostate gland occurs during an acute or chronic bacterial infection. During acute bacterial prostatitis, the patient will exhibit a constant, dull perineal ache that becomes exquisitely tender on digital rectal examination. The discomfort is usually associated with systemic signs of infection, including fever and chills. The tenderness of acute prostatic inflammation can only be treated by antimicrobials that exhibit good penetration into the glandular tissue. Inflammation of the prostate gland during chronic bacterial prostatitis, chronic nonbacterial prostatitis, and prostatodynia is represented by intermittent, dull perineal discomfort of mild to moderate severity. These syndromes are not linked with any distinct constitutional symptoms and can only be differentiated through the analysis of expressed prostatic secretions (EPS) obtained by prostatic massage. The cardinal findings in the EPS of chronic bacterial prostatitis include greater than 10 leukocytes per high power field and the presence of fat-laden macrophages (oval bodies). The absence of these findings points to a nonbacterial etiology. Prostatic pain may be referred to broad areas, including the lumbosacral spine, lower extremities, and inguinal regions.[12]

The differential diagnosis of scrotal pain includes diseases of the testes and testicular appendages, epididymis, spermatic cord structures, and scrotal skin/soft tissue. Alternatively, scrotal tenderness may represent referred sensation from disorders of the upper urinary tract (e.g., ureteral obstruction) or groin (e.g., inguinal hernia). The ability to distinguish between these differing mechanisms of scrotal pain is integral to the competent urologic history and physical examination and often represents the difference between surgical exploration of the scrotum and medical management.

Orchitis, epididymitis, and blunt scrotal trauma are the most common causes of acute scrotal pain and must be differentiated from testicular torsion and torsion of an appendix testes or appendix epididymis. These conditions result in severe tenderness that is localized, continuous, sharp and exacerbated by scrotal palpation. Epididymo-orchitis may result in systemic symptoms of acute infection such as fever and chills. Torsion often produces GI reflexes such as nausea and vomiting. The pain of epididymo-orchitis can be palliated by treating the underlying disease (i.e., appropriate antimicrobials to treat probable organisms, including enterobacteriaceae, gonorrhea, and chlamydia). The tenderness of torsion of a testicular/epididymal appendage can be managed with nonsteroidal anti-inflammatory agents. Testicular torsion is a urologic surgical emergency and generally requires operative intervention. Blunt trauma to the scrotal contents can routinely be treated with expectant management. A severe injury may, however, result in testicular rupture or damage to cord structures, necessitating scrotal exploration.

Other processes involving structures of the spermatic cord (e.g., varicocele, hydrocele, spermatocele) can produce pain that is typically described as a constant, mild, vague ache. The discomfort is generally palliated by correction of the underlying anatomic abnormality. Primary disorders of the scrotal skin and soft tissues are uncommon causes of pain and are usually infectious in origin (e.g., cellulitis and Fournier's gangrene). These conditions are associated with severe, sharp, constant tenderness and concomitant high fever, malaise, and possible hemodynamic compromise.

Pain in the labia or vulva can represent a primary abnormality such as an infected Bartholin's cyst or squamous cell carcinoma. Discomfort of the female external genitalia of urologic significance can, however, reflect referred pain from an upper tract obstructive process.

A large percentage of patients seen by the general urologist complain of voiding disorders. Dysfunctional voiding can be divided into two rudimentary symptom complexes—irritative voiding and obstructive voiding.

The irritative voiding symptoms include urinary frequency, urgency, and dysuria. Urinary frequency, an abnormally large number of voids per day, can be a manifestation of several urologic and nonurologic problems and, in general, is caused by either a high urine output or a low bladder capacity. Increased urinary volume can be a result of systemic disease such as diabetes mellitus (DM) or diabetes insipidus (DI). Diabetes mellitus produces polyuria because excess glucose filtered by the glomerulus is not completely resorbed and acts as an osmotic diuretic. In nephrogenic DI, the formation of antidiuretic hormone by the posterior pituitary gland in response to an increase in serum osmolality is intact. The physiologic defect lies in the response of the collecting duct to this hormone. Comparatively, in central DI, there is inadequate production or release of antidiuretic hormone (ADH) by the pituitary.[13]

Both forms of DI result in an increased plasma osmolality and an extremely dilute urine. Nephrogenic and central DI can be differentiated by the patient's response to exogenous ADH. Central DI will exhibit a response to synthetic antidiuretic hormone with a concentrating effect on the urine and a decrease in serum osmolality. Conversely, no effect on urine or plasma osmolality is seen during nephrogenic DI.[13]

Polyuria can also be related to the ingestion of substances such as alcohol or caffeine, which have known diuretic effects. Additional causes of increased urine output are the voluntary consumption of excess fluid in certain dietary plans and the psychogenic polydipsia/polyuria syndrome.

Reduced bladder capacity has a number of etiologies, including inflammation, infravesical obstruction, neuropathic bladder dysfunction, anxiety, and extrinsic compression of the bladder. Inflammatory processes such as bacterial and nonbacterial cystitis, tumor, calculi, foreign bodies, and radiation damage amplify the sensitivity of the bladder and decrease vesical compliance, provoking an urge to void at lower than normal intravesical volumes. Infravesical obstruction is commonly caused by benign prostatic hyperplasia, urethral stricture disease, detrusor/sphincter dyssynergia, and carcinoma of the prostate. In bladder outlet obstruction, frequency occurs secondary to detrusor hypertrophy, which causes vesical instability (compensatory phase) or ancillary to detrusor atony, in which case high residual volumes result in a reduced functional capacity (decompensatory phase).

Neuropathic bladder dysfunction can, in addition to the possibility of detrusor/sphincter dyssynergia, result in urinary frequency if the nerve injury generates a hyperreflexic, poorly compliant bladder. Extrinsic compression of the bladder can occur with large pelvic tumors, ovarian cysts, uterine fibroids, and pregnancy. The emotional status of the patient can also affect bladder function. Anxiety in particular has been shown to increase bladder irritability and cause urinary frequency.[14]

Urinary frequency is comprised of two distinct subtypes—nocturnal frequency (nocturia) and daytime frequency. Though at times induced by the same pathophysiologic mechanisms, nocturia and daytime frequency may not always occur synchronously. The pattern of presentation of these symptoms can help the clinician determine the underlying abnormality. Daytime frequency in the absence of nocturia may be psychogenic. Nocturnal frequency can, however, occur without daytime frequency in several clinical situations. First, patients who develop large amounts of interstitial tissue edema during the day tend to mobilize this fluid when recumbent. The resultant increased intravascular volume leads to greater renal plasma flow, glomerular filtration, and subsequent urine volume. Second, patients who take long-acting diuretics or a diuretic dose in the evening tend to have nocturia in the absence of clinically significant daytime frequency. In urinary frequency of urologic significance, nocturia and daytime frequency should, in some degree, occur simultaneously.

Urgency, the sudden intense desire to urinate, is the result of conditions that contribute to bladder instability. As with urinary frequency, urgency develops when the functional capacity of the bladder is diminished (i.e., infravesical obstruction) or when the sensitivity of the bladder to distention is augmented (i.e., inflammation). Dysuria, as described in the section on lower urinary tract pain, is discomfort during the act of urination. Dysuria signifies an inflammatory process of either the bladder or urethra. Common causes of painful micturition include infection, calculi, tumor, and foreign bodies (e.g., ureteral stents). Pain occurring at the start of urination typically indicates a urethral source, whereas terminal dysuria denotes intravesical pathology.

The obstructive voiding symptoms include hesitancy, decreased force of the urinary stream, terminal dribbling of urine, intermittency, and the sensation of incomplete emptying of the bladder. Hesitancy is difficulty in initiating urination and is an early symptom of obstructive uropathy. When questioned, patients often describe a situation where they must either wait several minutes before micturition will occur or where they must strain to void. A decreased force of the urinary stream, often occurring over several years, is an insidious indicator of a gradually evolving process of bladder outlet obstruction. Terminal dribbling also represents early infravesical obstruction and is marked by an uncontrollable postvoid loss of urine.

Intermittency, the interruption of urination, signifies severe bladder outlet obstruction. Intermittent micturition occurs during the stage of detrusor decompensation or atony when bladder contractions are inadequate to overcome urethral resistance. The increased intra-abdominal pressure generated during straining cannot be sustained indefinitely, giving rise to a "start-and-stop" pattern of voiding. Incomplete emptying of the bladder also reflects more severe obstructive uropathy and is presumptive evidence of a significant postvoid residual volume. In general, patients describe a situation in which they must return several minutes after urination in order to void to completion.

Obstructive voiding is typically the result of conditions such as benign prostatic hyperplasia, urethral stricture disease, and neurogenic bladder dysfunction. Other possible etiologies include prostatic carcinoma and bladder calculi. In cases where the history and physical examination is ambiguous, cystoscopy, cystometry, uroflowmetry, and pressure/flow studies can be useful means to delineate the underlying disease process, to outline the extent of bladder dysfunction, and to follow the course of treatment.

Urinary incontinence, the unintentional loss of urine, can be categorized into four distinct pathophysiologic entities—total, stress, urge, and overflow. In total incontinence (TI), the patient has a continuous loss of urine without relief. The mechanism of total incontinence is the circumvention, either anatomically or functionally, of the external urinary sphincter. Continuous incontinence is the result of either an aberrant urinary fistula (e.g., vesicovaginal), an ectopic ureter, or an ineffective urethral sphincter complex.

Stress urinary incontinence (SUI) is the intermittent leakage of urine during activities that result in an increase in intra-abdominal pressure (e.g., Valsalva, cough, sneeze, exercise). This momentary increase in intra-abdominal pressure causes a concomitant rise in detrusor pressure that overcomes urethral resistance. Three subtypes of SUI have been identified. Type I is defined as stress incontinence with minimal urethral hypermobility and a leak point pressure greater than 20 cm H_2O. Type II is characterized by marked urethral hypermobility, a horizontally positioned urethra at peak intra-abdominal pressure, and a leak point pressure greater than 20 cm H_2O. Type III occurs when the urethra and bladder neck are open at rest with a leak point pressure less than 20 cm H_2O.[15]

Physiologically, SUI can be separated into two broad categories—anatomic incontinence and intrinsic sphincteric dysfunction. Anatomic incontinence (i.e., type I and type II SUI) occurs when there is loss of the pelvic support of the bladder and urethra. Intrinsic sphincteric dysfunction (i.e., type III SUI) results from damage to the urethral urinary sphincter unit.

Urge incontinence (UI) is the periodic loss of urine that follows an intense urge to void. Urge incontinence develops under the conditions of extreme bladder irritability found in obstructive uropathy (e.g., anatomic or neurogenic), bladder inflammation, and neuropathic hyperreflexic bladder dysfunction. Urge and stress urinary incontinence are often found together as part of a mixed picture of voiding dysfunction. These conditions must be differentiated because, whereas a number of surgical options exist for SUI, the treatment of UI is principally medical.

Overflow incontinence (OI) is defined as the leakage of small amounts of urine past a significant infravesical outflow obstruction. Physiologically, overflow incontinence represents the endpoint of extremely severe obstructive uropathy in which the patient, already in urinary retention, develops chronic vesical overdistention and a decompensated hypotonic bladder. In this condition, high residual urine volumes reduce the functional capacity of the bladder and eventually result in intravesical pressures that can overcome the intrinsic resistance of the urethral sphincter. The treatment of overflow incontinence relies on the effective management of the bladder outlet obstruction and the eventual return of intrinsic detrusor tone.

Enuresis is the involuntary loss of urine at night. This phenomenon is quite common in young children and usually resolves over time. Enuresis—particularly when it coexists with daytime incontinence, frequency, fecal soiling, or obstructive voiding symptoms—can signify an anatomic urinary tract defect. In general, children with isolated enuresis without evidence of urinary tract infection do not require a full-scale evaluation.[16] If enuresis coincides with the presence of recurrent infections or occurs in conjunction with any of the aforementioned conditions, laboratory and radiographic investigation of the upper and lower urinary tract is warranted to rule out the possibility of congenital anomalies such as vesicoureteral reflux, neurogenic bladder dysfunction, and ectopic ureter.

Male sexual dysfunction includes erectile impotence, the loss of libido, the absence of seminal emission/orgasm, and premature ejaculation. Erectile impotence can be organic or functional in origin. Organic impotence has a true pathophysiologic mechanism based on a defect in either the neurologic or vascular pathways leading to normal erection. Disease states that can contribute to the development of organic impotence include peripheral vascular disease, diabetes mellitus, spinal cord injury, and hypertension.[17] Essentially, any process that affects penile arterial inflow (e.g., atherosclerosis), cavernosal sinus and penile venous outflow (e.g., Peyronie's disease), or penile neurologic function (e.g., multiple sclerosis) can produce erectile impotence. Functional impotence is generally due to psychogenic factors such as performance anxiety and stress. This type of sexual dysfunction is characterized by the intermittent presence of normal erections that often occur during sleep and are noted in the morning or that develop under conditions where the pressure of adequate performance is allayed.

The loss of libido commonly occurs with advancing age and can be attributed to both psychogenic and hormonal perturbations. Sexual desire is stimulated by adequate plasma levels of androgenic hormones such as testosterone. The release of testosterone, principally by the testes, is regulated by the hypothalamic–pituitary–gonadal axis. Thus, androgen deficiency and, consequently, loss of libido may be caused by diseases of the pituitary or hypothalamus (e.g., tumor or infarction). More commonly, low circulating androgen levels are the result of testicular atrophy. Psychogenic loss of libido can occur at any age and is typically the result of life stresses.

The absence of seminal emission has several possible etiologies. Retrograde ejaculation, which occurs after transurethral resection of the prostate or with the use of alpha receptor blocking antihypertensive medication, can lead to a marked decrease in seminal volume. Further, processes affecting the sympathetic autonomic innervation of the prostate and seminal vesicles that can occur in systemic disease such as diabetes mellitus, after spinal cord injury, or during retroperitoneal surgery can result in an alteration of seminal emission.[18,19] Moreover, circulating androgen levels have a direct effect on prostatic and seminal vesicle glandular function. Androgen deficiency can therefore result in a low semen volume.

The mechanism of orgasm, while still not clearly understood, is thought to be under central nervous system control. The absence of orgasm may be functional, and its treatment should include a thorough psychologic evaluation. Premature ejaculation is generally thought to be psychogenic in nature and may be the result of generalized stress, performance anxiety, or unrealistic expectations regarding the sexual experience.[20]

External genital dermatologic disorders in the male and female are routinely treated by the practicing urologist. Dermatologic problems of the male genitalia include infection (balanitis) involving the glans, penile shaft, scrotum, or labia/vulva. Genital infections may be bacterial, fungal, viral (i.e., condyloma acuminata or herpes simplex), or parasitic. Neoplastic lesions rarely occur on the male genitalia but include precancerous growths such as leukoplakia and balanitis xerotica obliterans as well as benign processes such as giant cell condyloma (Buschke-Lowenstein tumor). Carcinoma in situ (Bowen's disease and Erythroplasia of Queyrat) and frank squamous cell carcinoma are extremely uncommon in both the male and female populations in the Western Hemisphere. Their appearance ranges from small erythematous plaques to large papillary or ulcerative lesions. Other inflammatory disorders of the external genitalia can be seen such as contact/atopic dermatitis, intertrigo, lichen sclerosis et atrophicus, and drug reactions.

UROLOGIC SIGNS

A number of signs of genitourinary disease, often detected by the patient, can be confirmed and evaluated at the time of the initial history and physical examination. These signs include changes in the character of the urine, abnormalities in the appearance of the seminal fluid, urethral discharge, abdominal masses, scrotal masses, gynecomastia, and virilism.

Changes in the character of the urine primarily involve color. Discoloration of the urine often indicates underlying urologic abnormalities such as hematuria, pseudohematuria, pyuria, fecaluria, and chyluria. The urinalysis and microscopic examination of the urine are critical steps in the initial survey of the urologic patient and should be performed at the time of the history and physical exam.

Hematuria, red blood cells in the urine, is the most common alteration in urine character. Hematuria encompasses two main forms: gross and microscopic. Gross hematuria can be further described as initial, terminal, or total based on the timing of its appearance during micturition. Initial gross hematuria suggests a lesion in the anterior urethra (e.g., urethral stricture disease). Terminal gross hematuria routinely arises from the prostatic urethra, vesical neck or bladder (e.g., BPH, TCC of the bladder). Total gross hematuria reflects a source of bleeding in the bladder or upper urinary tract. Associated symptoms such as dysuria should be noted and can help to differentiate hematuria of infectious origin from other etiologies. An important caveat is that painful urination in conjunction with gross or microscopic hematuria, while often related to uncomplicated urinary tract infection, may indicate a more serious condition such as a secondarily infected tumor.

Blood in the urine is never a normal finding, and its presence should stimulate a thorough urologic investigation. The differential diagnosis of hematuria includes urolithiasis, upper and lower tract neoplasms, infection, trauma, hematologic dyscrasias (e.g., sickle cell anemia), polycystic kidney disease, and the glomerulonephritides. Several conditions, including menstruation and intense physical exercise, can produce hematuria that does not originate in the urinary tract. An adequate urologic evaluation for hematuria should include a microscopic examination of the urine for leukocytes, erythrocytes, bacteria, and casts. In addition, urine cytology to detect malignant cells should be obtained. The radiologic investigation should include studies of the upper tract (e.g., IVP or ultrasound) and cystopanendoscopy.

Pseudohematuria is reddish discoloration of the urine that mimics true hematuria. Pseudohematuria is caused by myriad agents, including food pigments (i.e., beets), phenazopyridine hydrochloride (pyridium) used to treat bladder irritability, rifampin for the treatment of tuberculosis, and the phenothiazine class of neuroleptic drugs.

Pyuria is white blood cells in the urine; it suggests an inflammatory process in the urinary tract and is often noted as "cloudy" urine macroscopically. Pyuria may accompany infections of the bladder and kidney. Approximately 50 percent of patients with clinically significant bacteriuria do not, however, exhibit pyuria.[21] A urine culture should always be sent when the clinical situation is consistent with urinary tract infection (UTI). Conversely, leukocyturia may be present in the absence of infection as a component of the inflammatory response propagated by tumor, urolithiasis, and foreign bodies. "Sterile pyuria" may also suggest urinary tuberculosis, and a culture for acid-fast bacilli should be done if a source of inflammation cannot be found, because active tuberculosis (TB) infections have displayed an epidemiologic resurgence in the last decade. A finding of more than three white blood cells (WBC) per high power field suggests clinically significant pyuria.

Fecaluria and chyluria are distressing causes of changes in urine character. Fecaluria describes the presence of macroscopic intestinal contents in the urine and is pathognomonic for a fistulous connection between the urinary tract and the bowel. Chyluria indicates a urinary-lymphatic fistula and is a result of lymphatic obstruction above the level of the kidneys. Chyluria is caused by such processes as filariasis, tuberculosis, and retroperitoneal tumors, and as a complication of surgery.

Pneumaturia, which is air in the urine, in the absence of an indwelling catheter, suggests the presence of an enterovesical fistula. These fistulas are commonly the result of a primary inflammatory process in the intestine such as

Crohn's disease or diverticulitis and require surgical correction. Malignancies typically originating in the sigmoid colon are another less common cause of this problem. Rarely, pneumaturia can represent infection in the urinary tract with gas-forming bacteria.

Abnormalities in the appearance of the seminal fluid comprise two major conditions—hematospermia and low semen volume. An abnormally low semen volume can result from a number of pathologic mechanisms, as described in the section on male sexual dysfunction. Hematospermia, gross blood in the ejaculate, typically reflects an inflammatory process within the prostate or seminal vesicles. Hematospermia occurring at the beginning of ejaculation is generally of prostatic origin, whereas terminal hematospermia typically arises from the seminal vesicles. Prostatitis is the most common cause of a bloody ejaculate. Other etiologies are rare and include prostatic carcinoma, transitional cell carcinoma of the prostatic ducts, and urinary tuberculosis.[22]

Urethral discharge is a common affliction and indicates infection of the lower urinary tract. The likely etiologies of purulent urethral discharge include urethritis caused by neisseria gonorrhea, chlamydia trachomatis, trichomonas vaginalis, and ureaplasma urealyticum. Urethritis by these sexually transmitted organisms may be accompanied by pruritis, dysuria, and hematuria. It is essential that urethral swab cultures be obtained and placed in appropriate media for growth and identification.

Abdominal masses can be the exclusive presenting complaint in a subset of patients, particularly in the pediatric population. The most common mass lesion of urologic significance in the neonate is congenital ureteropelvic junction obstruction. After the neonatal period, hydronephrosis becomes predominant. Other abdominal masses in childhood include multicystic and polycystic kidney, solid renal tumors (e.g., mesoblastic nephroma and Wilm's tumor), and neuroblastoma.[23] Abdominal masses are rarely the presenting complaint in adults. One exception, however, is a midline mass representing an overdistended bladder from chronic infravesical obstruction and urinary retention in the debilitated patient. Adults being evaluated for urinary tract masses should be questioned about the coexistence of hematuria, weight loss, and, in males, the sudden emergence of a varicocele indicating venous obstruction by a tumor thrombus typically originating in the kidney.

Scrotal masses within the testes are evidence of malignancy (i.e., seminoma or nonseminomatous germ cell tumor) until proven otherwise. Testicular torsion, especially in the newborn, may also display characteristics of a scrotal mass lesion. Varicoceles, spermatoceles, hydroceles, hematoceles, and inguinal hernias are benign scrotal masses that are distinct from the testes. These lesions can be differentiated by history, transillumination, and palpation. Malignant tumors of the spermatic cord structures such as rhabdomyosarcoma are extremely rare components in the differential diagnosis of a scrotal mass.

Gynecomastia and virilism are often evaluated by the urologist. Gynecomastia, the aberrant formation of breast tissue, can develop as part of the syndrome of germ cell and non–germ cell testicular tumors because of the circulation of estrogenic substances (i.e., choriocarcinoma and Sertoli/Leydig tumors). Gynecomastia is also often seen during hormonal treatment of advanced prostate carcinoma with a luteinizing hormone-releasing hormone (LHRH) agonist or diethylstilbestrol (DES). The complaint of virilism, the development of an abnormal male genital phenotype, should, in the pediatric population, prompt a search for congenital adrenal hyperplasia. In adults, the formation of atypical male secondary sexual characteristics can suggest the presence of an adrenal adenoma/adenocarcinoma or a non–germ cell testicular neoplasm. These syndromes can also be idiopathic and reflect abnormalities in the hypothalamic–pituitary–gonadal axis.

THE UROLOGIC PHYSICAL EXAMINATION

General Principles

A skillful physical examination is essential to the overall evaluation of the urologic patient. In combination with a competent history and astute use of appropriate laboratory and radiologic tests, the physical exam can define the urologic problem and lead to an accurate and precise diagnosis. The examination of the patient with a genitourinary problem should utilize the time-tested principles of inspection, percussion, auscultation, palpation, and transillumination.

Prior to beginning the specific genitourinary examination, the practitioner should assess the general medical condition of the patient. In particular, attention should be paid to the cardiovascular and respiratory systems, and any abnormalities during auscultation of the heart and lungs or on palpation of the peripheral arterial system should be noted. A brief neurologic evaluation should also be done. This abbreviated general survey will identify problems that may require further review before medical or surgical management of the urologic disorder is undertaken. Care should be taken at this time to record any systemic stigmata associated with genitourinary disease such as a sacral skin dimple, lymphadenopathy, cachexia, gynecomastia, and virilization.

The Abdominal Examination

During the abdominal examination, the kidneys, bladder, inguinal regions, and bony pelvis are surveyed. The abdominal examination begins with a general inspection. During this stage any evidence of abdominal, retroperitoneal, or pelvic surgical scars or ostomies should be noted. If the patient has a surgical problem, the choice of operative approach may be dictated by these landmarks.

The kidneys are generally examined by palpation, auscultation, and percussion. Palpation of the kidneys is performed with the patient in the supine position. In this position, one hand is placed in the costovertebral angle and the other on the anterior abdomen inferior to the costal margin.

Upon deep inspiration, palpation of the kidneys is achieved as they are pushed caudad by the diaphragmatic excursion. Direct palpation of the kidneys in the adult is extremely difficult owing to the developed layer of subcutaneous fat and the flank musculature. This exercise is executed primarily to elicit tenderness of renal origin and to identify large flank masses. In contrast, palpation of the kidneys in the child is easily done with this maneuver. Auscultation of the abdomen is performed, again in the supine position, in the midclavicular line just inferior to the tenth rib to identify vascular bruits that may indicate an aneurysm, stenosis, or arterial-venous malformation involving the renal vasculature. Percussion of the kidneys is enacted with the patient sitting upright and is done by gently striking the closed fist upon the costovertebral angle. Percussion can serve to localize flank pain to the kidney or ureter and is a sensitive test for identifying upper urinary tract inflammatory and obstructive processes.

The urinary bladder can be surveyed by inspection, percussion, and palpation in the supine position. In an adult, the normal bladder does not become identifiable abdominally until it reaches a volume of 150 mL. At normal adult capacity (approximately 400 mL), the bladder may be visualized as a mass or as mild distention superior to the pubic symphysis. In instances of chronic urinary retention, the distended bladder can reach the level of the umbilicus. In the child, the distended bladder is essentially an abdominal organ lying outside the true pelvis. Therefore in cases of outlet obstruction (e.g., posterior valves and neurogenic bladder dysfunction), the bladder can be readily inspected as a midline abdominal mass. Percussion of an abdominal mass perceived to be the urinary bladder should begin at the level of the pubis and should proceed toward the umbilicus. The distended bladder can be identified by its dull pitch. The bladder outline can be delineated by comparing this dullness to the resonant pattern of gas-filled bowel. Palpation of the bladder is best executed under general anesthesia using a bimanual technique to feel the bladder between the anterior abdominal wall and vagina (female) or rectum (male). In this fashion, the wall thickness and degree of mobility of the organ can be elucidated.

When indicated, the bony pelvis should be palpated with the patient in the supine position. In most cases, suspicion of a bony injury occurs after blunt abdominopelvic trauma. The pelvis is evaluated by placing the hands on the anterior superior iliac crests and inflicting even downward pressure. In this way, an attempt is made to elicit pain or crepitance that may distinguish a pelvic fracture.

The External Genital Examination

The male external genitalia are examined by inspection and palpation in the supine and standing positions. First, the glans and shaft are visually surveyed. Inflammation of the glans and foreskin (balanoposthitis), phimosis (the inability to retract the prepuce), paraphimosis (the inability to replace the prepuce), and any external lesions are noted. The inspection should proceed carefully and should allow the clinician to clearly identify the lesions of condyloma acuminata, syphilis, chancroid, lymphogranuloma venereum, granuloma inguinale, and genital herpes simplex as well as the erythematous lesions of carcinoma in situ and frank squamous cell carcinoma. Any urethral discharge should be cultured and the meatus should be inspected and its position described in relation to the tip of the glans.

In the male child, epispadias (dorsal positioning of the meatus) and hypospadias (ventral positioning of the meatus) should be recorded along with any torsion of the shaft or chordee (ventral curvature). The degree of hypospadias should be determined and characterized in terms of its position on the penile shaft (i.e., glanular, coronal, distal shaft, mid-shaft, proximal shaft, penoscrotal, scrotal, and perineal). In addition, the size of the penis in relation to age, the distribution of pubic hair, and any other congenital phenotypic defects should be ascertained.

Palpation of the penis should include a separation of the urethral meatus to evaluate meatal stenosis. The shaft of the penis must be palpated and cavernosal plaques indicating Peyronie's disease should be recognized. Further, the ventral urethra should be examined. Pain in this area may be secondary to infection of the periurethral glands subsequent to acute urethritis.

Examination of the scrotum and inguinal regions should next be performed. Inspection of the scrotal skin will reveal dermatologic disorders such as dermatitis, eczema, seborrhea, and intertrigo as well as infected sebaceous cysts and interstitial edema. The lesions of condyloma acuminata can be hidden by the scrotal folds. A dilute ascetic acid solution (3 to 5%) will often turn these lesions white and allow identification. The hernia exam should be executed with the patient standing. During the hernia examination, the index finger is gently inserted via the lateral scrotum into the external inguinal ring. The patient is then asked to perform a Valsalva maneuver and the hernia sac, if present, is palpated projecting through the inguinal canal at the level of the external ring.

The examination of the testes and spermatic cord is done in both the supine and standing positions. These structures are evaluated principally through palpation and transillumination. First, the presence of paired testes should be demonstrated. If a testis is not present in the scrotum, a clear determination between a retractile testis and true cryptorchidism (undescended testis) must be made. A retractile testis can usually be found inferior to the external ring and can easily be brought into the base of the scrotum. An undescended testis may be impalpable (i.e., abdominal or congenitally absent) or may be found either in the inguinal canal, along the course of the spermatic cord inferior to the external inguinal ring or in an ectopic location (e.g., suprapubic, femoral, perineal, etc.).

The testicular examination should begin by palpating each testis between the thumb and forefinger using the other hand to stabilize the spermatic cord. The size of the testis should be compared to age-matched controls (adult size approximately 3 to 4.5 cm in longest dimension). The consistency of the normal testis is firm, smooth, and rubbery. Any deviation from a smooth contour and any focal nodularity should be regarded as a mass lesion. Testicular appendages may also be palpable. The cremasteric reflex should be elicited, particularly in the evaluation of testicular torsion. This reflex is evoked by stroking the medial skin of the thigh with the examiner's thumbnail. In an intact cremasteric reflex, this action should stimulate a brief contraction of the cremasteric fibers and cause retraction of the testis. Although its presence cannot be relied on to rule out a torsion completely, the absence of this reflex does add contributory evidence that torsion of a testis has occurred.

The spermatic cord, from the epididymis to the external inguinal ring, should be examined sequentially. Epididymal appendages may be palpable emanating from the head and body of the structure. The epididymis should be distinct from the testis. This separation is of primary importance in distinguishing epididymal pain (i.e., epididymitis) from torsion. If this distinction is not clear, a scrotal ultrasound may be warranted, in the appropriate clinical setting, to clarify the situation.

Masses arising from the epididymis and proximal spermatic cord are generally benign. The most common mass lesions in this area are hydroceles, spermatoceles, varicoceles, and hematoceles. If a mass is felt, transillumination should be accomplished with a concentrated light source in a darkened room. Fluid-filled masses will glow red, whereas a solid lesion will fail to illuminate. The existence of a varicocele (dilated spermatic vein), usually on the left owing to the venous drainage of the left spermatic vein into the renal vein, should be noted. The classic description of a varicocele as an engorged "bag of worms" is quite accurate. The presence of a varicocele can be confirmed by palpation in the supine position, which should result in a diminution of the venous dilation produced when the patient is standing. Finally, the vas deferens should be found in the scrotum by gently squeezing the spermatic cord structures between the thumb and index finger. The vas should be identified bilaterally and traced to its origin in the tail of the epididymis.

The female external genital and pelvic examinations are done in the dorsal lithotomy position. First, the external genitalia are inspected for congenital anomalies such as fused labia and clitoromegaly as well as for dermatologic disorders such as infected Bartholin's cysts. Next, the bimanual examination is executed to detect cervical motion tenderness (i.e., pelvic inflammatory disease) and any adnexal masses. The vaginal speculum is then placed and any urethral or cervical exudate is cultured. A Papanicolaou (PAP) smear can be taken at this point. The urethra is then palpated through the anterior vaginal wall to detect the presence of diverticula and urethral prolapse. Any evidence of a cystocele, rectocele, enterocele, or vaginal prolapse should be noted; a Marshall test or Valsalva maneuver also can be done to reveal the presence of stress urinary incontinence.

The digital rectal examination (DRE) is integral to the complete physical examination of the urologic patient and must be performed in both male and female patients. This portion of the urologic physical examination can be effected in either the lateral decubitus position or the standing position with the patient leaning on the elbows. The anus should be visually inspected, and external hemorrhoids, fissures, fistulas, and anal sensation should be noted.

A well-lubricated, gloved index finger should then be inserted into the rectum gently and the sphincter tone assessed. The bulbocavernosus reflex should be elicited in any patient being evaluated for neurogenic urinary tract dysfunction. This reflex is based upon the shared sensory innervation of the glans/clitoris and the anal sphincter. Afferent somatic fibers travel from these anatomic structures via the pudendal nerve to sacral spinal levels 2 to 4. With an intact spinal reflex arc, gentle compression of the glans or clitoris should result in contraction of the anal sphincter. The absence of this reflex indicates a sacral nerve injury such as spina bifida occulta. A stool sample should be tested for occult blood, and any palpable rectal masses should be further appraised with proctoscopy.

In males, the prostate is examined by sequential palpation of the lateral lobes from apex to base. Although it is difficult to assess the size of the gland accurately by DRE, the classification of prostatic enlargement as either mild, moderate, or severe is advisable. The anterior and median lobes are not palpable during the digital rectal examination and may give rise to symptomatic benign prostatic hyperplasia (BPH) in the presence of a normal-sized gland. The contour of the gland should be smooth, and any irregularity should be recorded. The consistency of the normal prostate resembles that of the thenar muscles. The normal architecture of the prostate includes the lateral sulci and a median furrow. The loss of these elements may indicate either BPH or extension of cancer to the periprostatic region. A boggy, exquisitely tender gland usually indicates acute bacterial prostatitis. Induration of the gland is suggestive of early prostatic cancer but may also represent scarring from chronic prostatitis. A "rock-hard" prostate nodule is generally pathognomonic for adenocarcinoma. Any clinically significant irregularity or nodule should be biopsied to detect prostatic carcinoma at an early stage.

Dedication

This chapter is dedicated to my parents, Alyce and Robert Stovsky.

REFERENCES

1. Stamey T, McNeal J: Adenocarcinoma of the prostate. In Walsh P, Retik A, Stamey T, Vaughan E, eds.: *Campbell's Urology*, 6th ed. Philadelphia: WB Saunders, 1992;1159–1160.

2. Levien D: The History and Physical Examination. *Introduction to Surgery*. Philadelphia: WB Saunders, 1987;4–5.
3. Warwick R, Williams P: The urogenital system. *Gray's Anatomy*, 36th ed. Philadelphia: WB Saunders, 1980;1385–1409.
4. Kabalin J, Tanagho E: Surgical anatomy of the genitourinary tract. In: Walsh P, Retik A, Stamey T, Vaughan E, eds. *Campbell's Urology*, 6th ed., Philadelphia: WB Saunders, 1992;39–45.
5. Tanagho E: Surgical anatomy of the genitourinary tract. In: Walsh P, Retik A, Stamey T, Vaughan E, eds. *Campbell's Urology*, 6th ed. Philadelphia: WB Saunders, 1992;40.
6. Mclellan A, Goodell H: Pain from the bladder, ureter and kidney pelvis. *Res Publ Assoc Nerv Ment Dis* 1942;23:252.
7. Wyker A: Standard diagnostic considerations. In: Gillenwater J, Grayhack J, Howards S, Duckett J, eds. *Adult and Pediatric Urology*, 2nd ed. St. Louis: Mosby Year Book, 1991;66.
8. Wyker A: Standard diagnostic considerations. In: Gillenwater J, Grayhack J, Howards S, Duckett J, eds. *Adult and Pediatric Urology*, 2nd ed. St. Louis: Mosby Year Book, 1991;67.
9. Hinman F Jr: Differential diagnosis of flank pain. *Probl Urol* 1989;3:179.
10. McAninch, J: Symptoms of Disorders of the Genitourinary Tract. *Smith's Urology*, 13th ed. Norwalk, CT: Appleton and Lange, 1992;30.
11. Tanagho E: Surgical anatomy of the genitourinary tract. In: Walsh P, Retik A, Stamey T, Vaughan E, eds. *Campbell's Urology*, 6th ed. Philadelphia: WB Saunders, 1992;45.
12. Lowe F, Brendler C: History, physical examination and urinalysis. In: Walsh P, Retik A, Stamey T, Vaughan E, eds. *Campbell's Urology*, 6th ed. Philadelphia: WB Saunders, 1992;308.
13. Verney E: The antidiuretic hormone and the factors which determine its release. *Proc R Soc Lond* (Biol), 1947;25:135.
14. Straub L, Ripley H, Wolf S: Disturbances of bladder function associated with emotional status. *JAMA* 1949;141:1139.
15. Blaivas J, Olsson C: Stress incontinence: classification and surgical approach. *J Urol* 1988;139:727.
16. Kass E, Diokno A, Montealegre A: Enuresis: principles of management and result of treatment. *J Urol* 1979;121:794–796.
17. Newman H, Marcus H: Erectile dysfunction in diabetes and hypertension. *Urology* 1985;26:135.
18. Kedia K, Markland C: The effect of pharmacologic agents on ejaculation. *J Urol* 1975;114:237.
19. Kedia K, Markland C, Fraley E: Sexual function following high retroperitoneal lymphadenectomy. *J Urol* 1975;114:237.
20. Masters W, Johnson V: Principles of the new sex therapy. *Am J Psychol* 1976;133:548.
21. Kass E: Asymptomatic infections of the urinary tract. *Trans Assoc Am Physicians* 1956;69:56.
22. Lowe F, Brendler C: History, physical examination, and urinalysis. In: Walsh P, Retik A, Stamey T, Vaughan E., eds. *Campbell's Urology*, 6th ed. Philadelphia: WB Saunders, 1992;311.
23. Elder J, Klacsmann P, Sanders R, et al: Clinicopathological conference: flank mass in the neonate. *J Urol* 1981;126:94.

2 Laboratory Evaluation of the Urologic Patient

Lee Anne Matthews, Martin I. Resnick

Laboratory studies are an integral part of the urologist's diagnostic armamentarium for solving clinical problems. While the urinalysis and the determination of renal function have remained the cornerstones of the urologic evaluation, laboratory studies for prostate cancer have continued to evolve. Serum acid phosphatase, once considered the gold standard tumor marker for prostate cancer, has now been replaced by prostate specific antigen (PSA). This chapter will review laboratory studies available to the urologist and the role PSA has assumed in the evaluation and management of prostate cancer.

URINALYSIS

The complete urinalysis consists of a chemical and microscopic analysis. Its reliability depends on careful collection technique, prompt and proper preparation, and experience of the examining physician.

Collection Technique

Since most urethral bacteria are voided in the initial stream, a midstream voided specimen should be obtained to reduce contamination of the bladder urine. In the adult female patient, the labia are spread with the fingers and the urethral meatus is cleansed with soap and water in a front-to-back motion. In the uncircumcised male, the foreskin is retracted and the glans is washed with soap and water. Urethral catheterization should not be used routinely for collection of a urinary specimen, as there is a 1 to 2% risk of introducing bacteria and subsequently causing an infection.[1] However, when catheterization is necessary (i.e., when the patient cannot void after hydration or is debilitated), aseptic technique is mandatory.

Suprapubic bladder aspiration is another technique available for urine collection, particularly in a neonate or a young child in whom a reliable, clean voided specimen cannot be obtained. It is helpful to have a full bladder, then a site 2 cm above the pubic symphysis is anesthetized and a 20-gauge needle is inserted directly into the bladder. Ultrasound guidance is helpful when the bladder cannot be palpated.

Gross Inspection of Urine

The urinalysis should be performed on a fresh urine specimen or one that has been refrigerated. Urine that has been sitting for more than an hour at room temperature will result in lysis of cells. Fresh voided urine is usually clear; however, cloudy urine is common and is usually caused by excessive crystals. In alkaline urine, these are usually amorphous phosphates, and in acid urine they are amorphous urates. These crystals are clinically insignificant and can be dissolved readily by adding acid to alkaline urine with amorphous phosphates or by heating acid urine with amorphous urates. Pyuria is another important cause of cloudy urine.

Specific Gravity

Specific gravity is a measure of urine's tonic state, and it reflects the kidney's ability to concentrate or dilute urine. The presence of other substances in the urine such as glucose or protein will also have an effect on its value. The specific gravity of urine ranges between 1.003 and 1.040. Its value should be determined prior to microanalysis because a specific gravity of less than 1.007 may cause lysis of red blood cells (RBCs). Therefore, the microanalysis can be negative even though the dipstick will detect the free hemoglobin.[2]

Dipstick Analysis

The dipstick analysis uses chemical assays to determine urine pH and to detect the presence of protein, glucose, ketones, bilirubin, blood, nitrites, and leukocyte esterase. The dipstick is immersed in fresh uncentrifuged urine and is then held horizontally to prevent mixing of adjacent reagents. Urinary pH is useful in the evaluation of urinary tract infections and stone disease. An alkaline pH (greater than 7.5) with concurrent infection suggests a urea-splitting organism, most commonly *Proteus*. These patients are more likely to have struvite calculi.

Acid urine favors cystine and uric acid calculi. Alkalinization of the urine plays an important therapeutic role in managing these patients. Urine pH also helps confirm the diagnosis of renal tubular acidosis. Inability to acidify one's urine below 5.5 despite an acid load is indicative of this disorder.

Protein, bilirubin, glucose, and ketones should not be detected on dipstick analysis. Although the kidney does excrete small amounts of protein and glucose, the amounts are below the sensitivities of the dipstick. If any of these substances are detected in the urine, a medical evaluation should be performed. The dipstick for blood detects intact erythrocytes, free hemoglobin from lysed cells, and myoglobin. Since normal individuals excrete approximately 1000 RBCs per milliliter of urine, a high urine specific gravity may cause a false-positive in the dipstick by concentrating the normal volume of RBCs.[3]

Two biochemical tests have been developed to aid in the detection of bacteriuria and pyuria. The Griess test identifies bacteriuria by detecting nitrites, which are normally absent in urine. Many gram-negative bacteria convert nitrates to nitrites. The specificity (true negative) of the Griess test has been reported to be between 92 and 100%. But the sensitivity (true positive) is only 35 to 85%.[4] Bladder incubation time is needed for the bacteria to convert the nitrates to nitrites; therefore a first morning urine sample is recommended. This test is not good for detecting staphylococci.

The presence of leukocytes in urine indicates inflammation of the urinary tract. Dipstick analysis can detect leukocytes indirectly by measuring the esterases bound to their membranes. The sensitivity of this test has been reported at 72 to 97%, and the specificity is 64 to 82%.[4] Combining the nitrite and leukocyte esterase dipstick as a screening alternative to microscopy has been advocated by some.[5] Studies using both dipstick tests report sensitivities ranging from 70 to 100% and specificities ranging from 60 to 98%.[4] Pyuria does not necessarily equal bacteriuria, and the nitrite test is poor detecting staphylococci. Several studies have shown that dipstick screening is not adequate in certain populations.[4,6]

Urinary Sediment Examination

There is no uniform standard for preparing a urinary specimen. Roughly 10 mL of fresh urine should be centrifuged 3 to 5 minutes at 2000 rpm. The force and duration of centrifugation as well as the volume of urine centrifuged affect the number of cells in the sediment. The supernatant is discarded by inverting and pouring off the liquid. Ideally, the volume of sediment remaining should be between 0.01 and 0.02 mL, which is the maximum volume that will fit under a standard coverslip. After the supernatant is discarded, the tube should be tapped to resuspend the cellular pellet in the remaining supernatant.[3] The urine should be examined for the presence of red blood cells, white blood cells, casts, crystals, bacteria and other microorganisms (Fig. 2–1).

Casts

Urinary casts are formed within the lumen of the renal tubules. Tamm-Horsfall mucoprotein that originates from tubular epithelial cells is the basic matrix of all renal casts. If this mucoprotein is the only component of the cast, it is a hyaline cast with little significance. Casts that also contain erythrocytes signify glomerular injury, usually glomerulonephritis. Leukocyte casts are pathognomonic of pyelonephritis. Epithelial casts represent sloughed tubular epithelial cells and are indicators of nonspecific nephron damage. Granular casts are considered a more advanced degenerative stage of cellular elements.

Crystals

Crystals may be found in stone formers as well as normal patients. The cystine crystal is diagnostic of cystinuria. Uric acid, oxalate, and cystine crystals are more often precipitated in acidic urine, whereas phosphate crystals are more commonly seen in alkaline urine.

Erythrocytes, Leukocytes, and Bacteria

Hematuria is a sign of disease in the urinary tract, and it deserves a full urologic workup. Causes of hematuria include infection, stones, tumors, trauma, sickle cell disease, and benign prostatic hyperplasia. Gross hematuria is associated with tumors approximately 20% of the time, while asymptomatic microscopic hematuria is associated with tumors around 12% of the time.[2] A diagnosis of microscopic hematuria can be made if more than two erythrocytes are seen per high-power field (hpf) in a centrifuged specimen. As stated earlier, if urine specific gravity is less than 1.007, red cells may not be seen on microscopic examination secondary to osmotic rupture. However, the dipstick will be positive for hemoglobin. Pyuria represents an inflammatory response that may be related to infection, tumor, interstitial cystitis, stones, tuberculosis, or trauma. Pyuria may be defined as more than 5 WBCs per hpf. In centrifuged urine, 2 to 5 bacteria per hpf represents approximately 10^5 bacteria per milliliter because each hpf view represents between 1/20,000 and 1/50,000 mL.[3]

URINE CULTURE

During passage through the urethra, urine can be contaminated with bacteria from the skin or vagina. Squamous epithelial cells on microscopy suggest contamination. Urine that is initially sterile in the bladder will grow fewer than 10,000 colonies of contaminant bacteria in culture. On the other hand, urine that contains multiplying bacteria usually has colony counts greater than 100,000. Therefore 10^5 is accepted as the standard for significant bacteriuria.[7] In symp-

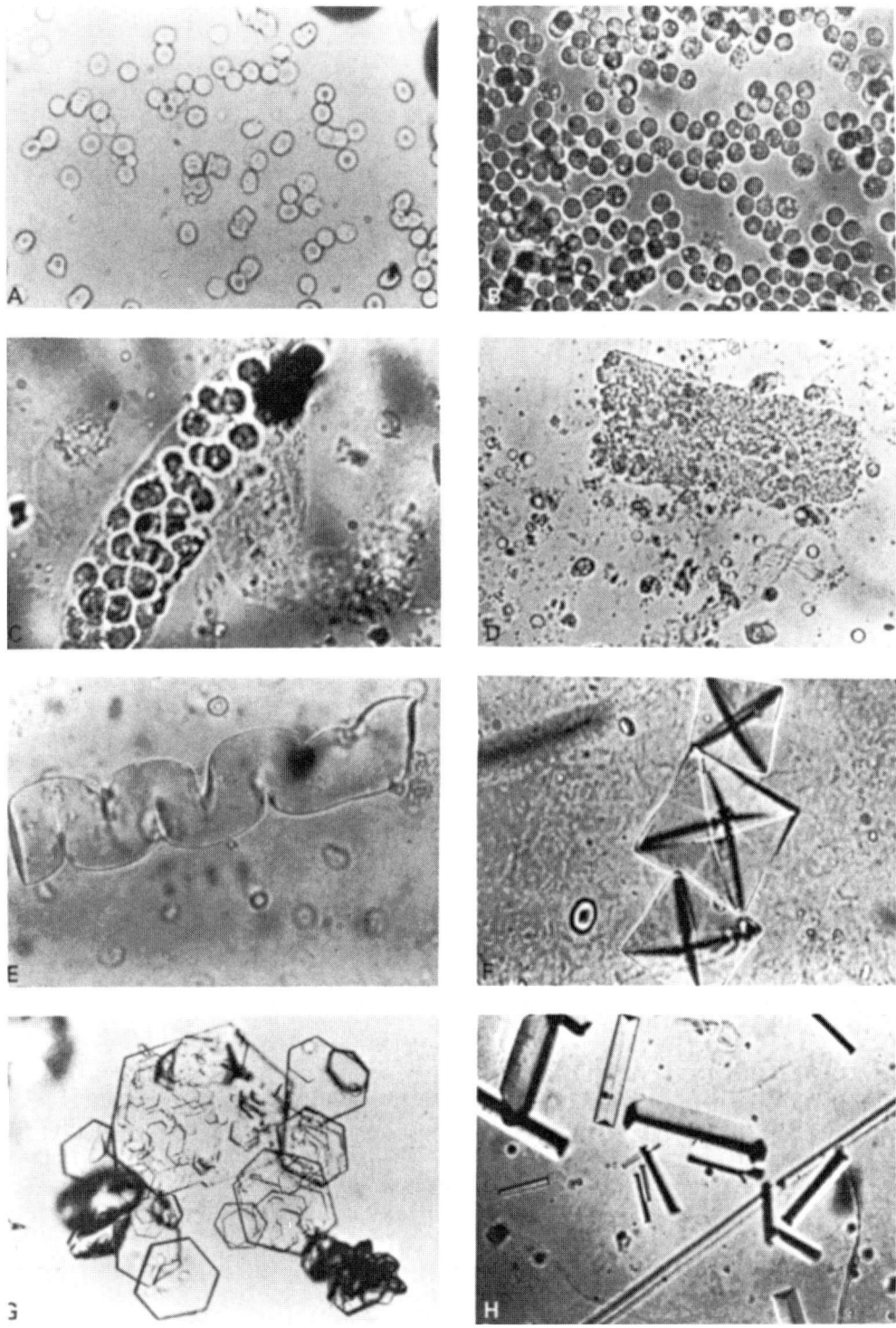

Figure 2–1. (**A**) Erythrocytes, (**B**) Leukocytes, (**C**) Leukocyte cast, (**D**) Granular cast, (**E**) Waxy cast, (**F**) Calcium oxalate crystals, (**G**) Cystine crystals, (**H**) Struvite crystals. (From Kelalis PP, King LR (eds): *Clinical Pediatric Urology.* 1976, Philadelphia, PA: WB Saunders Co.)

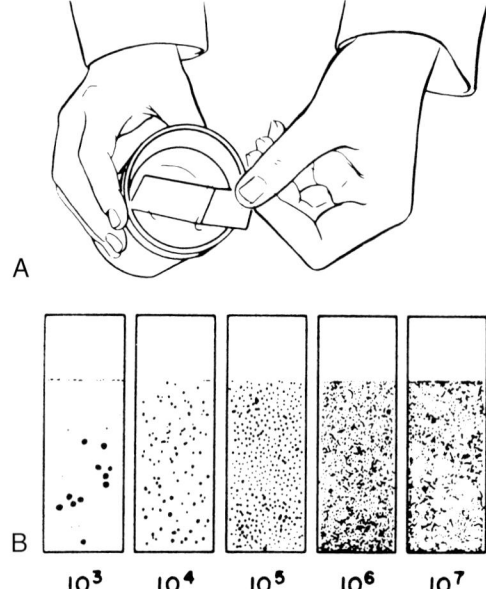

Figure 2–2. (A) Inoculation of dip slide in urine, (B) Interpretation of density of bacterial colonies on the dip slide. (From *Urology Clinics N A*, vol. 2, no. 3, 1975, Philadelphia, PA: WB Saunders Co.)

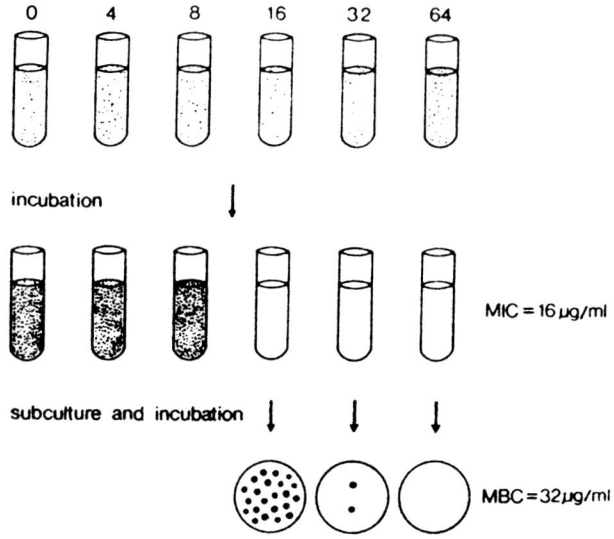

Figure 2–3. Broth dilution method of antimicrobial susceptibility testing. Note that bacterial growth is inhibited by the drug at a concentration of 16 ug/mL (the minimal inhibitory concentration [MIC]). However, a concentration of 32 ug/mL (the minimal bactericidal concentration [MBC]) is required to kill most of the inoculated bacteria. (From Fowler JE, Jr: *Urinary Tract Infection and Inflammation*. 1989, Chicago, IL: Year Book Medical Publishers, p. 52).

tomatic patients bacterial counts as low as 10^2 to 10^4 may represent a true bacterial infection.[8]

There are several different methods for performing a quantitative urinary culture. One of the most widely used methods in bacteriology laboratories is the streak plate method, which utilizes a calibrated wire loop to deliver a fixed amount of urine to an agar plate (0.001 mL). One hundred colonies represents more than 100,000 colonies per milliliter of urine. This technique, although easily performed and inexpensive, is too time-consuming for the average urology practice. A more practical method is the dip-slide culture (Fig. 2–2). This technique utilizes commercially available glass slides coated with agar on one side and a selective medium such as eosin methylene blue (EMB) on the reverse side. Gram-positive organisms are inhibited by EMB; therefore growth on both sides of the slide suggests a gram-negative organism. The dip slide is inoculated by immersion into a urine specimen or by holding the slide in a urine stream. The slide is then incubated for 24 hours and the quantitation is performed by comparing the slide to pictures of standardized colony densities that accompany the kits.[7]

Susceptibility Tests

After a urinary tract infection has been diagnosed, the physician needs to determine the antimicrobials to which the bacterial strain is susceptible. The concentration of the antibiotic in urine, not serum, is the important factor for successful therapy. Susceptibility tests are expressed either as the minimal inhibitory concentration (MIC) or as ''sensitive'' or ''resistant.'' Three basic in vitro tests are available:

(1) broth dilution, (2) plate dilution, (3) disc diffusion (Kirby Bauer method).

The broth dilution method inoculates serial dilutions of antibiotic solutions with the infecting organism (Fig. 2–3). After a 24-hour incubation period, the broths are examined for turbidity, which indicates bacterial growth. The first tube to remain clear on visual inspection is considered the MIC,

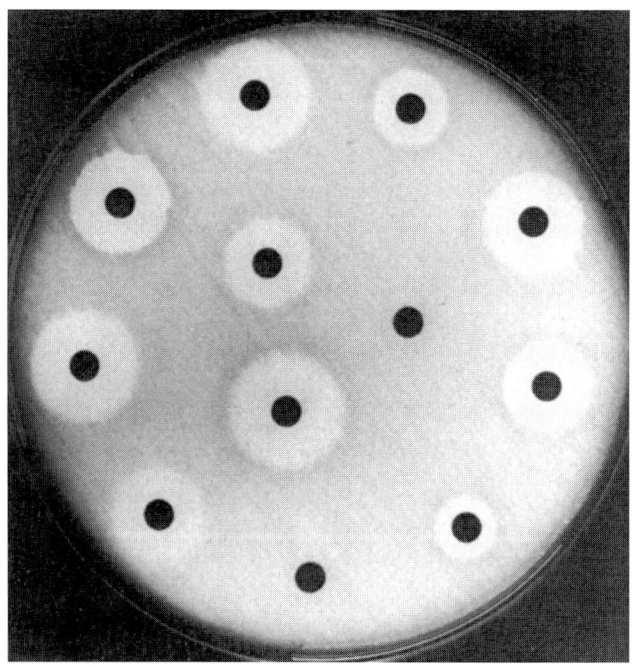

Figure 2–4. Antimicrobial discs utilized for sensitivity testing.

or the lowest concentration of drug that inhibits bacterial growth. The mean bactericidal concentration (MBC) is the lowest concentration of drug that is lethal to the bacteria and it is determined by subculture of the nonturbid tubes onto an agar medium. In most cases, the MBC will exceed the MIC by one or two dilutions. The plate dilution method is very similar, but instead of antibiotic solutions, agar mediums with antibiotics added to them are used. The bacterial inoculum is streaked onto the surface and the MIC is determined from that plate without bacterial growth.

The disc diffusion method (Kirby Bauer assay) is the simplest method of antimicrobial testing now available (Fig. 2–4). For this technique an entire surface of agar is inoculated with the infecting organism. Discs impregnated with antibiotic solution are laid on the agar. Antibiotic diffuses from the disc and inhibits bacterial growth in a ring around the disc. The further the antibiotic diffuses, the less its concentration becomes. Therefore the size of the inhibitory ring around the disc is proportional to the susceptibility of the organism to that particular antibiotic.

RENAL FUNCTION

Serum creatinine and blood urea nitrogen (BUN) provide an estimate of overall renal function. Neither provides information about the quantitative function of an individual kidney. The patient may have a nonfunctioning kidney but, given a normal contralateral kidney, may have a completely normal serum creatinine and BUN.

In the normal adult, serum creatinine ranges from 0.7 to 1.5 mg per 100 mL. Creatinine is a metabolic product of creatine, which is derived primarily from muscle. Therefore the muscle mass of the patient is an important determinant of the absolute serum creatinine level. BUN represents one of the end products of protein metabolism, and it varies from 5 to 25 mg per 100 mL. BUN is dependent on several factors, including state of hydration, protein intake, and catabolic state. The ratio of BUN/CR is usually 10:1; however, with prerenal azotemia the ratio may approach 20:1 or 30:1 because renal perfusion is decreased and there is increased back diffusion of filtered urea from the renal tubules. In general, the GFR is maintained so that serum creatinine does not rise significantly. With severe hypoperfusion the serum creatinine will also rise.

Another method of evaluating renal function is to estimate the glomerular filtration rate (GFR). This is done by calculating the renal clearance of a substance that ideally is completely filtered by the glomerulus but is not secreted or reabsorbed by the renal tubules.

$$\text{Clearance} = \frac{U \times V}{P \times T}$$

U = urinary concentration of product measured
V = urinary volume during indicated time interval
P = plasma concentration of product measured
T = time interval of urine collection

Several substances may be used for this calculation. Inulin represents a foreign substance that is freely filtered and neither secreted nor reabsorbed; however, it must be infused intravenously at a constant rate and is therefore inconvenient to use routinely. Urea is a naturally occurring metabolite and therefore does not require a constant infusion; however, it is 40 to 70% reabsorbed by the renal tubules and therefore underestimates GFR. Creatinine is present at a relatively constant level in serum, and only a small amount is secreted by the renal tubules. Therefore, although it offers a slight overestimation of GFR, creatinine remains the standard by which most physicians estimate GFR. An average creatinine clearance for an adult male is 120 mL/min.

PROSTATE SPECIFIC ANTIGEN

Over the past decade, prostate specific antigen (PSA) has replaced acid phosphatase as the most important tumor marker for prostate cancer. Although there are still controversies about PSA's role in the screening and staging of patients with prostate cancer, it does have a solid role in monitoring treatment response.

PSA is a serine protease produced exclusively by the epithelial cells lining the acini and ducts of the prostate. At this time, only three PSA immunoassays are currently approved by the FDA, and they all incorporate monoclonal antibodies: the Hybritech Tandem-E and Tandem-R and the Abbott IMx PSA assay. Several other assays are available that are not yet FDA approved, including the Yang Pros-Check polyclonal immunoassay.[9] The reference ranges of these different assays are not standardized; therefore it is the responsibility of the physician to be aware of which assay is being used.

PSA as a Screening Test

Although PSA is specific for the prostate, it is not prostate cancer specific. PSA can also be elevated by benign prostatic hyperplasia (BPH), prostatitis, prostatic infarction, cystoscopy, transurethral resection of the prostate (TURP), and needle biopsy of the prostate. Digital rectal examination does not appear to have any clinically significant effect on PSA.[10,11] Finasteride, a 5-alpha reductase inhibitor that reduces prostate size also decreases PSA by as much as 50%.[12]

Both BPH and prostate cancer have their peak incidence in men more than 50 years old. It has been shown that BPH elevates serum PSA at a rate of 0.3 ng mL^{-1} g^{-1} of BPH tissue[13] and that 25% of men with BPH have PSA values above the normal reference range. In addition, not all prostate cancers cause a detectable elevation in PSA. In fact, 43% of men with prostate cancer have a PSA value within the normal range. Therefore the positive predictive value of PSA is 49% for PSA values greater than 4 and 75% for PSA values greater than 10 ng/ml. Because of the overlap in

PSA values between BPH and prostate cancer, PSA is not considered specific or sensitive enough to be used as a screening study.[14] In an attempt to enhance the predictive value of PSA, investigators have developed the concept of PSA density (PSAD), which is the quotient of PSA and prostatic volume.[15] PSA density may help distinguish between BPH and prostate cancer. One drawback is the error involved in determining prostatic volume by transrectal ultrasound.

PSA and Prostate Cancer Staging

Several studies have shown that PSA does increase proportionally with advancing clinical stage of prostate cancer[16,17]; however, there is significant overlap between stages. PSA therefore cannot determine clinical stage, nor can it distinguish extracapsular from organ-confined cancers. PSA may be helpful in predicting skeletal metastases. A recent study has shown that in asymptomatic prostate cancer patients with a PSA value of less than 10 ng/mL, there is only a 0.5% chance of having skeletal metastases on bone scan. Therefore it is recommended that bone scan no longer be routine in these patients.[18]

Monitoring Treatment Response with PSA

PSA does have a solid role in monitoring treatment response after radical prostatectomy, radiation, and hormonal therapy. Since PSA is produced exclusively by the prostate, PSA should theoretically become undetectable after a prostatectomy if all prostatic tissue is removed. Since PSA's half-life is approximately 3.2 days,[14] it is possible to detect a serum PSA for the first few weeks after prostatectomy. By 3 months the serum PSA should reach its baseline level. If the PSA does not become undetectable by 3 months postoperatively, the patient probably has residual disease.[19] Following serial PSAs after prostatectomy provides information about disease progression and offers the chance to initiate adjunctive therapy.

PSA is used in a similar manner to monitor patients after radiation therapy; however, PSA values rarely reach undetectable levels because remaining prostatic epithelium still secretes a measurable amount of PSA. Therefore after radiation therapy, the PSA will usually decline over several months until a nadir is reached. The nadir may be undetectable, in the normal PSA value range, or higher than normal range. Its value depends most on the pretreatment PSA value, the stage of the cancer, and the gleason grade.[20] Serial measurements of PSA can then be used to monitor disease course. A rising PSA has been shown to correlate with disease progression and positive biopsy results indicating treatment failure. Another finding is that PSA values of those patients who developed skeletal metastasis after radiation therapy were much lower than those untreated stage D2 patients.[21] In summary, physicians must be much more vigilant for skeletal metastases after radiation therapy than the PSA might indicate.

PSA appears to be very accurate in monitoring treatment response to hormonal therapy. PSA has been shown to decrease precipitously in patients with a good response to hormonal therapy.[22] If PSA remains undetectable or at normal levels at 6 months following initiation of hormonal therapy, a good long-term response can be expected from endocrine therapy. In contrast, a rising PSA predicts a hormone refractory cancer and a poor prognosis.

SERUM ACID PHOSPHATASE

Before assays for PSA were developed, the measurement of serum acid phosphatase was the mainstay in the staging of prostate cancer. In the prostate, acid phosphatase is secreted by the epithelial cells lining the acini. Isozymes of acid phosphatases are produced by other organ systems, and therefore a major drawback with serum acid phosphatase is not being able to measure the serum level reliably without interference from the acid phosphatases from other tissue. There are two different assays for the measurement of serum acid phosphatase: an enzymatic assay and a radioimmunoassay. The physician should be aware of which assay is being used, as there are different reference ranges.

Numerous studies have proven PSA to be a more sensitive tumor marker with respect to diagnosis, staging, and monitoring of patients for treatment response. Elevations in acid phosphatase have been shown to occur mainly in patients with advanced disease.[23] Measurements of serum acid phosphatases are no longer mandatory before radical prostatectomy but may add only confirmatory information in patients in whom advanced disease is suspected.

REFERENCES

1. Turck M, Goffe B, Petersdorf RG: The urethral catheter and urinary tract infection. *J Urol* 1962;88:834.
2. Wyker A: Standard Diagnostic Considerations. *Adult Urology and Pediatric Urology.* St Louis: Mosby Year Book, 1991.
3. Lowe F, Brendler C: Evaluation of the Urologic Patient. *Campbell's Urology,* 6th ed. Philadelphia: WB Saunders, 1992.
4. Pels R, Bor D, Woolhandler S, et al: Dipstick urinalysis screening of asymptomatic adults for urinary tract disorders. II. Bacteriuria. *JAMA* 1989;262:1221.
5. Flanagan P, Davies E, Rooney P, Stout R: Evaluation of four screening tests for bacteriuria in elderly people. *Lancet* 1989; 1:1117.
6. Propp D, Weber D, Ciesla ML: Reliability of a urine dipstick in emergency department patients. *Ann Emerg Med* 1989; 18:560.
7. Kunin C: The concept of significant bacteriuria. *Detection, Prevention and Management of Urinary Tract Infections,* 4th ed. Philadelphia: Lea & Febiger, 1987.

8. Stamm W, Counts G, Running K, et al: Diagnosis of coliform infection in acutely dysuric women. *N Engl J Med* 1982; 307:463.
9. Vessella R, Lange P: Issues in the assessment of PSA immunoassays. *Urol Clin North Am* 20;4:607–619.
10. Crawford E, Schutz M, Clejan S: The effect of digital rectal examination on prostate specific antigen levels. *JAMA* 1992; 267:2227.
11. Yaun J, Coplen D, Petros J, et al: Effects of rectal examination, prostatic massage, ultrasonography and needle biopsy on serum prostate specific antigen levels. *J Urol* 1992;147:810–814.
12. Guess HA, Heyse JF, Gormley GJ: The effect of finasteride on prostate specific antigen in men with benign prostatic hyperplasia. *Prostate* 1993;22:31.
13. Stamey TA, Yang N, Hay AR et al: Prostate specific antigen as a serum marker for adenocarcinoma of the prostate. *N Engl J Med* 1987;317:909.
14. Oesterling J: Prostate specific antigen: a critical assessment of the most useful tumor marker for adenocarcinoma of the prostate. *J Urol* 1991;145:907.
15. Benson M, Whang IS, Pantuck A, et al: Prostate specific antigen density: a means of distinguishing benign prostatic hypertrophy and prostate cancer. *J Urol* 1991;147:815–816.
16. Hudson M, Bahnson R, Catalona W: Clinical use of prostate specific antigen in staging patients with newly diagnosed prostate cancer. *J Urol* 1989;142:1011.
17. Stamey T, Kabalin J: Prostate specific antigen in the diagnosis and treatment of adenocarcinoma of the prostate. I. Untreated patients. *J Urol* 1989;141:1070.
18. Oesterling J, Martin S, Bergstralh E, Lowe F: The use of prostate-specific antigen in staging patients with newly diagnosed prostate cancer. *JAMA* 1993;269:57.
19. Stamey T, Kabalin J, McNeal J, et al: Prostate specific antigen in the diagnosis and treatment of adenocarcinoma of the prostate. II. Radical prostatectomy treated patients. *J Urol* 1989; 141:1076.
20. Goad J, Chang S, Ohori M, Scardino P: PSA after definitive radiotherapy for clinically localized prostate cancer. *Urol Clin North Am* 1993;20;4:727.
21. Stamey T, Kabalin J, Ferrari M: Prostate specific antigen in the diagnosis and treatment of adenocarcinoma of the prostate. III. Radiation treated patients. *J Urol* 1989;141:1084.
22. Stamey T, Kabalin J, Ferrari M, Yang N: Prostate specific antigen in the diagnosis and treatment of adenocarcinoma of the prostate. IV. Anti-androgen treated patients. *J Urol* 1989; 141:1088.
23. Walsh P: The value of serum enzymatic acid phosphatase in staging of localized prostate cancer. *J Urol* 1992;148:1832.

3 Urodynamic Studies

Stephen D. Mark, George D. Webster

Urodynamics is the study of the physiologic and pathologic factors involved in the storage, transportation, and evacuation of urine. The lower urinary tract comprises the bladder and urethra, each of which has dual functions, the bladder to store and void, the urethra to control and convey. Abnormalities of these functions may be caused by neurologic and psychologic disturbances, muscular dysfunction, and structural abnormalities. Customarily, the investigatory armamentarium used for evaluating lower urinary tract problems leans strongly on the patient's history, physical examination, radiologic studies, and endoscopy. Urodynamics, however, is the only test of function; endoscopy and radiologic studies are only able to identify structural abnormalities.

LOWER URINARY TRACT FUNCTION

The micturition cycle involves two discrete phases, that of bladder storage and bladder emptying. Normal bladder storage requires the accommodation of increasing volumes of urine at low pressure with appropriate sensation, a competent bladder outlet and the absence of involuntary contractions. Bladder emptying requires a coordinated bladder contraction of adequate magnitude and duration, the coordinated relaxation of both smooth and striated sphincters, and an absence of any anatomic urethral obstruction. In lower urinary tract evaluation, a detailed history and physical examination are essential, and a voided volume diary is indispensable to indicate the volume of urine customarily stored (functional bladder capacity), to show the diurnal pattern of urine output, and to document episodes of urinary incontinence (Fig. 3–1). The bladder chart helps identify patients with diurnal frequency due to excessive fluid intake and those with nocturia due to physiologic nocturnal diuresis; it also helps to anticipate the fill volume when cystometry is performed.

The physical examination includes a routine urologic exam and should also try to identify gross and subtle neurologic signs that may suggest a neuropathic bladder. Abnormalities of the peripheral nervous system may manifest with impaired peripheral power, coordination and sensation, and alteration in peripheral reflexes.

The diagnosis of bladder dysfunction using clinical evaluation alone is both difficult and unreliable, and it has been shown that treatment based on urodynamic findings provides for better outcome when compared with therapy based on clinical findings alone.[1]

It is essential that clinicians performing urodynamic studies standardize their terminology to allow for the accurate exchange and comparison of data. This official terminology is summarized by the International Continence Society (ICS) in their publications on standardization of lower urinary tract function.[2]

HISTORY

In 1876, Dubois first measured intravesical pressure, observing the desire to void was associated with a rise in intravesical pressure.[3] Subsequently, in 1882 Mosso and Pellacici showed that this rise in pressure was unrelated to intra-abdominal pressure and thus was due to bladder contraction alone.[4] Rose, in 1927, coined the term *cystometer*, describing its development and a clinical usefulness.[5] In 1948, Drake pioneered the use of uroflow measurements where previously a record of timing of micturition was utilized.[6] This instrument measured the increasing weight of urine against time on a kymograph, producing graphic uroflowgrams. Eight years later von Garrelts used electronics to report flow rate.[7] In 1962, Gleason and Lattimer reported the use of cystometry and uroflow in combination to determine bladder outlet obstruction indirectly.[8] The term *urodynamics* was coined by Davis in 1954 but was not used in publication until 1962.[9] Miller subsequently popularized the use of cinefluoroscopy in conjunction with lower urinary tract urodynamic studies, now recognized as videourodynamics.[10] In 1970, Bates, Whiteside, and Turner-Warwick reported more than 220 cases of videourodynamic evaluation, showing these studies provided excellent objective data necessary for the evaluation of a variety of lower urinary tract disorders.[11] This history and other important events are reported by this author.[12]

The Urodynamic Society was formed in 1965; through its own journal, *Neurology and Urodynamics*, it reports all major advances in the field. Urodynamics has now cemented its role in urology and is pivotal in the assessment of neurogenic bladder, is important in the diagnosis of bladder outlet obstruction, and is useful in classifying female stress urinary incontinence.

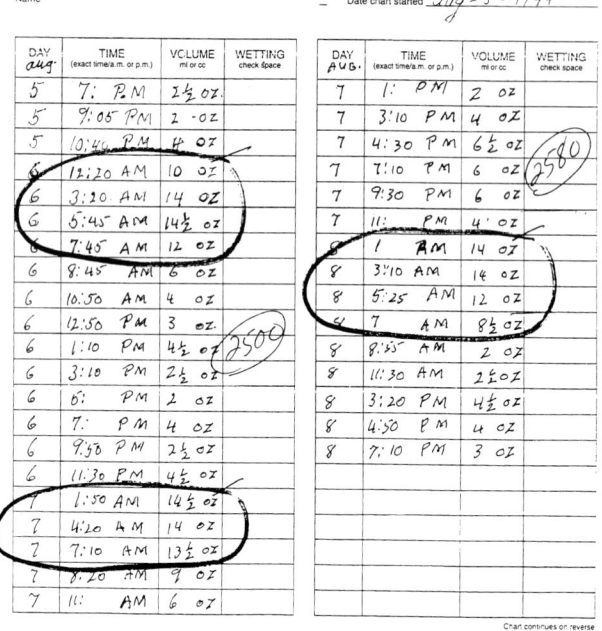

Figure 3–1. A voided volume chart (bladder diary) in an elderly woman with nocturia. The study confirms nocturnal diuresis.

ROLE OF URODYNAMICS

The role of urodynamics includes (1) the characterization of detrusor function; (2) the evaluation of voiding function; (3) the evaluation of the outlet; (4) the diagnosis and characterization of neuropathy.

The urodynamic armamentarium is extensive; however, the majority of patients may be evaluated adequately by the use of relatively simple studies. To be of maximal value, testing should be performed by experienced personnel, who should attempt to reproduce the storage and voiding symptoms being evaluated.

Patient Preparation

Prior to the study the procedure performed should be explained to the patient along with completion of an adequate history and clinical examination. It is our custom to mail patients an information brochure along with a further history questionnaire and bladder chart to be completed for the 3 to 5 days prior to their studies.

Studies should be deferred in the presence of acute urinary infections and, ideally, should not be performed after recent instrumentation (e.g., cystoscopy) or with catheters in place. Many drugs will also affect lower urinary tract function, and their impact should be taken into account. Parenteral antibiotic prophylaxis is not necessary in the majority of patients; however, those with prosthetic implants such as heart valves or orthopedic joints should receive antibiotic chemoprophylaxis. We do use antibiotic prophylaxis for 48 hours after completion of the study in those patients undergoing multiple lower urinary tract instrumentation.

CYSTOMETRY

Cystometry evaluates the filling and storage phases of bladder function by measuring bladder pressure during artificial filling. The filling phase of the micturition cycle is usually characterized by the bladder accommodating increasing volumes of urine at low pressure until capacity is reached.

The cystometrogram (CMG) may be performed using a variety of techniques. The most common involves urethral access and a liquid filling medium (either contrast or sterile saline), instilled at a medium fill rate (50 to 100 mL/min). Liquid fill is more physiologic, facilitates the observation of incontinent episodes, and allows voiding studies to be performed. CO_2 may be used as the filling medium; however, it is not as ideal as it is compressible and may leak without being seen. It may also irritate the bladder mucosa because of its dissolution in water, which produces carbonic acid, and it prevents voiding studies from being performed. However, CO_2 is clean and allows a study to be performed quickly; occasionally, it is useful in the office setting. Overall, we feel CO_2 cystometry is inferior to fluid cystometry and should be looked on as historic.

Urethral catheterization and suprapubic catheterization give similar results. Because of the ease of urethral catheterization and the risk and discomfort of suprapubic catheter insertion, urethral access is customary. Controversy exists over fill rate, with medium fill rate being looked on as provocative and therefore being used in an attempt to unmask detrusor instability. Too fast a fill rate may cause an elevation in pressure during fill, described as reduced compliance. Should this occur the cystometrogram should be repeated at a slower fill rate. Slow fill rates of less than 25 mL/min are desirable for neuropathic patients, particularly if bladder hyperactivity is suspected, for involuntary contractions may otherwise be triggered early in the filling study and it may be impossible to get an appreciation of true capacity or compliance. In children the fill rate is even slower—10 mL/min sufficing in the neonate.

Overall, cystometry gives specific information about the following aspects of detrusor behavior: (1) bladder compliance; (2) bladder stability (the presence or absence of involuntary contractions); (3) bladder sensation; and (4) bladder capacity. The important variable is detrusor pressure (P_{det}) which is not directly measurable. To obtain this measure, total bladder pressure (P_{ves}) is recorded and abdominal pressure (P_{abdo}), approximated by rectal pressure, is subtracted from it by the instrument electronics. Recording P_{det}

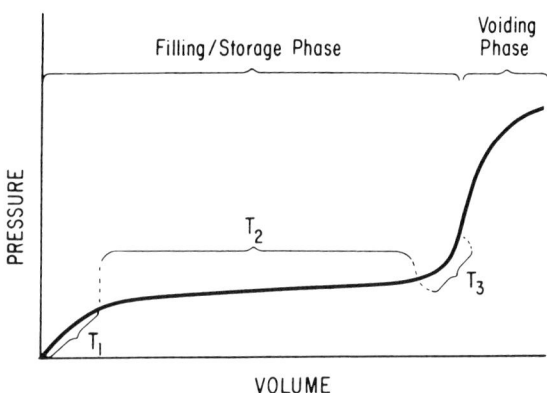

Figure 3–2. A schematic normal cystometrogram.

(or subtracted bladder pressure) avoids the interpretation difficulties that result from abdominal pressure changes due to movement or straining.

Communication between the patient and the personnel performing urodynamic studies is important, especially during cystometry. At the commencement of cystometry the patient is asked to cough and to strain to ensure that complete subtraction of P_{abdo} is occurring and that P_{det} is being measured. During filling patients are asked to "hold their urine" (suppress any bladder activity) and not to attempt to void. Wein describes four specific phases of cystometry (Fig. 3–2). Phase 1 presents an initial pressure rise in response to filling. This is an initial myogenic response to filling together with the elastic and viscoelastic response of the bladder wall to stretch. Phase 2 is called the tonic phase, and compliance ($\Delta v/\Delta P$) is normally high, uninterrupted by any detrusor contractile activity. Because of the unphysiologic nature of this study, compliance is always lower than that during physiologic bladder filling. Phase 3 represents bladder activity when the elastic and viscoelastic properties of the bladder wall have reached their limit. Phase 4 represents voiding and will be discussed later.

Bladder capacity represents the subjective measure of maximal volume and should be compared with voided volumes noted on the frequency–volume chart to check its validity. In children bladder capacity may be estimated by using the formula (age + 30 × 2) as described by Koff.[13] In adults the range for cystometric capacity is approximately between 300 and 700 mL. Measurement of this volume is operator dependent; it is our practice to stop filling when the patient has a strong desire to void or once the functional volume seen on the voiding diary is achieved and exceeded by a small amount.

Bladder compliance represents the bladder's ability to accommodate increasing volumes without a rise in pressure, as represented by the slope of phase 2 on the filling curve. Low or reduced bladder compliance implies a poorly distensible bladder in which the pressure–volume curve is steep (Fig. 3–3). Compliance will also be affected by the rate of filling, the type of filling medium, and the temperature of the filling medium. It is difficult to find normal values for compliance. Abrams stated that a pressure of 3.3 cm H_2O or less at 100 mL volume would represent normal compliance,[14] whereas McGuire stated bladder pressures should not exceed 6 cm of water during normal filling.[15] Both of these represent an arbitrary assessment; compliance should be described as being either grossly normal or abnormal. If an

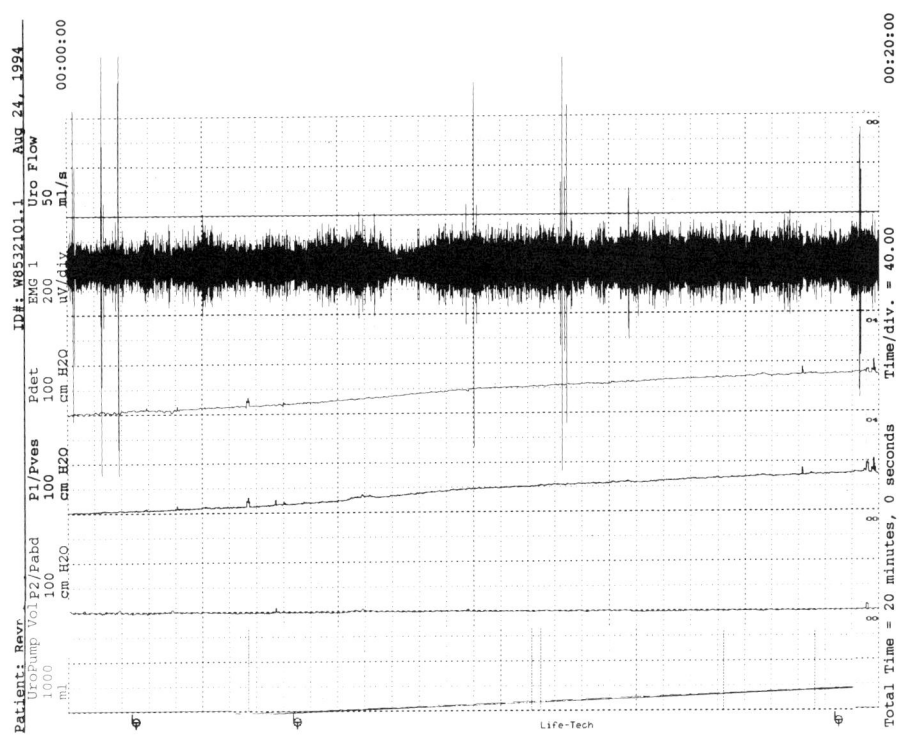

Figure 3–3. Reduced bladder compliance in a patient with neurogenic bladder dysfunction. The steep cystometrogram is evidence (P_{det} tracing).

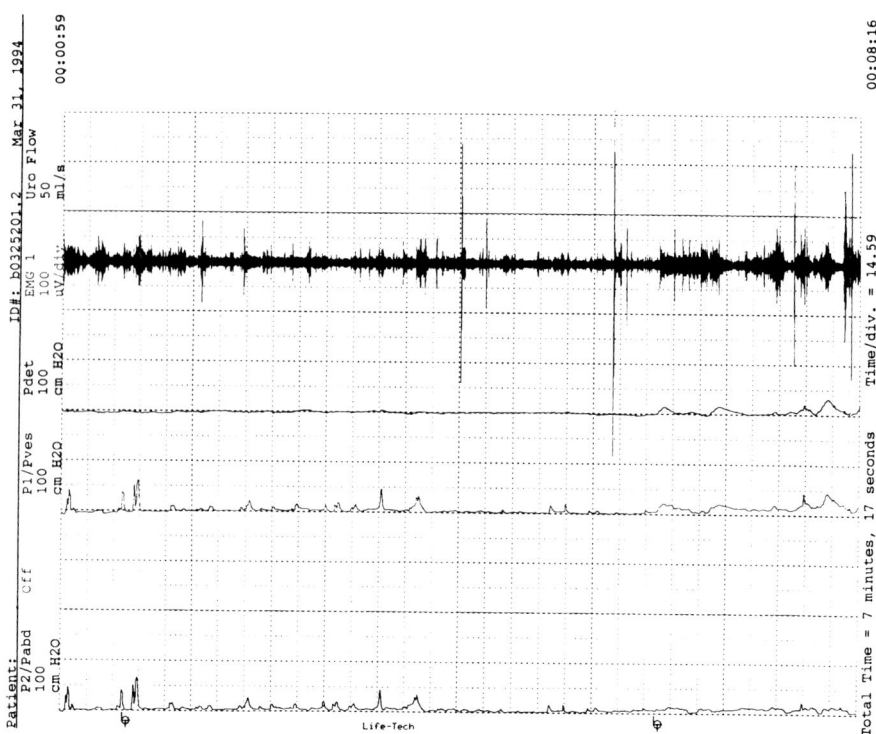

Figure 3–4. Idiopathic detrusor instability in an adult woman with urinary incontinence. The P_{det} tracing shows numerous involuntary detrusor contractions.

abnormal pattern occurs one should describe whether it is early or late in the fill and what the numerical value of $\Delta v/\Delta P$ is.

Involuntary contractions during filling are always significant. Originally, the ICS has restricted its definition of bladder instability to phasic rises of detrusor pressure greater than 15 cm H_2O, but in practice symptomatic unstable contractions are often smaller. Currently, the ICS recognizes as abnormal any involuntary phasic contraction occurring during filling cystometry (Fig. 3–4).[2,16] Detrusor overactivity includes both detrusor hyperreflexia where involuntary detrusor contractions are a result of neurologic disease and detrusor instability where the etiology of these contractions is nonneurogenic and due to such etiologies as obstruction or unknown causes.

The description of sensory phenomenon during bladder filling is subjective. A significant degree of pain on bladder filling at low volume is described as hypersensitivity, and it often implies inflammatory changes within the wall of the bladder. This is commonly seen in the patient with interstitial cystitis. Early sensation of filling and urgency is customarily seen in those patients with detrusor instability, and delay sensation may be seen in those with diabetes or in habitual infrequent voiders.

A number of factors may alter the appearance of the CMG and lead to misinterpretation. An incompetent bladder outlet will allow the urine or filling medium to leak around the catheter before adequate distension is achieved. Thus low bladder compliance and/or detrusor overactivity, which may not have been provoked, may be missed. To evaluate the

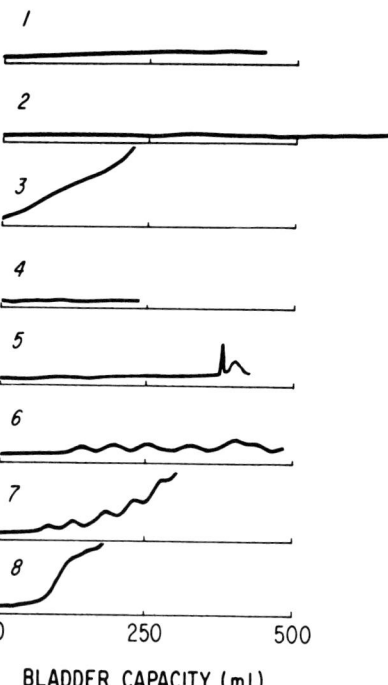

Figure 3–5. Schematic representation of the more commonly seen CMG curves. (1) normal; (2) high compliance, large capacity; (3) low compliance, low capacity; (4) hypersensitive with low functional capacity; (5) cough-induced bladder instability; (6) spontaneous detrusor instability; (7) high-pressure cumulative involuntary contractions; (8) high-pressure involuntary contraction at low capacity in a neurogenic bladder.

storage phase of cystometry in such patients the bladder outlet may be occluded with a Foley balloon to provide some outlet resistance. Reflux of urine, especially into wide, capacious ureters, may also mask poor compliance because of the sequestration of fluid into these reservoirs. Using contrast media to fill the bladder and screening with fluoroscopy (videourodynamics) should make this obvious.

Noncooperative patients, some children, or the mentally ill may invalidate the study because of a lack of understanding of the requirements during cystometry. Urodynamics, however, has been shown to be reliable and reproducible within the pediatric and specifically neonatal population with spinal dysraphism.[17] Urinary infection and long-term indwelling catheterization may falsely decrease the functional bladder capacity, reduce compliance, and cause bladder overactivity. Infection should be eliminated prior to urodynamic studies. In those who require catheter drainage, clean, intermittent catheterization would be preferable.

Provocative maneuvers may unmask an overactive bladder. These include a faster fill rate, postural changes, coughing, performance of the study in the standing position, and handwashing. Figure 3–5 represents the various types of CMGs that may be obtained.

UROFLOWMETRY

Uroflowmetry is the simplest and least invasive urodynamic test and is a measure of the integrated activity of the bladder and outlet during the emptying phase of the micturition cycle. The measured flow rate (mean and maximum), the voided volume, and the graphic display of the voiding pattern are the usual recorded variables. Although uroflowmetry may produce a high index of clinical suspicion for bladder outlet obstruction, it does not permit accurate diagnosis or localization of a suspected abnormality. Unfortunately, a normal flow rate does not rule out obstruction as defined by the relationship between detrusor pressure and uroflow.

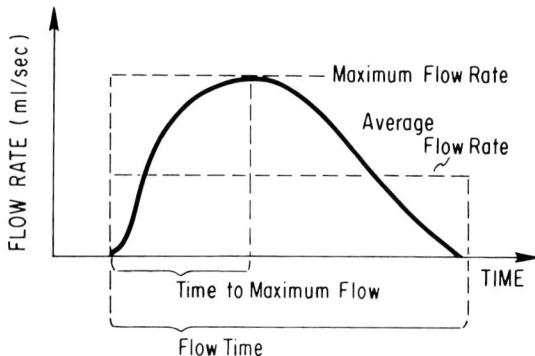

Figure 3–6. Idealized uroflow curve identifying frequently measured variables.

The procedure for uroflow examination should be performed in a socially appropriate environment with the patient voiding in the usual position. It is important that the flow measured be thought by the patient to be representative of the normal voiding pattern and that the volume voided be recorded. A volume of more than 150 mL usually gives a reliable uroflow, but it is important to note that low and very high voided volumes may not give representative flow rates (Fig. 3–6).

The maximum flow rate is the most frequently recorded variable during uroflowmetry. Consistently low flow rates despite adequate volume generally indicate increased bladder outlet resistance, decreased bladder contractility, or both. Flow rates considerably in excess of normal may indicate decreased outlet resistance.

The pattern of the flow curve varies in different voiding dysfunctions. An abnormally broad plateau with a low mean and maximum flow rate generally indicates obstruction, decreased contractility, or both. Intermittent or "stacato" flow is generally seen in patients who are using abdominal strain to void, who have sphincter dyssynergia, or who display voluntary inhibition.

As normal flow rates vary with age, sex, and voided vol-

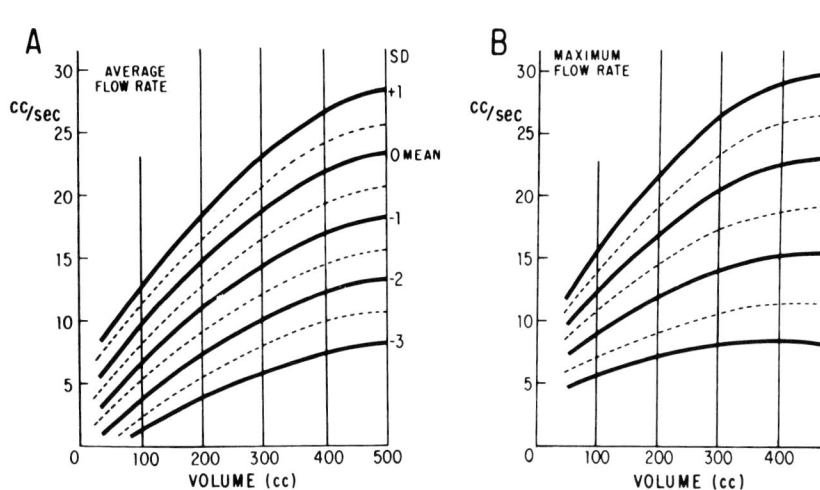

Figure 3–7. Flow rate nomogram relating average flow rate and maximum flow rates to volume voided. (From Siroky BM, Olsson CA, Krane RJ. The flow rate nomogram: 1. Development. *J Urol* 1979;122:665.

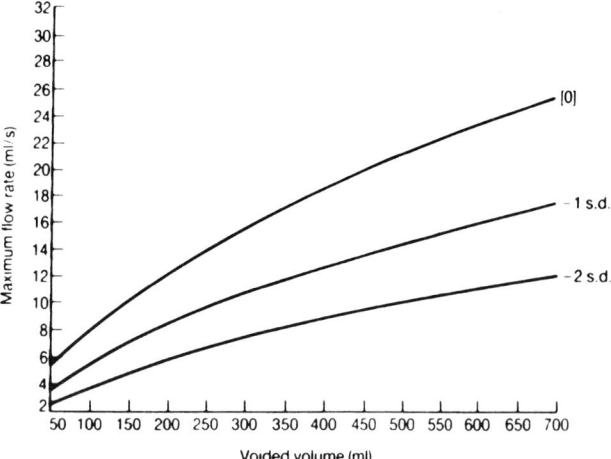

Figure 3–8. The Bristol flow nomogram for men over 50 years of age.

umes, flow rate nomograms have been published in an attempt to provide normal baseline data independent of these variables.[18–20] The flow rate nomograms developed by Krane and that by Abrams allow the flow rates on different voided volumes to be compared (Figs. 3–7, 3–8).[14,18]

It is important when interpreting uroflow to be sure that the flow measured closely approximates the usual voiding event of the patient. Ideally, two flow events should be measured, one of which may be a spontaneous "free" flow rate, the other of which follows the pressure-flow study. Clinically, uroflow remains a good screening test; however, a more definitive and complete evaluation of the lower urinary tract requires further urodynamic study.

Residual Urine Volume

Residual urine volume indicates voiding efficiency and is best considered with the voided volume and the peak flow rate. It may be estimated indirectly by ultrasound or measured by catheterization during urodynamics. Negligible residual urine is expected if lower urinary tract function is normal. Increased residual urine may be due to increased bladder outlet resistance, decreased bladder contractility, or both. It is important to note that the magnitude of the residual urine has been shown by some workers to bear no relationship to the magnitude of outlet obstruction (Fig. 3–9).[21]

VOIDING STUDIES

The study of the bladder's "voiding" function requires the concurrent recording of detrusor pressure (P_{det}) and uroflow (Q). Because the bladder and urethra have independent functional properties but act together during micturition, the combination of these characteristics determines the pressure–flow relationship of micturition (Fig. 3–10). By measuring both factors both normal and obstructed voiding may

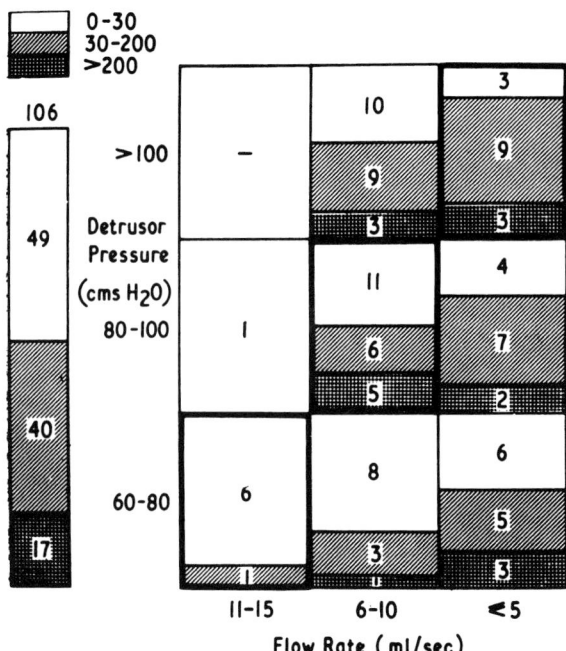

Figure 3–9. Residual urine volume related to the severity of prostatic obstruction; 106 pts with prostatic obstruction are grouped according to urodynamic micturition study results and the volume of their residual urine. It is evident that the degree of outlet obstruction as assessed by the voiding pressure and that urine flow rate does not correlate with the volume of residual urine. (From Turner-Warwick R, Whiteside CG, Arnold EP, et al. A urodynamic view of prostatic obstruction and the results of prostatectomy. *Br J Urol* 1973;45:631.

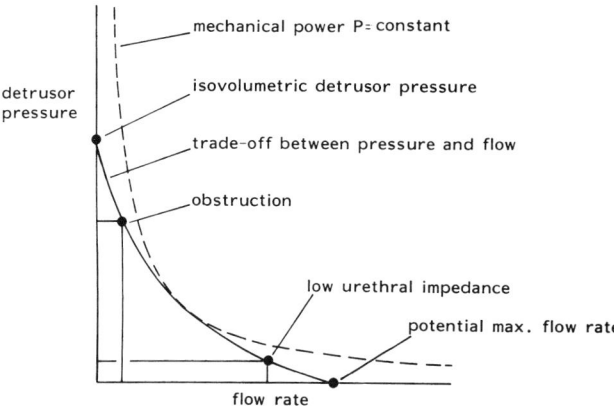

Figure 3–10. Relation showing the trade-off between pressure and flow rate produced by a contracting detrusor (unbroken curve). The operating point on this curve depends on the resistance of the urethra (see points marked *obstruction* and *low urethral impedance*). If flow is interrupted the detrusor pressure rises from the operating point to the isovolumetric value. The broken curve shows the hypothetical relation between pressure and flow rate that would be valid if the mechanical point generated by the contracting detrusor were constant. (From Griffiths DJ. Hydrodynamics and mechanics of the bladder and urethra. In: Mundy AR, Stephenson TP, Wein AJ, eds. *Urodynamics: Principles, Practice and Application.* London: Churchill Livingstone; 1994.)

be characterized. Some patients find it difficult to void in the urodynamic laboratory, and every attempt should be made to ensure a socially appropriate environment and to reduce such inhibition. Additionally, the presence of the urethral pressure line, the rectal recording catheter/balloon, and the periurethral EMG electrodes further influences the study outcome adversely and renders the pressure–flow study less reliable in characterizing detrusor function. The normal adult male generally voids with a P_{det} of between 40 and 60 cm H_2O. The normal adult female voids with a lower pressure. During many studies women void with no apparent contraction at all; however, this is due to the fact in women bladder outlet resistance is often very low during voiding. It does not indicate that no bladder contraction is occurring.

Voiding studies may define a number of variables useful for clinical application (Fig. 3–11). The opening time is the time that elapses from the initial time of P_{det} rise to the onset of flow. Detrusor opening pressure is the P_{det} at the onset of micturition. It is high in patients with infravesical obstruction, and a pressure of 80 cm H_2O or greater may be diagnostic of obstruction. Detrusor pressure at maximal flow is the magnitude of the micturition contraction when the flow rate is maximal. When this pressure is greater than 100 cm H_2O, it implies the presence of outlet obstruction even when flow rates are good. Urethral resistance may be calculated from the P_{det} at maximal flow and the maximum flow rate; however, this does not appear to be a valuable measurement, for the urethra does not behave like a rigid tube. The maximum P_{det} is the maximum pressure recorded regardless of flow at the time. The maximum P_{det} may exceed that recorded at the time of the maximum flow, perhaps because outlet relaxation is incomplete other than at the time of peak flow. The P_{iso}, or isometric maximum detrusor contraction, is a "stop test" contrived to determine the pressure the bladder can achieve when contracting against a closed outlet. This study is an attempt to quantify maximum detrusor activity. However, results are not always reproducible, for some patients find it difficult to stop voiding in midstream, and the maximum pressure will vary at different bladder volumes; consequently, it has not been found to have great clinical usefulness. A postmicturition after-contraction is seen as a detrusor contraction after all flow has ceased. It was previously thought this would represent an abnormality in patients with overactive bladders; however, this does not appear to be so.

A number of factors may interfere with normal voiding studies, including the nonphysiologic test environment, urethral instrumentation, overdistention of the bladder, and medications that may alter detrusor contractility. Additionally, there are no absolute pressure–flow criteria that are diagnostic of bladder outlet obstruction. There is, however, usually little debate among urodynamicists about the general features of both urethral fluid dynamics and detrusor contractility and therefore of normal and obstructed voiding function. There is agreement that the plot of P_{det} against flow rate is the optimum way to display the data. There is also agreement on how these pressure–flow curves should be interpreted. There is, however, considerable debate regarding the most reliable procedure for abstracting this information for both clinical and research purposes. The ICS P–Q graph and Abrams-Griffiths nomogram distinguish only between the clearly obstructed and the clearly unobstructed.[22] Schafer has described the passive urethral resistance relationship (PURR) and the dynamic urethral resistance relationship (DURR), which provide information related to the opening pressure and to the effect of luminal size as well as the dynamic changes during voiding.[22,23]

The computerization of urodynamic data and subsequent analysis are known as advanced urodynamics, which, it is hoped, may better identify patients with infravesical obstruction. Attempts have been made to reduce this complex information to a single factor, and the urethral resistance factor (URA) currently appears to correlate best with infravesical obstruction. A number of these advanced urodynamic packages are available as optional software when purchasing urodynamic equipment.[24] Unfortunately, there is a lack of reliable data for the role of advanced urodynamics, but it is hoped that ongoing studies will clarify its position in the urologic armamentarium. It is, however, important to recognize that the accuracy of computer analysis must be matched by accurate signal recording.

Ambulatory Urodynamics

Ambulatory monitoring of the physiologic function of the lower urinary tract is the ideal. Conventional cystometry is unphysiologic not only because of fast fill rates, short duration of the test, urethral catheterization, and clinical setting, but also because of the degree of immobility resulting

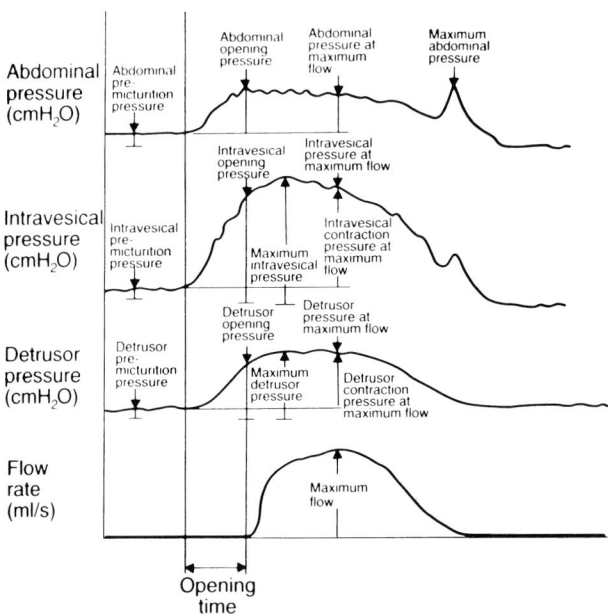

Figure 3–11. Frequently measured variables during pressure flow micturition studies.

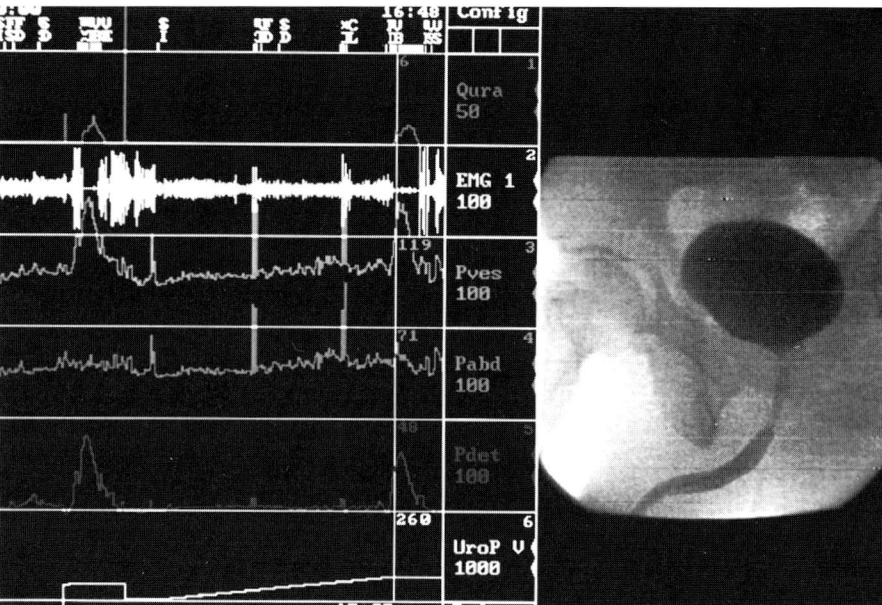

Figure 3–12. A typical screen for a patient undergoing videourodynamic study. The electronic data and fluoroscopic image of the bladder and outlet are simultaneously depicted.

from the test environment. Methods for performing ambulatory urodynamics are still, however, not ideal, and it is looked on as a research tool. Current techniques require long-duration urethral catheterization, for the monitoring of intravesical pressure and the measurement of intra-abdominal pressure are by rectal transducer, with the data being stored on a small portable device for later evaluation. Patients may document episodes of urgency or incontinence, for example, with an event marker for closer scrutiny later.

Neal et al[25] have shown differences between the result for physiologic fill (ambulatory) versus conventional fill cystometry. As expected, with conventional cystometry there is a higher P_{det} rise on filling as compared with natural fill, and there is an increased bladder volume with conventional studies. Ambulatory studies also demonstrate detrusor instability more frequently. An increased voiding pressure is also noted. This may be due to some functional or anatomic obstruction resulting from the lengthy period of urethral catheterization. These changes are seen not only in patients with lower urinary tract pathology but also in asymptomatic controls.

Current application of ambulatory urodynamics appears to be in those patients whose symptoms do not match conventional cystometric findings. As the role of ambulatory studies increases and technology advances, mechanisms of evaluation may become less invasive and may use an electronic "pill" or suprapubic access, thereby making ambulatory studies more amenable to current practice.

VIDEO URODYNAMICS

Video urodynamics combines the fluoroscopic screening of the bladder and outlet and the electronic urodynamic data during portions of the bladder storage and voiding study, adding an anatomic "dimension" to the urodynamic study (Fig. 3–12). It does, however, require a larger investment in equipment because of the need for fluoroscopy (Fig. 3–13). A key advantage of simultaneous imaging is that it allows one to localize the obstruction in patients with voiding dysfunction as resulting from the prostate, a dyssynergic sphincter, a urethral stricture, or in women, a distorted outlet. A second clinical situation in which videourodynamics is invaluable is in the classification of stress urinary incontinence. Fluoroscopy helps distinguish between those with "anatomic" stress incontinence who have significant vesical neck hypermobility and those in whom intrinsic sphincter deficiency predominates and there is minimal pelvic floor descent. It is important to recognize that in most women the two factors coexist and that the degree to which this occurs determines largely what type of surgical procedure is most appropriate. In the evaluation of the neuropathic bladder, fluoroscopic screening allows one to determine the presence of and pressure at which the vesicoureteral reflux occurs and to evaluate sphincter events that may interfere with voiding dysfunction.

The major disadvantage of video urodynamics is the large investment in equipment, the cost of contrast material, and the x-ray exposure necessary. Its selective use, however, allows improved diagnosis and yields maximal information.

URETHRAL PRESSURE STUDIES

Information about the function of the bladder outlet is obtained in a variety of urodynamic tests, including static urethral pressure profilometry, stress urethral pressure profiles, leak point pressures, and micturitional urethral pressure profiles (UPP).

The UPP is a recording of the intraluminal pressure along

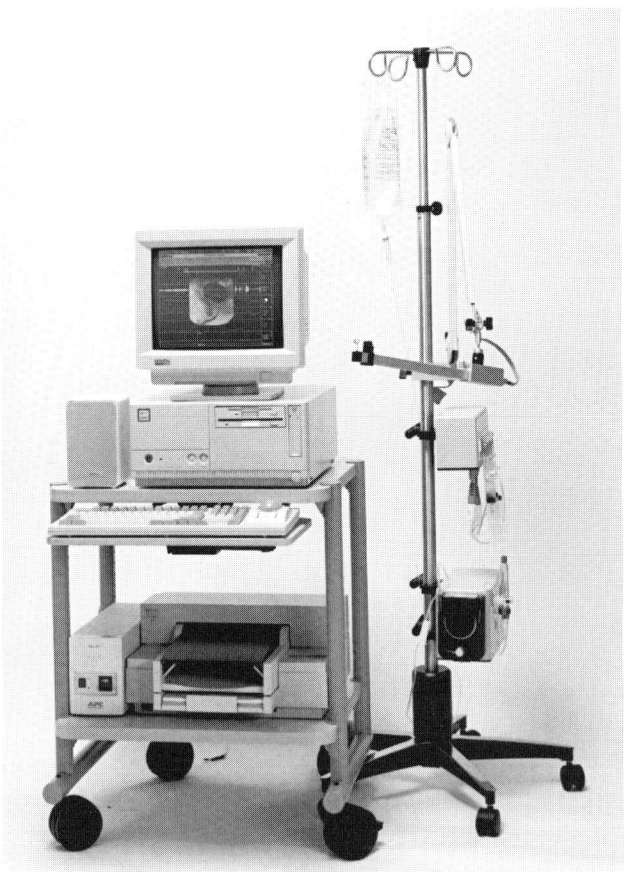

Figure 3–13. Videourodynamic equipment (Courtesy of Life-Tech, Inc., Houston, TX.)

the length of the urethra. The study is performed using slow retraction of a catheter that has radially drilled side holes and is perfused with liquid. An automatic pulling device is used to advance the catheter at a rate of 0.5 mm/sec. Functional urethral length is represented by the length of urethra where the intraluminal pressure exceeds intravesical pressure (Fig. 3–14). The maximum urethral pressure profile (MUPP) denotes the maximal pressure of the UPP, whereas maximum urethral closure pressure (MUCP) is the difference between the MUPP and the intravesical pressure. Whenever UPP is considered, bladder pressure and volume should be measured simultaneously to exclude an associated detrusor contraction. The subtracted pressure of the bladder from the urethral pressure is the urethral closure pressure profile. In addition to these measures some have measured and interpreted the area beneath the curve to represent a continence zone. Normal values for female urethral closure pressure decline with age. With the upper edge of the symphysis pubis used as a zero reference, premenopausal mean profiles of more than 50 cm H_2O are usual, whereas postmenopausal women have average MUCP of 35 cm of water.

Urethral pressure profilometry has not found widespread clinical use as a method to quantify the bladder outlet resistance. It is unfortunately highly subject to artifact variation and measures show wide variation within normal patients and in those presenting with symptoms suggestive of bladder outlet weakness such as stress incontinence. Both MUCP and functional urethral length tend to be lower in patients with genuine stress incontinence, but enough overlap exists between these patients and continent women to prevent these measures from being diagnostic.[26,27] Sorensen provided an exhaustive review of urethral function in healthy women, showing again that urethral pressure profilometry provides accurate measures, that urethral pressure measurements decrease with age, but that as a single measure it is not accurate to define a subgroup of patients with stress incontinence versus those without outlet weakness.[28]

Although urethral pressure profiles provide little useful information on their own, they may, in conjunction with a full urodynamic evaluation, assist in categorizing the quality of a patient's outlet, for it is certainly true that the profile represents the summation of static forces active upon the urethra. McGuire, however, argues that static UPP provides little information on the efficiency with which the urethral sphincter resists abdominal pressure.[29] The static infusion urethral profile may be useful for testing the function of an artificial urinary sphincter. Needless to say, the role of UPP measurement remains controversial.

The stress urethral pressure profile involves the simultaneous measurement of urethral and bladder pressure as the urethral catheter is withdrawn and as the patient intermittently stresses (coughs), allowing a pressure transmission ratio to be recorded. If urethral hypermobility is present, pressure transmission from the intra-abdominal zone to the urethra is altered. This study is widely used in gynecologic practice but has few urologic proponents. The test is difficult to perform and interpret, and it is prone to artifact.

Leak point pressure as described by McGuire represents an alternative assessment of urethral function.[29,30] The abdominal or Valsalva leak point pressure is that pressure required to cause leakage in the absence of a bladder contraction. The test may be performed during cystometry (preferably standing) when the bladder has been filled to approximately 150 ml. The patient is asked to strain, and if no leakage occurs, to cough, and the urethra observed (di-

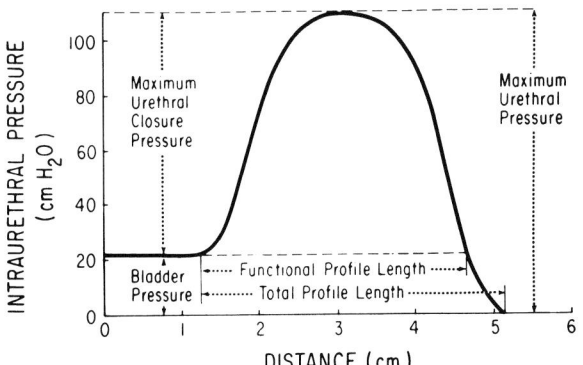

Figure 3–14. An idealized urethral pressure profile curve with frequently measured variables.

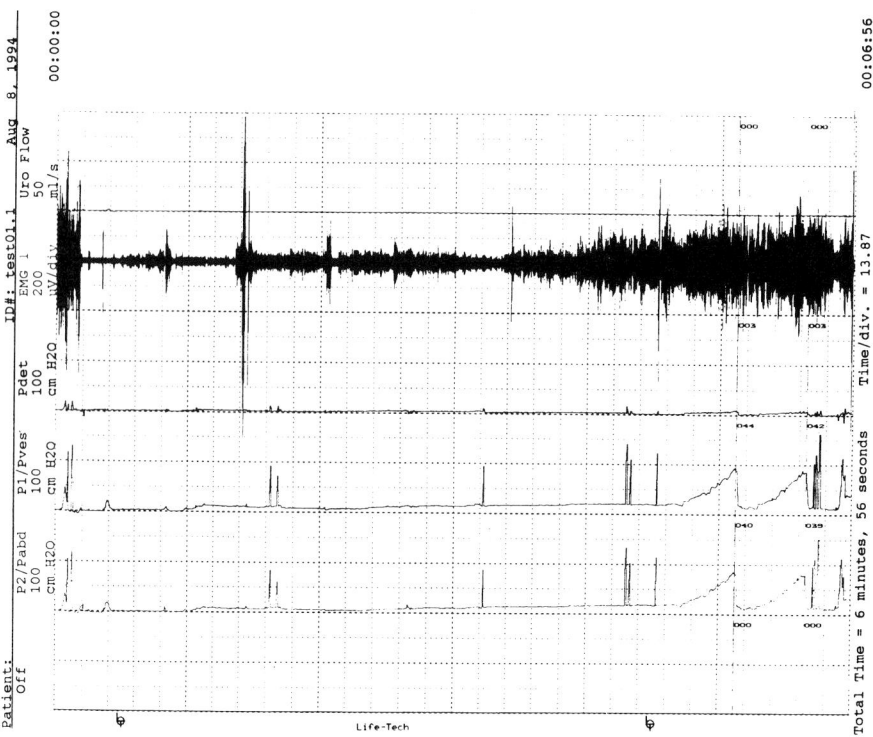

Figure 3–15. Valsalva leak point pressure is depicted in the P_{ves} tracing of this cystometrogram. The brief duration spikes are due to cough. The prolonged pressure elevation is due to Valsalva, and leak occurred at 44 cm H_2O pressure.

rectly or radiographically) for leakage around the catheter. The pressure at which leakage occurs is the leak point pressure (LPP) (Fig. 3–15). The LPP, which appears reproducible, correlates well with the magnitude of incontinence; those with high volume incontinence due to intrinsic sphincter weakness (type III incontinent women) have low LPPs. A number of factors may interfere with the study including the presence of significant cystocele, detrusor instability or the patient involuntarily contracting the striated sphincter during the test. The test has also not yet been standardized with respect to catheter size, catheter location (bladder/vaginal/rectal), and bladder volume, nor indeed have normal values been established. This author currently uses a LPP of 100 cm as the lower limit of normal; certainly pressures of less than 60 cm H_2O imply profound outlet weakness. McGuire has shown that maximum urethral pressure was unrelated to abdominal LPP in incontinent patients, once again calling into question urethral pressure profilometry.[29]

SPHINCTER ELECTROMYOGRAPHY

Sphincter electromyography (EMG) studies the bioelectric potentials generated in the distal striated sphincter mechanism. Such studies are performed at two different levels of sophistication, each with distinct goals and requiring different instrumentation. The first, termed *kinesiologic* studies, are commonly performed in the urodynamic laboratory and simply examine sphincter activity during bladder filling and voiding. The second are neurophysiologic tests that require considerable expertise and elaborate equipment, and are designed to examine the integrity of innervation of the muscle.

Kinesiologic Studies

Kinesiologic studies may be performed using a variety of electrodes and display methods. The signal is usually recorded using surface electrodes (stick-on skin EKG electrodes) or preferably hooked wire electrodes introduced into the periurethral muscle. The advantage of the latter is that their more proximate location to the muscle being recorded renders the information more interpretable. Although in many patients the recordings obtained from periurethral pelvic floor and perianal sphincter is the same, dissimilar information may be obtained, particularly in patients with lower spinal cord injury[31] and in those who have had pelvic surgery or who have demyelinating disease. Hence it is always preferable to record from the periurethral area. The signal is generally recorded onto a chart strip recorder and/or the signal is amplified and recorded as sound on an audio monitor. Chart strip recording of the signal shows characteristic changes in sphincter activity during bladder filling and voiding (Fig. 3–16). As bladder filling proceeds progressive recruitment of sphincter activity is demonstrated by increased amplitude and frequency of firing. During voiding, sphincter activity should cease; failure to do so is termed *detrusor–sphincter dyssynergia*. This feature is seen in certain neurologic diseases, particularly suprasacral spinal cord injury. Normal sphincter EMG activity has a recognizable audio quality, whereas in neurologic conditions abnormal EMG waveforms, which include complex polyphasic potentials, fibrillation potentials, and complex repetitive discharges result in characteristic identifiable sounds. Many urodynamic investigators will simultaneously monitor the chart strip and audio recordings for improved interpretability.

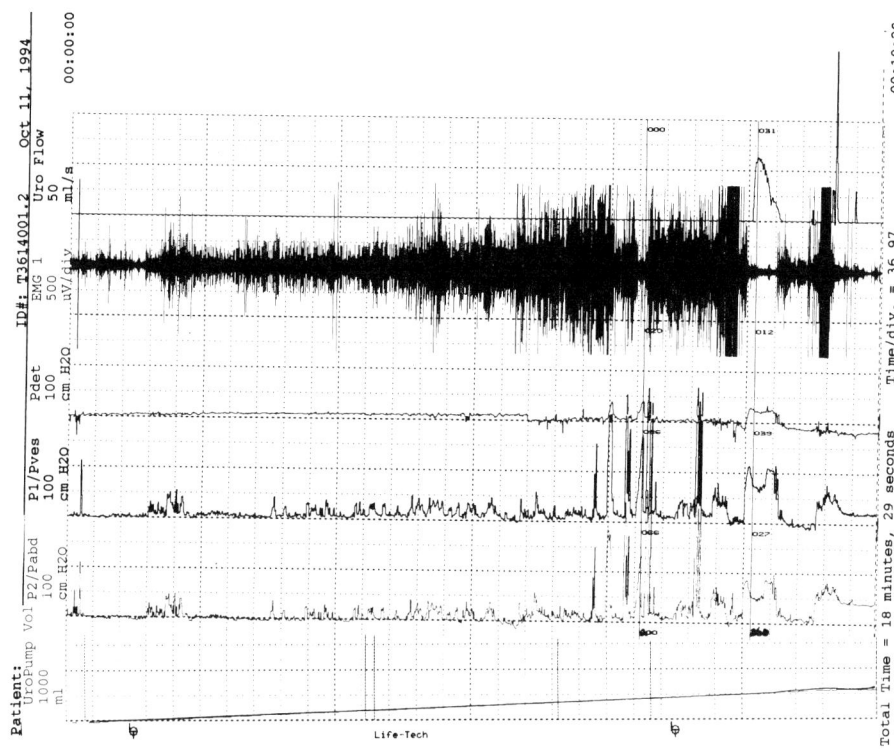

Figure 3–16. A multichannel filling and voiding study. The P_{det} tracing shows a stable bladder during the filling study and a small detrusor contraction (12 cm H_2O pressure) during micturition. This detrusor contraction achieves a flow of 31 mL/sec. The EMG tracing shows progressive recruitment of activity during fill identified by the increased amplitude of excursion of the cursor. During voiding there is "electrical silence" of the sphincter.

Neurophysiologic Recordings

These studies require more sophisticated instrumentation and investigator expertise, and are designed to actually diagnose and characterize the presence of neuropathy. Action potentials generated during sphincter activity may be recorded using a specialized needle electrode inserted directly into the muscle to be tested, with the individual waveforms being recorded on an oscilloscope. Motor unit action potentials (MUAP) in health and disease differ, and so, within certain limitations, the expert observer may use these studies to determine whether neuropathy is present or not. Normally, the MUAP recorded from the distal urethral sphincter muscle has a biphasic or triphasic waveform with an amplitude of 50 to 300 μv and a firing frequency of 10 to 100 discharges per second (Fig. 3–17). Simplistically, when the motor neuron or nerve to a muscle is damaged, the muscle responds in a characteristic fashion. Those muscle fibers that have lost their nerve supply become reinnervated by adjacent healthy nerves and the motor unit action potential changes. The waveform becomes larger in amplitude and increases in complexity and duration (Fig. 3–18). These changes may infer the presence of neurologic injury; further refinement of study may imply whether the injury is ongoing or old.

Nerve Conduction Studies

Nerve conduction studies are performed by the stimulation of a peripheral nerve and the monitoring of the time taken for a response to occur in its innervated muscle (Fig. 3–19). The time from stimulation to response is termed the *latency*. These studies are a test of the integrity of a reflex arc and can be relatively sensitive indicators of the presence of

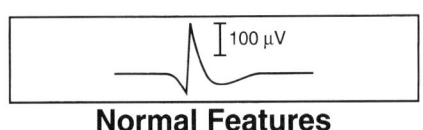

Normal Features

Characteristic configuration	
Amplitude	50 - 300 μv
Duration	3 - 5 m.secs.
Frequency	1 - 4 per sec.

Figure 3–17. Motor unit action potentials

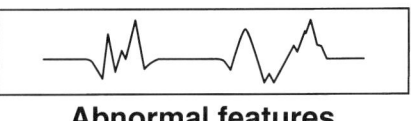

Abnormal features

Increase in amplitude, duration, complexity of wave form.

Polyphasic potentials (>5 deflections)
Fibrillation potentials
Positive sharp waves
Bizarre high frequency forms

Figure 3–18. Motor unit action potentials

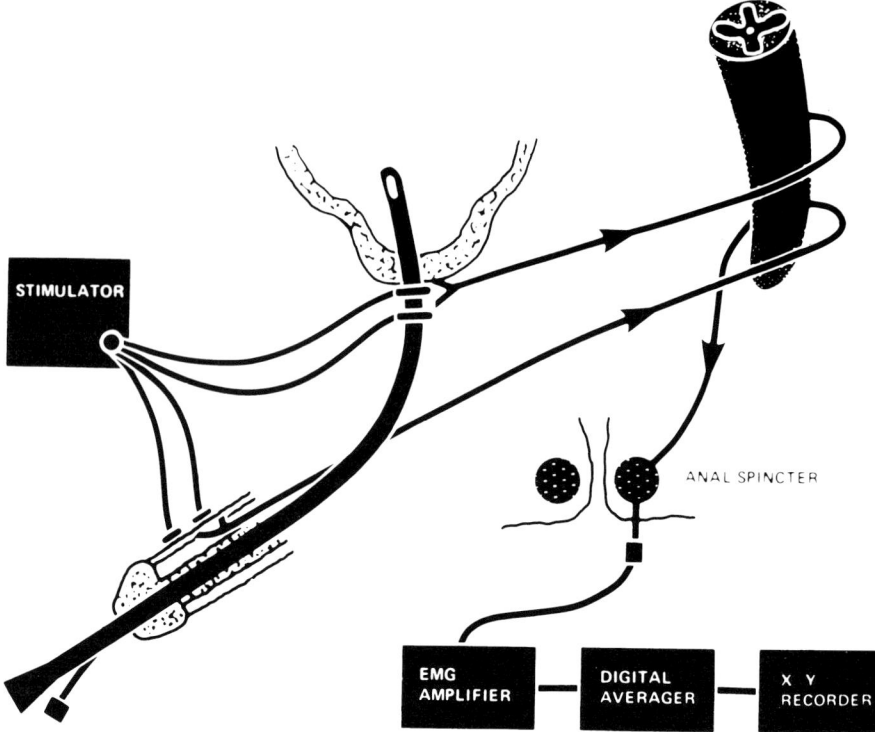

Figure 3–19. A schematic depicting pathways and equipment used for nerve conduction studies (sacral latency study).

neurologic disease. In urologic practice these studies are most often performed as bulbocavernosus reflex latency determinations. These studies require elaborate instrumentation and careful user interpretation. Abnormal responses occur in a variety of situations and are particularly diagnostic in patients with diabetes and peripheral neuropathies. In patients with conus medullaris or cauda equina lesions one may find normal, prolonged, or absent latencies, and asymmetrical responses are not uncommon. Patients with suprasacral lesions may have normal or low latencies (26 to 30 msec) because of loss of inhibitory neural pathways from higher centers.

Evoked Responses

Evoked responses are potential changes in the central nervous system neurons that have resulted from distal (often electrical) stimulation. They are used to test the integrity of peripheral, spinal, and central nervous pathways, and in urology they are performed as genitospinal and genitocortical evoked-response recordings. They require sophisticated instrumentation using averaging techniques, and their performance is confined to specialized centers.

COMMON URODYNAMIC USAGE

Urodynamic study finds valuable use in many clinical scenarios, some of which we summarize below.

Spinal Dysraphism

In recent decades there has been a marked change in the management of children with spinal dysraphism (bladder preservation and rehabilitation have been performed in preference to urinary diversion). It has been recognized that urodynamic study performed soon after birth can predict those children who are at risk for upper tract deterioration; hence the study is now performed as soon after back-closure as possible.[32] The technique of study requires little modification and has led to the categorization of lower urinary tract dynamics into those with dyssynergic systems, synergic systems, and complete lower tract denervation. It has been noted that 71% of newborns with dyssynergia will develop deterioration of the upper urinary tract in the first 3 years of life, whereas this occurs in only 17% of the synergic group and in 23% of the completely denervated group.[17] Low bladder compliance is also a potent predictor of future deterioration, occurring in 63% of cases.

The institution of a clean intermittent catheterization program together with the addition of anticholinergic medications in the newborn period in those individuals with high-risk systems can almost completely reverse this trend to deterioration. Although some have used simple cystometry and LPP to identify the high-risk group, we have preferred multifunction testing and the use of "hostility score."[33,34] This latter system recognizes the fact that features other than low bladder compliance are also hazardous to the developing upper tracts. It is also important to recognize that in this group of patients the neurologic lesion may change with time and that sequential urodynamic study is therefore necessary, particularly if incontinence, recurrent infections, or upper tract deterioration supervene despite a seemingly acceptable management program. In a series reported by Spindel et al, 15 of 79 children developed worsening urodynamics with time.[35]

Spinal Cord Injury

As in the child with spinal dysraphism, spinal cord injury will result in neurogenic bladder dysfunction, and increases in intravesical pressure due to alterations in bladder compliance, reflex contractility, and outlet resistance may also lead to the deterioration of the upper urinary tracts. Here too the management of such patients has become less expectant and more active. Baseline urodynamic evaluation is indicated as soon as reflex activity has returned following cord injury; again, sequential study is necessary because of the possibility of changing lesions. The early introduction of clean intermittent catheterization and anticholinergic medication to suppress involuntary detrusor activity predictably leads to continence and appears to prevent the progressive loss of bladder capacity due to increasingly high-pressure involuntary contractions or loss of compliance, which seemed to accompany expectant management alone. Based on a study of 105 patients with spinal cord injury in whom bladder pressure data were carefully monitored and managed, McGuire et al suggested that periodic upper tract radiographic evaluation is not essential, providing bladder pressures remain controlled.[36]

Women with Stress Urinary Incontinence

As noted earlier, women with the symptom of stress urinary incontinence frequently have associated bladder instability symptoms. The CMG may show involuntary bladder contractions, in which event motor urgency is diagnosed; alternatively, the CMG may be stable and the patient may be diagnosed as having sensory urgency. Both motor and sensory urgency frequently coexist with anatomic incontinence, but they may not influence its management. It is important that an attempt be made to improve symptoms with anticholinergic management and behavioral therapy (bladder drill); however, the anatomic problem will generally cause continuing incontinence and will still require surgical correction. In this event, there is an approximately 75% chance that the urge component will also resolve following surgery for the stress component. Resolution is less common in elderly patients; in those with high-pressure, low-volume, involuntary contractions; and in those with bladder instability of long standing. In the woman with a history of primary stress urinary incontinence without urgency symptoms, in whom physical examination confirms anterior vaginal wall hypermobility, cystometry may be dispensed with prior to surgery. However, in patients with recurrent incontinence, those with associated neurologic dysfunction, and those with significant bladder instability symptoms, formal urodynamic testing with fluoroscopy is valuable. Urodynamic evaluation in this patient population includes LPP to identify the presence of intrinsic sphincter deficiency, which will significantly alter management. Videourodynamics is also invaluable in this regard.

Obstructive Voiding Symptoms

The hierarchy of study techniques and the limitations of urodynamic evaluation in patients with voiding symptoms have been elaborated earlier. Despite diagnostic limitations, the study remains invaluable, particularly in the elderly male, in whom at least 25% considered for prostatectomy on symptom evaluation alone prove to be unobstructed by urodynamic evaluation.[37] Symptoms in this nonobstructed group are generally due to bladder instability, bladder hypersensitivity, or impaired contractility. It is notable that in those patients with obstruction the severity of symptoms does not correlate well with the degree of obstruction.

REFERENCES

1. Blaivas JG: Management of bladder dysfunction in multiple sclerosis. *Neurology* 1980;30:12.
2. Abrams PH, Blaivas JG, Stanton SL, et al: The standardization of terminology of lower urinary tract function. *Scand J Neurol Nephrol (Suppl)* 1988;115–119.
3. Dubois P: Uber den Druck in der Blaharnblase. *Arch Klin Med* 1876;17:148.
4. Mosso A and Pellacini P: Sullagiunzione Della Vesica. *R Accad Nazzllincei (Rome)* 1881;12:1.
5. Rose DK: Cystometric bladder pressure determinations: their clinical importance. *J Urol* 1927;17:487–501.
6. Drake WM: The uroflowmeter: an aid to the study of the lower urinary tract. *J Urol* 1948;59:650–658.
7. von Garrelts B: Analysis of micturition: a new method of recording the voiding of the bladder. *Acta Chir Scand* 1956;112:326–340.
8. Gleason DM, Lattimer JK: The pressure flow study: a method for measuring bladder neck resistance. *J Urol* 1962;87:844–852.
9. Davis DM, Zimskind P: Progress in urodynamics in conjunction with lower urinary tract urodynamic studies. *J Urol* 1962;87:243–248.
10. Miller ER: Techniques of simultaneous display of X-ray and physiologic data. In: Boyaski S eds. *The neurogenic bladder*. Baltimore: Williams & Wilkins, 1967;79–85.
11. Bates CP, Whiteside BM, Turner-Warick R: Synchronous cine-pressure-flow-cystourethrography with special reference to stress and urge incontinence. *Br J Urol* 1970;42:714–723.
12. Perez LM, Webster GD: The history of urodynamics. *Neurourol Urodyn* 1992;11(1):1.
13. Koff SA: Relationship between dysfunctional voiding and reflux. *J Urol* 1992;148:1703–1705.
14. Abrams PH, Blaivas JG, Stanton SL, Anderson JT: Standardization of terminology of lower urinary tract function. *Neurourol Urodyn* 1988;7:403–428.

15. McGuire EJ: Neuromuscular dysfunction of the lower urinary tract. In: Walsh PC, Gittes RF, Perlmater AD, Stamey TA, eds. *Campbell's Urology*, 5th ed. Philadelphia: WB Saunders, 1986.
16. Bates P, Bradley WE, Melkeor H, Rowan D, Sterline A, Harold T: The first report on the standardization of terminology of lower urinary tract function. Urinary incontinence. Procedures related to the evaluation of urinary storage. Cystometry urethral closure pressure profiles units of measurement. *Br J Urol* 1976;48:39.
17. Bauer SB, Hallot M, Khoshbin S, et al: The predictive value of urodynamic evaluation in the newborn with myelodysplasia. *JAMA* 1984;152:650–652.
18. Siroky MB, Olsson CA, Krane RJ: The flow rate nomogram: 1. Development. *J Urol* 1979;122:665–668.
19. Beckman KA: Urinary flow during micturition in normal women. *Acta Chir Scand* 1965;130:357–370.
20. Cierup J: Micturition studies in infants and children: Normal urinary flow. *Scand J Urol Nephrol* 1974;191–207.
21. Turner-Warwick RT, Whiteside CG, Worth PHL, et al: A urodynamic view of bladder neck obstruction. *Br J Urol* 1973;45:44–59.
22. Schafer W: Principles and clinical application of advanced urodynamic analysis of voiding function. *Urol Clin North Am* 1990;17(3):553–566.
23. Schafer W: Urethral resistance? Urodynamic concepts of physiological and pathological bladder outlet function during voiding. *Neurourol Urodyn* 1985;4:161–201.
24. Rollema JH, Mastrigt R: Objective analysis of prostatism: clinical application of the computer program CLIM. *Neurourol Urodyn* 1991;10:71–76.
25. Robertson AS, Griffiths CJ, Ramsden PD, Neal DB: Bladder function in healthy volunteers: ambulatory monitoring and conventional urodynamic studies. *Br J Urol* 1994;73:242–249.
26. Asmussen M, Ulmsten U: Simultaneous urethrocystometry and urethral pressure profile measurement with a new technique. *Acta Obstet Gynecol Scand* 1976;54:385.
27. van Geelen JM: The urethral pressure profile in continent women. Thesis Schriks: Drukker IJ, Asten, 1983.
28. Sorensen S: Urethral pressure variations in healthy and incontinent women. *Neurourol Urodyn* 1992;11:549–591.
29. McGuire EJ, Fitzpatrick CC, et al: Clinical assessment of urethral sphincter function. *J Urol* 1993;150:1452–1454.
30. McGuire EJ, Woodwide JR, Boarding TA, Weiss RM: Prognastic value of urodynamic testing in myelodysplastic patients. *J Urol* 1981;126–205.
31. Perkash I: Urodynamic evaluation: periurethral striated EMG vs. perianal striated EMG. *Paraplegia* 1980;18:275–282.
32. Bauer SB: Early evaluation and management of children with spina bifida. In King LR, ed. *Urologic Surgery in Neonates and Young Infants*. Philadelphia: WB Saunders, 1988;252–264.
33. McGuire EJ, Woodside JR, Borden TA, Weiss RN: The prognostic value of urodynamic testing in myelodysplastic patients. *J Urol* 1981;126:205–209.
34. Galloway NTM, Mekras JA, Helms M, Webster GD: An objective score to predict upper tract deterioration in myelodysplasia. *J Urol* 1991;145:535–537.
35. Spindel MR, Bauer SB, Dyro FM: The changing neurourologic lesion in myelodysplasia. *JAMA* 1987;258:1630–1633.
36. McGuire EJ, Noll F, Maynard F: A pressure management system for neurourogenic bladder after spinal cord injury. *Neurourol Urodyn* 1991;10:223–230.
37. Abrams PH, Feneley RCL: The significance of the symptoms associated with bladder outlet obstruction. *Urol Int* 1978;33:171.

4 The Abdominal Radiograph

Robert A. Older

THE NORMAL ABDOMINAL RADIOGRAPH

The technical factors in abdominal radiography vary depending upon the size of the patient and the equipment available. We employ a 60- to 70-kVp range with MAS dependent on patient size. The abdominal radiograph is a potential source of invaluable information. Understanding of the normal abdominal structures that can be identified on an abdominal radiograph provides a greater awareness of pathologic changes.

Evaluation of the normal abdominal radiograph can be difficult not only for beginning physicians, but also for those with more experience. The multiple overlying structures with varying appearances are a challenge to all. Normal abdominal radiographs are shown in Figure 4–1 and reveal a vast amount of normal anatomy. The four basic radiographic densities of calcium (white), soft tissue (gray), fat (dark gray), and air (black) provide natural contrast for the abdominal contents. The lumbar spine, sacrum, lower ribs, and a portion of the bony pelvis are seen in most patients. The tip of the spleen is visible in the left upper quadrant, and the right lobe of the liver is seen in the right upper quadrant. The renal outlines are seen because of surrounding lower density fat between the kidneys and other soft-tissue structures. Surrounding fat, darker than soft tissue, outlines not only the kidneys, but most of the abdominal soft-tissue structures, including the psoas muscles. The properitoneal fat stripes are seen laterally. The pelvic soft tissues are more difficult to separate into distinct structures, but muscles outlined by fat are symmetrically present and the bladder is partially visualized because of perivesical fat. Gas outlines portions of the stomach, small intestine, and colon. Calcium, incorporated in bone, provides the natural contrast for the skeletal structures.

A systematic review of the abdominal radiograph is important. Although some abnormalities will "stand out," many will be appreciated only if searched for carefully. A relatively simple approach in viewing the abdominal radiograph is as follows:

1. Review the skeletal structures, including the lower ribs, lumbar spine, sacrum, pelvis, and those portions of the hips that are visualized.
2. Evaluate the intestinal gas pattern, looking for regions of abnormally increased gas, such as those seen in an obstruction or ileus. Abnormally decreased gas is seen in bowel atresia or from mass effect that displaces the intestines.
3. Evaluate the abdominal soft tissues, to include both the intraperitoneal and the retroperitoneal organs and the surrounding fat stripes. Look for increased size, displacement, or loss of outline.
4. Observe the soft tissues for abdominal calcifications.
5. Evaluate the soft tissues for abnormal extraluminal gas collections.

In the following sections we will discuss the evaluation of the abdominal soft tissues, calcifications, and retroperitoneal gas collections. Review of the skeletal structures and various intestinal gas patterns is peripheral to the focus of this chapter.

THE PATHOLOGIC ABDOMEN

Soft-Tissue Abnormalities

"Positive" findings are typified by two observations: (1) mass effect (soft-tissue mass and/or displacement of surrounding structures) and (2) viceromegaly—liver, spleen, kidneys.

"Negative" findings are typified by the *absence* of normal structures and may be (1) localized—loss of psoas or renal outline due to inflammation, hemorrhage, or tumor, or (2) generalized—loss of all soft-tissue planes as in ascites or edematous states such as the nephrotic syndrome.

"Positive" soft-tissue abnormalities such as the masses in Figures 4–2 and 4–3 are easier to detect, as they tend to catch the eye. Negative abnormalities such as the localized loss of a psoas or renal margin are less apparent unless the normal structures are systematically looked for and identified. The obliteration of the psoas margin is obvious in the inflammatory process shown in Figure 4–4 but is more subtle in Figure 4–5, where localized adenopathy is the cause. A generalized loss of soft-tissue planes is often due to ascites, which can produce a striking radiographic appearance (Fig. 4–6) or, less commonly, to a generalized edematous state in which the normal fat planes become indistinct.

The soft-tissue abnormalities discussed earlier are primarily related to changes in the shape of structures, but changes in density can also be diagnostic. Obliteration of the

36 Diagnosis of Genitourinary Disease

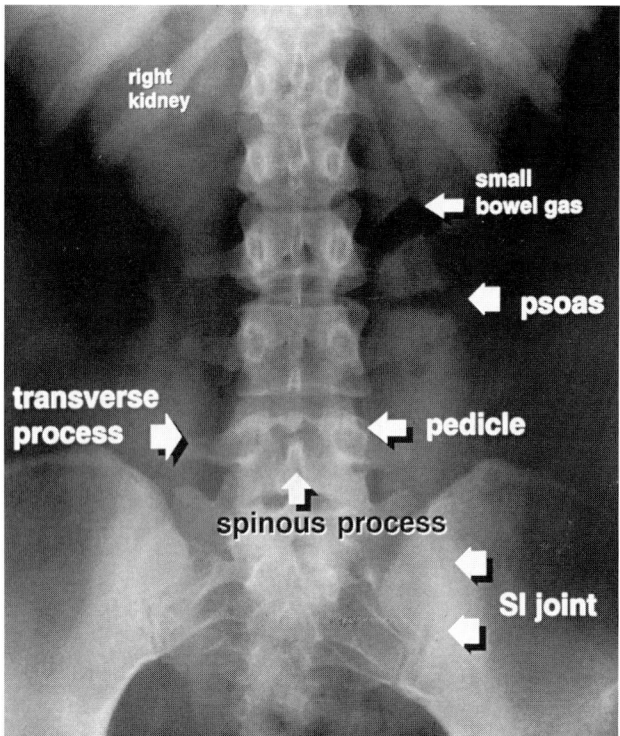 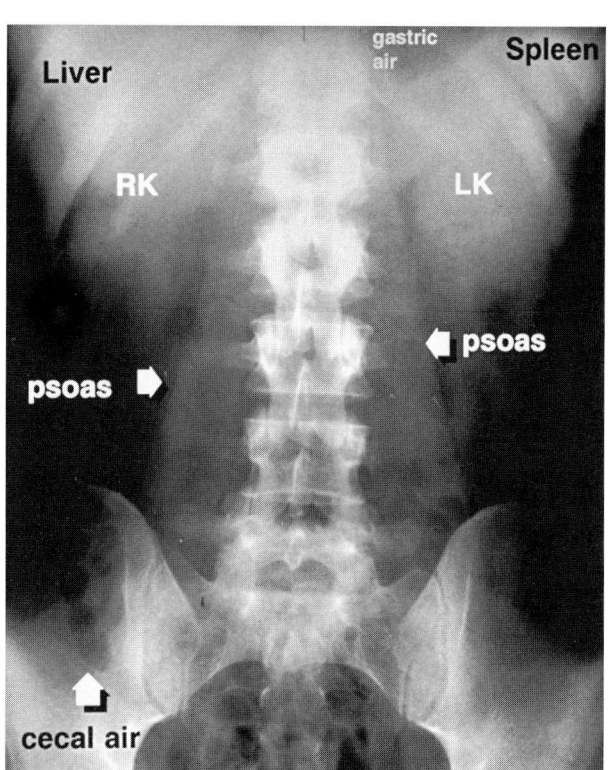

Figure 4–1. Normal abdominal radiographs.

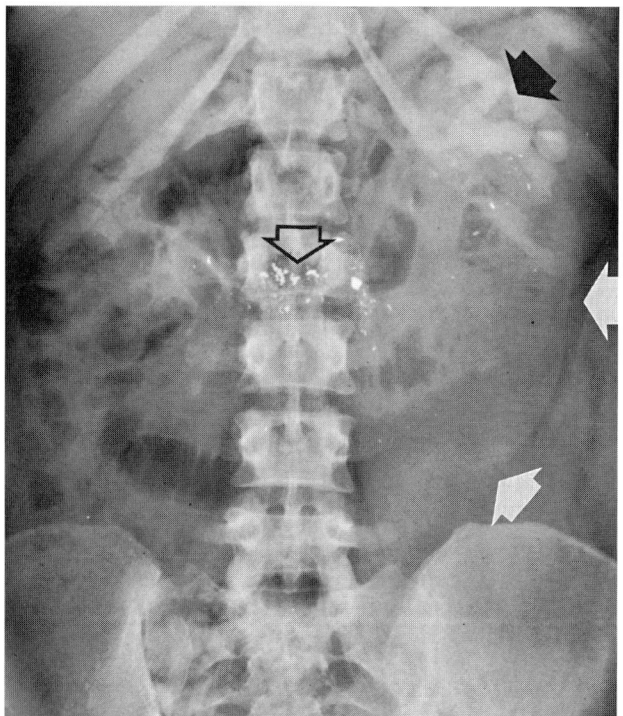 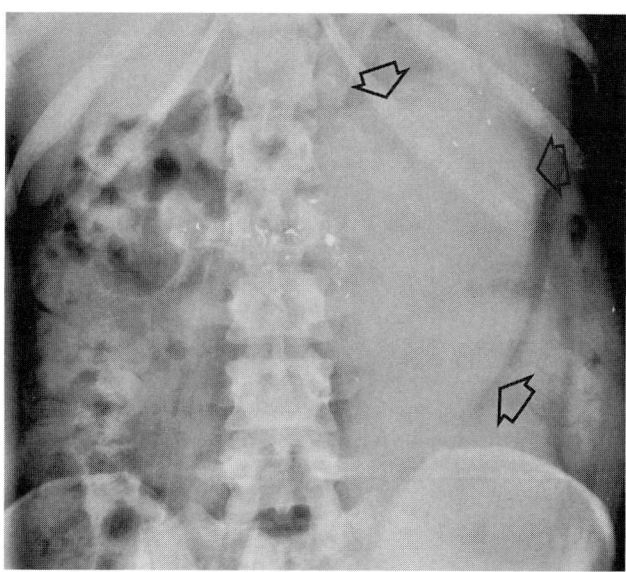

Figure 4–2. (A) Urinoma due to gunshot injury produces a soft-tissue mass (white arrows), displacing bowel and left kidney (black arrow) on an early radiograph from a urogram. Metallic bullet fragments (open arrow) overlie the spine. (B) Urinoma (open arrows) later fills with contrast and is more obvious.

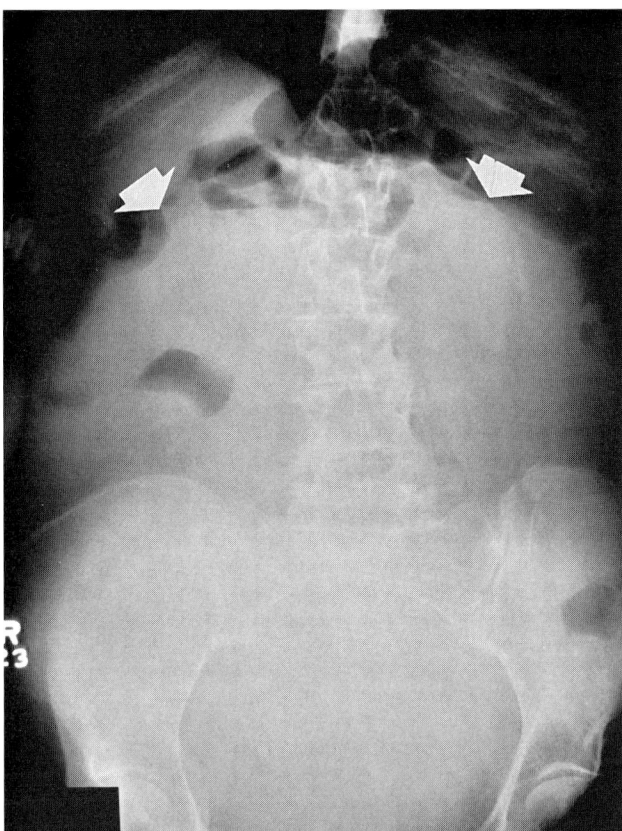

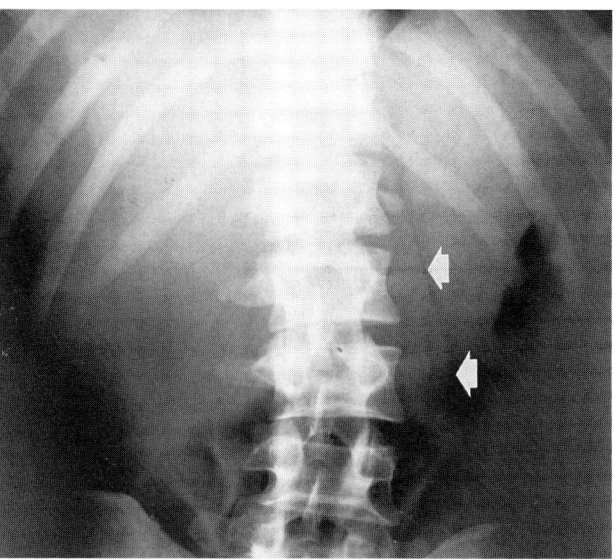

Figure 4–3. Large abdominal mass (arrows) displaces intestinal contents and produces a relatively gas-free central abdomen. The mass also obscures the abdominal structures.

Figure 4–4. Retroperitoneal abscess obscuring the right psoas margin and right renal outline. Left psoas clearly seen (arrows). Scoliosis away from the abscess is present. (Reprinted with permission from Older RA. *Excretory Urology*. Update 1980. Copyright The Chemical Rubber Co., CRC Press, Inc.)

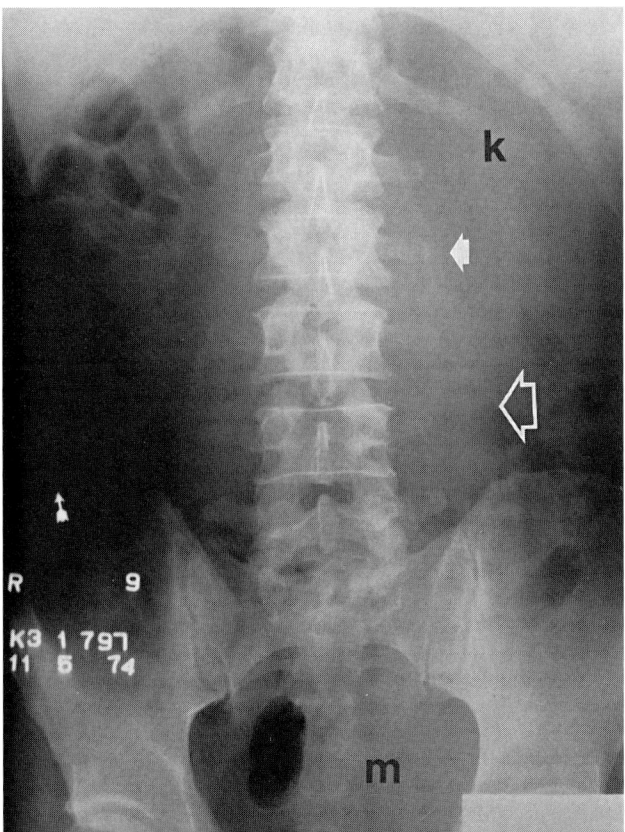

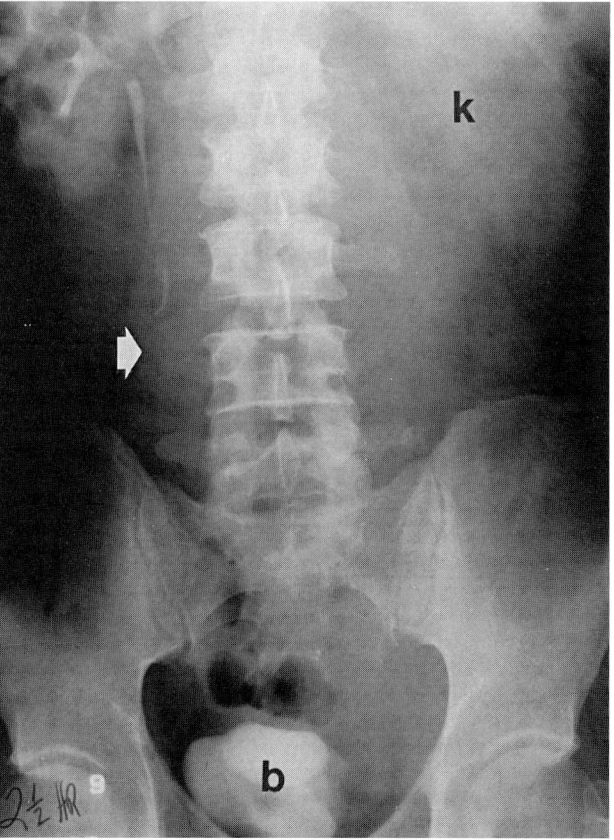

Fig. 4–5. (A) Retroperitoneal adenopathy obliterating portions of the left psoas outline. The left psoas is seen proximally (white arrow) but is obscured distally (open arrow). Adenopathy also displaces the left kidney (K) laterally, and pelvic adenopathy produces a mass (M) displacing the intestines to the right. Following contrast administration (B), the obstructed and displaced left kidney is more easily seen, as is the displaced bladder (B). Deviation of the right midureter by a nodal mass is also present (white arrow).

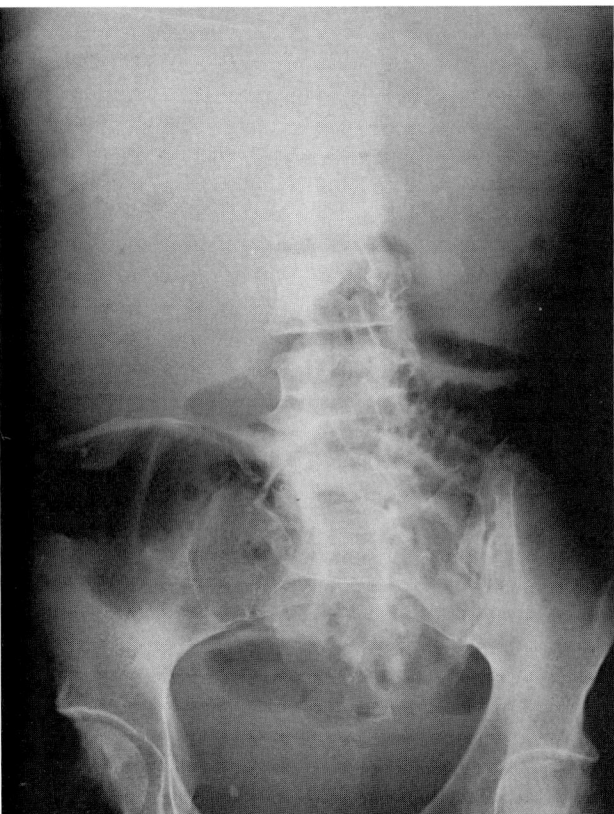

Figure 4–6. Ascites. All normal soft-tissue structures are obscured by the ascitic fluid. In the supine position the air-filled intestines are floating on top of the peritoneal fluid and thus are located centrally at the highest point in the abdomen.

right psoas is present in Figure 4–7, but the mass causing the loss of the psoas margin is darker than the liver above and indicates that the mass contains either fat or air, both of which are darker than the soft-tissue (water) density of most abdominal structures.

Abdominal Calcification

Calcium is a natural contrast agent appearing in a host of abnormalities within the abdomen. It is beyond our scope to discuss in detail all the types of abdominal calcification that can occur. We will concentrate primarily on those related to the urinary tract. If we consider both urologic and nonurologic calcifications, a healthy list can be produced. Nonurologic calcifications include those in the

1. Arteries (atherosclerosis)
2. Pancreas (chronic pancreatitis)
3. Gallbladder (gallstones and porcelain gallbladder)
4. Liver (granuloma, abscess, calcified cysts)
5. Spleen (granuloma, hematoma)
6. Lymph nodes

Urologic calcifications include

1. Parenchymal
   a. Cortical (acute cortical necrosis, chronic glomerulonephritis)

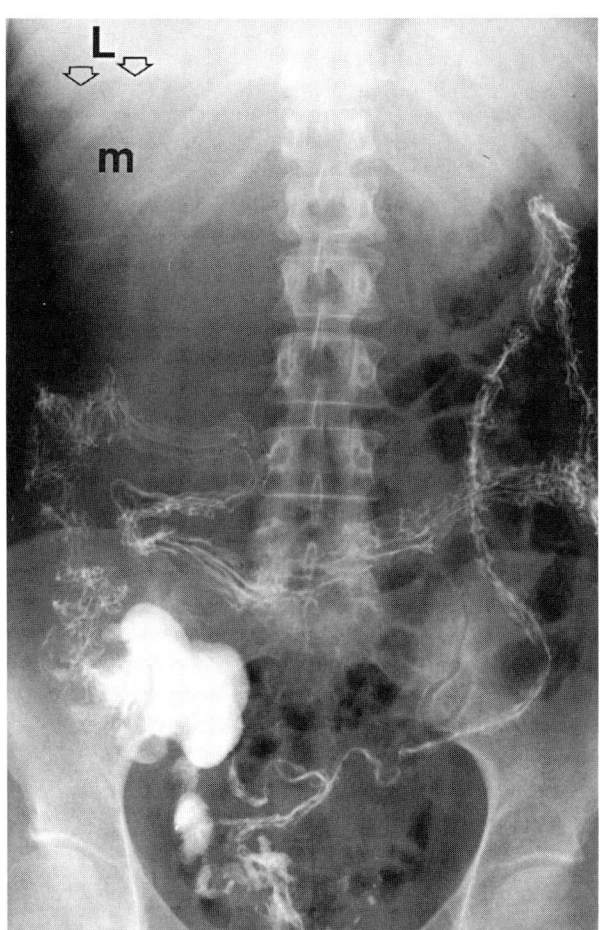

Figure 4–7. Liposarcoma obliterating the right psoas and renal outlines. The mass that fills the right retroperitoneum and displaces the bowel appears "darker" than the adjacent liver, as it contains large amounts of fat. A sharp interface (arrows) between "White" liver (L) and "Gray" mass (m) is present. The mass is also confirmed by the absence of gas on the right and the downward displacement of the hepatic flexure. Contrast in the colon is from a prior barium enema.

   b. Medullary (hypercalcemic conditions, renal tubular acidosis, medullary sponge kidney)
2. Collecting structures ("stones")
3. Mass calcifications (tumor, cyst, abscess)

In dealing with renal calcifications it is important to separate, whenever possible, parenchymal calcification from calcification occurring in the collecting structures because their etiologies differ. Cortical calcification is rare and occurs in acute cortical necrosis (postpartum), chronic glomerulonephritis, and oxalosis (Fig. 4–8). The radiographic appearance is similar to an early nephrogram phase after a bolus injection of contrast, when the cortex exhibits its greatest radiodensity. Medullary calcification occurs in renal tubular acidosis, hyperparathyroidism, or other hypercalcemia states, producing linear or globular calcifications in the medullary area. This presents a different radiographic appearance (Fig. 4–9A,B). Medullary sponge kidney can produce

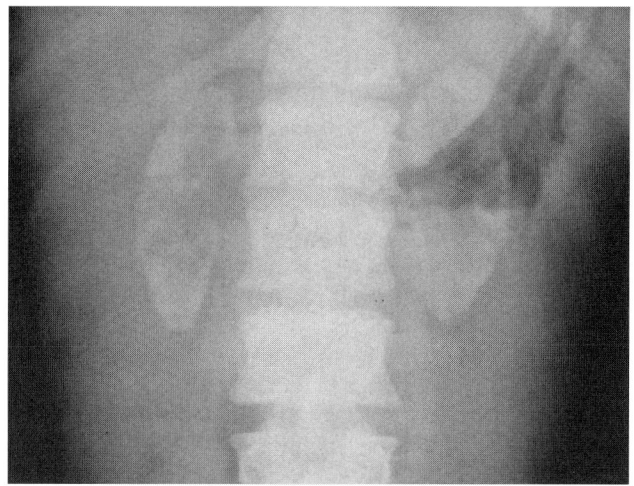

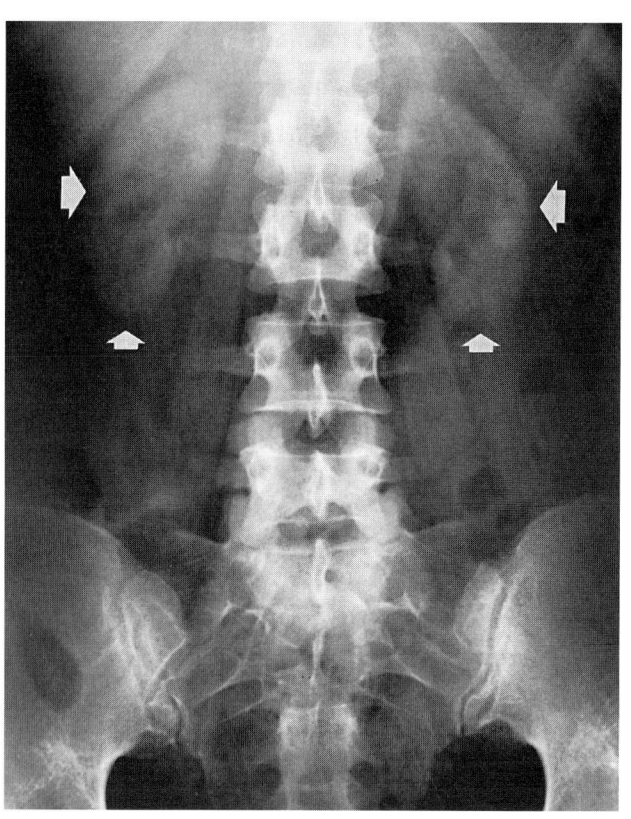

Figure 4–8. (A) Chronic glomerulonephritis with diffuse cortical calcification producing a dense rim in the periphery of each kidney. Note the small size of these chronically diseased kidneys as compared to the size of the vertebral bodies. (Reprinted with permission from Older RA. *Excretory Urology*. Update 1980. Copyright The Chemical Rubber Co., CRC Press, Inc.) (B) Bilateral diffuse thick cortical calcification (arrows) secondary to oxalosis. Kidneys are also small.

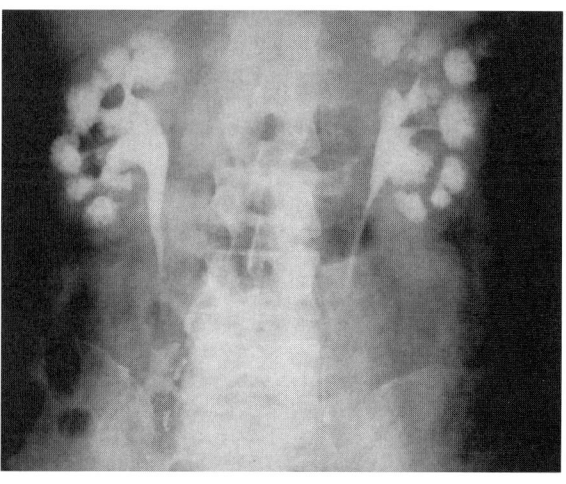

Figure 4–9. Medullary nephrocalcinosis due to renal tubular acidosis. (A) Typical ''popcorn''-type calcification throughout the medulla bilaterally. Retrograde pyelograms confirm (B) that the calcifications are outside the normal-appearing calyces. (Reprinted with permission from Older RA. *Excretory Urology*. Update 1980. Copyright The Chemical Rubber Co., CRC Press, Inc.) (C) Medullary calcification in ''sponge'' kidney.

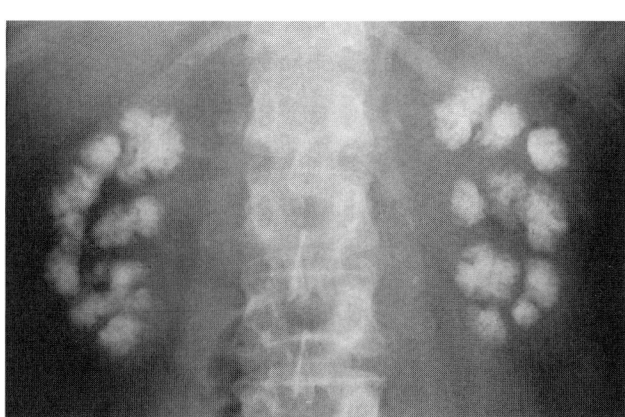

40 Diagnosis of Genitourinary Disease

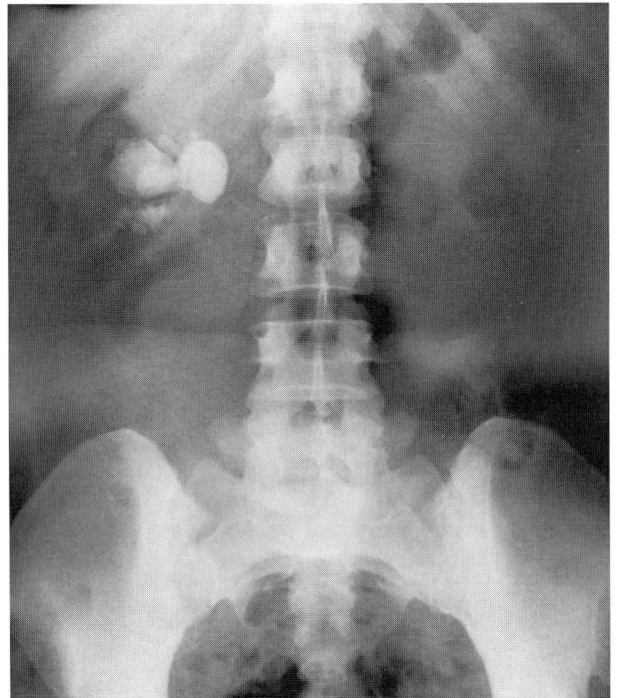
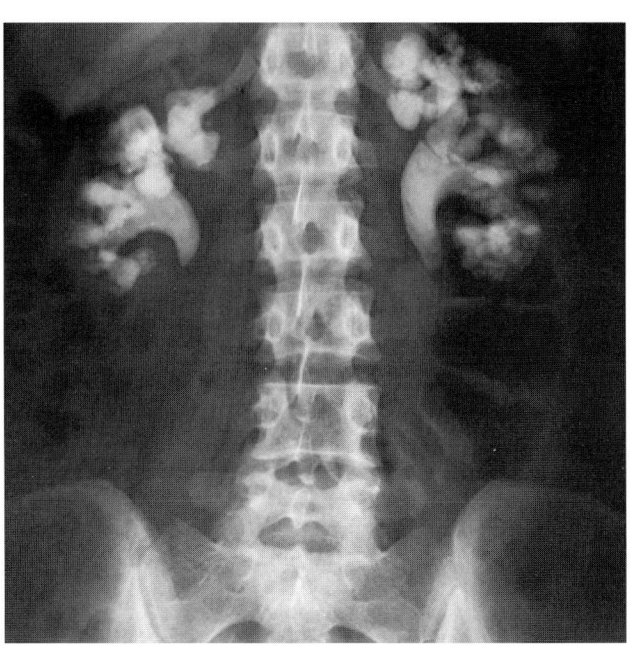

Figure 4–10. (A) Partial staghorn calculus with separate fragments in the right lower pole. (B) Bilateral staghorn calculi filling both collecting systems in a patient with renal tubular acidosis.

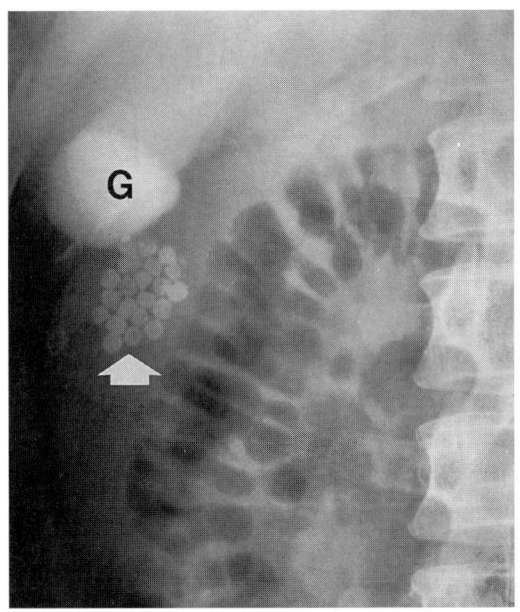
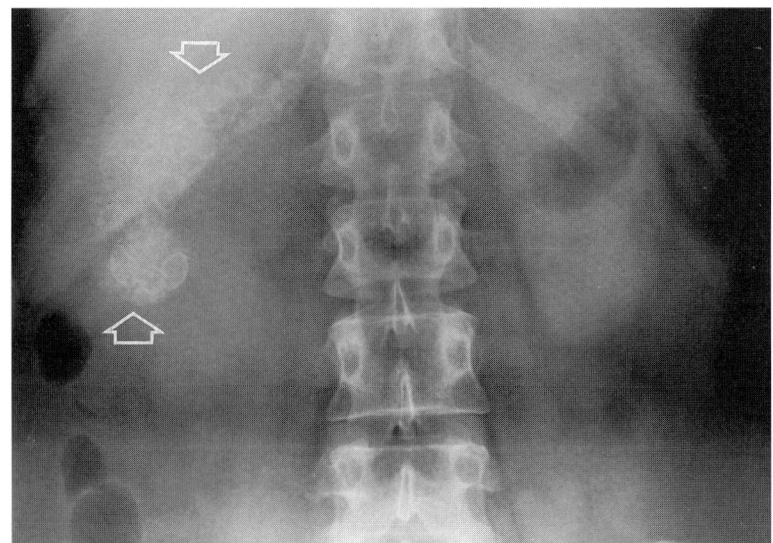

Figure 4–11. (A) Multiple laminated small stones (arrow) in the right upper quadrant have an appearance identical to gallstones but are clearly outside the opacified gallbladder (G). These were in a hydronephrotic calyx. (From Ref. 1) (B) Typical gallstones filling the gallbladder (arrows).

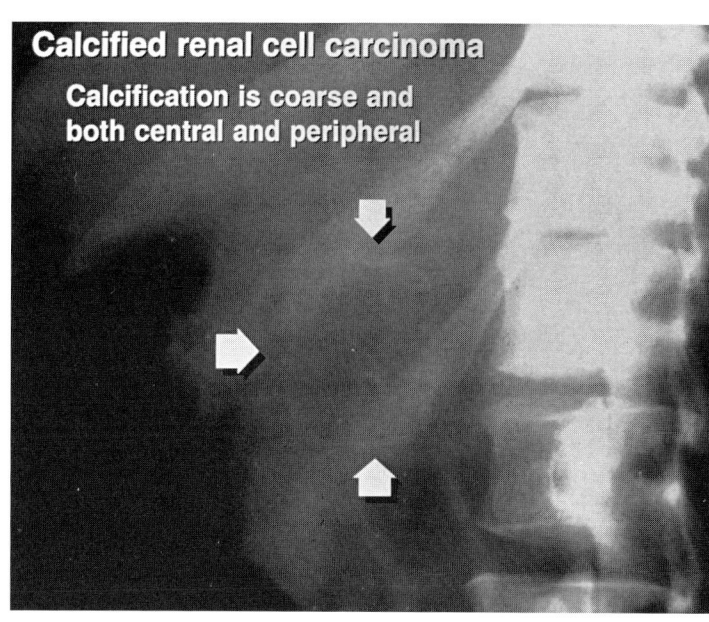

Figure 4–12. (A) Small, densely calcified hemorrhagic renal cyst. The differential would include renal cell carcinoma, complex cyst, trauma, tuberculosis, or old abscess. (B) Calcified renal cell carcinoma.

an appearance radiographically similar to that seen in hypercalcemic states because of the underlying tubular dilatation, but the calcification is usually not as extensive (Fig. 4–9C).

The most common type of renal calcification is the typical renal stone that forms in the collecting structures. These range from small calyceal calculi to large dendritic or staghorn calcifications that fill the entire collecting system (Fig. 4–10). Occasionally, renal stones can have an appearance that suggests calcification in another organ. Calcifications in a hydronephrotic kidney (Fig. 4–11) can appear to be more typical of gallstones than renal stones. This occurs because facetted stones such as those typically seen in the gallbladder can occur in any saccular structure. This can be a hydronephrotic kidney or a large calyceal diverticulum.[1]

Calcification in a renal mass is a significant finding, especially if the calcification is punctate or located centrally within the mass (Fig. 4–12). This appearance strongly suggests carcinoma.[2] Curvilinear calcification in the periphery of a mass can represent either cyst or tumor. Thin, smooth calcification is often found in a benign cyst, whereas thick or irregular calcification is more suggestive of carcinoma. This differentiation is further discussed in Chapter 17.

Abnormal Gas Collections

Like calcium, gas is a natural contrast agent and when present in areas other than the bowel lumen can provide significant information regarding pathologic processes. Probably the best known abnormal abdominal air pattern is pneumoperitoneum, where free air is present within the peritoneum. This is typically seen collecting under the hemidiaphragms on the upright radiograph. Less well known, because they are less common, are abnormal abdominal gas collections related to the urinary tract (see Table 4–1).

Table 4–1. Abnormal Gas Collections Related to the Urinary Tract

Calyceal gas	Pyonephrosis with gas production; fistula to intestine or skin
Parenchymal gas	Emphysematous pyelonephritis (gas produced by fermentation of sugar in diabetics)
Perirenal gas	Infection, fistula, or retroperitoneal perforation of the intestine
Bladder gas	Emphysematous cystitis (diabetic with fermentation of sugar in the bladder)
Postoperative gas	Retroperitoneal gas with a linear or bubbly appearance

42 Diagnosis of Genitourinary Disease

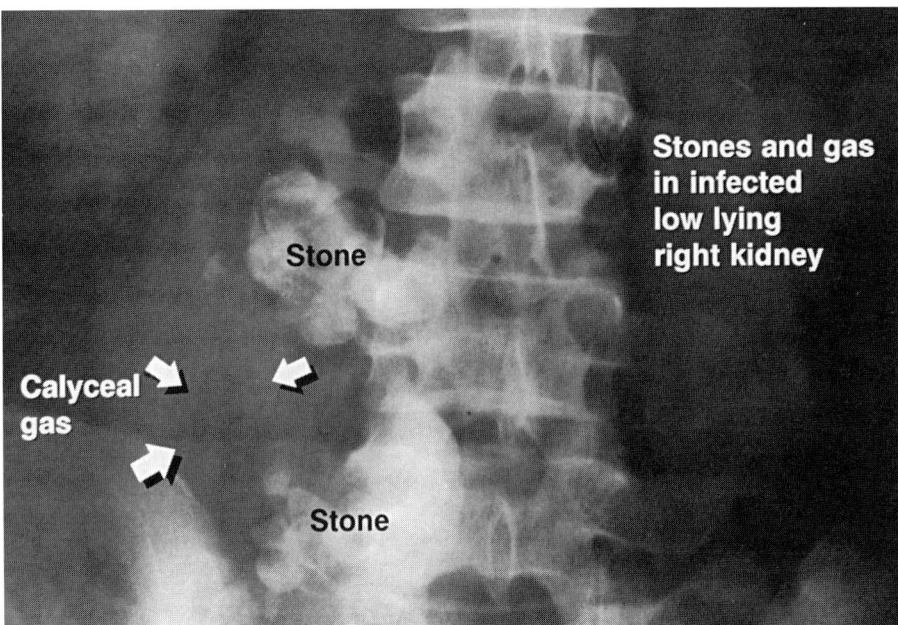

Figure 4–13. Pyonephrosis with gas in the calyces (arrows).

Gas within the calyces generally implies a severe pyonephrosis with gas production (Fig. 4–13), although a fistulous communication with the bowel or the skin could also produce this appearance. A more ominous radiographic sign is seen in emphysematous pyelonephritis, where gas dissects through the parenchyma of the kidney. This severe and life-threatening infection is most often found in diabetics with urinary stasis (Fig. 4–14). This gas is produced by *Escherichia coli*, which ferments the sugar. Gas around the kidney in the perinephric space can be due to a local infection such as perinephric abscess or to a perforation of a retroperitoneal viscus (Fig. 4–15).

Emphysematous cystitis is the term used when gas is found within the bladder lumen and bladder wall (Fig. 4–16). This gas is produced by fermentation of sugars in diabetic urine by *E. coli*. As with emphysematous pyelonephritis this finding generally implies a severe infection, usually associated with urinary tract obstruction. After surgery,

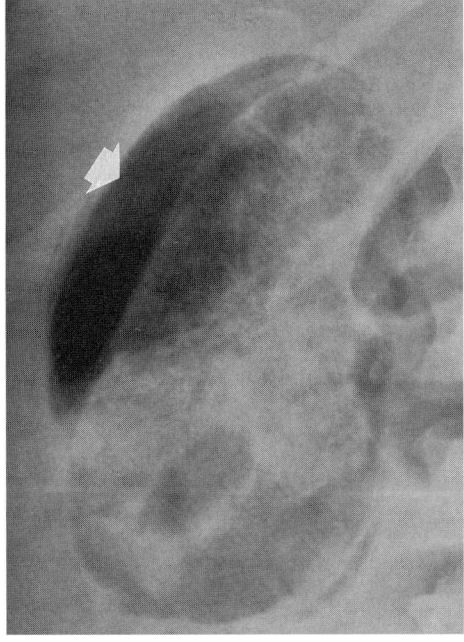

Figure 4–14. Emphysematous pyelonephritis. Gas dissects through the entire renal parenchyma producing a sponge-like appearance. Gas extends to the subcapsular space (arrows). (Reprinted with permission from Older RA. *Excretory Urography*. Update 1980. Copyright The Chemical Rubber Co., CRC Press, Inc.)

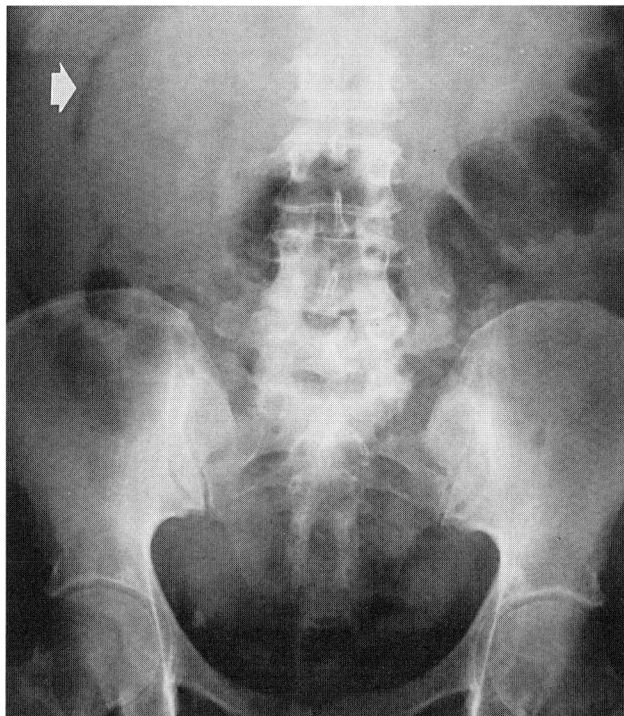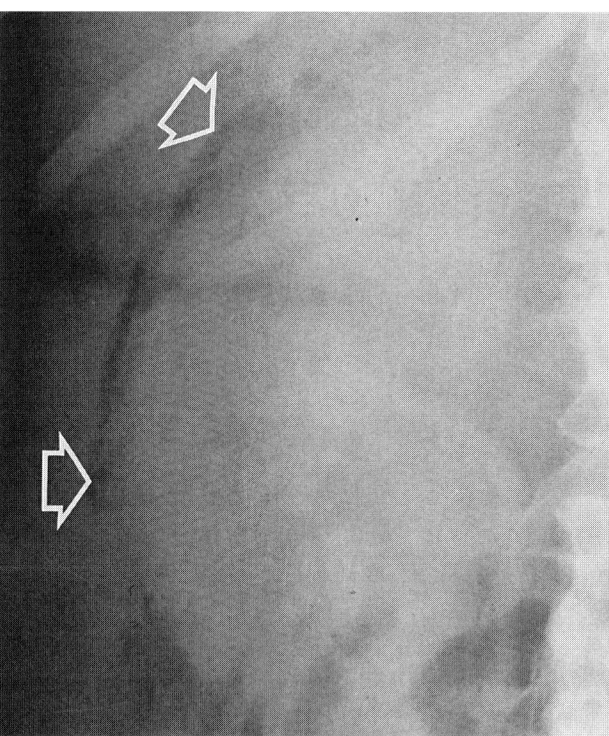

Fig. 4–15. (**A**) Perirenal gas (arrow) caused by retroperitoneal perforation of a cecal abscess. No gas is present within the kidney parenchyma. (**B**) Coned radiograph of right kidney during urogram shows the perirenal gas (arrows) more clearly.

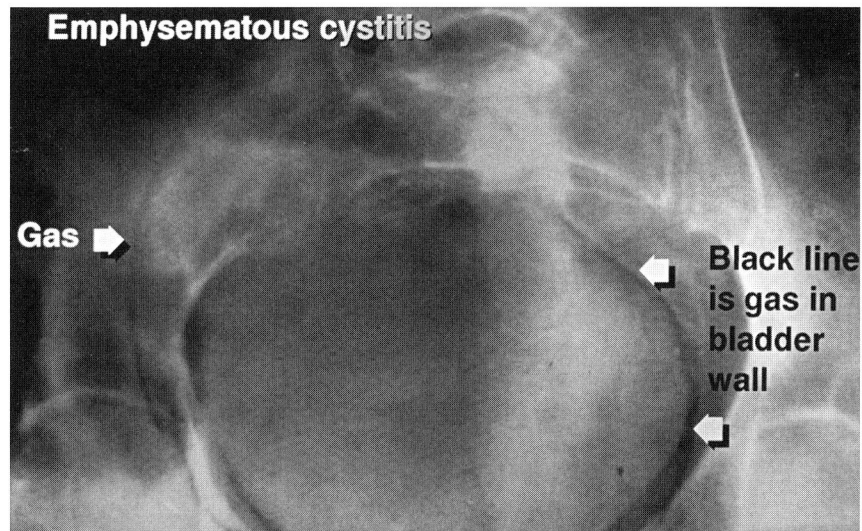

Figure 4–16. Emphysematous cystitis. The well-defined black line (arrows) outlining the bladder represents gas which has dissected into the bladder wall.

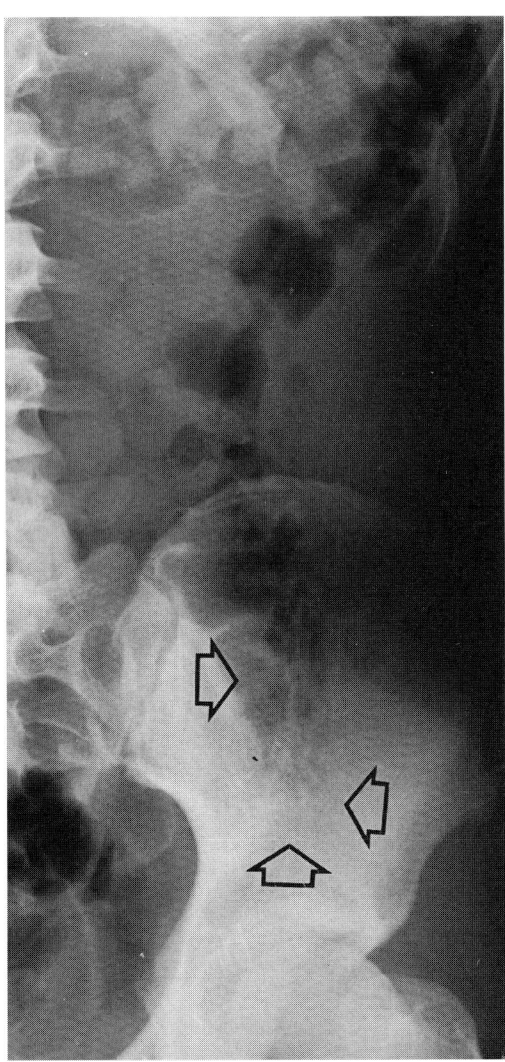

Figure 4–17. Postoperative gas. Abdominal radiograph 3 days following a left nephrectomy shows "bubbly" gas in the left flank (arrows) which is indistinguishable from gas due to a retroperitoneal abscess. (Reprinted with permission from Older RA. 1978, The Williams & Wilkins Co., Baltimore.)

particularly following a nephrectomy, gas can remain within the retroperitoneum for days to weeks. The appearance may be irregular, bubbly, and indistinguishable from an abscess (Fig. 4–17).[3]

REFERENCES

1. Hewitt MJ, Older RA. Calyceal calculi simulating gallstones. *Am J Roentgenol* 1980;134:507–509.
2. Daniels WW, et al. Calcified renal masses: a review of ten years experience at the Mayo Clinic. *Radiology* 1972;103:503–508.
3. Older RA, Rice RP, Kelvin FM, Thompson WM, Weinerth JL. Extraperitoneal gas following nephrectomy: patterns and duration. *J Urol* 1978;120:24–27.

5 Basic Radiologic Techniques for Imaging the Urinary Tract

Robert A. Older

UROGRAPHY

Excretory urography provides a major tool for urologic diagnosis. The urographer's basic philosophy toward excretory urography and how it should be performed determines the diagnostic results obtained. An examination monitored closely by a radiologist with specific radiographs determined by the needs of the particular patient is best. Excretory urography consisting of a predetermined number of radiographs to be reviewed later often provides inadequate diagnostic information and frequently entails unnecessary patient irradiation. More important, the ratio of information gained to radiation given is lower. When performing urography, the radiologist should examine each radiograph and determine which questions have been answered and which questions remain unanswered. The radiologist should then determine which radiographs are most likely to answer the needed questions and have these executed. A question unanswered during urography will often remain unanswered when the films are later reviewed. When this is done, regrets later surface for not having pursued a particular problem further while the patient was on the radiographic table.

Accurate uroradiologic diagnosis depends on an optimal urogram. Diagnosis is often relatively easy if the appropriate radiographs are obtained and the anatomic urinary tract is demonstrated. There are a limited number of ways in which the urinary tract can respond to pathology. The most important feature of any urogram is to display the anatomy so that these pathologic changes can be detected. An optimal urogram minimizes diagnostic errors.

In each clinical urographic setting there may be minor variations in the speed with which decisions regarding additional radiographs can be made. This will depend on film-processing time and physician availability. It is reasonable therefore to obtain certain standard radiographs in the immediate postinjection phase of the examination, with further radiographs determined on the basis of the initial findings.

In the following sections we will discuss multiple aspects of excretory urography, including patient selection, patient preparation, contrast media, radiographic sequencing, and positioning and technical factors important in producing optimal excretory urograms.

Patient Selection

Generally, selection of patients will be determined by the referring physician, but close communication between the radiologist and the referring physician is important. There are multiple imaging techniques that can provide information similar to urography. The radiologist should act as a consultant to the referring physician to optimize the use of these studies.

There are three groups of patients in whom the use of urography should be carefully considered. First are those patients with low diagnostic yield indications. During the past decade considerable attention has been paid to this group, and many previously accepted indications are no longer considered justified. Evaluation for hypertension is generally not considered the realm of urography,[1,2] although recently some have advocated it because of the multiple renal abnormalities other than renovascular disease that can relate to hypertension.[3] Uncomplicated urinary tract infections, preoperative studies for prostatic hypertrophy,[4] gynecologic surgery, and enuresis fall into this group.[1,2] Some indications such as trauma have become more controversial; others have been taken over by other imaging studies and comprise group 2.

The second group contains patients in whom alternate methods of diagnostic imaging may be more appropriate for the clinical problem. Here a broad knowledge of the capabilities of other available imaging modalities is important. Excretory urography is still used extensively for suspected obstruction, but ultrasound has become the primary screening study to rule out hydronephrosis and possible obstruction. Renewed interest in the diuretic renogram also encroaches upon what was previously the realm of urography. Urography, however, continues to be used because of its availability and unique combination of anatomy and function. Urography and ultrasound are often complementary, with each providing information not obtainable from the other. This is true in suspected obstruction related to stone disease. Although replacement of the urogram by a combination of ultrasound and an abdominal film has been advocated,[5] each case needs to be considered individually because not all will require the same study. Ureterovesicle junction stones are usually easily seen on ultrasound, but stones slightly more proximal are difficult to detect and can be more easily demonstrated with excretory urography. Availability and experience in interpretation favor urography.[6] Ultrasound requires an experienced sonographer,[6] and in the case of small ureteral stones, considerable experience and patience. Urography and ultrasound are both complementary and competitive, and knowledge of the advantages and disadvantages of each modality is important in choosing the best examination.

Abdominal masses and retroperitoneal disease, once the province of urography, are now studied with CT or ultrasound. Adrenal lesions are studied with CT, isotope studies, or MRI. Extensive abdominal trauma warrants CT, but for injuries suspected to involve only the urinary tract, urography is still used,[1] but controversial.[7] The urogram is still used as a primary screening study for hematuria, as it provides not only parenchymal information, but also detailed visualization of the collecting system. It is excellent for lesions such as transitional cell carcinoma or papillary necrosis, but the sensitivity of excretory urography for detection of mass lesions is significantly less than CT,[8] and CT is recommended if a mass is suspected. Transplant evaluation no longer involves urography and is usually provided by a combination of ultrasound and nuclear medicine studies.

The third and probably most important group comprises those patients in whom excretory urography is associated with an above-average risk of complication. This complication may result from allergic reactions, abnormal cardiovascular responses, and toxic reactions from the contrast medium. Each of these complications will be dealt with in more detail in the following sections, but it is important that the risk of urography be balanced against its potential benefit. Alternate imaging methods become more important in the higher-risk patient.

Although urography is often performed in patients with prior allergic reactions, the use of an alternate method such as ultrasound, computed tomography without contrast, or radioisotope scanning should be considered in any patient with a previous severe allergic reaction. Patients with significant heart disease as manifested by arrhythmias or congestive heart failure are also at higher risk during excretory urography, and the indications for the study should be thoroughly considered before it is performed. Often a postponement of the examination will allow the patient to be studied under better clinical conditions.

Evaluation of renal failure is no longer within the realm of urography. There are two main reasons for this. First are the advances in diagnostic ultrasound, with its refinement to the point where it can accurately detect the presence and often cause of an obstructive process. The presence or absence of obstruction is often the most important factor in a patient with renal failure, and ultrasound can make this determination without the use of iodinated contrast material.[5,9–12]

Second, the past 20 years have given us a much greater awareness of the potential renal toxicity of iodinated contrast media. The tri-iodinated contrast material used for urography and arteriography are capable of producing significant renal dysfunction, and patients at highest risk are those with preexisting renal disease.[13–23] Contrast-induced renal failure is in fact the second leading cause of renal failure developing in the hospital situation.[24]

It is therefore no longer justifiable to study patients in renal failure with excretory urography. Alternate methods such as ultrasound, nonenhanced CT, MRI, and nuclear medicine studies will provide the necessary information without the inherent risks of iodinated contrast. Even with the development of nonionic contrast agents this problem still exists.

With the alternative procedures available, which indications remain for urography? The answer to this may not be the same for every institution, depending on local experience and preference. Availability will also affect choice. Acute abdominal pain suspected of being ureteral colic can be easily resolved by urography any time of the day or night, but the expertise to detect small ureteral stones with ultrasound may not always be available.

The following are current indications for excretory urography. Some of these, such as obstruction, also use other technology, and others such as trauma are controversial.[1,7]

Stone disease
Pre-op ESWL
Acute abdominal pain (colic)
Suspected obstruction
Blunt trauma (thought to involve only the urinary tract)
Hematuria (especially if abnormality of the collecting structures is suspected)
Complicated or unusual infection (including TB)
Postoperative evaluation of urologic procedures
Preoperative for endourologic procedures
Suspected transitional cell carcinoma
Questionable abnormality on isotope or ultrasound studies

Contrast Media

At the time of this writing there is an ongoing debate regarding contrast media for both intravenous and intra-arterial use. This centers on the increasing use of the newer nonionic media as opposed to the tri-iodinated ionic contrast material that has been in use for many years. As will be discussed, the nonionic contrast media provide a substantial increase in patient comfort, tolerance, and safety, but this is accompanied by a much higher cost.

MOLECULAR STRUCTURE AND PHYSIOLOGY

Contrast media can appear as a somewhat forbidding and confusing topic, though much of this confusion is due to a host of different products representing essentially identical or very similar chemical structures in varying concentrations. In addition to traditional ionic contrast media, nonionic media are commonly used, further increasing the options available. The following sections represent a distillation of the current data concerning radiographic iodinated contrast media available today. Our goal is to simplify this subject as much as possible with the complicated-appearing chemical structures presented as an aid in understanding the subject. The important basic physiologic concepts of contrast material will be considered to aid in understanding how contrast media works and why it is ineffective in certain patients. Although similar in many respects, there are differences in renal handling of ionic and nonionic contrast.

Ionic Contrast. The birth of organic urinary tract intravascular contrast media resulted from early attempts by Swick to formulate a bactericidal agent for the urinary tract. Contrast agent development and refinement produced the tri-iodinated intravascular contrast agents as we know them introduced early in the 1950s by Wallingford.[25] Since their introduction, a large number of tri-iodinated compounds have been developed for clinical use. The basic tri-iodinated anions most commonly used today are diatrizoate and iothalamate. These compounds are all tri-iodinated benzoic acid derivatives with the iodine atoms incorporated at positions 2, 4, and 6 on the benzene ring. Modification in the side chains attached at position 3 represents the only significant differences between the anions. Figure 5–1 illustrates the minor differences found in the chemical structure of these modifying side chains, whereas the basic molecular structure for diatrizoate and iothalamate remains unattended. There are numerous variations of these three common basic iodinated contrasts in clinical usage today.

Most ionic contrasts are associated with either a sodium or methylglucamine (meglumine) cation, employed singly or in combination, which is dissociated in solution from position 1. The ionic contrast agents available (Table 5–1) represent variations of concentration and cation(s) for either diatrizoate or iothalamate. The brand name of the contrast usually denotes a specific iodine concentration in the solution along with the cation(s) and anion employed. For practical purposes only the 50% or 60% agents need be considered for urography.

Glomerular filtrations is the primary means of excretion of the ionic contrast agents employed in excretory urography. Excretion or reabsorption of contrast material by the tubular mechanism contributes little in the overall process.[26] Glomerular filtration also is the predominant mechanism for contrast excretion in patients with abnormal renal function resulting from either primary renal disease or mechanical obstruction.[27] Urographic contrast media are administered intravascularly as hyperosmolar solutions. The amount of the solute load that will be excreted with the contrast will depend upon the contrast agent cation. Urine solute load represents the total amount of nonionic and ionic material in the urine. The primary difference in the variation of the urine solute load is detected when the contrast agent employed contains sodium as the cation. In this instance, a portion of the sodium from the contrast agent is reabsorbed by the tubular system. The sodium is returned into the intravascular compartment along with free water. Sodium reabsorption increases the iodine concentration and decreases the solute load of the urine.

In general, as urine solute load increases, the osmotic diuresis and urine flow rate increases. The tubular mechanism for sodium reabsorption is unaffected when methylglucamine is the cation of the contrast agent, as none of this cation is reabsorbed. Therefore with methylglucamine as the cation, the total solute load carried into the urine is greater. According to some investigators, this urine solute load difference is felt to represent the major difference in urographic contrasts that employ either the sodium or meglumine cat-

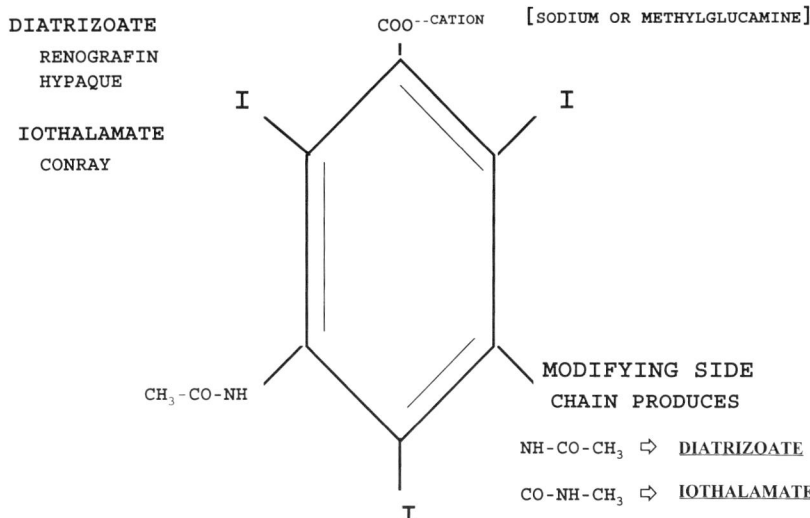

Figure 5–1. Chemical structure of the commonly used ionic contrast media.

Table 5-1. Comparative Physical Factors of Contrast Media for Urography

Product	Anion	Cation	Chemical Structure	% Salt Conc	%I Conc	Total Iodine (mg/mL)	Viscosity 37°C (cp)	Osmolality (mOsm/kg H$_2$O)	Ratio of Iodine Atoms to Particles in Solution
IONIC									
Reno-M-60 (Squibb)	Diatrizoate	Meglumine	Ionic	60.0	28.2	282	4.44	1505	3:2
Renografin 60	Diatrizoate	Meglumine (52%) Sodium (8%)	Ionic	60.0	29.2	292	4.27	1549	3:2
Hypaque (Sodium 50%) (Sanofi Winthrop)	Diatrizoate	Sodium	Ionic	50.0	30.0	300	3.43	1515	3:2
Conray 60 (Mallinckrodt)	Iothalamate	Meglumine	Ionic	60.0	28.2	282	4.13	1539	3:2
NONIONIC									
Omnipaque 300 (Sanofi Winthrop)	None	None	Nonionic (Iohexol)	None	30.0	300	6.30	672	3:1
Isovue 300 (Squibb)	None	None	Nonionic (Iopamidol)	None	30.0	300	4.70	616	3:1
Optiray 320 (Mallinckrodt)	None	None	Nonionic (Ioversol)	None	32.0	320	5.8	702	3:1

Excerpted from data by Winthrop Laboratories.

ions. This factor may determine to some extent the degree of pelvicaliceal opacification seen at urography and thus may be a primary variable used to evaluate the difference in urographic diagnostic quality.[28]

Nonionic Contrast. The currently used nonionic agents are shown in Figure 5–2. For urography the terms *nonionic* and *low osmolar contrast media* (LOCM) represent the same media. These show a similarity to the ionic contrast agents in that the central portion of the molecule is a tri-iodinated benzene ring. The carboxyl group at the number 1 position has been replaced by an amide,[29] therefore no cation such as sodium or methylglucamine is present. These compounds therefore do not dissociate into positive and negative ions in solution and do not double their osmolarity as do ionic agents. This is an important point in the increased tolerance and safety of these agents. This concept was first developed by a Swedish radiologist, Torsten Alman, and he is credited with the emergence of nonionic agents.[30]

Since the carboxyl group traditionally provided the high solubility of ionic contrast media, a solubility problem for the nonionic contrast arose. This was overcome by Alman and colleagues by providing multiple hydrophilic hydroxyl groups on the side chains.[30] Iohexol and Ioversol have six hydroxyl groups and Iopamidol has five.[29]

The nonionic agents show a marked decrease in osmolality (600–700 mOsm/kg) as compared to the ionic agents, although they are still hyperosmolar when compared to plasma. Because these agents do not dissociate in solution, the nonionic contrast media have a 3:1 ratio of iodine atoms to solute particles as compared to the ionic contrast in which the ratio is 3 iodine atoms per 2 particles in solution. Thus the iodine-containing particles compose a larger relative percentage of the solute load. Both ionic and nonionic media contain three iodine atoms per molecule, and thus nonionic agents have twice the iodine atoms per particle in solution (Table 5–1).[31] The urinary solute load in this situation is less and the urinary iodine concentration is increased as compared to ionic agents.[31] Osmotic diuresis and urine-concentrating mechanisms will oppose each other. With increasing dose increasing contrast is delivered to urine with a greater pyelographic density. At a certain dose, however, osmotic diuresis dominates the concentrating mechanism and pyelographic density cannot be further increased with increasing dose. With ionic contrast this is about 300 mg/kg. With nonionic contrast the diuretic effect is less marked and pyelographic density continues to increase until about 600 mg of iodine per kilogram. For an equivalent dose the nonionic media will give higher urinary concentrations.[32,33] As with the ionic agents, glomerular filtration is the primary method of excretion for the nonionic agents.

URORADIOGRAPHIC QUALITY

Ionic: Methylglucamine Cation Versus Sodium Cation. Several investigators have described objective differences in the pyelogram when comparing the cations sodium and methylglucamine.[28,34,35] In the laboratory the sodium salt produces higher urinary iodine concentrations. Methylglucamine, however, produces greater diuresis secondary to the osmotic effect and in theory provides better distention of the pelvicaliceal system. Translating these controlled experi-

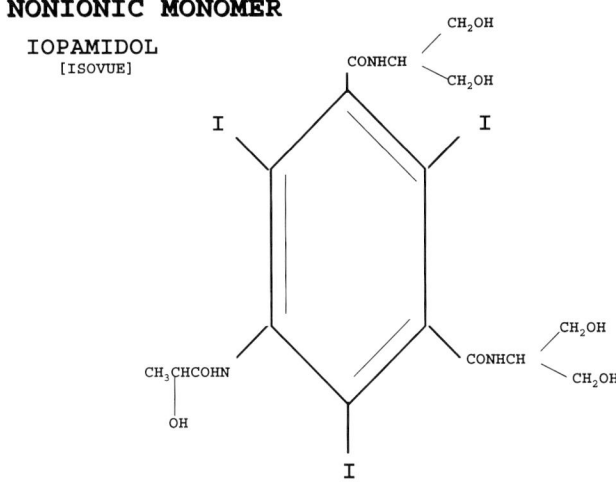
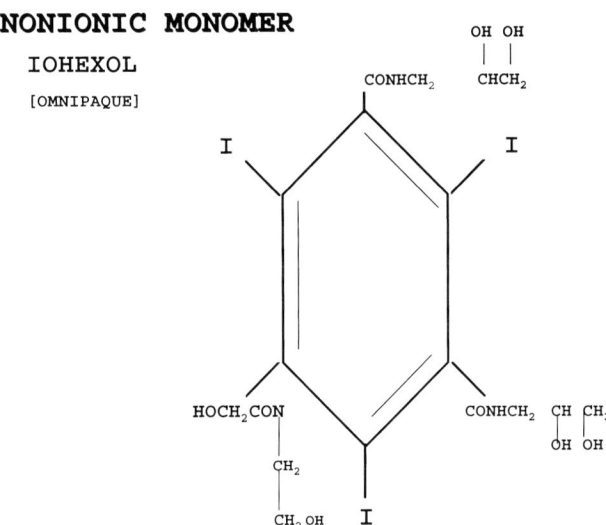
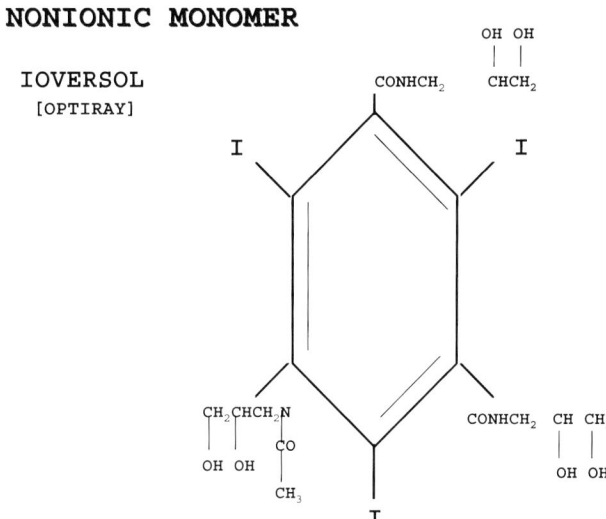

Figure 5–2. Chemical structure of the nonionic monomers. **(A)** Iopamidol, **(B)** Iohexol, **(C)** Ioversol.

mental differences to clinical uroradiography is difficult because of the wide variation in the degree of patient dehydration prior to urography. In strictly controlled clinical groups, differences may be seen between the urograms produced by the two cations. When these differences are reviewed they seem small, but they are nonetheless real. Overall, the sodium salt seems to produce better caliceal opacification for all degrees of dehydration, while methylglucamine provides better pelvicaliceal distention. Neither the methylglucamine nor the sodium salt produced any significant difference in the nephrogram phase.[34,36,37] The reason for the lack of a distinct difference in the opacification of the renal parenchyma may be that the filtered contrast media throughout the tubules is undergoing tubular reabsorption of the filtered plasma, whereas the contrast in the urine within the calyces and renal pelvis is the final result of the concentration process. Sequential computed tomographic studies have confirmed these clinical urographic observations by comparing the sodium and methylglucamine contrast agents in the renal cortex in the canine kidney.[38] The cortical CT density was not appreciably affected by changes in the chemical structure of the ionic contrast agents used. In clinical practice the choice of cation does not matter, as either sodium or methyglulamine will produce a diagnostic study.

Nonionic Versus Ionic Contrast. Numerous clinical studies have shown that the nonionic agents produce a urogram equal to ionic media,[29] and possibly better.[31] With a lower osmolality and solute load the nonionic agents produce a denser pyelogram with higher urinary iodine concentration.[31,39] There is a potential for decreased distention of the collecting system due to decreased diuretic effect, but with the use of abdominal compression this is avoided. No significant difference in nephrogram has been noted,[31,39] but the maximal nephrogram occurred at 3–4 minutes, rather than immediately following injection.[33] This may be related to a smaller total volume of distribution than with the ionic media.[36] Dray[37] compared Iohexol with Renografin and found all studies satisfactory, but 52% of the nonionic Iohexol studies were considered excellent as compared to 28% for the ionic agent. A similar comparison[40] compared not only equivalent doses of ionic and nonionic, but also a lesser fixed dose of nonionic contrast (17.5 g iodine of iohexol). No statistically significant difference was present in diagnostic quality among the three groups, although the nephrographic and ureteral quality were slightly lower in the lower-dose group. The use of nonionic contrast does not reduce the diagnostic efficacy of urography, and decisions as to use will be based on other factors such as cost or safety.

The increased concentration of contrast that occurs in the collecting tubules with nonionic media increased visualization of normal ducts in approximately 13% of cases,[41] and this should not be mistaken for tubular ectasia.

Table 5–2. Adverse Reactions During Urography

Study	No. of Patients		No. of Patients with Reactions	Percent Reactions
Intravenous urography	81,278		−4,589	5.65
		No therapy	−3,067	
		therapy	−1,439	
		Hospitalization necessary	−18	
		Fatal	−6	
Number of reactions relative to duration of intravenous urography injection				
0–2 min	60,654		3,094	5.10
3–10 min	18,603		1,385	7.45
11 min & over	2,021		110	5.56

Excerpted from Shehadi WH: *Am J Roentgenol* 1975;124:145, American Roentgen Ray Society.

ADVERSE REACTIONS TO CONTRAST MATERIAL

Many radiologists admit to some anxiety when injecting contrast material for excretory urography. This is justified, for there is always the potential for significant complications when iodinated contrast material is administered. Complacency, lack of awareness, or simply ignoring these potential problems will only aggravate a complication should one occur.

Allergic Reactions

Type and Incidence. Adverse contrast reactions can be placed into one of three major categories: (1) "allergic" reaction, (2) cardiovascular reactions, and (3) toxic effect, such as contrast-induced renal failure. The word *allergic* is in quotes because there is disagreement in the literature as to the etiology of these so-called allergic reactions.[42,43] The overall incidence of this type of reaction in patients with allergic histories in general is approximately twice that of the normal population.[44] Anxiety may play a role in the production of reactions, and as far as possible patients should not be unduly agitated.

A prospective study of adverse reactions related to urography revealed the overall incidence of reactions for ionic contrast media to be approximately 5%.[44,45] Most of these were mild reactions not requiring therapy (Table 5–2). Many were simply nausea and vomiting, and could well not be allergic reactions. Urticaria, or simple hives, is the next most common reaction and in some instances will require therapy in the form of an antihistamine. A small proportion of patients will have reactions severe enough to require hospitalization, including respiratory difficulty, circulatory collapse, hypotension, and other cardiovascular responses. Fatal reactions in the Shehadi study are definitely less common, occurring one in every 13,500 to 19,450 urographic examinations.[44,45] This number is considerably higher than that noted by Hartman, who studied 266,000 excretory urograms performed at the Mayo Clinic and its affiliated hospitals.[46] His reported mortality rate was only one in every 75,000 examinations. This lower rate probably reflects more effective therapy of severe reactions in this single institution study, as the rate of severe reactions was almost identical in the two studies. Other series have demonstrated mortality rates that have ranged between these numbers.[47]

Nonionic contrast show a significant decrease in the incidence of mild, moderate, and severe reactions, by a factor of approximately 5 (Table 5–3).[48–50] Although there has been controversy regarding the methodology of the initial studies, the data continue to indicate a markedly increased safety factor for the nonionic contrast,[51] and safety is no longer a controversial issue. Data on fatal reactions with the nonionic contrast are difficult to obtain due to the large number of patients who would need to be studied. It is reasonable to believe that the large decrease in severe reactions brought about by the use of nonionic contrast[51] will result in a decrease in fatal reactions.

In addition to reducing adverse reactions, nonionic agents reduce the side effects of intravenously administered contrast media. Uncomfortable sensations of warmth, nausea, and vomiting are markedly reduced. Overall, this has produced a dramatic change in the aura surrounding the excretory urogram. When nonionic agents are used there is no longer apprehension associated with the study. This is probably due to a combination of both physician and patient perception of the new media. Although fatal reactions are rare, they do occur with both ionic and nonionic media, and it is important that the equipment for prompt therapeutic measures be available.

Our approach to the performance of urography is to have the physician personally obtain the patient's history regard-

Table 5–3. Severe Adverse Reactions

	Ionic	Nonionic	Ratio
Wolf[50]	0.4%	0	
Katayama[48]	0.22%	0.04%	5.5
Palmer[49]	0.09%	0.02%	4.6

ing any previous radiographic studies employing iodinated contrast material and determine if the patient had any difficulty related to the contrast. The patient is also questioned regarding any other known allergies. We do not currently obtain written informed consent for intravenous contrast injections, but we realize that the issue of informed consent is a very controversial and complex one. At the present time we have a policy of universal use of nonionic contrast, and this plays a major role in our current position regarding informed consent. If an institution were to selectively use nonionic contrast for high-risk patients only, we would recommend that written informed consent be obtained. This consent should clearly explain the different risks of ionic and nonionic contrast. We do not use a routine test dose prior to giving the contrast material, as this has not been shown to be of any value.[44,52]

Premedication. In patients with a history of allergy to contrast material from a prior study or with a significant allergy history in general, our approach is to premedicate with steroids. The routine use of steroid premedication can reduce the risk of reaction for ionic contrast to a level close to that of nonionic contrast. Steroids, however, are not effective unless given for at least 12 hours prior to the administration of contrast media,[53,54] and the feasibility of routine premedication in most hospitals or outpatient settings is questionable.[55] The risk of an adverse reaction can be further reduced by using a steroid preparation in combination with a nonionic agent.[56] This is our approach to patients with previous adverse reactions. We use Decadron 4 mg po q 6 hr for 24 hours prior to the examination.

In patients who have had very severe prior reactions, the need for the examination should be reconsidered. Premedication and/or the use of nonionic contrast does not completely eliminate the risk of a severe reaction, and noncontrast methods of providing the desired information should be considered.

Treatment. Despite efforts to avoid contrast reactions they will inevitably occur with both ionic and nonionic media. It is important therefore to have a plan of therapy for these reactions.

1. Dermatologic manifestations such as hives or itching with no respiratory symptoms. These patients generally require no specific therapy. If hives do not resolve or become progressive, an antihistamine such as diphenhydramine 20 to 50 mg IM or IV can be given.
2. Bronchospasm (isolated). Initial therapy for isolated bronchospasm is an inhaled bronchodilator (albuterol, metaproterenol, or terbutaline). These can be obtained in preset metered dose inhalers. If the bronchospasm does not resolve with this therapy, subcutaneous epinephrine is used. Accelerating or severe bronchospasm should be treated with IV epinephrine given as 0.1 mg (1 mL) of 1:10,000 slowly over approximately 3 to 5 minutes, up to 0.3 mg (3 mL).[57]
3. More severe anaphylactoid reactions, including severe bronchospasm, laryngospasm, angioedema, and hypotension. These reactions require immediate administration of intravenous epinephrine.[57] This should be given as a slow incremental infusion of 0.1 to 0.3 mg (1 to 3 mL). IV epinephrine should be given as soon as a severe reaction is recognized but is a potent medication and should not be used casually for mild reactions. Table 5–4 provides a summary of therapeutic measures.

Cardiac Abnormalities. A number of studies have shown that electrocardiographic changes can occur during the injection of contrast media for excretory urography.[58–60] Although the majority of these are minor abnormalities, significant arrhythmias and ischemia occur. These are most likely to occur in patients with preexisting cardiac disease, but they also occur in normal patients.[60,61] It is more likely for cardiac abnormalities to occur following a rapid bolus injection of contrast, and although we generally recommend the use of the bolus technique, this injection should be given more slowly in patients with significant cardiac disease. Cardiac response may be related to dose per unit of time.[61] As with the other adverse reactions, cardiac abnormalities are also reduced with the use of nonionic contrast.[33,62]

Renal Toxicity. The third form of adverse reaction is renal toxicity. Renal toxicity is not a new concept, and complications of renal failure secondary to the administration of angiographic contrast media were well recognized in the 1950s.[63] With the advent of newer and safer contrast media, renal failure secondary to contrast material was somewhat forgotten and a number of retrospective studies appeared to document the safety of intravascularly administered iodinated contrast material.[64,65] In the late 1970s, however, radiologists again became aware of the potential toxic effects of contrast material.[14]

Although contrast toxicity has been an issue of some debate, recent studies have confirmed its existence and demonstrated an incidence similar to earlier work. Gomes reported a 7.1% incidence of renal dysfunction following arteriography,[23] and Lautin reported 26% for high osmolar contrast following arteriography,[22] as compared to an overall incidence of 10% in an earlier prospective study.[14] Variability in the incidence of contrast-induced renal failure is largely due to study design and the definition of contrast-induced renal failure. The incidence is clearly greater following angiography or cardiac catheterization,[66] but renal failure does occur with intravenous use such as that in urography (4.8%)[20] and body CT (2.8%).[67] The significance of this problem is exemplified by the fact that contrast-induced nephropathy is the second highest cause of hospital-induced renal insufficiency (12%).[24]

Contrast-induced renal failure is very unlikely to occur from an intravenous injection of contrast in a patient with normal renal function. Patients with preexisting renal disease, however, have consistently been shown to be at greater risk for contrast-induced nephropathy, especially if diabetic.[20–23] VanZee found a 0.6% incidence of renal failure following urography in patients with normal renal function, but the incidence increased to between 3.2% and 31%, depending on the severity of the preexistent renal disease.[20] Davidson found the baseline serum creatinine level to be a significant predictor of contrast-induced nephropathy.[68] Permanent renal damage can occur but is uncommon and often can be predicted by the patient's prestudy renal function.

Minimal elevations in serum creatinine should not dissuade us from administering contrast when it is necessary to establish a significant diagnosis. With preexisting renal disease the risk of the study is increased and should be balanced against potential gain. If studies not using contrast will provide the information at lesser risk, these should be used first.

Recent studies have been directed toward a comparison of the nephrotoxicity of high osmolar contrast media (HOCM) as compared to low osmolar contrast media (LOCM). Experimental studies[69] suggested that there would be a lower incidence of toxicity with LOCM, but initial clinical studies did not confirm this. In a review of 100 randomized trials, Kinnison found no difference in nephrotoxicity of the LOCM as compared to the HOCM.[70] Gomes found a 10% incidence of renal dysfunction following angiography with ionic media and 5.5% with nonionic contrast. This difference was not statistically significant.[71] More recently, however, studies have appeared showing a decrease in nephrotoxicity for the LOCM. Harris compared patients with abnormal serum creatinine levels undergoing CT and found a statistically significant decrease from 14% to 2%.[72] Lautin showed a decreased incidence of contrast-induced nephropathy following angiography for LOCM versus HOCM (7% versus 26% for all patients). A greater difference was noted in azotemic patients (10% versus 41%).[22] To evaluate these studies further and to pool the data into a larger base a meta-analysis was done by Barrett and Carlisle. A statistically significant benefit of LOCM was demonstrated in the group with prior renal impairment. The benefits of LOCM were greater with more sensitive determination of renal function.[21] Nonionic (low osmolar) contrast should be used in patients with preexisting renal disease.

It is important to identify patients with preexisting renal disease as high risk for contrast-induced renal failure prior

Table 5–4. Acute Reactions to Contrast Media: Treatment Outline

Urticaria:
   Mild: Observation
   Mod: Diphenhydramine 25–50 mg po/IM/IV
   Severe: Cimetidine 300 mg, diluted to 20 mL, slow IV
              (pediatric: 5–10 mg/kg diluted to 20 mL, slow IV)
           Ranitidine 50 mg, diluted to 20 mL, IV slowly
              (pediatric: use not established)

Bronchospasm (isolated):
   Oxygen (3 L/min)
   Beta-2-agonist metered dose inhaler: (2–3 deep inhalations)
      Metaproterenol (Alupent), terbutaline (Brethaire),
      Albuterol (Proventil)
   Epinephrine
      SubQ:1:1000, 0.1–0.2 mL (0.1–0.2 mg)
          (pediatric: 0.1–0.2 mg subQ)
      IV: 1:10,000, 1 mL (0.1 mg), slowly
          (e.g., over 3–5 min)
          (pediatric: 0.01 mg/kg, IV)

Anaphylaxis-like reaction (generalized):
   Oxygen (3 L/min)
   Suction, as needed
   Elevate patient's legs if hypotensive
   IV fluids: normal saline; Ringer's solution
   Epinephrine
      SubQ: 1:1000, 0.1–0.2 mL (0.1–0.2 mg)
          (pediatric: 0.1–0.2 mL subQ)
      IV: 1:10,000, 1 mL (0.1 mg), slowly
          (e.g., incrementally over 3–5 min)
          (pediatric: 0.01 mg/kg, IV)
   Avoid epinephrine for patients taking noncardioselective beta-adrenergic blocking drugs.
   Alternative drug therapy: isoproterenol 1:5000 solution (0.2 mg/mL), IV, 0.5–1.0 mL diluted to 10 mL with normal saline.

Anaphylaxis-like reaction (generalized) Continued:
   Antihistamines:
      H-1 blocker:
         Diphenhydramine 50 mg, IV (Caution: may exacerbate or cause hypotension)
      H-2 blocker:
         Cimetidine 300 mg, diluted to 20 mL, slow IV
            (pediatric: 5–10 mg/kg, diluted slowly)
         Ranitidine 50 mg, diluted to 20 mL, slow IV
            (pediatric: use not established)
   Beta-2 agonist metered dose inhaler (MDI):
      (2 or 3 inhalations)
      Metaproterenol (Alupent), terbutaline (Brethaire), albuterol (Proventil)
   Corticosteroids:
      Hydrocortisone 0.5–1.0 g IV
      Methylprednisolone 500 mg over 30 sec, or 2000 mg over 30 min

Hypotension (isolated)
   Elevate patient's legs
   Oxygen (3 L/min)
   IV fluids (primary therapy): rapidly, 0.9% sodium chloride for injection (normal saline) or Ringer's solution

Vagal reaction (hypotension and bradycardia):
   Elevate patient's legs
   Oxygen (3 L/min)
   IV fluids: rapidly, 0.9% sodium chloride for injection (normal saline) or Ringer's solution
   Atropine: 0.8–1.0 mg IV, repeat q 3–5 min to 2–3 mg total (adults)
      (pediatric: 0.02 mg/kg IV; max. 0.6 mg dose; may repeat to 2 mg total)

Reprinted with permission from the Society of Uroradiology Categorical Course 1994.

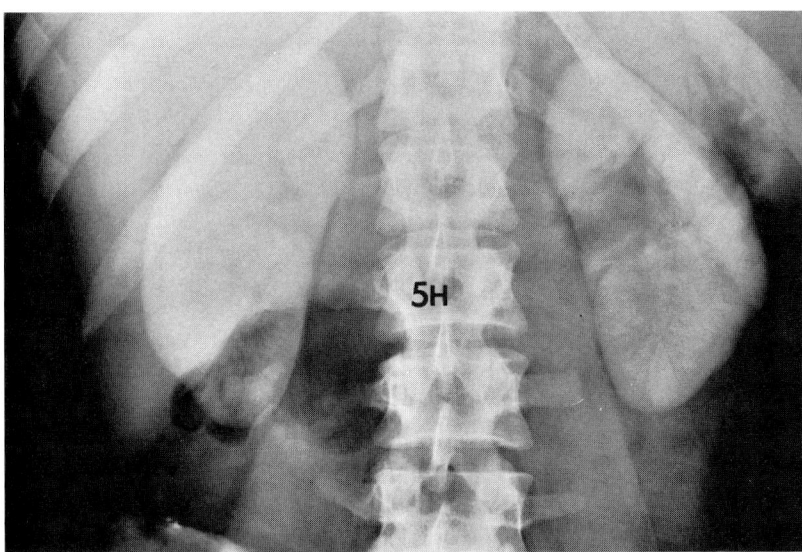

Figure 5–3. Delayed 5-hour radiograph shows a dense bilateral persistent nephrogram. This patient developed transient oliguric renal failure.

to urography. If urography is performed on a patient in this group, one should carefully observe the nephrographic pattern during the excretory urogram. A persistence or increase of the nephrogram on successive or delayed radiographs may be an early indicator of renal failure (Fig. 5–3) or hypotension.[13] A follow-up serum creatinine 36 hours following urography in high-risk patients for renal toxicity is a worthwhile precaution.

DOSAGE

The amount of contrast media used for urography is an important variable. A sufficient amount is needed to produce diagnostic visualization of the renal parenchyma and collecting structures. An excessive amount of contrast material is avoided because of the potentially toxic side effects. Dosage may be given as a standard amount in terms of total volume or total grams of iodine. The simplest way to formulate a dose of contrast material is to consider the grams of iodine administered. This method facilitates a quick means for comparison of the various commercial preparations. In Table 5–5 we have listed several of the commercially available media that are commonly used for urography, showing "routine dose" in different ways, including the dose in grams of iodine. For ionic media we recommend approximately 20 to 22 g of iodine for the "standard 150-lb" patient. For the ionic agents Hypaque 60, Renografin 60, or Conray 60 this is equivalent to 75 mL. The dose recommended in the categorical course on genitourinary tract radiology at the 1978 RSNA was 20 g of iodine,[73] and this dose has not changed significantly.[74] Doses for much smaller or larger patients can be adjusted by weight.

The drip-infusion contrast medium is marketed in single-dose bottles that contain 300 mL of a 30% iodine solution, approximately 42 g of iodine. This represents a considerably higher iodine dose, and although it is not necessary to administer the complete bottle when performing drip infusion, in practice this is usually done. The drip infusion technique is no longer commonly used.

Nonionic Contrast. With the introduction of nonionic contrast of similar iodine concentration to the ionic agents it was logical to use similar dosages. The use of 75 mL as an average dose, however, was not acceptable, given the significant wasted contrast media and expense. There is therefore a tendency to use either 100 or 50 mL as the standard dose. Packaging changes for nonionic contrast now allow a 75-mL dose without waste, but given cost considerations a 50-mL dose is most reasonable.

A 50-mL dose of iohexol when compared with a larger-weight-based dose of iohexol or diatrizoate in healthy outpatients showed no overall diagnostic difference, but the smaller dose did score slightly lower for the nephrographic and ureteral phases of the study.[40] Keenan evaluated low-dose urography with nonionic contrast using a dosage schedule based on age and weight and concluded that the amount of contrast could be reduced 42% and still produce diagnostic images. He found a decrease in nephrographic quality but

Table 5–5. Comparative Dosage Schedule

Product	"Routine" Dose for Average 150-lb Patient		Dose per Body Weight
	mL	Iodine (g)	mL/lb
Hypaque 50	75	22.5	0.5
Renografin 60	75	21.9	0.5
Conray 60	75	21.2	0.5
Conray 400	50	20.0	0.33
Omnipaque 300	50	15	0.33
Optiray 320	50	16	0.33
Isovue 300	50	15	0.33

compensated for this with tomography and delayed nephrogram films at 3 to 5 minutes rather than the traditional immediate postinjection film. Studies have shown peak plasma levels up to 5 minutes postinjection for nonionic contrast.[75] Dose reduction in urography may allow continued use of the safer nonionic agents and still maintain an acceptable cost.

Patient Preparation

Patient preparation concerns two primary aspects, bowel preparation and fluid restriction.

BOWEL PREPARATION

For many years bowel preparation was used to try and improve the image quality of the excretory urogram. Although helpful in some patients, bowel preparations were not uniformly successful. Recently, we have abandoned use of routine bowel preparation. Bowel preparation, which is often quite uncomfortable for the patient, has not consistently provided significant value in terms of improved visualization. A recent prospective randomized study to evaluate bowel preparation analyzed 90 patients receiving bowel preparation and 98 patients having no preparation. There was no difference between the groups in terms of number of films necessary, duration of procedure, visibility of the renal tracts, and overall quality.[76] Other studies have also shown no significant improvement in diagnostic quality by using any of several bowel preparations. These bowel preparations did, however, produce unpleasant side effects in a large number of patients.[77] The routine availability of tomography reduces the need for bowel preparation as the kidneys can be well visualized even with considerable bowel content present (Fig. 5–4). On occasion, however, a patient may have such a large amount of bowel content and gas on the preliminary film that a rescheduling of the study with a bowel preparation will be of help.

FLUID RESTRICTION

Fluid restriction for several hours prior to excretory urography is a controversial issue. The controversy revolves around these points:

1. What does fluid restriction or dehydration prior to excretory urography really mean?
2. Is it effective?
3. Is it dangerous?

Before considering these three points, certain basic physiologic concepts regarding contrast material should be reviewed to understand the rationale behind the use of fluid restriction and its effects in the normal and the azotemic patient. Currently employed tri-iodinated contrast media enter the renal tubule through the process of glomerular filtration. There is no significant tubular secretion or reabsorption. As the contrast medium passes through the proximal tubule it is concentrated approximately 5 to 10 times through the reabsorption of sodium and water. Approximately 85% of water in the glomerular filtrate is reabsorbed in the proximal tubules.[32,78] Reabsorption of water in the proximal tubule is independent of the patient's state of hydration. The final concentration of contrast material is determined in the distal tubule, where there is some regulation by antidiuretic hormone (ADH). Fluid deprivation will increase serum levels of antidiuretic hormone and thus increase the concentration of contrast medium in the distal tubule and collecting structures. In the patient with renal insufficiency, especially when it is advanced, the kidney is incapable of concentrating the urine in response to dehydration. This may be due either to a urea-induced osmotic diuresis or to an increased rate of sodium excretion by the tubules. In either case, fluid deprivation will not be effective in producing the increased concentration of contrast medium due to antidiuretic hormone.[78] Fluid deprivation therefore will not be beneficial in this group of patients, and it may be harmful.

Using these basic physiologic principles, it would seem that in the patient with normal renal function the use of dehydration prior to excretory urography would be helpful. Dunbar compared a group of normal human volunteers with approximately 15 hours of dehydration to a group without dehydration.[79] He concluded that with dehydration there was a slight and consistent improvement in calyceal opacification, which usually occurred later in the course of the study. Cattell found the urine concentration of iodine to be markedly increased by dehydration prior to urography (approximately 14 hours), while full hydration produced lower urinary iodine levels.[26]

The actual effectiveness of currently used methods of fluid deprivation in producing dehydration is an important issue. McClennan found marked urine osmolality variations prior to excretory urography in patients who had essentially the same fluid deprivation.[80] Individual patients had variation of the urine osmolality on different days after the same fluid restriction program. Therefore to produce a reproducible, effective state of dehydration, a very controlled clinical situation would be necessary.

Bell[81] compared 50 patients with fluid restriction of 550 mL for 24 hours prior to urography with 50 patients having no fluid restrictions. The fluid-restricted group had slightly better radiographic scores, but the difference in quality of the urograms was not statistically significant. These authors recommended elimination of fluid restriction, as have others.[32]

In most clinical uroradiological situations, significant dehydration is probably not achieved. Fluid and food restriction after midnight, however, limits the intake of fluid prior to urography and avoids the possibility of diuretic substances such as coffee. This can avoid a state of excessive hydration or increased urine flow rates.[74,82] It is my own observation

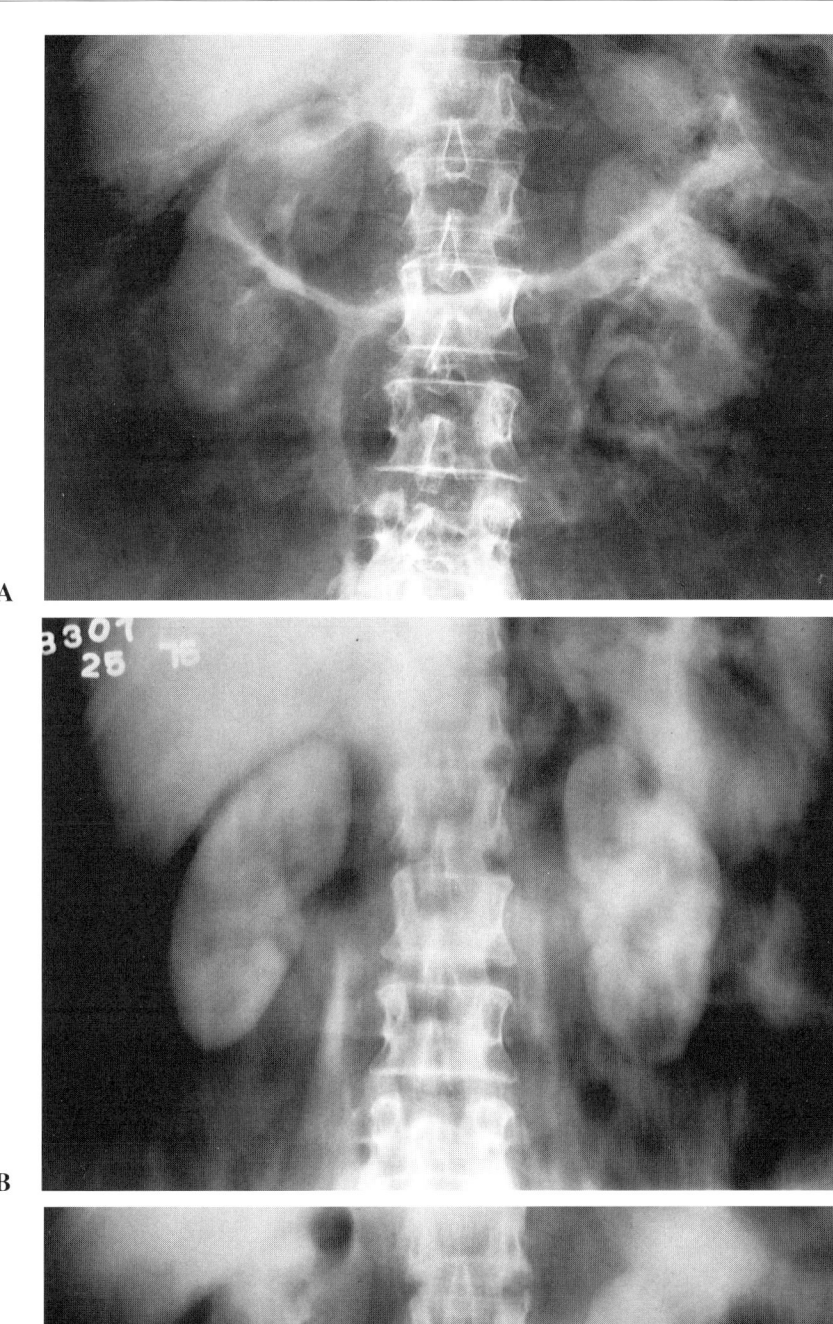

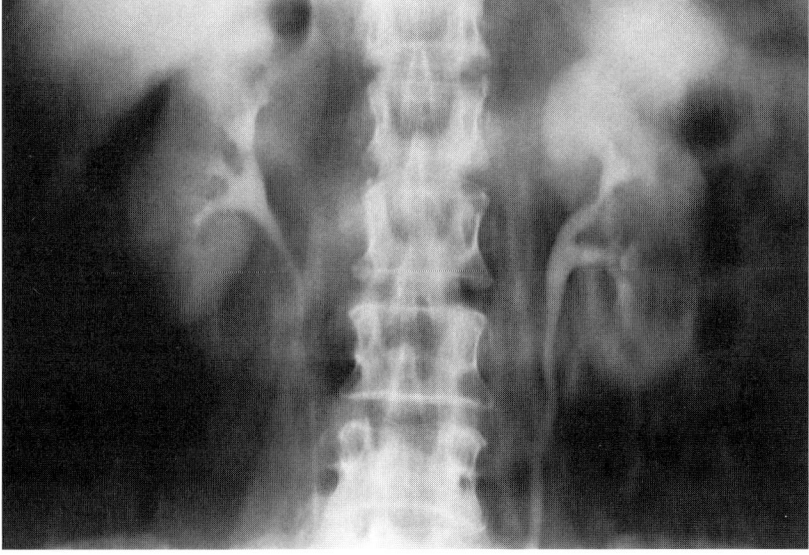

Figure 5–4. Use of tomography to salvage a study in a patient with a large amount of overlying bowel content. **(A)** Nontomographic film is nondiagnostic. Tomography during the nephrographic **(B)** and calyceal **(C)** phases provides excellent visualization of the kidneys. (Reprinted from Older RA, with permission of Professional Medical Services Company.)

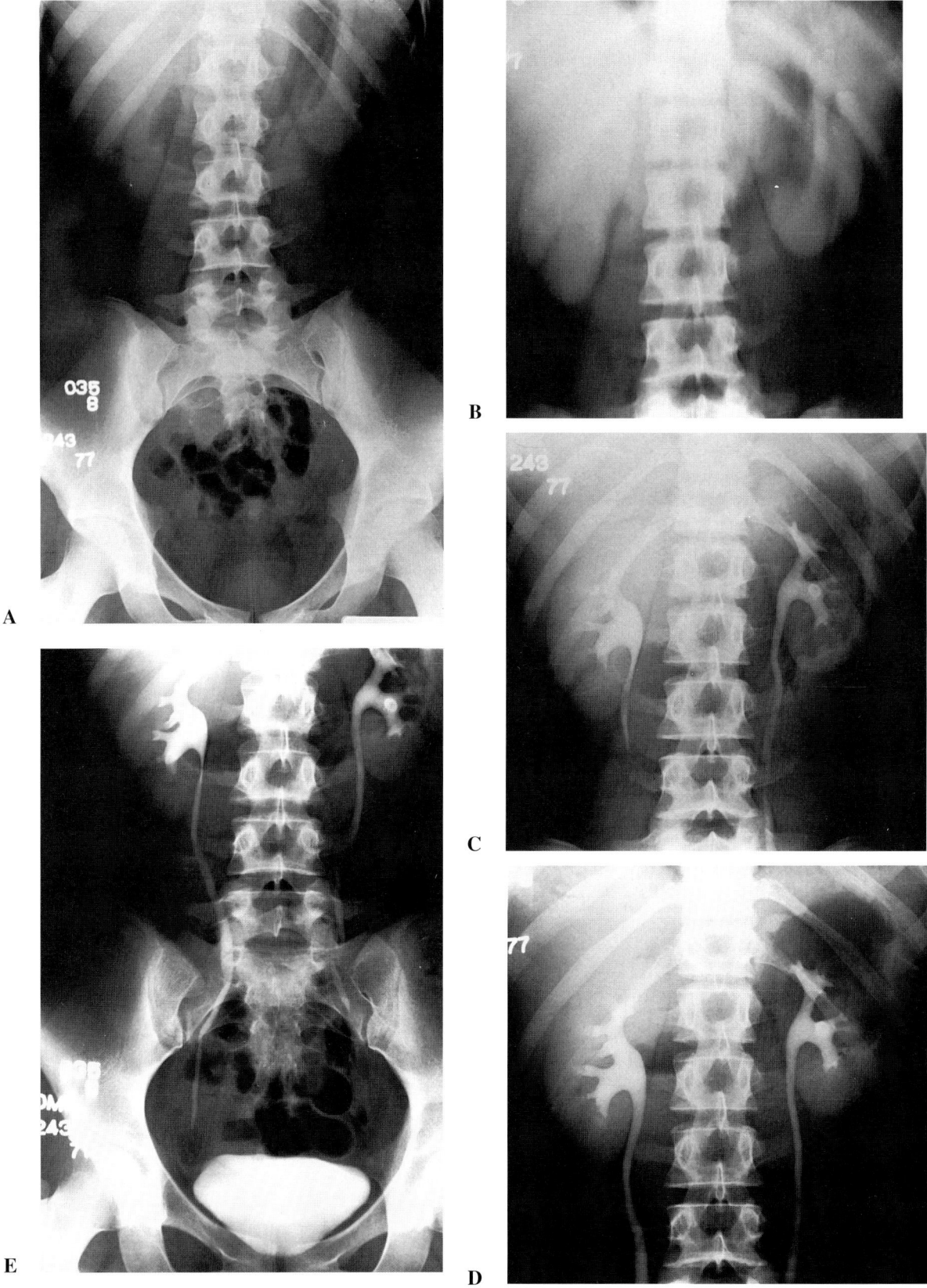

Figure 5–5. (A) Preliminary radiograph. (B) Immediate postinjection tomogram. (C) Nontomographic 5-min film. (D) Nontomographic film with abdominal compression. (E) Full abdominal radiography following release of compression.

that these urograms are generally of better quality than those with no fluid restriction.

The primary danger of dehydration is an increased risk of nephrotoxicity in patients with preexisting renal disease. For these patients fluid restriction is ineffective and dangerous. In clinical situations, where patients cannot have a careful evaluation of renal function prior to urography or are at risk for contrast-induced renal failure for any other reason, the routine use of fluid deprivation should be avoided because the risk of contrast-induced renal failure may outweigh any potential diagnostic benefits. For patients with normal renal function, overnight fluid restriction may avoid an inadequate urogram due to excessive hydration.

Excretory Urography: Performance

OVERVIEW

Excretory urography includes the visualization of both the renal parenchyma and the collecting structures. Therefore a uroradiographic examination should include sufficient radiographs to evaluate each phase. Before discussing details related to the performance of urography, a normal example will be shown to provide an overview of the subject (Fig. 5–5). The preliminary radiograph (Fig. 5–5A) shows no significant abnormalities of the soft tissues or intestinal gas pattern, and no pathologic calcifications are present. A preliminary tomogram (not shown) is used to determine the optimal tomographic levels. This tomogram is obtained in as full and reproducible a phase of expiration as possible. An arc of 20 degrees, producing a tomographic field thickness of approximately 0.5 cm, is used. With experience, technicians can determine the best level for the test tomogram.

If the preliminary tomogram is satisfactory, then 50 to 100 mL of contrast medium is injected through a 19-gauge needle. At the end of the injection the patient holds the same deep expiration as on the test tomogram and the middle level tomogram is obtained (Fig. 5–5B). This immediate postinjection tomogram clearly demonstrates the renal parenchyma. A smooth outline is present, with no evidence of a mass or other parenchymal abnormality. The entire renal outline must be visualized clearly to totally exclude a lesion. The second and third tomograms (not shown) are obtained as soon as possible after the first.

The next radiograph obtained is collimated to the renal area at 5 minutes (Fig. 5–5C). Delicate calyces are present but not optimally distended. Abdominal compression is applied and a collimated radiograph of the kidneys is obtained approximately 5 minutes later, 10 minutes after injection. Compression distends the calyces and provides better visualization (Fig. 5–5D). Although the calyces can have many anatomic variations and numbers, they should have sharp outlines without filling defects, extrinsic compression, or extensions of the contrast into the surrounding parenchyma. Following the release of the compression device a full abdominal radiograph is obtained to demonstrate the ureters and the bladder (Fig. 5–5E).

METHOD OF INJECTION

There are two basic techniques for the intravenous injection of contrast media: (1) syringe (bolus) technique and (2) drip infusion technique. In recent years the bolus technique has become the dominant method used. Contrast injection using a syringe allows one to vary both the dose and the injection time. The rapid bolus technique (used in Fig. 5–5) is one variation of this technique. Slower injection rates can be used, but they will not produce the initial intense nephrogram. The drip infusion technique employs a continuous drip of a dilute contrast medium from an infusion bottle. The standard manufacutred infusion bottle contains 300 mL of a 30% solution. This gives the equivalent of 150 mL of a 60% contrast solution in a bolus technique.

Fry and associates provided an equivalent dose comparison by giving 80 mL of Hypaque-45 either by drip infusion or by bolus injection.[83] No significant difference was found in the radiographs obtained from the two groups, and they therefore concluded that technique had no significant effect on the diagnostic quality of the examination. McClennan has pointed out that it is only the amount of contrast material that makes the difference in the diagnostic quality of the urogram and not the way it is administered.[73,84]

In general, this statement is true, but there is an advantage to the rapid bolus technique in terms of nephrographic density. Immediately after the rapid bolus injection there is a combination of a vascular and a tubular nephrogram that provides the most radiodense nephrogram achieved during the study (Fig. 5–6).[73,85] The peak plasma concentration achieved with the rapid bolus injection exceeds that which is obtained with the infusion technique[86] (Fig. 5–7). Since the plasma concentration is the most important variable affecting the density of the nephrogram, the nephrogram will be maximal during this period of peak plasma concentration, which occurs almost immediately after the bolus injection of contrast.

Most published data indicate therefore that for an equivalent dose of contrast, a more radiodense nephrogram can be achieved with a bolus injection. The calyceal visualization will be essentially the same.

RADIOGRAPHIC SEQUENCE

In determining the radiographs to be used during a urographic examination the goal, which should be kept in mind, is to provide optimal visualization of the renal parenchyma during the nephrographic phase followed by optimal visualization of the collecting structures, ureters, and bladder during the pyelogram phases of the examination.

The Preliminary Abdominal Radiograph. The preliminary abdominal radiograph or scout film is an indispensable part of excretory urography. There are several methods for obtaining this film. Our own preference is a single preliminary supine abdominal radiograph to include both the kid-

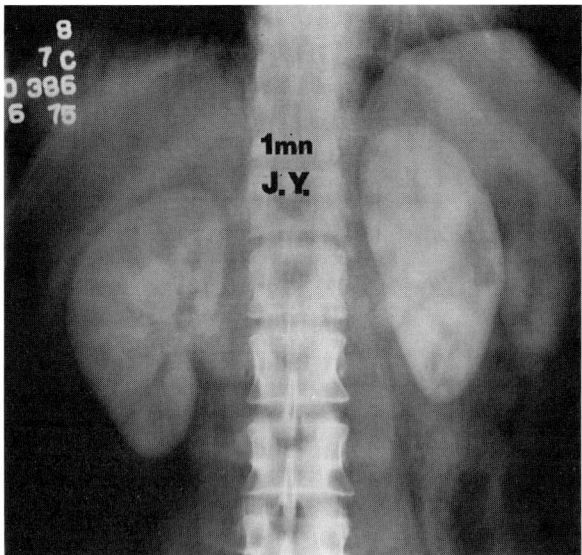
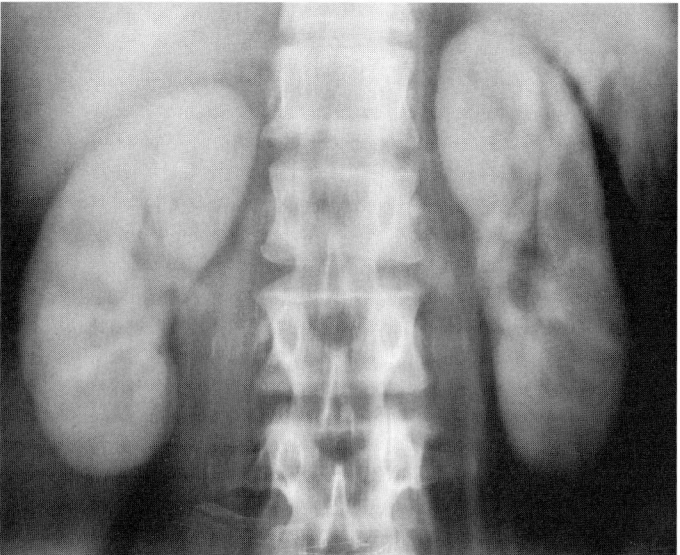
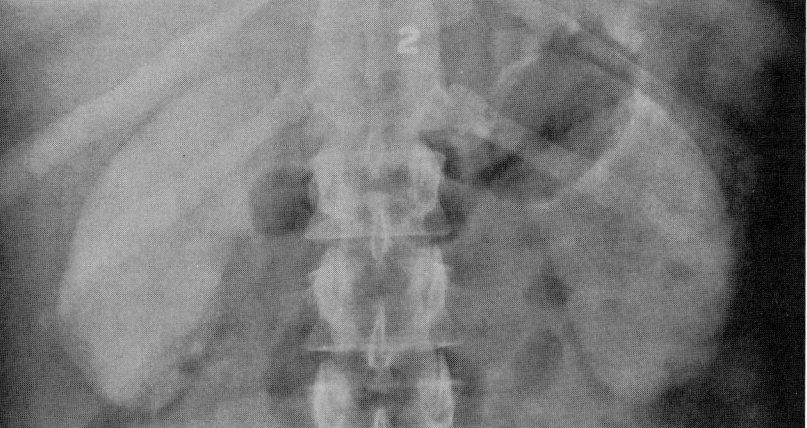

Figure 5–6. Immediate postinjection tomograms. (Reprinted from Older RA, with permission of Professional Medical Services Company.) **(A)** and **(B)** Intense nephrograms obtained postinjection. Parenchymal visualization is maximal at this time. **(C)** Nontomographic nephrographic radiograph in a patient with limited overlying bowel content.

neys and bony pelvis to the level of the symphysis pubis. In instances where the patient is too large to accomplish this, a second coned radiograph of either the kidneys or the bony pelvis can be added. We prefer coning to the kidneys in most cases to reduce the radiation burden on the gonads. When using routine tomography, a preliminary tomogram coned to the kidney area is added to establish the proper tomographic plane. Two routine preliminary radiographs with high–low centering and angled or oblique views can be used to eliminate the problem of calcified cartilage overlying the renal area. Our approach has been to obtain these additional radiographs only when necessary.

Radiographs of the Renal Parenchyma. A radiograph demonstrating the renal parenchyma at the height of contrast enhancement is extremely important in providing the best visualization of the renal parenchyma during excretory urography (Fig. 5–6). The renal parenchyma can be visualized throughout a considerable portion of the excretory urogram, but its density relative to surrounding structures diminishes with the passage of time following the injection of contrast (Fig. 5–8). Both clinical and experimental data indicate that

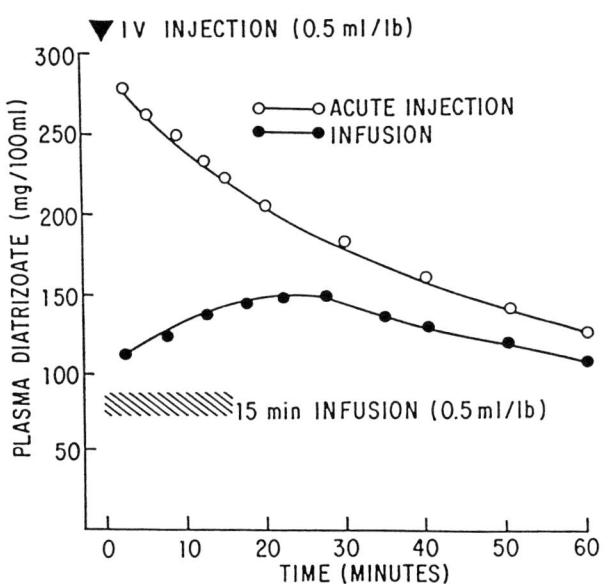

Figure 5–7. Plasma diatrizoate concentration as a function of time and type of injection (Reproduced with permission from Cattell WR, *Investigative Radiology*. Philadelphia: JB Lippincott.

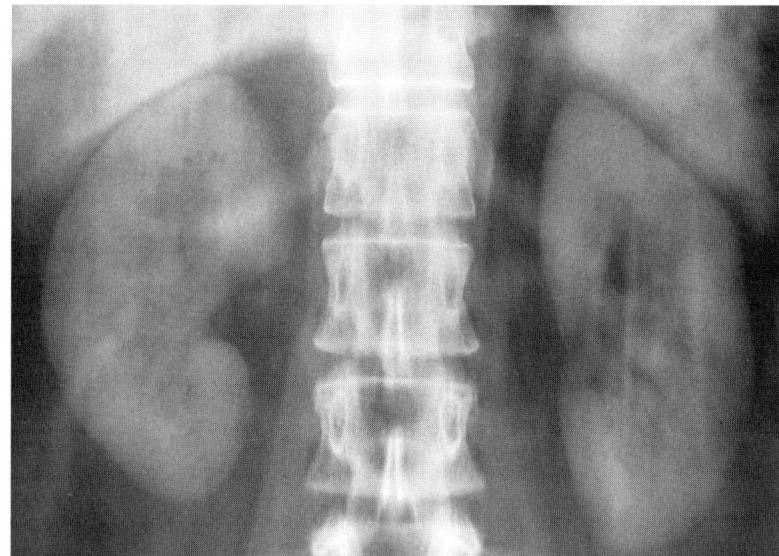

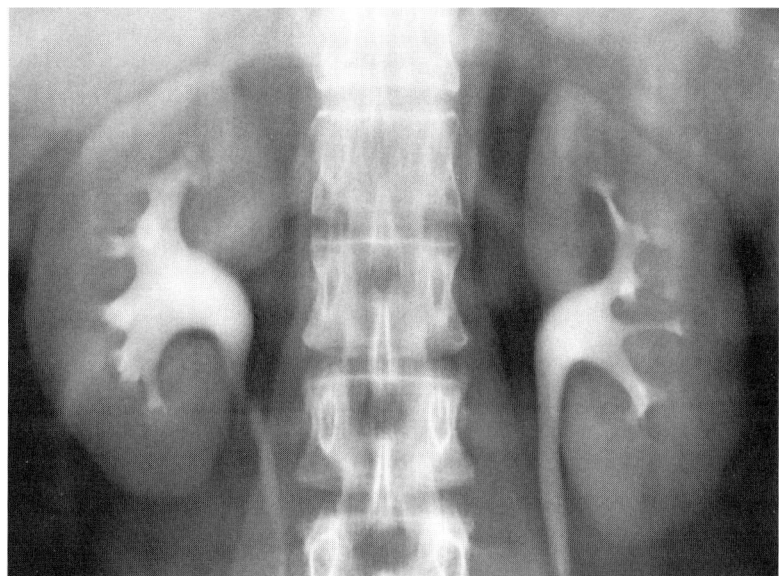

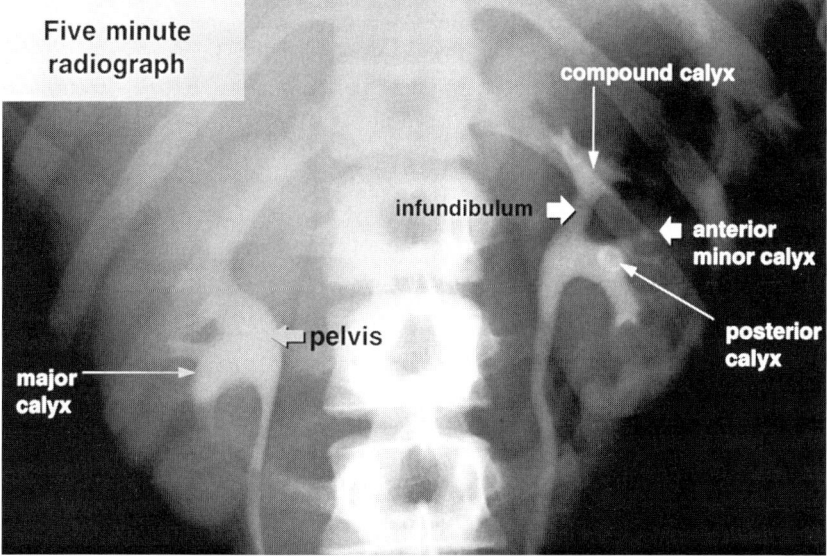

Figure 5–8. (A) Immediate postinjection tomogram and (B) 5-minute tomogram. Both provide excellent parenchymal visualization, with the nephrogram slightly decreased on (B). The latter tomogram, however, also provides clear visualization of the collecting structures. (C) Labeled collimated 5-minute nontomographic radiograph. (Same patient as Fig. 5–5.)

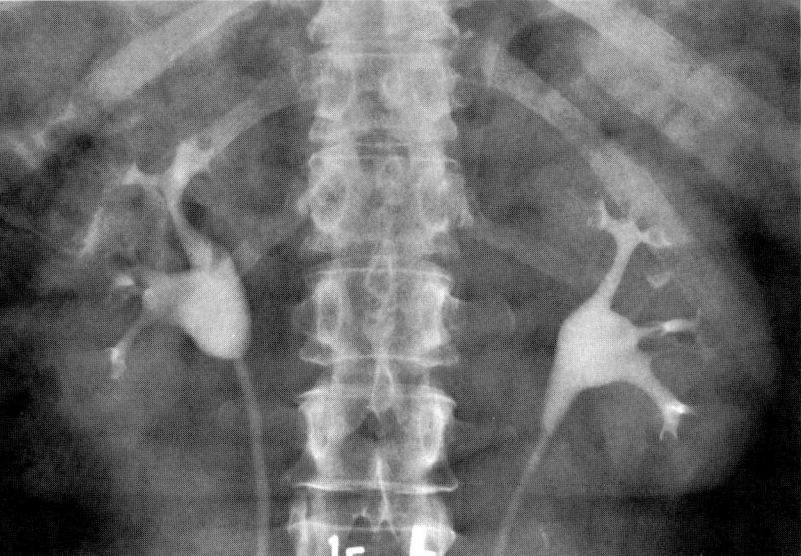

Figure 5–9. (A) Five-minute nontomographic radiograph. Renal parenchyma no longer fully visualized. Prompt filling of delicate calyces, pelvis, and proximal ureter. (B) Abdominal compression significantly improves filling and visualization of the collecting structures.

immediately following a rapid bolus injection of ionic contrast media there will be a peak in plasma concentration and therefore nephrographic density.[26,38,85,87,88] For nonionic contrast the nephrogram appears to be delayed slightly. The reasons for this are not fully understood.[36,39]

Hamilton described the vascular nephrogram phase of excretory urography and included a method of timing the nephrogram based on the patient's sensations.[89] A very rapid bolus injection over a period of 3 to 4 seconds was used with a relatively large 16-gauge needle. We initially used a similar method but found that the vascular information obtained with this extremely fast injection was not generally necessary and have slowed our injection of ionic media to approximately 30 to 60 seconds through a 19-gauge needle. This produces an intense nephrogram that often demonstrates the corticomedullary junction.[85] When using nonionic contrast, injection time is slightly longer because of the increase in viscosity of the nonionic contrast media. A nephrogram demonstrating corticomedullary separation is therefore not usually obtained.

Radiographs of the Collecting Structures. At 5 minutes there is generally good calyceal filling and the nephrogram, although not as intense, is still satisfactorily visualized (Fig. 5–8B,C). Although there may be slight differences in peak calyceal opacification for ionic and nonionic contrast media, we have not found it necessary to alter our basic radiographic timing. Comparisons of ionic and nonionic contrast media have not shown a significant difference in the time required for maximal opacification of the pyelocalyceal system.[90]

Coned Kidney Radiograph with Abdominal Compression. If the 5-minute kidney radiograph shows no evidence of obstruction, a compression device can be applied immediately. Contraindications to the use of abdominal compression include suspected ureteral or intestinal obstruction, recent surgery, abdominal aneurysm, general debilitation, or severe pain. The compression provides greater distention of the calyceal structures and is especially helpful when calyceal filling is less than optimal on the initial 5-minute radio-

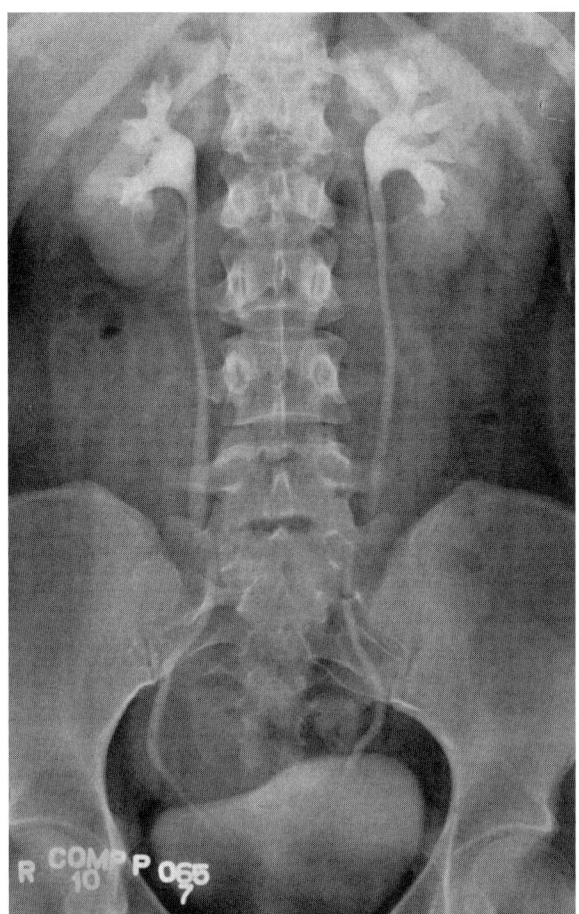

Figure 5–10. Immediate postcompression radiograph shows the majority of both ureters.

graph (Fig. 5–9). The compression radiograph is coned to the kidneys and proximal ureters and is obtained after approximately 5 minutes of compression. Modern compression devices provide a belt that encircles the patient's abdomen and two separate inflatable balloons that are positioned so that they are centered over the iliac crests. Having the compression belt around the patient instead of being attached to the table allows variation in patient positioning while compression is maintained.[91] When compression is applied carefully and is used in the routine urographic setting so that technicians maintain familiarity with the compression device, it becomes a very effective method of providing optimal distention of the calyceal structures. Compression can produce spontaneous calyceal extravasation and has rarely been implicated in more severe complications such as hypotension.[92] Calyceal extravasation is not considered significant clinically and the hypotension reverses with release of compression.

Postcompression Full Abdominal Radiograph. Immediately following the release of abdominal compression there is generally excellent opacification of the ureters. In most cases, sufficient contrast medium has already entered the bladder as well (Fig. 5–10). This radiograph should be centered low enough to include the base of the bladder, for it is usually not necessary to demonstrate the entire upper system again.

Accessory Radiographs. In addition to the preceding routine radiographs, several accessory radiographs may be used. These radiographs may not be needed, but they frequently aid in answering diagnostic questions.

1. Oblique views are frequently used, especially when tomography is not used in the calyceal phase. We prefer our oblique radiographs coned to the kidneys to provide better renal detail. The kidney that is nearest the table will be in a posterior oblique position, whereas the opposite kidney will be in a "reverse oblique."

   The posterior oblique position profiles more of the anterior surface of the kidney, whereas the reverse oblique profiles more of the posterior surface. The posterior oblique view provides a sharper renal image because of the closeness of the kidney to the film. A primary role of the oblique view is to evaluate the calyceal structures, and it is particularly helpful in further evaluating potential filling defects and in clarifying pseudo-filling defects related to overlapping calyces or crossing vessels (Fig. 5–11). Oblique views with tomography are also helpful in confirming a mass lesion suspected on other radiographs.

2. Postvoid radiographs are most often used in the older male population, where bladder outlet obstruction from prostatic hypertrophy is a diagnostic consideration. Postvoid radiographs may also be helpful in evaluating obstructive processes of the upper urinary tract. Having the patient stand up, walk to the bathroom, and empty his or her bladder will aid greatly in evaluating the ability of the upper urinary tract to drain.

3. Prone radiographs are used primarily to evaluate the ureters when they are not adequately opacified on the postcompression radiograph. The prone position will place the ureters in a more dependent position and facilitates emptying the contrast material from the renal pelvis and calyces into the ureters. This same position can be used to facilitate more rapid filling of the ureters when a distal obstruction is present.

4. Upright radiographs are occasionally used in urinary tract obstruction where gravity may facilitate movement of the contrast to the point of obstruction. Upright radiographs can be helpful in severe hydronephrosis where contrast is very poorly concentrated because of mixing with the nonopacified urine. In these instances upright radiographs may reveal contrast-fluid levels and clearly outline the collecting structures.

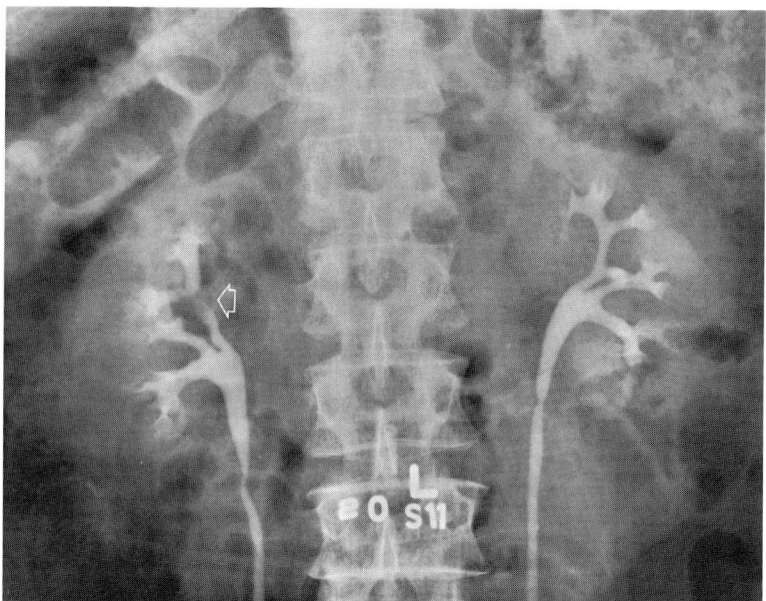

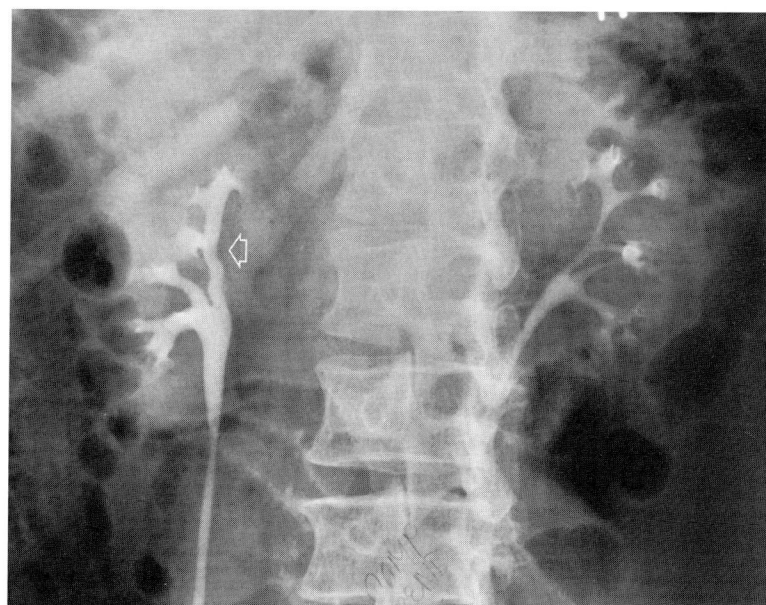

Figure 5–11. (A) Collimated AP view shows a vague filling defect (arrow) in the right upper infundibulum as well as overlapping calyces. (B) Right posterior oblique view clearly shows an extrinsic vascular impression (arrow) on the infundibulum and separates overlapping calyces.

Technical Factors

A range of approximately 60 to 70 kVp is optimal for the preliminary abdominal radiograph as well as for routine and tomographic radiographs of the urinary tract. The use of higher kVp will decrease the visibility of the contrast media. With the use of a relatively low kVp it is necessary to have generators that can produce sufficient milliamperage (mA) without prolonging the exposure time. A 500 mA or greater three-phase generator is preferable.[82] Using a 600-mA three-phase generator and using a kVp of 65, sufficient mA can be achieved with relatively low exposure times. With generator capabilities of only 300 mA, kVp may have to be increased to 70, and even at this level, exposure times will be longer.

Multiple types of film-screen combinations are available, and use will depend to some extent on personal preference. Use of a high-speed system can reduce radiation dose and still produce high-quality urograms. We use high-speed Fuji-HR-H film that, when combined with Fuji GH-1 intensifying screens, gives a relative speed of 600. This is a high-contrast film well suited for stone detection.

Collimating to the area of interest is crucial to eliminate degradation of the image from scattered radiation. Failure to collimate properly can significantly affect image quality (Fig. 5–12); technologists should be encouraged to collimate closely.

Tomography and Nephrotomography

Because of its ability to blur out the surrounding structures and provide greater visualization of the kidney, tomography

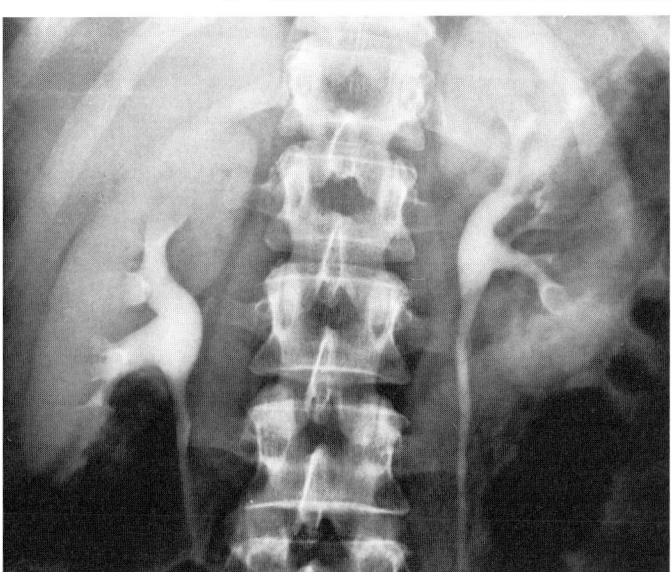

Figure 5–12. Collimated versus noncollimated films. The non-collimated film (A) is markedly degraded by scattered radiation with a generalized "grayness" to the radiograph. Collimation (B) produces a much improved image.

is one of the most important advances in the refinement of excretory urography. Tomography need not be sophisticated. Simple linear tomography is sufficient. We prefer to use a relatively short arc of 20 degrees, which produces a tomographic cut of approximately 0.5 cm. Using three of these tomographic cuts during the nephrographic phase, we can cover the majority of the kidney in most cases.

There are a number of terms related to tomography that are used in different ways and can therefore be confusing. The term *nephrotomography* as used by Evans in 1954 and 1957 described a secondary procedure used to further evaluate a "known" renal mass.[93,94] Multiple thin tomographic sections were obtained after a large bolus of contrast medium was given and an intense nephrogram was produced. The purpose of the nephrotomogram in these cases was to determine the etiology of the mass (i.e., cyst versus tumor). This was "nephrotomography" in its original sense, and for a number of years it was used as a primary method of separating a cyst from a solid tumor. With the development of ultrasound and computed tomography, nephrotomography as a method to determine the etiology of a renal mass became obsolete. True nephrotomography in its original sense, therefore, is no longer performed. What has occurred, however, is an incorporation of the use of tomography into the routine urogram, so that tomography has moved from a secondary procedure used to determine the etiology of the mass to a first-line procedure used in the detection of not only masses but other renal abnormalities.

Two issues regarding tomography are the needs to decide (1) the most effective time during urography to use tomography and (2) whether it should be used routinely. Tomography's major contribution is in evaluating the renal parenchyma. Tomograms should be obtained when the nephrogram is most intense, which is immediately after the bolus injection of ionic contrast media (Fig. 5–6) and possibly slightly later for nonionic.[33] Our routine tomograms are therefore obtained at the completion of the contrast injection. Previous studies have demonstrated the increased detection of renal masses with tomography[95,96] and have demonstrated that this is best performed during the nephrographic phase (Fig. 5–13).[85] We have not delayed this timing for nonionic contrast. Tomography later in the urogram, to better visualize the collecting structures, is used selectively and is most helpful when there is considerable overlying bowel content or poor concentration of contrast in the pelvocalyceal structures.

The routine use of tomography provides more than the detection of renal masses. It frequently salvages a study that would otherwise be nondiagnostic and increases diagnostic confidence (Fig. 5–4). Visualization of the kidneys, including their internal architecture, is improved overall and abnormalities are more easily detected. Evaluation of abnormalities is more precise and diagnosis is more definitive.

Routine use of tomography will be unnecessary in some patients. In young patients and, in particular, in patients who have relatively classic symptoms of urinary tract stone disease we will often forgo tomography initially and only obtain it later in the study if necessary. Our standard urogram includes tomography, but each case is considered individually and tomography can be eliminated if the expected benefits do not warrant the additional radiation.

DIGITAL RADIOGRAPHY

Two distinct types of digital radiography systems are currently available.

1. A system based on imaging plates with photostimulable substances such as phosphorus and barium-flurohalide europium-doped crystals (digital luminescent radiography)
2. A system based on digital image amplification of conventional x-ray fluoroscopy.[51,52]

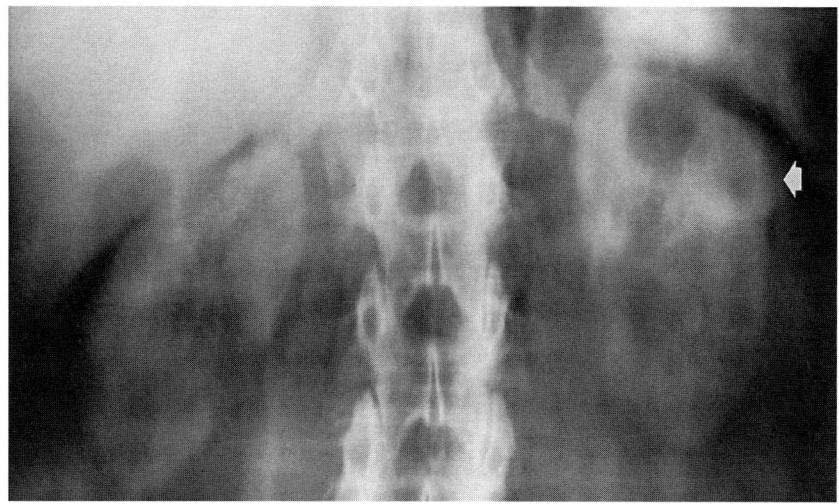

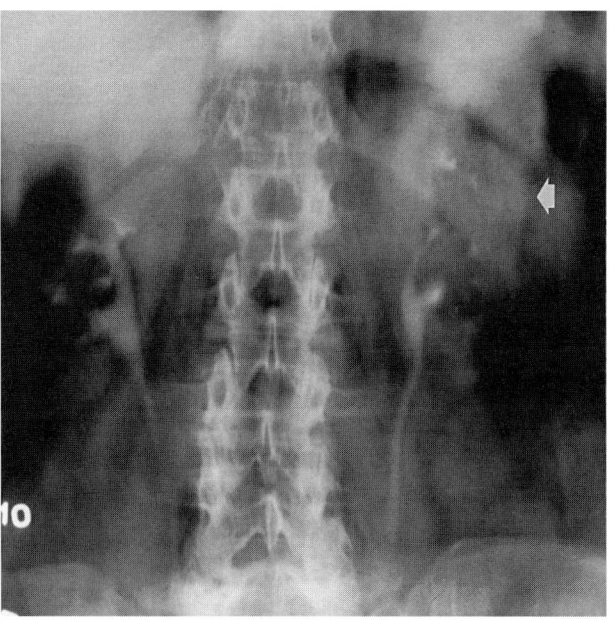

Figure 5–13. Immediate postinjection tomography (**A**) demonstrates the "blush" (arrow) of a small vascular renal cell carcinoma. The lesion (arrow) becomes isodense and is more difficult to see with tomography later in the study (**B**). (Reprinted from Older RA,[85] with permission of Professional Medical Services Company.)

Basic Radiologic Techniques for Imaging the Urinary Tract 65

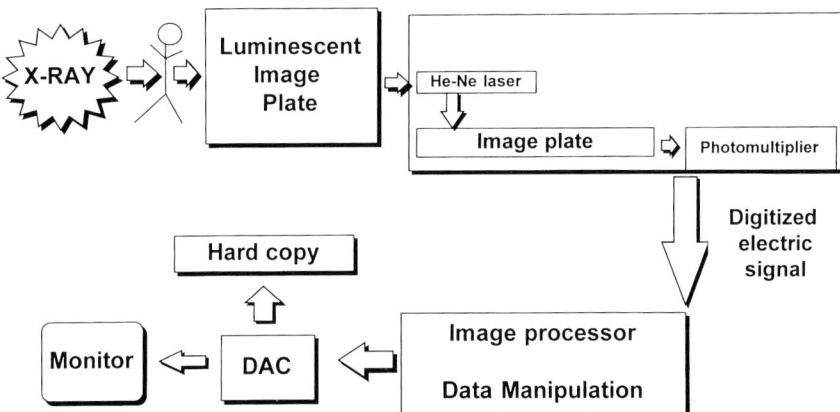

Figure 5–14. Photostimulable digital system.

With digital luminescent radiography (Fig. 5–14) the initial exposure is made not to film, but to a reusable luminescent image plate containing photostimulable phosphorus.[97] The exposure is made with standard radiographic equipment, including portable equipment.[98] The x-ray beam hits the luminescent image plate just as it would conventional film, but instead of producing a direct film image, it raises the energy state of the photostimulable phosphorus crystals in the plate. This energy is stored until the plate is scanned with a helium-neon laser beam.[97,99] Initial laser scanning is done with a low-power beam to determine exposure. The plate is then rescanned by a high-intensity laser beam that releases luminescent radiation corresponding to the absorbed x-ray energy. This luminescent radiation is sent to a photomultiplier tube and converted into an electric signal that is then digitized into 10 bits, or 1024 gray levels.[97,99] The digital image is then processed and converted back to an analog image that can be used to generate a hard copy on film or be displayed on a CRT console. During processing two image types are usually produced. One uses an algorithm that is similar to a conventional film and the other provides an edge-enhanced image.[99]

A major advantage of the digital system is radiation dose reduction. Imaging plates with photostimulable phosphorus have a much wider linear dynamic range than conventional screen-film combinations, allowing imaging to be obtained at a significantly decreased radiation dose.[97–99] Dose reduction of up to 50% has been achieved for urography,[99] and reductions of as much as 90% have been achieved in urethrocystography.[97] The independence of film density to dose also will eliminate most repeat examinations caused by exposure errors.

Comparison of digital urography with conventional films has shown no significant difference in diagnostic accuracy or image quality.[99,100] For some features such as renal margins, digital images have produced better results than conventional films.[101] This has occurred despite the fact that spatial resolution is decreased to approximately 2.5 to 3.5 line pairs/mm as compared to 4 to 6 line pairs/mm in conventional film-screen radiography.[97] This may be due to greater contrast resolution of the digital image, or it may be because high spatial resolution is not as critical in urographic diagnosis.[99]

Other potential advantages of this type of digital system include (1) reduced cost of each examination, (2) potential for transmission and storage in digital form, (3) no modification of existing radiographic equipment, and (4) automatic image processing.[98] Disadvantages are limited throughput, complex equipment, initial cost, and smaller image format.[98]

The second type of digital system is digital fluororadiography (Fig. 5–15). The x-ray image is converted by the image intensifier into an optical image projected onto the

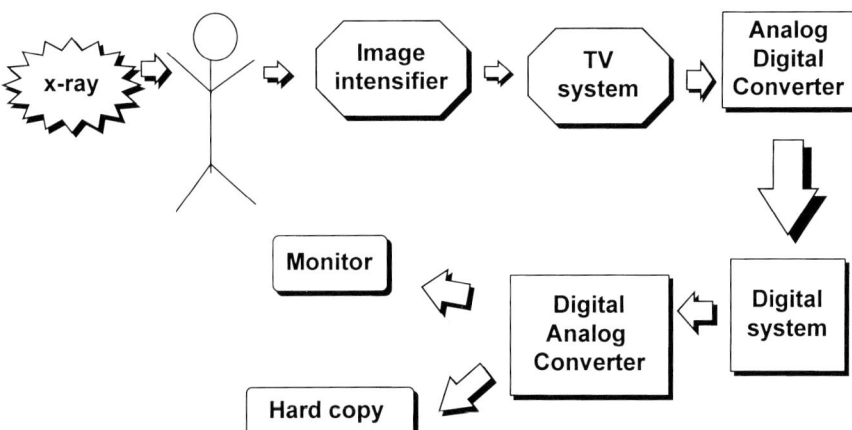

Figure 5–15. Digital fluoroscopy system.

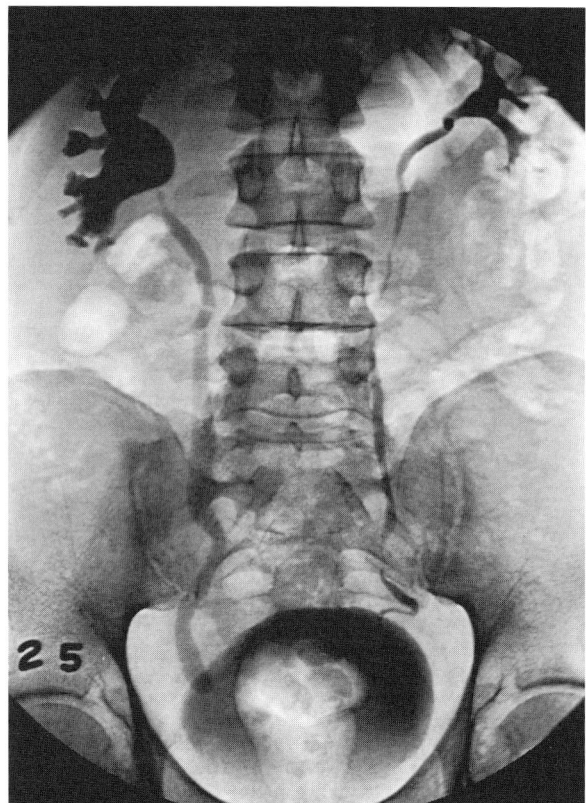 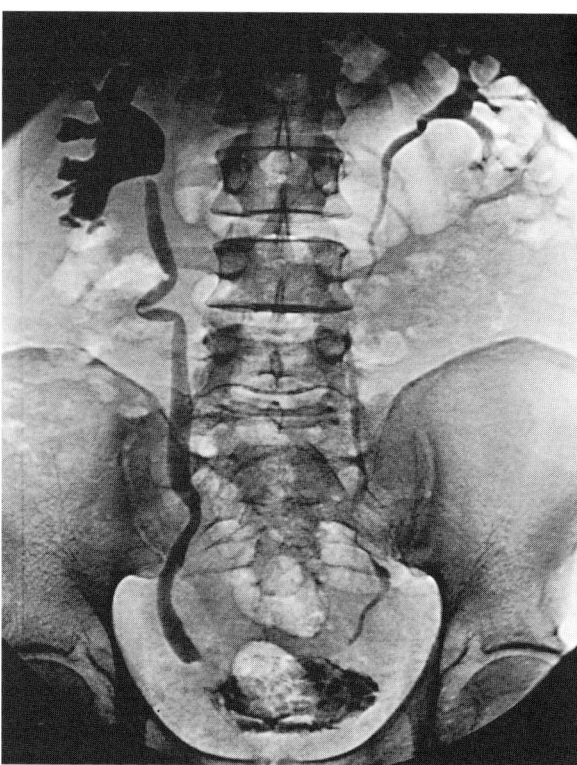

Figure 5-16. Comparison of full digital radiograph with **(A)** minimal edge enhancement (10%) and **(B)** 31% edge enhancement.

input screen of the TV tube. Within the TV system the image is converted into a series of electrical signals. The digital x-ray image is produced by conversion of the electrical signal into a digital image. The stored digital image is converted back to an analog image through a digital analog converter and is sent immediately to the monitor for review. Images can later be selected for data manipulation such as edge enhancement, window settings, brightness, or image reversal (Figs. 5-16, 5-17). Hard-copy printing by a laser camera can be obtained on any images pre- or postdata manipulation.[102]

CYSTOGRAPHY

Retrograde cystography is a relatively simple procedure with limited applications in adults. A preliminary abdominal film of the pelvis is first obtained. Following this, catheterization of the urethra is performed using sterile technique. A soft rubber catheter or Foley catheter is used in adults. A balloon-type catheter is avoided in young children. Following catheterization, contrast medium is instilled by gravity drip until the patient has a sensation of bladder fullness and discomfort. This usually requires approximately 200 to 400 mL of contrast material but can vary, depending upon patient size and any pathologic states present in the bladder. When the patient has a sensation of fullness, the catheter is removed and radiographs are obtained. This technique is varied for the trauma patient or postoperative patient. In these instances a smaller volume of contrast (50 mL) is instilled and checked for extravasation before complete filling.

At a minimum an anterior posterior (AP) radiograph with the bladder full and a postvoid radiograph are obtained (Fig. 5-18). These are often supplemented by both oblique views to better visualize the bladder margins and to detect extravasation or fistulas that might be hidden on the AP view. One of the oblique views can be obtained during voiding or straining to aid in detection of contrast extravasation. Although we do not routinely use fluoroscopy in our adult patients, fluoroscopy is essential to detect intermittent reflux in children.[91,103] Fluoroscopy permits dynamic evaluation of the bladder, urethra, and ureters, and may detect reflux not seen on standard overhead films. For adults this is not a major concern.

Contrast media used during cystography are iodinated aqueous solutions similar to those used for intravenous urography. Various concentrations of these contrast media can be employed. The suspected abnormality is important in determining the concentration of contrast medium used. In instances where reflux or extravasation are suspected, a more concentrated contrast medium may be of value to detect small degrees of reflux or extravasation. A more dilute con-

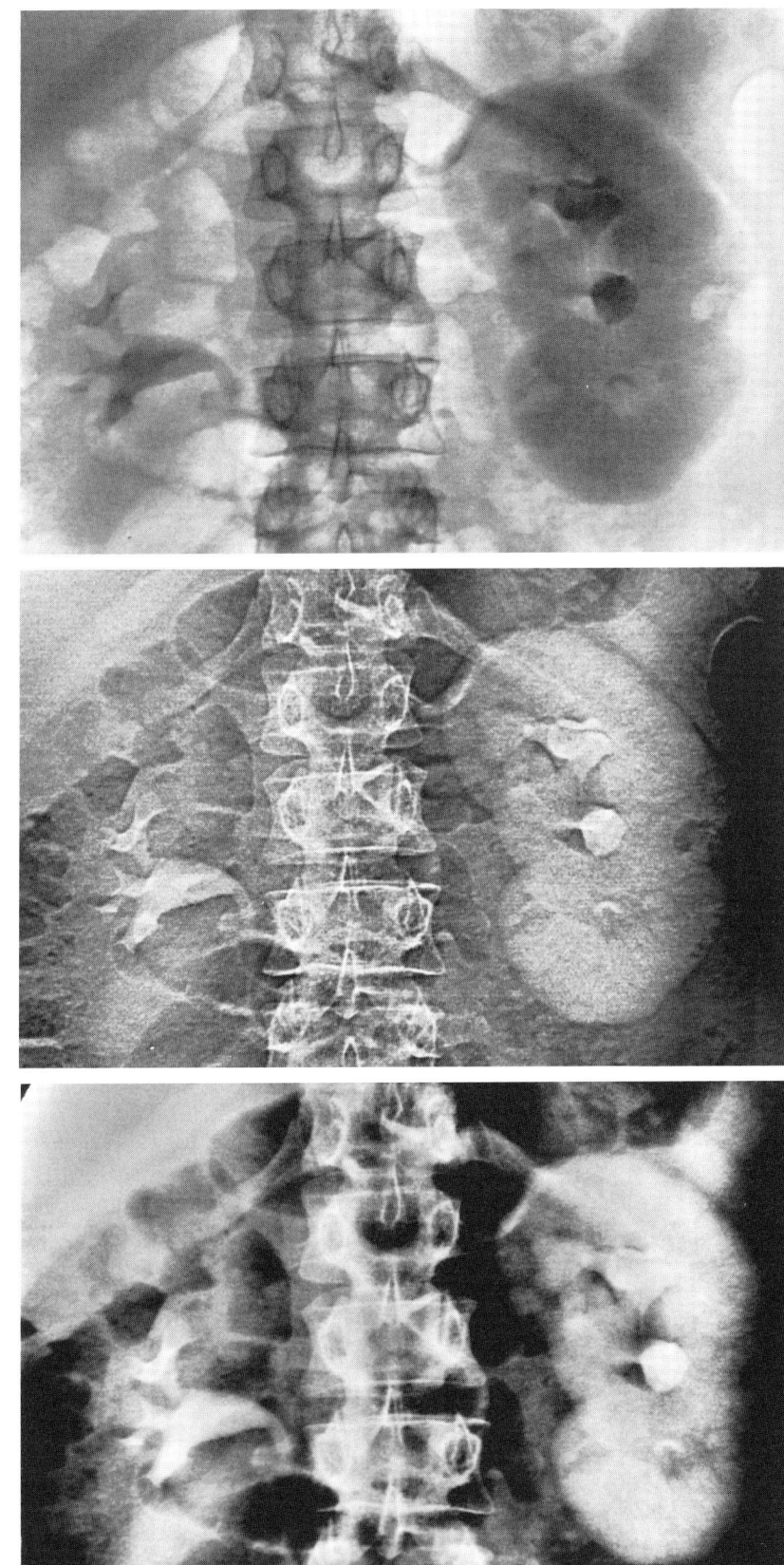

Figure 5–17. Digital manipulation on a patient with acute left-sided obstruction. **(A)** Original digital image shows delayed filing of dilated calyces and delayed intense nephrogram. **(B)** Image reversal and use of edge-enhanced algorithm. **(C)** Image manipulation with alteration of window settings to enhance contrast.

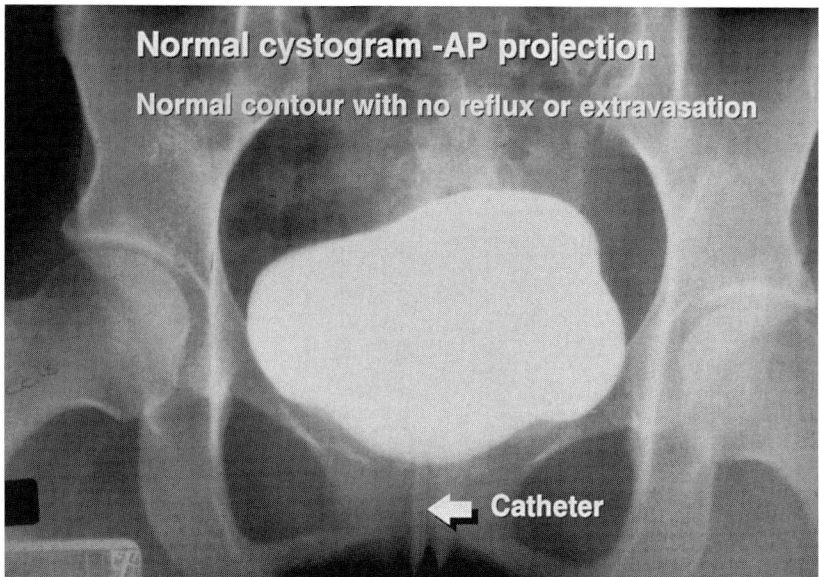

Figure 5–18. Normal cystogram AP projection. Normal contour with no reflux or extravasation.

trast medium, however, may be advantageous when examining the bladder for possible filling defects or other intrinsic abnormalities. We routinely use a 15 to 17% solution that contains approximately 70 to 81 mg of iodine per milliliter. Dilution of commercially available 30% cystographic agents can produce a 15% solution or prepackaged bottles of approximately 17% (81 mg/mL) Cysto-Conray II (Mallinckrodt Pharmaceutical) can be used. This dilute contrast medium is less irritating to the bladder.[104]

A major question about cystography involves its indications. As will be discussed in other chapters, there is general agreement that cystography, or more specifically voiding cystourethrography (VCUG), plays an important role in children with urinary tract infections and is the prime method to detect vesicoureteral reflux in this group of patients. In the adult population, however, cystography to detect reflux is not generally indicated. Although vesicoureteral reflux does occur in the adult population, its incidence in adults with urinary tract infection is not as clear.[105–111] In 1966, Baker studied 210 adult patients and found a 5.2% incidence of reflux.[111] Amar found a 13.7% incidence of reflux in 190 patients but in neither of the preceding studies was the patient population clearly defined.[106] In a high percentage of the patients described in the preceding studies the upper urinary tracts were abnormal, that is, small, scarred kidneys; nonfunctioning kidneys; hydronephrosis; mucosal striations; or ureteral dilation.[105,107–110] The efficacy of cystography and of the value of upper tract abnormalities in predicting reflux was evaluated in a series of 249 patients having cystography for both infectious and noninfectious indications.[112] With a previous history of reflux, previous surgery for reflux, or urographic abnormalities suggesting reflux 14.7% of patients showed reflux. If, however, the patient had no upper tract urographic abnormalities or history other than infection, then the incidence of reflux detected was only 3.4%. The finding of reflux in this second group was not particularly significant, altering therapy in only one patient.

If reflux is the primary clinical concern, it appears that cystography should generally be confined to patients with upper tract abnormalities (including congenital abnormalities often associated with reflux), history of reflux, or previous reflux surgery.

Cystography in adults does play a role in both pre- and postoperative assessment. Preoperative cystography is often performed in patients undergoing renal, pancreatic, or combined transplantation to exclude preexisting abnormalities that could impact surgery. Postoperative cystography is used in these patients as well for detection of anastamotic leaks or extravasation.

The increase in radical prostatectomies for prostatic carcinoma has produced an increase in the use of cystography for postoperative management. The cystogram is used primarily to detect extravasation at the anastamotic site and to determine if the indwelling catheter can be removed (Fig. 5–19). Cystography can be used to direct early decatheterization. Patients with no extravasation can have their catheters removed while those with extravasation require follow up cystograms.[113]

Cystography is indicated in patients with pelvic trauma to exclude intraperitoneal or extraperitoneal bladder rupture as well as in patients suspected of having fistulas or leaks due to pelvic surgery, malignancy or inflammatory disease.

URETHROGRAPHY

Urethrography, or examination of the urethra, is performed in several ways. Knowledge of the various procedures available and of the advantages and disadvantages of each will allow selection of the proper study for the clinical problem. Urethrography is divided into two major categories: (1) antegrade, descending, or voiding urethrography, which refers to a study during the act of voiding; and (2) retrograde, or ascending, urethrography, which implies radiographic ex-

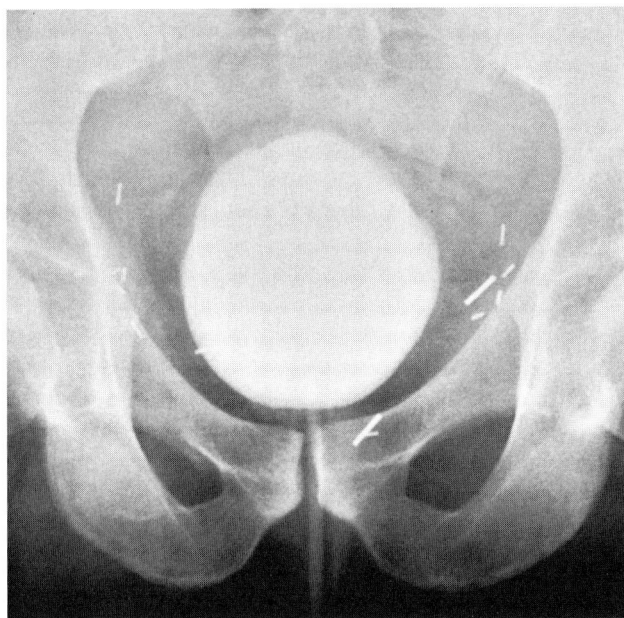
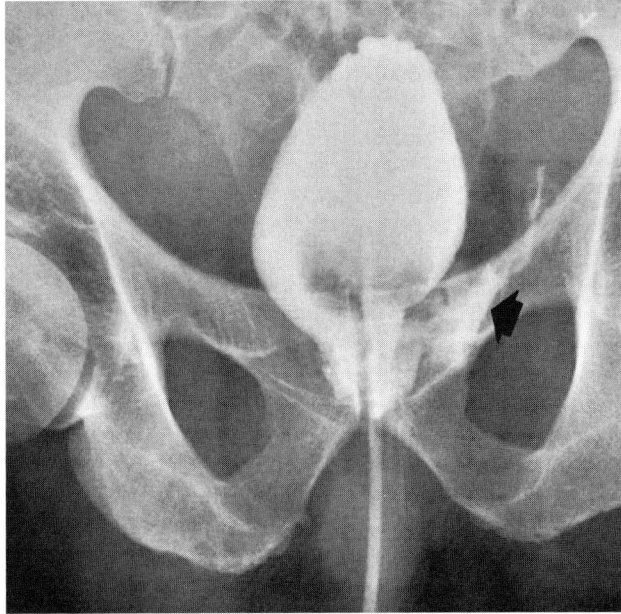
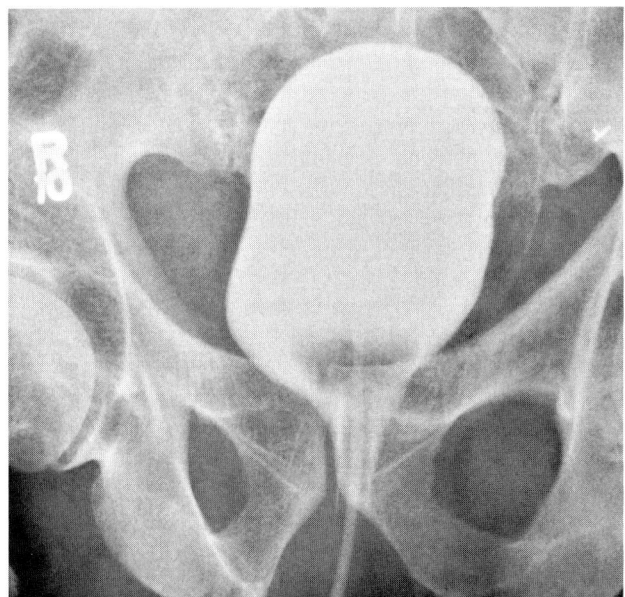

Figure 5-19. Postprostatectomy cystograms. **(A)** No extravasation. **(B)** Different patient with extravasation at anastomosis (arrow). **(C)** Follow-up showing almost complete resolution of extravasation.

amination during or following retrograde injection of contrast into the urethra.

Antegrade Descending–Voiding Urethrography

Antegrade descending–voiding urethrography is accomplished in three ways: (1) excretory voiding urethrography (EVU) using the contrast that has been excreted by the kidneys during urography and that accumulates in the bladder, (2) use of contrast material instilled into the bladder [usually combined with cystography and referred to as voiding cystourethrography (VCUG)] following catheterization of the bladder, and (3) use of either the contrast that has reached the bladder during a retrograde injection or further contrast through the same route after retrograde urethrography.

EXCRETORY VOIDING URETHROGRAPHY

Excretory voiding urethrography (EVU) uses contrast material accumulated from excretion of the kidneys and is performed during the act of voiding. This form of urethrography has been used for a number of years, and although some of the earlier investigations were not uniformly successful, others have had success with this technique in obtaining diagnostic images of the urethra.[114-116] Some of the success of the later investigators may have been related to larger volumes of contrast material (up to 150 mL) used intravenously.[116] EVU involves more than just the addition of radiographs at the end of a routine excretory urogram. Care must be taken to have the bladder empty prior to excretory urography to maximize the concentration of contrast medium. Varying doses for the excretory urogram associated with this study have been used up to 1 mL/lb with a maximum of 150 mL of 60% contrast medium.[116] This is higher than a standard dose for excretory urography. Following the excretory urogram, the patient is given fluids until there is a strong desire to void. This may require as much as an additional 1500 mL of water.[116] At this point, voiding radiographs are obtained. The simplest study will include only a right posterior oblique voiding film with the patient in the supine position. AP, as well as left posterior obliques can also be obtained but are often not necessary.[114,116] A standing film can be used.[115] Fluoroscopy is often used when children are being evaluated.[104]

A variation of EVU is the addition of a penile clamp to produce greater distention of the anterior urethra during voiding. Either a Brodney or a Zipser clamp can be used to produce greater distention of the urethra with improved visualization of both the anterior and posterior urethra.[117,118]

EVU depends on good concentration of contrast media within the bladder and is therefore limited by renal function and the concentrating ability of the kidneys. Fluid restriction, if used prior to the excretory urogram, may reduce the ability of the patient to void, and the study can be time-consuming if the patient is not totally cooperative.[115] The advantage of EVU is the lack of catheterization, which makes this a relatively noninvasive procedure. The visualization obtained is not generally as good as would be obtained with catheterization and instillation of a more concentrated contrast material. It is, however, a simple noninvasive method for urethral visualization and can be used as a screening study in selected situations.

VOIDING CYSTOURETHROGRAPHY

Voiding cystourethrography is an examination of the bladder and urethra following the retrograde instillation of contrast medium into the bladder through a catheter within the bladder, a catheter in the urethra, or a suprapubic catheter. The absence of the word *excretory* in its title separates it from the previous category of urethrography. The need for catheterization to place the contrast material into the bladder is the primary disadvantage of this technique. The major advantages are a greater concentration of contrast media than can be achieved following EVU and the ability to evaluate for vesicoureteral reflux.

The patient is placed in the supine position on the radiographic table and a preliminary radiograph in the right posterior oblique position is obtained. To minimize overlying soft tissue, the leg nearest the table should have the thigh flexed and knee bent, as this will move soft tissue away from the urethra.[119] Using sterile techniques, catheterization is performed. A straight rubber catheter can be passed into the bladder or a Foley catheter can be used. When this technique is used in young children, as is often the case, a non-balloon-type catheter such as a feeding tube is used to reduce risk of injury caused by overdistention of the bladder.

Through either type of catheter the bladder is filled with relatively dilute contrast media (15 to 30%). Contrast medium is a bladder irritant, and this increases with concentration.[104] The end point of bladder filling is determined by patient sensation, that is, when the urge to void is felt. This usually requires approximately 200 to 400 mL of contrast medium in an adult. The contrast medium is instilled under gravity drip from a height of approximately 2 to 3 feet above the tabletop. If there is any history of trauma or reason to suspect a perforation, filling should be monitored either by fluoroscopy or by the use of a radiograph after approximately 25 to 50 mL has been instilled. This will prevent excessive extravasation. With the bladder full, the patient is placed in the right posterior oblique position and a radiograph is obtained during voiding (Fig. 5–20).

Prior to voiding, the catheter is removed in adults. In small children the small-caliber feeding tube used does not need

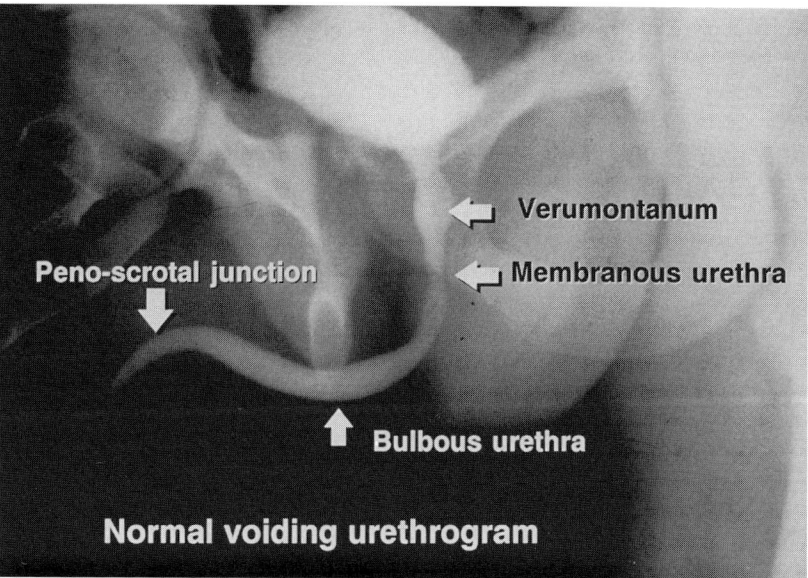

Figure 5–20. Normal voiding urethrogram.

to be removed. If the patient is able to cease voiding voluntarily after exposure of the first radiograph, then a second film can be obtained either in the same projection or in the left posterior oblique. Fluoroscopy with spot filming of the urethra can be used in place of overhead films if the equipment is available. Fluoroscopic monitoring with a limited number of spot films is considered the standard when evaluating young children. This technique allows visualization of the area to be radiographed and is particularly important in children, where overhead films may miss significant portions of the voiding sequence. Fluoroscopy with limited spot films also provides limited radiation. A postvoid film is obtained to access the completeness of emptying.

As with excretory voiding urethrography, this study is most important for evaluation of the posterior urethra. This area is usually well distended with good visualization of the bladder neck and prostatic urethra. With the use of any of the penile clamps greater distention of the anterior urethra can also be obtained. Indications in males, other than reflux, include congenital abnormalities such as suspected urethral valves, postoperative evaluation, suspected stricture (either traumatic or inflammatory), or voiding dysfunction. As with males the VCUG is primarily used in female children to evaluate possible reflux (Fig. 5–21). Urethral abnormalities are less common in females, but this study has had excellent results in evaluating urethral diverticuli (Fig. 5–22).[120,121]

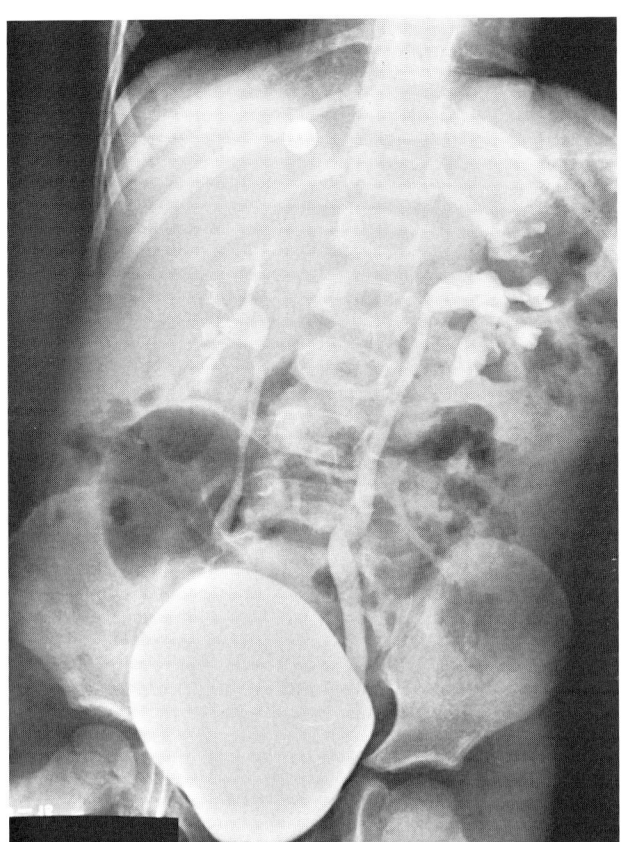

Figure 5–21. VCUG showing bilateral reflux, grade 2 on the right and grade 3 on the left.

Retrograde Urethrography

There are two basic methods of retrograde urethrography, static and dynamic. Static urethrography is performed by retrograde injection of contrast medium into the urethra followed by placement of a penile clamp with radiographs obtained after the injection of contrast has been completed. Contrast generally will be in the anterior urethra but not in the posterior urethra. The degree of urethral filling can vary

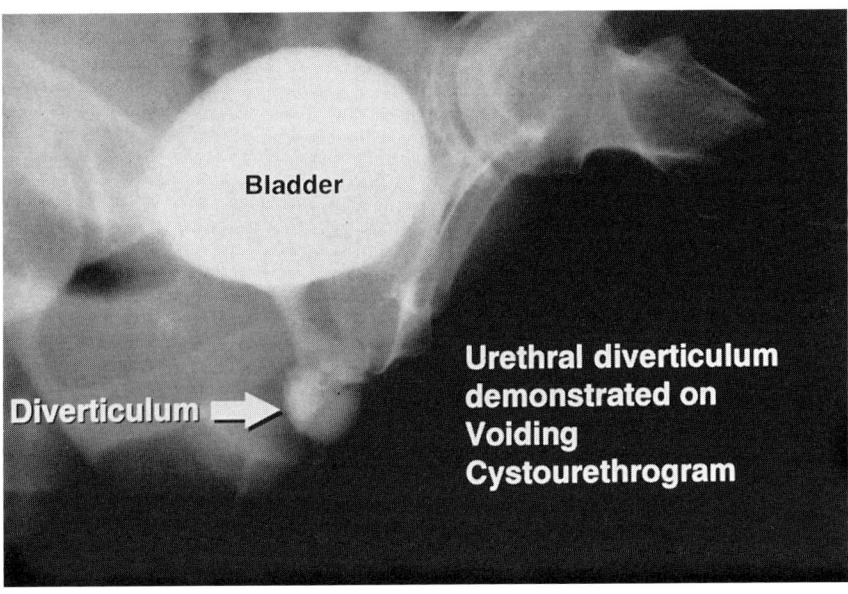

Figure 5–22. VCUG demonstrating a urethral diverticulum (arrow).

and does not provide the information that can be obtained with dynamic retrograde urethrography.[122,123] The dynamic study is performed while contrast is still being injected,[124] producing greater distention of the anterior urethra as well as some visualization, in many cases, of the posterior urethra. Dynamic or ascending retrograde urethrography is often combined with voiding cystourethrography to produce total visualization of both the posterior and anterior urethra.[119,123,125]

Dynamic retrograde urethrography can be performed either with a 50-mL syringe and an adaptor, a Brodney clamp, or a Foley catheter. A Foley catheter (size 8 to 10) offers the advantage of keeping the physician's hand away from the x-ray beam.[119,123–125] One to 2 mL of saline is placed into the Foley balloon with the balloon positioned in the fossa navicularis. With the balloon snugly in the fossa, mild traction can be used to straighten the urethra during the injection. Thirty percent aqueous contrast medium is then injected through the Foley catheter with gentle pressure. No additional materials such as oily or lubricating substances are used. There is always a possibility of extravasation into the venous system, and if this occurs, the safest course is to have used contrast material that is safe to administer intravenously.[126] Mild resistance to flow will occur at the external urethral sphincter, but this can be overcome with gentle pressure. If significant resistance is encountered, the injection is stopped and a radiograph is obtained. With no abnormal resistance, one to three films are obtained during the injection of contrast. It is important that contrast is still being injected when the radiographs are obtained. This distends the bulbous urethra, outlines the "cone" of the normal bulb, and allows some contrast to enter the posterior urethra so that anatomic landmarks can be determined.[123] Films are generally obtained in the right posterior oblique position (Fig. 5–23). If available, fluoroscopy can be used to monitor the injection of contrast and is most important in cases of trauma or other suspected extravasation. Following completion of the retrograde urethrogram the bladder can be filled through the same catheter and voiding cystourethrography obtained as outlined earlier. The combination of these two studies provides excellent visualization of the entire urethra, particularly the region of the membranous urethra.[123,126]

In addition to a Foley catheter or syringe, a 9-cm-long catheter with a flared end to fit over a toomy syringe can be used. The flared end occludes the urethra, although digital pressure is also used. Because of the short catheter, close collimation is necessary to keep the physician's hands out of the x-ray beam.[127]

Another technique uses the patient to inject the contrast. A size 8- to 10-F foley is placed with the balloon at the fossa navicularis and inflated with 1.5 mL of water. The catheter is taped to the glans and attached to a 50-mL syringe. The patient is placed in the posterior oblique position and instructed to inject the contrast slowly. The study is monitored under fluoroscopy. This technique resulted in greater success in filling the posterior urethra and bladder, probably because of decreased patient anxiety and resultant relaxation of the external sphincter. There is no radiation to the radiologist or urologist.[128]

With the current increase in radical prostatectomies, there is an increase in postoperative evaluation of the anastamotic site either by cystography or retrograde urethrography. A simple technique for evaluating the urethra while the Foley is still in place is to use a small sheath-type catheter to inject around the Foley (Fig. 5–24). An 8-F feeding tube gives a good flow rate and keeps the injector's hands further from the x-ray beam than a small sheath-type catheter.[129] Knoll recently described a new device that fits around a Foley catheter and allows contrast to be injected without catheter removal. This comes in two sizes and is thought to give better

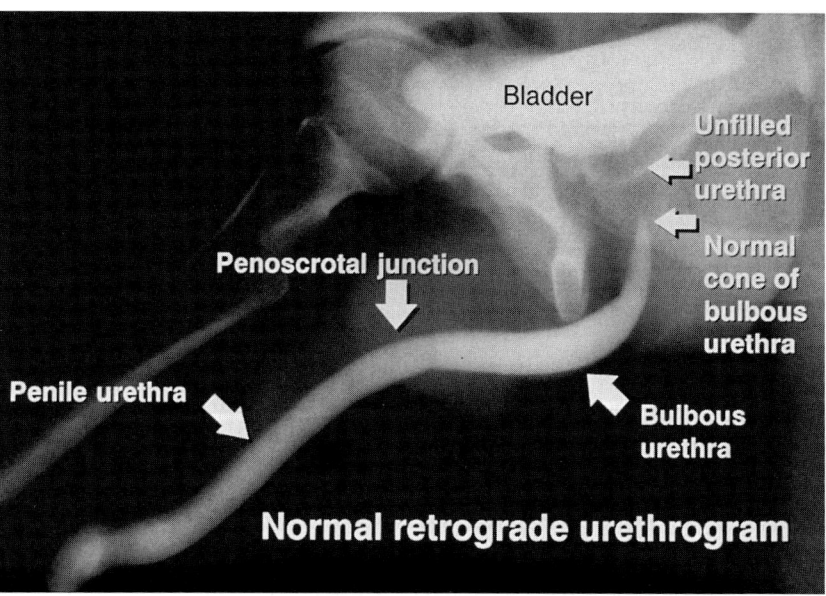

Figure 5–23. Retrograde urethrogram.

Basic Radiologic Techniques for Imaging the Urinary Tract 73

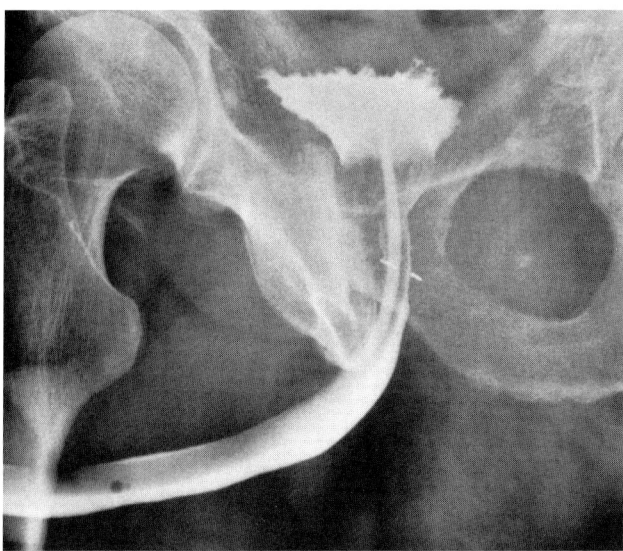

Figure 5–24. Retrograde urethrogram injected around a Foley catheter with a small sheath-type catheter. No extravasation is seen in this postprostatectomy patient. Surgical clips are at the urogenital diaphragm.

visualization of the urethra than the use of small catheters to inject next to the Foley.[130]

NORMAL ANATOMY

Analysis of the anatomy visualized on the voiding and retrograde studies shows the importance of their combined use. The retrograde study (Figs. 5–23, 5–25) distends and fills the anterior urethra with contrast, reaching but not distending the posterior urethra. Sufficient contrast, however, may be present to identify the verumontanum as a "filling defect" (Fig. 5–25). The membranous urethra lies between the verumontanum and the "cone" of the bulbous urethra, which is normally a smoothly tapered conical structure. The bulbar urethra extends from this cone to the penoscrotal junction. From this point to the external meatus is the penile urethra.

The voiding study complements the retrograde examination by distending the posterior urethra and further demonstrates its anatomy. With voiding there is opening of the bladder neck and subsequent filling of the urethra. Both the bladder base and the posterior urethra descend approximately 2 cm during the act of voiding (Fig. 5–20). The bladder neck, verumontanum, membranous urethra, and anterior urethra can all be well visualized. The membranous urethra is the narrowest portion of the urethra and is usually 3 to 4 cm from the bladder neck.

Double Balloon Technique. Retrograde urethrography in the female is uncommonly performed, as most urethral abnormalities will be detected with the VCUG or ultrasound. When necessary, a double balloon technique can be used to demonstrate the urethra. A Trattner catheter is used that has an inner inflatable balloon within the bladder and a second inflatable balloon to press against and occlude the external meatus. Contrast is injected through a separate channel in the catheter, which opens into the urethra and fills this with contrast. AP and oblique radiographs are then obtained.[124,131]

SEMINAL VESICULOGRAPHY (SV)

Seminal vesiculography is an examination that has largely been replaced by other studies, including ultrasound and

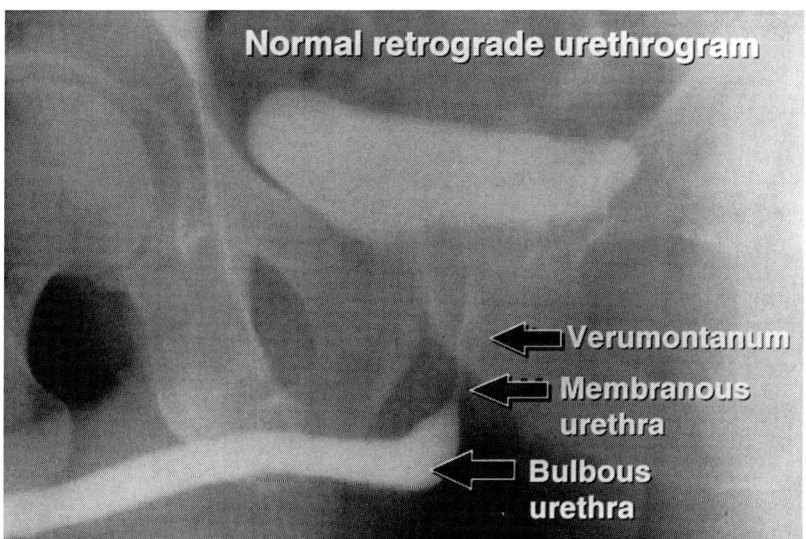

Figure 5–25. Normal retrograde urethrogram. Some contrast reaches the posterior urethra and identifies the verumontanum.

magnetic resonance imaging. In most institutions this is probably performed on a very limited basis, if at all.

Patency of the vas deferens, seminal vesicles, and ejaculatory ducts is the main determination in these cases. The preferred method of SV is direct injection of contrast into the vas deferens through a small scrotal incision. Fifty to 60% iodinated aqueous contrast media is injected through a 23- or 25-gauge needle. Approximately 2 mL is used for each side.[132,133] At the completion of the injection one or more radiographs are obtained. We obtain a coned AP film after completion of the injection. Banner evaluated several views and found an AP view with 30-degree caudal angulation provided the best visualization by projecting the seminal vesicles off the pubic ramus.[133] Measurements of the various structures, however, were obtained from the straight view to limit distortion. Herbert also used a combination of a straight AP view and a radiograph with 30- to 35-degree angulation toward the feet.[132]

Normal Vasogram

The vas deferens is a narrow tube arising from the epididymis and extending 30 to 45 cm.[132] Most have a diameter of approximately 1 mm with a range of 0.5 to 1.5 mm. The distal segment of the vas deferens is called the ampulla. The ampulla can have a variable size, but certain constant relationships have been determined. Most begin at the fundus of the seminal vesicle (Fig. 5–26). Banner found the ampullae to begin within 1.5 cm of the most lateral aspect of the seminal vesicles in all his cases.[133] Most ampullae have a tubular appearance, but they can also be serrated, producing a feathery appearance. This appearance is found in approximately 20% of cases.

The seminal vesicles have a variable appearance. They occasionally appear tubular but usually have many closely spaced convolutions. The seminal vesicles consist of the neck, which continues into the excretory duct; the body, or corpus; and the fundus, which is the most lateral portion (Fig. 5–26). The fundus is almost as wide as the body, which is the widest part, and there is rapid tapering in the region of the neck.[133] Although symmetry of the seminal vesicles was considered one indication of normality, a significant number of normal patients can have asymmetric vesicles in terms of length or width.[132,133]

The ejaculatory duct is formed by the junction of the ampullae of the vas deferens and the most proximal portion of the seminal vesicles, which is called the excretory duct. The ejaculatory duct passes through the prostate and opens on either side of the verumontanum.

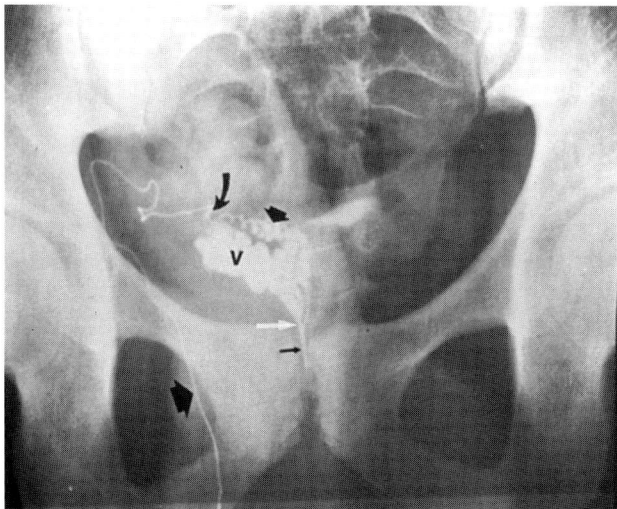

Figure 5–26. Normal vasogram. The tubular-appearing vas deferens (large black arrowhead) follows a midly tortuous course to the lateral aspect of the seminal vesicle (V), where it becomes more dilated and forms the ampulla (small black arrowhead). This junctional point is indicated by the curved black arrow. The normal convoluted appearance of the seminal vesicle is present. A confluence of the duct (white arrow) of the seminal vesicle and the ampulla leads to the ejaculatory duct (small black arrow), which opens on the verumontanum.

REFERENCES

1. Pollack HM, Banner MP: Current status of excretory urography: a premature epitaph? *Urol Clin North Am* 1985; 12(4):585–601.
2. Kumar R, Schreiber MH: The changing indications for excretory urography. *JAMA* 1985;254(3):403–405.
3. Cameron HA, Close CF, Yeo WW, et al: Investigation of selected patients with hypertension by the rapid-sequences intravenous urogram. *Lancet* 1992;339:658–661.
4. Talner LB: Routine urography in men with prostatism. *AJR* 1986;147:960–961.
5. Haddad MC, Sharif HS, Shahed HS, et al: Renal colic: diagnosis and outcome. *Radiology* 1992;184:83–88.
6. Choyke PL: The urogram: are rumors of its death premature? *Radiology* 1992;184:33–36.
7. Burbridge BE, Groot GG, Oleniuk FF, et al: Emergency excretory urography in blunt abdominal trauma. *Journal de l'Association Canadienne des Radiologistes* 1991;42:326–328.
8. Warshauer DM, McCarthy SM, Street L, et al: Detection of renal masses: sensitivities and specificities of excretory urography/linear tomography, US, and CT. *Radiology* 1988; 169:363–365.
9. Ellenbogen PH, Scheible FW, Talner LB, Leopold GR: Sensitivity of gray scale ultrasound in detecting urinary tract obstruction. *Am J Roentgenol* 1978;130:731–733.
10. Scheible W, Talner LB: Gray scale ultrasound and the genitourinary tract: a review of clinical application. *Radiol Clin North Am* 1979;17:281–300.
11. Sanders RC, Conrad MR: The ultrasonic characteristics of the renal pelvicalyceal echo complex. *J Clin Ultrasound* 1977;5:372–377.
12. Hasch E: Ultrasound in the diagnosis of hydronephrosis in infants and children. *J Clin Ultrasound* 1974;2:21–25.
13. Older RA, Korobkin M, Cleeve DM, Schaaf R, Thompson W: Contrast-induced acute renal failure: persistent nephrogram as clue to early detection. *Am J Roentgenol* 1980; 134:339–342.
14. Older RA, Miller JP, Jackson DC, Johnsrude IS, Thompson

WM: Angiographically induced renal failure and its radiographic detection. *Am J Roentgenol* 1976;126:1039–1045.
15. Byrd L, Sherman RL: Radiocontrast-induced acute renal failure: a clinical and pathophysiologic review. *Medicine* 1979; 58:270–279.
16. Krumlovsky FA, Simon N, Santhanam S: Acute renal failure: association with administration of radiographic contrast material. *JAMA* 1978;239:125–127.
17. Ansari Z, Baldwin D: Acute renal failure due to radio-contrast agents. *Nephron* 1976;17:28–40.
18. Alexander RD, Berkes SL, Abuelo JG: Contrast media-induced oliguric renal failure. *Arch Intern Med* 1978;138:381–384.
19. Shafi T, Chou S, Proush JG, Shapiro WB: Infusion intravenous pyelography and renal function: effects in patients with chronic renal insufficiency. *Arch Intern Med* 1978;138:1218–1221.
20. VanZee BE, Hoy WE, Talley TE, Jaenike JR: Renal injury associated with intravenous pyelography in nondiabetic and diabetic patients. *Ann Intern Med* 1978;89:51–54.
21. Barrett BJ, Carlisle EJ: Metaanalysis of the relative nephrotoxicity of high- and low-osmolality iodinated contrast media. *Radiology* 1993;188:171–178.
22. Lautin ME, Freeman NJ, Schoenfeld AH, et al: Radiocontrast-associated renal dysfunction: a comparison of lower-osmolality and conventional high-osmolality contrast media. *AJR* 1991;157:59–65.
23. Gomes AS, Baker JD, Martin-Paredero V, et al: Acute renal dysfunction after major arteriography. *AJR* 1985;145:1249–1253.
24. Hou SH, Bushinsky DA, Wish JB, Cohen JJ, Harrington JT: Hospital-acquired renal insufficiency: a prospective study. *Am J Med* 1983;74:243–248.
25. Wallingford VH: The development of organic iodine compounds as x-ray contrast media. *J Am Pharm Assoc* (Scient Ed) 1953;42:721.
26. Cattell WR, Fry IK, Spencer AG, Purkiss P: Excretion urography. I—Factors determining the excretion of Hypaque. *Br J Radiol* 1967;40:561–571.
27. Miller RE, Skucas J: *Radiographic contrast agents*. Baltimore: University Park Press, 1977;273.
28. Pearson MC, Gilkes R, Hall JH, Boulpec JE, Saxton HM: Sodium or methylglucamine? A comparison of iothalamate in urography. *Br J Radiol* 1974;44:55.
29. Amin MM, Cohan RH, Dunnick NR: Ionic and nonionic contrast media: current status and controversies. *Appl Radiol* 1993;41–54.
30. Dawson P: The physiology and toxicology of low osmology contrast media. *Diagn Imag* 1987; Dec(suppl):3–8.
31. Spataro RF: New and old contrast agents: pharmacology, tissue opacification, and excretory urography. *Urol Radiol* 1988;10:2–5.
32. Dawson P: Intravenous urography revisited. *Br J Urol* 1990; 66:561–567.
33. Dawson P: A new look at intravenous urography. *Australas Radiol* 1988;32:309–312.
34. Dacie JE, Fry IK: A comparison of sodium and methylglucamine diatrizoate in clinical urography. *Br J Radiol* 1971; 44:51.
35. Benness GT: Urographic contrast agents: a comparison of sodium and methyglucamine salts. *Clin Radiol* 1970;21:150.
36. Golman K: Urography: physiological considerations on the excretion of contrast media. *J Belge Radiol-Belg Tijdschr Radiol* 1977;60:229–238.
37. Dray RJ, Winfield AC, Muhletaler CA, Kirchner FK Jr: Advantages of nonionic contrast agents in adult urography. *Urology* 1984;24:297–299.
38. Brennan RE, Curtis JA, Pollack HM, Weinberg I: Sequential changes in the CT numbers of the normal canine kidney following intravenous contrast administration. I: The renal cortex. *Invest Radiol* 1979;14:141–148.
39. Dawson P, Heron C, Marshall J: Intravenous urography with low-osmolality contrast agents: theoretical considerations and clinical findings. *Clin Radiol* 1984;35:173–175.
40. Gavant ML, Ellis JV, Klesges ML: Diagnostic efficacy of excretory urography with low-dose, nonionic contrast media. *Radiology* 1992;182:657–660.
41. Ohlson L: Normal collecting ducts: visualization at urography. *Radiology* 1989;170:33.
42. Lalli AF: Urographic contrast media reactions and anxiety. *Radiology* 1974;112:267.
43. Lalli AF: Contrast media reactions: data analysis and hypothesis. *Radiology* 1980;134:1.
44. Shehadi WH: Adverse reactions to intravascularly administered contrast media: a comprehensive study based on a prospective survey. *Am J Roentgenol* 1975;124:145.
45. Shehadi WH, Toniolo G: Adverse reactions to contrast media. *Radiology* 1980;137:299–302.
46. Hartman GW, Hattery RR, Witten DM, Williamson BW: Mortality during excretory urography: Mayo Clinic experience; *AJR* 1982;139:919–922.
47. Palmer FG: morbidity and mortality with intravenous contrast media: ionic and nonionic. *Invest Radiol* 1990;25(suppl):18–19.
48. Katayama H, Yamaguchi K, Takshima T, Seez P, Matsuura K: Adverse reactions to ionic and nonionic contrast media. *Radiology* 1990;175:621–628.
49. Palmer FJ: The RACR survey of intravenous contrast media reaction: final report. *Australas Radiol* 1988;32:426–428.
50. Wolf GL, Arenson RL, Cross AP: A prospective trial of ionic vs nonionic contrast agents in routine clinical practice: comparison of adverse effects. *AJR* 1989;152:939–944.
51. Caro JJ, Trindade E, McGregor M: The risks of death and of severe nonfatal reactions with high vs low osmolality contrast media: a meta-analysis. *AJR* 1991;156:825–829.
52. Fischer HW, Doust MB: An evaluation of pretesting in the problem of serious and fatal reactions to excretory urography. *Radiology* 1972;103:497–501.
53. Lasser EC, Berry CC, Talner LB, Santini LC, et al: Pretreatment with corticosteroids to elevate reactions to intravenous contrast. *N Engl J Med* 1987;317:845–849.
54. Lasser EC: Pretreatment with corticosteroids to prevent reactions to IV contrast material: overview and implications. *AJR* 1988;150:257–259.
55. Dunnick NR, Cohan RH: Cost, corticosteroids, and contrast media. *AJR* 1994;162:527–529.
56. Lasser EC, Berry CC, Mishkin MM, Williamson B, Zheutlin N, Silverman JM: Pretreatment with corticosteroids to prevent adverse reactions to nonionic contrast media. *AJR* 1994; 162:523–526.
57. Bush WH: Treatment of systemic contrast medium reactions. Syllabus. The Society of Uroradiology, January 1994;160–161. Laguna Niguel, California.
58. Berg GR, Hutter AM, Pfister C: Electrocardiographic changes with intravenous pyelography in healthy individuals. *Urology* 1977;9:88.
59. Kappelman NB, Putman CE, Rosenfield AT, Ulreich S: Electrocardiographic changes with intravenous pyelography in healthy individuals. *Urology* 1977;9:88.
60. Stadalnik RC, et al: Electrocardiographic response to intravenous urography: prospective evaluation of 275 patients. *Am J Roentgenol* 1977;129:825.
61. Pfister RC, Hutter AM: Cardiac alterations drug intravenous urography. Presented in part at the XVI International Con-

ference of Radiology, Symposium on Contrast Media. Rio de Janeiro, Brazil, Oct. 21–29, 1977.
62. Higgins CB, Berber KH, Mattrey RF, Slutsky RS: Evaluation of the hemodynamic effects of intravenous administration of ionic and nonionic contrast materials. *Radiology* 1982; 142:681–686.
63. Miller GM, Wylie EJ, Hinman F Jr: Renal complications from aortography. *Surgery* 1954;35:885.
64. Davidson AJ, Abrams HL, Stamey TA: Renal extraction of PAH in man following abdominal aortography. *Radiology* 1965;85:1043.
65. Wollowick HE, Foster JH, Snyder HE, Younger R, Killen DA: Effect of abdominal aortography on proximal renal tubule function. *J Surg Res* 1966;6:346.
66. Schwab SJ, Hlatky MA, Pieper KS, et al: Contrast nephrotoxicity: a randomized controlled trial of a nonionic and an ionic radiographic contrast agent. *N Engl J Med* 1989; 320:149–153.
67. Moore RD, Steinberg EP, Powe NR, et al: Frequency and determinants of adverse reactions induced by high-osmolality contrast media. *Radiology* 1989;170:727–732.
68. Davidson CJ, Hlatky M, Morris KG, et al: Cardiovascular and renal toxicity of a nonionic radiographic contrast agent after cardiac catheterization. *Ann Intern Med* 1989;110:119–124.
69. Humes HD, Cieslinski DA, Messana JM: Pathogenesis of radiocontrast induced acute renal failure: comparative nephrotoxicity of diatrizoate and iopamidol. *Diagn Imag Suppl* May 1987;12–18.
70. Kinnison ML, Powe NR, Steinberg EP: Results of randomized controlled trials of low-versus-high-osmolality contrast media. *Radiology* 1989;170:381–389.
71. Gomes AS, Lois JF, Baker JD, et al: Acute renal dysfunction in high-risk patients after angiography: comparison of ionic and nonionic contrast media. *Radiology* 1989;170:65–68.
72. Harris KG, Smith TP, Cragg AH, et al: Nephrotoxicity from contrast material in renal insufficiency: ionic versus nonionic agents. *Radiology* 1991;179:849–852.
73. McClennan BL: Syllabus: Categorical course in genitourinary tract radiology. Chicago: Radiology Society of North America, Nov 26–Dec 1, 1978.
74. McClennan B: Urography: anatomy and technique. In: Putman CE, Ravin CE, eds. *Textbook of Diagnostic Imaging*. Philadelphia: WB Saunders, 1988:1161–1168.
75. Kennan RJ, List A, Kengsakul C: Low dose intravenous urography: results and technique modifications. *Aust Radiol* 1990; 34(2):137–141.
76. George CD, Vinnicombe SJ, Balkissoon ARA, Heron CW. Bowel preparation before intravenous urography: is it necessary? *Br J Radiol* 993;66:17–19.
77. Bailey SR, Tyrell PNM, Hale M: A trial to assess the effectiveness of bowel preparation prior to intravenous urography. *Clin Radiol* 1991;44:335–337.
78. Talner LB: Urographic contrast media in uremia: physiology and pharmacology. *Radiol Clin North Am* 1972;10(3):421.
79. Dunbar JS, MacEwan DW, Herbert F: The value of dehydration in intravenous pyelography—an experimental study. *Am J Roentgenol* 1960;84:813.
80. McClennan BL, Becker JA: Excretory urography: choice of contrast material. *Clin Radiol* 1971;100:591.
81. Bell KE, McIlrath EM: Dehydration in urography: is it really necessary? *Clin Radiol* 1985;36:311–312.
82. Hattery RR, Williamson B, Hartman GW, et al: Intravenous urographic technique. *Radiology* 1988;167:593–599.
83. Fry IK, Cattell WR, Spencer AG, Perkiss P: The relation between hypaque excretion and the intravenous urogram. *Br J Radiol* 1967;40:572–580.
84. McClennan BL: Optimal evaluation at intravenous urography. *CRC Crit Rev Radiol Sci* 1971;2:577–594.
85. Older RA, McClelland R, Cleeve DM, Moore AV, Webster GD: Importance of routine vascular nephrotomography in excretory urography. *Urology* 1980;15:312–317.
86. Cattell WR: Excretory pathways for contrast media. *Invest Radiol* 1970;5:473–492.
87. Dure-Smith P: The dose of contrast medium in intravenous urography: a physiologic assessment. *AJR* 1970;108:691–697.
88. Brennan RE, et al: Sequential changes in the CT numbers of the normal canine kidney following intravenous contrast administration II: The renal medulla. *Invest Radiol* 1979; 14:239–245.
89. Hamilton G: The vascular nephrogram phase of excretory urography and its implications. *Radiology* 1974;102:37–40.
90. Gavant ML, Ellis JV, Klesges LM: Maximizing opacification during excretory urography: effect of low-osmolality contrast media. *Can Assoc Radiol J* 1992;43:111–115.
91. Witten DM, Myers GH, Utz DC: *Emmett's Clinical Urography*, Philadelphia: WB Saunders, 1977, Ch. 1.
92. Svendsen P, Wilson J: Adverse reactions during urography and modification by atrophine. *Acta Radiol* 1971;2:427–433.
93. Evans JA, Dubilier W Jr, Monteith JC: Nephrotomogram: preliminary report. *Radiology* 1955;64:655–663.
94. Evans JA: Nephrotomography in investigation of renal masses. *Radiology* (Lond) 1957;23:684–689.
95. Greene LF, Segura JW, Hattery RR, Hartman GW: Routine use of tomography in excretory urography. *J Urol* 1973; 110:714–720.
96. Lloyd LK, Witten DM, Bueschen AJ, Daniel WW: Enhanced detection of asymptomatic renal mass with routine tomography during excretory urography. *Urology* 1978;11:523–528.
97. Zoeller G, May C, Vosshenrich R, et al: Digital radiography in urologic imaging: radiation dose reduction in urethrocystography. *Urol Radiol* 1992;14:56–58.
98. Merritt CR, Tutton RH, Bell KA, et al: Clinical application of digital radiography: computed radiographic imaging. *Radiographics* 1985;5:397–414.
99. Fahardo LL, Hillman BJ, Hunter TB, et al: Excretory urography using computed radiography. *Radiology* 1987; 162:345–351.
100. Fahardo LL, Hillman BJ: Image quality, diagnostic certainty, and accuracy: comparison of conventional and digital urograms. *Urol Radiol* 1988;10:72–74.
101. Cervi PM, Bighi S, Merlo L, et al: Digital radiography versus conventional radiography during excretory urography: our experience. *Ann Radiol* 1990;33:321–328.
102. Siemens Medical Division: *Digital Fluid-Radiography Reference Manual*. Erlanden, Germany: Siemens Marketing Roentgensysteme, 1993.
103. Sane SM, Worsing RA Jr: Voiding cystourethrography: recent advances. *Minnesota Medicine* 1975;58:148–155.
104. McAlister WH, Shackelford GD, Kissane J: The histologic effects of 30% cystokon, hypaque 25%, and renografin-30 in the bladder. *Radiology* 1972;104:563–565.
105. Lipsky H, Chisholm GD: Primary vesico-ureteric reflux in adults. *Br J Urol* 1971;43:277–283.
106. Amar AD, Singer B: Vesicoureteral reflux: a 10 year study of 280 patients. *J Urol* 1973;109:999–1001.
107. Berquist TH, Hattery RR, Hartman GW, Kelalis PP, De Weerd JH: Vesicoureteral reflux in adults. *Am J Roentgenol* 1975;125:314–321.
108. Kern HB, Malament M: Vesico-ureteral reflux and the adult male. *Br J Urol* 1969;41:295–306.
109. McAninch JW, Campbell PM: Primary vesicoureteral reflux in adult patients. *Urology* 1973;2:393–395.

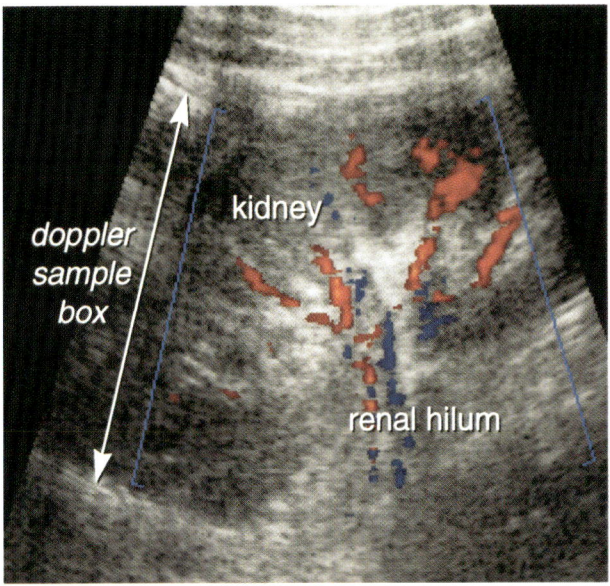

Plate 1. Normal renal vascularity. The vigorous blood supply of the normal kidney permits easy color Doppler visualization of the intrarenal arterial and venous trees.

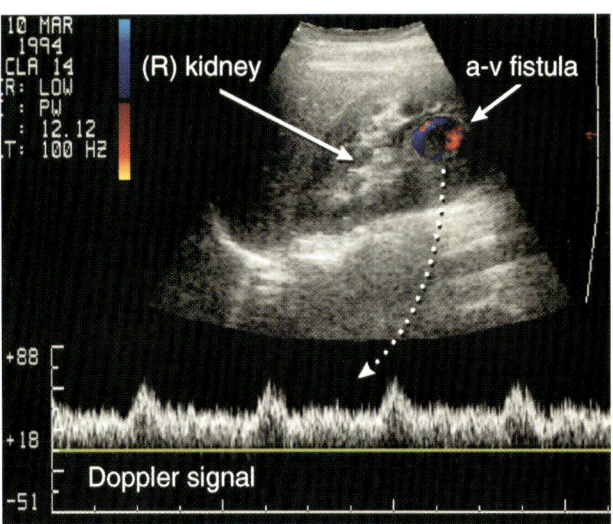

Plate 2. Renal arteriovenous fistula. The Doppler spectral trace at the bottom of this image shows the arterialized nature of the dramatic, biopsy-induced swirl of color in the mid-kidney. Without the benefit of Doppler, this arteriovenous fistula may have been misinterpreted as a parapelvic cyst.

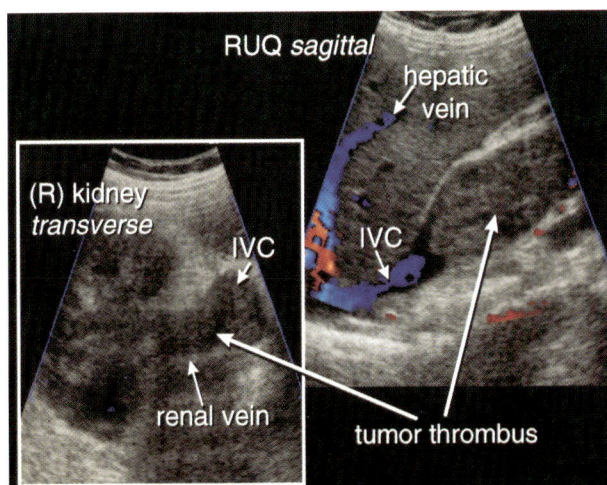

Plate 3. Tumor thrombus in the renal vein and inferior vena cava (IVC). The inset image of a kidney with renal cell cancer shows solid material within an expanded renal vein and IVC. In the main image, a sagittal view in the right upper quadrant (RUQ), color Doppler graphically demonstrates IVC occlusion by thrombus.

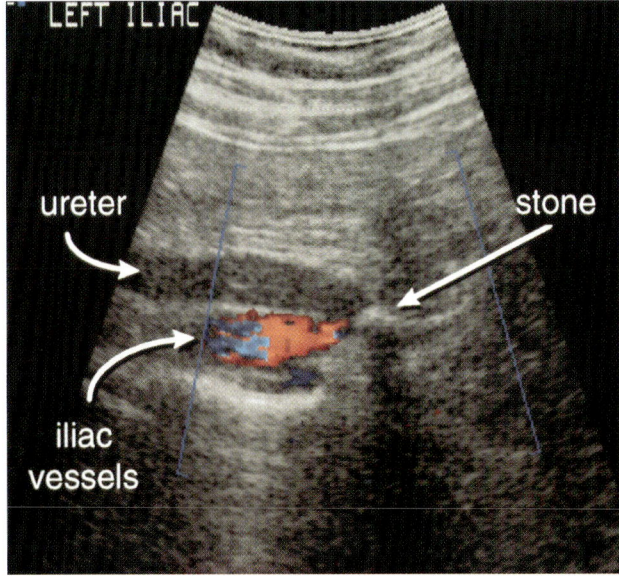

Plate 4. Midureteral stone. A dilated ureter may be followed distally to the point of calculus impaction. In this case, made graphic by the use of color Doppler, a midureteral stone is held up at the crossing point of the iliac vessels.

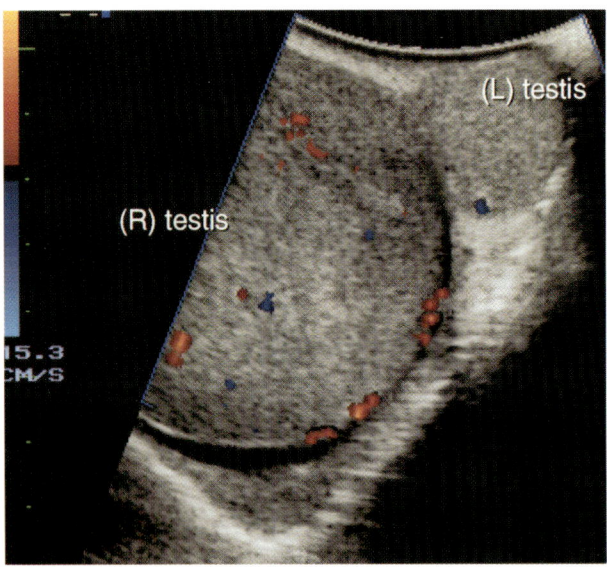

Plate 5. Plasma cell infiltrate. In this example, the right testis exhibits marked but uniform enlargement. There is relative hyperemia on color flow imaging. Lymphoma may give rise to focal abnormality.

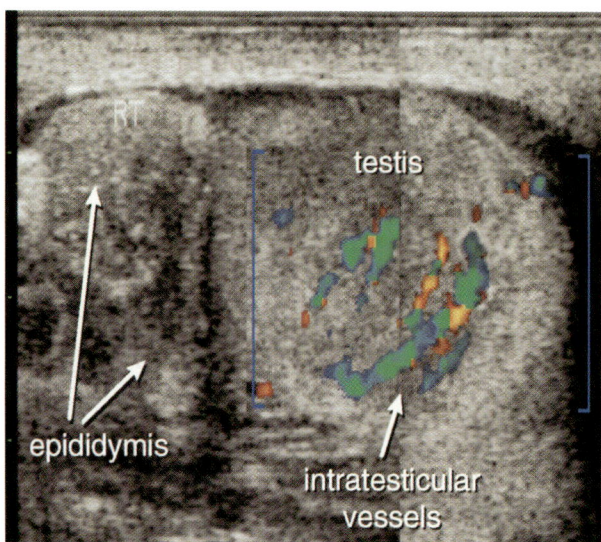

Plate 6. Epididymoorchitis. In this long-axis view through the right hemiscrotum, there are several signs of inflammation: The epididymis appears enlarged, the gray-scale pattern of the testis is mildly disturbed, there is intratesticular hyperemia and a small hydrocele is present.

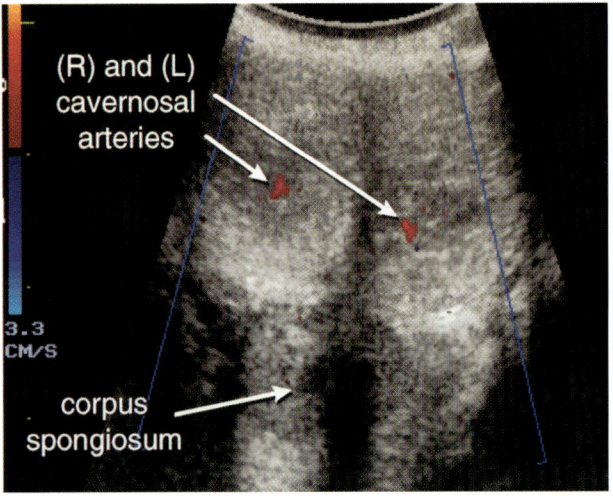

Plate 7. Deep cavernosal arteries. Within each corpus cavernosum runs a centrally located artery. Viewed here in cross section, each artery is readily identified as a centrally located focus of color. Quantitative Doppler measurements are generally made with each cavernosal artery viewed in longitudinal section.

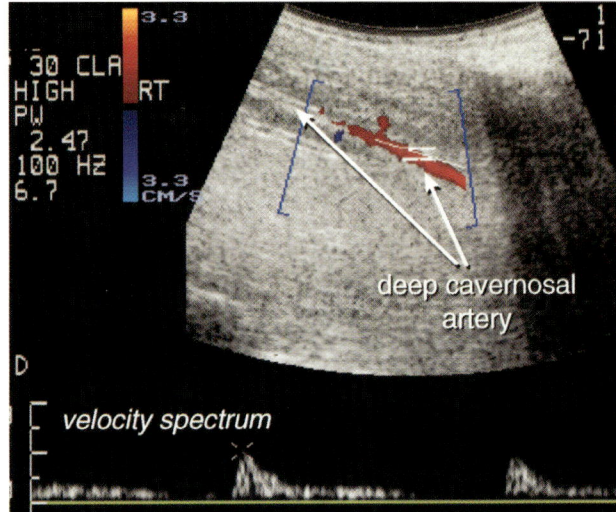

Plate 8. Doppler evaluation of the cavernosal arteries. Seen here in longitudinal section, the cavernosal artery is readily identified with color Doppler. Velocity and spectral analyses are made at a point on the artery at which the beam angle favors a strong Doppler signal.

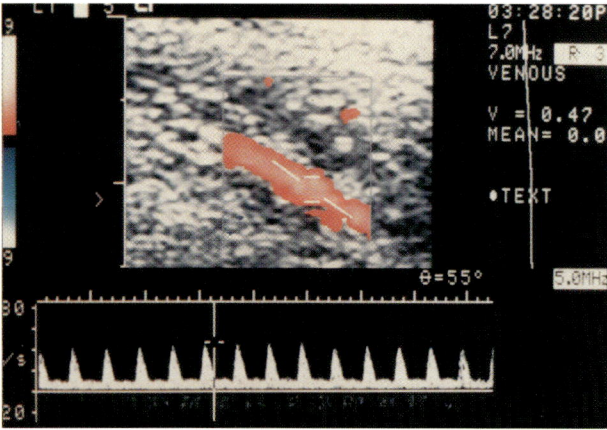

Plate 9. Normal color Doppler examination of the left cavernosal artery showing color flow in the artery with a pulsed Doppler gate positioned over the artery. Normal pulsed Doppler arterial tracing is shown below with peak systolic velocity of 0.47 m/sec.

110. Watsubo KE, et al: Non-obstructive vesicoureteral reflux in adults: value of conservative treatment. *J Urol* 1976;2:566–570.
111. Baker R, et al: Relation of age, sex, and infection to reflux: data indicating high spontaneous cure rate in pediatric patients. *J Urol* 1966;95:27–32.
112. Older RA, et al: Cystography in adults: an assessment of its efficacy. Atlanta, GA: Radiology Society of North America, Nov. 24–30, 1979.
113. Dalton P, Schaeffer AJ, Garnett JE, Grayhack JT: Radiographic assessment of the vesicourethral anastomosis directing early decatheterization following nerve-sparing radical retropubic prostatectomy. *J Urol* 1989;141:79–81.
114. Pearman RO, Miller J: Choke voiding cystourethrography. *J Urol* 1963;90:481–488.
115. Fumerton WR, MacEwan DW: Excretory micturition cystourethrography (EMCU) in the adult age group. *Journal de l'Association Canadienne des Radiologistes* 1970;21:90–97.
116. Fitts FB Jr, Herbert SG, Mellins HZ: Criteria for examination of the urethra during excretory urography. *Radiology* 1977;125:47–53.
117. Boltuch RL, Lalli AF: A new technique for urethrography. *Radiology* 1975;115:736.
118. Fitts FB Jr, Mascatello VG, Mellins HZ: The value of compression during excretion voiding urethrography. *Radiology* 1977;125:53–56.
119. Brooks V, Bateson EM: Cysto-urethrography in the University Hospital of the West Indies. *Clin Radiol* 1968;19:278–286.
120. Summit RL Jr, Stovall TG: Urethral diverticula: Evaluation by urethral pressure profilometry, Cystourethroscopy and the voiding cystourethrogram. *Obstet Gynecol* 1992;80:695–9.
121. Leach GE, Bavendam TM: Female urethral diverticula. *Urology* 1987;30:407–415.
122. McCallum RW, Colapinto V: *Urologic Radiology of the Adult Male Lower Urinary Tract*. Springfield, IL: Charles C. Thomas, 1976;37.
123. McCallum RW: The adult male urethra: normal anatomy, pathology, and method of urethrography. *Radiol Clin North Am* 1979;17(2):227.
124. Yoder IC, Papanicolaou N: Imaging the urethra in men and women. *Urol Radiol* 1992;14:24–28.
125. McCallum RW, Colapinto V: The role of urethrography in urethral disease. Part I: Accurate radiological localization of the membranous urethra and distal sphincters in normal male subjects. *J Urol* 1979;122:607–611.
126. McClennan BL, Becker JA, Robinson T: Venous extravasation at retrograde urethrography: precautions. *J Urol* 1971;106:412–413.
127. McLellan GL, Turetsky DB, Swartz DA: New catheter for retrograde urethrography. *Urology* 1991;37:582–583.
128. Kirshy DM, Pollack AH, Becker JA, Horowitz M: Auto-urethrography. *Radiology* 1991;180:443–445.
129. Brown RC, Thompson BH, Williams RD, et al: Two new uses of 8-F feeding tube in performing injecting urethrograms. *Urology* 1991;37:347–349.
130. Knoll LD, Furlow WL, Karsburg W: Pericatheter retrograde urethrography: introduction of a new device and technique. *J Urol* 1989;142:1533–1535.
131. Greenberg M, Stone D, Cochran ST, et al: Female urethral diverticula: double-balloon catheter study. *AJR* 1981;136:259–264.
132. Hebert G, Bouschard R, Charron J: Vasoseminal vesiculography. *AJR* 1971;113:735–740.
133. Banner MP, Hassier R: The normal seminal vesiculogram. *Radiology* 1978;128:339–344.

6 Ultrasound of the Genitourinary Tract

William Horstman, Laurence Watson

Ultrasound (US) has become a common imaging procedure for many types of genitourinary (GU) disorders. Initially, its major role was to detect urinary obstruction and to determine if a renal mass was cystic or solid. As the technology improved, its usefulness increased, especially in the evaluation of the female pelvis and the scrotum. With the development of pulsed Doppler ultrasound and even more recently color Doppler ultrasound (CDU), blood flow evaluation is now easily performed. Technological advances continue to improve the resolution, and all other aspects of US imaging,[1] keeping it on the forefront of GU diagnosis.

INSTRUMENTATION AND TECHNIQUES

Ultrasonic waves are generated by piezoelectric crystals that are most commonly made of a thin sheet of lead zirconate titanate. When the crystal is subjected to an electric pulse, the crystal changes shape and begins to vibrate. This vibration causes the generation of an ultrasonic wave that is directed into the patient by the transducer housing. After the initial burst of sound energy, the transducer housing damps the vibrations to allow the crystal to receive the returning sound waves during its listening phase. The returning sound waves cause the crystal to deform, which generates a very subtle electric voltage. This voltage is electronically amplified and is modified into the signal that is displayed on the monitor. The US unit determines the depth of the structure being imaged by the length of time it takes for the reflected sound wave to reach the transducer. The deeper the structure, the longer it takes the reflected sound wave to return to the transducer. The thickness of the crystal determines the frequency at which the crystal resonates. A thicker crystal has a lower resonance frequency, which generates a lower-frequency ultrasonic wave. Higher-frequency transducers have the advantage of giving better resolution, especially in the shallow areas near the transducer surface, called the "near field." The higher-frequency transducers have the disadvantage of decreased tissue penetration, and they cannot effectively image deeper structures, since the sound energy is rapidly absorbed in the superficial tissues. Generally, it is best to use as high a frequency as possible to image the desired structures. For most applications a 3- or 5-MHz transducer is used. Evaluation of the scrotum is generally performed with a 7.5- or 10-MHz transducer.

The commonly used transducers are divided into linear and sector formats. Linear transducers emit ultrasonic waves from a linear crystal face. This format gives better resolution in the "near field" and is useful for imaging shallow objects, but it decreases the depth of penetration of the sound energy. Linear transducers are mainly used to image the scrotum and other shallow objects. The sector format emits sound waves in a triangular-shaped region from a smaller crystal face. These transducers are useful for imaging deeper objects, such as the kidneys. Modern transducers also can be focused at certain depths, which increases the resolution at that depth but decreases the resolution in the region outside the point of focus.

Doppler US is a recently developed imaging technique that allows the display of real-time images, along with blood flow assessment. Doppler imaging is based on the Doppler effect, which changes the frequency of the sound wave reflected off a moving object. Sound waves reflected off an object [usually a red blood cell (RBC)] moving toward the transducer will increase in frequency, whereas those reflected off an RBC moving away from the transducer will have a lower frequency. The magnitude of the frequency difference between the transmitted sound wave and the reflected sound wave is the *Doppler shift*, and this change in frequency can be quantified. The Doppler shift frequency is usually within the frequencies detectable to the human ear; this frequency can be amplified, giving rise to the familiar audible signal produced by Doppler equipment. Continuous wave Doppler has been used for many years to detect faint pulses and to detect fetal heart motion. Pulsed wave Doppler is used in ultrasound imaging. Pulses of sound energy are transmitted into the patient, and the transducer listens for the returning echoes when it is not transmitting sound. The transmitter listens for the Doppler shift only during a certain time interval after emitting the sound wave and determines the depth of the object being imaged by the amount of time it takes for the reflected wave with the Doppler shift to return. Combining this depth sensitivity with real-time images allows the examiner to evaluate the blood flow in selected small areas (such as a blood vessel seen on real-time images).

Ultrasound imaging is carried out in real time, with the examiner evaluating a constantly changing image on the video screen. The screen produces a series of static images that change faster then the eye can perceive them, thus giving the appearance of smooth real-time motion. A flicker-free image requires a frame rate of greater than 16 frames per second. The real-time image is the key to a good ultrasound examination and is the reason ultrasound is very operator dependent. If the sonographer does not recognize an abnormality during a real-time examination, he or she will not make an image of the abnormality, and significant pathology will be missed.

NORMAL ANATOMY

The adrenal glands are paired organs that lie within the retroperitoneum adjacent to the kidney. The right gland generally is located superior and medial to the kidney, and a portion lies adjacent to and behind the inferior vena cava (IVC). The left adrenal gland lies anterior and medial to the upper pole of the left kidney. Unlike the right adrenal, the left adrenal usually does not extend above the upper pole of the left kidney and in some cases it extends inferior to the left renal hilum. The left adrenal is bordered anteriorly by the tail of the pancreas, splenic vein, and lesser sac. Both right and left adrenal lie within the perirenal fascia. In neonates and children the adrenals are usually well visualized.[2] Nomograms of the normal adrenal size have been developed beginning in the fetus and neonate. The normal neonate's adrenal demonstrates a prominent hypoechoic cortex and a thinner hyperechoic medulla.[3] During the first weeks of life the cortex becomes less prominent and smaller. The adrenal size decreases by up to 60% in the first week of life in a normal infant. The differentiation between cortex and medulla also becomes much less prominent.[4]

The normal kidney measures 9 to 12 cm in length, although there is significant variability, and the length generally depends on the size of the patient. The renal cortex is generally smooth, and the cortical thickness is uniform except for slightly increased thickness in the polar regions (Fig. 6–1). The renal cortex is usually homogeneous and hypoechoic. In most patients the renal cortex is less echogenic then the liver or spleen. The adult renal cortex can also be isoechoic to liver, and still be normal.[5] The renal sinus is very echogenic, mainly due to the sinus fat. The intrarenal portion of the renal pelvis is generally not seen, although this is extremely variable. Patients with an extrarenal pelvis can have a large renal pelvis with the intrarenal portion easily visualized within the renal sinus. The size of the renal pelvis also depends on the patient's state of hydration and degree of bladder filling. The medullary pyramids are small, rounded, hypoechoic structures adjacent to the renal sinus. They are more prominent in neonates, and because of the surrounding anechoic urine the pyramids can occasionally be well visualized in patients with hydronephrosis.[6]

The ureters are muscular tubes that transport urine from the kidneys to the bladder. They arise from the renal pelvis posterior to the main renal vessels, and travel in the retroperitoneum along the psoas muscles into the pelvis. The middle portions of the ureters are almost never sonographically

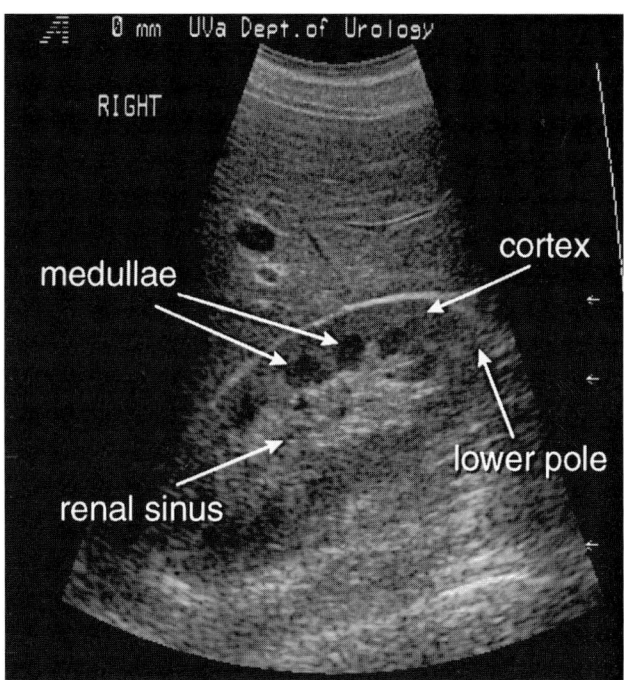

Figure 6–1. Normal kidney. With good renal access, the medullae are well differentiated from the cortex. The renal sinus appears hyperechoic. The echogenicity of the cortex is slightly less than that of liver or spleen.

visible. They empty into the bladder at the level of the trigone. The ureters actually enter the bladder wall higher and more laterally, and travel in an intramural tunnel prior to the ureteral orifice. Ureteral jets are a common occurrence and represent reflections from the fluid–fluid interface of a jet of urine entering the bladder.[7] Ureteral jets are best seen with CDU, when the urine emptying into the bladder has a different specific gravity from the urine already in the bladder. A partially filled bladder and a well-hydrated patient also make visualization easier.[8]

The bladder is a muscular organ that stores urine prior to voiding. Normally, the bladder has a smooth, thin wall, which is thicker when it is empty.[9] The wall should be no more than 3 mm thick when full and 5 mm thick when empty. The anterior wall of the bladder is usually difficult to visualize because of the ring down artifact. This can give the appearance of debris in the bladder. Visualization of the anterior wall can be improved by using a linear high-frequency transducer, which improves evaluation of objects in the near field. The position of the trigone, interureteric ridge, and ureteral orifices can usually be distinguished with gray scale, but the position is better demonstrated by using CDU to visualize the ureteral jets.[8] The internal urethral orifice can also be demonstrated in most patients.

NORMAL RENAL DOPPLER ULTRASOUND

The distal renal vessels that course through the renal hila are usually visualized on transverse views. Pulsed Doppler and

Ultrasound of the Genitourinary Tract   81

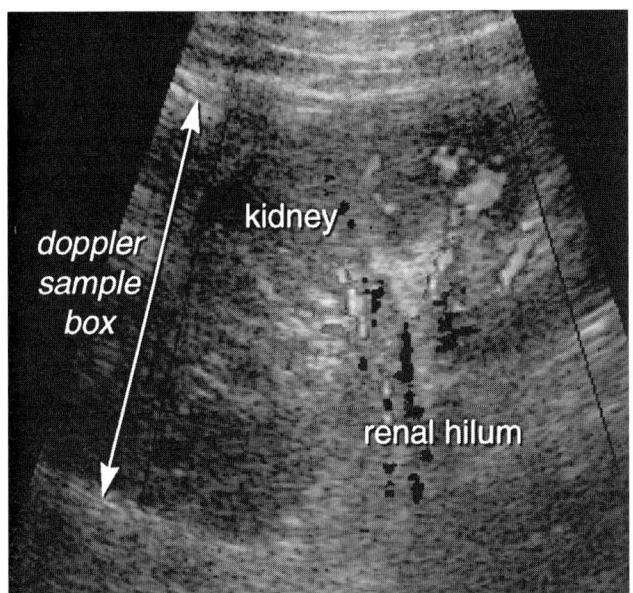

Figure 6–2. Normal renal vascularity. The vigorous blood supply of the normal kidney permits easy color Doppler visualization of the intrarenal arterial and venous trees. (See Plate 1)

multiple renal arteries are present. CDU makes examination of renal vasculature much easier, since smaller vessels not seen with gray scale sonography will be demonstrated with CDU. Normal arterial waveforms show low impedance flow, with a large amount of continuous forward diastolic flow. The resistance to flow is generally measured by the resistive index (RI). RI is peak systolic velocity minus end diastolic velocity divided by peak systolic velocity.[10,11] The normal RI of the renal vessels is less than 0.7, with most being approximately 0.6. Normally, the RIs of the two kidneys are within 0.1 of each other.[11] Another commonly used measurement is the pulsatility index, which is peak systolic frequency minus end diastolic frequency divided by the mean frequency.

CDU greatly improve the visualization and characterization of the renal vessels (Fig. 6–2). Occasionally, prominent renal vessels will be seen in the renal sinus that simulate mild hydronephrosis. CDU will quickly reveal the nature of these hypoechoic structures. Portions of both renal veins and arteries can usually be visualized, but in most cases the entire course of these vessels cannot be examined because of overlying bowel gas.[10] It is often very difficult to visualize the aortic origin of the renal arteries where much atherosclerotic disease occurs. It is also difficult to determine if

ADRENAL GLANDS

Computed tomography (CT) is the best modality for evaluating the adult adrenal gland, with magnetic resonance imaging (MRI) also being used more frequently.[12] In neonates and children US can often evaluate the adrenal glands better then CT, because of the lack of fat in the retroperitoneum.

Reports of discovery of prenatal neuroblastoma exist in the literature. The nature of the lesion is suggested by the location.[13] In the child adrenal hemorrhage, neuroblastoma, pheochromocytoma, and adrenal cortical carcinoma can present as mass lesions. Neonatal adrenal hemorrhage is seen as unilateral or bilateral enlargement of the adrenal glands (Fig. 6–3). Soon after the hemorrhage the adrenal gland is often homogeneously hyperechoic.[14] As the blood liquefies it becomes less echogenic. Eventually, the lesion will appear cystic and can demonstrate septations and internal debris.[15]

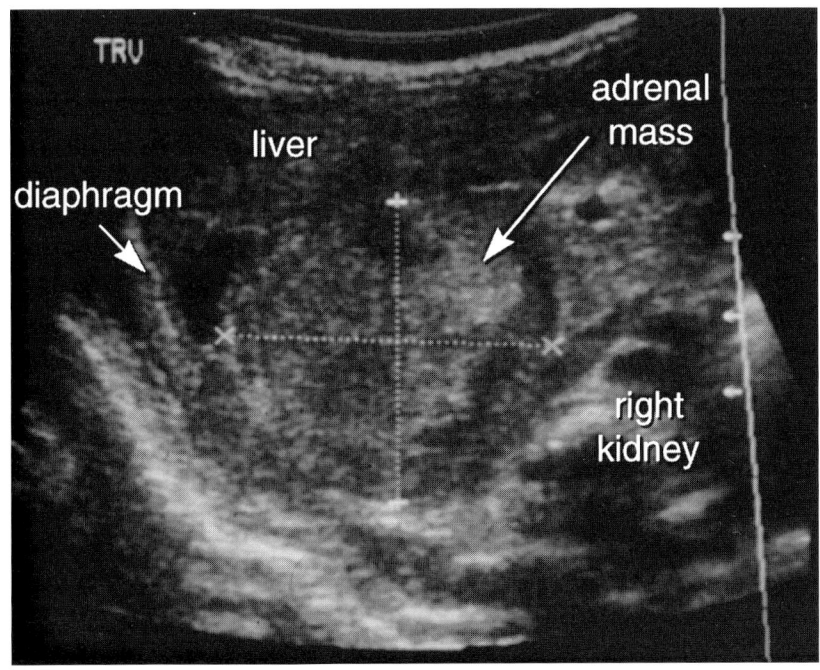

Figure 6–3. Neonatal adrenal hemorrhage. In this sagittal view of a relatively acute hemorrhage, the adrenal has enlarged to about the same size as the kidney. The adrenal appears quite echogenic, with little apparent organization of the hematoma.

Coarse calcifications often develop later. Neuroblastoma is the most common adrenal lesion in the neonate and infant, and most originate in the adrenal gland. The US appearance is nonspecific, except for the location of the lesion, which suggests the diagnosis. Many times the lesion will demonstrate sonographically visible calcifications and will encase the aorta and IVC, and cross the midline. Differentiating a neuroblastoma from a large exophytic Wilms' tumor can occasionally be difficult. Differentiating a pheochromocytoma, adrenal cortical carcinoma, or lymphoma of the adrenal gland cannot be done by US criteria and is best done clinically.

Adult adrenal glands are difficult to visualize, but good sensitivity for detecting adrenal masses has been demonstrated.[16,17] Differential diagnosis of an adult adrenal mass includes adrenal adenoma, metastasis, myelolipoma, lymphoma, pheochromocytoma, and adrenal cortical carcinoma. The ultrasound appearance is nonspecific in all these cases. Myelolipomas tend to be hyperechoic because of the fat content.[18] Most adrenal cortical carcinomas present as huge lesions. Pheochromocytomas usually cause typical symptoms and can be suggested by clinical criteria. Adenomas are usually less than 3 cm; however, they can become larger.[19,20] Metastasis and lymphomas usually occur in patients with known primary lesions. CT is used most commonly to evaluate an adrenal mass and to guide biopsy.[21] MRI has shown promise of being more specific in the diagnosis of pheochromocytoma and adenomas. CT or MRI will generally demonstrate the fat in a myelolipoma.

KIDNEYS

Normal Variants

The renal cortex can have a wavy appearance due to fetal lobation. The cortex should still have symmetric thickness, with the exception of small external indentations. A column of Bertin is a localized cortical thickening that projects into the renal sinus at the junction of the upper one-third and lower two-thirds of the kidney. A junctional parenchyma defect is often associated with a column of Bertin or can be seen without a column of Bertin. This is an echogenic defect in the cortical margin that can extend into the renal sinus (Fig. 6–4). Both the column of Bertin and the junction parenchyma defect are thought to be residua of the renunculi that joined to form the metanephros in fetal life.[22] The column of Bertin should also be isoechoic with the rest of the cortex and not cause a mass effect on the renal sinus; commonly, it has a medullary pyramid associated with the cortical tissue.[23,24]

URINARY OBSTRUCTION

Ultrasound is very sensitive in diagnosing obstruction by demonstrating hydronephrosis. Unfortunately, it is not very specific because previous obstruction, reflux nephropathy, overdistention of the bladder, papillary necrosis, renal sinus cysts, congenital megacalicosis, diabetes insipidus, and even

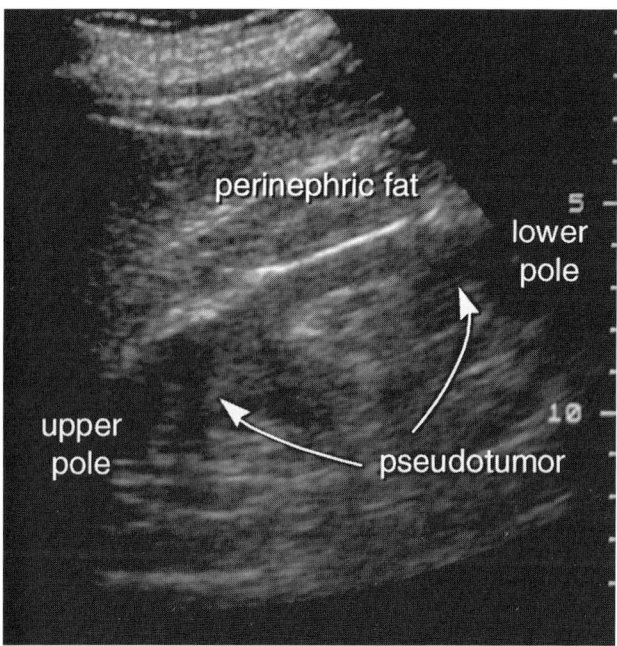

Figure 6–4. Hypertrophied column of Bertin. This anatomic variant gives rise to the commonly encountered renal pseudotumor effect. The keys to correct diagnosis are experience and the basic sonographic normality of the architecture.

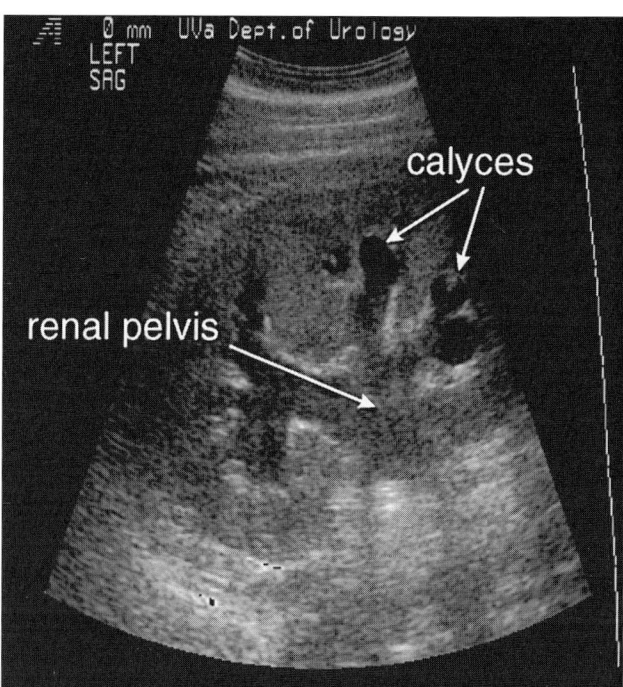

Figure 6–5. Mild hydronephrosis. The renal pelvis and calyceal system become apparent as the collecting system distends with urine. On this image, a papilla is just discernible in a lower pole calyx.

brisk diuresis can cause collecting system dilation without obstruction.[25,26]

Hydronephrosis is graded as mild (grade 1), moderate (grade 2), or severe (grade 3).[27] Mild cases demonstrate minimal separation of the central sinus echo complex by tubular anechoic urine-filled renal pelvis and calyces (Fig. 6–5). Mild hydronephrosis can be simulated by prominent renal vessels, but with prominent vessels CDU will demonstrate flow in the tubular structures. Moderate hydronephrosis is diagnosed when there is definite anechoic separation of the entire renal sinus, which is easily seen to extend into the calyces. Severe hydronephrosis involves marked dilation of the collecting system with parenchymal thinning (Fig. 6–6).[27]

False-positive studies for obstruction are common in patients suspected of having mild hydronephrosis. In fact, false-positives occur in up to 25% of ultrasound examinations that have evidence of hydronephrosis. Most false-positives are in patients diagnosed with mild hydronephrosis, where up to 50% of cases may be normal.[28] Voiding can occasionally cause mild separation of the central sinus echoes to resolve as the collecting system is decompressed. Doppler (or CDU) will distinguish prominent renal vessels from a mildly dilated collecting system. Patients with US findings of moderate or severe hydronephrosis are much more likely to have obstruction, but false-positive studies still do occur. Comparison with old ultrasounds is always helpful. Increased or new hydronephrosis makes the diagnosis of obstruction much more likely. When hydronephrosis is seen, every effort should be made to determine the level of obstruction. Proximal and distal obstructing lesions will often be visualized, whereas obstruction in the midureter is difficult to delineate.

False-negative ultrasounds in patients with obstruction are uncommon, occurring in approximately 1% of cases. Usually this occurs early in the course of obstruction, before the renal collecting system has become dilated.[29,30] Occasionally, forniceal rupture will decompress the collecting system, or the urinary output will be low, and dilation will not occur. Other uncommon false-negatives occur in patients with retroperitoneal fibrosis, where the ureter and renal pelvis are encased and cannot become distended.

Doppler ultrasound has been suggested as a means to separate obstructive from nonobstructive hydronephrosis. Some investigators have demonstrated up to 92% sensitivity and 88% specificity by measuring renal arterial RI.[11,31,32] The resistance to blood flow in the kidney increases when the patient becomes obstructed, causing an increased RI (Fig. 6–7). The RI normally is less then 0.7, but in obstructed kidneys it usually increases above this level. Additionally, there will be a difference of more than 0.1 in the RI between the obstructed and the contralateral nonobstructed kidney.[11,31,32] The RI increases in many pathologic processes, but in the correct clinical situation in which the ultrasound demonstrates hydronephrosis the elevation of the RI may help separate obstructive from nonobstructive hydronephrosis.[33] Other centers have not shown comparable accuracy, and definitive evaluation will require further study. The RI may take some time to become elevated, and if the scan is performed early in the course of obstruction, the RI may not have increased. In that case serial ultrasounds may show the increasing RI along with increasing hydronephrosis.

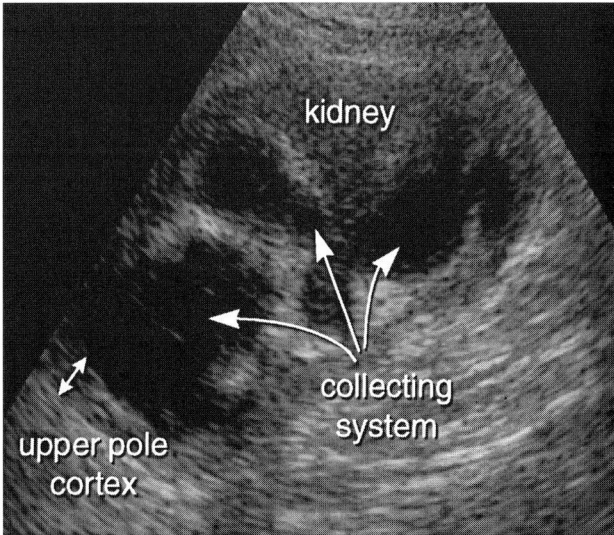

Figure 6–6. Chronic hydronephrosis. This condition is characterized by moderate or severe distention of the collecting system, with thinning of the cortical parenchyma.

Evaluation of ureteral jets has also been suggested to help diagnose obstruction. Ureteral jets occur normally in the bladder and are best demonstrated with CDU. The jet is caused by color being assigned to the moving urinary stream as it exits the ureteral orifice into the bladder. Studies have shown that ureteral jets are normally seen in the bladder, but they are not seen or are decreased in patients with high-grade obstruction. Patients with low-grade partial obstruction will usually have normal ureteral jets.[8]

Ureteropelvic Junction Obstruction

The ureteropelvic junction (UPJ) obstruction is a relatively common congenital anomaly with a variable presentation. Most severe cases will present in childhood as a palpable abdominal mass; however, less severe cases are often not diagnosed until adulthood. Most adults will complain of intermittent flank pain. The US findings include a dilated renal pelvis that ends abruptly at the UPJ (Fig. 6–8). The ureter distal to the UPJ is collapsed and not visible. The amount of residual renal parenchyma will be variable and depends on the degree of obstruction. In some cases the parenchymal thickness will be near normal, and in others no discernible parenchyma will remain.

Hydronephrosis of Pregnancy

Sixty to 80% of pregnant patients will develop hydronephrosis on the right, and 30% have hydronephrosis on the

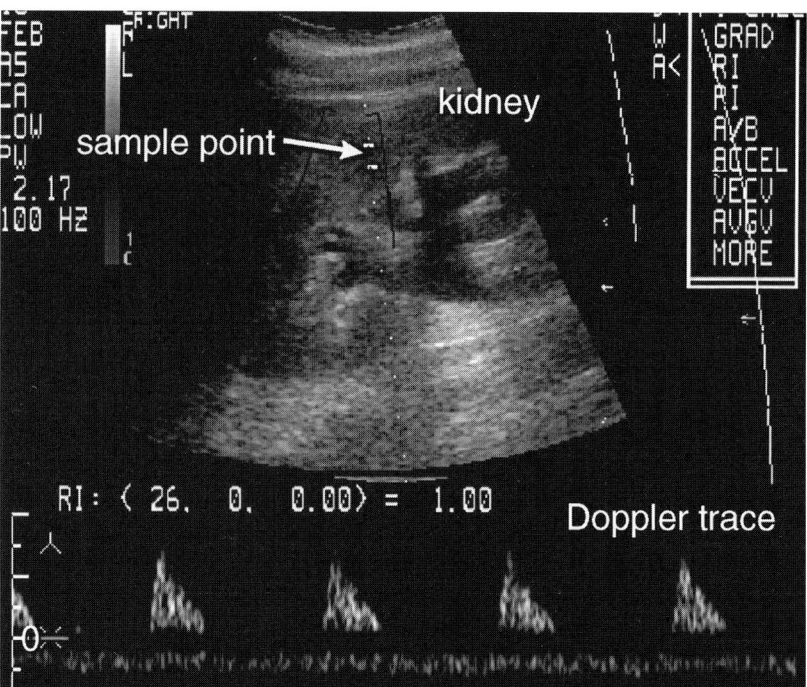

Figure 6–7. Hydronephrosis and arterial resistive index. A Doppler signal is sampled from an intrarenal artery. Resistive index is derived from the values of the peak systolic and end-diastolic velocities. In this case of mild hydronephrosis, vascular resistance is very high, giving rise to a positive result.

left.[34] The dilation begins late in the first trimester and usually plateaus at 24 to 28 weeks. The dilation usually resolves by 6 to 8 weeks postpartum.[34] Differentiating normal hydronephrosis of pregnancy from obstruction can be clinically and sonographically difficult. The right side is normally dilated earlier and more significantly than the left. If the left is more dilated, an obstructing lesion such as stone should be suspected. A recent study demonstrated that the RIs of the kidneys in pregnant patients were less then 0.7 and symmetric, even if the right side was significantly more dilated than the left. Further study to determine if Doppler will be helpful in pregnant patients is needed.[35]

Renal Stone Disease

Plain radiography, renal tomography, and intravenous urography remain the methods of choice in evaluating patients with suspected urolithiasis.[36] US demonstrates stones as an

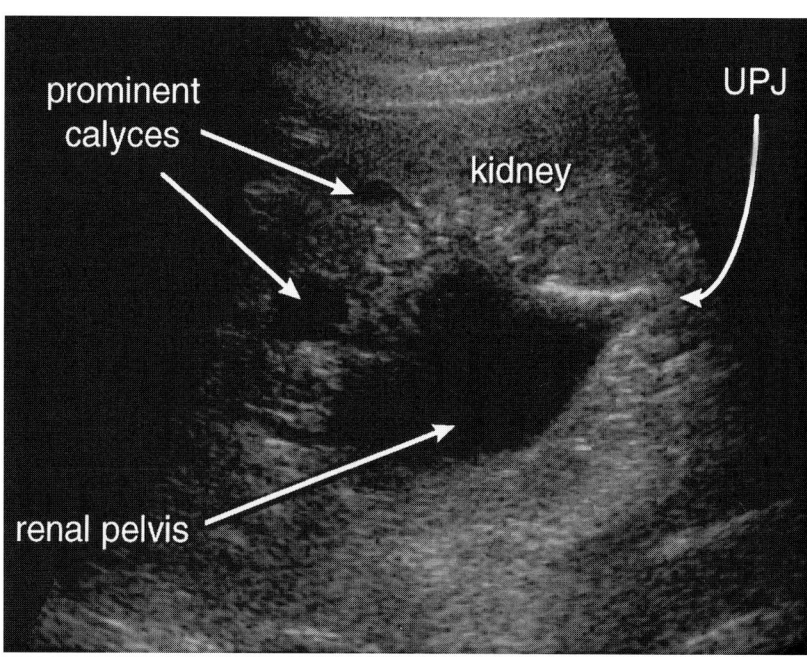

Figure 6–8. Congenital ureteropelvic junction obstruction. In this case of mild UPJ obstruction, a capacious renal pelvis gives off slightly dilated calyces. The collecting system distention ends abruptly at the UPJ.

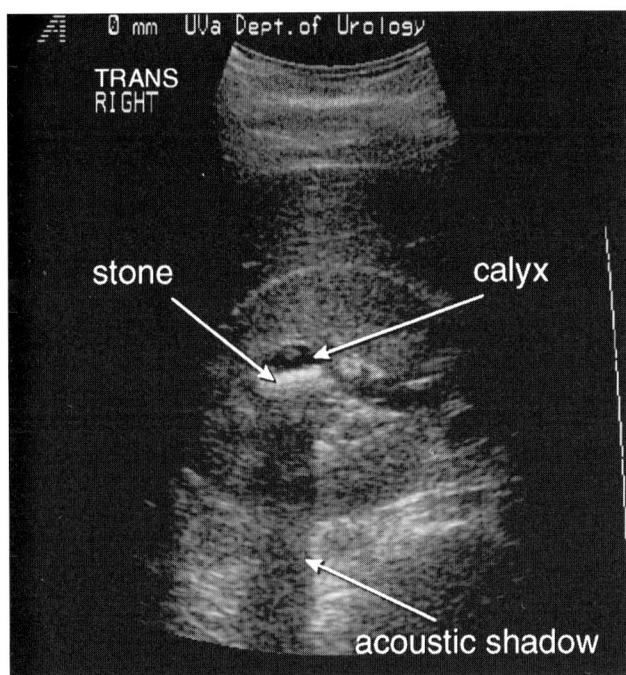

Figure 6–9. Kidney stone. The stone appears hyperechoic and casts a discrete acoustic shadow. In this view, there is some distention of the associated calyx.

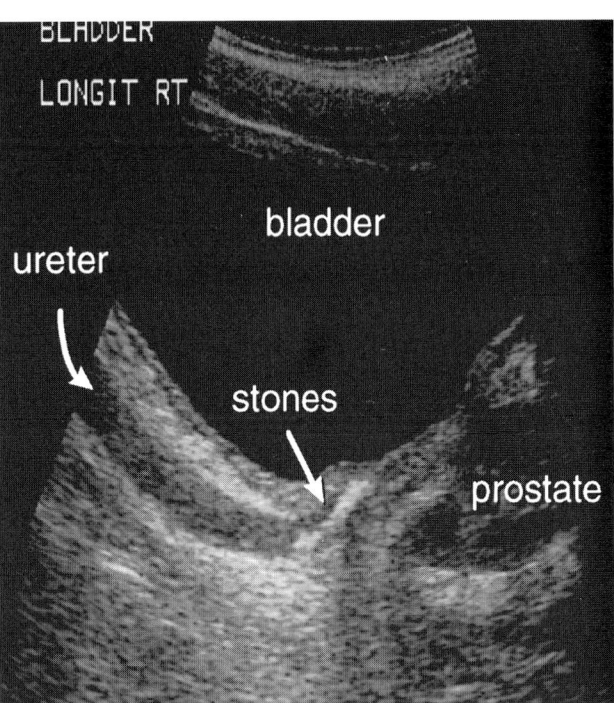

Figure 6–10. Distal ureteral stone. After lithotripsy, a small steinstrasse has formed in the distal ureter at the ureterovesical junction. The upstream ureter is distended.

echogenic focus with distal acoustic shadowing (Fig. 6–9). Multiple interfaces with vessels and fat in the normal renal sinus often cause echogenic structures, but these should not cast an acoustic shadow. Recent studies have demonstrated approximately 80% sensitivity to detecting stones.[37,38] US can detect noncalcified stones that cannot be seen on plain abdominal radiographs. The composition of the stone has no effect on the US appearance.[39] US sensitivity depends mainly on the size of the stone and the patient's body habitus. Renal vascular calcifications can simulate stones. Haddad et al recently reported that US combined with plain radiography may be able to replace intravenous urography in the evaluation of patients with suspected urolithiasis. US will document hydronephrosis, and the plain film can be used to evaluate and follow a suspected stone.[40] US can also visualize the stone in many cases, especially those calculi lodged at the UPJ or at the ureterovesical junction (UVJ) (Fig. 6–10). The bladder and the region of the UVJ should be evaluated in every patient with suspected obstruction. Transvaginal ultrasound can also be helpful in evaluating this portion of the ureter. The dilated distal ureter will often be seen terminating at an echogenic stone.[38] A well-distended urinary bladder is needed as a sonic window.

Staghorn calculi will be demonstrated as multiple highly echogenic structures in the expected position of the calyces. The posterior shadowing will often mask the hydronephrosis that occurs in these patients.

Nephrocalcinosis

Nephrocalcinosis is generally divided into medullary and cortical types. Medullary nephrocalcinosis is more common and can be due to medullary sponge kidney, renal tubular acidosis, hyperparathyroidism, or any cause of systemic hypercalcemia. Cortical nephrocalcinosis is most commonly caused by oxalosis, acute cortical necrosis, or long-term chronic renal disease. Both medullary and cortical nephrocalcinosis are usually bilateral and diffuse.

Sonographically, medullary nephrocalcinosis presents as mild to marked increased medullary echogenicity (Fig. 6–11). Posterior shadowing can occur, but more often it does not, and shadowing is not needed to make the diagnosis. The medullary pyramids are identified mainly by the location of the echogenic foci and the absence of the hypoechoic normal pyramids.[41,42] Calculi can form in the collecting system causing the typical findings of renal stone disease.

Cortical nephrocalcinosis presents as increased echogenicity of the renal cortex. In some cases there will be dense distal shadowing that may obscure the rest of the kidney. In other cases little or no shadowing will be present, and it can be difficult to distinguish cortical nephrocalcinosis from other causes of increased cortical echogenicity. Primary oxalosis tends to cause the most dense cortical calcification.[43,44] End-stage tuberculosis (putty kidney) can also have dense cortical calcification and be indistinguishable from primary oxalosis.

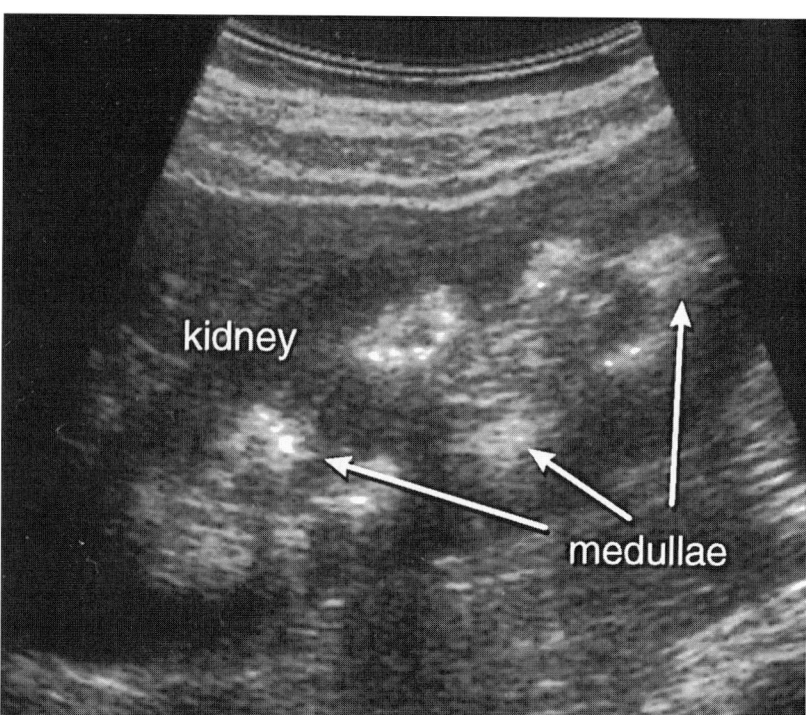

Figure 6–11. Medullary nephrocalcinosis. Dramatically echogenic areas in the anatomical location of the renal medullae characterize this disease. Punctate, parenchymal calculi may just be discerned in this image.

RENAL CYSTIC DISEASE

Simple Cysts

Simple renal cysts are extremely common, occurring in approximately one half of patients more than 50 years old.[45] The ultrasound criteria for diagnosis of simple cysts have been well established and include: (1) anechoic structure, (2) well-defined back wall, (3) imperceptible cyst wall thickness, (4) enhanced through transmission, (5) round or oval shape (Fig. 6–12). A mass that meets all these criteria can be diagnosed as a simple cyst, and no further diagnostic evaluation is needed.[45,46] If the mass does not meet all the preceding criteria, then further evaluation should be performed. CT and occasionally MRI are used for this further evaluation, and in most cases a cyst can be classified as simple using these other modalities in combination with US. Diagnostic cyst aspiration is rarely needed today. These different imaging modalities are often complementary when evaluating renal cysts.

A mass that does not meet all the criteria for a simple cyst is sonographically indeterminate. As many as 40% of simple cysts may lack one or more characteristics of a simple renal cyst. This high number is often due to operator uncertainty.[47] This number probably is lower today because of the significant improvement in sonographic technology. Hemorrhage into a cyst or an infection can give scattered internal echoes to the cyst fluid. CT in this case will usually show a fluid attenuation mass that does not enhance following contrast, and the diagnosis of a cyst can be made.[48] A single septation that is thin walled (<1 mm) or a small amount of rim calcification is also common in simple cysts. CT will show these lesions to be sharply marginated, water dense with no enhancment after contrast. Thin, smooth calcification of the cyst wall can also be well demonstrated with CT. Lesions with thick walls or nodularity, or dense, thick calcification cannot be diagnosed as simple cysts, and further evaluation or biopsy is needed.[47] US will occasionally be needed to evaluate cysts that have an atypical appearance on CT, such as a hyperdense cyst or one in which volume-averaging artifact is present.[49] US will often show that these lesions are simple cysts.[50] Care must be taken to be sure all the US

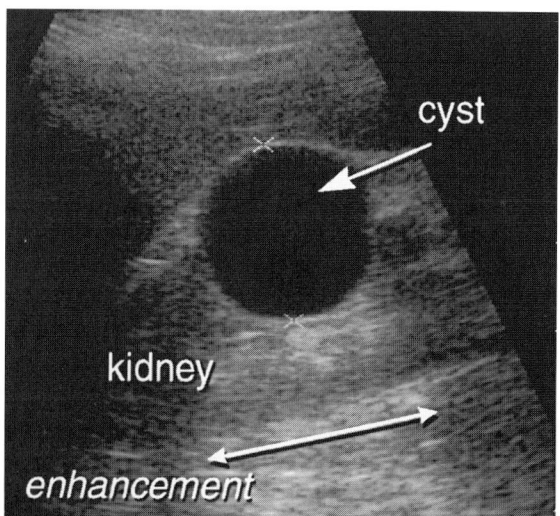

Figure 6–12. Simple renal cyst. Thin-walled, anechoic lesion with posterior enhancement of the ultrasound beam.

criteria of a cyst are met, since some hypercellular lesions such as lymphoma can appear nearly anechoic, but they will not demonstrate a well-defined back wall or enhanced through transmission. If the mass cannot be proven to be a simple cyst, then surgical intervention or very close follow-up are needed.[47]

Renal Sinus Cysts

Cysts of the renal sinus are common, occurring in approximately 1.5% of autopsy cases. The terminology is very confusing, and peripelvic cysts, parapelvic cysts, and parapelvic lymphatic cysts have all been used to describe this entity. These lesions are clinically insignificant except that they may simulate a renal mass compressing the collecting system during an intravenous urogram (IVU). Amis suggests the use of the term *renal sinus cysts* to describe these lesions.[51] The etiology of these cysts is thought to be due to dilation of the renal sinus lymphatics. Some parenchymal cysts can protrude into the renal sinus and give a similar sonographic appearance. US will demonstrate cystic structures within the renal sinus. Occasionally, they will be multiple and large, simulating hydronephrosis. Careful coronal views will usually demonstrate that these cystic structures do not communicate with each other or with the collecting system.[51,52] If needed, IVU will demonstrate a compressed distorted collecting system rather than a hydronephrotic collecting system.[51] CT can also be useful to evaluate these patients, especially if the cysts have an atypical US appearance.[53] Rarely, renal sinus cysts will cause obstruction in which case cyst aspiration and sclerosis can be performed.

CYSTIC RENAL DISEASES

Autosomal Dominant Polycystic Kidney Disease

Autosomal dominant polycystic kidney disease (ADPKD), also called adult polycystic kidney disease, is the most common renal cystic disease. Many other organs, including the liver and pancreas, can be involved and have multiple cysts. Up to 16% of patients also have berry aneurysms, and death from intracerebral hemorrhage can occur. Most patients with ADPKD present in early adulthood with hypertension and renal failure. The age of presentation is variable, and cases presenting in utero and infancy have been documented. One report using CT demonstrated renal stones in 36% of patients with ADPKD, but stones can be difficult to distinguish from cyst wall calcification.[54] These patients also have a high incidence of hemorrhage into cysts and infection, both of which can cause flank pain.[54] The cysts can also cause acute obstruction if the cyst enlarges due to hemorrhage. Moreover, there is some evidence of an increased risk of renal cell carcinoma (RCCA), compared with the general population.[55]

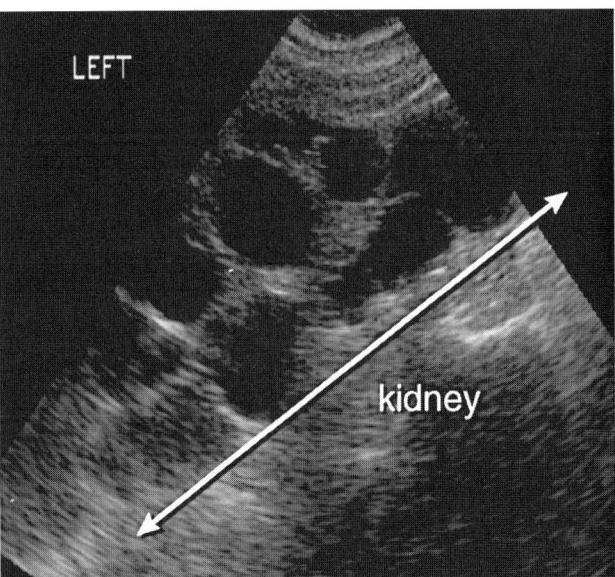

Figure 6–13. Adult polycystic kidney disease. Over time, the kidneys enlarge considerably, with numerous, variably sized cysts replacing the normal parenchymal pattern. Hemorrhage into cysts may complicate the usual cystic pattern. The overall picture of the disease is best appreciated at real-time examination.

Sonographic diagnosis is usually easy to make. The kidneys are bilaterally enlarged, with multiple cysts of varying sizes (Fig. 6–13). The remaining renal parenchyma is usually hyperechoic. The patient may not have a family history of ADPKD.[56,57] Frequently one or more cysts will have an atypical appearance with scattered internal echoes or irregular margins, caused by cyst hemorrhage, infection, or proteinaceous debris. CT can be helpful but often renal failure will not allow contrast administration. Additionally, it is often difficult to know if the same cyst seen on ultrasound is being evaluated with CT. In these cases close US follow-up is probably the best management.[58] Hemorrhagic or infected cyst fluid should eventually clear. Hyperdense cysts seen on CT can be evaluated with ultrasound, but a similar problem in determining which cyst was abnormal on CT exists with ultrasound.[49] In some cases aspiration of the cysts to diagnose infection or tumor is needed. In these cases ultrasound is an excellent method to guide the procedure.

Autosomal Recessive Polycystic Kidney Disease

Autosomal recessive polycystic kidney disease (ARPKD) has often been called infantile polycystic disease. It usually presents in utero or during infancy. The disease also is associated with hepatic fibrosis. The degree of renal involvement is variable, with some patients presenting in utero with renal failure and oligohydramnios, and dying soon after birth from pulmonary hypoplasia. Patients with mild renal involvement often present late in the first or early in the second decade because of hepatic fibrosis. Sonographs of severely affected patients show enlarged hyperechoic kidneys. Multiple small cysts that are too small to resolve with ultrasound have multiple reflecting interfaces within the renal cortex, causing increased echogenicity. Single cysts large enough to delineate are uncommon.[57]

Medullary Cystic Disease

Medullary cystic disease is an uncommon disease that can present in children or young adults. Small cysts are present in the medullary portion of the kidney. The patients present with azotemia and have a salt-wasting nephropathy. Sonographically, the kidneys are of normal size to small. Individual cysts can be seen in the medullary portion of the kidney. Most of the cysts are below the resolution limits of the US, and increased medullary echogenicity will be noted. The increased echogenicity can cause the medulla to blend with the renal sinus echogenicity, which makes the diagnosis difficult to make with US.[57,59] Biopsy is needed in these cases.

Multicystic Dysplastic Kidney

Multicystic dysplastic kidney (MCDK) is a congenital abnormality thought to be caused by arrest of ureteral growth before it completely arborizes to form the distal intrarenal collecting system. A reniform mass of multiple nonconnected cysts will be present in the renal fossa. This usually presents during infancy as an abdominal mass. Recent reports of the natural history have suggested that these lesions commonly regress, and MCDK may be a cause of adult renal agenesis.[60,61] US demonstrates multiple cysts of varying size within the renal fossa (Fig. 6–14). No normal parenchyma is usually seen. A UPJ obstruction with marked hydronephrosis and parenchymal loss can simulate a MCDK. Careful coronal views that document that the cystic spaces do not interconnect make the correct diagnosis. Since these lesions often resolve, sonographic follow-up rather than resection is considered appropriate.[60]

Aquired Renal Cystic Disease

Aquired renal cystic disease (ARCD) occurs in most patients who have been on chronic hemodialysis. The changes usually occur after 3 years, but can occur earlier.[62–64] Chronic stimulation of the few remaining functioning nephrons is thought to cause hyperplasia leading to cyst and neoplasm formation. A recent study using CT to evaluate the natural history of ARCD demonstrated 87% developing cysts after 7 years. Fifty percent developed hemorrhagic cysts, 17% of which were greater than 2 cm; 13% developed perinephric hematomas; and 7% developed renal cell carcinoma. Smaller solid lesions probably representing adenomas are also very common, occurring in up to 40 to 50%. The malignant potential of these lesions is unknown, and some authors have suggested careful follow-up of lesions less than 3 cm, since lesions of this size rarely metastasize. If the lesion is larger than 3 cm or if it is growing, then resection should be considered.[65]

Sonographically the kidneys are usually small in size reflecting the chronic renal disease. Multiple cysts of varying sizes are present in the cortex. Frequently, atypical cysts are present because of hemorrhage. The renal cortical margins are often irregular, and the common occurrence of small solid masses makes evaluation very difficult.[63,65,66] CT can be helpful to image these patients.[65,67] It is uncertain at this time if prolonged screening of these patients will help detect developing RCCA early and improve patient survival.

RENAL MASSES

Renal Cell Carcinoma

Renal cell carcinoma (RCCA) is the most common solid renal tumor in adults. The lesions usually present with flank pain or hematuria, although they are occasionally discovered as incidental findings on cross-sectional imaging techniques. The incidence of RCCA is increased in von Hippel–Lindau disease, and also in ADPCKD and ARCD. Most RCCAs are large when they are discovered, although there has been a trend toward discovering smaller tumors because of the increased use of cross-sectional imaging techniques.[68] When the lesions are less than 3 cm, the question of whether the lesion is a renal cell carcinoma or an adenoma has been debated.[69] These small lesions have the same histologic ap-

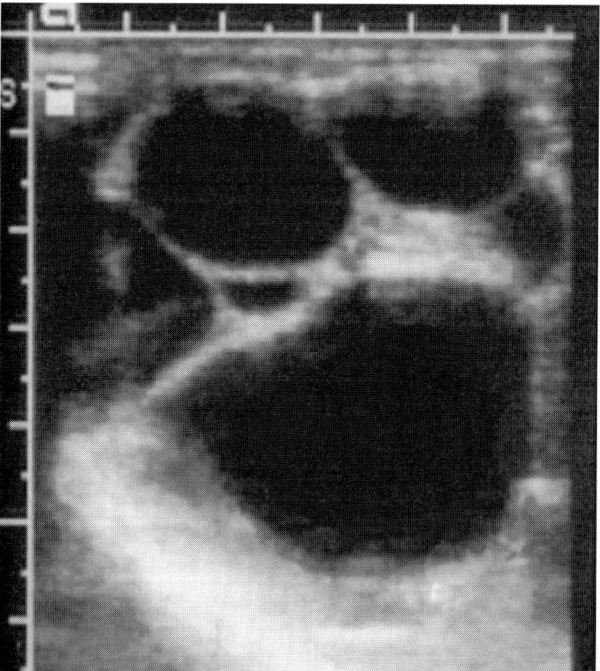

Figure 6–14. Multicystic renal dysplasia. In this neonatal study, the renal bed contains a multicystic complex with a prominent central cyst. Little renal parenchyma is apparent.

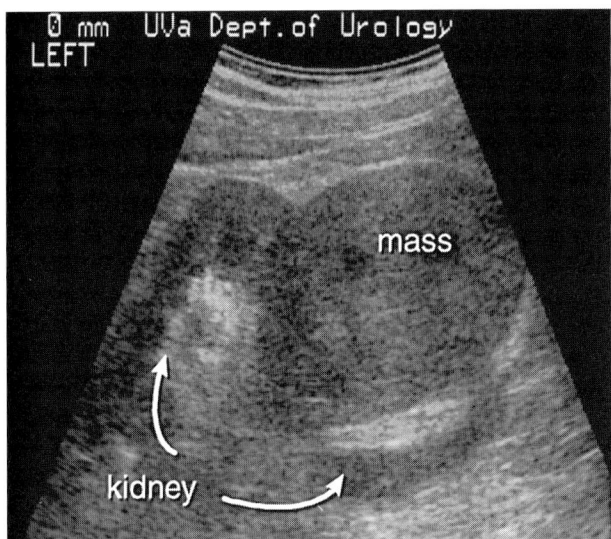

Figure 6–15. Renal cell carcinoma. A solid mid-kidney mass forms an eccentric contour defect and is distorting the central sinus pattern.

pearance as RCCA and are usually asymptomatic. Renal adenomas have been discovered in up to 15% of patients in autopsy series; they are usually less than 1 cm, and 25% are multiple.[70] Some investigators have said that renal adenoma is an early-stage renal cell carcinoma of low malignant potential; others believe they are truly benign.

Sonographically RCCA is usually a large mass that protrudes beyond the renal margin (Fig. 6–15).[71] The echogenicity is usually inhomogeneous and hypoechoic. One to 2% are mainly cystic, or present as a mural nodule, or adjacent to a simple cyst. When the lesion is large and hypoechoic, there is little difficulty making the correct diagnosis. The appearance of an oncocytoma or other benign lesion cannot be distinguished from RCCA by US criteria, but RCCA is much more common, and any mass with this appearance must be considered malignant until proven otherwise. Renal metastasis or lymphoma can also give a similar US appearance, but the clinical situation can usually help make the diagnosis. Early ultrasound literature stated that approximately 5% of RCCAs were hyperechoic, but more recent studies have demonstrated that a much higher percentage of tumors are hyperechoic.[72] In fact, Forman et al recently reported that 50% of RCCAs were hyperechoic.[73] Twelve percent were markedly hyperechoic and simulated angiomyolipomas (AML). Hyperechogenicity is more common in small tumors, including 77% of tumors smaller than 3 cm.[73] Hyperechogenicity also appears to be more common in tumors with tubular or papillary histology.[72,73] A recent study by Yamashita also points out how commonly small RCCAs can present as hyperechoic lesions, and demonstrated that small RCCAs often have a subtle hypoechoic ring surrounding the mass, and areas of internal inhomogeneity. The hypoechoic ring and inhomogeneity were not seen in the small hyperechoic AMLs.[74] CT should be performed with thin sections to look for fat in any hyperechoic lesion. If no fat is detected, the lesion probably represents an RCCA. Whenever a suspicious renal mass is detected with US, every effort should be made to visualize the renal vein and IVC. Evaluation of the retroperitoneum, liver, and contralateral kidney should also be performed. If tumor is detected in the renal vein, it is likely to be malignant thrombus because bland thrombus is uncommon in a patient with RCCA. Malignant thrombus tends to enlarge the vein and extend into the IVC, hepatic veins, and occasionally the right atrium.[75] Doppler evaluation of the thrombus can occasionally detect arterial blood flow within the thrombus, confirming that it is malignant.

Doppler evaluation of RCCA has demonstrated visible vascularity in more than 90% of lesions in some series.[76–78] High systolic flow velocity and high diastolic velocities that occur in arteriovenous shunting are commonly seen, although the findings do vary, making the findings nonspecific in individual cases.[79] Inflammatory lesions such as abscesses can also produce high flow velocities.

Renal metastases cannot be distinguished by their US appearance. Although metastases are common in autopsy studies, they rarely present clinically. RCCA is the most likely diagnosis in a solitary renal mass lesion even if the patient has another primary cancer. Lung carcinoma and melanoma are probably the most commonly detected renal metastasis.

Renal Lymphoma and Leukemia

Most lymphomas involving the kidney are metastatic or direct spread from other primary lesions. Primary renal lymphoma is rare, and non-Hodgkin's lymphoma is much more common in the kidney than Hodgkin's disease. In most patients who have renal involvement at autopsy, the renal lesions were not radiographically detected.[80,81] Renal involvement can take several forms, including unilateral or bilateral infiltrating disease, or multiple masses. A single unilateral mass is uncommon. Sonographically, renal lymphoma can demonstrate enlarged, diffusely hypoechoic kidneys with no definable masses. Histologically, this usually represents the infiltrative type. Multiple renal masses can also be seen.[82] When discrete masses are present they tend to be very hypoechoic, and some will simulate cysts.[82] These lesions are very cellular, with little intervening stroma, and thus have very few echogenic interfaces. Usually, the lesions have some low-level echoes and do not demonstrate a well-defined back wall or enhanced through transmission. CT is very helpful in patients with renal lymphoma to demonstrate the extent of renal disease and to detect extrarenal disease.

Leukemia also commonly involves the kidneys. Like lymphoma, the lesions are usually bilateral. Most cases demonstrate an infiltrative pattern of involvement. The involved kidneys are usually enlarged and hypoechoic, although discrete hypoechoic masses lesions can also occur. Occasionally, uninvolved kidneys are mildly enlarged in patients with leukemia.[83]

Transitional Cell Carcinoma and Squamous Cell Carcinoma

Transitional cell carcinoma (TCC) is the most common tumor in the bladder, but it is a much less common renal lesion than RCCA. The lesion originates in the renal pelvis and usually causes hematuria relatively early in its course. Therefore it does not become nearly as large as most RCCA. Most lesions in the renal pelvis and ureter are small and difficult to visualize sonographically, unless the patient has a large lesion and moderate hydronephrosis. The lesions can be bilateral and synchronous, or metachronous.[84,85] US can often be normal with a small TCC, unless it has caused hydronephrosis.[85] When they are detectable the lesions are usually hypoechoic. Uroepithelial thickening may be the only finding. When TCC involves the renal parenchyma it usually has an invasive pattern, unlike the discrete masses seen with RCCA. Unlike lymphoma or RCCA, invasive TCC usually does not enlarge the kidney or distort the external contour.

Squamous cell carcinoma of the kidney is very rare. It originates in the renal pelvis and invades the kidney early in its course. Sonographic findings are similar to TCC.

BENIGN RENAL NEOPLASMS

Angiomyolipoma

Angiomyolipoma (AML) is the most common benign renal neoplasm in adults. The lesion is composed of angiomatous, smooth-muscle, and lipomatous elements. The amount of each of these tissue types varies in each lesions. Some lesions will be almost totally fatty, whereas others will have very little fat. Solitary AMLs occur mostly in females in the fifth through seventh decades but can be found in any patient. Multiple bilateral AMLs occur in patients with tuberous sclerosis.[86,87] AMLs are usually small and asymptomatic, but they can become very large; occasionally, they cause hematuria and life-threatening retroperitoneal hemorrhage.

The radiographic appearance of an AML depends on the proportion of the various tissue types in the individual tumor. A typical AML is hyperechoic, well defined, and homogeneous (Fig. 6–16).[88] A hypoechoic ring around the lesion or inhomogeneity of small lesions should not be present. The hyperechoic appearance is thought to come mainly from the fat in the lesion.[74] The tumors are often small, but they can be very large and distort the external renal contour. Larger lesions can be less echogenic than the renal sinus, or inhomogeneous. When an echogenic mass is detected, a CT is the test of choice to evaluate the lesion. Usually fat is easily visualized on 10-mm-thick CT sections.[86] In some cases the amount of fatty tissue will be very small, making its detection by CT very difficult. Thin sections through the lesion to eliminate volume averaging are needed to demonstrate small amounts of fatty tissue. If the lesion is extremely small (<1 cm), it will be difficult to detect the fatty component even with thin-section CT, and the lesion can be followed with US.[89]

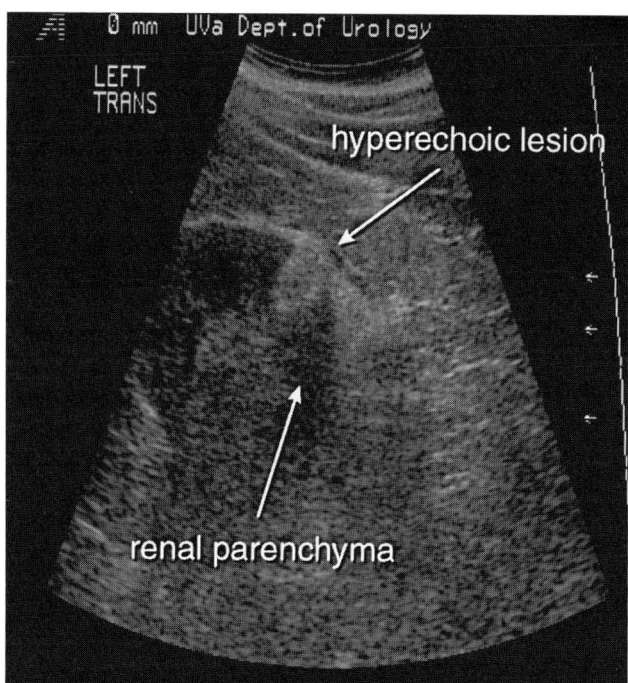

Figure 6–16. Angiomyolipoma. This well-defined, uniformly hyperechoic lesion exhibits typical properties of this benign tumor.

Oncocytoma

Oncocytomas are an uncommon type of renal adenoma that has a distinctively eosinophilic cytoplasm. Oncocytomas occur in the thyroid, adrenals, salivary glands, and kidneys. The size varies from 1-cm to huge lesions. Large renal lesions tend to have a well-defined central scar. Oncocytomas with benign cytological features display clinically benign courses. Some lesions with less benign histologic features have been reported to metastasize. Adding to the confusion is the fact that some RCCAs have some oncocytic cells within the tumor. The lesion is more common in men and tends to present between the ages of 50 and 70 years.

The US appearance of a small lesion is usually well defined, homogeneous, and hypoechoic.[90,91] The stellate central scar can be seen in larger lesions, but US is not as sensitive for detection of the central scar as CT or MRI. The angiographic findings can be characteristic, with vessels radiating in a spoke–wheel pattern. Unfortunately, all the imaging findings are nonspecific because RCCA can have any of these findings.[92] Because RCCA often has oncocytic cells, even percutaneous biopsy is not specific enough to exclude RCCA, and most lesions are surgically resected. If there is a strong preoperative suspicion that the lesion is an oncocytoma, the urologist may use a renal-sparing surgical technique.

Multilocular Cystic Nephroma

Multilocular cystic nephroma (MCN) is a rare tumor with a bimodal incidence. Some occur in young boys, and the rest usually occur in adult females.[57] The lesion tends be a multilocular cystic mass with many septations. The septations are often thick and irregular, and can enhance on CT scanning. In children the septations may contain Wilms' tumor cells, and some argue that the lesion is a benign variant in the Wilms' tumor spectrum. The lesion tends to invade the renal collecting system.[93] The US findings include a mass that is usually large, with multiple echogenic septations. Calcification within the lesion is common. CT can also be helpful to characterize the lesion. Since RCCA can also be a multiseptated cystic mass, the US is not specific, and most of these lesions are surgically resected.[94]

RENAL INFECTIONS

Pyelonephritis and Focal Bacterial Nephritits

Pyelonephritis is a common infection that affects primarily women of child-bearing age. *Escherichea coli* is the most common bacterial pathogen, and most cases are thought to be caused by ascending bacteria from an infected or colonized bladder. Most cases are unilateral and respond well to antibiotic therapy. The diagnosis is usually made clinically, and imaging in the acute situation is used to exclude obstruction or a complication such as an abscess. US will be normal in most uncomplicated cases. Renal enlargement, possibly with diffusely decreased cortical echogenicity, may be present.[95] A severe infection can lead to development of emphysematous pyelonephritis. This most commonly occurs in diabetics or other patients with decreased immunocompetency. Emphysematous pyelonephritis is considered a surgical emergency, with nephrectomy the treatment of choice. Sonographically, ill-defined areas of bright echogenicity, often with posterior "dirty shadowing," are seen.[95] The ringdown artifact, which is a bandlike area of markedly increased echogenicity posterior to the air collection, can also be seen. A plain abdominal radiograph should be obtained if there is a suspicion of emphysematous pyelonephritis.

Focal bacterial nephritis (FBN) (also known as acute lobar nephronia) can be diagnosed when focal areas of decreased echogenicity, often with mass effect, are seen in the renal cortex (Fig. 6–17). Occasionally, the affected area may also show slightly increased echogenicity.[95–97] The area of decreased echogenicity typically has a wedge shape, characteristic of a lobar distribution. FBN may be an intermediate step between acute pyelonephritis and an abscess. Close US follow-up or CT should be performed to watch for development of an abscess. CT scanning usually shows more areas of involvement than were suspected on US.[95,96] The appearance of FBN can be simulated by an acute infarction or an infiltrating neoplasm. The clinical history will differentiate these possibilities.

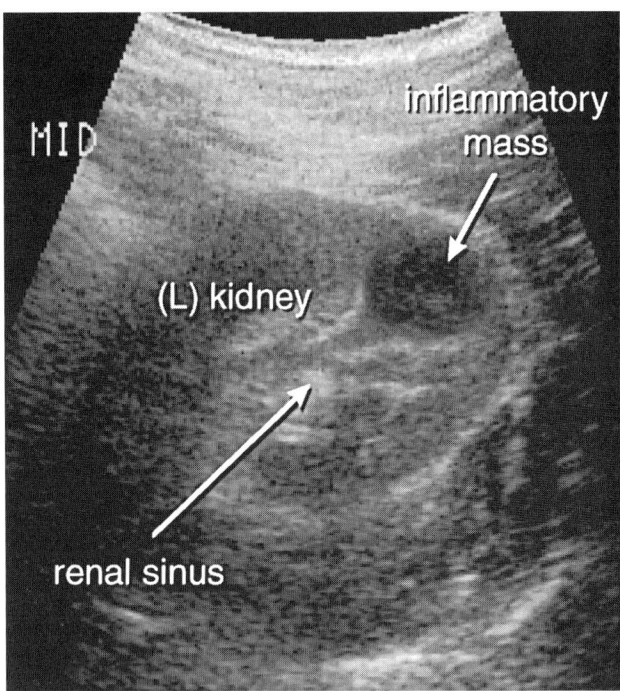

Figure 6–17. Focal bacterial nephritis (lobar nephronia). The hypoechoic mass in the lateral aspect of this kidney is consistent with an inflammatory focus. There may be little to distinguish between a focal nephritis, such as this, and a frank abscess.

Renal Abscess

Renal abscesses are most commonly due to ascending infections and are often the end result of progression from acute pyelonephritis and FBN. Hematogenous renal abscesses are uncommon. The abscess can progress and involve the perinephric space.[95] US usually shows a poorly defined area of decreased echogenicity with some mass effect and posterior acoustic enhancement (Fig. 6–18). The central portion of the lesion usually has a fluidlike component, but that area often has internal echoes and debris. A fluid/debris level or small, brightly echogenic foci (representing small gas bubbles) increase the likelihood of an abscess. In most situations these findings, along with the clinical picture, allow the diagnosis to be made. CT sometimes displays the abscess and surrounding tissues better. US or CT can be used to guide percutaneous aspiration or drainage.[95,98]

Pyonephrosis

Pyonephrosis is present when purulent material is in the collecting system. This rarely occurs unless collecting system obstruction is present. The most common US finding is echogenic debris, with or without a fluid/debris level in a dilated collecting system. Pyonephrosis requires emergent treatment, and usually percutaneous nephrostomy drainage is performed.[95] Unfortunately, US is not very sensitive and

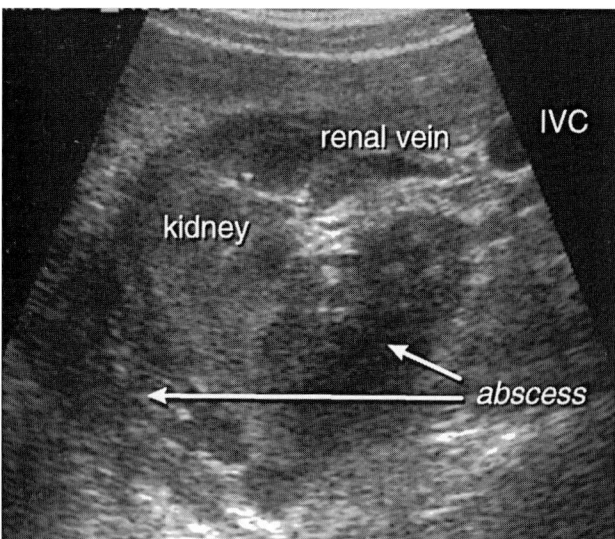

Figure 6–18. Renal abscess. In this transverse view of the right kidney, the hypoechoic region in its inferomedial aspect is an abscess. The echogenic material of the abscess can be seen extending toward the flank.

percutaneous aspiration should be performed if clinical suspicion is high. Blood within a dilated collecting system will simulate pyonephrosis, and correlation with the clinical situation will be needed.

Xanthogranulomatous Pyelonephritis

Xanthogranulomatous pyelonephritis (XGP) is an uncommon type of chronic renal infection, which usually occurs in diabetic patients who have renal calculi and chronic obstruction.[95,99] The entire kidney is usually involved, although focal XGP can occur, especially when a stone causes focal obstruction. Many patients with XGP have staghorn calculi, and the kidney or affected portion of the kidney usually does not function.[95,100] The renal parenchyma is infiltrated by lipid-laden macrophages, which grossly give the affected kidney a yellowish color. The lesion frequently invades the surrounding tissues.

Sonographically, a large calculus is present. The kidney itself is enlarged and often hydronephrotic. The remaining renal parenchyma is hypoechoic, and because of the infiltrative nature of the lesion the cortical margins may be difficult to define. Large cystic spaces with smaller calcifications are also commonly seen. CT is the test of choice for evaluation in suspected cases. CT will better display the global picture and invasion of the perinephric tissues.[95,100]

Focal cases of XGP can be very confusing since the inflammatory mass usually demonstrates polar involvement and cannot be radiographically distinguished from RCCA. The clinical history and association with a stone and localized hydronephrosis will suggest the diagnosis.

Malacoplakia and Leukoplakia

Malacoplakia is an uncommon type of inflammatory lesion that most commonly occurs in the GU tract, although it has been reported in the gastrointestinal tract, testes, prostate, and ovaries. The lesion usually occurs in the bladder, but the ureters, renal pelvis, and kidneys can also be involved. The disease is most common in older females and is probably due to altered host immunity. Macrophages cannot digest the ingested bacteria in patients with chronic E. coli infections. Multifocal disease is common when the upper urinary tract is involved. Sonographically, the lesion is often echogenic and indistinguishable from other mass lesions.[101] The diffuse type can cause renal enlargement and invade the perinephric tissues.[102] CT will better demonstrate the perinephric changes if they are present.[103] IVU and US findings are nonspecific and mimic TCC.

Leukoplakia is a descriptive term that describes the gross anatomic feature (white patches on the urinary epithelium) of squamous metaplasia of the transitional epithelium.[104] It is thought to be due to chronic infection. The term *cholesteatoma* describes a sloughed ball of keratinous material that can occur in patients with squamous metaplasia. Some feel leukoplakia is a precursor to squamous cell carcinoma, but the association is probably weak. The imaging findings often include flat, plaquelike lesions with ridges that have been termed a "corduroy" appearance on IVU. Little has been written about the US appearance, although these flat, plaquelike lesions would likely be difficult to image. If a cholesteatoma forms it would be likely to simulate a mass within the collecting system.[105]

Reflux Nephropathy

Vesicoureteral reflux (VUR) most commonly affects young girls and has a tendency to resolve as the patient gets older. VUR without infection probably does not cause serious consequences. Reflux can be unilateral or bilateral and is graded from mild to severe, grade I through grade V. Patients with severe bilateral reflux nephropathy often develop azotemia and severe hypertension requiring renal transplantation. Unilateral reflux nephropathy causes the affected kidney to become small, scarred, and nonfunctional. The affected kidney is shrunken, with irregularly scarred margins, and a dilated collecting system. Sonography will show the small, irregular, scarred kidneys with diffuse irregular cortical loss (Fig. 6–19).[95,106] The remaining renal parenchyma is usually hyperechoic. In some less severe cases only a single scar, which will be demonstrated as an area of decreased parenchymal thickness, and an underlying dilated calyx will be seen.[106]

Renal Tuberculosis

Renal tuberculosis (TB) usually presents as a unilateral disease despite the hematogenous nature of the infection.[95] The

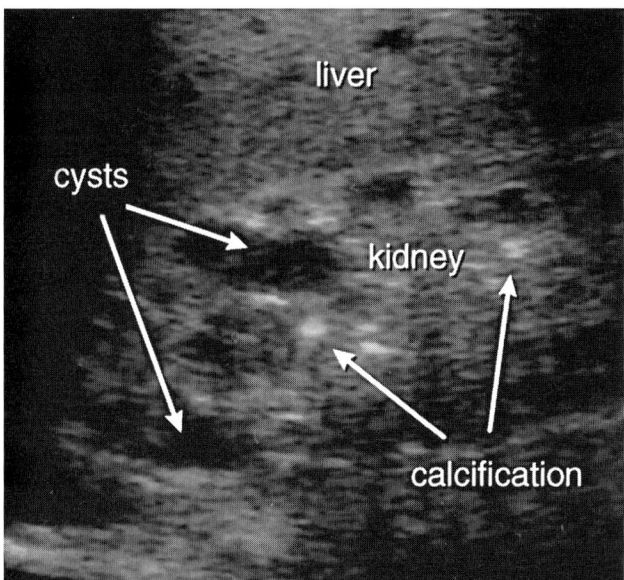

Figure 6–19. Chronic pyelonephritis. In severe cases, loss of normal parenchyma to scar tissue, and the common findings of calcification and cyst formation, may make the chronic pyelonephritic kidney difficult to define.

infection usually begins in the polar cortex and then extends into the medullary region; eventually it can involve the entire kidney.[83] Descending infection involving the ureter, bladder, testes, and epididymis is also common. The earliest radiographically visible manifestation of renal involvement is papillary necrosis and an infundibular stricture. The infundibular stricture commonly leads to focal dilation of the calyx. Calcification is also very common in the kidney but less common in the ureter and bladder. When the entire kidney becomes involved a so-called autonephrectomy can occur, forming a putty kidney that can become diffusely calcified.[83,95]

The sonographic findings in renal TB are as varied as the manifestations of the disease. The kidney can appear normal even if severely infected. Calcifications and focal hydronephrosis are common findings. Abscesses and fluid collections within the kidney and perinephric spaces are also seen. A diffusely calcified "putty kidney" will be echogenic and indistinguishable from oxalosis except that TB is usually unilateral, and no history of oxalosis is present. IVU and CT are also helpful in making the diagnosis. Growing the acid-fast bacilli in culture is the ultimate proof of diagnosis.[83,107]

Renal Fungal Infection

Renal fungal infection is usually due to renal deposition of *Candida albicans* in immunocompromised patients or to infection of long-term indwelling stents. The lesions can be indistinguishable from acute pyelonephritis of FBN. Occasionally, a fungus ball forms in the collecting system, which will appear as an echogenic focus without posterior shadowing. The diagnosis of fungus ball is difficult to make unless hydronephrosis is present.[95,108]

AIDS

A significant percentage of AIDS patients develops renal involvement during the course of their illness. Generally, AIDS nephropathy occurs late in the course of the disease, and patients who become azotemic have an average life expectancy of approximately 6 months.[109] Histologically, AIDS nephropathy involves glomerular sclerosis and tubular abnormalities. It is thought that a primary infection with the HIV virus is the etiology.[109] Sonographically, the kidneys are usually enlarged, with markedly increased echogenicity. In fact, the increased echogenicity in AIDS nephropathy is often more prominent than with other end-stage medical renal diseases.[110] Disseminated *Pneumocystis carinii* infection can also involve the kidney. Sonographically, multiple round brightly echogenic foci with or without shadowing are seen. Lymphoma and Kaposi's sarcoma are both common in AIDS patients, and either can involve the kidney. The sonographic appearance of AIDS-related lymphoma of the kidney is similar to that described for non-AIDS-related lymphoma.

DIFFUSE RENAL DISEASE

Renal Failure

US is very well suited for evaluating patients with both acute and chronic renal failure. In patients with acute renal failure, US is often the first examination performed to exclude bilateral obstruction. Although acute bilateral obstruction is uncommon in patients without a suggestive clinical history, US is a noninvasive way to exclude this easily treatable cause of renal failure. In patients with chronic renal failure ultrasound can document renal size and echogenicity. Ultrasound is also commonly used to guide renal biopsy. Ultrasound findings in prerenal azotemia are generally nonspecific, but obstruction can be excluded.

Glomerulonephritis

Multiple different diseases will cause glomerular pathology. Primary autoimmune glomerulopathies along with collagen vascular disease and vasculitis can lead to acute or chronic azotemia. In the acute stage renal swelling is often present, whereas patients with chronic disease have small, smooth kidneys with normal collecting systems. Sonographically, in acute disease the kidney is often enlarged with increased cortical echogenicity and very prominent corticomedullary differentiation.[111] Chronic disease from any cause will demonstrate small, smooth echogenic kidneys, with the corticomedullary differentiation maintained.[83,112]

Acute tubular necrosis (ATN) is a common cause of acute renal failure. Hypotensive episodes, toxins, antibiotics, and intravenous contrast can all cause ATN.[83] Sonographically, acute ATN will often demonstrate renal enlargement and increased cortical echogenicity with prominent corticomedullary differentiation.[83] The increased echogenicity is more prominent in toxin-induced ATN than in hypotension-induced ATN. Patients with chronic renal failure from ATN have diffusely hyperechoic small kidneys similar to those seen with other causes of chronic azotemia.

RENAL VASCULAR DISEASE

Obstructive Nephropathy

Renal vascular resistance increases in most renal diseases. Platt et al have performed several studies, demonstrating an increased RI (>0.7) in obstructed kidneys. The RI will also have a greater than 0.1 difference between the obstructed and the contralateral nonobstructed kidney.[10,11,31–33] The elevated RI helps differentiate acute or chronic obstruction from other nonobstructive causes of hydronephrosis. A recent study also demonstrated that pregnant patients with hydronephrosis do not have increased renal vascular resistance and that even if the right kidney were significantly more hydronephrotic than the left, the RI was similar in both kidneys.[35] Further study of pregnant patients with obstruction or other renal pathology is needed to determine if Doppler ultrasound could be helpful in this subgroup of patients. Unfortunately, most acute and chronic renal diseases will cause an elevated RI, making the finding nonspecific, but in the proper clinical setting Doppler ultrasound may be helpful. Other studies have not confirmed the high sensitivity and specificity for differentiating obstructive and nonobstructive hydronephrosis, and more study may be needed before definitive recommendations for use of Doppler can be made.

Renal Artery Stenosis

A noninvasive method of diagnosing renal artery stenosis (RAS) has long been sought. Doppler sonography has met with varying success. Evaluation is difficult because the renal arteries are not usually visible throughout their entire course. Additionally, visualizing multiple renal arteries is very difficult, as is measuring accurate Doppler shifts, because angle correction and angles of less than 60 degrees are needed. CDU is helpful to locate and determine the flow direction of the vessels being evaluated. The criteria for detecting RAS has varied. Some investigators have used a peak systolic velocity of more than 180 cm/sec; others have compared the peak systolic velocity in the renal artery to that in the adjacent aorta.[113,114] A ratio exceeding 3.5 indicates a significant stenosis is likely.[113] Recently, the use of the tardus-parvus waveform has been suggested.[115,116] The systolic upstroke will be slowed and the time to peak systolic velocity will increase in patients with RAS. The slope of the upstroke and the frequency of the transducer are incorporated into an acceleration index, which Handa et al reported to be 100% sensitive in diagnosing significant RAS.[115] The ability to evaluate intrarenal distal branches of the renal artery would make the technique much less difficult technically because these vessels can be seen in almost all patients. The problem of multiple renal arteries may also be alleviated because sampling of peripheral intrarenal arterial branches could be performed in all parts of the kidney. Doppler ultrasound is still investigational in the evaluation of RAS. If the study is abnormal in a patient with the appropriate clinical history, it may increase the chance of true positive arteriogram.

Renal Artery Aneurysms, Arteriovenous Fistulas, and Arteriovenous Malformations

Renal artery aneurysms can be detected with CDU because they demonstrate swirling flow patterns and a Doppler bruit is often seen. Most aneurysms are atherosclerotic in origin and occur at branch points in the renal hilum.[117] Pseudoaneurysms usually occur in patients who have undergone percutaneous renal biopsy, nephrostomy tube drainage, or other penetrating renal trauma. Aneurysms often simulate a renal cyst because most occur in the renal parenchyma, and the flowing blood within them is anechoic. CDU is also the best way to evaluate patients with suspected pseudoaneurysms because it shows a characteristic swirling flow pattern in the anechoic structure. Arteriovenous fistula (AVF) also typically occurs following renal biopsy or percutaneous nephrostomy placement. CDU will demonstrate turbulent flow with increased velocity and increased turbulent diastolic flow in the feeding artery (Fig. 6–20). Pulsed Doppler will demonstrate pulsatile arterial flow in the affected branch of the renal vein. CDU can show arterial flow moving in opposite directions in two adjacent vessels. Spectral broadening and a soft-tissue bruit are also helpful signs. Arteriovenous malformations are uncommon causes of hematuria. Angiography is the gold standard for diagnosis, and neither gray-scale US nor CT has proven sensitive for their detection. A recent study by Takebayashi et al has shown that CDU can be successful in visualizing these malformations. In six cases diagnosed by angiography they noted focal areas of increased flow with increased peak systolic velocities detected by duplex Doppler examination.[118]

Renal Vein Thrombosis

Renal vein thrombosis (RVT) can occur in patients with RCCA, dehydration, membranous glomerulonephritis, and several other diseases. Acute thrombosis often causes flank pain and hematuria. The degree of symptomatology depends on how complete the thrombosis is and the amount of col-

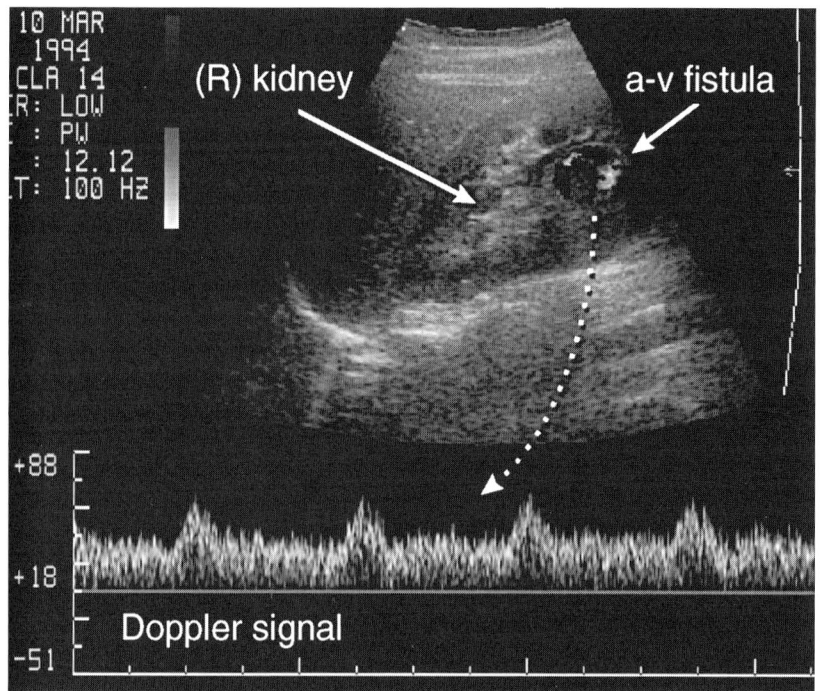

Figure 6–20. Renal arteriovenous fistula. The Doppler spectral trace at the bottom of this image shows the arterialized nature of the dramatic, biopsy-induced swirl of color in the mid-kidney. Without the benefit of Doppler, this arteriovenous fistula may have been misinterpreted as a parapelvic cyst. (See Plate 2)

lateral vascularity. Patients with unilateral right-sided RVT often have worse symptoms and worse renal damage, since the left renal vein is longer and has a better collateral network, including the left adrenal and gonadal veins. US generally will demonstrate an enlarged hypoechoic kidney with decreased corticomedullary differentiation.[119,120] The renal vein may be enlarged and filled with echogenic material that can extend into the IVC (Fig. 6–21). CDU will help because acute thrombus can be very hypoechoic and difficult to differentiate from flowing blood on gray scale. CDU can visualize a partially occluding thrombus as a filling defect in the color-filled renal vein. High arterial RI and reversed diastolic flow have been reported in patients with RVT, especially in renal transplant patients.[121] This finding is nonspecific and needs to be evaluated in light of the clinical situation. RVT imaged late in the process can demonstrate fine punctate calcifications within the kidney.[122] In a recent study of children with RVT Laplante et al demonstrated that visualization of thrombus within the renal vein is the most sensitive and specific finding. The RI was elevated on the ipsilateral side in most cases, but only by 10%, and the RI usually normalized within 10 days. Several patients had no

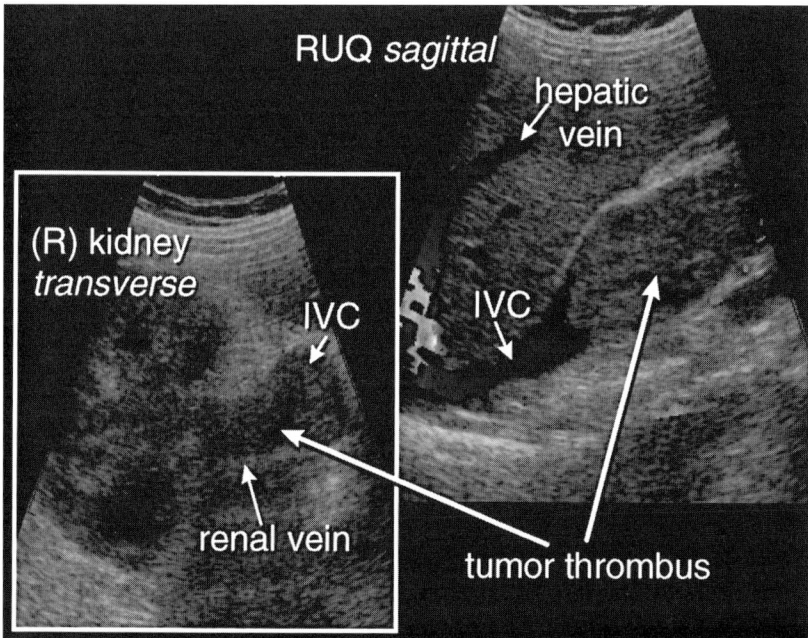

Figure 6–21 Tumor thrombus in the renal vein and inferior vena cava (IVC). The inset image of a kidney with renal cell cancer shows solid material within an expanded renal vein and IVC. In the main image, a sagittal view in the right upper quadrant (RUQ), color Doppler graphically demonstrates IVC occlusion by thrombus. (See Plate 3)

visible intrarenal venous flow with CDU very early in the course of the disease, but venous flow became visible within several days. Other helpful signs were loss of transmitted pulsations within the renal vein and visible capsular collateral vessels.[122]

RENAL TRANSPLANT EVALUATION

US has long been used to evaluate transplanted kidneys. Most allografts are placed in the right iliac fossa, which is close to the skin surface, allowing for easier US evaluation. Initially, US was used to evaluate for obstruction, and fluid collections in the perigraft tissues. Doppler and CDU have greatly increased the usefulness of US by allowing evaluation of the arterial and venous structures.[123]

Fluid Collections

Fluid collections in the region of the allograft are a very common postoperative finding. In some cases they have been reported in 50% of patients.[124] Hematomas are usually the earliest fluid collections arising in the perioperative period. Hematomas can form in the perigraft soft tissues or in the subcapsular region of the kidney. US will demonstrate a fluid collection with moderate internal echogenicity, often enhanced through transmission (Fig. 6–22). The hematoma will become less echogenic as it liquefies. Hematomas can have a significant mass effect compressing the bladder, the graft, or the ureter. Urinomas usually develop in the first few days to weeks after transplantation.[125] A leak of the ureteroneocystostomy is the usual cause. Occasionally, high-grade obstruction or ischemic necrosis of a portion of the collecting system will cause urinary extravasation. Radionuclide renal scans will often demonstrate the leak. Ascites is a common manifestation of urine leakage.[126] US evaluation of a urinoma will reveal an anechoic collection of fluid that often arises near the lower pole of the allograft. Blood or other debris mixed with the urinoma will give some internal echoes.

Lymphoceles are the most common fluid collection following transplantation. Most arise in the second to fourth weeks after surgery.[127] The collections are caused by leakage from the transected pelvic lymphatics. These fluid collections can be very large and usually occur medially or inferior to the kidney. They are a common cause of obstruction, especially when they occur between the kidney and bladder. Sonographically, most lymphoceles are hypoechoic to anechoic, although some do have debris, and many are septate.[128] Surgical resection is often needed because many lesions recur after aspiration.

Peritransplant abscesses are uncommon, but they can occur when another fluid collection, such as a lymphocele, becomes infected. A fluid collection with air is strong evidence for an abscess. Fluid with a large amount of debris or fluid/debris levels also is suggestive of an abscess.

Obstruction

Hydronephrosis of the allograft is easily evaluated with US. Often the ureter can be traced in its course to the bladder. Early in the perioperative period edema at the ureteroneocystostomy will often cause mild hydronephrosis that resolves with time. Strictures of the anastomosis can develop

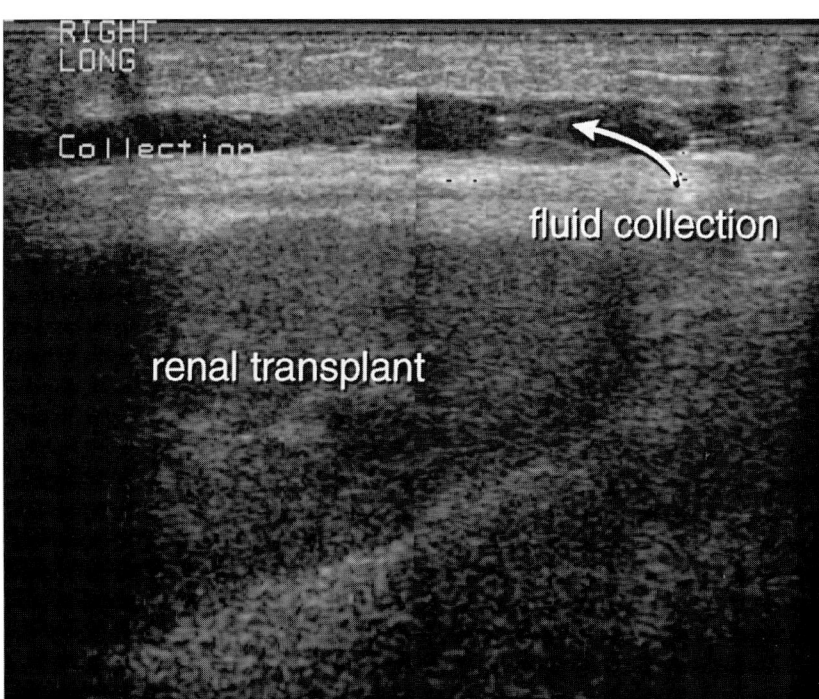

Figure 6–22. Fluid collection associated with renal transplant. In this image of a recently transplanted kidney there is an overlying, loculated, fluid collection. The fluid is clearly not intimately associated with the transplant and is most likely an incisional hematoma or seroma.

later as a result of scarring or ureteral ischemia. Perigraft fluid collections can also cause ureteral obstruction, especially large lymphoceles. If mild hydronephrosis is detected, obtaining images after voiding is important because an overdistended bladder can cause some collecting system dilation.[129] Recently, Platt et al have measured the RI of obstructed allografts and found it elevated in all cases. Unfortunately, there are multiple causes of elevated RI in this group of patients and it is a nonspecific finding. If the RI of a transplanted kidney is normal, it argues against obstruction.[130]

Acute Tubular Necrosis

ATN usually occurs in the first days after transplantation. Increased length of the graft ischemic time predisposes to ATN. This complication occurs almost exclusively in cadaveric kidneys.[131] The urinary output is low and the patient's creatinine levels do not decrease as expected. US findings in ATN are nonspecific and can include graft enlargement.[126] US will exclude obstruction, perinephric fluid collections, or urinary extravasation as the cause of oliguria. ATN cannot be distinguished from hyperacute or acute rejection. Doppler US is also nonspecific, and commonly an increased RI will be demonstrated, but the RI values and shape of the waveforms do not discriminate ATN from rejection, or from cyclosporin toxicity.[132–134]

Rejection

Four types of rejection can occur: (1) hyperacute, (2) accelerated acute, (3) acute, and (4) chronic. Hyperacute rejection is caused by preformed circulating antibodies and occurs almost immediately after transplantation. Often the rejection will be recognized intraoperatively. Hyperacute rejection usually leads to vascular thrombosis, and graft survival is rare. Accelerated acute rejection has the same immunologic mechanism and occurs during a similar time period as hyperacute rejection, but it is not as severe clinically. Treatment with immunosuppressive agents will salvage some grafts. Acute rejection can be vascular or interstitial, depending on the target site of the inflammatory response. It usually occurs within the first week after transplantation and is caused by antibodies produced in T-lymphocytes. Chronic rejection occurs after the first several postoperative weeks, but it can occur anytime after the transplantation.[131]

Sonographically, the renal abnormality is proportional to the severity of the rejection episode. The worse the rejection, the more pronounced the sonographic abnormalities. Hyperacute or accelerated acute rejection will usually produce an enlarged graft with loss of corticomedullary differentiation. Markedly abnormal Doppler waveforms or absent arterial and venous flow can be present. Edema and hemorrhage can give the renal parenchyma an inhomogeneous appearance. These findings usually suggest a poor prognosis.[128] Unfortunately, ATN can give similar features. Acute rejection will also demonstrate graft enlargement, but corticomedullary differentiation is often maintained. Thickening of the uroepithelium can occasionally be seen. Doppler evaluation can demonstrate a decrease in the diastolic flow velocity and an elevated RI.[132,133] The vascular form of acute rejection tends to have more profound Doppler waveform abnormalities and higher RI levels than the interstitial form, along with a worse prognosis.[134] The level of RI elevation does not differentiate ATN from acute rejection, although clinically acute rejection usually develops after several days to 2 weeks, and ATN usually develops in the early postoperative period.[132,133] Rejection is more likely to cause fever and perigraft tenderness, and ATN essentially occurs only in cadaveric transplants.

Chronic rejection is an antibody-mediated phenomenon that occurs weeks to months after transplantation. Little has been written about the sonographic features of chronic rejection. Decrease in the renal size, often with increased cortical echogenicity, and increase in the corticomedullary differentiation are seen.

Cyclosporin Toxicity

Patients are routinely treated with cyclosporin following renal transplantation. Cyclosporin does have well-recognized nephrotoxic effects that can occur in the early posttransplantation period. Gray scale US is not helpful in separating cyclosporin toxicity from acute rejection of ATN. Doppler US has been useful to separate acute vascular rejection (with a bad prognosis) from cyclosporin toxicity and cellular rejection (both with relatively good prognosis). Acute vascular rejection will cause increased resistance to flow in the small vessels. Buckley et al used the diastolic/systolic velocity ratios and found if this ratio was decreased, the patient was very likely to have acute vascular rejection. If the ratio was normal, then the patient could have cyclosporin toxicity or acute cellular rejection.[135] The latter two could not be separated by sonographic study, and biopsy is still needed to make this differentiation.

Vascular Complications

Vascular complications are a common cause of renal allograft dysfunction, occurring in up to 10% of patients.[123] Arterial and venous stenosis are the most common complications. Arteriovenous fistulas and pseudoaneurysms also occur frequently in patients who have undergone renal biopsy. Doppler sonography and CDU are the preferred noninvasive methods for imaging patients suspected of vascular complications. Often a specific diagnosis and triage of patients who need arteriography can be made.[123]

Normally, the cadaveric kidney is harvested with an intact renal artery and vein, along with a portion of the aorta and IVC. The renal artery is usually anastomosed end to side with the external iliac artery, or end to end with the internal iliac artery. The renal vein is nearly always anastomosed end to side with the external iliac vein. Often the entire course of the transplanted artery and vein can be visualized with CDU.[123] CDU should be used to screen the entire vascular system first, and any abnormal areas should be investigated further with pulsed Doppler. CDU will visualize smaller vascular structures not seen with gray scale US and graphically demonstrates flow disturbances as areas of turbulence and increased flow velocity. Normal CDU examination is strong evidence that no sonographically detectable vascular pathology exists. Pulsed Doppler will then be able to characterize any lesion that is visualized with CDU. Without CDU the examination is much more difficult because the entire vascular system must be surveyed with pulsed Doppler. This procedure is time-consuming and difficult because not all the vascular structures are visible with gray scale sonography.

Renal Artery Stenosis

Renal artery stenosis (RAS) is the most commonly reported vascular complication of renal transplantation. Cadaveric grafts have a higher incidence and usually occur within the first 3 years after transplantation.[136,137] Clinically worsening hypertension that cannot be medically controlled is the most common symptom. The stenosis can occur at the anastomotic site, the distal donor artery, and less commonly in the recipient's native artery. The anastomotic stenosis is usually a short-segment lesion, whereas the distal donor lesion can involve a longer segment. Rejection can also cause strictures at either site. The diagnosis of RAS is made by detecting an area of flow disturbance with CDU, often with a soft-tissue bruit. Pulsed Doppler US will show increased flow velocity distal to the stenosis.[123] Snider et al showed 94% sensitivity using Doppler shift of 7.5 MHz using a 3-MHz transducer.[138]

Renal Artery Thrombosis

Thrombosis of the main renal artery is very uncommon. The cases that occur early are probably due to a technical problem at surgery, or more commonly, to hyperacute or acute rejection.[137,138] No visible arterial flow with CDU or pulsed Doppler is highly specific for the diagnosis. Segmental arterial thrombosis is more difficult to diagnose, but CDU can also be helpful by showing segmental areas of nonperfusion.

Renal Vein Thrombosis and Stenosis

Renal vein thrombosis is also an uncommon complication.[139,140] Most cases occur early and are usually due to technical difficulties or to compression by surrounding fluid collections. The clinical symptoms are not specific and include graft swelling and tenderness, along with worsening renal function and proteinuria. Gray scale US will often show swelling of the graft.[123] CDU is helpful because most acute thrombi are hypoechoic and not visible with gray scale sonography. CDU will show absence of venous flow in completely obstructing thrombus or a filling defect within the vessel lumen with incomplete thrombus. The arterial flow is also abnormal, with marked increased RI, and often with reversal of diastolic flow.[141-143] Venous stenosis will have findings similar to arterial stenosis with turbulent flow patterns, and increased flow velocity distal to the stenotic area.

Arteriovenous Fistulas and Pseudoaneurysms

Arteriovenous fistulas (AVF) and pseudoaneurysms can occur within the renal parenchyma or in the extrarenal portion of the vessels. The intrarenal variety is much more common, and almost exclusively due to vascular trauma from percutaneous renal biopsies. These lesions are usually small and frequently thrombose without specific therapy. Significant graft dysfunction and bleeding are both uncommon. Catheter embolization or repair is indicated only if lesions become symptomatic.[123] Extrarenal AVFs and pseudoaneurysms are usually caused by technical problems with the vascular anastomosis and are similar to the pseudoaneurysms that occur with other vascular surgery.[144] These lesions are usually large and have a strong propensity to rupture and cause severe hemorrhage. Discovery of one of these lesions necessitates urgent surgical repair.

US findings in pseudoaneurysms and AVFs are the same as were discussed previously in the section on native kidney vascular lesions. CDU survey of the vascular structures will identify any areas of flow abnormality which can then be evaluated with pulsed Doppler. Intrarenal and extrarenal pseudoaneurysms usually are anechoic cystic structures on gray scale with a typical swirling flow pattern on CDU examination. The extrarenal lesions are usually significantly larger. Most AVFs are not visible with gray scale but show abnormal flow patterns with CDU. A pulsatile vessel flowing in the opposite direction of the other arterial structures, representing an arterialized vein, is demonstrated. Pulsed Doppler will demonstrate increased systolic and diastolic flow velocity in the involved artery, with turbulence and a soft-tissue bruit. The involved vein will be arterialized with pulsatile flow.[123]

URETERAL EVALUATION

The proximal ureter below the level of the UPJ can be visualized in most patients, especially if the patient has a large extrarenal pelvis. Additionally, the ureterovesical junction (UVJ) and the ureteral orifice can be seen in almost all patients with a full bladder. The distal ureter can be seen posterior to a filled urinary bladder if it is slightly dilated. The midportion of the ureter is usually not visible unless it is markedly dilated. Evaluation of the proximal and distal ureter should be part of every examination in which ureteral obstruction is suspected.

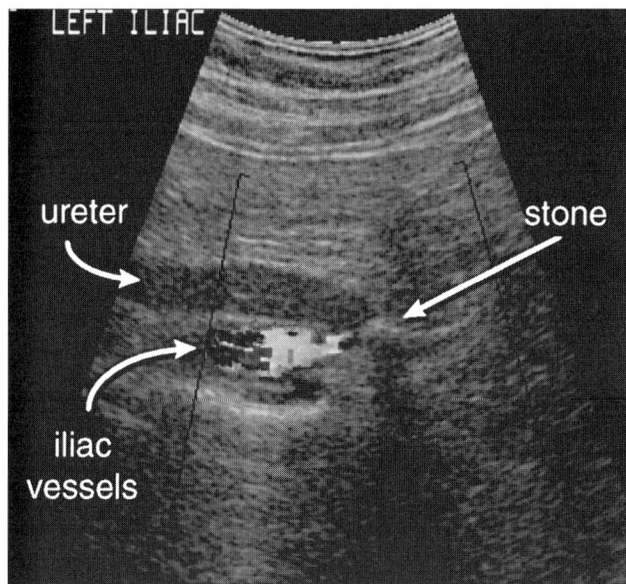

Figure 6–23. Midureteral stone. A dilated ureter may be followed distally to the point of calculus impaction. In this case, made graphic by the use of color Doppler, a midureteral stone is held up at the crossing point of the iliac vessels. (See Plate 4)

distal acoustic shadowing. Occasionally, stones in the mid-ureter and at the level of the vessel crossing can be seen with a graded compression technique that pushes the bowel gas out of the way and allows visualization of the ureter in the retroperitoneum (Fig. 6–23). Stones lodged at the UVJ can usually be demonstrated by careful scanning through a filled urinary bladder. Recently, transvaginal scanning has also been shown to help localize these UVJ stones in female patients.[145]

Extrinsic Ureteral Lesions

The differential diagnosis of masses causing extrinsic ureteral compression is extensive. Ultrasound is useful in evaluating these lesions (Fig. 6–24), especially in the female pelvis. Obstruction by ovarian masses, uterine masses, or masses from the cervix is common. Other lesions in the pelvis, including endometriosis and abscesses, can be easily evaluated with ultrasound. Lesions in the retroperitoneum such as metastatic adenopathy can usually be visualized, but CT provides a better method for evaluating these patients.

Intrinsic Ureteral Lesions

Intrinsic lesions of the ureter are difficult to evaluate with ultrasound. Transitional cell carcinoma (TCC), edema, strictures, and granulomas can all have a similar appearance, and most are relatively small and difficult to visualize. Hydronephrosis caused by these lesions is often the only abnormality that can be seen. Intravenous urography or retrograde pyelography is much better at demonstrating these abnormalities. CT can be used to evaluate the extraureteral extension of ureteral neoplasms such as TCC.

Ureteral Stones

Urinary stones in the proximal and distal ureters can usually be demonstrated with proper ultrasound techniques. The most common sites for stones to lodge are the UPJ, midureter where it crosses the iliac vessels, and the UVJ. The proximal ureter can be demonstrated by following the ureter as far distally as possible from the UPJ. The obstructed ureter is usually dilated, making it easier to follow caudally. A stone will be demonstrated as an echogenic structure with

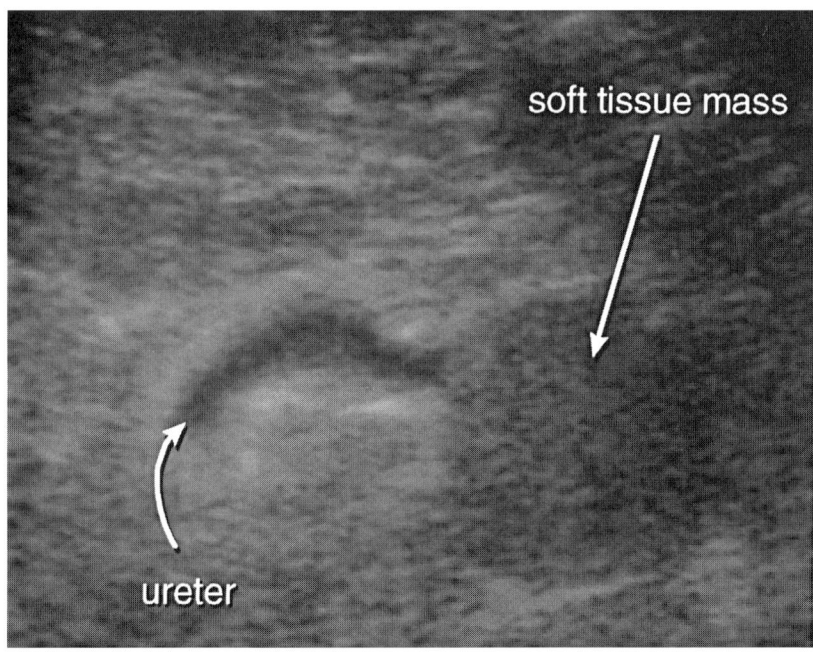

Figure 6–24. Extrinsic ureteral mass. In this magnified, longitudinal view of a slightly tortuous and dilated ureter, there is a soft tissue mass into which the ureter appears to terminate. There was moderate hydronephrosis (not shown). The lesion proved to be a benign tumor of neural origin.

Ureteroceles

Simple ureteroceles are common abnormalities that are usually asymptomatic and incidentally discovered in adults. These are round cystic structures that cover the ureteral orifice and project into the bladder. They intermittently fill and empty as a bolus of urine comes through the ureteral orifice. Occasionally, stones form within ureteroceles, and this can cause inflammation and obstruction. Some ureteroceles are associated with a dilated ureter because of chronic low-grade partial obstruction. Ectopic ureteroceles usually occur when the patient has a duplicated collecting system and the upper pole ureter inserts more medially and distally into the bladder. Ectopic ureteroceles are usually associated with obstruction of the upper pole of the duplicated collecting system.

EVALUATION OF THE URINARY BLADDER

Bladder Tumors

Evaluation of the bladder has less clinical utility because cystoscopy is usually used to evaluate bladder lesions. US can detect tumors but it will miss some early papillary lesions that are visible cystoscopically.[146,147] Most lesions larger than 5 mm are visible by transabdominal sonography (Fig. 6–25).[148,149] Transurethral intravesical sonography has also been used for evaluation of bladder tumors.[150] US has also been used to stage bladder tumors, with varied success.[151,152] Transitional cell carcinoma (TCC) is the most common type of bladder tumor. These tumors can be raised papillary lesions, or sessile masses; sometimes only bladder wall thickening is visible. Any focal or diffuse irregular thickening of the bladder wall, or mass seen on sonography could represent a TCC, but the finding is nonspecific and cystoscopy and biopsy are needed for further evaluation. Color Doppler ultrasound will demonstrate blood flow within some TCC lesions. The high-grade lesions (grade III) are more likely to have easily visible flow, but it is not specific for a neoplasm, and because there is overlap it cannot be used to determine the cytologic grade or stage of an individual tumor.[153] Other primary tumors of the bladder include squamous cell carcinoma, adenocarcinoma, and rhabdomyosarcoma in children. The bladder can also be invaded by other pelvic or metastatic neoplasms. Prostate cancer is the most common invasive neoplasm. Others include colon and rectal cancer, and cervical, uterine, or ovarian cancer. Endometriosis also commonly invades the bladder. Bullous edema of the bladder, which is often seen in patients with invasive lesions, appears sonographically as marked irregular thickening of the bladder wall.

Inflammatory and Infectious Lesions of the Bladder

Cystitis is a common problem especially in young and middle-aged females. The process can be acute or chronic. Bladder wall thickening is the most common finding, and it increases with increased duration of the inflammatory process (Fig. 6–26).[154] Eventually the bladder can become scarred and fibrotic, with markedly decreased capacity. Causes of cystitis are usually infectious, with *E. coli* the most common pathogen. Noninfectious causes include interstitial cystitis and cystitis secondary to cytoxan therapy. Sometimes the edema and wall thickening are focal and simulate TCC or other neoplasm. Hemorrhagic cystitis has a similar appear-

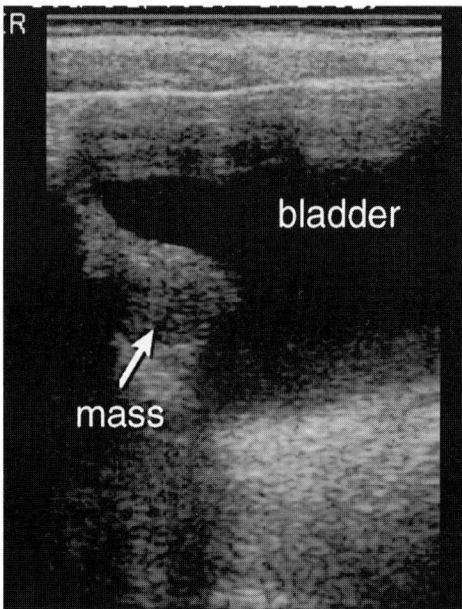

Figure 6–25. Bladder tumor. This suprapubic view shows a solid intravesical mass arising from the posterior bladder dome.

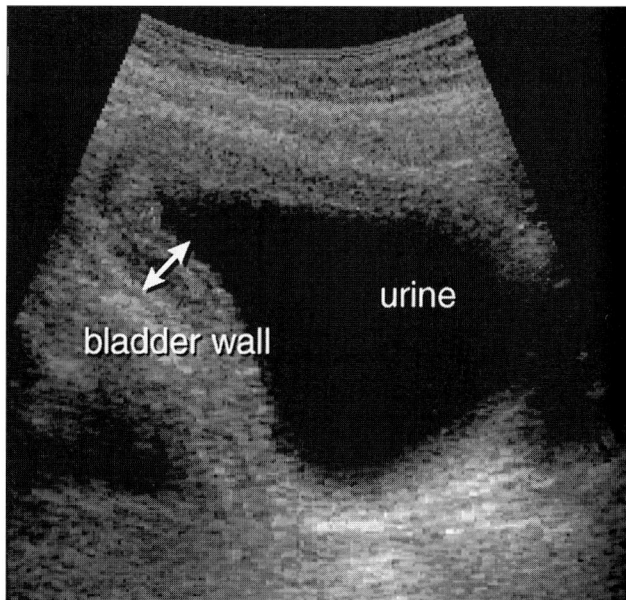

Figure 6–26. Bladder inflammation. As compared with trabeculation, in which discrete ridges of bladder wall hypertrophy are seen, grossly inflamed bladder mucosa appears as a uniform, circumferential thickening.

ance as uncomplicated cystitis except echogenic blood is often seen within the bladder lumen.[155] Emphysematous cystitis can be diagnosed if there is echogenic material that casts a typical "dirty shadow" within the bladder wall, or in the nondependent portion of the bladder lumen. Bladder wall calcification can be caused by a number of processes. Worldwide, infection with *Schistosoma haematobium* is the most common cause. Tuberculosis is another common cause of bladder calcification. Pelvic abscesses such as diverticular abscesses, appendiceal abscesses, or tubovarian abscesses can invade the bladder and cause inflammation.

Neurogenic Bladder

Neurogenic bladder is a very common abnormality whose most common cause is traumatic spine or head injuries. Other common causes include neuromuscular disorders, myelomeningoceles, cerebrovascular accidents, and multiple sclerosis. US will often visualize a thick-walled trabeculated bladder in the spastic types of neurogenic bladder, and a markedly dilated bladder in the flaccid type.

Miscellaneous Applications of Bladder Sonography

Bladder outlet obstruction of any etiology usually causes muscular hypertrophy of the bladder along with trabeculation (Fig. 6–27). Benign prostatic hypertrophy (BPH) is the most common cause. Severe cases can cause bladder decompensation, which will result in urinary retention and a markedly dilated urine-filled bladder.

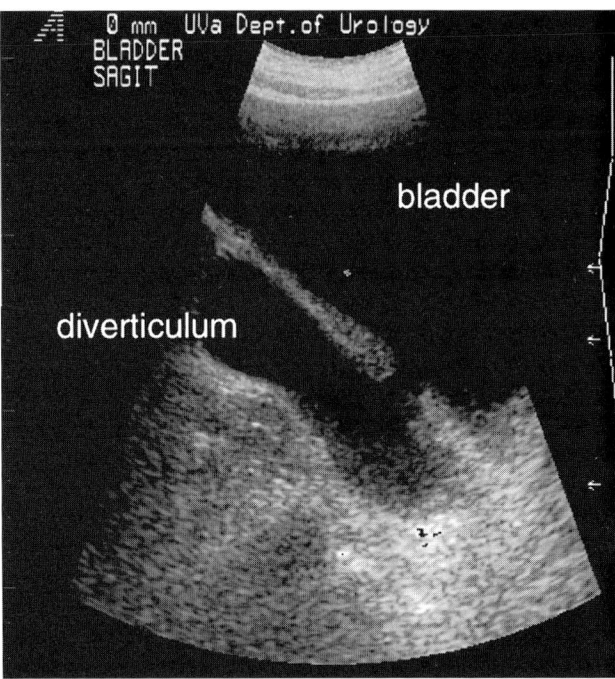

Figure 6–28. Bladder diverticulum. Diverticula are usually small, with openings into the bladder that may be difficult to discern. In this example of a large diverticulum off the posterior bladder, there is a wide throat. This diverticulum behaved as a dynamic reservoir during voiding.

Bladder diverticula are herniations of the mucosa and submucosa through areas of weakness in the bladder wall (Fig. 6–28). They usually occur in older men with bladder outlet obstruction due to BPH. A congenital form called a Hutch diverticulum can occur near the edge of the trigone in young patients. These diverticula are often associated with vesicoureteral reflux. Bladder calculi and bladder tumors can also occur within diverticula.

Measurement of bladder volume and determination of residual bladder volume after urination have been studied and found useful in children, patients with neurogenic bladders, and patients with bladder outlet obstruction in whom a residual urine volume needs to be quantitated.[156–161] Two formulas that have been used include (width $\times$ depth $\times$ height $\times$ 0.70) and (width $\times$ depth $\times$ height $\times$ 0.57).[162]

SCROTAL ULTRASONOGRAPHY

Scrotal ultrasound is a common procedure with many indications. Initially, the technique was used to study testis masses, hydroceles, and extratesticular structures such as the epididymis.[163–167] The introduction of CDU made assessment of scrotal blood flow possible, along with the ability to make specific diagnoses in cases of acute scrotal pain.[168–174] Other uses of ultrasound include evaluating infertile men, searching for an undescended testis, and evaluating the traumatized scrotum.

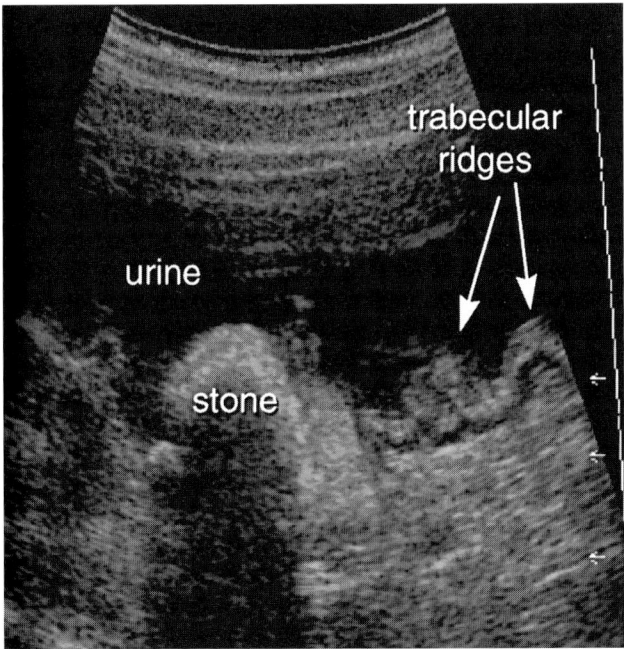

Figure 6–27. Bladder trabeculation. This is an example of gross trabeculation, in which the bladder cross-section shows prominent ridges of hypertrophied muscle. Diverticula are commonly seen. In this image, a large stone has formed in a posterior diverticulum.

The scrotal ultrasound examination is begun in the supine position with the scrotum supported between the legs with a towel. The highest-frequency transducer available should be used (10 or 7.5 MHz). Rarely, in cases with massive scrotal skin swelling, a 5.0-MHz transducer is needed. Real-time examination should be performed starting with the extratesticular structures. Longitudinal and transverse images of both testes should be obtained, along with images of any abnormalities. A transverse image showing both testes will allow comparison of the size and echogenicity of the testes. CDU should also be performed if there is a clinical indication or if an abnormality is seen on the gray scale examination. A careful history and physical examination are important because a scrotal abnormality often has a varied differential diagnosis, depending on the history and physical findings.

Normal Anatomy

The testes begin to form from the paired genital ridges along the posterior abdominal wall of the 6-week-old embryo.[175–177] The testes descend in the retroperitoneum during fetal life, maintaining their blood supply from the midabdominal aorta. The testes normally descend into the scrotum through an eversion of the peritoneum called the processus vaginalis during the seventh month of gestation. The vaginal process is then closed from the level of the inguinal canal down to the testes. Some of the peritoneal mesothelial lining remains in the scrotum as the tunica vaginalis. A testis that does not descend normally can be found anywhere along this course of migration.[175–177]

The scrotal sac consists of many layers, including the skin, dartos muscle, external spermatic fascia, internal spermatic fascia, and tunica vaginalis. These layers cannot be separated sonographically. The tunica vaginalis is a continuation of the peritoneal mesothial lining, and it has a parietal and visceral layer. The parietal layer lines the inner wall of the scrotal sac, and the visceral layer covers the testes, epididymis, and lower spermatic cord. The region, posterolaterally, where testis, epididymis, and spermatic cord join is not normally covered by the tunica vaginalis. The parietal and visceral layers of the tunica vaginalis are continuous and form a potential space that normally contains a small amount of fluid. The scrotum is divided into halves by a median septum, which is a continuation of the scrotal wall.[178]

The normal testis is approximately 4 to 5 cm in length and 2 to 3 cm thick. It is covered by a tough fibrous capsule called the tunica albuginea. The testis is divided into numerous lobules (up to 400) by septa that converge to form the mediastinum testis. Each lobule is occupied by multiple convoluted seminiferous tubules. The seminiferous tubules contain the germinal cells and the supporting cells. The supporting cells include sustentacular cells and Sertoli cells. The interstitium between the seminiferous tubules consists of androgenic hormone-producing Leydig cells, along with blood vessels and lymphatics. The seminiferous tubules converge at the rete testis. The rete testis then empties into the straight tubuli recti, which pierce the tunica albuginea in the superior posterolateral portion of the testis and join the head of the epididymis. Sonographically, the testes are homogeneous with a granular echotexture (Fig. 6–29). The mediastinum testis is an elongated echogenic structure extending craniocaudally on the posterolateral side of the testis. The appendix testis is attached to the upper pole of the testis and is not usually sonographically visible.[179,180]

The epididymis is divided into three sections called the head (also called the globus major), the body, and the tail (also called the globus minor). The tubuli recti join in the

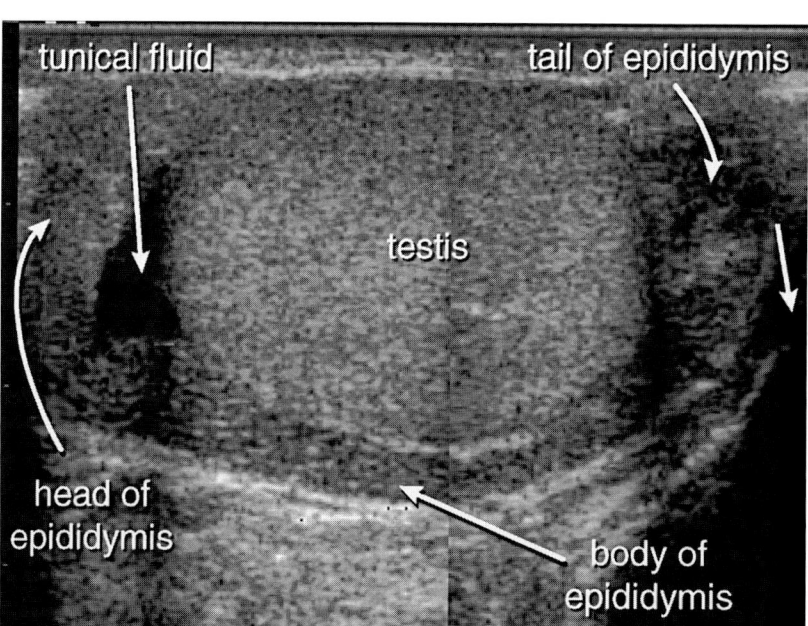

Figure 6–29. Normal scrotal anatomy. The testis has a uniform salt-and-pepper pattern. In this composite image, the epididymis can be seen running posterior to the testis from its superior pole. The convolutions of the epididymal duct within the body of the epididymis may just be appreciated.

epididymis to form the vas deferens. The vas deferens travels within the epididymis toward the tail and then joins the spermatic cord. It travels with the spermatic cord to the internal inguinal ring, where it turns medially and enters the prostate.[180] The epididymis itself is mainly composed of the tortuous and convoluted vas deferens, along with supporting tissues. The head is usually 10 to 12 mm in width. It is usually slightly more echogenic than the testis and is seen on the superolateral side of the testis. The body of the epididymis is often difficult to see, as it lies against the testis and is usually isoechoic. The tail is also difficult to identify in some cases, but when it is seen it lies on the inferolateral surface of the testis. The appendix epididymis is a small soft-tissue structure attached to the head. It is too small and isoechoic to be seen unless a hydrocele is present, or if it is enlarged.[180,181]

Vascular Supply of the Scrotum

The anterior scrotal wall is supplied by the external pudendal, and the posterior scrotal wall is supplied by branches of the internal pudendal. Collateral flow from the testicular and cremasteric vessels is also present.[180]

The testes are supplied by the testicular arteries, which are paired arteries arising from the aorta just inferior to the renal arteries. They course in the retroperitoneum and join the spermatic cord at the internal inguinal ring. These arteries are the major supply to the testis parenchyma and have low-resistance flow pattern similar to other parenchymal organs. Supply to the epididymis and other extratesticular structures comes from the deferential artery (a branch of the internal iliac) and the cremasteric (a branch of the external iliac). The cremasteric and deferential arteries have high-resistance flow patterns similar to the external iliac artery and other nonparenchymal vessels.[182,183] The testicular, cremasteric, and deferential arteries all travel in the spermatic cord; thus Doppler sampling of the spermatic cord can demonstrate both high- and low-resistance flow patterns. The testicular artery divides into branches that enter the testis in its posterosuperolateral portion. These vessels form the capsular arteries, which course along the periphery of the testis just deep to the tunica albuginea.[182,184,185] Each capsular artery supplies multiple centripetal arteries that course through the testis parenchyma toward the mediastinum testis. Prior to reaching the mediastinum the centripetal arteries branch into multiple smaller recurrent rami, which turn around and course away from the mediastinum testis and supply the testicular parenchyma.[182,184–186] All the branches of the testicular artery have low-resistance flow patterns with persistent diastolic flow. Normally, no vessels are large enough to be visible within the mediastinum testis. The improving sensitivity of modern CDU equipment may allow these small vessels to be visualized in the future. The venous flow from the testes is by way of the pampiniform plexus of veins within the spermatic cord. This plexus of vessels joins at the internal inguinal ring to form the testicular vein. The right testicular vein joins the IVC just below the right renal vein, while the left testicular vein joins the inferior surface of the left renal vein. Normally, no venous flow is seen within the testis or the epididymis. The flow in these vessels is too slow to be detected with today's Doppler equipment, although with increasing sensitivity of modern equipment this may change. Gray scale will demonstrate a linear anechoic structure coursing transversely through the testis in 10 to 25% of men.[187] Unlike other vessels, these transtesticular vessels can be visualized passing through the mediastinum testis. Middleton et al referred to these vessels as transmediastinal. He demonstrated a transtesticular artery in 52% of testes and a transtesticular vein in 26%. These vessels could be unilateral, bilateral, or absent. They almost always occur in the superior half of the testis. This anatomic variant has no pathologic significance.[188]

Blood flow to the epididymis is mainly supplied by the deferential artery. It has a high-resistance flow pattern with very little diastolic flow. Normally, no persistent arterial or venous flow is seen within the epididymis. This too may change with improved CDU technology. Some arterial flow occasionally will be seen in the scrotal wall.[182]

Scrotal Mass Lesions

The first major use of scrotal US was to detect and characterize scrotal mass lesions. Ultrasound is used to determine if the mass is intratesticular or extratesticular (Fig. 6–30). Because 95% of palpable intratesticular masses are malignant and almost all extratesticular masses are benign, this information is vital to patient management.[189]

Testis tumors represent only 1 to 2% of malignant tumors in men, but they are the most common solid malignancy in young adult males. Ninety-five percent of testis tumors are malignant germ cell neoplasms, the rest are tumors of the supporting cells and lymphomas. The germ cell neoplasms

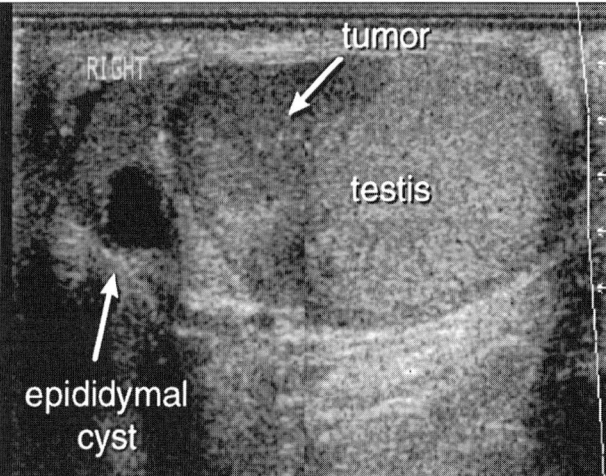

Figure 6–30. Mass at upper pole of testis. The clinical impression of upper pole testis tumor was complicated by a palpably contiguous, possibly related mass. Ultrasound shows the tumor to be confined to the testis, and the adjacent mass just a spermatocele.

are divided into two major histologic categories: seminomatous and nonseminomatous. Within these two categories are multiple subtypes of each. Up to 40% of germ cell tumors have mixed histology.[164,189,190]

Testis tumors usually cause nonpainful unilateral testis swelling. The tumors are commonly discovered after an episode of mild trauma draws the patient's attention to his scrotum, at which time he will palpate the mass. Approximately 10% of patients will present with metastatic disease, and physical examination will demonstrate the testis mass, or US will demonstrate a nonpalpable mass. Bilateral tumors are uncommon, but synchronous or metachronous lesions have been described in 1 to 5% of patients, most commonly seminomas. Patients with cryptorchidism are at increased risk of developing germ cell tumors, with seminomas being most common. Both the cryptorchid testis and the contralateral normal testis are at increased risk of developing a tumor.[164,189,190]

Germ cell tumors were the first neoplasms in which blood-borne tumor markers were clinically useful. Patients with nonseminomatous tumors have elevated alpha-fetoprotein (AFP) in 50 to 70% of cases and elevated human chorionic gonadotropin (hCG) in 40 to 60%. No patients with pure seminoma have elevated AFP, and 5 to 10% of pure seminomas will cause elevated human chorionic gonadotropin (hCG). Elevation of these markers is often the first sign of recurrence and can be a clue to the nature of metastatic disease when the primary lesion is not clinically obvious.[164,189,190]

Ultrasound has nearly 100% sensitivity for detecting testis masses.[191,192] Sonographically, most tumors are hypoechoic. The seminomas tend to be homogeneous, while the nonseminomatous lesions are more likely to be inhomogeneous because of internal hemorrhage, cystic changes and calcification.[193] The sonographic features of testis tumors are not specific, and tumors sometimes cannot be differentiated from benign conditions such as infarction, hematoma, or inflammatory conditions.[193–196] The most useful sign to suggest malignancy is the clinical history and physical examination. Most testis tumors are focal lesions, and some normal testis tissue remains; most nonmalignant abnormalities, on the other hand, involve the entire testis.[167] Scrotal skin thickening and enlargement of the epididymis are also common in benign disease.[194]

The non–germ cell tumors are a heterogeneous group representing approximately 5% of testis tumors. The most common tumors are Leydig and Sertoli cell tumors. Up to 10% of these lesions are malignant.[189]

Malignant Tumors

SEMINOMA

Seminoma is the most common type of germ cell tumor, representing approximately 40 to 50% of tumors with a single cell type. Seminomas are also present in up to 30% of mixed histology tumors. These tumors tend to occur in an older age group of patients than the nonseminomatous tumors.[189] They are also less locally invasive than nonseminomatous tumors, but metastases are present at the time of tumor diagnosis in 25%. Seminomas tend to metastasize to the retroperitoneal lymph nodes prior to the lungs and other parenchymal organs. Seminomas are highly radiosensitive and chemosensitive, and have the best long-term prognosis of the germ cell tumors. Seminomas are the most common tumor to occur bilaterally, and the contralateral testis can be affected synchronously or metachronously. Careful evaluation of the contralateral testis is important, as is long-term follow-up. They are also the most common tumor in patients with undescended testes. Most seminomas are homogeneous hypoechoic lesions. Some of the larger lesions are more inhomogeneous. Calcification or cystic areas within these tumors are less common than the nonseminomatous tumors.[193]

NONSEMINOMATOUS TUMORS

Embryonal Cell Carcinoma. Embryonal cell tumors represent approximately 25% of germ cell tumors, but most occur in combination with other cell types.[189,197] They tend to be more aggressive than seminomas and will metastasize and invade the tunica albuginea sooner. Unlike seminomas, embryonal cell and other nonseminomatous tumors are usually treated with retroperitoneal lymph node dissections and chemotherapy, rather than radiotherapy. Yolk sac tumors, which are a histologic variant of embryonal cell tumors, are the most common germ cell tumor in young children and infants. US examination of a patient with embryonal cell carcinoma generally demonstrates an irregular inhomogeneous lesion with areas of increased echogenicity caused by internal hemorrhage and calcification.[193] Cystic degeneration occurs in approximately 33%.[191] Invasion of the tunica albuginea and the spermatic cord occurs more often than with seminomas.

Teratoma and Teratocarcinoma. Teratomas contain more than one germ cell layer in varying stages of differentiation and maturation. Teratomatous elements are present in approximately 25% of adult malignant testis tumors.[189,198] Teratomas are classified as mature, immature, and grossly malignant. They are the second most common tumor in children. Teratomas in children often have mature histology and no other malignant cell types; consequently, they have a benign course. Teratomas in adults have immature elements, and almost all coexist with other malignant cell types; consequently, all teratomas in adults are considered malignant. (The term *teratocarcinoma* is often used instead of *teratoma*.) The prognosis of the tumor is determined by its most aggressive cell type. Sonographically, lesions with teratomatous elements are usually well-defined inhomogeneous masses. They usually have cystic areas and foci of calcification within the lesion (Fig. 6–31).[193]

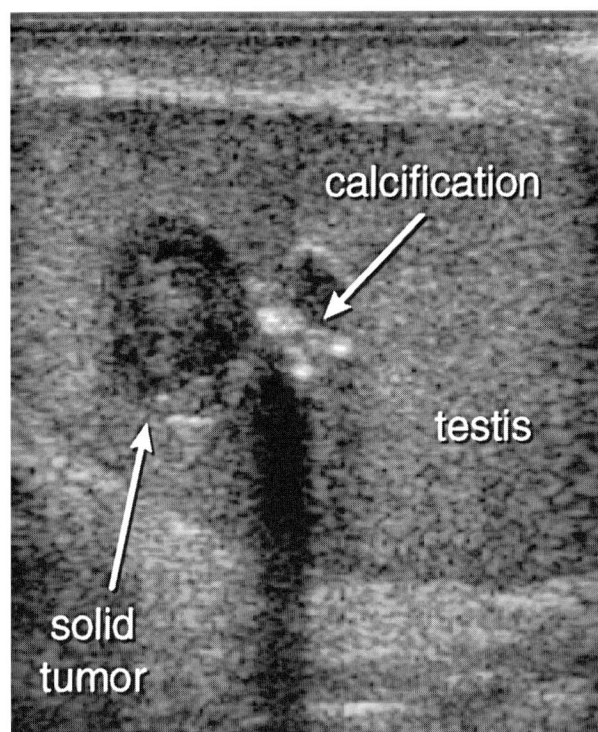

Figure 6–31. Teratoma of the testis. Testis tumor is usually well defined on ultrasound. In this example, there is a partially calcified tumor complex in the superior half of the testis. The margin of the testis appears normal, as does surrounding testicular tissue.

Choriocarcinoma. Choriocarcinoma is an uncommon lesion representing approximately 2% of primary germ cell tumors. It is rarely found in the pure form; usually it coexists with embryonal cell carcinoma and teratomatous elements.[199] Choriocarcinoma is highly malignant and metastasizes early via hematogenous routes. The hCG level is elevated in nearly 100% of patients.[189] Patients often present with symptoms of generalized metastatic disease.

Sonographically, these tumors are usually mixed with other cell types, and the appearance is usually dominated by the other cell type. The focus of choriocarcinoma often is represented by an area of inhomogeneity caused by hemorrhage and necrosis within the mass.

Mixed Germ Cell Tumors. Forty percent of germ cell tumors have mixed histology, including most nonseminomatous tumors. Teratomas and embryonal cell carcinomas are the most common, but any combination can occur.[199] The nonseminomatous tumors can also be mixed with seminomas. The prognosis of the lesion depends on the most aggressive cell type in the tumor.

Malignant Non–Germ Cell Tumors. Less than 1% of lymphomas involve the testes. The blood–testis barrier prevents adequate concentration of chemotherapeutic drugs in the testes, and they are a common site of recurrence.[200,201] Most testis lymphomas are non-Hodgkin's type. Rarely, a primary testis lymphoma occurs, but most patients have widespread disease when involvement is discovered. The prognosis for patients with disseminated lymphoma involving the testis is poor.[200] Unlike germ cell tumors, 80% of patients with testis lymphoma are older than 60, but because germ cell tumors are so rare in older men, lymphoma is the most common malignant testis tumor in men over age 50.[189,200,201]

Sonographically, testis lymphoma is usually large and often has invaded the epididymis and spermatic cord. Unlike most germ cell tumors, lymphoma tends to be infiltrative, and the margins are usually poorly defined.[203,204] The lymphoma can be isoechoic with the normal testis, and some masses can be difficult to define sonographically, even when the lesion is easily palpable. In these cases CDU will show hypervascularity in the lesion and make evaluation easier (Fig. 6–32).[171,205]

Leukemia commonly involves the testes during the course of the disease, including 65% of children with acute leukemia. Similar to lymphoma, the testes are often a site of recurrence, because of inadequate chemotherapeutic levels in the testes.[206–208] The sonographic appearance of leukemia is similar to that of lymphoma. The lesions are often diffusely infiltrative without well-defined margins; a diffusely enlarged hypoechoic testis is the most common sonographic finding.[209,210] Leukemia is not as likely as lymphoma to invade the epididymis and spermatic cord.

Metastasis to the testes is uncommon, rarely becoming clinically evident. The most common metastatic tumors are lung and prostate, followed by other intra-abdominal solid tumors and melanoma. Metastases are often multiple and bilateral, and most are discovered at autopsy.[211–213]

GONADAL STROMAL TUMORS

Gonadal stromal tumors are a heterogeneous group of lesions that account for approximately 5% of testis tumors. Leydig cell tumors and Sertoli cell tumors are by far the most common cell types. Gonadoblastomas and granulosa and theca cell tumors can also occur in the testes.[189,199]

Leydig cell tumors are the most common stromal tumor, making up 1 to 3% of testis tumors. They occur most commonly in men aged 20 to 60 but have been reported in younger patients.[186] Children usually present with precocious puberty, and approximately 33% of adults have feminizing symptoms such as gynecomastia, impotence, and decreased libido. These tumors commonly present as nonpalpable lesions discovered by US in patients with endocrine symptoms. Approximately 10% of Leydig cell tumors are malignant, and these are usually the larger lesions and occur in older men. Unfortunately, the light and electron microscopic features of the tumor cannot separate benign from malignant lesions. The presence of metastatic disease is the only definite indication of malignancy.[189,199] Ultrasound usually shows a small, well-defined hypoechoic lesion that is sonographically indistinguishable from a malignant germ

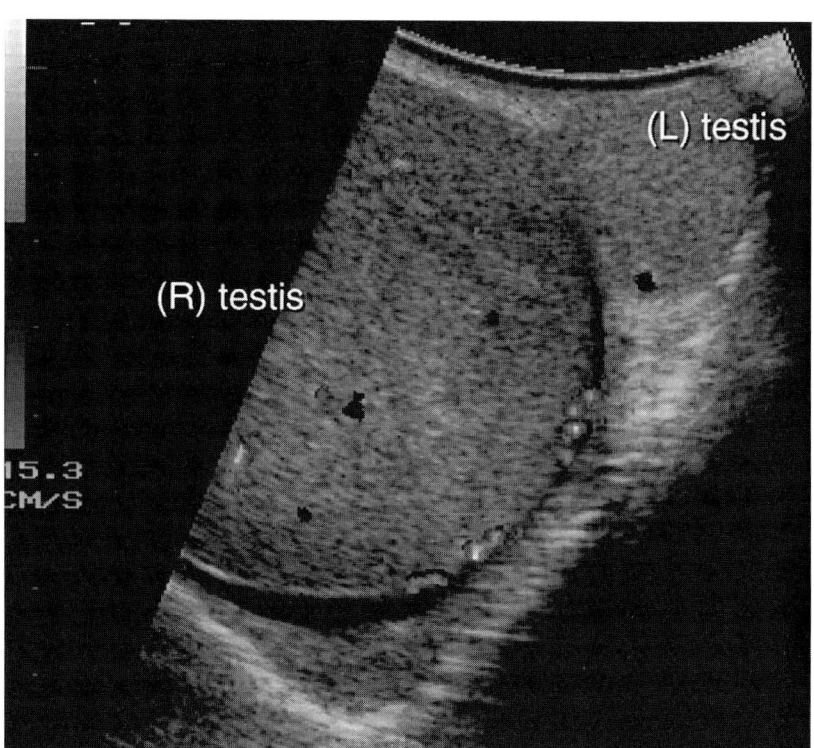

Figure 6–32. Plasma cell infiltrate. In this example, the right testis exhibits marked but uniform enlargement. There is relative hyperemia on color flow imaging. Lymphoma may give rise to focal abnormality. (See Plate 5)

cell tumor. Leydig cell tumors are the most common nonpalpable lesions discovered in clinically asymptomatic patients.[214–217]

Sertoli cell tumors represent less than 1% of testis tumors. Similar to Leydig cell tumors, they often present with feminizing endocrine manifestations.[189,199,215] Sertoli cell tumors are more likely to occur in children than are Leydig cell tumors. Ten percent of Sertoli cell tumors are malignant, and like Leydig cell tumors, the histologic features that determine malignancy are not established, and malignancy can only be diagnosed in patients with metastasis.[189,199] Ultrasound usually demonstrates a small, well-defined hypoechoic lesion indistinguishable from a malignant tumor.[215]

Gonadoblastomas are rare lesions occurring almost exclusively in patients with some form of gonadal dysgenesis.[218] The tumor usually has three cell types, including Sertoli cells, interstitial cells, and germ cells. In some cases the germ cells are recognizable as malignant seminoma or nonseminomatous germ cell tumors.[219] Nearly four of five patients with gonadoblastomas are phenotypic females who usually present with primary amenorrhea.[220] Most of the phenotypic males with gonadoblastomas have cryptorchidism, hypospadias, and some internal female genitalia.[219] The prognosis is determined by the malignant cells within the tumor.

NONPALPABLE TUMORS

Nonpalpable tumors discovered by US can be either clinically suspected lesions such as a nonpalpable tumor discovered in a patient with diffusely metastatic germ cell tumor or an incidentally discovered tumor. Patients who present with diffuse metastatic germ cell tumor without a palpable testis mass are very likely to have a small malignant intratesticular tumor discovered by US.[221–224] Occasionally, a patient will present with diffusely metastatic germ cell tumor, and scrotal US will only demonstrate a small, well-defined hyperechoic focus representing a primary tumor that has regressed.[224] These lesions often have no viable tumor cells on histologic section.[225]

Nonpalpable tumors that are discovered incidentally, such as a nonpalpable tumor in the contralateral testis of a patient with epididymitis or a spermatocele, are likely to be benign. In one study of patients with incidentally discovered nonpalpable lesions 78% were benign.[215] Most of these lesions were Leydig or Sertoli cell tumors.[215] Intraoperative ultrasound is helpful to localize a lesion in these cases,[226] and because they are usually benign, frozen-section diagnosis can be performed and the testis spared if the lesion is benign.

MISCELLANEOUS TESTIS LESIONS

The mesenchymal tissue of the tunica albuginea gives rise to several rare tumors, including fibromas, angiomas, neurofibromas, and mesotheliomas.[227,228] All are rare lesions that often cannot be sonographically differentiated from malignant lesions. Tunica albuginea cysts and calcifications are relatively common benign lesions and are usually easily distinguishable from intratesticular lesions. Most range from 2 to 4 mm in size.[229–231]

Intratesticular cysts occur in 4 to 8% of patients.[232] Discovery of an intratesticular cyst presents a diagnostic problem because testis tumors, especially teratomas, can be cystic. Benign testis cysts are usually single and occur near the margin of the testis. No other cysts are seen and there is no abnormal soft tissue surrounding the cysts. None of the 13 benign intratestis cysts described in one study were palpable. In the same study 12 of 13 malignant cystic lesions had multiple cysts that varied in size and diameter. Almost all the malignant lesions had abnormal solid elements surrounding or associated with the cystic lesion.[233]

Epidermoid cysts are uncommon lesions felt to be a benign tumor of germ cell origin.[234] They may represent monolayer teratomas, but the clinical behavior of these lesions has been uniformly benign.[235] Most cases occur in the second to fourth decade, but they can occur at any age.[236] Epidermoid cysts are often discovered incidentally, although they can become large enough to be palpable. Sonographically, epidermoid cysts are usually well-defined lesions with no abnormal surrounding soft tissue. The lesions often have an echogenic rim, and hypoechoic solid internal features.[237-239]

Tubular ectasia of the testis is a recently described benign condition of the testes that involves dilation of the seminiferous tubules in the region of the mediastinum, and rete testis.[240] Most instances occur in men older than 55, and most have an associated large spermatocele.[240] The process is bilateral in 70%. In one study by Tartar et al sonographically dilated fluid-filled spaces are seen in the region of the mediastinum testis and course in a craniocaudal direction following the mediastinum (Fig. 6–33).[241] In most cases the intratesticular process begins near the spermatocele. The sonographic appearance of this lesion is usually specific enough to make a diagnosis without resorting to surgical biopsy.[241]

Testicular microlithiasis is an uncommon entity that is usually discovered incidentally during US done for other reasons.[242] The microliths are laminated layers of collagenous material that form in the seminiferous tubules and calcify.[243] Testicular microlithiasis is associated with cryptorchidism, and these patients are at increased risk of developing testis tumors. Because the risk of malignancy

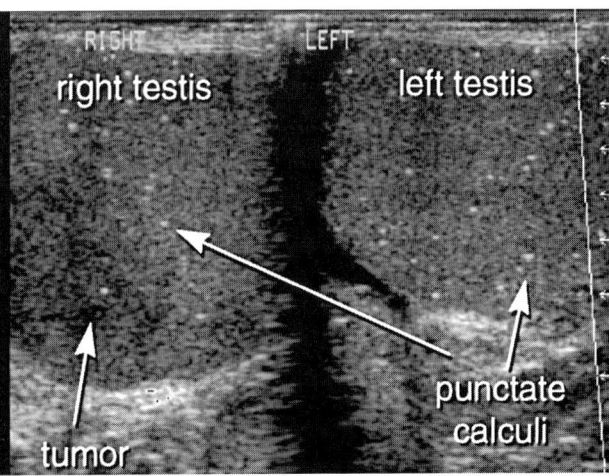

Figure 6–34. Testicular microlithiasis. In this example of cancer of the right testis, subtle bilateral punctate calcification is present.

with microlithiasis is not known, Janzen et al suggested that sonographic surveillance of patients with microlithiasis may be prudent. The condition does not appear to be progressive, nor does it cause symptoms by itself.[242] Sonographically, a diffuse speckled pattern with innumerable small brightly echogenic foci measuring 2 mm or less without posterior shadowing is seen throughout the testis (Fig. 6–34). The condition is usually bilateral.[242,243]

Color Doppler Ultrasound of Testis Tumors

Gray scale sonography is extremely sensitive and when combined with clinical data very specific for diagnosing testis tumors. The appearance of tumors with CDU depends on the tumor size. One study demonstrated that 20 of 21 tumors larger then 1.6 cm were hypervascular, compared with the residual normal testis, whereas six of seven tumors less than 1.6 cm were hypovascular.[205] The cell type of the tumor does not affect the vascularity. The visible vessels within the tumor can have a normal distribution throughout the testis or be distorted by the tumor. Lymphoma and leukemia are also hypervascular. CDU does not add clinically important information in most cases because the diagnosis can easily be made with physical examination and gray scale sonography. CDU can be useful in some cases of infiltrative lesions such as lymphoma. The infiltrative nature of the lesion makes it difficult to detect because it does not disturb the echo texture of the testis as much as a germ cell tumor. In these cases the hyperemia seen on CDU will increase the diagnostic confidence of the examiner.[171,205]

Extratesticular Scrotal Abnormalities

HYDROCELES

Normally a few milliliters of fluid are present between the parietal and visceral layers of the tunica vaginalis. The fluid is visible within the scrotum of 85% of asymptomatic pa-

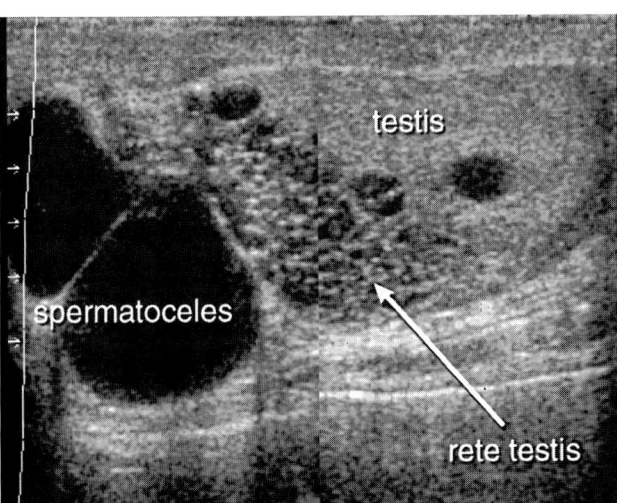

Figure 6–33. Tubular ectasia. Prominent tubules of the rete testis appear as cystic foci. This condition is almost invariably encountered, as in this example, in the presence of a spermatocele.

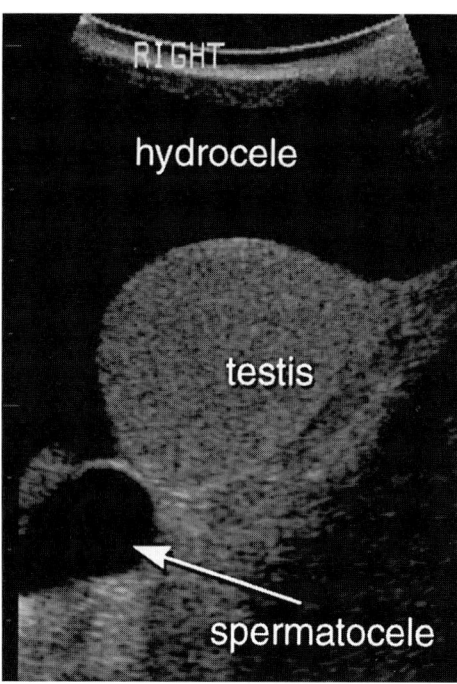

Figure 6–35. Hydrocele. Fluid in the tunica vaginalis lies anterior to the testis. On this image, a second cystic area toward the upper pole of the testis is a spermatocele.

tients who have scrotal ultrasound.[244] Hydroceles are an abnormal collection of fluid within this space, and they are a common cause of scrotal swelling (Fig. 6–35).[165] No well-accepted definition of the size or amount of fluid that defines a hydrocele is in common usage, and the diagnosis is usually made if the sonographer feels the amount of fluid is abnormal. Hydroceles only surround the anterior and lateral portions of the testis because the layers of the tunica vaginalis join on the posterolateral surface of the testis and no potential space exists there. Most hydroceles are echo-free fluid, although some hydroceles do have floating echogenic material within them.

Hydroceles can be congenital or acquired. The congenital type represents an open communication between the potential space within the scrotum and the peritoneum through the processus vaginalis. These hydroceles usually resolve by 1 to 2 years of age. Acquired hydroceles are more common and are usually idiopathic in origin. Hydroceles can be caused by trauma, epididymitis, torsion, or any inflammatory scrotal abnormality. Sixty percent of testis tumors are associated with small hydroceles.[245] Any patient with a hydrocele large enough to prevent adequate palpation of the testis should undergo an ultrasound to exclude a testis tumor. The etiology of some hydroceles can be determined clinically. Infrequently, US detects the etiology of the hydrocele, but most remain idiopathic.

Pyoceles and hematoceles are both uncommon. Hematoceles usually occur following trauma, in which case it is important to evaluate the testis to exclude testis rupture. Other causes include tumors that have invaded the tunica albuginea and torsion. Pyoceles usually result from an epididymal infection that spreads into the tunica vaginalis.[246] Sonographically, both hematoceles and pyoceles are usually complex fluid collections with internal echoes, fluid/debris levels, and internal septations. CDU often shows marked hyperemia in the affected scrotum and a rim of hyperemia around the fluid collection.[170,171]

SCROTOLITHS

Scrotoliths are freely movable calcified bodies that lie within the scrotum and that have no clinical significance. They may result from torsion and amputation of the appendix testis or appendix epididymis. Another cause could be inflammatory reaction of the tunica vaginalis. A hydrocele makes detection of scrotoliths easier.[247]

VARICOCELES

A varicocele is a group of dilated veins in the pampiniform plexus. The dilated veins course up the spermatic cord and join to form the spermatic vein. Normally, the veins of the pampiniform plexus are less then 2 mm and are not sonographically tortuous.[248,249] Varicoceles can be primary or secondary. Primary varicoceles are present in 10 to 15% of men and almost all involve the left side. Bilateral varicoceles occur in approximately 15%.[250,251] Primary unilateral right-sided varicoceles are rare. When one is encountered the possibility of a retroperitoneal mass obstructing the right spermatic vein should be investigated. The left-sided predominance may be related to the left spermatic venous drainage into the left renal vein and the compression of the left renal vein by the superior mesenteric vein. The right spermatic vein drains into the infrarenal IVC. Most varicoceles result from incompetent venous valves in the left spermatic vein that cause venous backflow and increased pressure in the pampiniform plexus. Primary varicoceles distend when the patient is erect or performs a Valsalva maneuver. They become less distended when the patient is supine.[251] Secondary varicoceles are caused by obstruction or increased pressure on the spermatic vein by a retroperitoneal mass or a hydronephrotic kidney. Secondary varicoceles usually occur in older patients and do not decompress when the patient changes positions.

Varicoceles can cause infertility and occasionally scrotal pain. The link to infertility is difficult to characterize because some men with large varicoceles have normal sperm counts whereas some men with small subclinical varicoceles have markedly abnormal semenalysis.[252] Varicoceles do occur more commonly in infertile men than in the rest of the population, and repair of varicoceles does improve semenalysis and fertility rates.[250] Additionally, varicoceles can be associated with abnormal testis histology.[251,253] On physical examination the large varicoceles are easily palpated as multiple tubular structures within the scrotum. Small varicoceles require palpation while the patient performs a Valsalva ma-

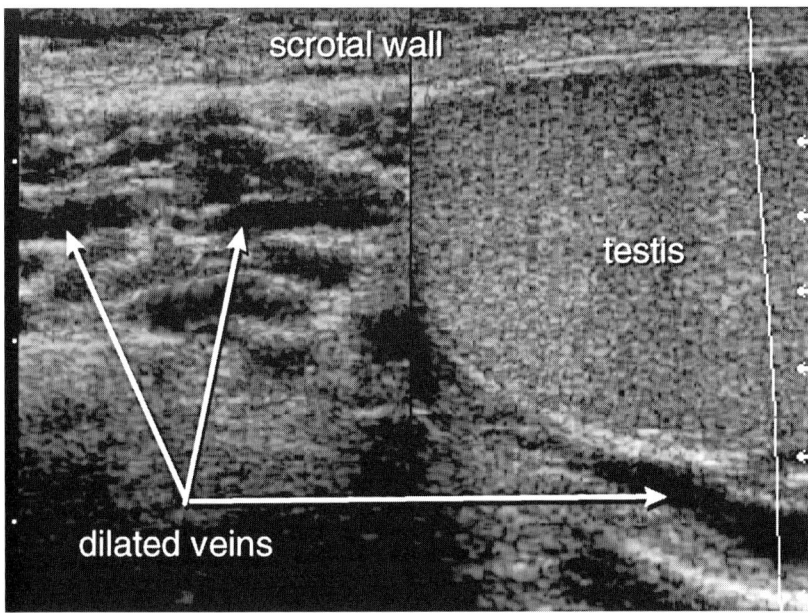

Figure 6–36. Varicocele. Dilated, serpiginous veins of the pampiniform plexus are seen in this gray scale image superior and posterior to the testis.

neuver standing in the erect position. Fertility rates and semenalysis improve with repair of both small and large varicoceles; thus the detection of even nonpalpable varicoceles is important in an infertile male.[254]

Sonographic detection of varicoceles depends on demonstrating intrascrotal veins larger than 2 mm (Fig. 6–36).[248,249] CDU is the best way to document the increased flow that occurs with Valsalva maneuver or with standing. The flow augmentation is often most dramatic when the patient is erect.[255] The flow augmentation should be prolonged and resolve with release of Valsalva. Mild transient flow enhancement can occur in patients without varicocele, but this will be represented as a ''flash'' of color that rapidly dissipates.[171]

Extratesticular Neoplasms

Solid neoplasms in the epididymis are very uncommon, and unlike testis masses they are usually benign. Cystic structures are present in the epididymis in 20 to 40% of asymptomatic subjects.[244] Spermatoceles are very common and represent dilated fluid-filled spaces that usually form in the head of the epididymis. The clinical diagnosis is easily made when a transilluminable nontender mass is present in the epididymal head. Sonographically, they are cystic spaces that occasionally have multiple internal septations and rarely have internal echoes (Fig. 6–37). Epididymal cysts are also very common and differ from spermatoceles only in the type of fluid within the cystic spaces.[256] Their US appearance is identical to spermatoceles. Chronic epididymitis can result in a fibrotic mass in the epididymis that simulates a solid neoplasm.

Sperm granulomas are a necrotizing granulomatous inflammatory response that usually occurs only after vasectomy. It is thought to be caused by extravasation of sperm into the scrotal soft tissues.[257,258] These granulomas are usually solid hypoechoic masses that occur along the course of the vas deferens.[258] Following vasectomy, changes can occur in the epididymis, including enlargement and inhomogeneity. Epididymal cysts can also develop after vasectomy.[259]

Adenomatoid tumors are the most common epididymal neoplasm. They usually occur in the epididymis but can occur in the spermatic cord and, very rarely, within the testis.[199,260] Most commonly, the mass is more echogenic than the testis and epididymis; however, some are hypoechoic. Other benign extratesticular tumors are extremely rare. Hemangiomas, lipomas, and fibromas have been described.

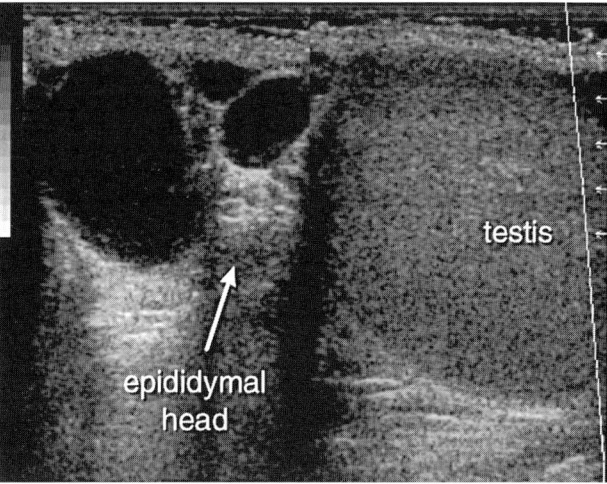

Figure 6–37. Spermatocele. Clustered around the head of the epididymis, most of these cysts are not true cysts but spermatoceles. Generally small in size, spermatoceles may sometimes become larger than the testis. They are readily distinguished from hydroceles by anatomic location and configuration.

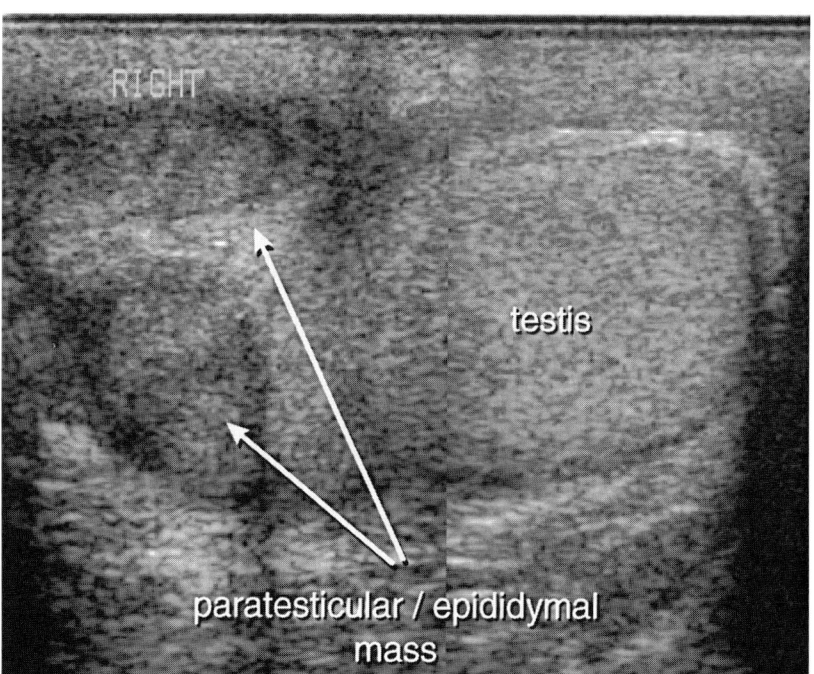

Figure 6–38. Paratesticular sarcoma. The testis appears essentially normal. There is a bizarre mass in the anatomical location of the epididymis. Sonographically, this condition may be difficult to distinguish from the far commoner condition of epididymitis. Possible clues to the correct diagnosis in this example are the absence of associated inflammatory signs such as hydrocele and scrotal wall edema.

Adrenal rests have been described in the scrotum and the testis of infants. They are thought to arise from adrenal cortical cells that migrate with the testis in utero.

Malignant epididymal tumors are exceedingly rare except for cases of invasion by primary testis tumors and lymphoma. Malignant mesotheliomas have been described along with fibrosarcomas and liposarcomas (Fig. 6–38). Papillary cystadenomas of the epididymis have been described in patients with von Hippel–Lindau disease.[261]

Scrotal and Testis Inflammation

Epididymitis and epididymoorchitis are the most common causes of acute scrotal pain and occur most commonly in postpubertal males.[262] Bacterial pathogens such as E. coli are the most common cause. Frequently no organism is demonstrated on routine cultures and viral or chlamydial pathogens are thought to be the cause.[262] Tuberculosis can also affect the epididymis and testis, and its incidence is increasing, probably because of the HIV epidemic. Clinically, most patients with epididymoorchitis are postpubertal, although the disease can affect prepubertal males. The inflammation usually starts in the epididymis and can spread to the testis. The onset of pain is usually insidious and increases slowly over 1 to several days, although a significant percentage of patients report a sudden onset of pain that simulates testis torsion. Fever, dysuria, and pyuria are common in bacterial epididymitis. Physical examination reveals an enlarged, tender epididymis and testis. Epididymitis and epididymoorchitis usually respond well to oral antibiotics and rest. Severe cases may need intravenous antibiotics. Occasionally, the inflammation and edema can become severe enough to compromise testis blood flow and cause infarction. Abscess formation in the epididymis or testis is another potential complication.

Gray scale US usually demonstrates enlargement and hypoechogenicity of the involved epididymis and testis.[170] The epididymis is usually diffusely involved, but focal involvement occurs in 20 to 30%. The testis is involved in 20 to 40% of cases. Involvement of the testis is usually diffuse, but focal involvement occurs in 10% of cases. CDU is now felt to be the optimal way to diagnose scrotal inflammation. CDU will demonstrate increased flow within the affected epididymis and testis (Fig. 6–39). Normally, no blood flow is sonographically visible in the epididymis, and any blood flow visible in the epididymis represents inflammation. Additionally, no venous blood flow is normally visible anywhere within the scrotum, except in patients with a transtesticular artery (a normal variant). In the future, as CDU equipment becomes more sensitive, normal arterial and venous flow may become visible in the epididymis. In one study of 51 cases of scrotal inflammatory disease the epididymis was hyperemic in all cases. Epididymoorchitis as diagnosed by hyperemia in the epididymis and testis was present in approximately 40%. The gray scale examination was normal in 20% of cases, and the hyperemia seen with CDU was the only evidence of inflammation.[170] Pulsed Doppler analysis is not needed to make the diagnosis, but when performed it will show increased flow with low RI. Venous flow will also be detectable in some cases. Testis and epididymal abscesses will be demonstrated as focal hypoechoic regions that usually have internal echogenic material and debris.[170] CDU will show "rim" hyperemia with no flow into the hypoechoic area. CDU is more sensitive and specific in the diagnosis of scrotal inflammation and can quickly exclude testis ischemia, making CDU an impor-

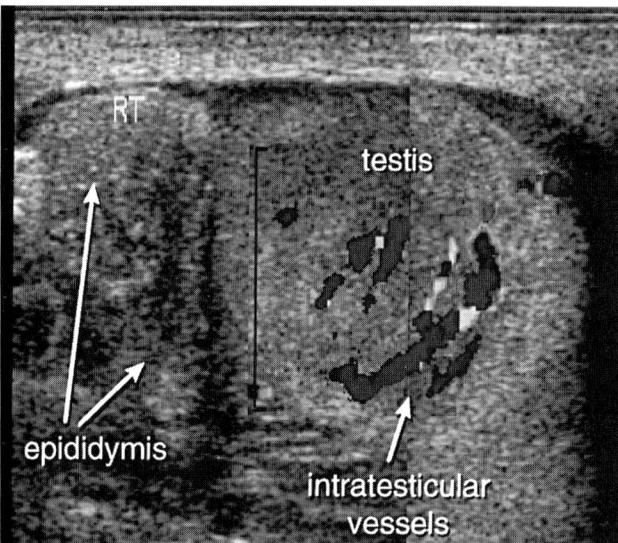

Figure 6–39. Epididymoorchitis. In this long-axis view through the right hemiscrotum, there are several signs of inflammation: The epididymis appears enlarged, the gray scale pattern of the testis is mildly disturbed, there is intratesticular hyperemia and a small hydrocele is present. (See Plate 6)

tant diagnostic tool in cases of suspected inflammatory disease.[170,171]

Testis Ischemia

Testis torsion is the most common cause of testis ischemia. Patients in whom the two layers of the tunica vaginalis do not fuse along the posterolateral side of the testis and scrotum (the bell clapper deformity) are at significant risk for torsion. The fusion of the layers of the tunica vaginalis anchors the testis to the scrotal wall, preventing free movement of the testis. In patients with the bell clapper deformity the testis is suspended freely in the scrotal sac and is more mobile than normal. Torsion can occur at any age but is most common in adolescent males. Torsion can also occur prenatally.[177]

Clinically, patients with torsion usually describe the sudden onset of severe scrotal pain and swelling. Often the patient describes being awakened from sleep.[263] Most patients also describe similar episodes in the past that resolved spontaneously. Reactive hydroceles, skin thickening, and erythema can also develop quickly. Rapid diagnosis and treatment are critical if the testis is to survive. If the torsion is relieved within 4 hours, most testes will remain viable, whereas most that are not detorsed within 10 hours will be infarcted. Between 4 and 10 hours the chance of testis salvage decreases.[263,264] The degree of torsion is also important because a 180-degree torsion causes less blood flow interruption and has a longer window of salvageability than a 360- to 720-degree torsion.[265] Work with a dog model has shown that torsion of 360 degrees or more will show absence of detectable blood flow after 1 hour. Torsion of 180 degrees or less will show decreased blood flow for up to 4 hours, followed by complete absence of sonographically detected blood flow.[265]

Physical examination usually reveals a swollen exquisitely tender testis. The epididymis is usually enlarged. The patient's white blood cell count is elevated in a significant number of cases, and surprisingly, 20 to 25% have fever and approximately 20% have positive urine cultures.[266] The physical findings and the clinical history make differentiation from epididymoorchitis very difficult in many cases.

Gray scale US is nonspecific in most cases of torsion. Early in the course of the disease, when the testis is still salvageable, the gray scale examination is often normal. Testis and epididymal swelling, along with slightly decreased echogenicity, may develop in the first 6 hours.[267] The longer the time after the torsion occurs, the more swollen and hypoechoic the testis will become. A testis with definite hypoechogenicity is usually not salvageable.

CDU allows for definitive early diagnosis of testis torsion.[168,171,173,174] In almost all cases no blood flow will be seen in the affected testis.[168,171] Some cases of partial torsion with less than 360-degree twists of the spermatic cord have been seen with decreased but detectable blood flow within the testis.[168] One case of torsion with normal blood flow has been reported.[173] One case of 180-degree torsion has been seen with decreased but visible blood flow within the testis and pulsed Doppler waveforms showing a high-resistance flow pattern with absent diastolic flow in the affected testis. More cases with a similar high-resistance blood flow pattern will need to be documented before this abnormal waveform in a torsed testis can be used as a helpful diagnostic sign.

The one pitfall in the diagnosis of testis torsion is the hyperemia that can occur with a recently detorsed testis. Presumably, the hyperemia is the result of an inflammatory response that occurs in the detorsed testis. Patients who had a resolved torsion are at extremely high risk of recurrence and should undergo orchiopexy.[171] Patients who have a clinical history suggestive of torsion with detorsion should not be diagnosed as having epididymoorchitis because CDU demonstrates hyperemia.

Scrotal Trauma

Testis trauma can be manifest as a contusion, hematoma, hematocele, or ruptured testis (Fig. 6–40). Testis rupture is extremely important to diagnose rapidly because surgical intervention prior to 72 hours will salvage approximately 90% of affected testes. Testis rupture that is untreated for longer than 72 hours has a salvage rate of 45%.[268–270] Scrotal swelling, hematoceles, and tenderness prohibit accurate physical examination. Direct evidence of testis rupture is often not seen on sonography. Jeffrey et al identified a discrete fracture plane in only 17% of 12 cases. Findings in his cases included focal areas of abnormal echogenicity that corresponded to areas of hemorrhage and infarction. Hematoceles

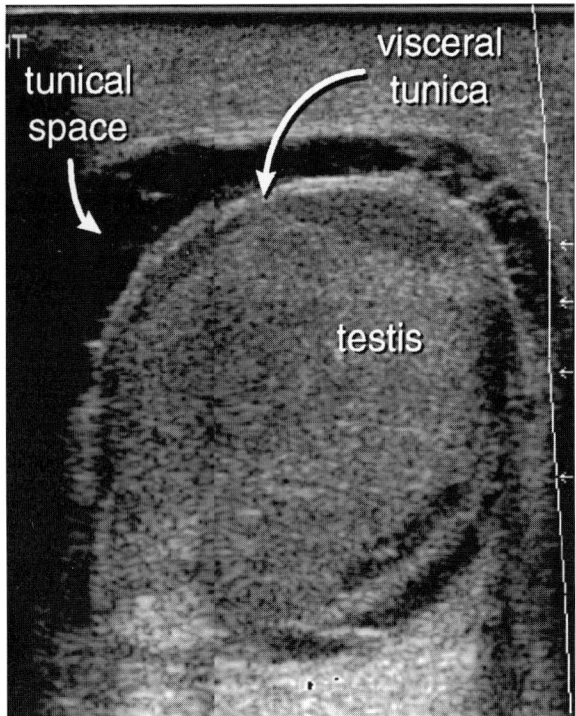

Figure 6–40. Testicular trauma. There is a rim of fluid under the tunica albuginea. Clearer, septate fluid is present in the tunical vaginalis. The testis itself appears to be essentially intact.

are another common finding. Because specific findings are not common, a high index of suspicion of testis rupture must be present in any case with a suggestive history and any abnormal findings on sonography.[268] CDU can be used to evaluate the perfusion of the testis because occasionally trauma can cause a contraction of the cremasteric muscle and cause torsion.[168,171]

Cryptorchidism

The testes form in the embryonic genital ridge and migrate to the scrotum through the retroperitoneum. Normally, the testes begin to descend into the scrotum at 36 weeks.[271] A testis is incompletely descended in 3–5% of boys at term, with up to 25% of cases being bilateral. The incidence of cryptorchidism at age 1 is 0.8%, and few testes spontaneously descend after 1 year.[272] The cryptoorchid testis should be localized and surgically brought into the scrotum or resected. The incidence of infertility is significantly higher if the testis remains outside the scrotum for more than 1 year.[273] The incidence of testis cancer is increased by 10 to 20 times above the normal population.[163] The increased risk occurs in the affected testis and to a lesser degree also in normally descended contralateral testes.[189,274] Even with orchiopexy the risk of carcinoma is increased and careful physical examinations should be performed serially.[189]

Sonographic detection of the cryptorchid testis should be performed with a high-frequency linear transducer. Eighty percent of cryptorchid testes are located within the inguinal canal, although the testis can be located anywhere from the retroperitoneum along the course of its embryonic descent. The cryptorchid testis is often slightly smaller and more echogenic than the normally descended testis. A lymph node or an enlargement of the gubernaculum testis can simulate a testis.[275] Visualizing the mediastinum testis confirms that the imaged structure is the cryptorchid testis. The success of US detection varies from 88% to 70%, depending on the series.[276,277] Nonpalpable testes are much more difficult to detect with ultrasound. MRI has recently been used to evaluate patients with a nonpalpable testis. MRI is better to evaluate retroperitoneal testis.[278,279] Anorchia occurs in only 4% of cases, and surgical exploration should be performed even if the testis is not seen with ultrasound or MRI.

ULTRASOUND EXAMINATION OF THE PENIS

US examination of the penis is a fast, noninvasive method for examining many penile disorders. Peyronie's disease, trauma, and congenital anomalies can all be evaluated. The addition of duplex Doppler and CDU has allowed examination of the physiology of penile blood flow and made it possible to study patients with vasculogenic impotence.

Anatomy

The major portion of the penis is made up of three corporal bodies. Two corpora cavernosa occupy the dorsal two-thirds of the penis. These are the main erectile bodies of the penis. The ventral one-third of the penis is made up of the corpus spongiosum. The urethra occupies the center of the corpus spongiosum. The corpus spongiosum does become engorged during erection but is less important in the erectile function of the penis than the paired corpora cavernosa. The corporal bodies are surrounded by a tough, nondistensible fascial sheath called the tunica albuginea, also known as Buck's fascia. The corporal bodies are made up of multiple sinusoidal spaces that are the erectile tissue and are lined by smooth muscle and vascular endothelium.

The blood supply to the penis is derived mainly from the paired pudendal arteries, which are branches of the internal iliac arteries. Each pudendal artery gives rise to a perineal branch, bulbar artery, and a dorsal artery, before it enters the base of the penis and forms the cavernosal arteries and the dorsal arteries. One cavernosal artery occupies the center of each corpus cavernosum. Multiple small helicine arteries emanate from the cavernosal arteries as they travel through the corpora, and these are the primary source of blood to the sinusoidal spaces. Although the corpora are separated by a fascial sheath, multiple small anastomotic channels are present that allow communication between the sinusoidal spaces of the two corpora cavernosa. The paired dorsal arteries travel in the subcutaneous tissues of the penis superficial to the corpora cavernosa and adjacent to the deep dorsal vein of the penis. They supply the skin and the erectile tissue in the glans penis. Multiple anastomotic channels connect the dorsal arteries with the cavernosal arteries.[280–282]

The venous drainage of the corporal bodies is primarily through emissary veins, which perforate the thick tunica albuginea. They drain into circumflex veins that ultimately drain into the deep dorsal vein of the penis. Drainage of the skin, subcutaneous tissue, and glans penis is via the superficial dorsal vein of the penis.[280–282]

Penile Physiology

Erection of the penis results from relaxation of the smooth muscle lining the walls of the helicine arteries and vascular sinusoids in the corporal bodies. This causes an increase in the arterial inflow to the penis. The progressive distention of the sinusoids increases intracavernosal pressure, compressing the emissary veins against the nondistensible tunica albuginea and causing venous outflow to be decreased, thereby increasing sinusoidal distention. Increasing sinusoidal distention and pressure increases penile rigidity. When the smooth muscle relaxation in the arterial supply decreases, the process reverses itself and the penis becomes flaccid.[281,283,284]

Examination Technique

A high-frequency (7.5- or 10-MHz) linear transducer is used for the examination. A standoff pad may be needed. The patient is supine, with the penis in the anatomic position. Examination is performed in both the transverse and the longitudinal planes. The corpora cavernosa are seen as paired symmetric rounded structures occupying the dorsal portion of the penis (Fig. 6–41). They are separated by the septum penis, which is a prominent hypoechoic band. The echotexture of the corpora is homogeneous. The corpus spongiosum is often compressed and not well seen when scanning on the ventral surface of the penis. Scanning with a standoff pad, scanning from the dorsal surface of the penis, or scanning with generous amounts of acoustic gel will improve evaluation of the corpus spongiosum. The penile urethra can be visualized by distending it with a viscous lidocaine jelly or other fluid. The cavernosal arteries are seen as hypoechoic bands in the center of the corpora cavernosa. CDU is useful to help find these arteries (Fig. 6–42). The internal diameter of the arteries should be measured with electronic calipers from the longitudinal gray scale image. The dorsal penile arteries are smaller and more easily seen when scanning from the dorsal surface of the penis. The penile veins are also seen better with CDU and from the dorsal surface of the penis.[281,283]

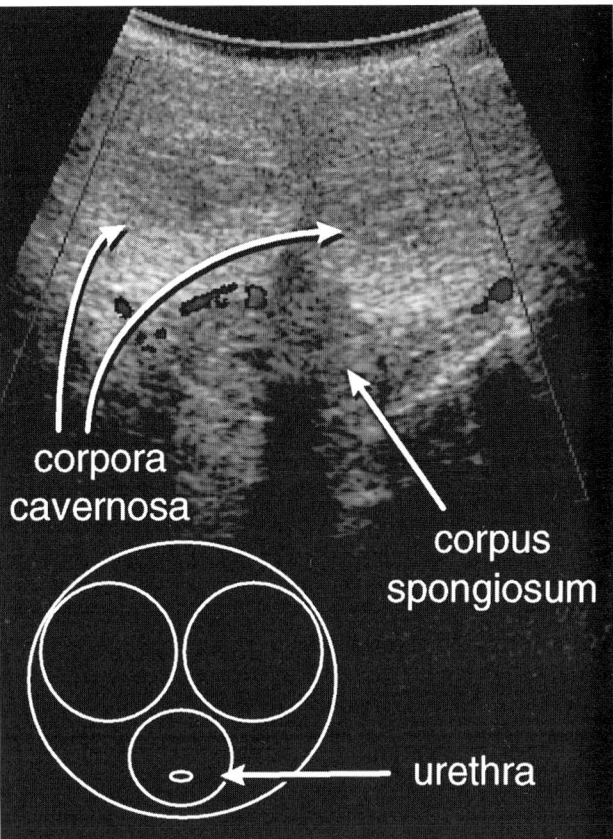

Figure 6–41. Normal penile anatomy. In this axial view of the penis, the three corporal bodies are seen from the dorsal surface of the penis, with the corpus spongiosum inferiorly.

Impotence

Male impotence may have vasculogenic, endocrinologic, neurogenic, or psychogenic factors. Until recently, most cases were thought to be secondary to psychogenic problems, but nocturnal penile tumescence studies have revealed that most cases are probably vasculogenic. Vasculogenic causes can be due to decreased arterial inflow to the penis (arteriogenic) or excessive venous leakage (venogenic). Dysfunction of the endothelium in the sinusoidal erectile tissue with decreased production of endothelium-derived relaxation factor has also been implicated.[285] Penile arteriography with selective internal iliac injection is the gold standard for evaluating arteriogenic impotence. Cavernosography is used to evaluate venogenic impotence.[286,287] Both are invasive and not suitable as screening techniques. Intracavernosal injection of vasodilating pharmacologic agents, including phentolamine, papaverine, and/or prostaglandin E-1, will bypass the normal psychoerotic and neurologic pathways that initiate an erection. The arterial inflow and venous outflow systems must be intact for adequate pharmacologically induced erection. Most investigators believe that if adequate erection occurs, then the impotence is not likely to be vasogenic. A poor response to

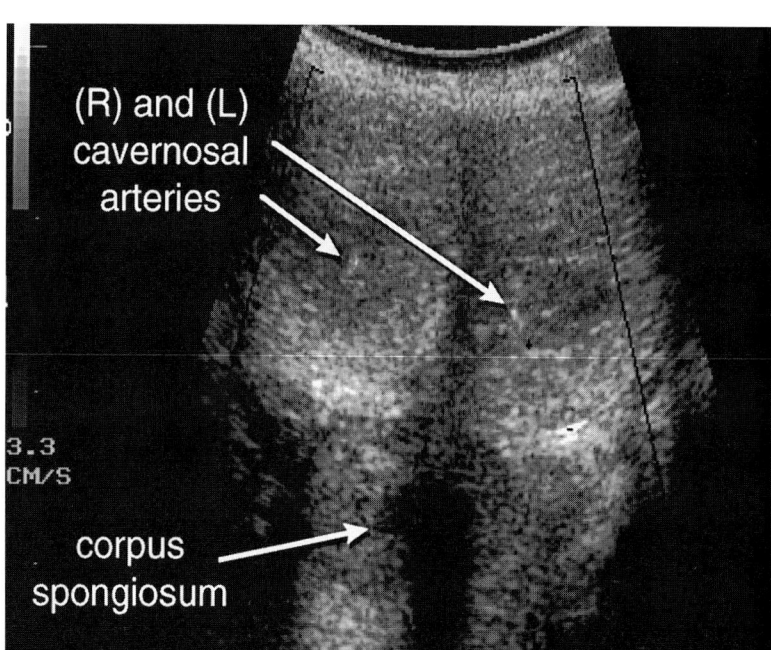

Figure 6–42. Deep cavernosal arteries. Within each corpus cavernosum runs a centrally located artery. Viewed here in cross section, each artery is readily identified as a centrally located focus of color. Quantitative Doppler measurements are generally made with each cavernosal artery viewed in longitudinal section. (See Plate 7)

injection of vasodilating agents indicates that vasogenic abnormalities are the most likely cause of impotence, but it does not differentiate arteriogenic from venogenic impotence. Recently, Doppler sonography has shown good results in evaluation of erectile dysfunction. It is relatively noninvasive and appears to be helpful in separating arteriogenic from venogenic impotence.

ARTERIOGENIC IMPOTENCE

The penis is initially scanned in the flaccid state in transverse and longitudinal planes. Any anomalies, echogenic plaques on the tunica, or inhomogeneous echotexture of the corpora are noted. The diameters of the cavernosal arteries are measured on the longitudinal scans. Next, a vasodilating agent is injected into the corpus cavernosa. Because of the multiple vascular anastomosis between the two corpora, the vasodilating agent has to be injected only on one side, and it rapidly diffuses to the other side. Care must be taken not to inject in the subcutaneous tissues or the corpora spongiosum. Several different vasodilating substances can be used. James uses triple agents consisting of papaverine (4.4 mg), phentolamine (0.15 mg), and prostaglandin E-1 (1.5 μg) in a 0.25 mL solution.[281] Fitzgerald et al use papaverine (60 mg)[284] and Schwartz et al use papaverine (45 mg) and phentolamine (2 mg).[288] The most common complication of vasodilator injection is priapism, which may occur in up to 5% of patients.[281] Patients should be warned of this possibility and should consult their urologist if they have a painful erection or one that lasts longer than 1 or 2 hours. After injection of the vasodilator the cavernosal arteries are again measured and spectral Doppler analysis is performed. CDU is very important because it helps identify the arteries quickly; it allows improved determination of flow direction and accurate measurement of the angle of insonation. The time at which the spectral Doppler analysis should be performed is controversial, but most examine every 5 minutes up to 30 minutes after injections.[281,283,284] Maximum effect can occur early, especially in normal patients, but it can be delayed in other patients. Many patients have maximum response in the 10- to 15-minute period. The peak systolic and peak diastolic velocities are measured with spectral Doppler. Care should be taken to have an angle of insonation less than 60 degrees. This angle is most easily obtained at the base of the penis, where the cavernosal artery changes from an anterior to a cephalad direction (Fig. 6–43). Valji et al and other investigators measure acceleration ([peak systolic velocity − end diastolic velocity]/pulse rise time) and have found this index to be more sensitive than measuring peak systolic velocities.[289–292] The appearance of the waveforms at the various stages of tumescence has been described by Schwartz et al[293] and Fitzgerald et al.[283,284] The arterial waveforms undergo a relatively constant sequence during erection or after injection of papaverine or other erection-stimulating drug. While the penis is flaccid monophasic flow is present with minimal diastolic flow. During the initial onset of erection an increase in both systolic and diastolic flow occurs. With the increase in intracavernosal pressure a dicrotic notch appears at the end of systole with a progressive decrease in diastolic flow. Next, the diastolic flow ceases; then diastolic flow reversal occurs. During the period of maximum rigidity the diastolic flow decreases to zero, and the intracavernosal pressure comes near or slightly exceeds systolic pressure, which causes a decrease in the peak systolic velocity and a narrowing of the systolic envelope.[283,284] The Doppler waveforms

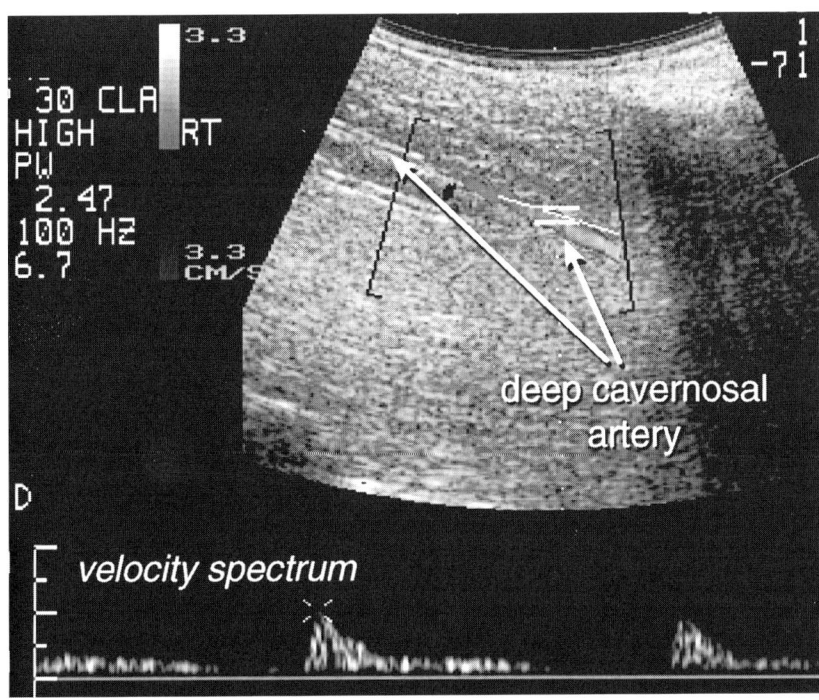

Figure 6–43. Doppler evaluation of the cavernosal arteries. Seen here in longitudinal section, the cavernosal artery is readily identified with color Doppler. Velocity and spectral analyses are made at a point on the artery at which the beam angle favors a strong Doppler signal. (See Plate 8)

obtained during the examination should be correlated with the stage of erection.

Some investigators have evaluated the change in size of the cavernosal arteries after vasodilator injection. Most investigators do not use these measurements because of the difficulty of accurate measurement.[281,283] The most important measurements are peak systolic and peak diastolic velocities. Lue et al[294] found that a peak systolic velocity measurement of less than 25 cm/sec was highly specific for arterial disease. Benson et al[295] felt 40 cm/sec was normal. Despite these differences most agree that a peak systolic velocity of less than 25 cm/sec is specific for arterial disease. Valji et al[289] found that this value is not sensitive and that measurement of an acceleration index of less than 400 cm/sec was much more sensitive for detecting arterial disease. A peak systolic velocity over 35 cm/sec is very likely to be normal, and a value between 25 and 35 cm/sec may indicate a borderline examination and suggest the need for further workup based on the clinical history. Visualization of collateral penile vessels may be a normal variant, but it could also be an indication of proximal arterial disease. Careful evaluation of patients who developed impotence following trauma to exclude arteriovenous or arteriosinusoidal fistulas should be performed.

VENOGENIC IMPOTENCE

Excessive venous leakage from the corporal bodies can also be a cause of vasculogenic impotence. Bookstein has noted that arteriogenic and venogenic dysfunction often co-exist.[289,296] The gold standard for diagnosis of venogenic impotence has been cavernosography. Doppler sonography has been found to be helpful in examining these patients. Immediately following the injection of vasodilators there is an increase in diastolic and systolic velocities that corresponds to the dilation of the cavernosal artery, helicine arteries, and sinusoidal spaces. When the sinusoidal spaces become distended enough to cause compression of the draining emissary veins, the vascular resistance increases and diastolic flow decreases and then reverses. If excessive venous leakage occurs, the intracavernosal pressure will not increase normally and prominent forward diastolic flow will continue. Patients who have end-diastolic flow rates of more than 5 cm/sec despite normal peak systolic velocities probably have venogenic impotence.[297] Fitzgerald et al[283,284] noted the importance of following the patients for at least 20 to 25 minutes after injection because the loss of diastolic flow can occur over a variable period, and terminating the examination after 10 minutes can cause a false-positive for venous leakage. Terminating the examination early also caused false-negative results because in some patients the increased end-diastolic velocity and venous leakage did not occur immediately. Fitzgerald also noted that persistent dorsal vein flow often indicated venous leakage, although occasional flow in the dorsal vein is often normal.[283]

Peyronie's Disease

Peyronie's disease is fibrosis of the tunica albuginea covering the corpora cavernosa. The cause is unknown, but it is thought to represent an inflammatory response or a vascu-

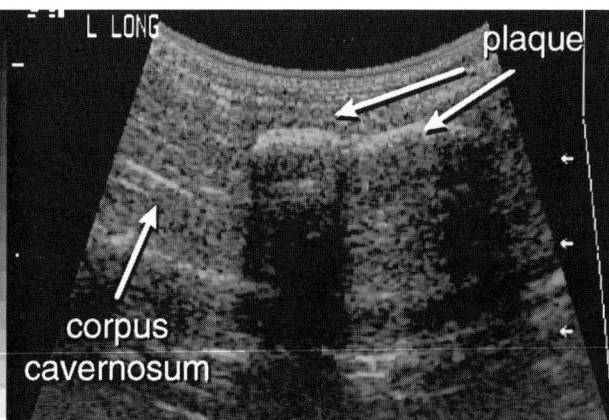

Figure 6–44. Peyronie's disease. In this longitudinally oriented view, scar tissue appears as linear, shadowing plaque at the tunical surface of the corpus cavernosum.

litis. The disease usually involves the dorsum of the penis, but it can involve any portion of the tunica albuginea, including the intercavernosal septum. During erection the penis bends toward the side of the fibrosis, since the involved portion of the corpora cannot lengthen normally. The condition can be painful, and it can be a cause of impotence.[298] Calcification can occur in the fibrous plaques. Sonographically, the plaques are hyperechoic linear structures (Fig. 6–44). Acoustic shadowing can occur. Sonography is useful to demonstrate the extent of the plaques, especially if they extend centrally into the erectile tissue.[299–301] Sonography can also demonstrate plaques that are not clinically palpable and demonstrate that some plaques are larger than expected. Sonography can also be used to follow patients who are treated medically.

Penile Trauma

Trauma usually occurs when the penis is erect such as a forceful thrust after the patient has inadvertently withdrawn the penis during intercourse. This is a common cause of penile fracture. Straddle injuries are another cause of penile and urethral injury. The corpus spongiosum is usually disrupted, and the urethra can also be injured. The injury is usually clinically obvious, but sonography can demonstrate the extent of cavernosal disruption and evaluate the penile vasculature.[302] Arteriovenous and arteriosinusoidal fistulas can also occur after penile trauma; CDU is especially useful in evaluating these patients. Arteriosinusoidal fistulas can cause persistent partial penile tumescence.[302]

Penile Carcinoma

Penile tumors usually involve the distal portion of the penis in uncircumcised men. The tumors often grow within the nonretractable foreskin. Ultrasound is useful to evaluate the local stage of the disease. A stage 1 lesion involves only the glans and foreskin, stage 2 lesions invade the corpora, stage 3 lesions have inguinal lymph node involvement, and stage 4 lesions have distant metastasis.[303,304] Sonography demonstrates the extent of the primary tumor involvement in the corporal bodies. The lesion can appear either hyperechoic or hypoechoic, and the margins are usually well demonstrated.[302]

Penile Urethral Evaluation

The anterior urethra can be evaluated with high-resolution sonography. The urethra is studied when it is distended with fluid or viscous lidocaine jelly. Indications include evaluation of penile urethral strictures, detection and localization of foreign bodies, evaluation of urethral trauma, and urethral diverticula.[303–306] The tissues around the urethra can be evaluated for thickening or fibrosis. The normal urethral lumen is 4 mm or less in size and has a smooth, thin wall. Strictures are demonstrated as segments that are narrowed with irregularity and thickening of the urethral wall.[307] Diverticula of the male urethra are rare and appear as fluid-filled outpouching from the urethral lumen.[306] Sonographic search for urethral foreign bodies should be performed prior to urethral distention because the retrograde instillation of fluid or gel can cause the foreign body to move proximally in the urethra.[307]

ULTRASOUND EXAMINATION OF THE PROSTATE AND SEMINAL VESICLES

Transrectal evaluation of the prostate to diagnose cancer and to facilitate core biopsy for histologic diagnosis has become a standard procedure in the last decade, displacing perineal core biopsy and transrectal fine-needle biopsy. As equipment has improved, so has the ability to extend diagnosis to include conditions other than cancer. Evaluation of the seminal vesicles, vasa deferentia, and even the terminal ureters for anatomic and functional disorder is now possible using transducers primarily designed for the prostate.

Anatomy

The prostate is a glandular organ that encloses the proximal urethra from its origin at the bladder neck to the urogenital diaphragm. It is broader along its base (the bladder aspect) than at its apex. Various anatomic and histologic models of the prostate have been devised. For all practical sonographic purposes, the gland may be divided into the peripheral zone posteriorly and laterally, and the transitional zone centrally. Although other areas may be discerned by ultrasound, this simplification works well because the majority of cancers

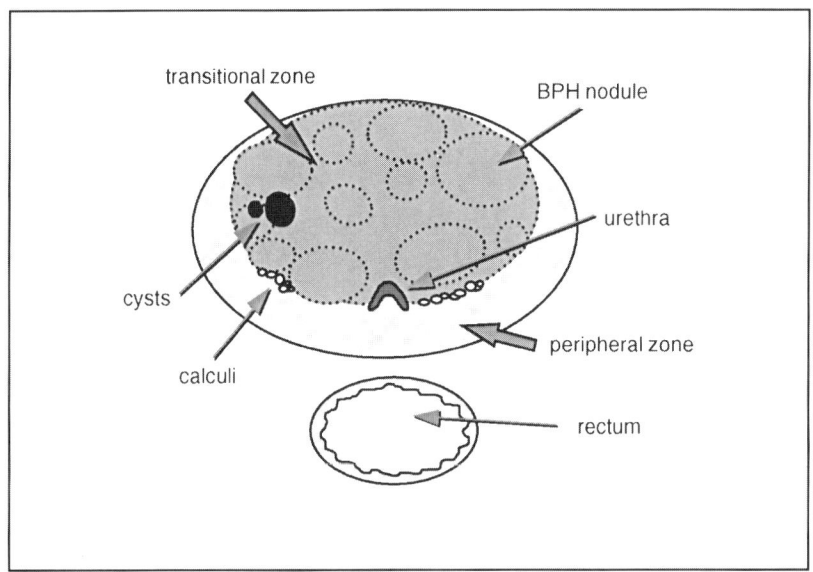

Figure 6–45. Prostate anatomy (axial plane). The centrally located transitional zone enlarges with the nodules and cysts of benign disease. The peripheral zone may become compressed. The urethra may be difficult to visualize.

arise in the peripheral zone, which is well evaluated sonographically. The transitional zone is where the changes of benign prostatic hypertrophy (BPH) occur and, although cancers certainly may arise here, this zone is problematic from a diagnostic point of view. In the younger man, the bulk of the gland is made up of peripheral zone tissue; the transition zone, as such, is not apparent. With the development of BPH in the fourth or fifth decades of life,[308,309] the transition zone enlarges, so that it may come to comprise the bulk of the prostate, with just a rim of peripheral zone visible (Fig. 6–45).

The position of the urethra on ultrasound cuts varies by plane, slice, and condition of the prostate; it is often not possible to define it with certainty on all cuts. The course of the urethra is better seen on sagittal views, although the verumontanum (where the ejaculatory ducts enter the urethra) is generally definable on transverse views, particularly in the younger patient. The left and right ejaculatory ducts curve up to enter the urethra from a medial position at the base of the prostate (Fig. 6–46). These too are often difficult to define and are generally easier to see on the younger patient or if they are obstructed. The left and right seminal vesicles and vasal ampullae enter the prostatic base near its midline. The vasa deferentia may be traced some little way proximally from their ampullae, particularly with forward-viewing transducers. Fluid within the seminal vesicles is readily appreciated and may be seen to flux as the transrectal transducer massages adjacent tissue. A certain variability in ap-

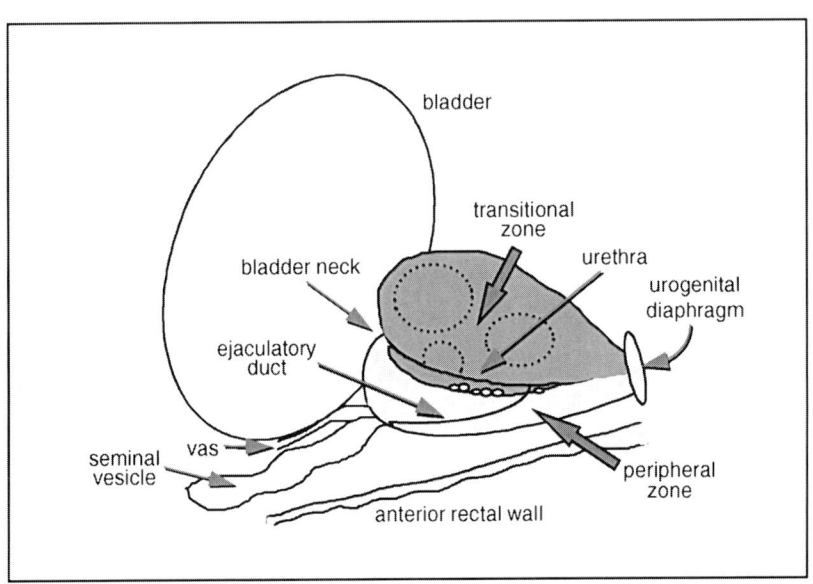

Figure 6–46. Transrectal anatomy (sagittal plane). The bladder neck, posterior bladder wall, terminal ureters, seminal vesicles, vasa deferentia, prostate and rectal wall may all be imaged with a transrectal probe.

pearance of the seminal vesicles is due partly to physiologic filling with seminal fluid and, probably more significantly, to the considerable variability in the amount of periprostatic fat and consequent sonographic access. On longitudinal views, the terminal ureters are often discerned, sometimes with great clarity.

Instrumentation and Technique

Early mechanical transrectal probes that produced 360-degree transverse views gave way to mechanical sector scanners capable of biplanar or multiplanar views. These too have largely been superseded by nonmechanical, linear and curved, phased-array transducers. Multidirectionality is achieved either by an end-fire design, where the transducer array is mounted in the tip of the transducer, giving a forward-looking sector, or by two separate arrays oriented to give switchable transverse and longitudinal views. Each has its advocates but both designs are capable of comprehensive imaging. A transducer frequency of about 7.5 MHz gives excellent detail on all but the deeper aspects of large prostates. Newer transducers are capable of multifrequency operation, permitting deep tissue to be imaged at 5 MHz. Attenuation at 7.5 MHz is less of a problem than it might seem because most prostates are not so large that the higher frequency does not penetrate them, and it is to the peripheral zone of the prostate that the search for cancer is primarily directed.[310] The prostate is examined from apex to base in more than one plane, and the seminal vesicles are included in the survey. Biopsy guides that accept an 18-gauge cutting needle attach to the shaft of the transducer. Depending on transducer design, the guide directs the needle parallel to the shaft or at an angular offset such that the needle passes through the anterior rectal wall just beyond the anus and into the prostate. The distance from first entering the rectal wall to penetration of the prostatic capsule is generally less than 10 mm. Software-generated guidelines overlie the real-time image so that a focus of interest may be aligned for the advancing needle. Different centers employ different biopsy strategies in terms of anatomic site and number of biopsies taken. Where a palpable or sonographic lesion is present, this will be sampled. In addition, random biopsies are obtained from the peripheral zone and, when prior peripheral zone biopsy has been negative for tumor, transitional zone and anteriorly directed cores are obtained. Clearly, the more samples that are taken, the greater the chance of sampling small-volume cancer. Attention to labeling of the cores will help in directing a subsequent biopsy to a site of equivocal cancer. Transient blood per rectum and per urethram are common sequelae of prostate biopsy, as hematospermia may also be. Frank hematoma formation is relatively uncommon and occurs most often in the rectal wall rather than periprostatically. If a rectal wall bleed is noted, 5-minute finger pressure to the rectal wall will generally mitigate against significant hematoma. Appropriate antibiotic cover is initiated prior to biopsy. Routine bowel preparation probably makes little difference to either imaging quality or infection rate. Complication rates are low and transient.[311]

Benign Prostatic Hypertrophy (BPH)

The hyperplastic and adenomatous nodules that characterize BPH form in the transitional zone of the prostate. They are frequently accompanied by cysts and the formation of small calculi. Calcifications typically occur at the junction of the transitional zone and the peripheral zone, the so-called surgical capsule. Cyst formation is quite common in BPH, most commonly present in the transition zone but also seen in the periphery. Sonographically, BPH nodules may be well defined and prominent, or they may be lost within a generalized pattern of areas of hypoechoic, hyperechoic, and mixed echogenicity (Fig. 6–47). It is this variability of pattern in BPH that mitigates against the detection of cancer in the transitional zone. Fortunately, only 20 to 25% of cancers arise primarily from this zone of the prostate.[310] The rich vascularity of the transitional zone in BPH may be appreciated by color Doppler, as may the vessels coursing anterior and lateral to the prostate. These lateral vessels mark the location of the neurovascular bundle within which run the nerves to the penis. Calculation of the size of the prostate is useful in deciding whether a prostate destined for resection for benign obstructive disease should be approached transurethrally or retropubically. Ultrasound measurements of the transverse (d_1), anteroposterior (d_2), and cephalocaudal (d_3) diameters

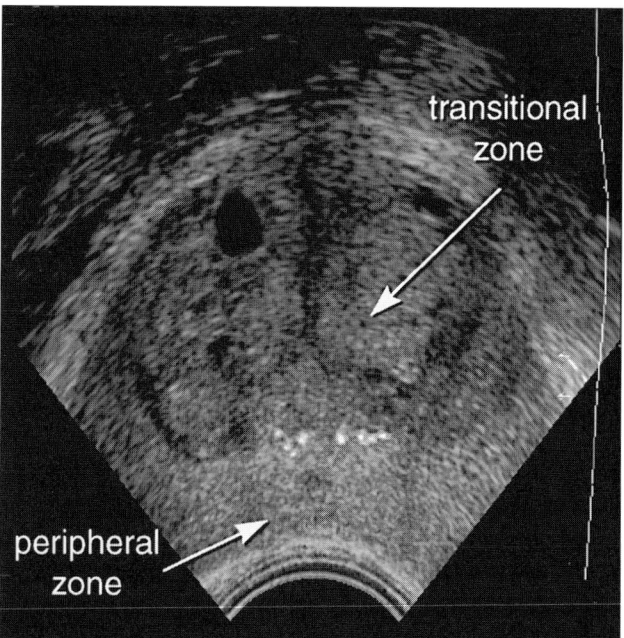

Figure 6–47. Benign prostatic hyperplasia. In this transverse view, the peripheral zone appears homogeneous, but there is enlargement of the transition zone by solid nodules and cysts. Note some punctate calculi at the junction of the two zones.

of the prostate may be entered into the formula for an oblate spheroid ($d_1 \times d_2 \times d_3 \times 0.524$) to give a volume in cubic centimeters or equivalent weight in grams.[312] The volume of the gland is also used in the calculation of the prostate specific antigen (PSA) density (PSAD), where serum PSA is interpreted in relation to the size of the prostate. PSAD is calculated according to the formula

$$\text{PSAD} = \frac{\text{PSA (ng/cm}^3)}{\text{Prostate volume (cm}^3)}$$

A PSAD of 0.15 or greater is considered suspicious for cancer.[313]

Prostate Cancer

In the United States the prostate is the commonest site of new cancer cases in men, with a probability of 1 in 8 of developing invasive disease between the ages of 60 and 79.[314] It is the second commonest cause of death by cancer in men.[314] In 1995, 244,000 new diagnoses of adenocarcinoma of the prostate were projected.[314] The main diagnostic tools are the digital rectal exam (DRE) and the serum PSA. The American Cancer Society currently recommends that all men from the age of 50—or age 40 for African Americans or anyone with a strong family history of prostate cancer—undergo annual DRE and PSA. Transrectal ultrasound-guided biopsy is generally reserved for those men having a palpable abnormality that is suspicious for cancer or for those with an elevated or rapidly rising PSA. The relatively low accuracy of ultrasound alone in detecting organ-con-

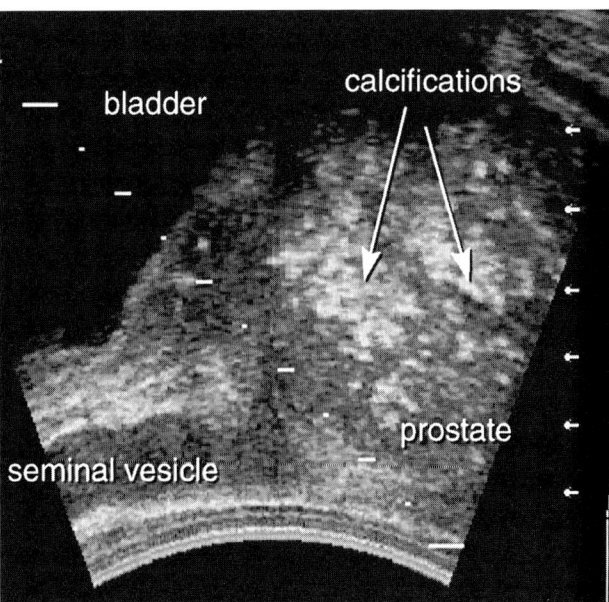

Figure 6–49. Chronic prostatitis. Sagittal transrectal image. Diffuse intraprostatic foci of calcification and fibrosis are common in chronic or resolved prostatitis.

fined cancer,[315,316] combined with the potential economic cost of ultrasound screening, has relegated it to a second-tier diagnostic tool. There have been conflicting reports on the advantage of ultrasound-guided biopsy over finger-guided biopsy of palpable defects,[317–319] with the more recent reports showing no clear advantage for ultrasound. However, when finger-guided biopsy of palpable defects has been negative for cancer but suspicion of cancer remains high, ultrasound-guided biopsy should be performed. For men with an abnormal PSA and benign DRE, ultrasound may detect impalpable cancer,[320,321] and it is clearly useful in guiding random biopsy.

The classic ultrasound prostate cancer is a reasonably well-defined lesion that is hypoechoic with respect to the surrounding peripheral zone.[322,323] There is generally good correlation with a palpable, firm nodule (the classic cancer on digital rectal exam) and the sonographic demonstration of a corresponding lesion (Fig. 6–48). Prostate cancer is often multifocal, may involve right and left lobes, and is extracapsular in approximately 31% of patients at the time of diagnosis.[314] Not all lesions that are firm by DRE are cancers. Foci of calcification are common in BPH and are often seen in chronic prostatitis (Fig. 6–49). Less commonly, a tense, peripherally situated cyst may mimic cancer. Although CDU may identify lesions that are inapparent on gray scale, it does not seem to increase the detection of prostate cancer significantly.[324,325]

The distinction between stage B disease (palpable, organ-confined cancer) and stage C disease (capsular invasion and/or seminal vesicular involvement) is clinically important.

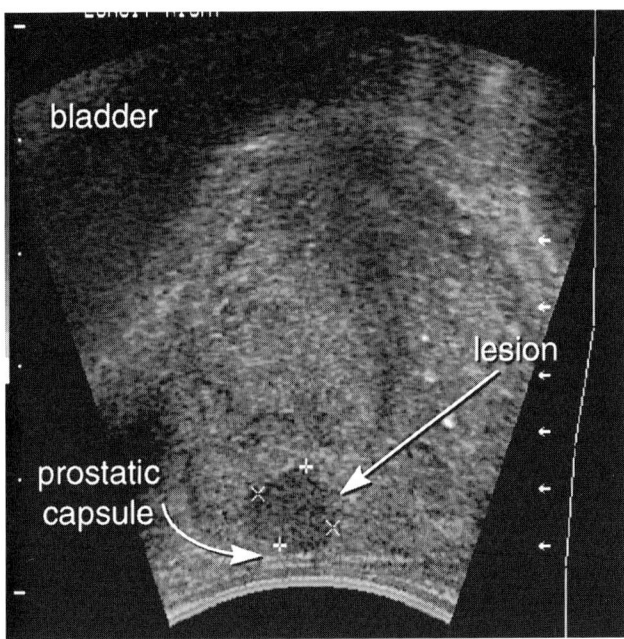

Figure 6–48. Prostate tumor. An easily discerned hypoechoic focus is seen in the periphery of the prostate. This is the classic location and appearance of prostate cancer.

120 Diagnosis of Genitourinary Disease

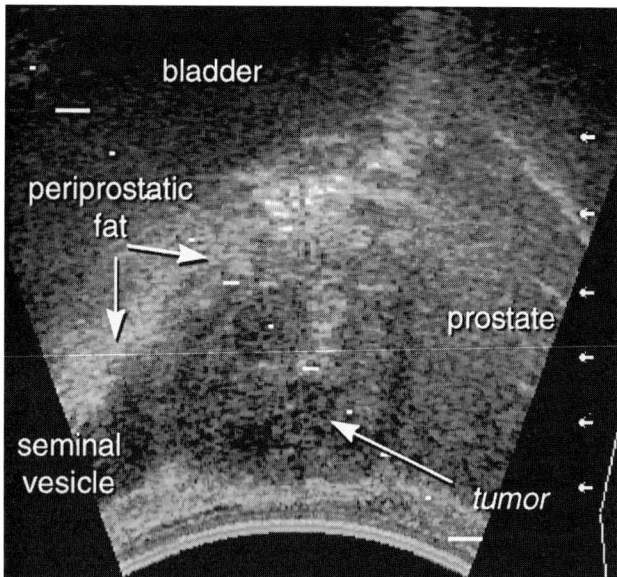

Figure 6–50. Locally invasive prostate cancer. In this transrectal sagittal view, irregular, hypoechoic tumor at the base of the prostate extends to the seminal vesicle. There is obliteration of usual fat planes.

the seminal vesicle insertion, even in the absence of identifiable seminal vesicle abnormality, should raise a strong suspicion of involvement. Many urologists include the seminal vesicles as part of routine prostate biopsy.

Local recurrence of prostate cancer after radical prostatectomy is usually confirmed by ultrasound-guided biopsy of the urethral anastomosis.[328,329] A frank tumor mass may be apparent at the anastomosis or in the anatomic location of the seminal vesicles. Frequently, however, the anastomosis may be unremarkable, and the role of ultrasound is merely to guide a needle accurately to the anastomosis.

Recent alternative treatments for prostate cancer have provided a new role for transrectal sonography. Cryoablation of the prostate, either as a primary surgical treatment for prostate cancer or as a surgical option for patients in whom radiation therapy has failed, requires extensive intraoperative ultrasound.[330] The critical placement of the cryoprobes through the perineum and subsequent monitoring of the ice ball within the prostate are monitored by ultrasound (Fig. 6–51). In similar fashion, transrectal ultrasound hyperthermia of the prostate also calls for transrectal guidance of thermocouples passed into the prostate through the perineum.[331]

Staging of prostate cancer by ultrasound has had mixed reports but is now generally agreed to be relatively inaccurate.[326,327] In practical terms, tumor that causes a distinct contour abnormality at the margin of the prostate is likely to be invading the prostatic capsule. Tumor at the base of the prostate may involve one or both seminal vesicles (Fig. 6–50) and may lead to visual blunting or obliteration of adjacent fat planes. Because the seminal vesicles are readily biopsied by transrectal ultrasound, prostate tumor at or near

Inflammatory Disorders

Acute and chronic prostatitis are conditions that are diagnosed by history, physical examination, and urinalysis. The role of ultrasound is reserved for the diagnosis and treatment of prostatic abscess. As with other parts of the body, the sonographic appearances of abscess vary. An abscess may be frankly fluid-looking or it may have the characteristics of soft tissue and may be difficult to appreciate sonographically (Fig. 6–52). Where visualized, a prostatic abscess may be

Figure 6–51. Cryosurgery of the prostate. In the photo inset, a perineally placed needle is guided to the base of the prostate. As the ice ball begins to form at the tip of the cryoprobe, its edge appears as a hyperechoic semicircle. The ice ball is not allowed to grow beyond the hyperechoic fat just anterior to the rectal wall.

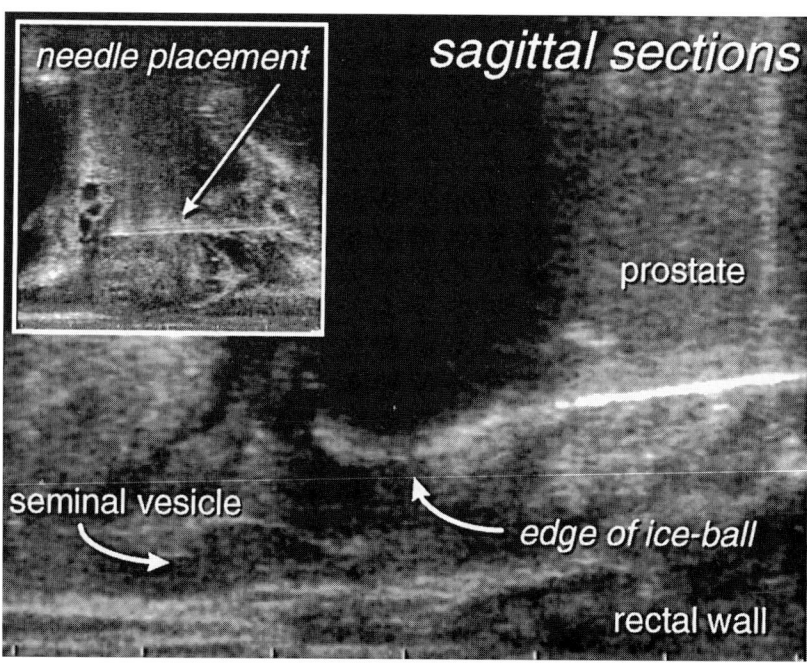

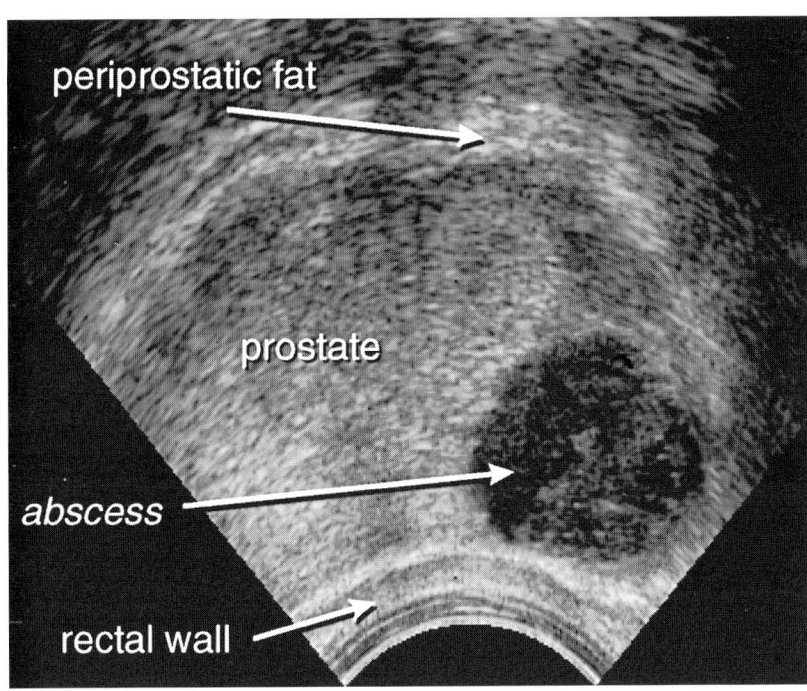

Figure 6–52. Prostatic abscess. Small abscesses in the central part of the gland may be masked by BPH changes. In this example, an obvious semi-fluid area in the left lobe was amenable to ultrasound-guided, transrectal aspiration.

drained by transrectally guided transperineal or transrectal placement of a wide-bore needle, or it may be resected transurethrally.[332]

Infertility

Infertile men with low ejaculate volume may have congenital absence or hypoplasia of the seminal vesicle or obstruction of an ejaculatory duct. Transrectal evaluation of the seminal vesicles is a quick, accurate, and well-tolerated test for these conditions.[333,334] In patients in whom a seminal vesicle appears absent, the ipsilateral flank should be evaluated for the associated condition of congenital absence of the kidney. Obstruction of the seminal vesicle is usually caused by obstruction of the ejaculatory duct, not uncommonly by a stone. A discrepancy in the relative size of the seminal vesicles, combined with a characteristic dilatation of the duct as it points toward the focus of obstruction, should lead to the correct diagnosis (Fig. 6–53). In view of the considerable variation in size and fullness of seminal vesicles, comparative discrepancy of left and right sides is of more value than measurement.

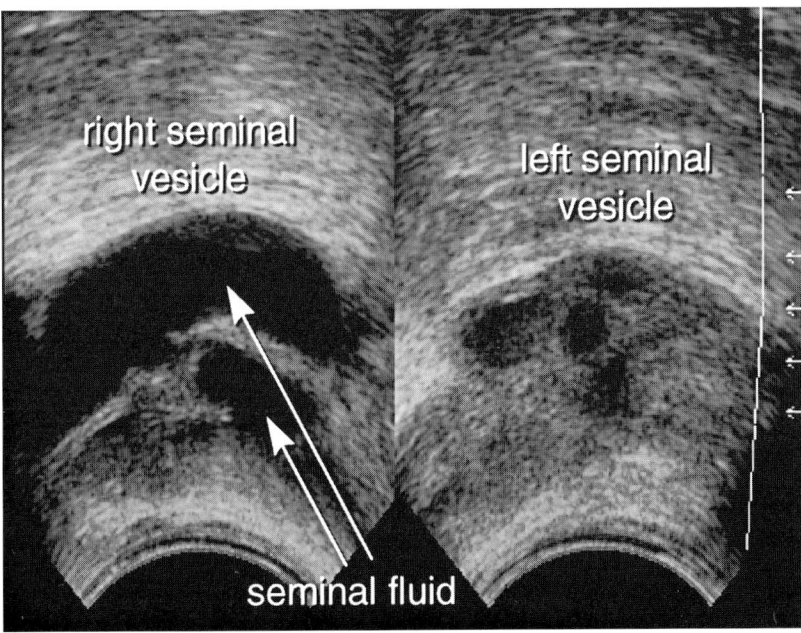

Figure 6–53. Ejaculatory duct obstruction. In this composite, transverse view of the seminal vesicles, the right vasal ampulla (anterior structure) and seminal vesicle (posterior structure) are distended with fluid. The comparison with the normal left side makes the diagnosis easier.

REFERENCES

1. Curry, III TS, Dowdey JE, Murray Jr. RC: Ultrasound. In: Curry, III TS, Dowdey JE, Murray Jr. RC, eds. *Christensen's Physics of Diagnostic Radiology*, 4th ed. Philadelphia: Lea & Febiger, 1990;323–372.
2. Yeh H: Ultrasonography of the adrenals. *Semin Roentgenol* 1988;23:250–258.
3. Hata K, Nagata H, Nishigaki A, et al: Ultrasonographic evaluation of adrenal involution during antenatal and neonatal periods. *Gynecol Obstet Invest* 1988;26:29–32.
4. Kangarloo H, Diament MJ, Gold RH, et al: Sonography of the adrenal glands in neonates and children: changes in appearance with age. *J Clin Ultrasound* 1986;14:43–47.
5. Platt JF, Rubin JM, Bowerman RA, et al: The inability to detect kidney disease on the basis of echogenicity. *AJR* 1988; 151:317–319.
6. Hricak H, Slovis TC, Callen PW, et al: Neonatal kidneys: sonographic anatomic correlation. *Radiology* 1983;147:699–702.
7. Cox IH, Erickson SJ, Foley WD, et al: Ureteric jets: evaluation of normal flow dynamics with color Doppler sonography. *AJR* 1992;158:1051–1055.
8. Baker SM, Middleton WD: Color Doppler sonography of ureteral jets in normal volunteers: importance of the relative specific gravity of urine in the ureter and bladder. *AJR* 1992; 159:773–775.
9. Jequier S, Rousseau O: Sonographic measurements of the normal bladder wall in children. *AJR* 1987;3:566–568.
10. Taylor KJW, Rosenfield AT: US of the kidney. In: Rifkin MD, Charboneau JW, Laing FC, eds. *Ultrasound 1991* Syllabus for categorical course. Chicago, IL: Radiological Society of North America, 1991.
11. Platt JF, Rubin JM, Ellis JH, et al: Duplex Doppler US of the kidney: differentiation of obstructive from nonobstructive dilation. *Radiology* 1989;171:515–519.
12. Davidson AJ, Hartman DS: Imaging strategies for tumors of the kidney, adrenal gland, and retroperitoneum. *Cancer J Clin* 1987;37:151–164.
13. Ferraro EM, Fakhry J, Aruny JF, et al: Prenatal adrenal neuroblastoma: a case report with review of the literature. *J Ultrasound Med* 1988;7:275–278.
14. Heij HA, Taets Van Amorangen AMH, Ekkelkamp S, et al: Diagnosis and management of neonatal adrenal hemorrhage. *Pediatr Radiol* 1989;19:391–394.
15. Wu CC: Sonographic spectrum of neonatal adrenal hemorrhage: report of a case simulating a solid tumor. *J Clin Ultrasound* 1989;17:45–49.
16. Wan YL, Lee TY, Tsai CC: Ultrasonography of adrenal lesions. *J Formos Med Assoc* 1991;90:392–397.
17. Paivansalo M, Merikanto J, Kallioinen M, et al: Ultrasound in the detection of adrenal tumors. *Eur J Radiol* 1988;8:183–187.
18. Thornhill BA, Morehouse HT, Hoffman-Tretin JC: Adrenal and pseudoadrenal masses: CT and US findings. *Crit Rev Diagn Imaging* 1988;28:1–22.
19. Hubbard MM, Husami TN, Abumirad NN: Non-functioning adrenal masses: dilemmas in management. *Am J Surg* 1989; 5:516–522.
20. Silverman ML, Lee AK: Anatomy and pathology of the adrenal glands. *Urol Clin North Am* 1989;16:417–432.
21. Glaser HS, Weyman PJ, Sagel SS, et al. Nonfunctioning adrenal masses: incidental discovery on computed tomography. *AJR* 1982;139:81–85.
22. Hsu-Chong Y, Halton KP, Shapiro RS, et al: Junctional parenchyma: revised definition of hypertrophy of column of Bertin. *Radiology* 1992;185:725–732.
23. Lafortune M, Constantin A, Breton G, et al: Sonography of the hypertrophied column of Bertin. *AJR* 1986;146:53–56.
24. Mahony BS, Jeffrey RB, Laing FC: Septa of Bertin: a sonographic pseudotumor. *J Clin Ultrasound* 1983;11:317–319.
25. Ellenbogen PH, Scheible FW, Tanner LB, et al: Sensitivity of gray-scale ultrasound in detecting urinary tract obstruction. *AJR* 1978;130:731–733.
26. Stuck KJ, White GM, Granke DS, et al: Urinary obstruction in azotemic patients: detection by sonography. *AJR* 1987; 149:1191–1193.
27. Kriegshauser JS, Carroll BA: The urinary tract. In: Rumack CM, Wilson SR, Charboneau JW, eds. *Diagnostic Ultrasound* St. Louis: Mosby Year Book, 1991;242.
28. Kramholtz RG, Cronan JJ, Dorfman DS: Obstruction and the minimally dilated collecting system: ultrasound evaluation. *Radiology* 1989;170:51–53.
29. Goldford CR, Ongseng F, Chokski V: Nondilated obstructive uropathy. *Radiology* 1987;162:879.
30. Naidich JB, Rackson ME, Mossey RT, et al: Nondilated obstructive uropathy: percutaneous nephrostomy performed to reverse renal failure. *Radiology* 1986;160:653–657.
31. Rogers PM, Bates JA, Irving HC: Intrarenal Doppler ultrasound studies in normal and acutely obstructed kidneys. *Br J Radiol* 1992;65:207–212.
32. Bude RO, Platt JF, Rubin JM: Dilated renal collecting systems: differentiation of obstructive from nonobstructive dilation using duplex Doppler ultrasound. *Urology* 1991; 37:123–125.
33. Platt JF, Rubin JM, Ellis JH: Intrarenal arterial Doppler sonography in patients with nonobstructive renal disease: correlation of resistive index with biopsy findings. *AJR* 1990; 154:1223–1228.
34. Fried AM, Woodring JH, Thompson OJ: Hydronephrosis of pregnancy: a prospective sequential study of the course of dilation. *J Ultrasound Med* 1983;2:244–247.
35. Hertzberg BS, Carroll BA, Bowie JD, et al: Doppler US assessment of maternal kidneys: analysis of intrarenal resistivity indexes in normal pregnancy and physiologic pelvicaliectasis. *Radiology* 1993;186:689–692.
36. Laing FC, Jeffrey RB, Wing VW. Ultrasound vs. excretory urography in evaluating acute flank pain. *Radiology* 1985; 154:613–616.
37. Kimme-Smith C, Perrella RP, Kaveggia LP, et al: Detection of renal stones with real-time sonography: effects of transducers and scanning parameters. *AJR* 1991;157:975–980.
38. Erwin BC, Carroll BA, Sommer FG, Renal colic: the role of US in initial evaluation. *Radiology* 1984;152:147–150.
39. Kino W, Kimme-Smith C, Winder J: Renal stone shadowing: investigation of contributing factors. *Radiology* 1985; 154:191–196.
40. Haddad MC, Sharif HS, Shahed MS, et al: Renal colic: diagnosis and outcome. *Radiology* 1992;184:83–88.
41. Glazer GM, Callen PW, Filly RA: Medullary nephrocalcinosis: Sonographic evaluation. *AJR* 1982;138:55–57.
42. Paivansalo MJ, Kallioinen MJ, Merkanto JS, et al: Hyperechoic rings in the periphery of renal medullary pyramids as a sign of renal disease. *J Clin Ultrasound* 1991;19:283–287.
43. Villamora PE, Fabian TM, Schultz EE, et al: Aquired renal oxalosis. *J Can Assoc Radiol* 1983;7:158–160.
44. Shurman WP, Mack LA, Rogers JU: Diffuse nephrocalcinosis: hyperechoic sonographic appearance. *AJR* 1981; 136:830–832.
45. Bosniak MA: The current radiologic approach to renal cysts. *Radiology* 1986;158:1–10.

46. Pollack HM, Banner MP, Arter PH, et al: The accuracy of gray-scale renal ultrasonography in differentiating cystic neoplasms from benign cysts. *Radiology* 1982;143:741–745.
47. Hartman DS, Aronson S, Frazer H: Current status of imaging indeterminate renal masses. *Radiol Clin North Am* 1991; 29:475–496.
48. Bosniak MA: The current radiologic approach to renal cysts. *Radiology* 1986;158:1–10.
49. Zirensky K, Auh YH, Rubenstein WA, et al: Computed tomography of the hyperdense renal cyst: sonographic correlation. *AJR* 1984;143:151–156.
50. Foster WL, Roberts L, Halvorsen RA, et al: Sonography of small renal masses with indeterminate density characteristics on computed tomography. *Urol Radiol* 1988;10:59–63.
51. Amis ES: Cysts of the renal sinus: In: Pollack HM, ed. *Clinical Urography*. Philadelphia: WB Saunders, 1990;1185–1192.
52. Cronan JJ, Amis ES, Yoder RO, et al: Peripelvic cysts: an impostor for sonographic hydronephrosis. *J Ultrasound Med* 1982;1:229–236.
53. Hildago H Dunnick MR, Rosenberg ER, et al: Parapelvic cysts: appearance on CT and sonography. *AJR* 1982; 138:667–671.
54. Levine E, Grantham J: Calcified renal stones and cyst calcifications in autosomal dominant polycystic kidney disease: clinical and CT study in 84 patients. *AJR* 1992;159:77–81.
55. Bernstein J, Evan AP, Gardner KD: Epithelial hyperplasia in human polycystic kidney disease: its role in the pathogenesis of neoplasia. *Am J Pathol* 1987;129:92–101.
56. Rosenfield AT, Lipson MH, Wolf B, et al: Ultrasonography and nephrotomography in presymptomatic diagnosis of dominantly inherited (adult onset) polycystic kidney disease. *Radiology* 1980;135:423–427.
57. Grossman H, Rosenberg ER, Bowie JD, et al: Sonographic diagnosis of renal cystic diseases. *AJR* 1983;140:81–85.
58. Goldman SM, Hartman DS: Autosomal dominant polycystic kidney disease. In: Pollack HM, ed. *Clinical Urography*. Philadelphia: WB Saunders, 1990;1092–1112.
59. Rego JD, Laing FC, Jeffrey JB: Ultrasonographic diagnosis of medullary cystic disease. *J Ultrasound Med* 1983;2:433–436.
60. Avni EF, Thoua Y, Lalmand B, et al: Multicystic dysplastic kidney: natural history from in utero diagnosis and postnatal follow-up. *J Urol* 1987;138:1420–1424.
61. Pedicelli G, Jequier S, Bowen A, et al: Multicystic dysplastic kidneys: spontaneous regression demonstrated on ultrasound. *Radiology* 1986;160:23–26.
62. Jabour BA, Ralls PW, Tang WW, et al: Aquired cystic diseases of the kidneys: computed tomography and ultrasonography appraised in patients on peritoneal and hemodialysis. *Invest Radiology* 1987;22:728–732.
63. Mindell HJ: Imaging studies for screening native kidneys in long term dialysis patients. *AJR* 1989;153:768–769.
64. Anderson BL, Curry NS, Gobien RD: Sonography of evolving renal cystic transformation associated with hemodialysis. *AJR* 1983;141:1003–1004.
65. Levine E, Slusher SL, Grantham JJ, et al: Natural history of acquired renal cystic disease in dialysis patients: a prospective longitudinal CT study. *AJR* 1991;156:501–506.
66. Breton PN, Busch WP, Hricak H, et al: Chronic renal failure: a significant risk factor in the development of acquired renal cysts and renal cell carcinoma: case reports and review of the literature. *Cancer* 1986;57:1871–1879.
67. Taylor AJ, Cohen EP, Erickson SJ, et al: Renal imaging in long term dialysis patients: a comparison of computed tomography and sonography. *AJR* 1989;153:765–767.
68. Mevorach RA, Segal AJ, Tersegno ME, et al: Renal cell carcinoma: incidental diagnosis and natural history: review of 235 cases. *Urology* 1992;39:519–522.
69. Levine E, Huntrakoon M, Wetzel LH, et al: Small renal neoplasms: clinical pathological and imaging features. *AJR* 1989; 153:69–73.
70. Levine E: Malignant renal parenchymal tumors in adults. In: Pollack HM, ed. *Clinical Urography*. Philadelphia: WB Saunders, 1990;1216–1217.
71. Levine E: Malignant renal parenchymal tumors in adults. In: Pollack HM, ed. *Clinical Urography*. Philadelphia: WB Saunders, 1990;1251–1254.
72. Yamashita Y, Matsumarasa T, Watanabe O, et al: Small renal cell carcinoma: pathologic and radiologic correlation. *Radiology* 1992;184:493–498.
73. Forman HP, Middleton WD, Melson GL, et al: Hyperechoic renal cell carcinomas: increase in detection at US. *Radiology* 1993;188:431–434.
74. Yamashita Y, Sukeyoshi U, Oasmu M, et al: Hyperechoic renal tumors: anechoic rim and intratumoral cysts in US differentiation of renal cell carcinoma for angiomyolipoma. *Radiology* 1993;188:179–182.
75. Vale JA, Hendry WF, Kirby RS, et al: Diagnostic and surgical aspects of renal carcinoma with involvement of the inferior vena cava. *Br J Urol* 1991;68:345–348.
76. Shiamato K, Sadanke S, Ishigaki I, et al: Intratumoral blood flow: evaluation with color Doppler echography. *Radiology* 1987;165:683–685.
77. Taylor KJW, Ramos I, Carter D, et al: Correlation of Doppler US tumor signals with neovascular morphologic features. *Radiology* 1988;166:57–62.
78. Kier R, Taylor KJW, Feyock AL, et al: Renal masses: characterization with Doppler US. *Radiology* 1990;176:703–707.
79. Dubbins PA, Wells I: Renal cell carcinoma: duplex Doppler evaluation. *Br J Radiol* 1986;59:231–236.
80. Richmond JJ, Sherman RS, Dearmond HD, et al: Renal lesions associated with malignant lymphoma. *Am J Med* 1962; 32:184–207.
81. Hartman DS, Davis LJ, Goldman SM, et al: Renal lymphoma: radiologic pathologic correlation in 21 cases. *Radiology* 1982;164:759–766.
82. Gash JR, Zagorra RJ, Dyer RB: Imaging features of infiltrating renal lesions. *Crit Rev Diagn Imag* 1991;33:293–310.
83. Green D, Carroll BA: Ultrasound of renal failure. In: Hricak H, ed. *Clinics in Ultrasound*. Vol 18. New York: Churchill Livingstone, 1986;55–58.
84. Grant DC, Dee GJ, Yoder IC, et al: Sonography of transitional cell carcinoma of the renal pelvis. *Urol Radiol* 1986;8:1–5.
85. Yousum DM, Gatewood OMB, Goldman SM, et al: Synchronous and metachronous transitional cell carcinoma of the urinary tract: prevalence incidence and radiographic detection. *Radiology* 1988;167:613–618.
86. Hartman DS, Goldman SM, Friedman AC, et al: Angiomyolipoma: ultrasonic pathologic correlation. *Radiology* 1981; 139:451–458.
87. Chonko AM, Weiss SM, Stein JH, et al: Renal involvement with tuberous sclerosis. *Am J Med* 1974;56:124–127.
88. Arenson AM, Graham RT, Shaw P, et al: Angiomyolipoma of the kidney extending into the inferior vena cava: sonographic and CT findings. *AJR* 1988;151:1159–1161.
89. Zappasodi F, Sanna G, Fiorentini G, et al: Small hyperechoic nodules of the renal parenchyma. *J Clin Ultrasound* 1985; 13:321–324.
90. Charboneau JW, Hattery RR, Ernst EC, et al: Spectrum of sonographic findings in 125 renal masses other than benign cysts. *AJR* 1983;140:87–94.

91. Goiney RC, Goldenberg C, Cooperberg PL, et al: Renal oncocytoma: sonographic analysis of 14 cases. *AJR* 1984; 143:1001–1004.
92. Ball DS, Friedman AC, Hartman DS, et al: Scar sign of renal oncocytoma: magnetic resonance imaging appearance and lack of specificity. *Urol Radiol* 1986;8:46–48.
93. Banner MP, Pollack HP, Chatten J, et al: Multilocular renal cysts: radiologic pathologic correlation. *AJR* 1981;136:239–247.
94. Feldberg MAM, VanWaes PFGM: Multilocular cystic renal cell carcinoma. *AJR* 1982;138:953–955.
95. Piccirillo M, Rigsby CM, Rosenfield AT: Sonography of renal inflammatory disease. *Urol Radiol* 1987;9:66–78.
96. Johnson JR, Vincent LM, Wang K, et al: Renal ultrasonographic correlates of acute pyelonephritis. *Clin Infect Dis* 1992;14:15–22.
97. Rigsby CM, Rosenfield AT, Glickman MG, et al: Hemorrhagic focal bacterial nephritis: findings on gray-scale sonography and computed tomography. *AJR* 1986;146:1173–1177.
98. Kuligowska E, Newman B, White SJ, et al: Interventional ultrasound in detection and treatment of renal inflammatory disease. *Radiology* 1983;147:521–526.
99. Golomb J, Solomon A, Peer G: Bilateral metachronous xanthogranulomatous pyelonephritis and end stage renal failure. *Urol Radiol* 1986;8:95–97.
100. Subrumanyam, BR. Megibow AJ, Raghavendra N, et al: Diffuse xanthogranulomatous pyelonephritis: analysis by computed tomography and sonography. *Urol Radiol* 1982;4:5–9.
101. Charboneau JW, Hattery RR, Williamson JR, et al: Malacoplakia of the urinary tract and renal parenchymal involvement. *Urol Radiol* 1980;2:89–93.
102. Gold RP, McClennen BL, Kenney PJ, et al: Renal inflammation. In: Pollack HM, ed. *Clinical Urography*. Philadelphia: WB Saunders, 1990;835.
103. Gold RP, McClennen BL, Kenney PJ, et al: Renal inflammation. In: Pollack HM, ed. *Clinical Urography*. Philadelphia: WB Saunders, 1990;836–838.
104. Gold RP, McClennen BL, Kenney PJ, et al: Renal inflammation. In: Pollack HM, ed. *Clinical Urography*. Philadelphia: WB Saunders, 1990;838–840.
105. Gold RP, McClennen BL, Kenney PJ, et al: Renal inflammation. In: Pollack HM, ed. *Clinical Urography*. Philadelphia: WB Saunders, 1990;840–842.
106. Kay CJ, Rosenfield AT, Taylor KJW, et al: Ultrasonographic characteristics of chronic atrophic pyelonephritis. *AJR* 1979; 132:47–49.
107. Premkumar A. Lattimer J, Newhouse JH: Computed tomography and sonography in advanced urinary tract tuberculosis. *AJR* 1987;148:65–69.
108. Stuck KJ, Silverton TM, Jaffee MH: Sonographic demonstration of renal fungal balls. *Radiology* 1981;142:473–474.
109. Miller FH, Parikh S, Gore R, et al: Renal manifestations of AIDS. *Radiographics* 1993;13:587–596.
110. Hamper UM, Goldblum LE, Hutchins GM, et al: Renal involvement in AIDS: sonographic pathologic correlation. *AJR* 1988;150:1321–1325.
111. Lesoos I, Thomas RG: The value of ultrasound in the diagnosis of renal failure. *Br J Urol* 1986;58:358–360.
112. Paivansola M, Huttunen K, Suramo I: Ultrasonographic findings in renal parenchymal diseases. *Scand J Urol Nephrol* 1985;19:119–123.
113. Kohler TR, Zierler RE, Martin RL, et al: Noninvasive diagnosis of renal artery stenosis by ultrasonic duplex scanning. *J Vasc Surg* 1986;4:450–452.
114. Desberg AL, Pauscter DM, Lammont GK, et al: Renal artery stenosis: evaluation with color Doppler flow imaging. *Radiology* 1990;177:749–753.
115. Handa N, Fukanaga R, Etani H, et al: Efficacy of echo-Doppler examination in the evaluation of renovascular disease. *Ultrasound Med Biol* 1988;14:1–5.
116. Patriquin HB, Lafortune M, Jeguire JC; et al: Stenosis of the renal art: assessment of the slowed systole in the downstream circulation with Doppler sonography. *Radiology* 1992; 184:479–485.
117. Vaughn TJ, Barry WF, Jeffords DL, et al: Renal artery aneurysms and hypertension. *Radiology* 1971;99:287–293.
118. Takebayahi S, Aida N, Matsui K: Arteriovenous malformations of the kidneys: diagnosis and follow-up with color Doppler sonography in six patients. *AJR* 1991;157:991–995.
119. Braun B, Weilmann LS, Weigand W: Ultrasonographic demonstration of renal vein thrombosis. *Radiology* 1981; 138:157–158.
120. Rosenfield AT, Xeman RK, Cronan JJ, et al: Ultrasound in experimental and clinical renal vein thrombosis. *Radiology* 1980;137:735–741.
121. Reuther G, Wanjura D, Bauer H: Acute renal vein thrombosis in renal allografts: detection with duplex Doppler ultrasound. *Radiology* 1989;170:557–558.
122. Laplante S, Patriquin HB, Robitaille P, et al: Renal vein thrombosis in children: evidence of early flow recovery with Doppler US. *Radiology* 1993;189:37–42.
123. Dodd GD, Tublin ET, Shah A, et al: Imaging of vascular complications associated with renal transplants. *AJR* 157:449–459.
124. Letourneau JG, Day DL, Feinberg SB: Ultrasound and computed tomographic evaluation of renal transplantation. *Radiol Clin North Am* 1987;25:267–279.
125. Coyne SC, Walsh JW, Tisnado J, et al: Surgically correctable renal transplant complications: an integrated clinical and radiologic approach. *AJR* 1981;136:1113–1119.
126. Becker JA: The role of radiology in evaluation of the failing renal transplantation. *Radiol Clin North Am* 1991;29:511–526.
127. Silver TM, Campbell D, Wicks JD, et al: Peritransplant fluid collections. *Radiology* 1981;138:145–151.
128. Kriegshauser JS, Carroll BA: Diagnostic ultrasound. In: Rumack CM, Wilson SR, Charboneau JW, eds. *The Urinary Tract in Diagnostic Ultrasound*. St. Louis: Mosby Year Book, 1991;251.
129. Becker JA, Kutcher R: Urologic complications of renal transplantation. *Semin Roentgenol* 1978;13:341–351.
130. Platt JF, Ellis JH, Rubin JM: Renal transplant pyelocaliectasis: role of duplex Doppler US in evaluation. *Radiology* 1991;179:425–428.
131. Becker JA, Kutcher R: The renal transplant: rejection and acute tubular necrosis. *Semin Roentgenol* 1978;13:352–362.
132. Genkins SM, Sanfilippo FP, Carroll BA: Duplex Doppler sonography of renal transplants: lack of sensitivity and specificity in establishing pathologic diagnosis. *AJR* 1989; 169:367–370.
133. Kelcz F, Pozniak MA, Pirsch JD, et al: Pyramidal appearance and resistive index: insensitive and nonspecific indicators of acute renal transplant rejection. *AJR* 1990;155:531–535.
134. Taylor KJW, Morse SS, Rigsby CM, et al: Vascular complications in renal allografts: detection with duplex Doppler US. *Radiology* 1987;162:31–38.
135. Buckley AR, Cooperberg PL, Reeve CE, et al: The distinction between acute renal transplant rejection and cyclosporine nephrotocity: value of duplex sonography. *AJR* 1987;149: 521–525.
136. Roberts JP, Ascher NL, Fryd DS, et al: Transplant renal artery stenosis. *Transplantation* 1989;4:580–583.
137. Rijksen JFWB, Koolen MI, Walaszewski JE, et al: Vascular

complications in 400 consecutive renal allograft transplants. *J Cardiovasc Surg* 1982;23:91–98.
138. Snider JF, Hunter DW, Moradian GP, et al: Transplant renal artery stenosis: evaluation with duplex sonography. *Radiology* 1989;172:1027–1030.
139. Palleschi J, Novick AC, Braun WE, et al: Vascular complications of renal transplantation. *Urology* 1980;16:61–67.
140. Jordan ML, Cook GT, Cardella CJ: Ten years of experience with vascular complications in renal transplantation. *J Urol* 1982;128:689–692.
141. Reuther G, Wanjura D, Bauer H. Acute renal vein thrombosis in renal allografts: detection with duplex Doppler ultrasound. *Radiology* 1989;170:557–558.
142. Kaveggia LP, Parrella RR, Grant EG, et al: Duplex Doppler sonography in renal allografts: the significance of reversed flow in diastole. *AJR* 1990;155:295–298.
143. Warshauer DM, Taylor KJW, Bia MJ, et al: Unusual causes of increased vascular impedance in renal transplants; duplex Doppler evaluation. *Radiology* 1988;169:367–370.
144. Tobben PJ, Zajko AM, Sumkin JH, et al: Pseudoaneurysms complicating organ transplantation: roles of CT, duplex sonography and angiography. *Radiology* 1988;169:65–70.
145. Laing FC, Benson CB, Disalvo DN, et al: Detection of distal ureteral calculi with vaginal sonography. Abstract. Chicago, IL: Radiological Society of North America, 1993.
146. Brun B, Sammelgaard J, Christoffersen J: Transabdominal dynamic ultrasonography in detection of bladder tumors. *J Urol* 1984;132:19–20.
147. Vallancien G, Veillon B, Charton M, et al: Can transabdominal ultrasonography of the bladder replace cystoscopy in the follow-up of superficial bladder tumors. *J Urol* 1986;136:32–34.
148. Abu-Yousef MM, Narayana AS, Franken EA, et al: Urinary bladder tumors studied by cystosonography. Part 1: Detection. *Radiology* 1984;153:223–226.
149. Denkhaus H, Crone-Munxebrock W, Hulund H: Non-invasive ultrasound in detecting and staging bladder carcinoma. *Urol Radiol* 1985;7;121–131.
150. Akdas A, Turkeri D, Ersev D, et al: Transurethral ultrasonography, fiberoptic cystoscopy and bladder washout cytology in the evaluation of bladder tumors. *Int Urol Nephrol* 1992;24:503–508.
151. Abu-Yousef MM, Narayama AS, Brown RC, et al: Urinary bladder tumors studied by cystosonography. Part II: Staging. *Radiology* 1984;153(1):227–231.
152. Dershaw DD, Sceer H: Sonography in evaluation of carcinoma of the bladder. *Urology* 1987;24:454–457.
153. Horstman WG, Gorman JG, Mcfarland R: Evaluation of bladder and renal pelvic transitional cell tumors with color Doppler ultrasound. Unpublished data.
154. Lamki N, Ruppert D, Madewell JE. Bladder diseases and imaging methods. *Crit Rev Diagn Imag* 1989;29:13–99.
155. Kauzianc D, Varmeir E: Sonography of emphysematous cystitis. *J Ultrasound Med* 1985;4:319–320.
156. Mainprize TC, Drutz HP: Accuracy of total bladder volume and residual urine measurements: comparison between real-time ultrasonography and catheterization. *Am J Obstet Gynecol* 1989;160:1013–1016.
157. Bis KG, Slovis TL. Accuracy of ultrasonic bladder volume measurements in children. *Pediat Radiol* 1990;20:457–460.
158. Hendrikx AJM, Diesborg WH, Stappen W, et al: Ultrasonic determination of the residual bladder volume. *Urol Int* 1989; 44:96–102.
159. Willot P, McLorie GA, Gilmour RF, et al: Accuracy of bladder volume determinations in children using a suprapubic ultrasonic bi-planar technique. *J Urol* 1989;141:900–902.
160. Massagli TL, Jaffe KM, Cardenas DD: Ultrasound measurement of urine volume in children with neurogenic bladder. *Dev Med Child Neurol* 1990;32:314–318.
161. Patitieli Y, Degani S, Ahorani A, et al: Ultrasound assessment of the bladder volume after anterior colporrhaphy. *Gynecol Obstet Invest* 1989;32:314–318.
162. Stam HJ, Rijst HVD, Bangma BD. Ultrasonic determination of bladder volumes in patients with spinal cord injury. *Int J Rehab Res* 1991;14:256–260.
163. Krone, KD, Carroll BA: Scrotal ultrasound. *Radiol Clin North Am* 1985;23:121–139.
164. Carroll BA, Gross DM: High frequency scrotal sonography. *AJR* 1983;140:511–515.
165. Vick W, Bird KI, Rosenfield AT, et al: Ultrasound of scrotal contents. *Urol Radiol* 1982;4:147–153.
166. Hricak H, Filly RA: Sonography of the scrotum. *Invest Radiol* 1983;18:112–121.
167. Rifkin MD, Kurtz AB, Pasto ME, et al: The sonographic diagnosis of focal and infiltrating intrascrotal lesions. *Urol Radiol* 1984;6:20–26.
168. Middleton WD, Melson GL: Testicular ischemia: color Doppler sonographic findings in five patients. *AJR* 1990; 152:1237–1239.
169. Ralls PW, Jensen MC, Lee KP, Mayekawa DS, Johnson MB, Halls JM: Color Doppler sonography in acute epididymitis and orchitis. *J Clin Ultrasound* 1990;18:383–386.
170. Horstman WG, Middleton WD, Melson GL: Scrotal inflammatory disease: color Doppler ultrasound findings. *Radiology* 1991;179:55–59.
171. Horstman WG, Middleton WD, Melson GL, Siegel BA: Color Doppler US of the scrotum. *Radiographics* 1991; 11:941–957.
172. Ralls PW, Larsen D, Johnson MB, Lee KP: Color Doppler sonography of the scrotum. *Semin Ultrasound CT MR* 1991; 12:109–114.
173. Learner RM., Mevorach RA, Hulbert WC, et al: Color Doppler ultrasound in the evaluation of acute scrotal disease. *Radiology* 1990;176:355–358.
174. Burks DD, Markey BJ, Burkhard TK, et al: Suspected testicular torsion and ischemia: evaluation with color Doppler sonography. *Radiology* 1990;175:815–821.
175. Rifkin MD: Embryology and anatomy. In: Rifkin MD, ed. *Diagnostic Imaging of the Lower Genitourinary Tract.* New York: Raven, 1985;7–26.
176. George FW, Wilson JD: Embryology of the genital tract. In: Walsh PC, Gittes RF, Perlmutter AD, Stamey TA, eds. *Campbell's Urology*. 5th ed. Philadelphia: WB Saunders, 1986; 1804–1817.
177. Rajfer J: Congenital anomalies of the testis. In: Walsh PC, Gittes RF, Perlmutter AD, Stamey TA, eds. *Campbell's Urology*. 5th ed. Philadelphia: WB Saunders, 1986;1947–1968.
178. Bloom W, Fawcett DW: The male reproductive system. In: Bloom W, Fawcett DW, eds. *A Textbook of Histology*, 10th ed. Philadelphia: WB Saunders, 1975;805–857.
179. Behre HM, Nashan D, Neischlag E: Objective measurement of testicular volume by ultrasonography: evaluation of the technique and comparison with orchidometer estimates. *J Androl* 1989;12:395–403.
180. Tanagho EA: Anatomy of the lower urinary tract. In: Walsh PC, Gittes RF, Perlmutter AD, Stamey TA, eds. *Campbell's Urology*, 5th ed. Philadelphia: WB Saunders, 1986;65–68.
181. Stewart R, Carroll BA: The scrotum. Rumack CM, Wilson SR, Charboneau JW, eds. In: *Diagnostic Ultrasound*. St. Louis: Mosby Year Book, 1989.
182. Middleton WD, Thorne DA, Melson GL: Color Doppler ultrasound of the normal testis. *AJR* 1987;152(2):293–297.
183. Harrison RG: The distribution of vasal and cremasteric arter-

ies to the testis and their functional importance. *J Anat* 1949; 83:267–282.
184. Trainer TD: Histology of the normal testis. *Am J Surg Pathol* 1987;11:797–809.
185. Kormano M, Suoranta H: An angiographic study of the arterial pattern of the human testis. *Anat Anz* 1971;128:69–76.
186. Harrison RG, Barclay AE: The distribution of the testicular artery (internal spermatic artery) to the human testis. *Br J Urol* 1948;20:57–66.
187. Fakhry J, Khoury A, Barakat K: The hypoechoic band: a normal finding on testicular sonography. *AJR* 1989;153:321–323.
188. Middleton WD, Bell MW: Analysis of intratesticular arterial anatomy with emphasis on transmediastinal arteries. *Radiology* 1993;189:157–160.
189. Morse MJ, Whitmore WF: Neoplasms of the testis. In: Walsh PC, Gittes RF, Perlmutter AD, Stamey TA, eds. *Campbell's Urology*, 5th ed. Philadelphia: WB Saunders, 1986;1947–1968.
190. Hill MC, Sanders RC: Sonography of benign disease of the scrotum. In: Sanders RC, Hill MC, eds. *Ultrasound Annual*. New York: Raven Press; 1986.
191. Benson CB, Doubilet PM, Richie JP: Sonography of the male genital tract. *AJR* 1989;153:705–713.
192. Rifkin MD, Kurtz AB Pasto ME, et al: Diagnostic capabilities of high-resolution scrotal ultrasonography: prospective evaluation. *J Ultrasound Med* 1985;4:13–19.
193. Schwerk WB, Schwerk WN, Rodeck G: Testicular tumors: prospective analysis of real time US patterns and abdominal staging. *Radiology* 1987;164(2):369–374.
194. Arger PH, Mulhern CB, Coleman BG, et al: Prospective analysis of the value of scrotal ultrasound. *Radiology* 1981; 141:763–768.
195. Tackett RE, Ling D, Catalona WJ, Melson GL: High resolution sonography in diagnosing testicular neoplasms: clinical significance of false positive scans. *J Urol* 1986;135:494–496.
196. Fournier GR, Laing FC, Jeffrey RB, Macanninch JW: High resolution scrotal ultrasonography: a highly sensitive but nonspecific diagnostic technique. *J Urol* 1985;134:490–493.
197. Talerman A, Roth LM: Pathology of the testis and adnexa. New York: Churchill Livingstone, 1986.
198. Jacobsen GK, Talerman A: *Atlas of Germ Cell Tumors*. Copenhagen: Munsgaard, 1989.
199. Mostofi FK, Price EB Jr: Tumors of the male genital system. In: *Atlas of Tumor Pathology*, 2nd series, Fascicle 8. Washington, DC: Armed Forces Institute of Pathology, 1973.
200. Paladugu, RR, Bearman RM, Rappaport H: Malignant lymphoma with primary manifestation in the gonads, a clinicopathologic study of 38 patients. *Cancer* 1980;45(3):561–566.
201. Portalez D, Song MY, Marty MH, et al: Ultrasonographic features of testicular non-Hodgkins lymphoma: a report of five cases. *Eur J Radiol* 1982;2:222–225.
202. Doll DC, Weiss RB: Malignant lymphoma of the testis. *Am J Med* 1986;81:515–523.
203. Moorjani V, Mashankar A, Goel S, et al: Sonographic appearance of primary testicular lymphoma. *AJR* 1991; 157:1225–1226.
204. Damjanov I: Tumors of the testis and epididymis. In: Murphy WM, ed. *Urologic Pathology*. Philadelphia: WB Saunders, 1989;314–379.
205. Horstman WG, Melson GL, Middleton WD, et al: Color Doppler ultrasound findings in testicular tumors. *Radiology* 1992;185:733–737.
206. Setchell BP: The functional significance of the blood testis barrier. *J Androl* 1980;1:3–7.
207. Rayor RA, Scheible W, Brock WA et al: High resolution ultrasonography in the diagnosis of testicular relapse in patients with acute lymphoblastic leukemia. *J Urol* 1982; 128:602–603.
208. Lupetin AR, King W, Rich P, et al: Ultrasound diagnosis of testicular leukemia. *Radiology* 1983;146:171–172.
209. Phillips G, Kumari-Subaiya S, Sawitsky A: Ultrasonic evaluation of the scrotum in lymphoproliferative disease. *J Ultrasound Med* 1987;6:169–175.
210. Stoffel TJ, Nesbit ME, Levitt SH: Extramedullary involvement of the testis in childhood leukemia. *Cancer* 1975; 35:1203–1206.
211. Werth V, Yu G, Marshall FF: Nonlymphomatous metastatic tumors to the testis. *J Urol* 1981;127:142–144.
212. Dahnert WF, Rifkin MD, Kurtz AB: Ultrasound case of the day. *Radiographics* 1989;9:554–558.
213. Grignon DJ, Shum DT, Hayman WP: Metastatic tumors to the testes. *Can J Surg* 1986;29:359–361.
214. Caldamone AA, Alterbarmakian V, Frank IN, et al: Leydig cell tumors of the testis. *Urology* 1979;14:39–42.
215. Horstman WG, Haluszka MM, Burkhard TB: Management of testicular masses incidentally discovered by ultrasound. *J Urol* (in press).
216. Corrie D, Norbeck JC, Thompson I. et al: Ultrasound detection of bilateral Leydig cell tumors in palpable normal testes. *J Urol* 1987;137:747–750.
217. Haas GP, Pittaluga S, Gormella L, et al: Clinically occult Leydig cell tumor presenting as gynecomastia. *J Urol* 1989; 142:1325–1327.
218. Bolen JW: Mixed germ cell–sex cord stromal tumor: a gonadal tumor distinct from gonadoblastoma. *Am J Clin Pathol* 1981;75:565–568.
219. Talerman A: A distinctive gonadal neoplasm related to gonadoblastoma. *Cancer* 1972;30:1219–1221.
220. Hart WR, Burkons DM: Germ cell neoplasms arising in gonadoblastomas. *Cancer* 1979;37:1770–1772.
221. Powell S, Hendry WF, Peckham MJ: Occult germ-cell testicular tumors. *Br J Urol* 1983;55:440–441.
222. Glazer HS, Lee JKT, Melson GL, McClennen BL: Sonographic detection of occult testicular neoplasms. *AJR* 1982; 138:673–674.
223. Moudy PC, Makhija JS: Ultrasonic demonstration of a nonpalpable testicular tumor. *J Clin Ultrasound* 1983;11:54–55.
224. Grantham JG, Charboneau JW, James EM, et al: Testicular neoplasms: 29 tumors studied by high-resolution ultrasound. *Radiology* 1985;775–780.
225. Kirschling RJ, Kvols LK, Charboneau JW, et al: High resolution ultrasonographic and pathologic abnormalities of germ cell tumors in patients with clinically normal testes. *Mayo Clin Proc* 1983;58:648–653.
226. Peterson LJ, Catalona WJ, Koehler RE: Ultrasound localization of a nonpalpable testis tumor. *J Urol* 1979;122:843–844.
227. Belis JA, Post GJ, Rochman SC, et al: Genitourinary leiomyomas. *Urology* 1979;13:424–425.
228. Kasdon EJ: Malignant mesothelioma of the tunica vaginalis propria testis: report of two cases. *Cancer* 1969;23:1144–1145.
229. Warner KE, Noyes DT, Ross JS: Cysts of the tunica albuginea testis: a report of three cases and review of the literature. *J Urol* 1984;132:131–132.
230. Turner WR, Derrick RD, Sanders P, et al: Benign lesions of the tunica albuginea. *J Urol* 1977;117:602–604.
231. Mancilla JR, Matsuda GT: Cysts of the tunica albuginea: report of four cases and a review of the literature. *J Urol* 1975; 114:730–733.
232. Gooding GAW, Leonhardt W, Stein R: Testicular cysts: US findings. *Radiology* 1987;163:537–538.
233. Hamm B, Fobbe F, Loy V: Testicular cysts: differentiation

with ultrasound and clinical findings. *Radiology* 1988; 168:19–23.
234. Shah KH, Maxted WC, Chun B: Epidermoid cysts of the testis: a report of three cases and an analysis of 141 cases from the world literature. *Cancer* 1981;47:577–582.
235. Price EB: Epidermoid cysts of the testis: a clinical and pathological analysis in 69 cases from the testicular tumor registry, *J Urol* 1969;102:708–713.
236. Talerman A, Roth LM: *Pathology of the Testis and Its Adnexa.* New York: Churchill Livingstone, 1986.
237. Buckspan, MB, Skeldon SC, Klotz PG, et al: Epidermoid cysts of the testicle. *J Urol* 1985;134:960–961.
238. Maxwell AJ, Mamtora H: Sonographic appearance of epidermoid cyst of the testis. *J Clin Ultrasound* 1990;18:188–190.
239. Bahnson RR, Slasky BS, Ernstoff MC, et al: Sonographic characteristics of epidermoid cysts of the testicle. *Urology* 1990;35:508–510.
240. Brown DL, Benson CB, Doherty FJ, et al: Cystic testicular mass caused by dilated rete testis: sonographic findings in 31 cases. *AJR* 1992;158:1257–1259.
241. Tartar VM, Trambert MA, Balsara ZN, Mattrey RF: Tubular ectasia of the testicle: sonographic and MR imaging appearance. *AJR* 1993;160:539–542.
242. Janzen DL, Mathieson JR, Marsh JI, et al: Testicular microlithiasis: sonographic and clinical features. *AJR* 1992; 158:1057–1060.
243. Smith WS, Brammer HM, Henry M, et al: Testicular microlithiasis: sonographic features with pathologic correlation. *AJR* 1991;157:1003–1004.
244. Leung ML, Gooding GAW, Williams RD: High resolution sonography of the scrotal contents in asymptomatic subjects. *AJR* 1984;143:161–164.
245. Worthy L, Miller EI, Chin DH: Evaluation of the extratesticular findings in scrotal neoplasms. *J Ultrasound Med* 1986; 5:261–263.
246. Cunningham JJ: Sonographic findings in clinically unsuspected acute and chronic scrotal hematoceles. *AJR* 1983; 141:775–779.
247. Linkowski GD, Avellone A, Gooding GAS: Scrotal calculi: sonographic detection. *Radiology* 1985;156:484.
248. Rifkin MD, Foy PN, Kurtz AB et. al: The role of diagnostic ultrasonography in varicocele evaluation. *J Ultrasound Med* 1983;2:271–275.
249. Wolverson MK, Houttuin E, Heiberg E. et al: High-resolution real-time ultrasonography of scrotal varicocele. *AJR* 1983; 141:775–779.
250. Greenberg SH: Varicocele and male infertility. *Fertil Steril* 1977;28:699–706.
251. Belker AM: The varicocele and male infertility. *Urol Clin North Am* 1981;8:41–51.
252. Nilsson S, Edvinssson A, Nilsson B: Improvement of semen and pregnancy rate after ligation and division of the internal spermatic vein: fact or fiction? *Br J Urol* 1979;51:591–596.
253. Dubin L, Amelar RD: Varicocele. *Urol Clin North Am* 1978; 5:563–572.
254. Dubin L, Amelar RD: Varicocele size and results of varicocelectomy in selected subfertile men with varicocele. *Fertil Steril* 1970;21:606–609.
255. Middleton WD: Genitourinary US: testes and scrotum. In: Rifkin MD, Charboneau JW, Laing FC, eds. *Ultrasound 1991.* Syllabus for categorical course. Chicago, IL: Radiological Society of North America, 1991.
256. Rifkin MD, Kurtz AB, Goldberg BB: Epidymis examined by ultrasound: correlation with pathology. *Radiology* 1984; 151:187–190.
257. Dunner PS, Lipsit ER, Nochomovitz LE: Epididymal sperm granuloma simulating a testicular neoplasm. *J Clin Ultrasound* 1982;10:353–355.
258. Ramanathan K, Yaghoobian J, Pinck RL: Sperm granuloma. *J Clin Ultrasound* 1986;14:155–156.
259. Jarvis LJ, Dubbins PA: Changes in the epididymis after vasectomy: sonographic findings. *AJR* 1989;14:155–156.
260. Horstman WG, Sands JP, Hooper D: Adenomatoid tumor of the testis. *Urology* 1992;40:359–361.
261. Gruber MB, Healey GB, Toguri AG, Warren MM: Papillary cystademona of the epididymis: component of von Hippel–Lindau syndrome. *Urology* 1980;16:305–306.
262. Mittemeyer BT, Barger RE, Borsatti AA: Epididymitis: a review of 610 cases. *J Urol* 1966;95:390–398.
263. Williamson RCN: Torsion of the testis and allied conditions. *Br J Surg* 1976;20:465–476.
264. Skoglund RW, McRoberts JW, Ragde H: Torsion of the spermatic cord: a review of the literature and an analysis of 70 new cases. *J Urol* 1970;104:604–607.
265. Sonda LP, Lapides J: Experimental torsion of the spermatic cord. *Surg Forum* 1961;12:502–504.
266. Cass AS, Cass BP, Beeraraghavan K: Immediate exploration of the unilateral acute scrotum in young male subjects. *J Urol* 1980;124:829–832.
267. Bird K, Rosenfield AT, Taylor KJW: Ultrasonography in testicular torsion. *Radiology* 1983;147:527–534.
268. Jeffrey RB, Laing FC, Hricak H, et al: Sonography of testicular trauma. *AJR* 1983;141:993–995.
269. Lupetin AR, King W, Rich PF, et al: The traumatized scrotum: ultrasound evaluation. *Radiology* 1983;148:203–207.
270. Peters PC, Sagalowsky AI. Genitourinary trauma. In: Walsh PC, Gittes RF, Perlmutter AD, Stamey TA, eds. *Campbell's Urology*, 5th ed. Philadelphia: WB Saunders, 1986.
271. Langman J: Genital system. In: *Medical Embryology*, 3rd ed. Baltimore: Williams & Wilkins, 1975.
272. Elder JS: Cryptorchidism: isolated and associated with other genitourinary defects. *Pediatr Clin North Am* 1987;34:1033–1053.
273. Kogan SJ: Cryptorchidism and infertility: an overview. *Dialog Pediatr Urol* 1982;4:2–3.
274. Friedland GW, Chang P: The role of imaging in the management of the impalpable undescended testis. *AJR* 1988; 151:1107–1111.
275. Rosenfield AT, Blair DN, McCarthy S, et al: The pars infravaginalis gubernaculi: importance in the identification of the undescended testis. *AJR* 1989;153:775–778.
276. Wolverson MK, Houttuin E, Helberg E, et al: Comparison of computed tomography with high-resolution real-time ultrasound in the localization of the impalpable undescended testis. *Radiology* 1983;146:133–136.
277. Weiss R, Carter AR, Rosenfield AT: High-resolution real-time ultrasound in the localization of the undescended testis. *J Urol* 1986;135:936–938.
278. Fritzshe PJ, Hricak H, Kogan BA, et al: Undescended testis: value of magnetic resonance imaging. *Radiology* 1987;169–173.
279. Kier R, McCarthy S, Rosenfield AT, et al: Nonpalpable testes in young boys: evaluation with magnetic resonance imaging. *Radiology* 1988;169:429–433.
280. Tanagho EA: Anatomy and surgical approach to the urogenital tract. In: Walsh PC, Gittes RF, Perlmutter AD, Stamey TA, eds. *Campbell's Urology*, 5th ed. Philadelphia: WB Saunders, 1986;68–70.
281. James EM: Penile US. In: Rifkin MD, Charboneau JW, Laing FC, eds. *Ultrasound 1991.* Syllabus for categorical course. Chicago, IL: Radiological Society of North America, 1991.
282. King BF: Doppler sonography of the penis. In ultrasound

categorical course syllabus. American Roentgen Ray Society, 1993.
283. Fitzgerald SW, Erickson SJ, Foley DW, et al: Color Doppler sonography in the evaluation of erectile dysfunction. *Radiographics* 1992;12:3–17.
284. Fitzgerald SW, Erickson SJ, Foley DW, et al: Color Doppler sonography in the evaluation of erectile dysfunction: patterns of temporal response to papaverine. *AJR* 1991;157:331–336.
285. Saenz de Tejada I, Goldstein I, Azodzoi K, et al: Impaired neurogenic and endothelium-mediated relaxation of penile smooth muscle from diabetic men with impotence. *N Engl J Med* 1989;320:1025–1030.
286. Rosen MP, Schwartz AN, Levine FJ, et al: Radiologic assessment of impotence: angiography, sonography, cavernosography, and scintigraphy. *AJR* 1991;157:923–931.
287. Bookstein JJ, Karin V: The arteriolar component in impotence: a possible paradigm shift. Commentary. *AJR* 1991;157:932–934.
288. Schwartz AM, Lowe M, Berger R, et al: Assessment of normal and abnormal erectile function: color Doppler flow sonography versus conventional techniques. *Radiology* 1911;180:105–109.
289. Valji K, Bookstein JJ: Diagnosis of arteriogenic impotence: efficacy of duplex sonography as a screening tool. *AJR* 1993;160:65–69.
290. Velcek D, Sniderman KW, Baughan ED, et al: Penile flow index utilizing a Doppler wave analysis to identify penile vascular insufficiency. *J Urol* 1980;123:669–672.
291. Meuleman EJH, Bemelmans BLH, vanAsten WNJC, et al: The value of combined papaverine testing and duplex scanning in men with erectile dysfunction. *Int J Impotence Res* 1990;2:87–98.
292. Mellinger BC, Fried JJ, Vaughan ED. Papaverine-induced penile blood flow acceleration in impotent men measured by duplex scanning. *J Urol* 1990;144:897–899.
293. Schwartz AN, Wang KY, Mack LA, et al: Evaluation of normal erectile function with color flow Doppler sonography. *AJR* 1989;153:1155–1160.
294. Lue TF, Hricak H, Marich KW, et al: Vasculogenic impotence evaluated by high-resolution ultrasonography and pulsed Doppler spectrum analysis. *Radiology* 1985;155:777–781.
295. Benson CB, Vickers MA. Sexual impotence caused by vascular disease: diagnosis with duplex sonography. *AJR* 1989;153:1149–1153.
296. Bookstein JJ: Penile angiography: the last angiographic frontier. *AJR* 1988;150:47–54.
297. Krane RJ: Sexual function and dysfunction. In: *Campbell's Urology*. 5th ed. Walsh PC, Gittes RF, Perlmutter AD, Stamey TA, eds. Philadelphia: WB Saunders, 1986;712–713.
298. Balconi G, Angelli E, Nessi R, et al. Ultrasonic evaluation of Peyronie's disease. *Urol Radiol* 1988;10:85–88.
299. Fleischer AC, Rhamy RK: Sonographic evaluation of Peyronie's disease. *Urology* 1981;17:290–291.
300. Gelbard M, Sarti D, Kanfman J: Ultrasound imaging of Peyronie's plaques. *J Urol* 1981;125:44–45.
301. Dierks PR, Hawkins H: Sonography and penile trauma. *J Ultrasound Med* 1983;2:417–419. 24. Schellhammer PF, Gravstald H: Tumors of the penis. In *Campbell's Urology*. 5th ed. Walsh PC, Gittes RF, Perlmutter AD, Stamey TA, eds. Philadelphia: WB Saunders, 1986;1588–1603.
302. Rifkin M: Urethra and penis. In: *Diagnostic Imaging of the Lower Genitourinary Tract*. New York: Raven Press, 1985.
303. McAnnicch JW, Laing FC, Jeffrey RB: Sonourethrography in the evaluation of urethral strictures: a preliminary report. *J Urol* 1988;139:294–297.
304. Gluck CD, Bundy AL, Fine C, et al: Sonographic urethrogram: a comparison to roentgenographic techniques in 22 patients. *J Urol* 1988;140:1404–1408.
305. Merkle W, Wagner W: Sonography of the distal male urethra: a new diagnostic procedure for urethral stricture: results of a retrospective study. *J Urol* 1988;140:1409–1411.
306. Kauzlaric D, Barmeir E, Peyer P, et al: Sonographic appearances of urethral diverticulum in the male. *J Ultrasound Med* 1988;7:107–109.
307. King BF: The penis. In: Rumack CM, Wilson SR, Charboneau JW, eds. *Diagnostic Ultrasound*. St. Louis: Mosby Year Book, 1991;604.
308. Garraway W, Russell E, Lee R, et al: Impact of previously unrecognized benign prostatic hyperplasia on the lives of middle-aged and elderly men. *Br J Gen Pract* 1993;43:318–321.
309. Chute C, Panser L, Girman C, et al: The prevalence of prostatism: a population-based survey of urinary symptoms. *J Urol* 1993;150:85–89.
310. McNeal JE: Origin and development of carcinoma of the prostate. *Cancer* 1969;23:24–34.
311. Desmond PM, Clark J, Thompson IM, et al: Morbidity with contemporary prostate biopsy. *J Urol* 1993;150:1425–1426.
312. Jones DR, Roberts EE, Griffiths GJ, et al: Assessment of volume measurement of the prostate using per-rectal ultrasonography. *Br J Urol* 1989;64:493–495.
313. Benson MC, Whang IS, Olsson CA, et al: The use of prostate-specific antigen density to enhance the predictive value of intermediate levels of serum prostate-specific antigen. *J Urol* 1992;147:817–821.
314. Cancer statistics 1995. *CA: A Cancer Journal for Clinicians* (American Cancer Society) 1995;45(1):8–30.
315. Sheth S, Hamper UM, Walsh PC, et al: Stage A adenocarcinoma of the prostate: transrectal ultrasound and sonographic-pathologic correlation. *Radiology* 1991;179:35–39.
316. Hamper UM, Sheth S, Walsh PC, et al: Stage B adenocarcinoma of the prostate: transrectal ultrasound and pathologic correlation of nonmalignant lesions. *Radiology* 1991;180:101–104.
317. Weaver RP, Noble MJ, Weigel JW: Correlation of ultrasound guided and digitally directed transrectal biopsies of palpable prostatic abnormalities. *J Urol* 1991;145:516–518.
318. Rifkin MD, Alexander AA, Pisarchick J, et al: Palpable masses in the prostate: superior accuracy of ultrasound-guided biopsy compared with accuracy of digitally guided biopsy. *Radiology* 1991;179:41–42.
319. Harris JM, Watson LR, Kolbeck SC, et al: A comparison of digitally guided and ultrasound-guided core biopsy of palpable defects of the prostate. Proceedings of the Mid-Atlantic Section American Urological Association, Southampton, Bermuda 1991.
320. Lee F Jr, Bronson JP, Lee F, et al: Nonpalpable cancer of the prostate: assessment with transrectal ultrasound. *Radiology* 1991;178:197–200.
321. Lee F, Torp-Pedersen ST, Siders DB: Use of transrectal ultrasound in diagnosis, guided biopsy, staging, and screening of prostate cancer. *Urology* 1989;33(suppl):7–12.
322. Rifkin MD: *Ultrasound of the Prostate*. New York: Raven Press, 1988;157–178.
323. Cooner WH, Mosley BR, Rutherford CL, et al: Clinical application of transrectal ultrasonography and prostate specific antigen in the search for prostate cancer. *J Urol* 1988;139:758–761.
324. Rifkin MD, Sudakoff GS, Alexander AA: Prostate: techniques, results and potential applications of color Doppler scanning. *Radiology* 1993;186:509–513.

325. Kelly IMG, Lees WR, Rickards D: Prostate cancer and the role of color Doppler ultrasound. *Radiology* 1993;189:153–156.
326. McSherry SA, Levy F, Schiebler ML, et al: Preoperative prediction of pathological tumor volume and stage in clinically localized prostate cancer: comparison of digital rectal examination, transrectal ultrasonography, and magnetic resonance imaging. *J Urol* 1991;146:85–89.
327. Andriole GL, Coplen DE, Mikkelsen DJ, et al: Sonographic and pathologic staging of patients with clinically localized prostate cancer. *J Urol* 1989;142:1259–1261.
328. Wasserman NF, Kapoor DA, Hildebrandt WC, et al: Transrectal ultrasound in evaluation of patients after radical prostatectomy: Part II. Transrectal ultrasound and biopsy findings in the presence of residual and early recurrent prostatic cancer. *Radiology* 1992;185:367–372.
329. Foster LS, Jajodia P, Fournier G, et al: The value of prostate specific antigen and transrectal ultrasound in detecting prostatic fossa recurrences following radical prostatectomy. *J Urol* 1993;149:1024–1028.
330. Onik GM, Cohen JK, Reyes GD, et al: Transrectal ultrasound-guided percutaneous radical cryosurgical ablation of the prostate. *Cancer* 1993;72:1291–1299.
331. Fosmire H, Hynynen K, Drach GW, et al: Feasibility and toxicity of transrectal ultrasound hyperthermia in the treatment of locally advanced adenocarcinoma of the prostate. *Int J Radiat Oncol Biol Phys* 1993;26:253–259.
332. Kinahan TJ, Cooperberg PL, Goldenberg SL, et al: Transurethral resection of prostatic abscess under sonographic guidance. *Urology* 1991;37:475–477.
333. Abbitt PL, Watson L, Howards S: Abnormalities of the seminal tract causing infertility: diagnosis with endorectal sonography. *AJR* 1991;157:337–339.
334. Kuligowska E, Baker CE, Oates RD: Male infertility: role of transrectal ultrasound in diagnosis and management. *Radiology* 1992;185:353–360.

7 Practical Use of Radionuclides in the Evaluation of Urinary Tract Disease

David Teates, Jayashree S. Parekh

RADIOPHARMACEUTICALS FOR GENITORENAL IMAGING

Genitorenal imaging using radionuclides is attractive because it allows noninvasive and low-risk functional evaluation. The dynamic vascular sequence of the renal area can assess the perfusion, and the static acquisition allows measurement of differential renal function with the aid of a computer. Additional information about parenchymal transit and clearance are also obtained. Renal imaging has come a long way since the introduction of mercury-labeled radioisotopes in the early 1950s. With the advent of technetium-labeled tracers, good-quality pictures are obtained. The wide availability of SPECT cameras and renal cortical agents has made it possible to define renal pathology accurately. In this chapter we will review the commonly used tracers.

Technetium-99m is the most widely used nuclide in nuclear medicine. An ideal renal radiopharmaceutical would be the one that is tagged to Tc-99m, has a high extraction rate, is excreted primarily through the kidneys, and is fairly stable in vivo and in vitro. Several pharmaceuticals are widely available. An excellent review of the renal radiopharmaceuticals excluding MAG3 was done by Chervu and Blaufox.[1] Technetium is produced in the laboratory by elution of a generator containing a parent nuclide, molybdenum 99. The eluate is water-soluble and contains Tc-99m pertechnetate. Pertechnetate behaves biologically and chemically like iodide and is not suitable for genitorenal imaging except for a vascular flow study of kidneys or testes, or for cystograms.

Tc-99m DTPA (diethylene triaminopenta-acetic acid) is the agent that is cleared exclusively by glomerular filtration. Very little is bound to plasma proteins, and that makes it ideal for estimating the GFR. It is available in a ready-to-use kit containing a reducing agent. It is fairly stable in vitro and is relatively inexpensive. It is used routinely to assess renal perfusion and function, and to evaluate hydronephrosis and obstruction in diuretic renography. The usual adult dose is 10 to 15 mCi given as a rapid intravenous bolus. The activity peaks in the kidney at 3 to 4 minutes and appears in the bladder by 5 to 6 minutes. About 3 to 4% of the injected dose is present in the kidneys at 1 hour, and approximately 50% of the activity is excreted in the urine at 2 hours. The kidneys receive a radiation dose of about 0.05 rad/mCi.

Tc-99m glucoheptonate is a multipurpose agent that is also cleared by glomerular filtration. There is some retention of radioactivity in the renal cortex (about 5% at 1 to 6 hours) permitting delayed imaging to look for cortical lesions. It is also used to evaluate hydronephrosis and obstruction. The radiation dose to the kidneys is about 0.1 to 0.2 rad/mCi.

Iodine-131 or iodine-123 are the radionuclides used for labeling ortho-iodohippuran (OIH), which has similar biological properties to para-aminohippurate (PAH), used to measure effective renal plasma flow (ERPF). Hippuran is secreted by the tubules and is filtered by the glomeruli, and its clearance is faster than the previously mentioned radiopharmaceuticals. I-131 emits high-energy gamma as well as beta radiation, thus limiting its dose to less than 400 μCi. Renal perfusion therefore cannot be evaluated. I-123 has a more favorable dosimetry because of its 159-KeV photon and lack of beta, but commercially labeled OIH is currently unavailable in the United States. The radiation dose to the kidney from I-131 OIH is 0.1 to 0.4 rad and is significantly increased in renal failure and obstruction. The thryoid must be protected from free radioiodide by administration of drugs such as saturated solution of potassium iodide.

Tc-99m mercaptoacetyltriglycine, or MAG3, as it is commonly known, has been available for routine use for about 3 years as an alternate to OIH. The images obtained are excellent. Renogram curves are nearly identical to those from hippuran, and vascular sequence can also be obtained with a 10 to 15-mCi dose.[2] The liver is usually visible, and occasionally the gallbladder is as well. The physiologic handling of MAG3 has been reported in a number of articles.[3] MAG3 has higher plasma protein binding and slower plasma clearance than OIH (about 50 to 65%), and for this reason it cannot be used for measurement of ERPF directly. Recently, Eshima and Taylor provided a review of the literature along with some clinical trials.[4]

The kit formulation with MAG3 requires one heating step in boiling water. Pharmaceutical quality control includes use of a small ion-exchange column and several solvents, but the process is simple to perform. Labeling efficiency is high and multiple doses can be drawn and used for up to 6 hours.[5] The advantages of MAG3 outweigh its cost in instances where renal function is poor. In infants with immature kidneys, the renal image with DTPA is suboptimal because of poor renal concentration ability.[6] We use MAG3 routinely in these children. Renal transplant scanning permits the evaluation of perfusion as well as tubular function while identifying other complications such as urinary extravasation, rejection, or lymphocele formation. Taylor et al have compared renal transplant imaging with MAG3 and DTPA and noted the improvement in image quality and diagnostic capability with MAG3.[7]

INSTRUMENTATION

The scintillation camera devised by Hal Anger in 1957 is the commonly used imaging device in the nuclear medicine department. Performance has improved tremendously compared to the original camera. Dual- and three-detector systems are now available and the capability of performing emission computed tomography has improved. The wide availability of fast computers also allows rapid renal function quantitation.

The camera mechanics are composed of a large sodium iodide thallium crystal, which is about 1/4 in. to 3/8 in. thick and about 20 in. in diameter. Rectangular and "jumbo" cameras have larger surface areas. On the inner surface of the crystal is an array of photomultiplier tubes, usually numbering from 37 to 91. The photomuliplier (PM) tubes detect the amount of light produced by the gamma ray interaction with the crystal measuring not only the intensity, but also the location. The PM tubes thus convert the light into an electronic pulse. The pulse height analyzer then amplifies the pulse and distinguishes the primary photons from scatter radiation. On the outer surface of the crystal is a lead collimator with multiple parallel holes separated by septa. The thickness of the septa can be variable (Fig. 7–1). For low-energy radiotracers like Tc-99m, thallium-201, or I-123 (energy around 80–160 KeV) collimators with relatively thin septa are used. Medium-energy collimators are used for In-111 or Ga-67. High-energy collimators with thicker septa are reserved for I-131. Pinhole collimators are used when the imaged object is very small. It gives a magnified image, depending on the distance of the object from the pinhole. Pinhole images of the kidneys can be obtained with DMSA scans to improve the lesion detection but have now been replaced almost entirely by single photon emission computed tomography (SPECT) images. SPECT consists of angular sampling of the data with single or multiple cameras rotating around the object in circular or elliptical orbits. The raw data are then filtered, back projected, and attenuation corrected to be displayed in three imaging planes. SPECT imaging improves the study sensitivity by improving the target-to-background ration and also helps determine the exact location of the lesion.

IMAGING PROCEDURES

Renal Imaging

Imaging is usually performed with the patient lying supine and the camera positioned posteriorly. Supine imaging slows the emptying of the collecting system, but it is difficult for the patient to remain still in the upright position for a long time. Imaging with technetium-labeled compounds consists of a rapid bolus injection of 10 to 15 mCi of activity. This vascular sequence is simultaneously acquired on films by the gamma camera and on a computer interfaced to the camera every 2 seconds for the first 20 seconds. Static images are then recorded every 5 minutes for the next 30 minutes or longer. A postvoid film is then obtained to assess upper tract emptying.

Tc-99m DTPA and MAG3 are cleared from blood rapidly by the normal kidneys. On the vascular sequence, the kidneys are visualized at the same time as the spleen and within

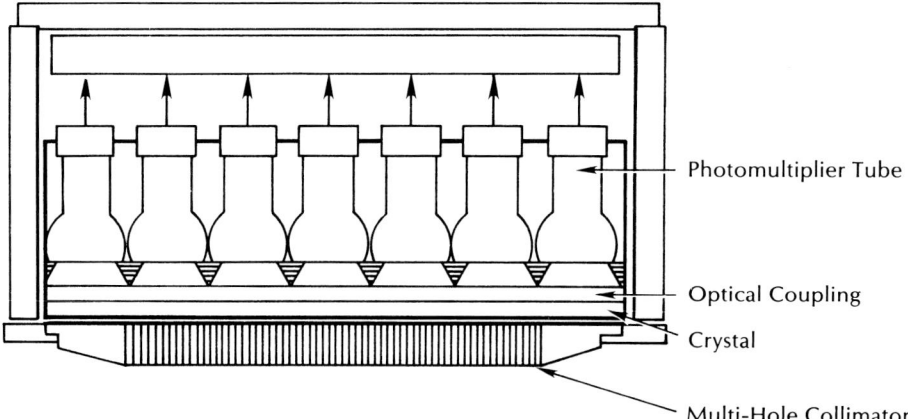

Figure 7–1. Diagram of a cross section through a 37 PM tube gamma camera. The PM tubes detect the amount of light produced by the gamma ray interaction with the crystal, converting the light into an electronic pulse. The pulse height analyzer amplifies the pulse, which is sent to the cathode ray tube. (From Croft BY, Joyce J, Parekh Jk, Teates CD: Nuclide studies. In: Gillenwater JY, Grayhack JT, Howards SS, et al, eds: *Adult and Pediatric Urology*. St. Louis: Mosby–Year Book, 1996; 198. With permission.)

2 seconds of visualization of the aorta. A nephrogram is seen at 3 to 5 minutes with activity seen in the collecting systems shortly thereafter. The bladder starts filling by 5 minutes, and at the end of 30 minutes very little tracer is seen in the kidneys unless ureteral obstruction is present. Delayed imaging is therefore not indicated in most patients. Tc-99m GH and Tc-99m DMSA have delayed cortical accumulation and imaging at 4 hours can assess cortical lesions.

Activity in the kidneys can be monitored by the camera or single system probes (Fig. 7-2). The renogram curve reflects the increasing activity during the vascular phase (phase I), gradual accumulation in the parenchyma and collecting system in phase II, and washout during phase III (Fig. 7-3).

Renal transplant imaging is performed anteriorly since the transplant is located in the iliac fossa. We routinely use MAG3 for transplant evaluation. Fifteen millicuries of activity is injected rapidly. On the vascular sequence, the kidney is seen at the same time as the iliac artery. Data are acquired on the computer for 30 minutes, at the end of which renogram curves are generated and a bladder-to-kidney ratio is calculated. Renal clearance can be estimated based on kidney activity at 2 minutes. Renograms using I-131 hippuran can also be performed to evaluate tubular function. Because the activity injected is in the range of 200 to 400 µCi, vascular sequence cannot be performed. Static images are obtained every 5 minutes for 30 minutes. Thyroid blockade with Lugol's solution or potassium perchlorate is done to protect the thyroid from free radioiodine. Hippuran reno-

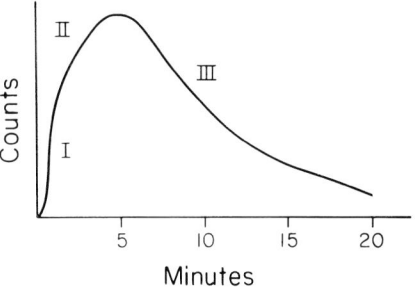

Figure 7-3. Renogram curve showing count rate versus time. The curve represents an ideal curve following OIH injection in a moderately hydrated patient. Phase I is vascular content in the kidney and background. As the kidney extracts the tracer, activity rises in phase II. When the collecting system starts emptying through the ureter, activity falls in phase III. (From Croft BY, Joyce J, Parekh Jk, Teates CD: Nuclide studies. In: Gillenwater JY, Grayhack JT, Howards SS, et al, eds: *Adult and Pediatric Urology*. St. Louis: Mosby–Year Book, 1996; 200. With permission.)

grams have been replaced by MAG3 or DTPA at least in major medical centers.

Renal Function Quantitation

Renal function evaluation techniques can be categorized into 2 main divisions: those that involve quantitation with a camera and those that are nonimaging techniques that require collection of single or multiple blood samples.

Renal function quantitation with a camera is done in the 2- to 3-minute phase of the renogram when activity is localized to the renal parenchyma. Correction of background activity is usually needed to avoid artifactually elevated estimates of function. This is done by drawing crescentic regions of interest (ROIs) laterally at the inferior poles of both kidneys. The computer then subtracts normalized activity from the renal ROIs. The renal function is then expressed as a percentage relative to the other kidney. This method of function assessment is not truly quantitative because it measures relative renal function by comparing one kidney to another. Since the drawing of the ROIs is operator dependent, potential errors may occur by this method and reproducibility may vary. Cortical agents such as DMSA or GH allow delayed fractionation of function because renal tubular binding is present.

Schlegel was the first to describe the method to quantitate renal function using a gamma camera and I-131 OIH.[8] The method for attenuation correction was inaccurate and was later modified by Gates using Tc-DTPA.[9] By the Gates method, the uptake in the kidneys in the first 2- to 3-minute interval after injection was noted to be highly correlative of creatinine clearance. After intravenous injection of DTPA, posterior images of the kidneys are obtained. Pre- and postinjection counts from the syringe are acquired to calculate the exact amount of radioactivity injected in the patient. Attenuation correction for renal depth is then applied and GFR is calculated. Gates found good reproducibility, as well as correlation with the creatinine clearance by this method. The

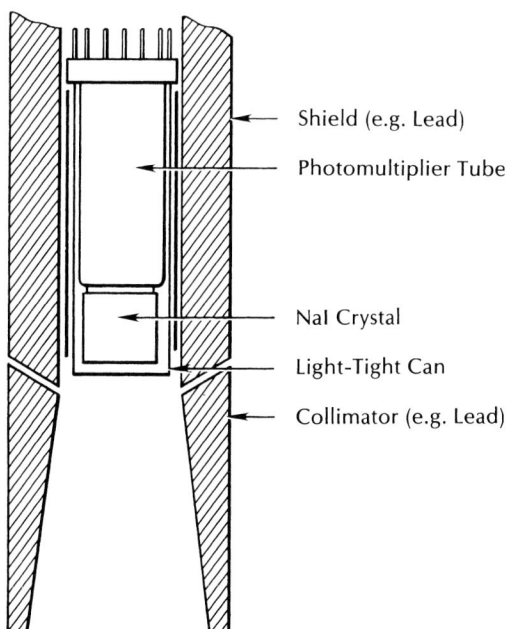

Figure 7-2. Single probe detector. Sodium iodide crystal and the PM tube are shielded by lead to restrict the field of view to a desired organ system. The crystal is enclosed in a polished can to increase the reflection of light to the PM tube and protect the crystal from degradation by moisture. (From Croft BY, Joyce J, Parekh Jk, Teates CD: Nuclide studies. In: Gillenwater JY, Grayhack JT, Howards SS, et al, eds: *Adult and Pediatric Urology*. St. Louis: Mosby–Year Book, 1996; 198. With permission.)

potential advantages for this include ease, rapidity, and lack of a need to draw blood samples. This method may exaggerate the glomerular filtration rate (GFR) in poor renal function because of delayed clearance of the tracer from the blood pool. Varying results have been reported using Gates's technique. Ginjaume et al found very poor correlation, whereas Chachati et al had good correlation with inulin clearance.[10,11] These camera-based methods of renal function measurement have been applied in the pediatric population by Piepsz[12] and Shore.[13] Attenuation correction is less problematic in this age group, as expected.

Nonimaging Renal Function Quantitation

Renal function is measured routinely by creatinine clearance. It is a tedious procedure and requires 24-hour urine collection. Nuclear medicine techniques have been available for a long time to calculate GFR and effective renal plasma flow (ERPF). Accurate renal function determination is essential before giving chemotherapy with nephrotoxic agents and other clinical situations. The nonimaging methods are based on monitoring the tracer kinetics and its disappearance from the plasma by assaying multiple blood samples for radioactivity.

Tc-99m DTPA is used for calculating GFR. Its clearance correlates well with clearance of inulin, iothalamate, and Cr-EDTA. I-131 hippuran is used for ERPF calculation. Several different methods are available for quantitation and are discussed later.

Constant infusion technique is based on the principle that in a steady state of tracer concentration in the plasma, clearance equals excreted tracer divided by plasma tracer concentration. If the plasma clearance is total on each passage through the kidney, then the clearance is equivalent to the flow. Accurate urine collection is necessary and the flow can be calculated by the formula $U \times V/P$, where U is the concentration of the substance in the urine, V is the urine volume excreted, and P is the concentration of the substance in the plasma.

The two compartmental analysis techniques utilize the method described by Sapirstein, where a single intravenous injection of radioisotope equilibrates between the vascular compartment and the extracellular space and is simultaneously excreted in the urine. Depending on the tracer used, either GFR or ERPF can be calculated. In this method, disappearance of radioactivity is plotted against time, and rate constants are determined (Fig. 7–4). This method also requires that serial blood samples be drawn and is time-consuming.

The single-injection, single-blood-sample technique has replaced the constant-infusion technique in many institutions because of its convenience and accuracy. For ERPF, the optimum sampling time reported is 44 minutes,[14,15] whereas for GFR it is 180 minutes.[16,17] Recently, Ham and Piepsz applied the single-sample method for GFR determination in children and found good correlation with a 2-hour blood

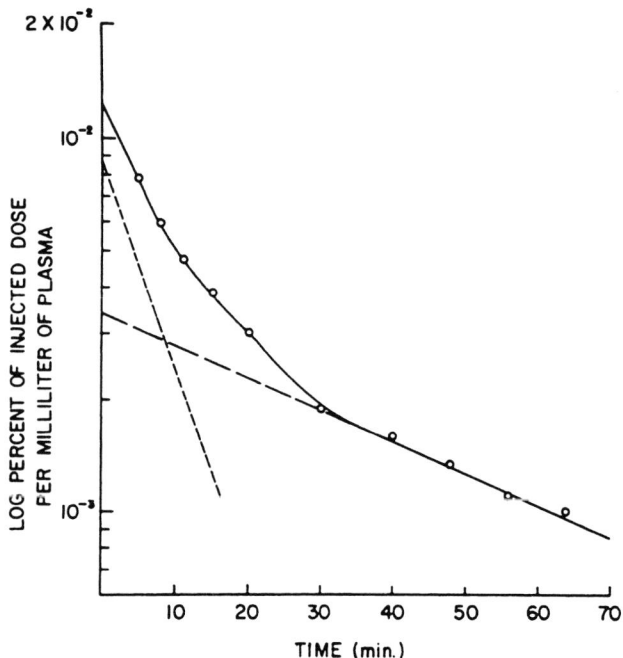

Figure 7–4. The semilog graph of percent of injected dose per milliliter of plasma versus time shows a biexponential functionality. The two exponential parts are shown. (From Croft BY, Joyce J, Parekh Jk, Teates CD; Nuclide studies. In: Gillenwater JY, Grayhack JT, Howards SS, et al, eds: *Adult and Pediatric Urology*. St. Louis: Mosby–Year Book, 1996; 201. With permission.)

sample.[18] This method appears to be ideal in children when multiple blood samples may be difficult to obtain. Several studies are needed to validate these data.

The nonimaging methods for renal function determination are very accurate overall. Nonetheless, they are time-consuming and require special skills for wet laboratory techniques that are typically available only at major university centers. The gamma camera methods do not require blood or urine collection, are quick, and are able to quantitate individual renal function with reasonable accuracy.

Cystograms

Radionuclide cystography was introduced by Winter in 1959 to assess vesicoureteral reflux.[19] About 1 mCi of Tc-pertechnetate is instilled in the urinary bladder via a catheter connected to a bag full of sterile saline, no more than 36 in. above the bladder. If possible, the patient sits on a "potty chair" with the back to a gamma camera and the bladder region in the field of view. Computer acquisition is started at the same time as bladder filling. The volume of fluid entering the bladder is recorded every 30 seconds. When the bladder is full or the patient tolerance is reached, the volume of fluid is noted and a static image is acquired. The computer recording is again stated when the patient voids. The total volume of fluid voided is also noted. Computer images are reviewed to determine time of reflux and extent (Fig. 7–5). This method is sensitive for small volumes of reflux, allows

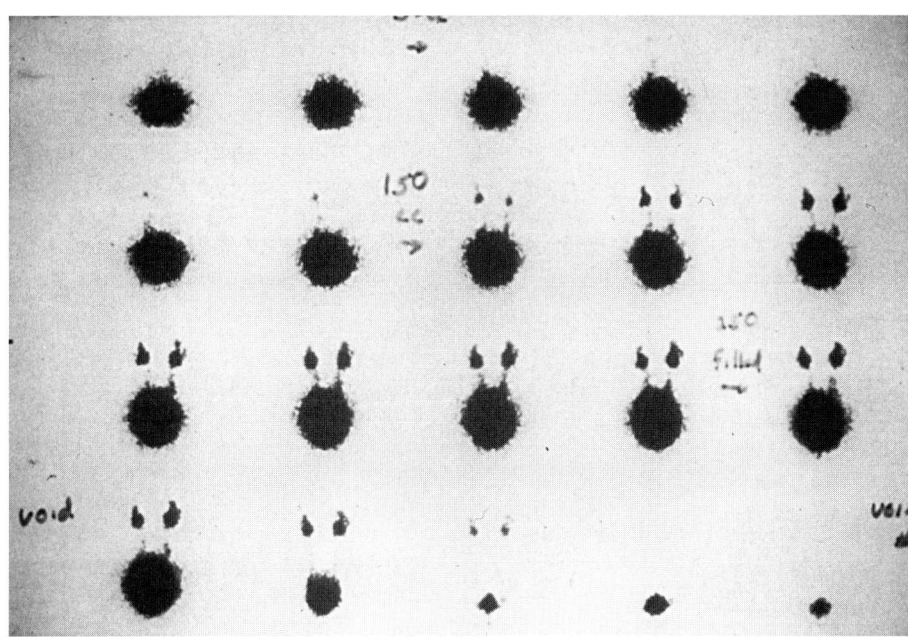

Figure 7–5. Radionuclide cystogram using 1 mCi of Tc-99m pertechnetate and sequential dynamic imaging demonstrates the presence of bilateral vesicoureteral reflux, right greater than left, occurring at a volume of 150 mL.

the measurement of the volume at which reflux occurred, and gives less radiation than contrast VCUG. It can therefore be used as a follow-up study in patients with known reflux and after corrective surgery. The major drawback of this method is its inability to demonstrate anatomic detail of the urinary tract.

Diuretic Renograms

Hydronephrosis of varying degrees may be present because of congenital abnormalities of the urinary tract. It is important to identify obstruction in a dilated collecting system because corrective surgery such as pyeloplasty or ureteral reimplantation may be necessary. Previously, only invasive tests such as the Whitaker test were used to identify obstruction.[20] This test involves percutaneous puncture of the renal pelvis and calculating resistance to flow while increasing the pressure. It was realized that this test had indeterminate readings and was not reliable in large hydronephrosis and complete obstructions, where dilatation may be minimal. It also does not measure function, which may deteriorate in long-standing uncorrected obstruction.

O'Reilly et al described the use of diuretic renography to differentiate mechanical from functional obstruction in 1978.[21] This test has become very popular, especially in the pediatric population, since it is noninvasive and reliable. Quantitative measurement of the clearance half-times ($T_{1/2}$) of the tracer after intravenous furosemide (Lasix) administration is done to evaluate obstruction. The $T_{1/2}$ of less than 10 minutes indicate no obstruction, and those of more than 20 minutes indicate significant obstruction. Values of 10 to 19 minutes are equivocal.

Either Tc-DTPA or Tc-MAG3 can be used for the diuretic renogram. Since Tc-MAG3 use is somewhat limited by cost, it can be restricted to infants with immature kidneys and in patients with poor renal function. Patients can be imaged either in the supine or in the upright position. Sedation is usually necessary in younger children. After a rapid intravenous bolus, static images are obtained every 5 minutes for 30 minutes. Computer data are continuously acquired. Diuretic administration is delayed until the appearance of activity in the renal collecting system. Lasix is given intravenously (1 mg/kg in children; 0.4 mg/kg in adults), and imaging is continued for 30 minutes more. We calculated the $T_{1/2}$ by curve fit to the steepest slope of the responsive curve, usually in the first 15 minutes after injection.

False-positive tests due to prolonged $T_{1/2}$ occur in a number of situations, as mentioned later. Poor renal function causes inadequate diuretic response. In sedated infants, a full bladder may prevent emptying of the dilated upper tracts. Extremely dilated and atonic collecting systems holding large volumes of urine produce longer emptying times. Dehydration also causes slow drainage of the collecting systems. Conway has discussed the technical aspects, pitfalls, and standardized technique for diuretic renography recently because of a number of variations of the technique.[22] Despite the problems listed earlier, the diuretic renogram still remains the initial diagnostic test to evaluate ureterohydronephrosis.

Scrotal Imaging

Imaging is performed after an intravenous injection of 10 to 15 mCi of Tc-99m pertechnetate. An anterior vascular sequence is followed by static images for the next 10 minutes. The scrotum can be supported on a sling and a midline lead marker is used to outline the raphe. Good imaging technique is critical and computer storing of the data adds a margin of filming reliability. Pinhole imaging may occasionally be necessary in infants. Timing of imaging is critical because the image quality deteriorates after more than 10 minutes.

CLINICAL APPLICATIONS IN PEDIATRICS

Congenital Renal Anomalies

HORSESHOE KIDNEY

Horseshoe kidney is the most common anomaly of renal fusion and consists of fusion of the inferior poles across the midline by an isthmus. The isthmus usually consists of functioning renal parenchyma but may occasionally consist of fibrous tissue. The axis of the kidneys is directed downward and medially. The ureters descend anterior to the isthmus and are displaced medially. The renal vessels also pass anteriorly and may occasionally be anomalous. The malrotation and anomalous vasculature make these kidneys prone to myriad problems, including ureteropelvic junction (UPJ) obstruction, nephrolithiasis, infections, and renovascular hypertension. Other associated anomalies are duplication of the upper tracts, reflux, and ureteroceles.

Anterior imaging using either Tc-99m, DTPA, MAG3, or DMSA clearly demonstrates the midline isthmus (Fig. 7–6). The use of Lasix helps determine if obstruction is present in association with caliectasis (Fig. 7–7). Similarly, Tc-99m DMSA SPECT imaging may be performed to assess scarring and clearly demonstrates anatomy better than planar view.

RENAL DYSPLASIA

The multicystic dysplastic kidney is a severe form of renal dysplasia usually encountered in a newborn infant who presents with an abdominal mass. The involved kidney is enlarged and consists of multiple cysts of various sizes with intervening connective tissue. The dysplasia can be unilateral, bilateral, or focal. It is associated with other urinary tract anomalies like ureteral atresia or UPJ obstruction. Histologically, multiple cysts lined with cuboidal epithelium are present. Immature stromal elements, primitive tubules, and glomeruli may be present.

Tc-99m DTPA or MAG3 scan usually demonstrates a photopenic defect in the region of the mass, indicative of a nonfunctioning kidney (Fig. 7–8). Occasionally, a small amount of tracer localization may be seen on delayed images because of the presence of some primitive glomeruli and tubules. However, renal excretion of the tracer is not seen. A similar picture may be seen in cases of severe hydronephrosis caused by high-grade UPJ obstruction. The early images usually show a functioning cortical rim with progressive excretion of radioactivity in the collecting system on delayed images.

HYDRONEPHROSIS AND OBSTRUCTION

Congenital ureteral obstruction is commonly diagnosed prenatally or in a newborn with a flank mass (Fig. 7–9). The obstruction may be unilateral or bilateral, with the latter being more common in males. About 10% to 30% of cases are bilateral. The obstruction may be functional because of deficiency of muscle fibers or mechanical because of stenosis or kinking of the ureter by fibrous bands or aberrant vessels, especially at the UPJ. Ureteral obstruction is also seen in a duplicated collecting system, where the obstruction occurs in the ureter draining the upper pole. Ureteral obstruction is an associated feature occasionally in malrotated and horseshoe kidneys. The obstruction leads to pelvicaliectasis and, if severe, may cause thinning of the renal parenchyma.

A diuretic renal scan using DTPA or MAG3 and Lasix is a simple and noninvasive way of differentiating functional from mechanical obstruction. A dilated nonobstructed collecting system responds to the diuretic challenge by showing a prompt washout of the tracer (Fig. 7–10), whereas an obstructed system shows poor or no washout (Fig. 7–11). It is

Figure 7–6. A 14-year-old child with recurrent urinary tract infections and proteinuria was evaluated with a DMSA scan to assess scarring. Reprojection images obtained after 4 mCi demonstrate a horseshoe kidney with a midline isthmus, with no evidence of scarring.

(text continues on page 142)

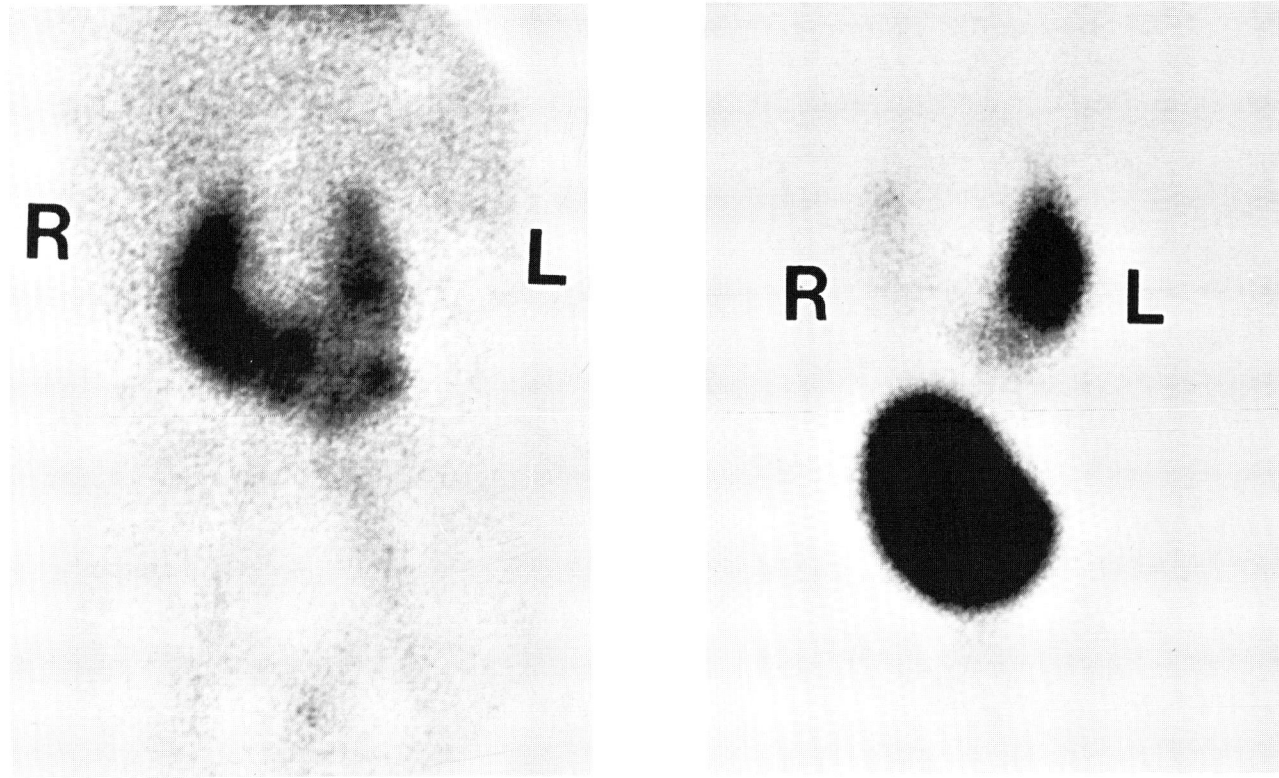

Figure 7–7. A 3-year-old child with a horseshoe kidney and hydronephrosis had a diuretic renogram to evaluate obstruction. Five mCi of Tc-99m DTPA was given and anterior imaging was performed. (**A**) The 3-minute image shows the fusion of the inferior poles by the isthmus. (**B**) After administration of Lasix, there is slow washout of the left collecting system with a $T_{1/2}$ of 17 minutes.

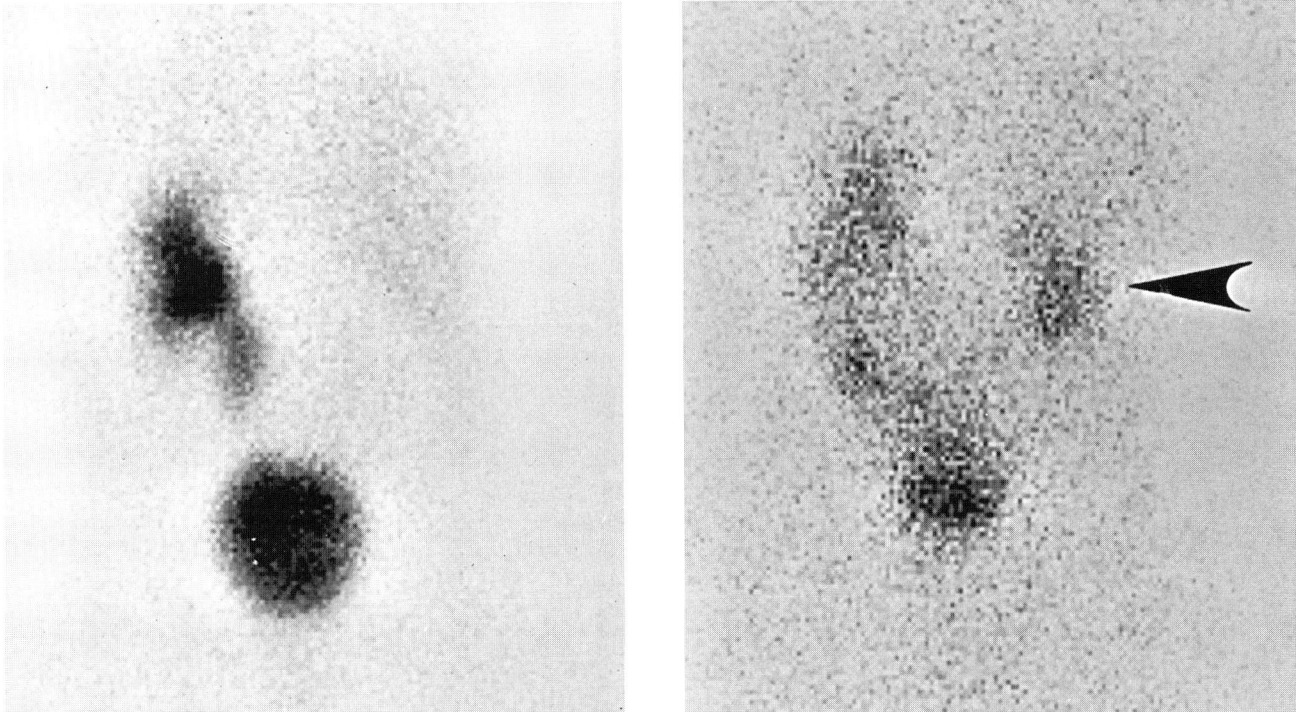

Figure 7–8. A newborn male infant with a right-sided abdominal mass. Tc-99m DTPA scan was performed. (**A**) The 10-minute posterior image shows nonvisualization of the right kidney and a normally functioning left kidney. (**B**) A delayed 4-hour image shows some tracer concentration in the right renal fossa caused by the presence of primitive nephrons.

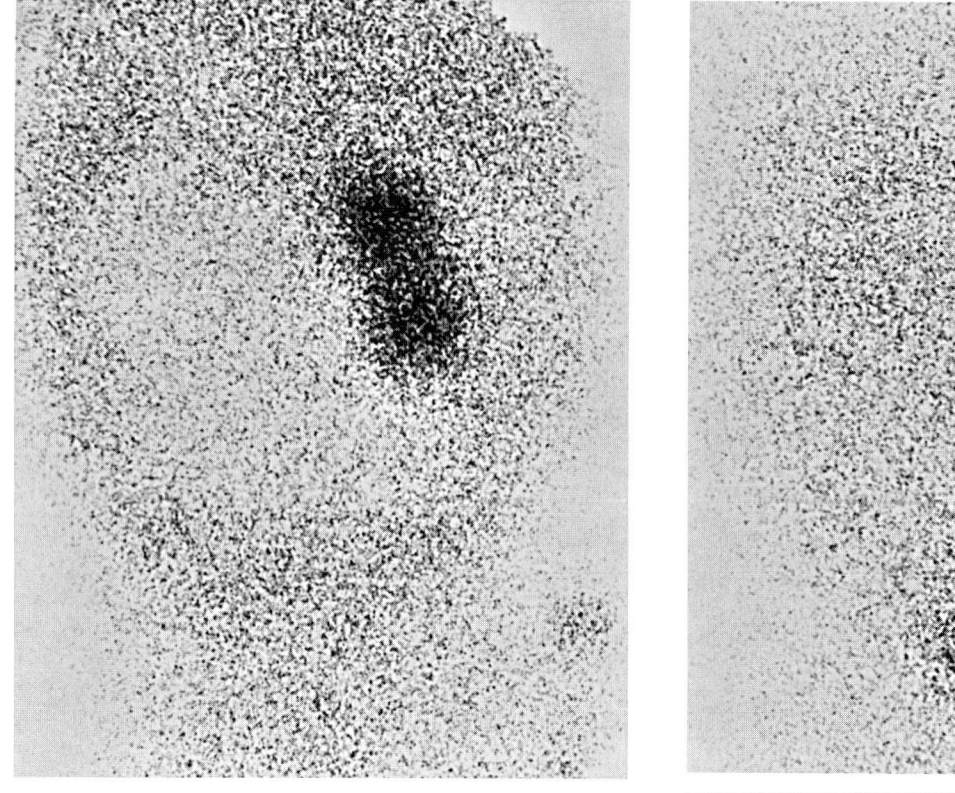
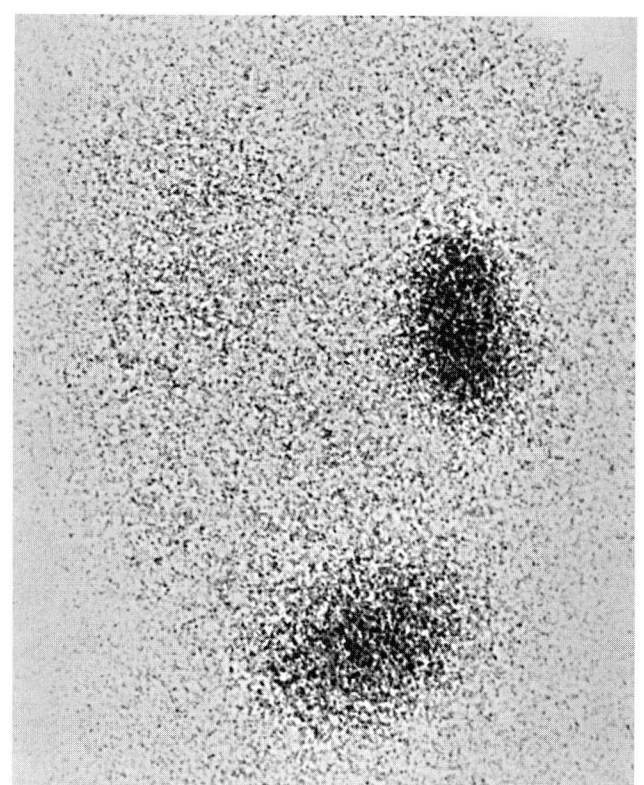
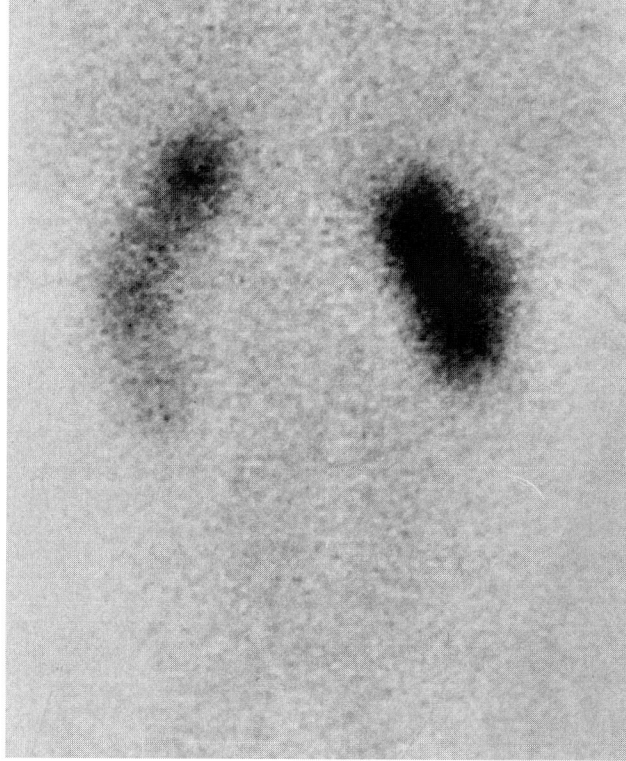

Figure 7–9. A 6-week-old baby girl presented with a left flank mass due to severe hydronephrosis. A diuretic renogram was performed to assess ureteral obstruction. (**A**) Initial 5-minute posterior image demonstrates a large photopenic defect in the left renal fossa, indicating severely reduced function resulting from high-grade obstruction. (**B**) Delayed image after Lasix administration shows some tracer accumulation in the left kindey. (**C**) Follow-up scan 6 months after left pyeloplasty. It shows diminished function of the left lower pole, but overall significantly improved function after the relief of obstruction. High-grade ureteral obstruction can significantly reduce renal function. There is potential for recovery of function if the relief of obstruction is prompt.

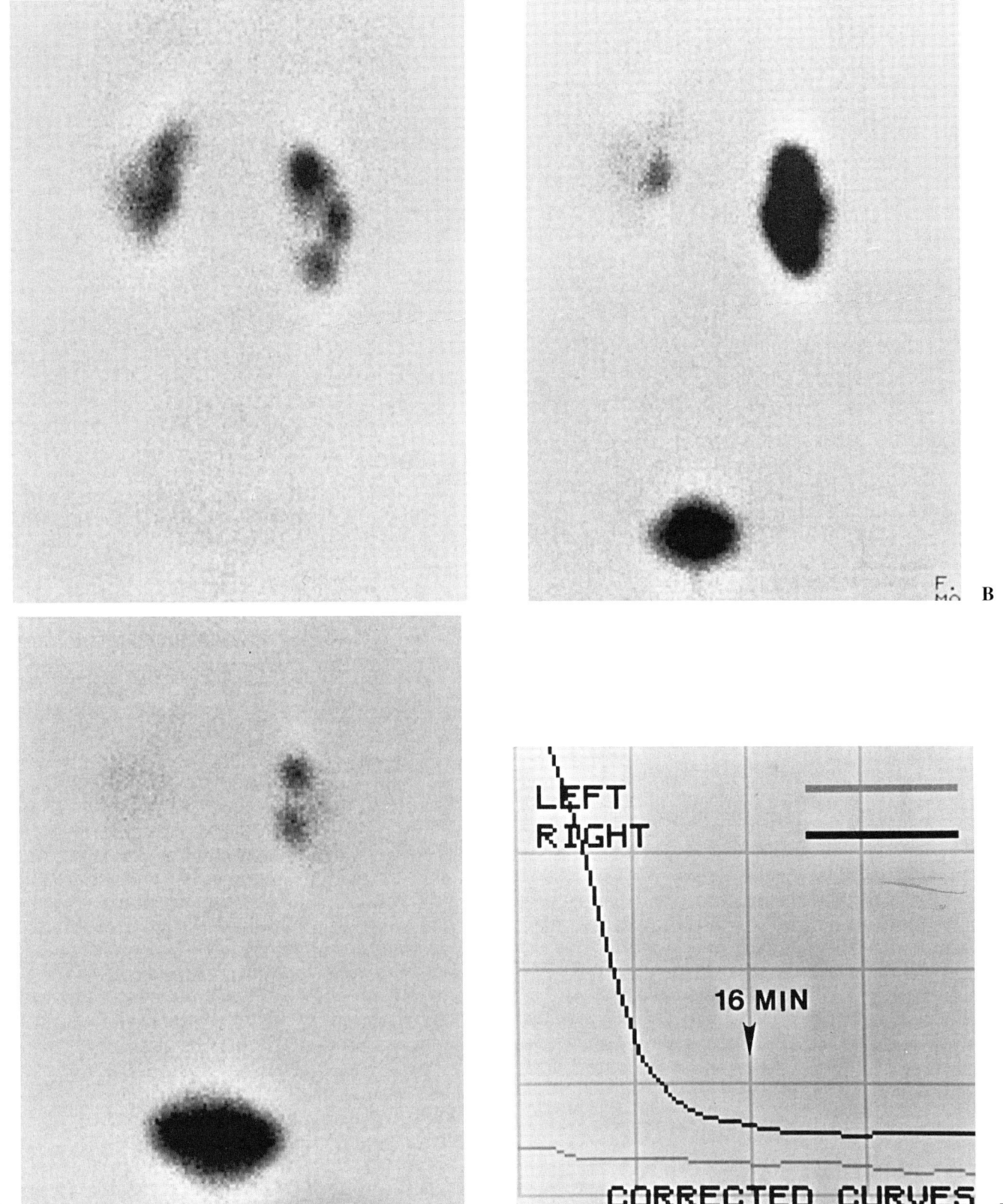

Figure 7–10. A 14-year-old girl is being followed for congenital ureteral obstruction with diuretic renal scans using DTPA. (**A**) Three-minute posterior image shows prominent calyceal system of the right kidney. (**B**) Retention of activity is seen in the right collecting system on the 25-minute image. The left kidney has normal washout of the tracer. (**C**) Fifteen minutes after intravenous Lasix administration, the right kidney shows almost complete washout of the tracer, indicating that it is a dilated but nonobstructed system. (**D**) Time activity curves generated by the computer after Lasix administration calculated the $T_{1/2}$ on the right to be 5 minutes. (Normal is less than 10 minutes.)

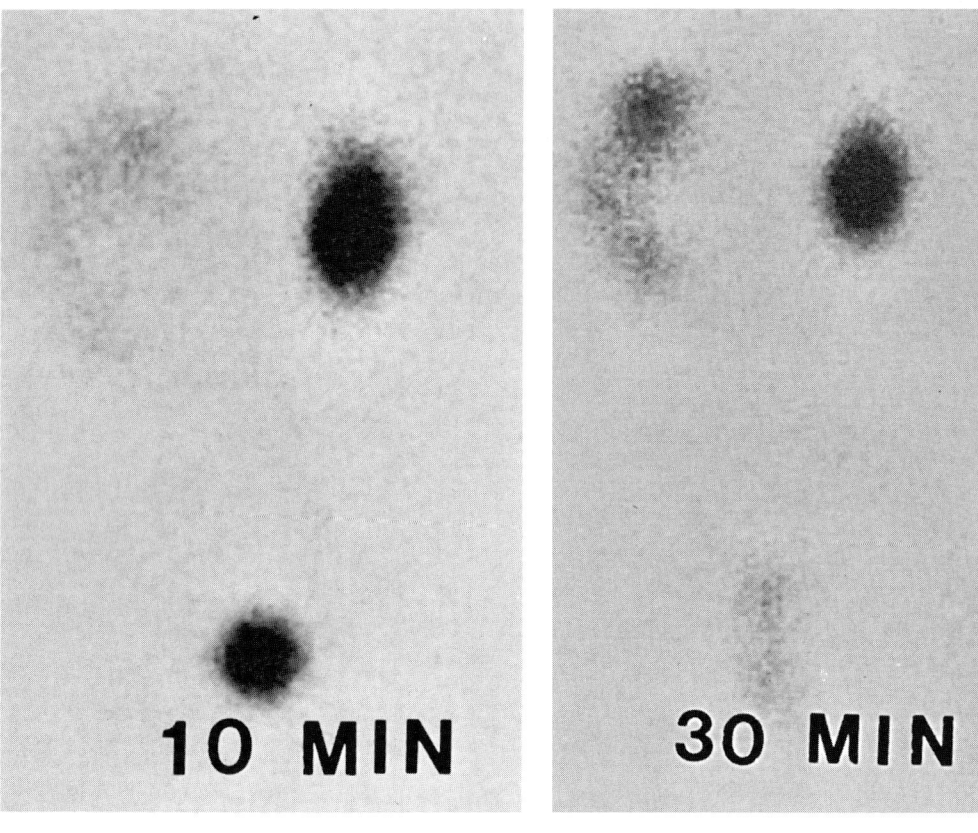

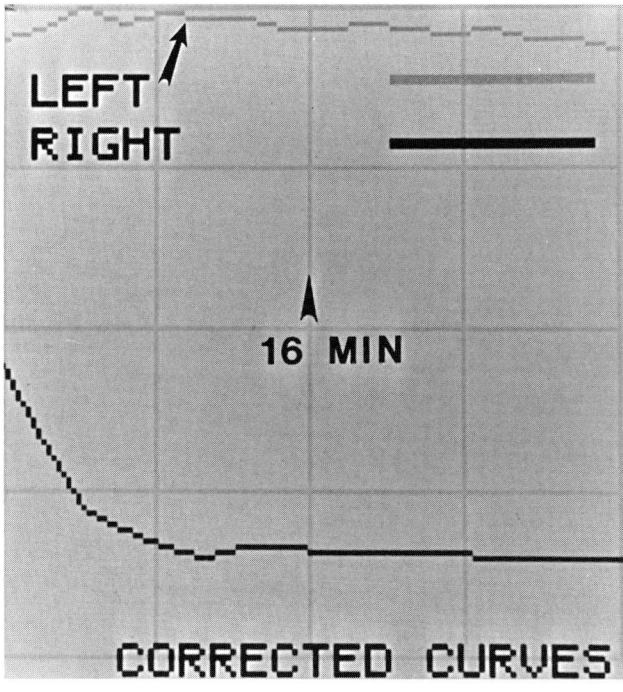

Figure 7–11. An 8-month-old boy with history of urinary tract infections, and left hydronephrosis was referred for a renal scan. The scan was performed using Tc-99m DTPA. The bladder was kept decompressed with a Foley catheter. (**A**) Posterior image at 10-minutes demonstrates a poorly functioning, large left kidney with a central photopenic region indicative of a dilated renal pelvis. (**B**) The left kidney has accumulated more tracer on the 30-minute pre-Lasix image especially at the upper pole. (**C**) The computer-generated curves after Lasix administration show a flat response resulting from ureteral obstruction on the left (arrow).

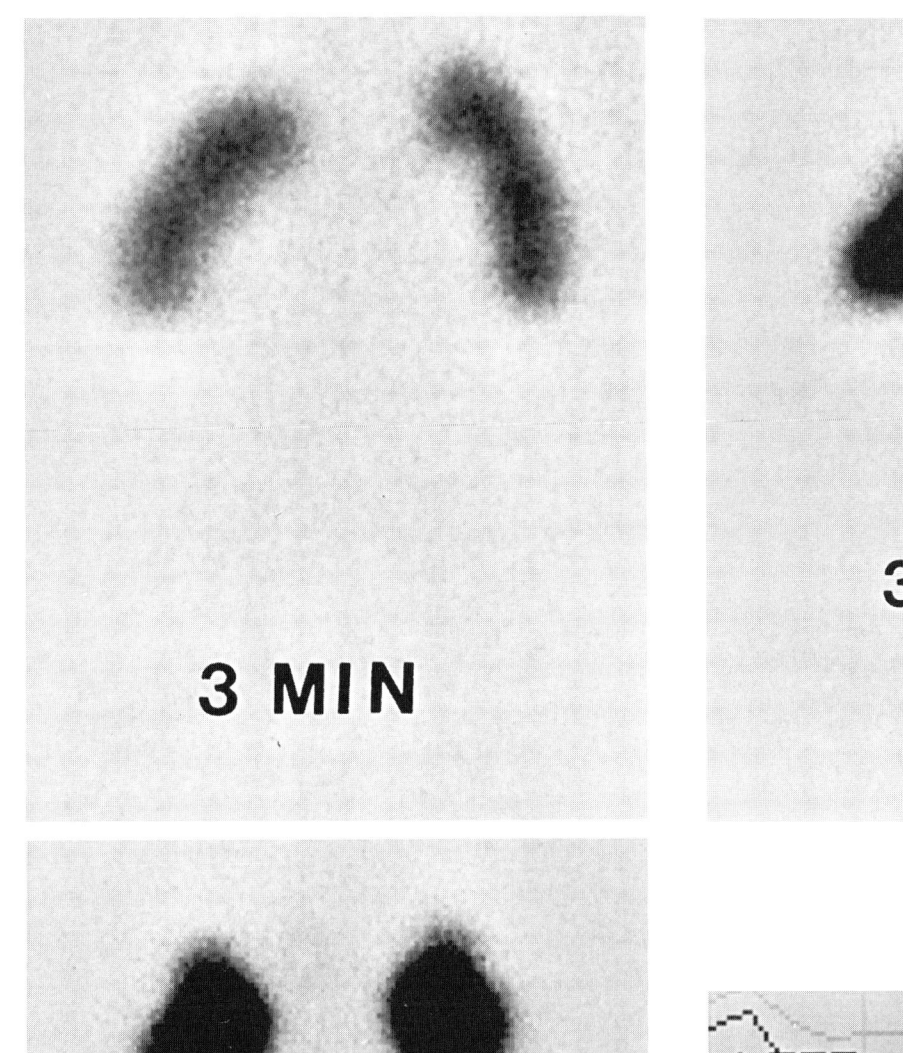

Figure 7-12. A 19-month-old boy with prune-belly syndrome, bilateral hydronephrosis and undescended testes returned for a sequential scan for evaluating worsening washout times. (**A**) Three-minute image shows symmetric nephrograms indicating balanced renal function. (**B**) There is bilateral hydronephrosis on the 30-minute pre-Lasix image. (**C**) There is very poor washout of the tracer 30 minutes after Lasix administration, indicating bilateral obstruction. The urinary bladder has some tracer excretion. (**D**) Renogram curves show slow washout bilaterally. The $T_{1/2}$s were more than 70 minutes bilaterally.

important to keep the urinary bladder decompressed by a Foley catheter to allow adequate drainage of the upper tracts. Additional information in the form of renal quantitation of function can also be obtained by calculating the percent uptake of the radiopharmaceutical on the initial 2- to 3-minute images. Deterioration of function on successive scans in the presence of obstruction indicates the need for pyeloplasty. We have reserved the use of MAG3 for cases with poor renal function and in newborn infants when the kidneys are immature.

Bilateral ureteral obstruction is more common in males and is associated with posterior urethral valves. The valvular obstruction of the posterior urethra causes dilatation of the ureters and hydronephrosis. The Lasix renal scan aids in determining the degree of obstruction and is also useful as a follow-up study, since the hydronephrosis improves or disappears after surgery.

Prune-Belly syndrome, or Eagle-Barrett syndrome, consists of a triad of deficiency of abdominal wall musculature, urinary tract abnormalities, and cryptorchidism. The urinary tract anomalies consist of dysplasia or hydronephrosis, hydroureters with kinking and sacculations, and megacystis. The bladder has poor contractility and may prevent drainage of the upper tracts (Fig. 7–12).

Vesicoureteral Reflux and Infection

Vesicoureteral reflux is a common childhood problem and is associated with renal infections. The common causes of reflux are infection, developmental anomaly at the ureterovesical junction, or the presence of bladder outlet obstruction, such as posterior urethral valves. VCUG is usually the initial imaging study performed because it helps define the anatomy, but subsequent follow-up studies may be performed with radionuclides. Radionuclide cystograms have the advantage of being more sensitive while administering a lower radiation dose.

Urinary tract infection is a common sequela of vesicoureteral reflux and can lead to scarring, nephropathy, and end-stage renal disease. Renal scarring, like urinary tract infections (UTIs), is more common in girls than in boys. Studies have reported that up to 50% of children with UTIs have reflux, and of these 33% will have reflux nephropathy.[23] It is therefore essential that the presence of reflux be documented and treated so that further complications are avoided. Intravenous pyelogram (IVP) was the standard method of evaluating renal cortex until the availability of ultrasound and renal scintigraphy using GH and, more recently, DMSA. Sty et al discussed the relative utility of different imaging modalities to detect inflammatory renal disease. GH was the cortical agent used. A statistical comparison of the imaging methods was not done, but the strengths and weaknesses of each were provided.[24]

Experimental data have also demonstrated high sensitivity for detection of renal damage using DMSA scanning. In a study by Majd et al, where piglets were screened for early renal damage caused by reflux and pyelonephritis, damage was seen in 87%.[25] Verber and Meller showed that 40 of 45 children under the age of 5 had definite scan defects after the first proven UTI. Eighty percent of these defects persisted on the repeat examination. They suggested that the outcome depended on the effect of the first infection and that grade 3 reflux may aggravate the damage.[26] Several clinical studies have demonstrated higher sensitivities for detection of renal cortical abnormalities with DMSA scintigraphy than those achieved with IVP[23] or ultrasonography.[27]

DMSA scan in pyelonephritis (Fig. 7–13) or scarring (Fig. 7–14) demonstrates loss of cortical tissue and photopenic defects. In acute pyelonephritis these defects may be transient and may resolve with therapy. SPECT images have dramatically improved the sensitivity for detection of cortical damage due to infection. Coronal images are by far the most helpful.

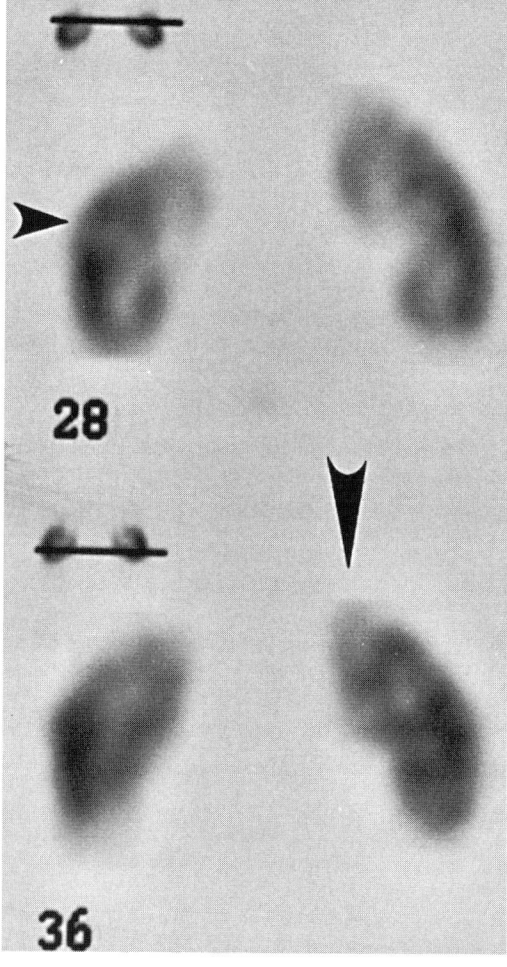

Figure 7–13. Coronal SPECT DMSA images in a patient with recurrent fever, flank pain, and urinary tract infection. Two cortical defects, one at the upper pole of the left kidney (large arrowhead) and the other at the lateral aspect of the right kidney (small arrowhead) are seen. Since the patient had evidence of acute infection clinically, these defects were most consistent with cortical damage associated with acute pyelonephritis.

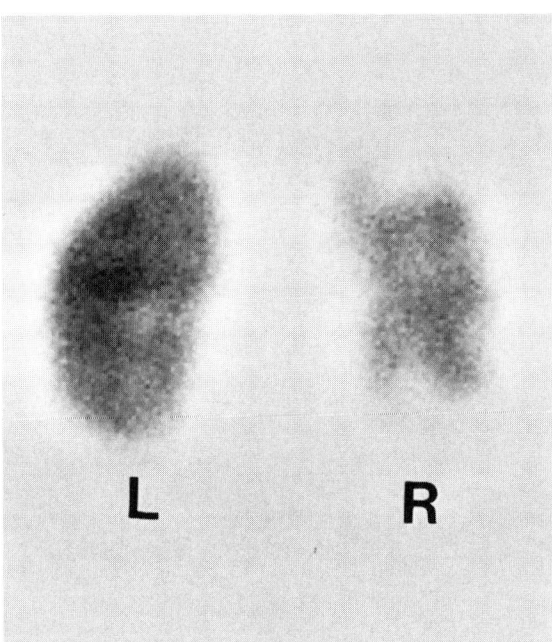

Figure 7-14. A 7-year old girl with recurrent urinary tract infections was referred for a DMSA scan. Posterior planar image shows multiple defects in the small right kidney. These were felt to be seondary to scarring from previous episodes of pyelonephritis.

Renal Imaging in Trauma

Renal trauma is usually a part of multiple injuries sustained as a result of vehicular accident. In the pediatric age group, it may be due to blunt trauma secondary to a fall or to sports-related injuries. Malrotated and ectopic kidneys are more vulnerable to trauma. In children renal injury is more common due to less perirenal fat, and a relatively large renal size. Because other visceral injuries are associated with the abdominal trauma, computed tomography is usually the examination of choice. Renal scintigraphy is usually performed to evaluate function when vascular injury has occurred (Fig. 7–15). Renal vascular injury may also occur as a result of abdominal surgery. Tc-99m DTPA, GH, or MAG3 can not only evaluate the perfusion and relative renal function, but also assess urinary extravasation. Renal arterial injury is manifested by lack of tracer localization in the angiogram as well as by the functional phase of the renogram. Renal vein injury may show mild to significant reduction in blood flow with a proportional reduction in function. The involved kidney is usually enlarged. Focal renal injury and associated infarct are seen as a wedge-shaped photopenic defect on the nephrogram phase of the renal scan. A significant reduction in tracer extraction and the presence of photopenia on the scan indicate irreversible renal damage; a nephrectomy is usually the outcome.

Renal Neoplasms

The most common pediatric renal tumor is Wilms' tumor. The child is about 2 to 3 years old and presents with an

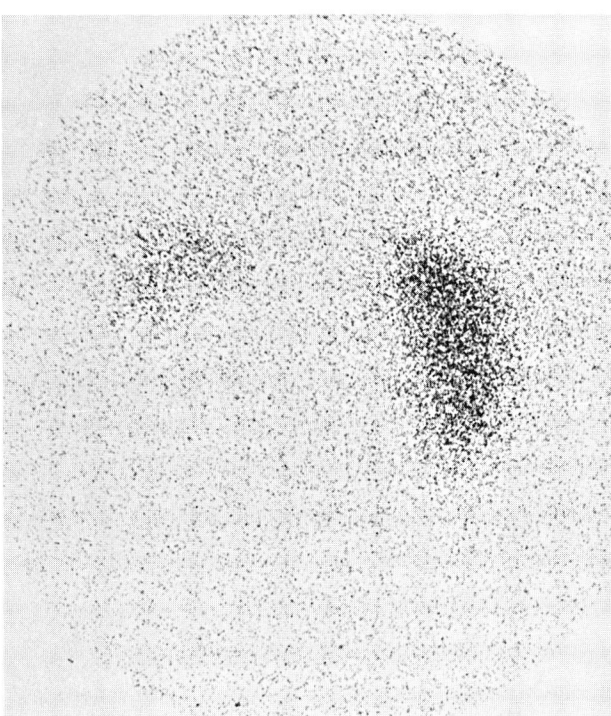

Figure 7-15. A young boy sustained multiple injuries in a vehicular accident. The left kidney had ruptured as a result of the trauma. A hippuran renal scan was performed to assess the extent of renal damage. Posterior 5-minute image shows loss of function of the left lower pole. The left kidney contributed to 16% of the global function.

abdominal mass. The tumor spreads via the lymphatics or blood vessels. Invasion into the right atrium as a direct extension from the cava may occasionally be seen. Diagnostic imaging modalities include US, CT, or MRI. Scintigraphy usually shows absence of uptake, poorly functioning tissue, and/or deformed or partially obstructed collecting system.

Neuroblastoma is the second most common abdominal tumor in children. It is a neuroendocrine tumor arising from the sympathoadrenal system. The adrenal medulla is the common site of occurrence in the abdomen. Extra-adrenal locations involve the sympathetic ganglion chains throughout the body. The age at presentation is 0 to 3 years. High levels of urinary catecholamine metabolites are present in the majority of cases. It is a highly malignant tumor with spread to the retroperitoneal lymph nodes, liver, bone marrow, and skeleton.

Along with ultrasound and computed tomography, skeletal scintigraphy is performed for staging of neuroblastoma. The tumor usually demonstrates uptake of Tc-99m methylene diphosphonate (Fig. 7–16) and may be related to the blood flow or calcification. The metaphyseal regions of the long bones, spine, and skull are the sites usually involved. Since the physes are usually the most active areas in the growing skeleton, subtle involvement of the metaphyses may not be easily appreciated. Not infrequently, the metastaseal involvement may be symmetric or occasion-

144 Diagnosis of Genitourinary Disease

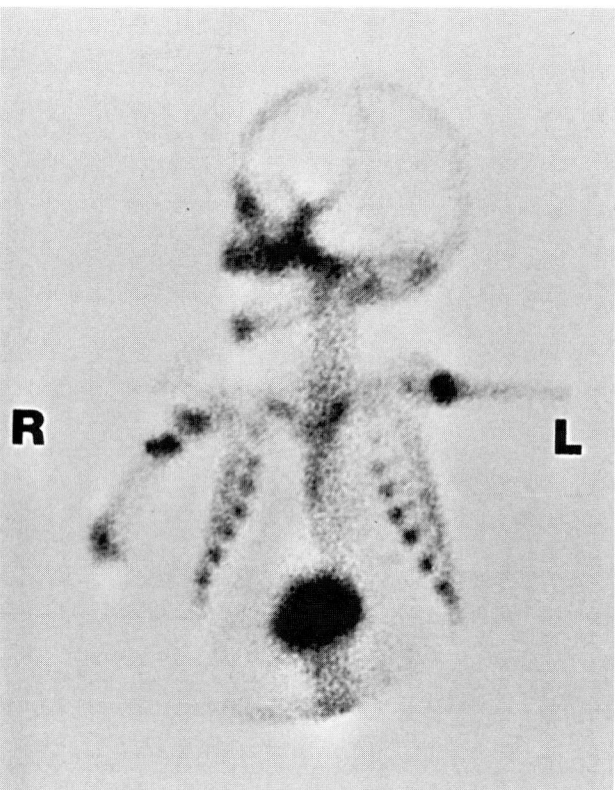

Figure 7–16. Prechemotherapy bone scan on a 1-year-old boy with neuroblastoma. Anterior image shows intense accumulation of Tc-99m MDP in the primary abdominal tumor. Subsequent bone scans after chemotherapy showed resolution of uptake in the primary tumor.

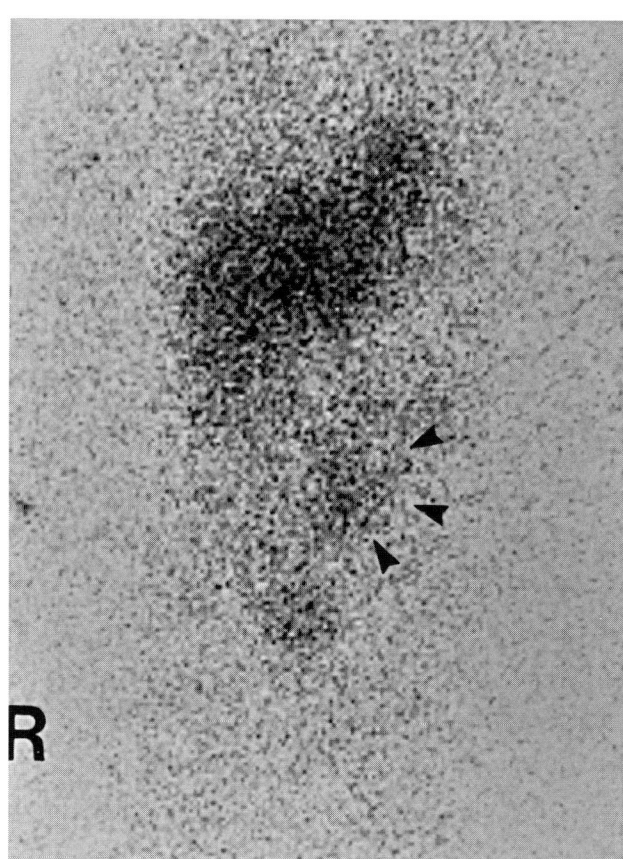

Figure 7–17. A 5-year-old boy with prior resection of neuroblastoma has I-131 MIBG scan for restaging. Anterior image of the abdomen illustrates uptake in the pelvic soft tissue mass (arrowheads) suggesting spread of tumor.

ally photopenic because of the presence of osteolytic lesions.[28]

Radio-iodinated meta-iodobenzylguanidine (MIBG) is a physiologic analog of norepinephrine and guanethidine. This radiopharmaceutical is concentrated in the neurosecretory granules of the adrenal medulla and has been used widely for the localization of adrenal and extra-adrenal pheochromocytomas. Since pheochromocytomas and neuroblastomas are derived from the same precursor cells, it was postulated that I-131 MIBG will also localize in neuroblastoma and its metastases. A number of studies have supported this.[29–31] The combined use of bone scan and I-131 MIBG scan leads to an overall increased detection rate of extraskeletal metastases (Figs. 7–17, 7–18). We use a dose of 1 mCi of I-131 MIBG intravenously for an adult. The pediatric dose is adjusted according to the age. Whole-body images are obtained at 24 and 48 hours. SPECT imaging of the abdomen and chest usually helps to delineate the extent of tumor involvement. I-131 MIBG has also been used for treatment of disseminated neuroblastoma.[32]

Scrotal Imaging

Scrotal imaging is usually performed in a child presenting to the emergency room with pain and swelling of the scrotum. The differential diagnosis is epididymitis, orchitis, torsion of the testis, or testicular appendages or trauma. Rare causes include abscess or testicular neoplasm.

Testicular torsion is most common in boys aged 10 to 17 years and is a surgical emergency. Prompt and accurate diagnosis is essential to avoid testicular infarction; at the same time, unnecessary surgical exploration should be avoided. Epididymo-orchitis also affects the same age group, and clinical presentation is similar, although fever and urinary tract infection may also be present. Radionuclide imaging is very useful, although color Doppler sonography has great potential.[33–36]

In acute testicular torsion (<24 hours' duration), the affected testis shows diminished blood flow on the nuclear angiogram, and the static images show a photopenic defect involving the entire hemiscrotum. Delayed or missed torsion (>24 hours' duration) shows a central photopenia surrounded by a hyperemic rim (Fig. 7–19). The hyperemia is due to the increased vascularity of the overlying dartos muscle, which is supplied by the pudendal vessels.[33,37] Other conditions that have a similar picture are abscess, hematoma, hydrocele, and hematoma.[33] History, physical examination, and ultrasonography may be helpful in these situations. The treatment of testicular torsion is emergent exploration and

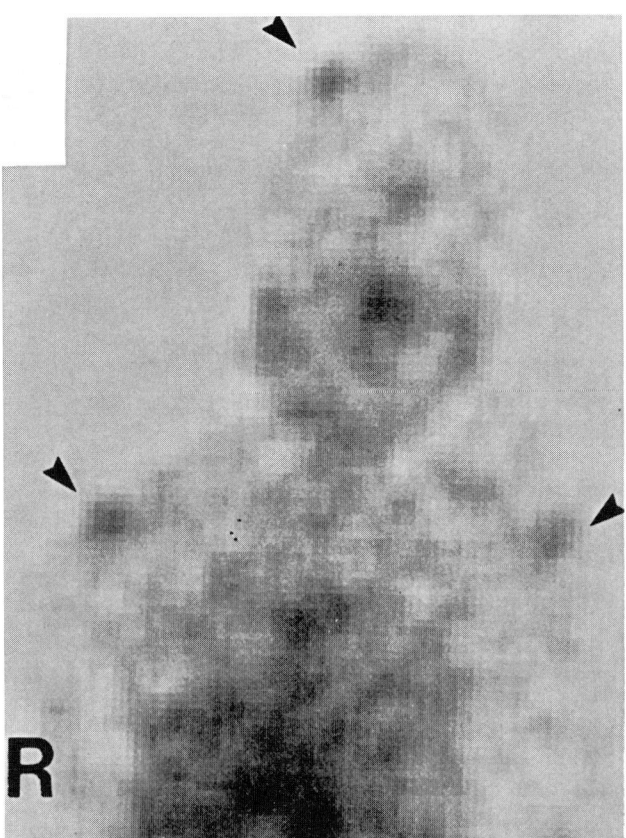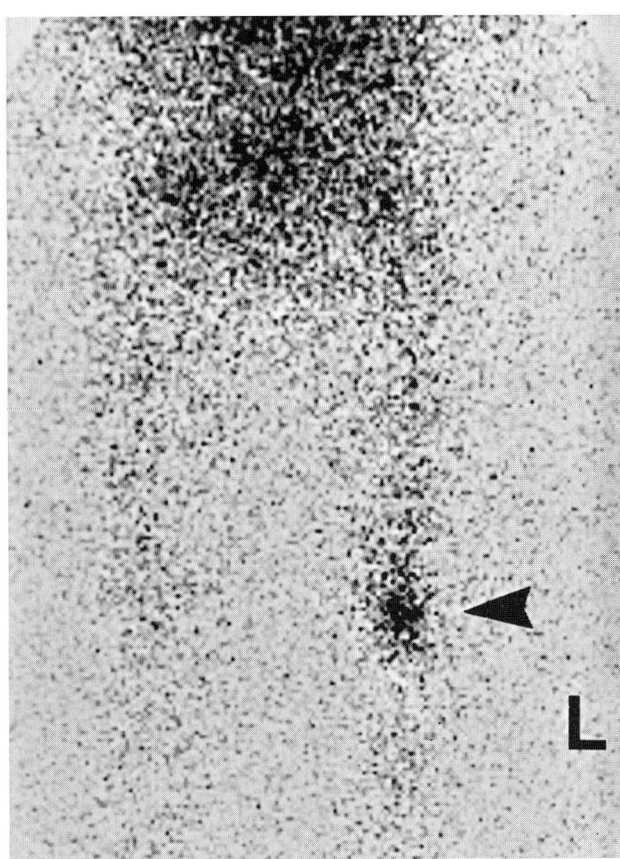

Figure 7–18. A 6-year-old boy with stage IV neuroblastoma in remission had I-131 MIBG scan. (**A**) Increased uptake is seen in the skull and both proximal humeri. These areas were normal by bone scan. (**B**) Metaphyseal region of the left tibia in the same patient also shows increased uptake on I-131 MIBG scan and is consistent with bony metastasis.

orchiopexy if the testis is viable. Exploration of the contralateral hemiscrotum is done because the predisposing condition to torsion is frequently bilateral. If spontaneous detorsion occurs by the time scrotal scintigraphy is performed, the study may be normal or mild hyperemia may be present on the affected side.

Epididymo-orchitis shows diffuse hyperemia of the affected hemiscrotum on the vascular sequence, as well as the static views. Infrequently, torsion of the appendix testis or transient torsion of the cord may cause mild hyperemia that may mimic epididymitis. Untreated or complicated infection that is chronic may not reveal the classic hyperemia typical of acute infection.

CLINICAL APPLICATIONS IN ADULT RENAL DISEASE

As in childhood situations with potential kidney dysfunction or disease, several modalities compete for clinical applications. Although these methods may supply important information, it is usual that the different modalities provide complemental image data, and an intelligent approach is to start with the study that is most likely to answer the prime clinical question. Other procedures may be needed, but considerations of cost effectiveness dictate that unnecessary steps or more expensive steps be avoided if possible. Often sonography is the cost-effective first step, but intravenous urography is more important than in childhood evaluation, where concern of radiation exposure is higher and image quality worse. Nuclear medicine tests provide more expensive secondary and occasional primary procedures. Improvements in nuclear equipment and radiopharmaceuticals have opened new possibilities. Computerized tomography, magnetic resonance imaging, and interventional procedures are reserved for specialized circumstances.

Acute Renal Disease

Several nuclear approaches are available for the patient who presents with acute renal failure. Early studies with I-131 hippurate showed that failure to visualize kidneys within 30 minutes of IV injection was a highly significant predictor of poor outcome, although some patients recovered life-sustaining function.[38,39] Faint visualization was more encouraging. The availability of technetium-labeled agents has offered more options, but the results are similar. Tc-99m DTPA is not as sensitive as OIH for detecting the severely damaged but viable kidney. MAG3 can be substituted for

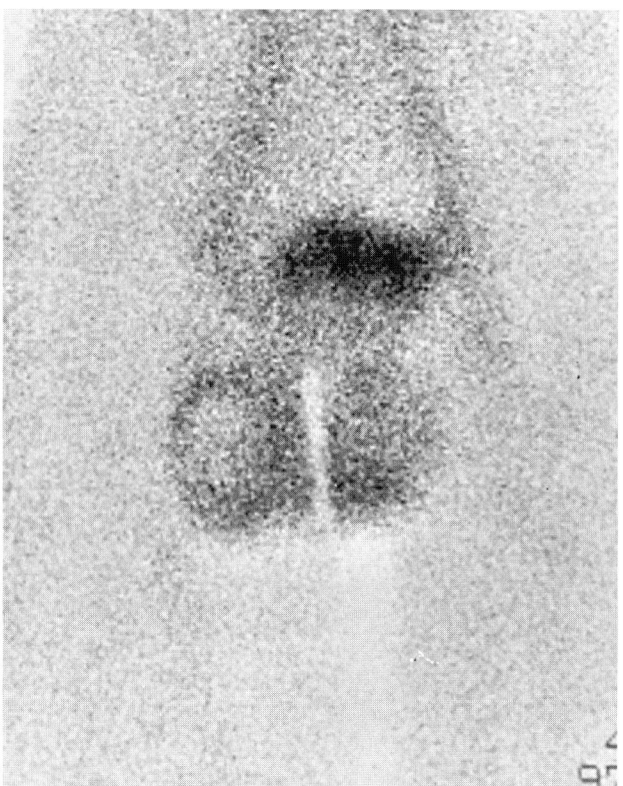

Figure 7–19. Adolescent presented to the emergency room with right testicular pain of 24 hours' duration. A testicular torsion was suspected and scintigraphy was performed with 20 mCi of Tc-99m pertechnetate. The static anterior image demonstrates a central photopenic defect in the right hemiscrotum surrounded by a hyperemic rim. A diagnosis of delayed torsion was made and confirmed at surgery.

OIH, and the millicurie-injected dosages make vascular imaging possible.[40] Dynamic vascular and static imaging to at least 30 minutes allows demonstration of blood flow and function. With impaired renal function, liver visualization is more intense than with either DTPA or OIH and must not be confused with a functioning kidney. Oblique or further delayed views may be needed to clarify that question.

Causes of acute renal failure include a number of common and unusual diseases. One of the more frequent reasons in hospitalized patients is damage from a nephrotoxic drug such as radiographic contrast, antibiotics, or chemotherapeutic agents. A MAG3 study usually shows progressively increasing activity in the kidneys with delayed excretion in the normal-size collecting system. This is the pattern of acute tubular necrosis (ATN). The more severe the damage, the worse the renal visualization. Although milder forms of ATN have little effect on renal blood flow, severe damage causes flow to decrease along with severely impaired or absent function (Fig. 7–20). When the kidneys have suffered ischemia because of hypotension, embolization, temporary surgical or interventional vascular occlusion, or a vascular event such as aortic dissection, fair to good visualization of renal flow and agent excretion reassures that return of life-sustaining function is likely. Rate of recovery is somewhat unpredictable. In renal cortical necrosis there is no flow or function evident, and there is no potential for renal recovery.

High-grade acute obstruction of a renal artery or vein causes acute damage of the involved tissue, as evidenced by a marked reduction or absence of nuclear tracer uptake. Arterial obstruction causes absence of activity and infarction, but with venous obstruction there may be minimal activity on delayed views because of collateral veins, which keep the kidney viable (Figs. 7–21, 7–22). The venous lesion may be associated with acute swelling, whereas the arterial lesion causes a small kidney, especially if chronic. A renal scan with DTPA or MAG3 can rapidly determine whether renal failure after aortic aneurysm repair is due to embolism and infarction or whether ATN is due to temporary vascular occlusion during surgery. Small branch vascular obstructions cause wedge-shaped damage that are best shown with DMSA scans with SPECT, but these lesions do not cause acute renal failure unless there is preexisting renal damage.

Medical causes of acute renal failure usually result in an ATN type of pattern (in patients with acute glomerulonephritis, for example). Nephrosis often has little effect on the excretion patterns, unless there is tubular as well as glomerular damage. If urine concentration is lowered by poor water resorption or hydration, the collecting system may be poorly visualized. It is important that the gamma camera include the lower ureters and bladder to demonstrate the amount of excretion of the radiopharmaceutical. In patients with more severe ATN or medical renal impairment, the imaging methods for quantitating renal function (Gates's method) tend to overestimate clearance of DTPA or MAG3 because of the blood pool activity present in the kidneys several minutes after IV injection. One of the blood-sampling or combined blood- and urine-sampling methods is needed for accurate clearance measurement.

Ureteral or bladder outlet obstruction also reduces renal function on nuclear studies, even if acute. Patients with an acute renal stone and near total ureteral obstruction will show only a nuclear nephrogram on that side. Delayed imaging may show activity in the collecting system as late as 24 hours after IV injection. Generally, bladder obstruction has less effect on renal function than ureteral obstruction unless chronically present. Sonography usually detects the dilated upper tracts prior to the nuclear renal scan, but tracer studies may help determine the level of obstruction as well as severity of dysfunction. Semiquantitative measurement of clearance with external imaging (Gates's method) helps to determine the effect of drainage procedures and to predict whether dialysis will be needed once the kidneys have been decompressed. At times, images may be misleading unless quantitation is done, because of a high output state with low urine concentration following decompression, which causes the collecting system to be faintly seen.

Acute infection of the kidneys may produce either unilateral or bilateral damage. Differentiating acute from chronic damage is uncertain using standard renal imaging agents un-

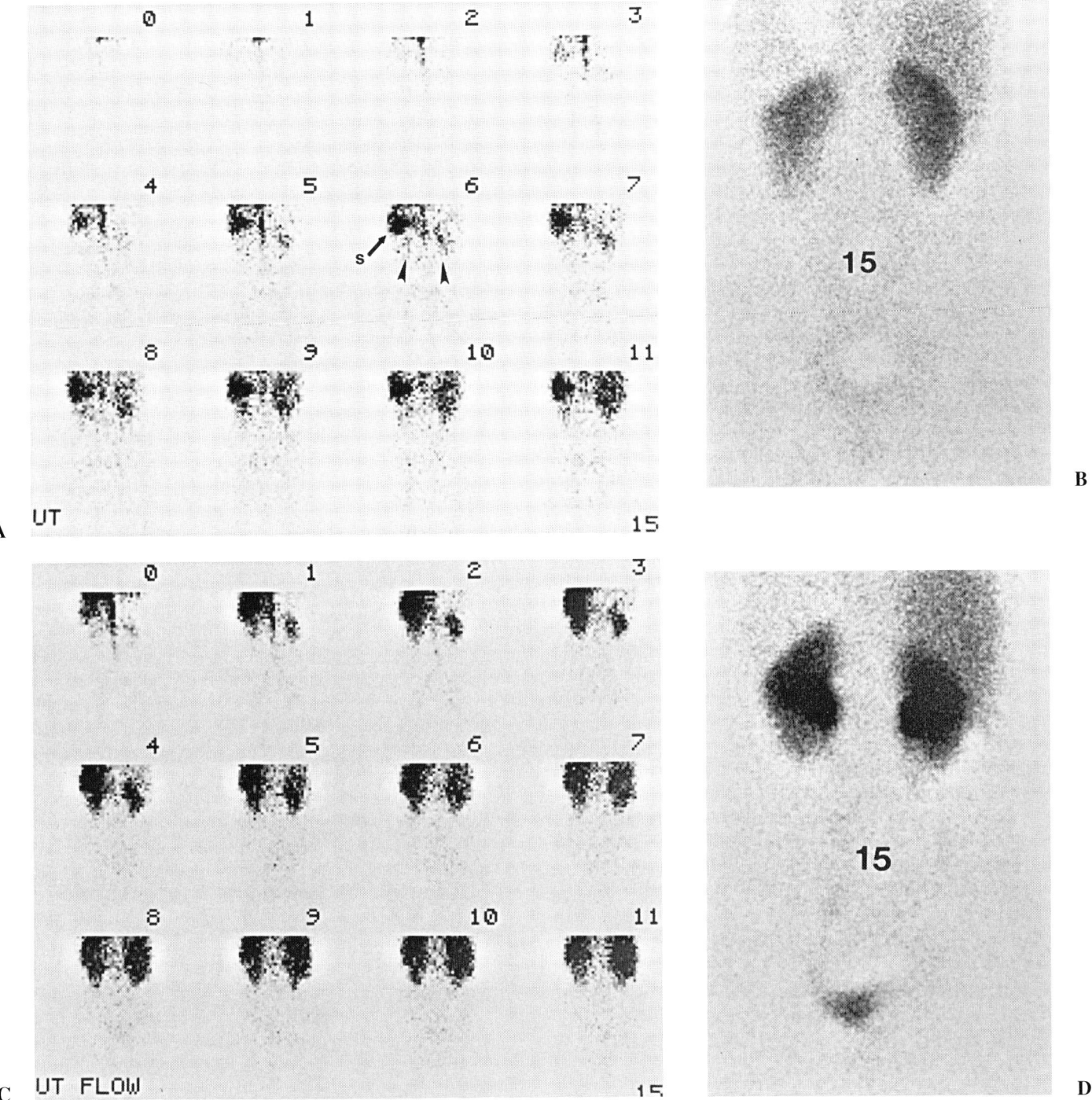

Figure 7–20. A 45-year-old woman suffered acute renal failure after a spider bite with profound hypotension. (**A**) Posterior vascular sequence with MAG3 shows some reduction in renal blood flow (arrowheads), compared to spleen flow (S). Liver activity is noted on the right on later views. (**B**) Static view at 15 minutes shows reduced renal activity and no bladder activity due to severe ATN. Even severely reduced renal activity is reassuring that function will improve. (**C**) Repeat study 10 days later shows improvement in blood flow to both kidneys. (**D**) Delayed static view at 15 minutes now shows activity in the renal pelvis and bladder. Function returned to normal.

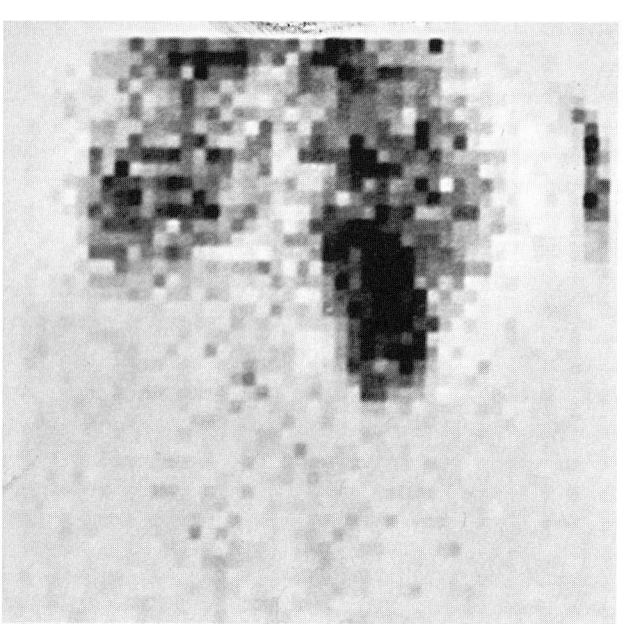
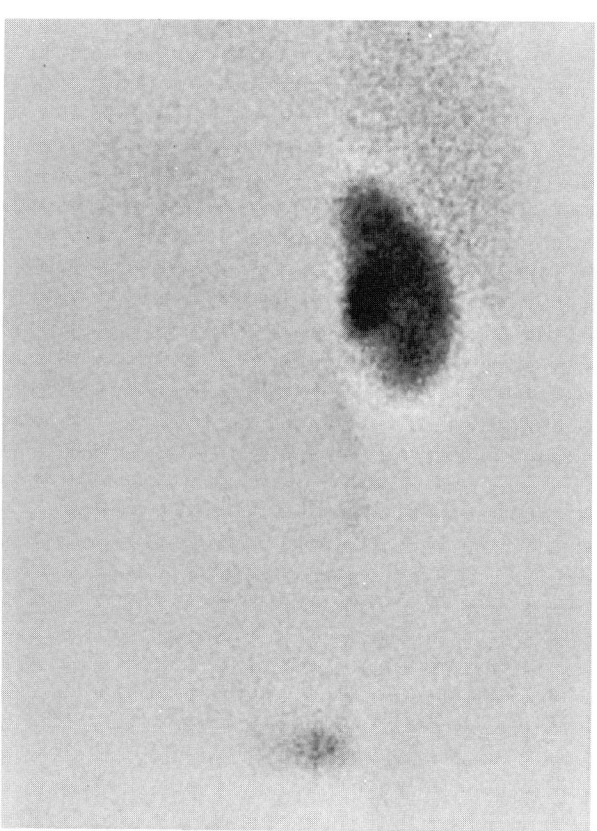

Figure 7–21. A 33-year-old woman suffered intraoperative injury to the left renal artery. (**A**) Posterior image 34 seconds after MAG3 injection shows good flow to the right kidney, liver, and spleen. (**B**) Ten-minute image confirms lack of function in the left kidney due to the arterial obstruction.

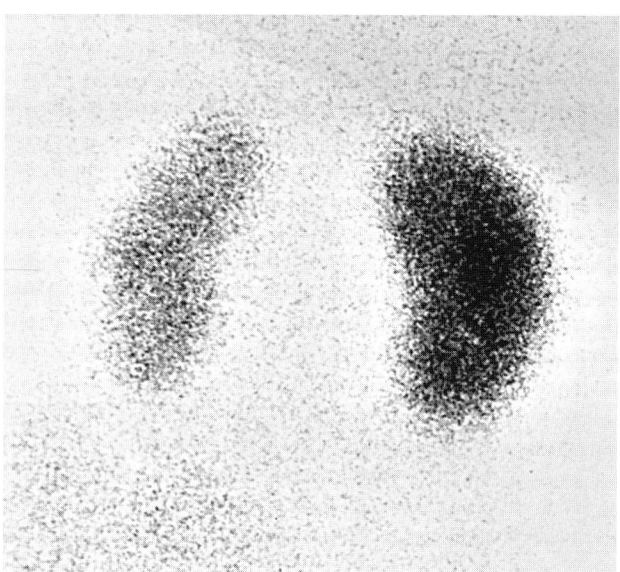

Figure 7–22. This 33-week-old premature baby boy had complications from an umbilical artery catheter, resulting in thrombosis in the lower aorta. The DMSA scan 3.5 hours after injection confirms reduced function in the left kidney. Computer analysis measured 28% activity in the left kidney and 72% in the right.

less there is significant kidney atrophy or serial studies are performed. DMSA scans in children have convincingly shown that nuclear studies are the most sensitive method of proving damage has occurred in the upper tracts. Initial studies show impaired regional uptake of Tc-99m DMSA, often followed by focal atrophy and scarring. Intravenous urograms and sonograms are less sensitive for both acute pyelonephritis and scarring.[27,41] Similarly, DTPA or MAG3 studies can be used to demonstrate functional damage, but cortical injury is best seen with DMSA.

In the acute situation, studies that demonstrate the inflammatory process more specifically include either gallium or labeled white cell (WBC) scans. Gallium-67 is excreted normally during the first 1 to 2 days, and blood pool activity clears slowly. Thus imaging of the kidneys is delayed at least 2 days, and further delays may be needed to clear the gallium excreted in bowel contents. SPECT may be helpful in localizing renal activity. Diffuse bilateral renal activity at 2 days usually indicates a nonbacterial inflammation or infiltration rather than pyelonephritis. Both acute and chronic infection show uptake of gallium.[42–44] Other inflammatory and neoplastic processess also show uptake of gallium, although primary renal cancers usually concentrate gallium poorly. WBC scans, whether labeled with In-111 or Tc-99m, more specifically demonstrate acute infection, but reported experience with renal infections is limited. Either tracer may be scanned in 24 hours or less, but there is a problem with normal excretion via urinary or gastrointestinal tracts.

Chronic Renal Disease

Chronic renal diseases are often suspected prior to nuclear imaging, and the diagnostic process may concentrate on whether the damage is acute, chronic, or a combination of both. As a general rule, small kidneys indicate a chronic process, but large kidneys may be seen in chronically involved organs. Examples of the latter include polycystic disease, amyloidosis, or other infiltrative diseases. Bilateral small kidneys result from many medical renal diseases such as diabetes, hypertension, and glomerulonephritis. A unilateral small kidney may indicate prior infection, perhaps with reflux; a hypoplastic kidney; and as discussed later, a renal vascular lesion. It is suggested that a congenitally hypoplastic kidney can be identified by the compensatory enlarged opposite kidney and a normal-shaped but small renogram curve,[45] although a captopril study might be needed if the patient is hypertensive.

Polycystic kidneys, or kidneys containing multiple simple cysts are usually followed with sonography or CT scans. At times, complications such as infection of cysts or neoplasm may be suspected and nuclear studies ordered. WBC or gallium scans help determine if a cyst is infected, but hemorrhage can cause WBC uptake also, complicating interpretation. Unfortunately primary renal cancers usually concentrate gallium poorly.[46] Thus, CT and needle aspiration often constitute the most appropriate procedure for both suspected cyst infection or neoplastic change. Other chronic renal diseases usually do not require nuclear studies other than quantitation of function, unless such complications as infection, infarction, or hypertension occur.

Suspected mass lesions in the kidney are typically studied initially with ultrasound or urograms. Most renal masses show decreased function on nuclear scans performed with DTPA, MAG3, or DMSA, although the vascular sequence can suggest hypervascularity in a primary renal carcinoma. Cystic lesions are best detected and evaluated with ultrasound or CT, as noted earlier. At times, a DMSA scan is needed to verify that a solid lesion seen on a sonogram is a column of Bertin, not a solid neoplasm.[47,48] The normal cortical tissue in the column or other variant shows high uptake of the tracer, contrasted with reduced activity in other lesions such as cysts, infection, or neoplasm. The nonspecific nature of gallium uptake, as well as low sensitivity for renal neoplasms, makes that scan unsuitable for primary cancer detection.[46]

Although, hypertension is not usually curable except for some infrequently encountered forms, control of blood pressure is usually possible. The challenge has been to develop a sensitive yet specific noninvasive study to detect those curable or correctable hypertensive individuals among the more than 95% of patients with essential hypertension. The early availability of several good renal radiopharmaceuticals led to widespread clinical applications of nuclear screening for renal artery stenosis (RAS), the most common curable hypertensive presentation. Agents such as radioactive mercurial diuretics, which labeled renal tubular cells in direct relationship with renal blood flow and OIH, were used for measurements of uptake and renograms, respectively. A positive test consisted of a significant asymmetry of renal cortical mass or function. The early nuclear medicine literature contains numerous studies showing the nuclear screening tests to be as good as or better than rapid sequence urograms, using arteriography and/or surgery as the gold standard. Sensitivities of 62% to 92% were reported,[49,50] but false-positive tests limited the usefulness in clinical practice. The development of effective antihypertensive drugs caused most clinicians to limit such imperfect screening methods to patients without a family history of hypertension, young patients, and patients difficult to control with drugs, because of higher pretest likelihood of renal artery stenosis in those groups. In the last decade, the availability of angioplasty as a nonsurgical method to treat renal artery stenosis made the need for an effective screening method more important[51] (Fig. 7–23). Majd and others noted an adverse effect on renal function of the new developed class of drugs used to treat hypertension, angiotensin-converting enzyme (ACE) inhibitors.[52] This effect has been confirmed in a number of clinical trials, although some technical differences in the test sequence have been tried. The use of renograms without and with ACE inhibitors has been reported to give sensitivities and specificities as high as 93% and 95%, respectively, for detecting renal vascular hypertension.[53–55]

It is now realized that the insensitivity of traditional renograms in many patients with renal vascular hypertension is due to compensatory physiologic changes in renal vasculature in response to the juxta-glomerular apparatus secretion of renin, which is converted to angiotensin II by ACE. Angiotensin II produces vasoconstriction of the efferent arterioles of the kidney, preserving glomerular filtration until such compensation is no longer sufficient to maintain function of the kidney. Thus a test looking for deterioration of function will be falsely negative in many patients unless ACE inhibitors are used.

The ACE inhibitor–augmented renal scintigraphic test has varied technically in various centers. All have agreed that some antihypertensive medications should be stopped if possible. Some simply stop ACE inhibitors for 1 day,[56] and others stop ACE inhibitors and diuretics for up to 14 days.[53,55] There is general agreement that good hydration is required. There are good reported results with I-131 hippurate, Tc-99m DTPA, and Tc-99m MAG3.[55] One- or 2-day protocols are employed, but most have relied on a 1-day method, using a low-dose–high-dose approach (Fig. 7–24). In the latter method, the first scintigram is usually a low-

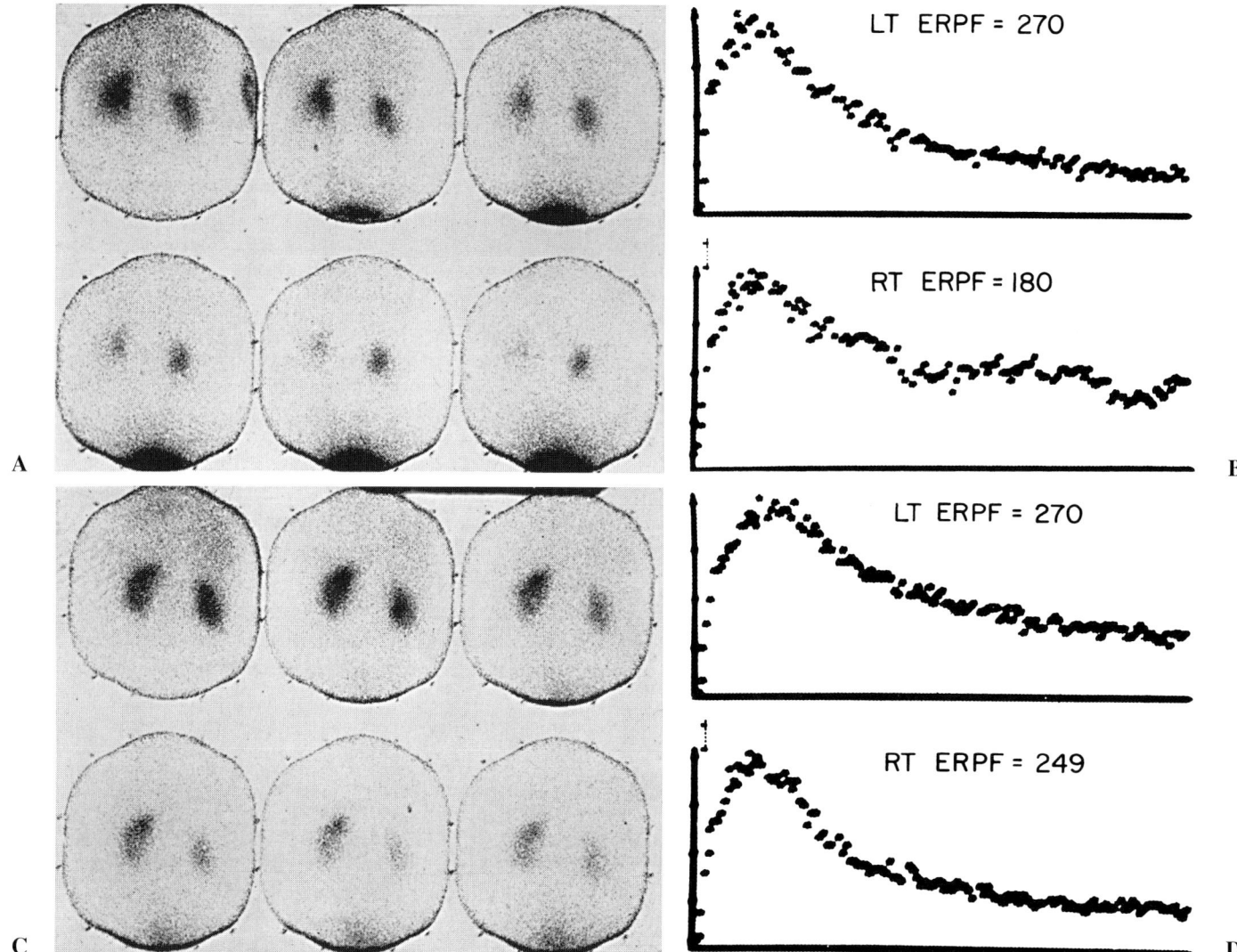

Figure 7–23. Pre- and postangioplasty of renal artery. **(A,B)** The preangioplasty renogram with OIH shows delayed washout from the right kidney on views every 5 minutes as well as the curve. The effective renal plasma flow (ERPF) is diminished on the right, based on blood sample analysis. Delayed washout is characteristic of renal artery stenosis (RAS), resulting from hyperconcentration of urine and reduced urine formation. **(C,D)** After right renal angioplasty the washout improved, as did the ERPF. (From Croft BY, Joyce J, Parekh Jk, Teates CD: Nuclear studies. In: Gillenwater JY, Grayhack JP, Howards SS, et al, eds: *Adult and Pediatric Urology*. St. Louis: Mosby–Year Book, 1991, 206. With permission.)

dose baseline study, followed 1 to 3 hours later with a repeat renogram an hour after giving captopril. Dosages of 25 or 50 mg captopril have both been successful, although some insist that 25 mg is not sufficient.[57]

Accurate results continue to be reported, indicating the captopril renogram to be the most reliable noninvasive test for renovascular hypertension. However, its use seems to be limited to patients with high clinical suspicion because of cost and some false-positive test results. The reliability in bilateral renal artery stenosis and renal failure is less well documented, but there is suspicion that results are less reliable than in patients with unilateral disease and normal creatinine levels. Regardless, the ACE inhibition intervention has dramatically improved the reliability of renograms for detecting renovascular hypertension, and some believe that this test is now the gold standard for determining which patients need intervention.

Other forms of correctable hypertension include adrenal cortical hypersecretion of cortisol and/or aldosterone and medullary hypersecretion of the catecholamines adrenaline and noradrenaline. Clinical investigators at the University of Michigan developed an effective cholesterol analog I-131 19-iodonorcholesterol (NP-59) for imaging functioning cortical lesions, based on the premise that cholesterol is a metabolic precursor to steroid synthesis. That agent successfully demonstrates bilateral adrenal uptake with hyperplasia and unilateral uptake with adenomas.[58] In the case of aldosterone overproduction, cortisol secretion needs to be

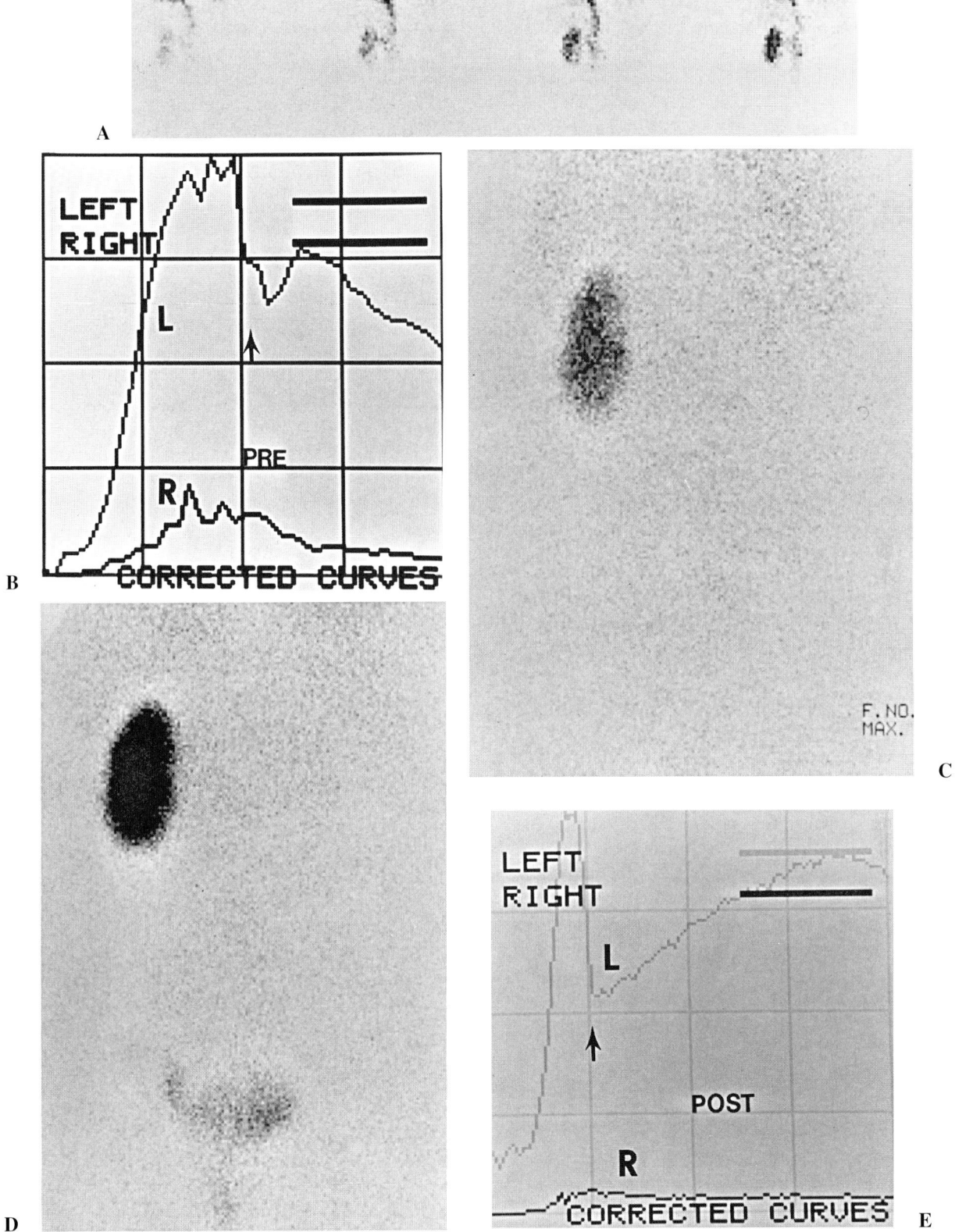

Figure 7–24. A 62-year-old woman with chronic hypertension and possible RAS. (**A**) Vascular sequence demonstrates good flow to the left kidney but no contralateral kidney. (**B**) DTPA histogram shows the 40-second vascular portion up to the arrow and 8 minutes into the renogram. The activity reaches a peak at about 3 minutes and washes out. There is no evidence of renal function on the right. The estimated clearance is 32 mL/min. (**C**) Image 1 hour after captopril administration and 3 minutes after DTPA injection. The renal activity is less with estimated clearance of 17 mL/min. (**D**) The image 30 minutes after captopril and repeat injection shows stasis in the left kidney and no right kidney uptake. (**E**) The postcaptopril histogram displays the prolonged retention in the left kidney for up to 30 min. The vascular sequence ends at the arrow. There is no evidence of right kidney function in this patient with a severely atrophied right kidney and RAS on the left.

stopped by administering dexamethasone, so that the hyperplasia or adenoma are not obscured by the much greater cortisol physiology. Adrenal carcinomas are included in the differential for Cushing's syndrome, and these lesions usually cause nonvisualization of both adrenals. At most institutions, the detection of the cortical lesions is currently done with CT because of accuracy and speed of results. The NP-59 scan can take up to 1 week, and the test is still investigational.

University of Michigan investigators later developed I-131 meta-iodobenzylguanidine (MIBG) for detecting pheochromocytomas and other functioning neuroendocrine tumors. This agent is not a precursor to adrenaline or noradrenaline, but it is transported across membranes of cells that have storage capability for such neurotransmitters. Because only 90% of pheochromocytomas are located in the adrenals and as many as 1% arise outside the abdomen, the value of MIBG scans continues despite continued improvement in CT and MRI quality. MIBG has found utility in demonstrating other tumors such as neuroblastomas, carcinoids, paragangliomas, and medullary cancers of the thyroid. With both MIBG and NP-59, the thyroid must be protected by administering loading doses of stable iodide, and scans may take 2 to 7 days to be completed.

Recent development of the somatostatin analog Octreotide, which can be labeled with In-111 has opened new possibilities for imaging such neuroendocrine tumors.[59] The imaging characteristics are clearly superior to I-131, allowing good-quality SPECT to be performed 1 or 2 days after injection. The specificity seems less than MIBG, because somatostatin receptors have been found of many cells such as small cell tumors, lymphocytes, and lymphomas. This new class of imaging agents, labeled peptides, has opened new doors for pharmaceutical development and disease imaging. Therapeutic potential is being investigated also.

A nonimaging test for gastrointestinal–genitourinary fistula has shown success in patients with suspected occult fistula. A number of other tests such as oral charcoal, contrast radiographs, and endoscopy have been devised to attempt to document a fistula as cause of recurrent infections, pneumaturia, fecaluria, and dysuria. Success has been low with occult fistulas. Lippert et al[60] noted that Cr-51 sodium chromate is nearly nonabsorbable by normal gastrointestinal mucosa and that nearly 100% of an oral dose is excreted in the stool. Clinical trials confirmed that less than 0.6% of the oral dose is normally detected in a 72-hour urine collection. Timing the appearance of activity in the urine samples helps determine the level of vesicoenteric leak. A few patients with apparent alteration in the mucosal barrier for chromium due to inflammatory bowel disease have had false-positive tests.

Transplant Evaluation

Renal transplant evaluation with radionuclides continues to have clinical utility despite improvements in sonography and Doppler studies. The availability of OIH helped start this approach soon after renal transplantation became feasible.[61,62] The renogram curves then available readily detected reduction of clearance and stasis in the parenchyma of a damaged kidney. Timing the appearance of transplant dysfunction helped differentiate acute tubular necrosis (ATN) of varying severity present in most cadaver organs shortly after surgery from subacute or chronic rejection that had onset a week or more after surgery[63] (Figs. 7–25, 7–26). Hyperacute rejection usually causes immediate failure of the transplant in the operative period and is rare with good tissue matching of donor and recipient. A number of methods have been used to quantitatively or semiquantitatively measure the kidney function, so as to document the onset of deterioration of function that usually signals rejection. A reliable method is the Gates' estimation of clearance,[9] but a simple, quick method is the bladder-to-kidney ratio of activity at 20 or 30 minutes after radiopharmaceutical injection.[64] The latter method assumes that there is no drainage from the bladder during the imaging sequence. Renal tubular dysfunction and stasis slow the clearance from the kidney to the bladder, and the camera images show whether dilatation of the collecting system is the cause. As the ATN clears, the bladder-to-kidney ratio and estimated clearance improve. Deterioration indicates rejection or one of the less common problems such as vascular occlusion, infection, or urine extravasation (Fig. 7–27). Extravasation of urine is readily detected by noting activity outside the kidney, ureter, and bladder, although at times delayed views are needed to verify the suspicion. Many centers have switched from OIH to Tc-99m DTPA or Tc-99m MAG3 to improve image quality and allow a vascular flow sequence as a routine part of the study. The vascular study is helpful because ATN usually causes only a mild decrease in renal blood flow in contrast to rejection. The vascular phase also permits an evaluation of the flow to a pancreas transplant that may be placed on the other side of the pelvis at the same surgical session (Fig. 7–28).

The use of cyclosporin to inhibit rejection has caused great difficulty in interpreting renal scintigraphic studies in transplant recipients. Cyclosporin is nephrotoxic and causes impairment of renal clearance and tubular stasis, and even decreased transplant blood flow that mimics rejection. This confusion is not surprising considering the similar pathology of the two conditions. A reliable method of differentiating these complications has not been found, other than stopping cyclosporin and increasing steroids, or perhaps biopsy.

Another complication that has been difficult to diagnose is renal artery stenosis. Acute vascular accidents at or soon after surgery are relatively easy to detect because the event is catastrophic and usually causes death of the kidney. Stenosis of the renal artery typically occurs months to years later and is associated with hypertension and kidney impairment. Many of the patients are already hypertensive, and detecting the stenosis is difficult short of angiogram.

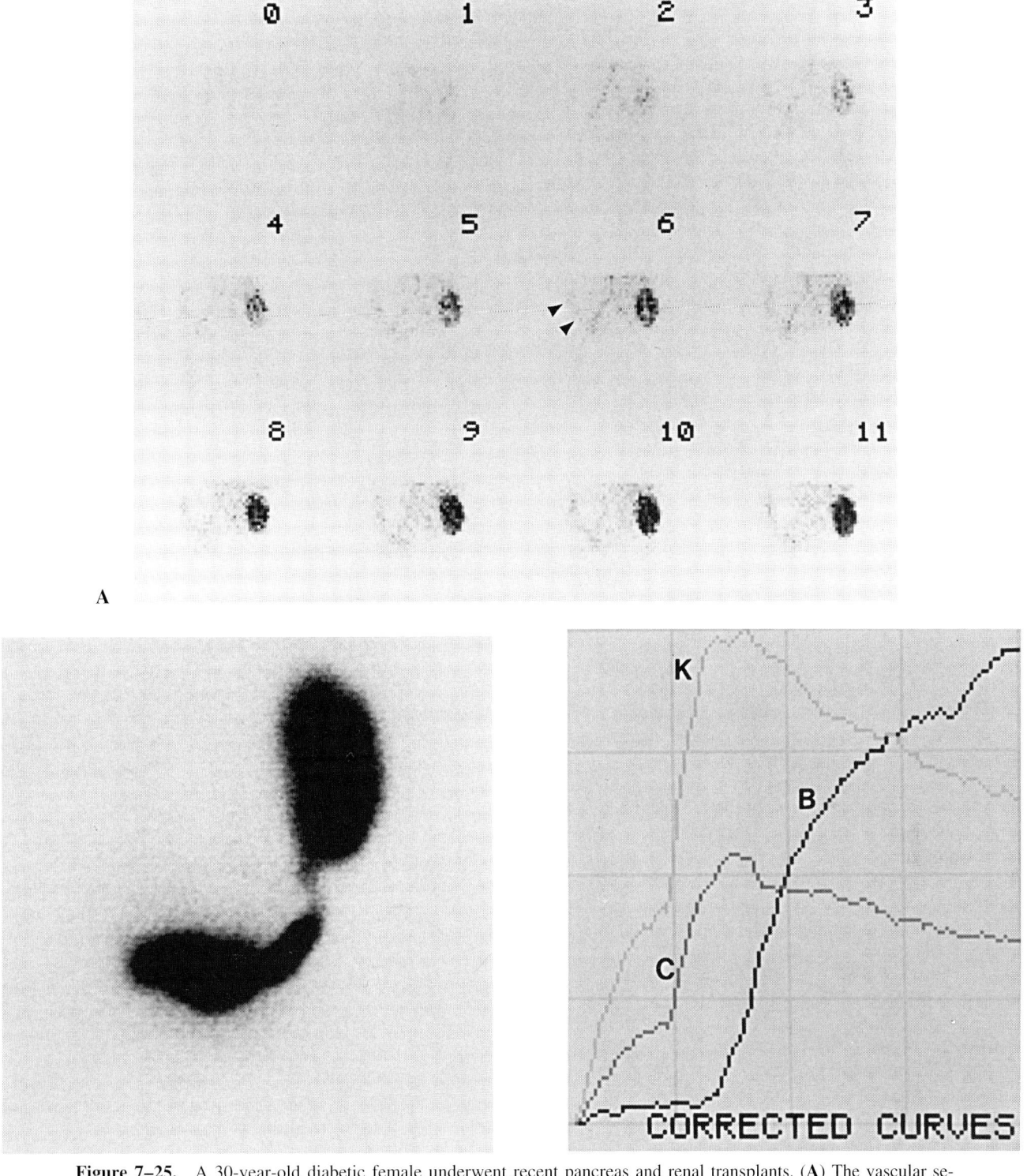

Figure 7–25. A 30-year-old diabetic female underwent recent pancreas and renal transplants. (**A**) The vascular sequence with MAG3 shows good flow in the pancreas (arrowheads) and the kidney in the left pelvis. (**B**) On the 30-minute image, activity in the kidney is intense because of tubular stasis. The bladder activity is low. (**C**) The histogram curves show reduced washout from the kidney (K) and kidney cortex (C), and show accumulation in the bladder (B). The bladder/kidney ratio (B/K) at 30 minutes is only 1.4 as a result of postoperative ATN. (From Teates CD, Parekh JS: New radiopharmaceuticals and new applications in medicine. *Curr Probl Diagn Radiol* 1993; 12(6):257. With permission.)

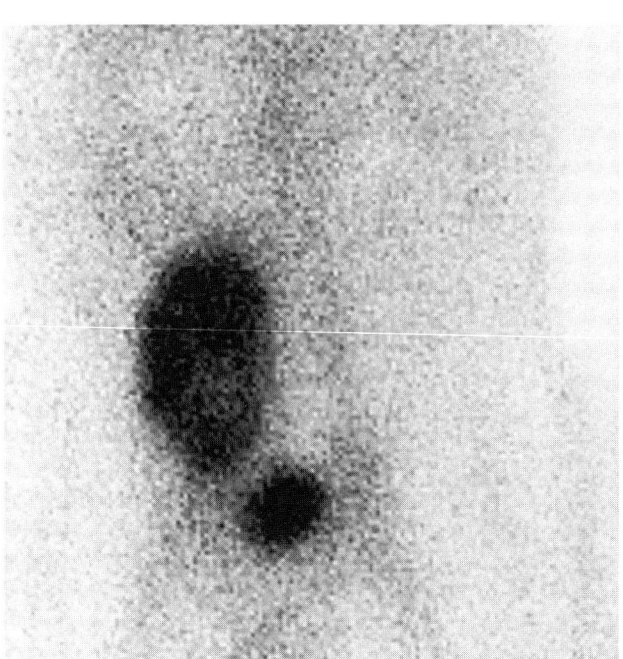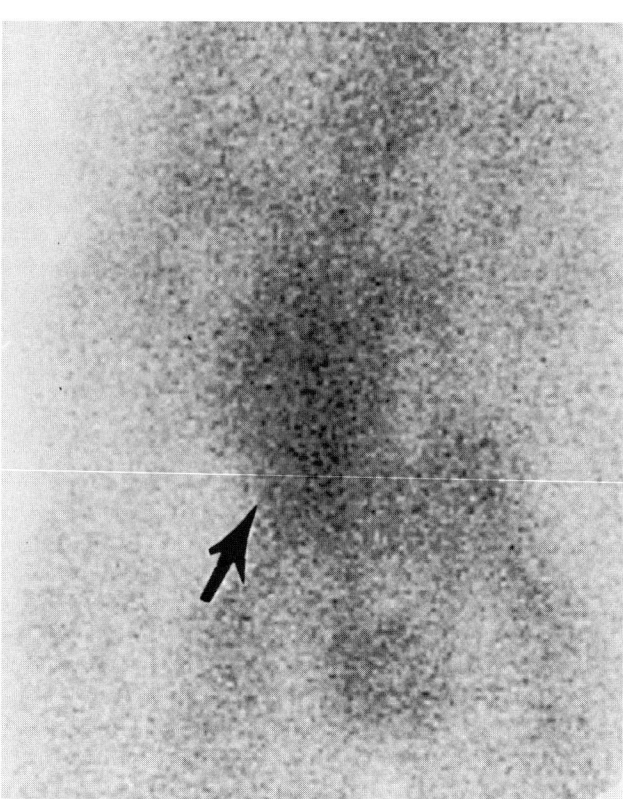

Figure 7–26. A 35-year-old patient 6 weeks after kidney transplant. After the initial renal function was established, a rising creatinine did not respond to antirejection therapy. (**A**) The 30-minute image after MAG3 injection shows high background and vascular activity, and suboptimal kidney and bladder activity. The B/K ratio is only 0.5:1 due to rejection and stasis. (**B**) Repeat study 12 days later shows worsening rejection and minimal MAG3 excretion. The arrow marks the kidney location. (From Teates CD, Parekh JS: New radiopharmaceuticals and new applications in medicine. *Curr Probl Diagn Radiol* 1993; 12(6):258. With permission.)

Generally, radionuclide studies have been unable to reliably differentiate chronic rejection from renal artery stenosis, but this appears possible now. The same test that is used for native renal artery stenosis, using captopril, seems to work well for transplants. In a small series, the response to captopril reliably predicted patients who would respond to angioplasty.[65] Other small series seem to confirm this success.

Other Nuclear Medicine Procedures

Many nuclear medicine studies are indicated in patients with genitourinary disease. Most are not particularly oriented to that group of patients, but the bone scan is one of the most frequently performed procedures in patients with prostate and other genitourinary malignancies. Prostate cancer has such a high propensity to spread to bone that the bone scan is frequently the first test thought of when metastatic disease would affect therapeutic options.

Metastases of prostate carcinoma usually cause radiopaque or sclerotic bone lesions when seen on radiographs. Sclerotic metastases are easier to perceive than lytic lesions, and radiographic films of the pelvis and lumbar spine have been routinely used in many practices as a first step in the workup for metastases. The lower spine and pelvis are often the first site of metastatic spread, and such radiographs have merit. However, a number of studies have shown that the bone scan detects many more lesions than radiographs. Therefore negative plain films have little significance and are only a first step. One of the advantages of the bone scan is that the entire skeleton is surveyed. Initial metastatic sites are often distant, and not limited to the pelvis or lumbar spine.

Harbert reviewed the literature and concluded that prostate cancer is the most common neoplasm metastatic to bone at the time of initial workup.[66] The incidence of positive scans is directly related to size of tumor and grade of malignancy. The frequency ranges from less than 10% in T1 lesions to more than 60% in T4 lesions, with an overall frequency of more than 50%. That frequency is in contrast with less than 1% for all stages of bladder cancer, less than 20% for kidney cancer, and less than 5% for testicular cancer. The incidence in patients with the early lesions now being diagnosed because of the prostate specific antigen test is unclear, but it is probably less than 10% overall.

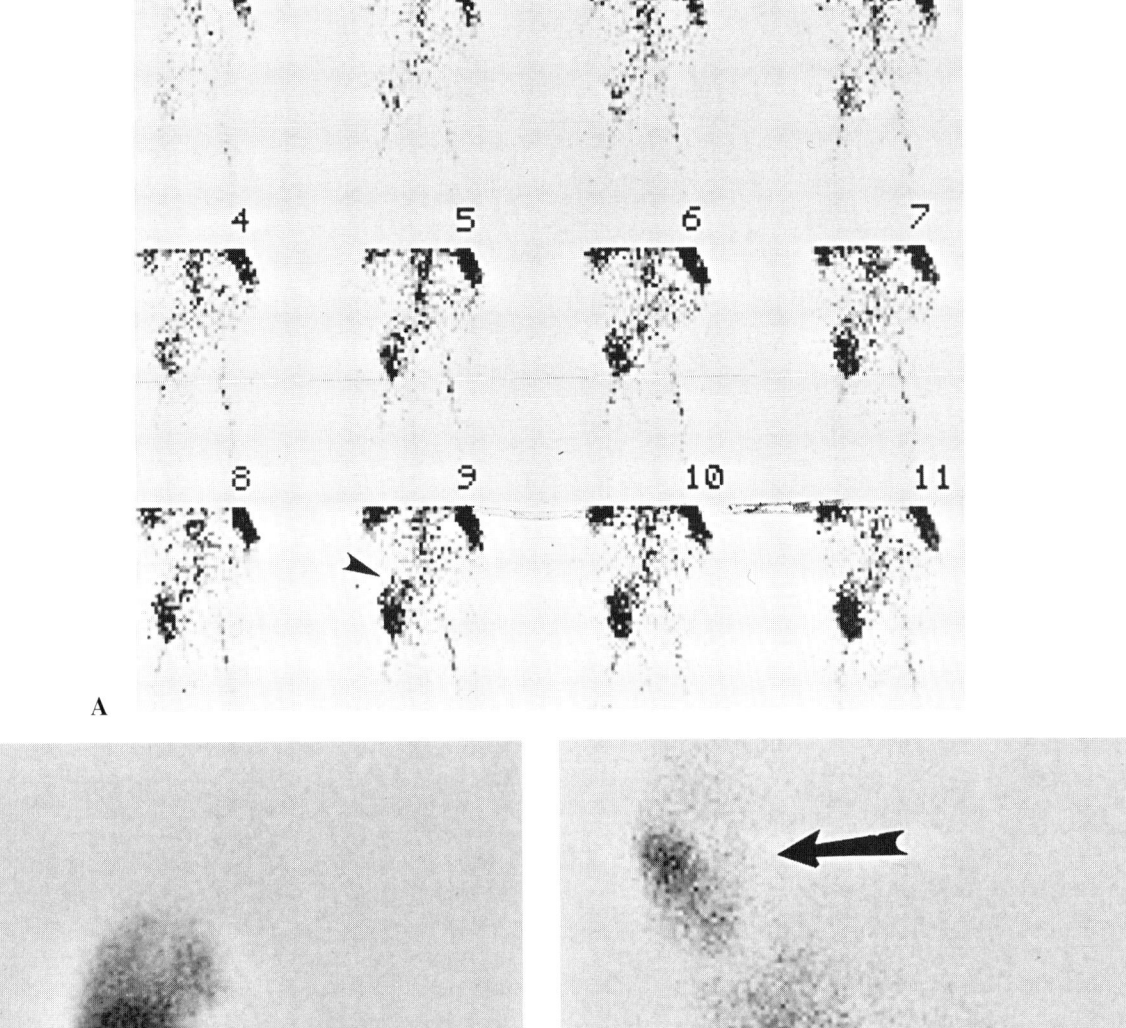

Figure 7–27. A 29-year-old with renal transplant a year ago and rising creatinine. (**A**) The MAG3 vascular sequence shows prompt flow to the kidney but decreased perfusion in the upper pole as a result of venous thrombosis. (**B**) The 3-minute image confirms the upper pole defect. Very slow filling of the collecting system followed because of ureteral obstruction, apparently caused by a clot. (**C**) A 7.5 hour image shows extravasation above the transplant (arrow) as well as retention in the renal pelvis (P) and bladder activity.

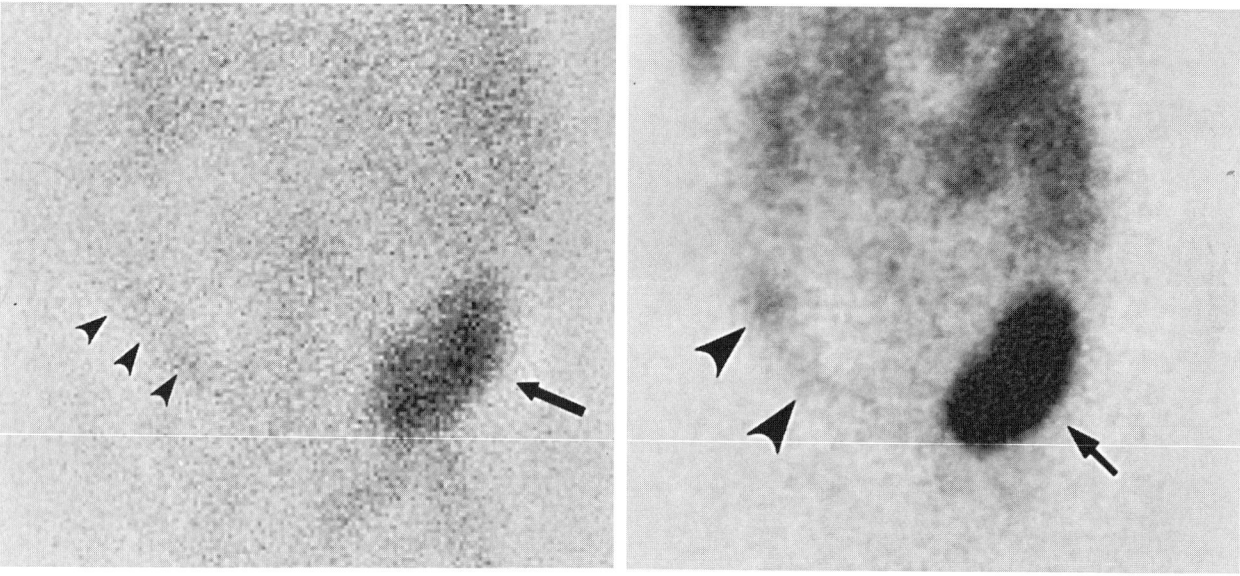

Figure 7–28. A 45-year-old diabetic received renal and pancreatic transplants several days ago. (**A**) The baseline study with DTPA shows normal renal (arrow) and pancreas (arrowheads) activity 3 min after injection. (**B**) A thallium study prior to the renal scan also shows uptake in the right iliac fossa (arrowheads), confirming the viability of the pancreas. With rejection or vascular compromise, the pancreas would show loss of uptake.

In most cases, metastases from prostate carcinoma and other genitourinary cancer are "hot" lesions on the bone scan. Some other tumors such as multiple myeloma have a tendency to produce little reparative bone and thus have a significant number of lesions with poor uptake or even "cold" areas on the scan. This has been noted with technetium-99m methylene diphosphonate (MDP) as with other bone imaging radiopharmaceuticals, which depend on deposition in newly formed bone crystals and increased blood flow. The "hot" lesions are easier to detect than "cold" ones, thus making the bone scan optimal for detection of prostate metastases to bone.

One striking pattern is strongly associated with prostate cancer, the so-called pseudonormal scan (Fig. 7–29). Some patients have widespread bony involvement and may be initially called normal if the reader is not aware that the central skeleton is much hotter than the peripheral skeleton. The metastases are usually dominantly in the central skeleton, because that is the area of hematopoietic marrow, which predisposes to tumor growth. Another name for the pseudonormal pattern is the "absent kidney sign." That pattern is produced because the skeleton is so active that the reduced excretion through the kidneys makes those organs difficult to detect on standard bone images.

More commonly, the lesions are seen as distinct focal areas of increased uptake and must be distinguished from other lesions. Older male patients often have degenerative joint and disc disease, and plain films or other correlative images may be needed to sort out the cause of the positive bone scan. Multiple lesions typical of prostate metastases can be confidently regarded as neoplastic spread. A single lesion usually needs tissue confirmation if the presence of metastasis is critical in treatment planning.

Even though the standard radionuclide bone scan is extremely sensitive for bone metastases, it is realized that not all lesions are detected. Recent magnetic resonance images (MRI) have demonstrated spinal lesions not detected by planar bone scans, lesions still limited to bone marrow with little or no reaction of surrounding bone. MRI does not lend itself to screening of large areas of the skeleton, although most of the spine can be included in one setup. Thus, the bone scan remains the main procedure for the initial screening. Recent experience with single photon emission computerized tomography (SPECT) using the same radiopharmaceutical, Tc-99m MDP, has shown that our standard planar bone scan is missing many lesions. SPECT needs to be incorporated into the bone scan, even if only in the lumbar spine and pelvis, unless the planar views show metastases. SPECT also helps determine if detected abnormalities are likely to be malignant.[67]

The bone scan is frequently used to indicate progression or regression of bone metastases, especially when hormone or chemotherapy is tried. Increasing activity or the appearance of new lesions usually means progression of disease. A well-recognized "flare" of activity may result from good response to a change in therapy, whether drugs, hormone change, or radiation therapy. The flare may last up to 3 months and can be mistaken for an adverse effect, if the recent therapeutic change is not known.[68] In general, plain films that show increasing sclerosis confirm that the pattern is a flare, a positive response to the therapeutic course.

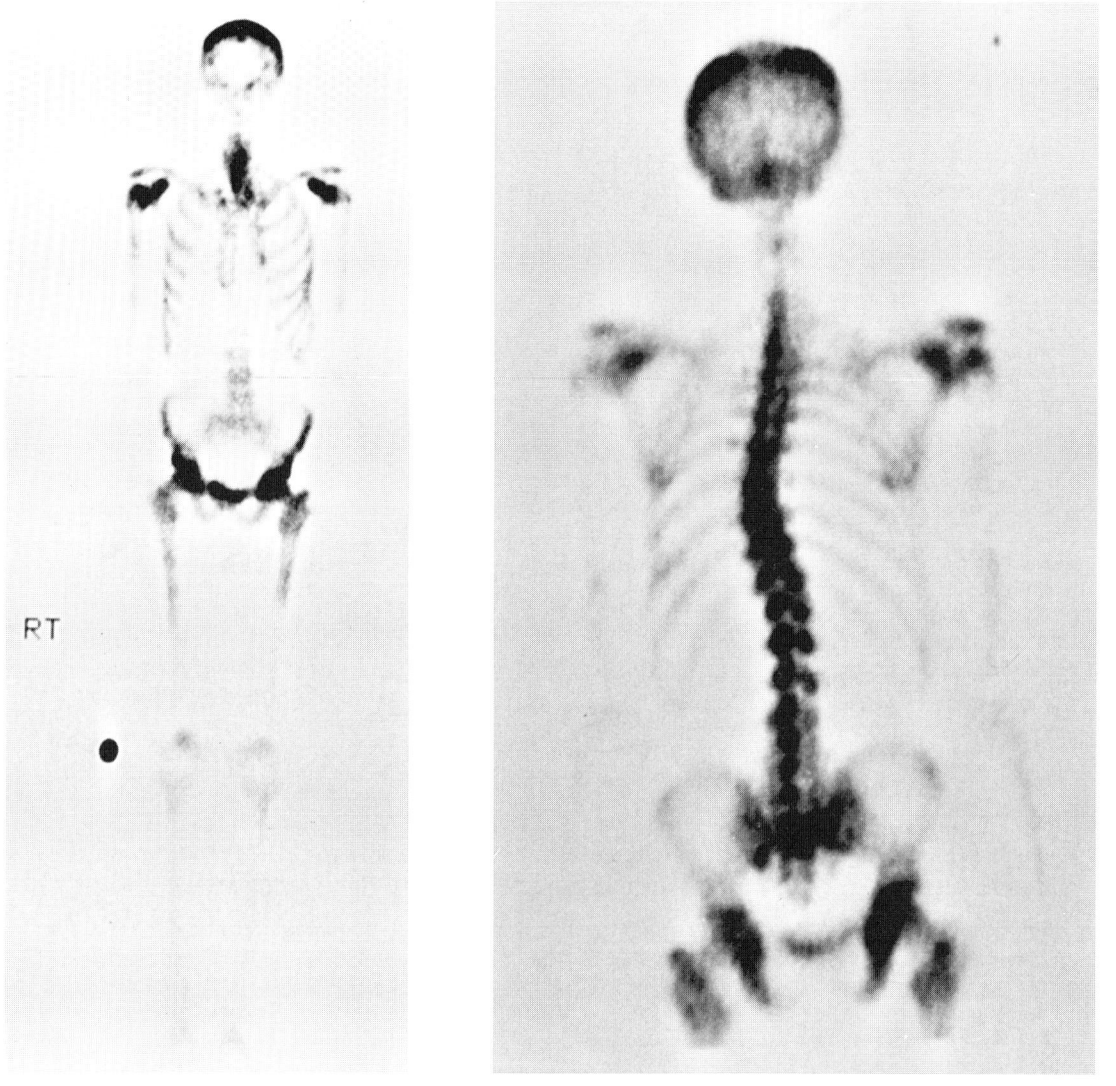

Figure 7–29. A 62-year-old with prostatic carcinoma and bone pain. (**A**) The whole body bone scan with Tc-99m methylene diphosphonate (MDP) shows the "pseudo-normal" or "superscan" pattern resulting from widespread bony metastases. Note the demarcation between the involved central skeleton and long bones at the midhumerus and midfemur on the anterior view. (**B**) The kidneys are poorly visualized on the posterior view because of avid bone uptake, the absent kidney sign.

REFERENCES

1. Chervu RL, Blaufox MD: Renal radiopharmaceuticals: an update. *Semin Nucl Med* 1982;12:224–239.
2. Taylor Jr. A, Eshima D, Fritzberg AR, et al: Comparison of iodine-131 OIH and technetium-99m MAG3 renal imaging in normal volunteers. *J Nucl Med* 1986;27:795–803.
3. Eshima D. Fritzberg AR, Taylor Jr A: Tc-99m renal tubular function agents: current status. *Semin Nucl Med* 1990;20:28–40.
4. Eshima D, Taylor A Jr: Technetium-99m mercaptoacetyltriglycine: update on the new Tc-99m renal tubular function agent. *Semin Nucl Med* 1992;22:61–73.
5. Taylor Jr. A, Eshima D, Christian PE, et al: A technetium-99m MAG3 kit formulation: preliminary results in normal volunteers and patients with renal failure. *J Nucl Med* 1988;29:616–622.
6. Taylor Jr A, Clark S, Ball T: Comparison of Tc-99m MAG3 and Tc-99m DTPA scintigraphy in neonates. *Clin Nucl Med* 1994;19:575–580.
7. Tayor Jr A, Ziffer JA, Eshima D: Comparison of Tc-99m MAG3 and Tc-99m DTPA in renal transplant patients with impaired function. *Clin Nucl Med* 1990;15:371–378.
8. Schlegel JU, Hamway SA: Individual renal plasma flow determination in 2 minutes. *J Urol* 1976;116:282–285.
9. Gates GF: Glomerular filtration rate: estimation from fractional renal accumulation of Tc-99m DTPA (stannous). *AJR* 1982;138:565–570.
10. Ginjaume M, Casey M, Barker F, et al: Measurement of glomerular filtration rate using technetium-99m DTPA (letter). *J Nucl Med* 1985;28:1347–1348.
11. Chachati A, Meyers A, Godon JP, et al: Repid method for the measurement of differential renal function: validation. *J Nucl Med* 1987;28:829–836.
12. Piepsz A, Denis R, Ham HR, et al: A simple method for mea-

suring separate glomerular filtration rate using a single injection of Tc-99m DTPA and the scintillation camera. *J Pediatr* 1987;93:769–774.
13. Shore RM, Koff SA, Mentser M, et al: Glomerular filtration rate in children: determination from the Tc-99m DTPA renogram. *Radiology* 1984;151:627–633.
14. Russel CD, Dubovsky EV, Scott JW: Estimation of ERPF in adults from plasma clearance of I-131 hippuran using a single injection and one or two blood samples. *Nucl Med Biol* 1989; 16:381–383.
15. Russell CD, Dubovsky EV: Measurement of renal function with radionuclides. *J Nucl Med* 1989;30:2053–2057.
16. Russell CD, Bischoff PG, Kontzen FN, et al: Measurement of glomerular filtration rate: single injection plasma clearance method without urine collection: *J Nucl Med* 1985;26:1243–1247.
17. Rowell KL, Kontzen FN, Stutzman ME, et al: Technical aspects of a new technique for estimating glomerular filtration rate using technetium-99m-DTPA. *J Nucl Med Tech* 1986; 14:196–198.
18. Ham HM, Piepsz A: Estimation of glomerular filtration rate in infants and in children using a single-plasma sample method. *J Nucl Med* 1991;32:1294–1927.
19. Winter CC: A new test for vesicoureteral reflux: an external technique for using radioisotopes. *J Urol* 1959;81:105.
20. Whitaker RH: Methods of assessing obstruction in dilated ureters. *Br J Urol* 1973;45:15–22.
21. O'Reilly PH, Lawson RS, Sheilds RA, et al: Idiopathic hydronephrosis—the diuretic renogram: a new non-invasive method of assessing equivocal pelvoureteral obstruction. *J Urol* 1979; 121:153.
22. Conway JJ: ''Well-tempered'' diuresis renography: its historical development, physiological and technical pitfalls, and standardized technique protocol. *Semin Nucl Med* 1992; 22:74–84.
23. Elison BS, Taylor D, Vanderwall H, et al: Comparison of DMSA scintigraphy with intravenous urography for the detection of renal scarring and its correlation with vesicoureteric reflux. *Br J Urol* 1992;69:294–302.
24. Sty JR, Wells RG, Schroeder BA, et al: Diagnostic imaging in pediatric renal inflammatory disease. *JAMA* 1986; 256:895–899.
25. Majd N, Rushton HG, Chandra R, et al: Accuracy of Tc-99m DMSA renal cortical scintigraphy in experimentally induced acute pyelonephritis in piglets. *J Nucl Med* 1988;29:778.
26. Verber IG, Meller ST: Serial Tc-99m dimercaptosuccinic acid (DMSA) scans after urinary infections presenting before the age of 5 years. *Arch Dis Child* 1989;64:1533–1537.
27. Shanon A, Feldman W, McDonald P, et al: Evaluation of renal scars by technetium-labeled dimercaptosuccinic acid scan, intravenous urography, and ultrasonography: a comparative study. *J Ped* 1992;120:399–403.
28. Weingrad T, Heyman S, Alavi A: Cold lesions on bone scan in pediatric neoplasms. *Clin Ncul Med* 1984;9:125–130.
29. Kimmig B, Brandeis WE, Eisenhut M, et al: Scintigraphy of neuroblastoma with I-131 MIBG. *J Nucl Med* 1984;25:773-775.
30. Geatti O, Shapiro B, Sisson JC, et al: Iodine-131 metaiodobenzylguanidine scintigraphy for the location of neuroblastoma: preliminary experience in ten cases. *J Nucl Med* 1985; 26:736–742.
31. Garty I, Friedman A, Sandler MP, et al: Neuroblastoma: imaging evaluation by sequential Tc-99m MDP, I-131 MIBG, and Ga-67 citrate studies. *Clin Nucl Med* 1989;14:515–522.
32. Hoefnagel CA, Voute PA, de Kraker J et al: Radionuclide diagnosis and therapy of neural crest tumors using iodine-131 metaiodobenzylguanidine. *J Nucl Med* 1987;28:308–314.
33. Chen DCP, Holder LE, Melloul M: Radionuclide scrotal imaging: further experience with 210 patients. Part I: Anatomy, pathophysiology, and methods. *J Nucl Med* 1983;24:735–743.
34. Chen DCP, Holder LE, Melloul M: Radionuclide scrotal imaging: further experience with 210 new patients. Part II: Results and discussion. *J Nucl Med* 1983;24:841–853.
35. Lerner RM, Mevorach RA, Hulbert WC et al: Color Doppler ultrasound in the evaluation of acute scrotal disease. *Radiology* 1990; 176:355–358.
36. Middleton WD, Siegel BA, Melson GL, et al: Acute scrotal disorders: prospective comparison of color Doppler ultrasound and testicular scintigraphy. *Radiology* 1990;177:177–181.
37. Tanaka T, Mishkin FS, Datta NS: Radionuclide imaging of scrotal contents. In: Freeman LM, Weissmann HS, eds: *Nuclear Medicine Annual*. New York: Raven Press, 1981:195–221.
38. Staab EV, Hopkins J, Patton DD, et al: The use of radionuclide studies in the prediction of function in renal failure. *Radiology* 1973;106:141–146.
39. Harwood TH, Hiesterman DR, Robinson RG, et al: Prognosis for recovery of function in acute renal failure. *Arch Intern Med* 1976;136:916–919.
40. Taylor A Jr, Eshima D, Christian PE, et al: Evaluation of Tc-99m mercaptoacetyltriglycine in patients with impaired renal function. *Radiology* 1987;162:365–370.
41. Rushton HG, Majd M. Dimercaptosuccinic acid renal scintigraphy for the evaluation of pyelonephritis and scarring: a review of experimental and clinical studies. *J Urology* 1992; 148:1726–1732.
42. Hurwitz SR, Kessler WO, Alazraki NP, et al: Gallium-67 imaging to localize urinary-tract infections. *Br J Radiol* 1976; 49:156–160.
43. Mendez G Jr, Morillo G, Alonso M, et al: Gallium-67 radionuclide imaging in acute pyelonephritis. *AJR* 1980;134:17–22.
44. Tsand V, Lui S, Moorhead J, et al: Gallium-67 scintigraphy in the detection of infected polycystic kidneys in renal transplant recipients. *Nucl Med Comm* 1989;10:167–170.
45. Whitley MA, Jacobson AF: Congenital or early developmental versus later acquired renal function asymmetry scintigraphic characteristics. *Clin Nucl Med* 1993;18:1020–1023.
46. Bekerman C, Hoffer PB, Bitran JD: The role of gallium-67 in the clinical evaluation of cancer. *Sem Nucl Med* 1984;14:296–323.
47. Older RA, Korobkin M, Workman J, et al: Accuracy of radionuclide imaging in distinguishing renal masses from normal variants. *Radiology* 1980;136:443–448.
48. Pollack HM, Edell S, Morales JO: Radionuclide imaging in renal pseudotumors. *Radiology* 1974;111:639–644.
49. Quinones JD, Varma V, Macal O: Radionuclide and pyelographic tests in screening for renovascular hypertension. *Arch Intern Med* 1972;129:570–577.
50. Meier DA, Beierwaltes WH: Radioisotope renal studies and renal hypertension. *JAMA* 1966;198:119–124.
51. Teates CD, Tegtmeyer CJ, Croft BY, et al: Effects of percutaneous transluminal angioplasty on renal plasma flow. *Sem Nucl Med* 1983;13:245–257.
52. Majd M, Potter BM, Guzzetta PC, et al: Effect of captopril on efficacy of renal scintigraphy in detection of renal artery stenosis. *J Nucl Med* 1983;24:23. Abstract.
53. Fommei E, Gjione S, Palla L, et al: Renal scintigraphic captopril test in the diagnosis of renovascular hypertension. *Hypertension* 1987;10:212–220.
54. Mann SJ, Pickering TG: Detection of renovascular hypertension; state of the art: 1992. *Ann Intern Med* 1992;117:845–853.
55. Nally JV, Black HR: State-of-the-art review: captopril renography—pathophysiological considerations and clinical observations. *Semin Nucl Med* 1992;22:85–97.
56. Chen CC, Hoffer PB, Vahjen G, et al: Patients at high risk for

renal artery stenosis: a simple method of renal scintigraphic analysis with Tc-99m DTPA and captopril. *Radiology* 1990; 176:365–370.
57. Cuocolo A, Esposito S, Volpe M, et al: Renal artery stenosis detection by combined Gates' technique and captopril test in hypertensive patients. *J Nucl Med* 1989;30:51–56.
58. Gross MD, Shapiro B: Scintigraphic studies in adrenal hypertension. *Semin Nucl, Med* 1989;19:122–143.
59. Lamberts SWJ, Krenning EP, Reubi J-C: The role of somatostatin and its analogs in the diagnosis and treatment of tumors. *Endocrine Rev* 1991;12:450–482.
60. Lippert MC, Teates CD, Howards SS: Detection of enteric-urinary fistulas with a noninvasive quantitative method. *J Urol* 1984;132:1134–1136.
61. Egleston TA, Acchiardo S, Rodriguez-Antunez A, et al: 131I hippuran in the evaluation of transplanted kidneys. *Radiology* 1969;93:1145–1148.
62. Davidson HD, Loken MK, Amplatz K: Isotope renography and renal arteriography in the evaluation of renal transplants. *AJR* 1969;105:682–688.
63. Freedman GS, Schiff M, Zager P, et al: The temporal and pathological significance of perfusion failure following renal transplantation. *Radiology* 1975;114:649–654.
64. Hayes M, Moore TC, Taplin GV: Radionuclide procedures in predicting early renal transplant rejection. *Radiology* 1972; 103:627–631.
65. Shamlou KK, Drane WE, Kawkins IF, et al: Captopril renography and the hypertensive renal transplantation patient: a predictive test of therapeutic outcome. *Radiology* 1994;190:153-159.
66. Harbert JC: Efficacy of bone and liver scanning in malignant diseases: facts and opinions. In Freedman LM, Weissmann HS, eds: *Nuclear Medicine Annual 1982*. New York: Raven Press, 1982;373–401.
67. Even-Sapir E, Martin RH, Barmes DC, et al: Role of SPECT in differentiating malignant from benign lesions in the lower thoracic and lumbar vertebrae. *Radiology* 1993;187:193–198.
68. Pollen JJ, Witztum KF, Ashburn WL: The flare phenomenon on radionuclide bone scan in metastatic prostate cancer. *AJR* 1984;142:773–776.

8 Computed Tomography in Urologic Disease: A Practical Guide to the Uses and Limitations of CT Scanning

Durba Dutta, John R. Haaga

Since inception, computed tomography has continued to be increasingly vital to urologic evaluation. It is a standard piece of diagnostic investigation in American medicine today and its uses are manifold. CT is used to assess trauma, evaluate calcifications, evaluate masses or suspected masses, and stage neoplasms. Particular utility is demonstrated when contrast is contraindicated or the kidney is nonfunctioning and intravenous urography cannot be performed. Palpable mass, unexplained pain, and paraneoplastic syndromes are also commonly accepted as indications for screening by CT. Hematuria alone is usually evaluated by urography first because of the many nonneoplastic entities that can cause it. The span of urologic disease cannot be covered in this chapter; therefore emphasis is placed on processess most frequently encountered or those for which CT is particularly useful.

ANATOMY

Axial images are ideal for defining the retroperitoneal fascial planes that limit certain pathologic processes, although the normal fascia itself may be difficult to see if there is little intra-abdominal fat. (For a brief review of anatomy as seen through the eyes of a CT scanner see Fig. 8–1.) The renal fascia defines the perirenal space by forming a cone that encloses the kidney, adrenal gland, and perirenal fat. This cone tapers caudally and opens into the pararenal space through which the ureter passes. The perirenal space is divided in the midline by connective tissue surrounding the aorta and vena cava. The lateral extension of the posterior lamina of the posterior leaf of renal fascia (Gerota's fascia, two layers) is called the lateroconal fascia. This divides the anterior pararenal from the posterior pararenal compartment. The anterior pararenal space extends from posterior parietal peritoneum to the anterior renal fascia (one layer) and contains the pancreas, duodenum, and ascending and descending colon. The posterior pararenal space is a potential space containing fat that continues as the properitoneal fat stripe in the flank. The medial boundary of this space is the lateral edge of the psoas and quadratus lumborum muscles. Effacement of this fat is usually related to hemorrhage.

The kidney is covered by a tight fibrous capsule. The right renal artery courses behind the vena cava and is longer than the left.

The adrenal glands are located anteromedial and superior to each kidney and are described as Y or V configuration. In the normal patient they may be quite thin.

TECHNIQUE

The patient is placed in the supine position for scanning, unless positioned for biopsy. Oral contrast is always preferable to delineate bowel loops from pathology, particularly when the patient is thin. Continuous 10-mm slices before and after intravenous contrast administration are optimal because 9% of lesions such as small stones or acute hemorrhage may be obscured by contrast.[1] The recommended amount and speed of contrast administration is 50 mL of 60% contrast at 2 mL/sec up to 150 mL maximum by mechanical injection.[2] This enables detection of small hypovascular lesions. An increase of 10 HU is considered "enchancing," but the average third- and fourth-generation scanner has a technical specification of 0.5 to 1.0%, and differences of up to 5 to 10 Hounsfield units may be due to machine variation.[2] Streak artifacts may simulate enhancement. A maximum milliampere setting decreases noise. A single breath-hold will decrease ventilatory motion artifact when patient cooperation is possible. Incremental slices are obtained during infusion of contrast into the arm, femoral vein, or foot. Respiration must be suspended for best results. Although technology dependent, scan time is usually less than 10 seconds. A second bolus with rapid-sequence scanning can delineate the corticomedullary junction. Localizing the renal hilum on the precontrast scan followed by 5- to 10-mm slices at that level during bolus contrast injection is ideal for evaluation of the renal veins and the inferior vena cava (IVC) at maximal enhancement.[3] This increases the sensitivity for detection of clot or tumor. Obviously, the study should be tailored to the individual patient. Most CT tables

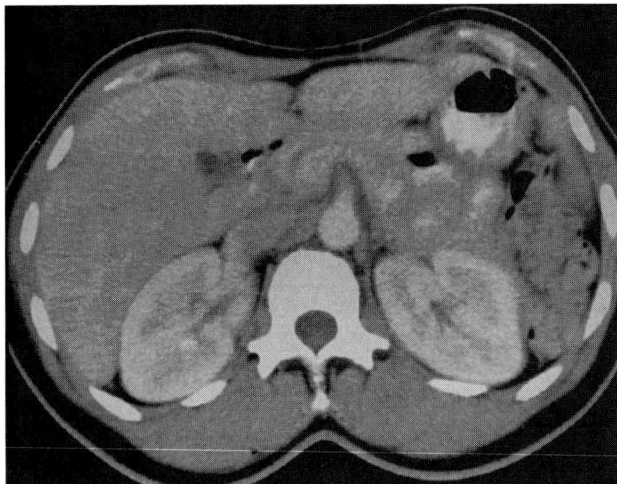

Figure 8–1. Normal contour and configuration of the kidneys at the level of the SMA. Note the crisp distinction of the cortex from the medulla following contrast administration. This patient is thin and very little intra-abdominal fat is present to separate tissues.

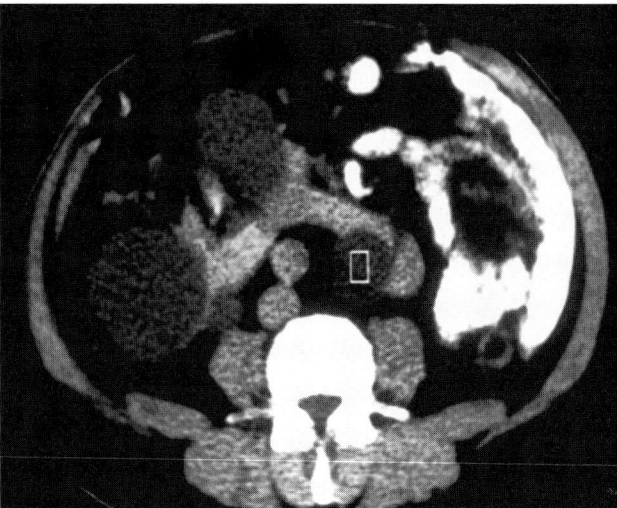

Figure 8–2. Horseshoe kidney. Fusion across the midline anterior to the great vessels is demonstrated. Several large low-attenuation cysts are also present.

have a weight limit of 300 lb. In patients where contrast is contraindicated, adjunctive studies such as MRI, US, or angiography may be helpful.

CONGENITAL AND ANATOMIC VARIANTS

Renal position and size are easily visualized by CT. Incomplete migration results in abnormal position or ectopia. These patients are at increased risk for developing pyelonephritis because of urinary stasis. Pyelonephritis often leads to the presenting symptoms. Forms of ectopia include simple ectopia, horseshoe kidney, crossed and crossed-fused ectopia. Horseshoe kidney refers to bilateral simple ectopia with fusion across the midline that usually occurs at the lower poles, anterior to the great vessels (Fig. 8–2). The position of the spine behind the kidney increases the susceptibility to trauma, and there is increased incidence of stones as well. Crossed ectopia is absence of lateralization, felt to be due to displacement of the ureteral bud across midline into the opposite nephrogenic ridge. The malpositioned kidney may be fused with the orthotopic one (Fig. 8–3). The heterotopic ureter crosses midline to drain into the bladder. Other variants that should be recognized because they may present as a pseudomass are hypertrophied Bertin's column, persistent fetal lobulation, and dromedary hump; however, contrasted CT easily demonstrates these as normal parenchyma. Surface grooves usually disappear by age 10, but up to 51% of adults have some persistent lobulation.[2] Renal sinus lipomatosis can be seen with aging or pathologic atrophy. This benign entity can be distinguished from angiomyolipoma by location (angiomyolipomas being parenchymal) or a peripelvic cyst by attenuation (cysts being fluid density).

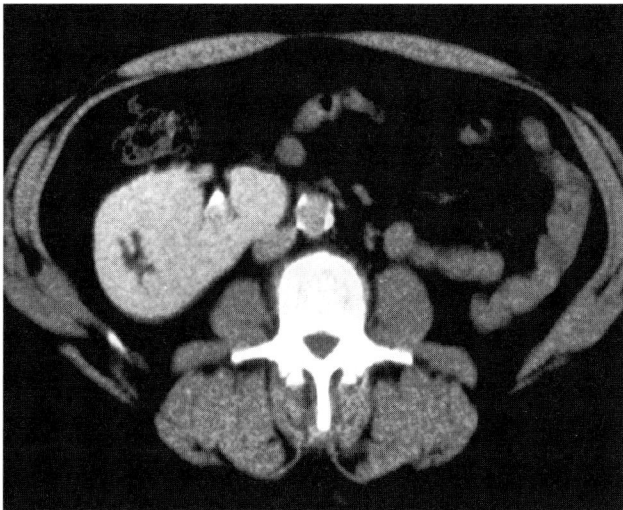

Figure 8–3. Crossed fused ectopia. The kidneys are adjoined and both pelvicocalyceal systems are to the right of midline.

TRAUMA

For the sake of accuracy and completeness a dynamic CT without and with contrast is the study of choice in the setting of acute abdominal trauma.[4] Acute hemorrhage (~60 HU) is readily identifiable on noncontrasted scans. The most frequent injury from blunt abdominal trauma is subcapsular hematoma (Figs. 8–4, 8–5).[5] Because of the tight fibrous capsule covering the kidney, subcapsular collections compress and flatten the adjacent parenchyma without affecting the perirenal fat. These are managed conservatively. As a hematoma retracts and the cellular components settle, it becomes low density peripherally with relative hyperdensity centrally.

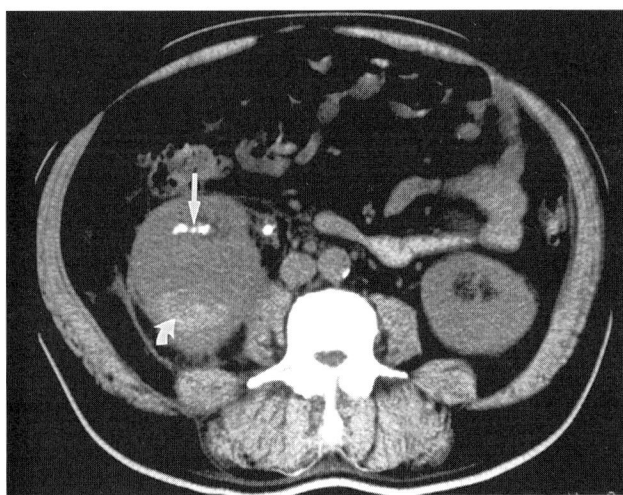

Figure 8–4. Subcapsular renal hematoma as a precontrast scan. The dense material is a stone (straight arrow). The patient had undergone extracorporal shock wave lithotripsy. Subcapsular hematoma is an acknowledged complication. The blood (curved arrow) is of intermediate attenuation (higher than that of the parenchyma). Inflammatory changes are present in the posterior pararenal fat and Gerota's fascia is made distinct. Also note that the kidney is anteriorly displaced.

Renal contusion may be focal, lobar, or diffuse and appears as patchy, moth-eaten enhancement of the parenchyma. Laceration or fracture of the parenchyma appears as a lucent defect extending through the parenchyma. Blood may be present in the perirenal space from disruption of the renal capsule. The "shattered kidney" is the extreme of renal fracture where multiple clefts and fragments are seen. The collecting system may be disrupted, causing contrast and urine to spill into the perirenal space and accumulating between the layers of anterior and posterior renal fascia.

Posttraumatic scarring often appears as a smoothly marginated cup-shaped (as a result of subcapsular bleeding) defect in renal contour. The calyces may extend to the edge of the defect from invagination of the cortex. Another picture of scarring is a grossly heterogeneous nephrogram with scattered bands of avascular scars between areas of normal parenchyma.

RENOVASCULAR DISEASE

If contrast is not seen in the kidney or collecting system, occlusion of the renal artery is suspected.[6] Occasionally, thrombus can be directly visualized. Other signs include the cortical rim and vermiform or spoke–wheel pattern of medullary enhancement unrelated to functional tissue. An intimal flap may be present, necessitating immediate surgery. Although embolism is more common, thrombosis from trauma is not unusual. Renal artery aneurysm is demonstrated as focal dilatation. Complications include microembolization to the kidney with subsequent destruction of parenchyma.

A wedge-shaped cortical defect of low attenuation with a subcapsular rim of high attenuation is classic for renal infarct (Fig. 8–6). Hyperemia of the cortical rim is due to the capsular artery, which receives collaterals from the retroperitoneum, sparing a rim of parenchyma.

Any distention of the renal vein is suspicious for thrombosis, but this is confirmed by visualizing the filling defect when contrast is administered. The most common site is below the SMA, where the renal vein becomes thin as it crosses.

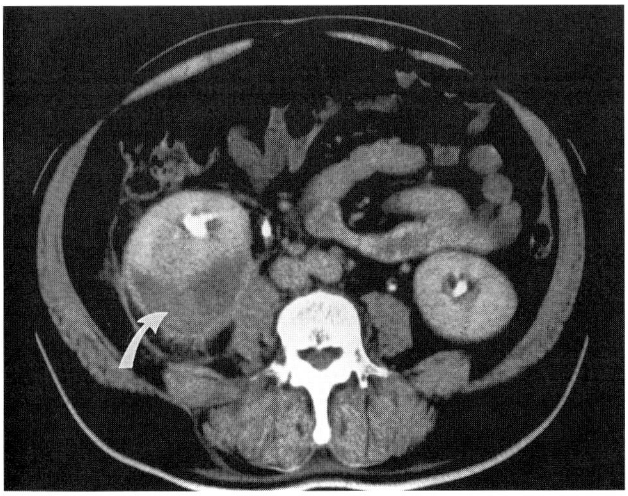

Figure 8–5. Subcapsular hematoma in a postcontrast scan. Now the mixed-attenuation hematoma (curved arrow) is lower than that of the parenchyma and the margins are distinct. The tight capsule has been lifted off the parenchyma. Secondary infection was shown on aspiration.

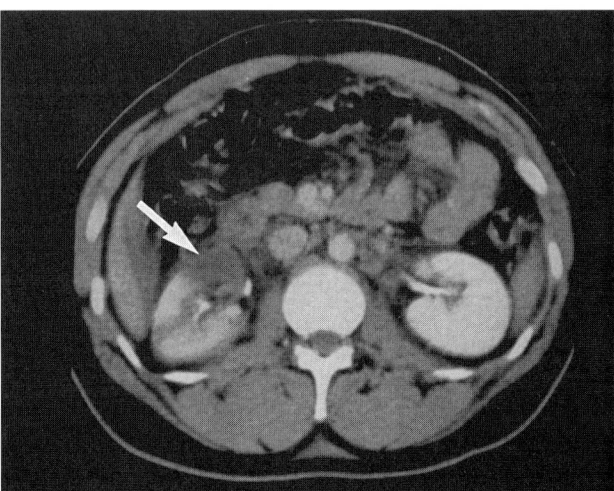

Figure 8–6. Renal infarct is demonstrated as a sharply marginated hypodense segment (arrow) anteriorly extending to the lower pole of the right kidney on this contrasted study. The patient had undergone a motor vehicle accident. Another band of hypodensity is present representing a previous fracture.

INFECTIOUS AND INFLAMMATORY DISEASE

Acute diffuse pyelonephritis in adults is a clinical diagnosis of fever, dysuria, frequency, and flank pain or a laboratory diagnosis of bacteriuria or pyuria. Pathologically, microabscesses of 1 to 5 mm are present throughout the parenchyma. CT rarely plays a role in evaluation unless there is inadequate response to treatment.[7] The "striated nephrogram" is the classically described appearance of acute pyelonephritis on CT (Fig. 8–7). After contrast administration, linear low-density bands are seen extending from medulla to cortex in a radial pattern. This is thought to be secondary to decreased function of nephrons from ischemia or obstruction. The pattern is not necessarily linear and may be patchy. Other findings are nonspecific but include impaired function (as demonstrated by decreased enhancement of parenchyma or delayed excretion), renal enlargement, nonobstructive calyceal dilatation, and fascial thickening. Findings are often not dramatic. Unless a baseline study is available for comparison, subtle changes in renal size and attenuation may be difficult to distinguish. Findings may be unilateral or bilateral. More pronounced findings are encountered when pyelonephritis has progressed to the suppurative form (renal phlegmon). This unusually severe form occurs most frequently in diabetic women who present septic with their initial urinary tract infection (UTI).[8]

Emphysematous pyelonephritis is associated with a mortality rate of 50% and is considered a surgical emergency (Fig. 8–8).[9] It is seen following acute pyelonephritis (frequently with *Escherichia coli*) in patients with a long history of diabetes, immunosuppressive therapy, or urinary tract obstruction. Here CT plays a vital role because gas can be specifically identified and early detection can improve mortality. Multiple collections of gas in the parenchyma and collecting system with destroyed parenchyma is diagnostic.

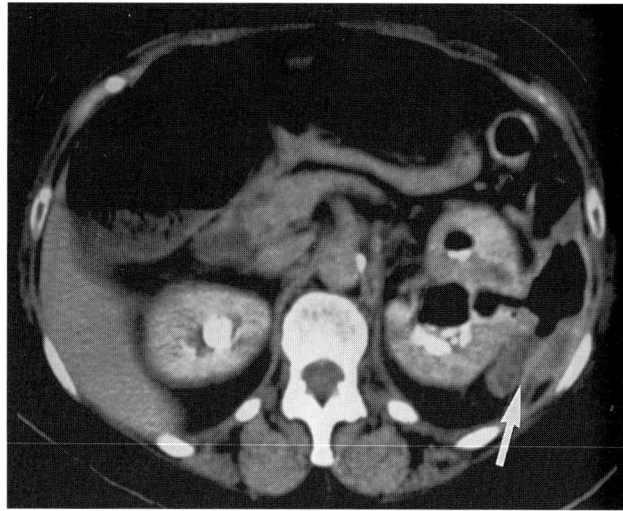

Figure 8–8. Emphysematous pyelonephritis (a surgical emergency) with staghorn calculus. Complications of perforation and fistula formation to the descending colon are demonstrated (air is black). Also a retroperitoneal abscess is seen as a low-density fluid collection of mixed attenuation (arrow).

The other findings of pyelonephritis may also be present, such as renal enlargement and loss of normal contour.

A form of indolent suppurative granulomatous infection known as *xanthogranulomatous pyelonephritis* is an unusual sequela of chronic obstruction by stone, stricture or tumor and infundibular stenosis.[10] Seventy-five to 80% are associated with staghorn calculus (Fig. 8–9). Infection by *Proteus* or *E. coli* organisms has been associated but urine cultures may be sterile. Females are three times more likely than males to develop XGP and usually present in their fifth to seventh decades. The parenchyma is replaced by lipid-laden macrophages, plasma cells and lymphocytes appearing as low-attenuation nephromegaly. Involvement is

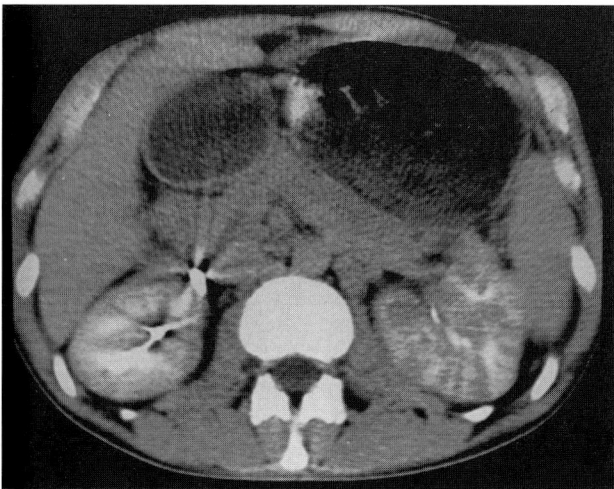

Figure 8–7. Striated nephrogram of the left kidney. This is the classically described spoke–wheel appearance associated with pyelonephritis.

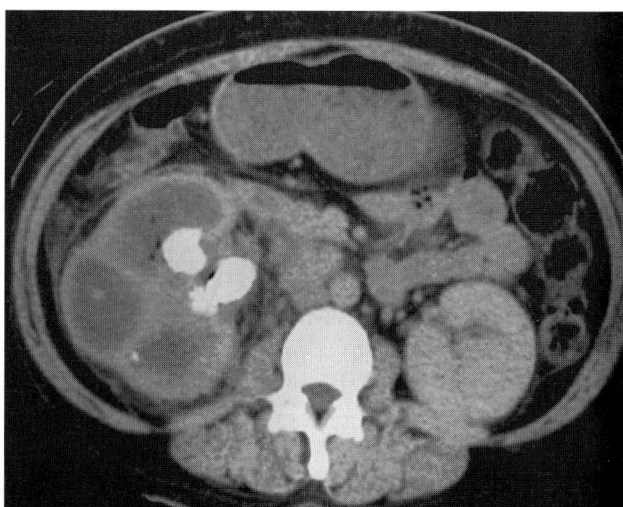

Figure 8–9. Xanthogranulomatous pyelonephritis is often associated with staghorn calculus, as seen here. The renal parenchyma is liquefied and suppurative. A few gas bubbles may also be present. The kidney is diffusely enlarged.

diffuse in 90%, segmental in 10%. Renal function is decreased or absent; therefore enhancement is marginal. Pelvicocaliectasis from obstruction can give the appearance of a "bear paw."

Nephronia, focal lobar nephritis, or acute bacterial nephritis is a stage between pyelonephritis and frank abscess, defined as acute focal infection without liquefaction (Hodgson). CT appearance is of a poorly marginated, slightly lower than normal density mass with patchy enhancement and no discrete wall. Focal enlargement is always present. The renal fascia may be thickened by edema. Usually, nephronias completely regress without scarring or calyceal clubbing, but occasionally they progress to abscess.

CT findings of abscesses are usually conclusive and include a complex renal mass, usually round and well demarcated, with a low attenuation (15 to 30 HU). CT is very effective in characterizing the abscess wall which may demonstrate surface irregularities or rim enhancement or may be thick and well defined (Fig. 8–10). Ultrasound may add complementary information on the cystic nature of such a lesion. Thickening of fascia and edema in perinephric fat are associated local inflammatory changes. Note that CT findings may lag behind clinical improvement for months. The presence of a localized collection of gas within a necrotic mass is usually diagnostic for abscess. An unusual exception was reported by Lenkey, Reece, and Herbert in a case of gas transformation in a renal cell carcinoma by *Bacteroides* species. The usual organisms in renal abscess are *E. coli, Enterobacter, Proteus,* and *Staphylococcus aureus.* Gram-negative infections occur by direct extension from an obstructed system. Gram-positive infections are caused by hematogenous spread, most often seen in intravenous drug abusers. *Candida* species can cause multiple abscesses in immunocompromised hosts. CT-guided percutaneous drainage of these collections is used to facilitate recovery or culture the organisms when therapy is not effective (Fig. 8–11).

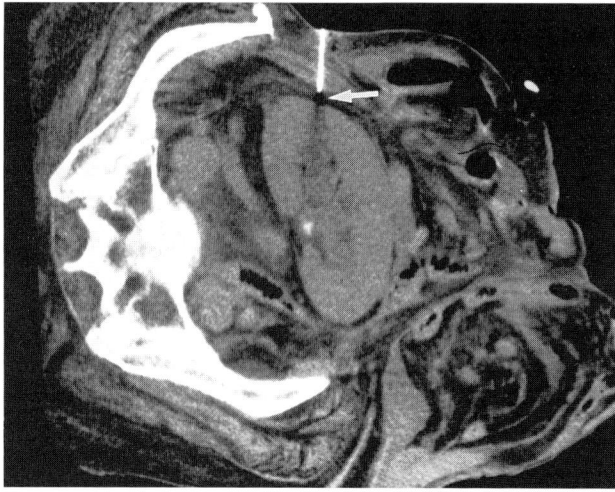

Figure 8–11. This large transplanted pelvic kidney developed pyohydronephrosis. The patient was placed in the left lateral decubitus position for sampling. The needle edge is defined by the black (arrow) at the end of the metal (white).

Vesicoureteral reflux with or without recurrent urinary tract infections in childhood can lead to end-stage renal disease and chronic atrophic pyelonephritis. Hypertension with renal failure is the most common presentation. Calyceal damage is better demonstrated by intravenous urography, but shrunken kidneys with hypertrophic parenchyma between scars can be seen on CT and functional tissue can be estimated.

AIDS

Viral nephritis, such as mumps, can cause initial swelling and ultimate shrinking of the kidney. Another increasingly important viral infection of the genitourinary tract is acquired immunodeficiency syndrome (AIDS). Thirty-eight to 68% of HIV+ patients present with azotemia, proteinuria, hematuria, or pyuria sometime during their course.[11] In addition, many drugs used in the treatment of AIDS are nephrotoxic. CT findings vary according to the various manifestations of the disease.

HIV nephropathy is a clinical syndrome of high proteinuria and rapidly progressive renal failure that occurs in 10% of cases (Fig. 8–12). The highest incidence is in black men with AIDS. Even with hemodialysis, death usually occurs within 6 months.[11] Findings on CT may include bilateral global nephromegaly with medullary hyperattenuation probably related to abnormality of the tubules.

Half of AIDS patients suffer from recurrent infections that cause pyelonephritis, cystitis, or abscesses from common or opportunistic pathogens. The CT findings are similar to those in patients without AIDS. In the population of intravenous drug abusers with AIDS, septic emboli are also encountered.

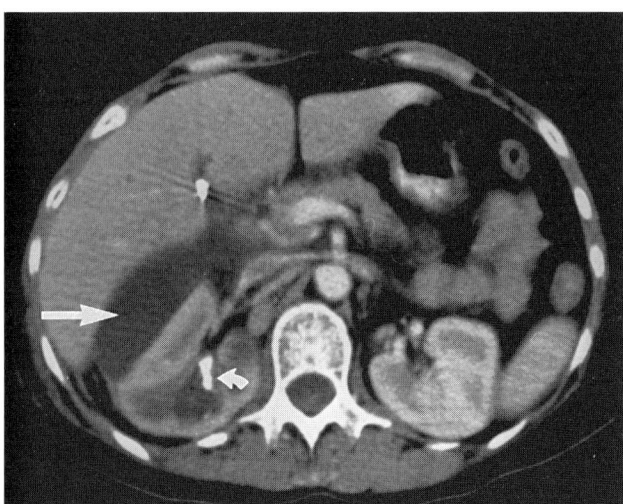

Figure 8–10. Pyonephrosis with perinephric abscess. The low-attenuation collection anterior to the right kidney (arrow) has compressed the parenchyma so that it is folded upon itself, causing the straight edge. This patient had undergone lithotripsy for the dense calculus (curved arrow).

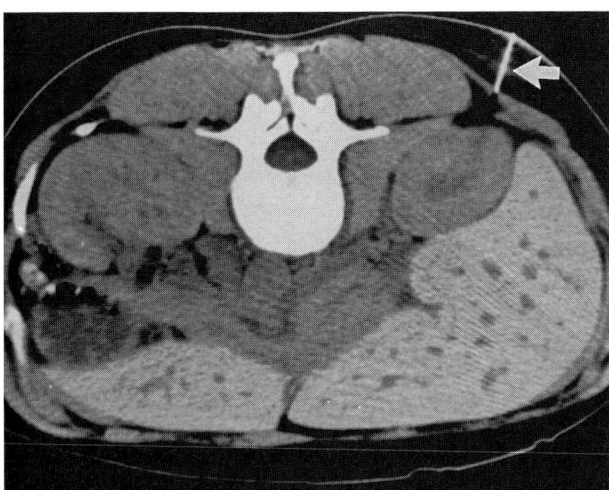

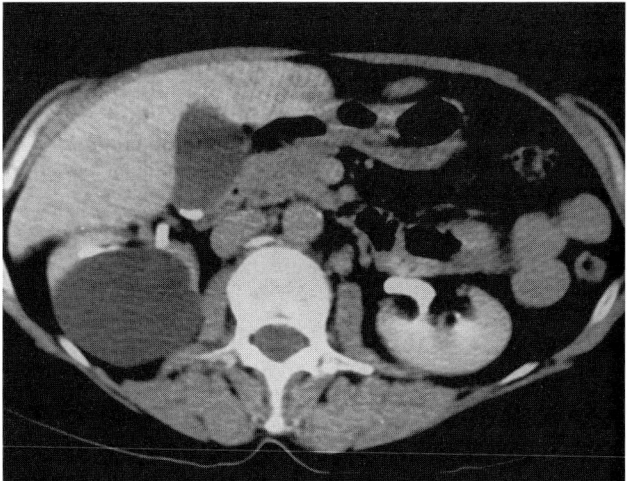

Figure 8–12. Biopsy-proven HIV nephropathy. Note that the renal appearance is nonspecific. The patient has been placed in the prone position for a direct, posterior approach of the needle (arrow) to the kidney.

Figure 8–13. The large, round low-attenuation lesion with smooth margins and an imperceptible wall is a simple cyst. The fluid is homogeneous and no septations are present. There is compression upon the right collecting system, which tapers medially, giving the appearance of "beaking." Also note that the kidneys are malrotated bilaterally, with the hila directed more anteriorly than medially. This is a congenital variant.

Hemorrhagic cystitis is common in the AIDS polulation. The etiologic agent can be usual gram-negative organisms or opportunistic organisms such as candida, B-hemolytic streptococcus, salmonella, cytomegalovirus (CMV) or cryptosporidia, which may fistulize from bowel.

CMV and hepatitis B virus induce high levels of circulating immune complexes that are deposited in the kidney, causing indirect renal disease. Directly, they can cause inflammatory and hemorrhagic cystitis. CMV is almost ubiquitous and is frequently cultured from the urine or kidneys of HIV-infected patients at autopsy.

Pneumocystis carinii infections of the kidneys have recently increased in frequency, possibly because of pneumonia prophylaxis by aerosolized pentamidine. This unique infection causes punctate cortical calcifications in the kidneys. Calcifications may also be present in the liver, spleen, lymph nodes, and adrenal glands. Calcification may be obscured by contrast, therefore a precontrast scan is recommended.

Disseminated mycobacterial infection has increased frequency in the AIDS population. *Mycobacterium avium* intracellulare is the most common of these pathogens found in the kidneys at autopsy; however, there is a growing incidence of mycobacterium tuberculosis. Focal renal lesions are not usually present on premortem CT scans, but partial cortical or medullary nephrocalcinosis can be seen. The most common CT finding is lymphadenopathy of the para-aortic, renal hilar, or mesenteric nodes.

CYSTIC DISEASES

Cysts are the most common renal masses present in up to 55% of the population over 50 years old on autopsy series.[12] A third of patients over 60 have renal cysts on CT.[13] Strict criteria must be upheld to make the diagnosis of simple cyst on CT because no further workup is required for simple cysts, whereas complicated cysts require further evaluation. Sonography is confirmatory (Fig. 8–13). Simple cysts are of cortical origin. The incidence of coexisting tumor is 1%.[13] They are filled with homogeneous transudate that has an attenuation coefficient of 0 to 25 HU and do not enhance. They are round and have smooth margins, a sharp interface with normal parenchyma, and a thin, imperceptible wall. They do not extend beyond Gerota's fascia or amputate calyces, although they may distort them, producing the "beak sign" as the calyx conforms to the convex border of the cyst. Size varies greatly. Those greater than 4 cm can cause hypertension, hematuria, pain, obstruction, or thickening of the renal fascia by compression. Lesions less than 1 cm in diameter can be lost to volume averaging.

Complex Cysts

CT plays an important role in distinguishing the liquid from the solid components of complicated cysts. These may be indistinguishable from necrotic or liquified carcinomas. The density of the contents should be measured before and after contrast administration to assess homogeneity and air–fluid or fluid–fluid levels. Enhancement is indicative of vascular, inflammatory, or neoplastic tissue. The wall visibility, thickness, and enchancement should be assessed as well as the presence of septations or papillary projections.

Some cysts have thin, linear septa that are comparable to the outer wall in thickness and are better visualized after contrast administration. Partial volume averaging and angle of scanning plan may limit detection of these septa. Because of the minute thickness of the septa, they are often averaged with the adjacent water density. Ultrasound is usually more sensitive to the detection of septa.

CT is the best modality for the evaluation of calcification. The most important thing to assess is the location of these calcifications.[14] Peripheral calcifications frequently occur in the walls of benign lesions such as simple cysts (only 3%), polycystic kidneys, multicystic kidney, echinococcal cysts, and remote hematomas. Central calcifications such as in septa can occur in benign processes, but malignancy is much more suspicious (8 to 18% of neoplasms calcify). Calcification always mandates more through evaluation. Calcification morphology may help distinguish the nature of the lesion. Thin, small, lamellar calcifications in septa or cyst walls may be dismissed as benign atypical cyst if all the other criteria for simple cyst are met and there is no evidence of solid tissue. If the calcifications are thick and irregular, malignancy must be excluded.

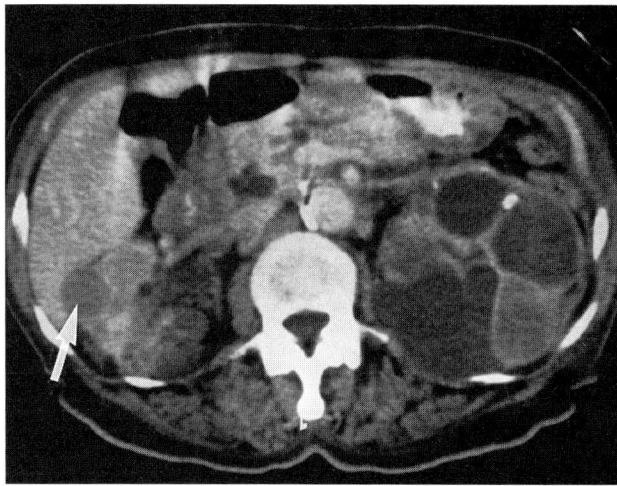

Figure 8–14. Adult polycystic kidney disease (APKD). Multiple cysts of varying sizes and densities are seen. Some contain hemorrhage (arrow); some are homogeneous. Calcification can also be seen in the septae. Note that cysts are also present in this pancreas.

HEMORRHAGIC AND PROTEINACEOUS CYSTS

Acute hemorrhage in a cyst is higher density than normal parenchyma but does not enhance with contrast. As a clot liquifies and hemoglobin is broken down, the periphery becomes hypodense compared to the center. Eventually, a previously hemorrhagic cyst may look like a simple cyst except that the wall may thicken or enhance. Mucoproteinaceous cysts are rare but also high in density.

Autosomal dominant polycystic kidney disease is a specific entity characterized by multiple cysts of variable size involving the kidneys, liver (30 to 50%), pancreas (10%), and spleen (Fig. 8–14). Ten to 15% of cases also have intracranial berry aneurysms in the circle of Willis.[15] Patients usually present with hypertension and uremia in their third to fifth decades. Hematuria or proteinuria can also occur. On CT the kidneys progressively enlarge as the cysts replace the parenchyma. These cysts may be complicated by bleeding or infection increasing the density of the fluid or the thickness of the walls. Up to 50% of polycystic kidneys are associated with cystic calcification or nephrolithiasis. Two-thirds of these patients are symptomatic with flank pain (62%) or hematuria (33%).[16] Cyst calcification usually occurs in older patients with large, severely cystic kidneys and poor renal function, but it is not associated with morbidity. The calcifications are usually flecks or lines in the wall, but luminal amorphous calcifications can occur in the setting or prior hemorrhage within a cyst. The high rate of renal stones may be due to metabolic abnormalities or stasis. Even when calices are displaced by multiple cysts, calculi can be identified in the collecting system. Calculi increase the risk for infection within the cyst (usually by *E. coli*).

Multicystic dysplastic kidney is a congenital but nonheredity form of renal dysplasia characterized by a greatly enlarged, functionless kidney at birth that shrinks and calcifies with age. On CT, the entire kidney is usually involved with multiple thin-walled cysts that are held together by connective tissue. If bilateral, it is fatal at birth. Thirty percent are associated with UPJ obstruction or anomalies of the opposite kidney.

Cystic neoplasms include multilocular cystic nephroma, clear cell, and papillary adenocarcinoma. They are predominantly fluid attenuation, occur in unilocular and multilocular forms, and are usually large and noticeable. They are distinguished from tumors that invade the wall of a cyst or arise from it.

CT is extremely useful in evaluating multilocular masses, because of improved visualization of wall irregularities, papillary projections, and calcifications. Malignant septa tend to be thicker and more enhancing than those in benign multilocular cystic nephroma. The limitations of CT include the inability to detect thin septa due to volume averaging and the similar appearance of a unilocular cystic tumor and an abscess. Both appear as round lesions with thick, irregular walls, and the distinction may depend on the presence of other signs.

SOLID MASSES

Bosniak et al have proposed a classification system for indeterminate renal masses primarily utilizing CT criteria.

Category I lesions meet all the criteria for simple cyst. They are nonenhancing, are well marginated, and have then smooth walls. No calcification, blood, septation, or opaque fluid is seen. The attenuation is usually less than 20 HU, but this is the least important factor because some proteinaceous cysts measure 20 to 50 HU. These lesions are very likely benign and do not require further evaluation or follow-up. Lesions of less than 1.0

cm often cannot be clearly characterized and are not usually pursued.

Category II lesions are primarily cystic, less than 3.0 in size, and may have thin wall calcifications, internal septations, or hyperdense fluid (50–90 HU). Less than 2-cm lesions are problematic because of partial volume averaging. These can be considered benign if the lesions are round and sharply marginated, homogeneous (using narrow window settings), nonenchancing, or extending outside the kidney so the smoothness of the wall can be seen. If they are greater than 3 cm or entirely intrarenal, ultrasound is indicated to confirm cystic nature. Approximately 50% of hyperattenuating cysts are anechoic on sonography, which is further evidence of benignity. Periodic CT follow-up (6 months to 1 year) is recommended to check for enhancement or growth.

Category III lesions are essentially indeterminate, and although most prove to be benign, they must be handled as if they are malignant. Features are thickening or enhancement of the walls or septa and irregular margins or thick calcifications. If the patient is more than 75 years of age or has other significant disease, conservative management is preferable, so as to avoid chronic hemodialysis. Otherwise, partial or total nephrectomy is warranted because of the significant number of malignancies. Needle aspiration for category II or III lesions is not useful if negative results are obtained.

Category IV describes the classic features of carcinoma, including solid enhancing abnormal tissue and central calcification from hemorrhage or necrosis. These should be resected despite a few false-positives. Fine-needle aspiration or biopsy is a reliable method.

Screening

High-resolution CT and improved enhancement techniques have increased the detection of small masses nearly fivefold in the last decade (Fig. 8–15). Fifteen percent of renal masses, particularly those in the poles, are missed by intravenous urography (IVU) (5 to 10% with tomograms). Five to 10% of the incidentally detected masses on IVU are malignant.[2] The average size of tumors at presentation is 7.5cm.[12] CT has a 94% sensitivity for lesions less than 3 cm compared with 79% by ultrasound, but widespread screening by CT is limited by availability, expense, and radiation.[13] Imaging criteria are the same regardless of size. Well-marginated homogeneous lesions tend to be less aggressive than irregular heterogeneous lesions. Needle apiration or biopsy is only useful when the results are positive. A diagnostic accuracy of 93% for FNAB has been reported, but small lesions are technically difficult and have a high sampling error.[17] Aggressivity cannot be determined by size; 8.5% of smaller than 4 cm lesions metastasize.[18]

High-risk patients that should be considered for serial routine screening examinations include patients with Von Hippel–Lindau syndrome, with a family history of renal cell carcinomas, and on chronic dialysis. Von Hippel–Lindau is an autosomal dominant disease expressed between the ages of 20 and 50 associated with central nervous system angiomas and cerebellar hemangioblastomas. Seventy-six percent have renal cystic disease; 35% have renal adenocarcinoma, which is frequently bilateral.[2] Small renal adenomas are also seen. Nine percent of patients on chronic dialysis, especially those with acquired renal cystic disease (ARCD), develop adenomas and carcinomas, which is seven times greater than the general population.

Most solid renal lesions are malignant and should be considered so until proven otherwise. Ninety percent of incidentally detected solid enhancing lesions of less than 3 cm are malignant or premalignant.[19] In an autopsy series of 100, 25% of lesions of less than 3 cm were malignant. In a series of 90 needle biopsies or aspirations 82% were renal cell carcinomas, 10% were oncocytomas, and 8% were benign adenomas, which have malignant potential.

RENAL CELL CARCINOMA

Renal cell carcinomas (RCCs)—also known as renal adenocarcinoma, renal clear cell carcinoma, hypernephroma, and Grawitz tumor—comprise 75% of all renal malignancies. In the United States, 15,000 new cases and 7500 deaths occur yearly.[20] The incidence is 2 to 3% greater in males than in females and increases with age (mean age is 55), smoking, high-fat diet, polycystic disease, and Von Hippel–Lindau. Clinical features are not specific. The triad of flank pain, hematuria, and palpable mass is only seen in 10% of cases when advanced. Fifty-five percent of nontraumatic renal hemorrhage is due to underlying RCC. Early detection allows cure.

Dynamic CT is the most cost-effective means of evaluation.[21] Accurate diagnosis by CT occurs in more than 95%, and more than 91% are accurately staged by CT alone.[22] In

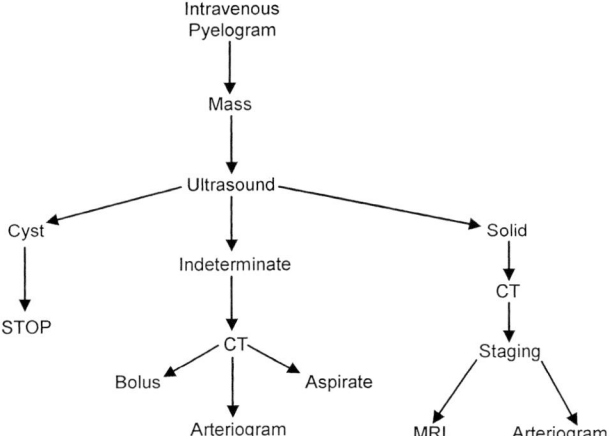

Figure 8–15. Algorithm for evaluation of renal mass.

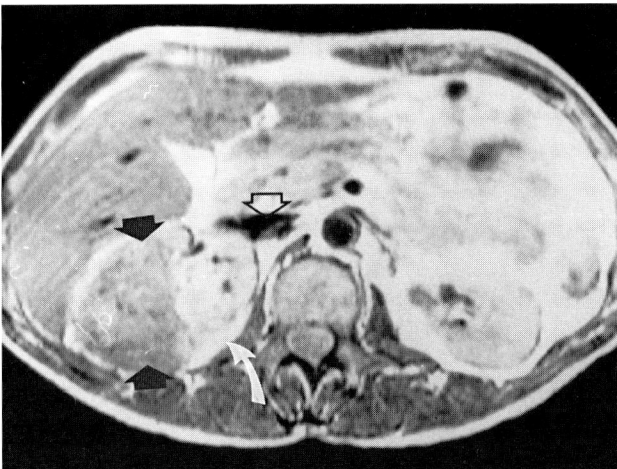

Figure 8–16. T1-weighted MRI image of renal cell carcinoma (arrows). The perinephric fat (curved white arrow) is bright. As in most cases, the tumor itself is intermediate signal intensity on T1. The renal borders are disrupted and there is infiltration of the perirenal fat, indicating state II disease. Normal flow void is seen in the renal vein and IVC (open arrow).[20]

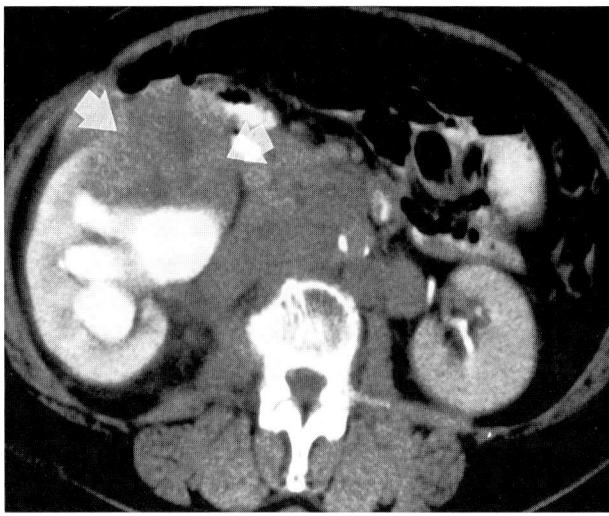

Figure 8–18. "Claw sign" of distorted collecting system associated with obstructing renal mass. In this case the tumor (arrows) is focal, is heterogeneous, and has relatively well-defined margins. The attenuation is lower than that of normal tissue (usual for neoplasm). The differential for the mass itself would include angiomyoma or adenoma; however, the dilated local venous structures are consistent with carcinoma.

1987 Johnson et al studied the sensitivity and specificity of specific criteria included in staging and found (1) 46% sensitivity/98% specificity for perinephric extension, (2) 78% sensitivity/98% specificity for venous invasion, (3) 83% sensitivity/88% specificity for metastatic lymphadenopathy, and (4) 60% sensitivity/100% specificity for involvement of adjacent organs. MR has the advantage of being multiplanar, and sagittal images may better identify extrarenal sources of a mass (Figs. 8–16, 8–17). A 96% accuracy of diagnosis and staging has been described, particularly in stage III or IV disease.[23]

CT appearance is greatly variable (Fig. 8–18). Ninety-four percent are exophytic, 6% infiltrating without disruption of renal contour. Seventy-eight percent are solid, 22% are predominantly cystic with thick walls. They can be homogeneous or heterogeneous and enhance but less than normal parenchyma (attenuation is to 15 to 50 HU without contrast and 50 to 90 HU with CE). The renal contour may be lobulated or irregular because of differences in the growth rate of larger lesions. The margins of the tumor, both inner and outer, are ill defined. When a large tumor outgrows its blood supply and undergoes central necrosis and involution, it is called a self-healed hypernephroma. Ten to 31% have calcifications, usually central and stippled, but the peripheral "eggshell" pattern is also seen. When infiltrating local tissue, sinus fat can be invaded or enveloped. Amputation of the collection system suggests malignancy. Secondary hemorrhage, abscess, or venous thrombosis can occur. Less than 2% are bilateral. The following are the characteristics of each stage:

I. Confined to renal parenchyma
II. Extending through capsule into perirenal fat but contained within Gerota's fascia
III. Renal vein involvement (low-attenuation thrombosis in enlarged renal vein) or lymphadenopathy
IV. Extent beyond Gerota's fascia, invasion of adjacent organs or distant mets (Fig. 8–19)

Discriminating stage I from stage II disease is problematic because the capsule cannot directly be visualized unless thickened. Currently, however, this distinction is only for prognostication and is not clinically relevant. The general policy is to perform partial or radical nephrectomy with semiannual or annual follow-up CT scans for any potentially curable malignancy regardless of size when the contralateral

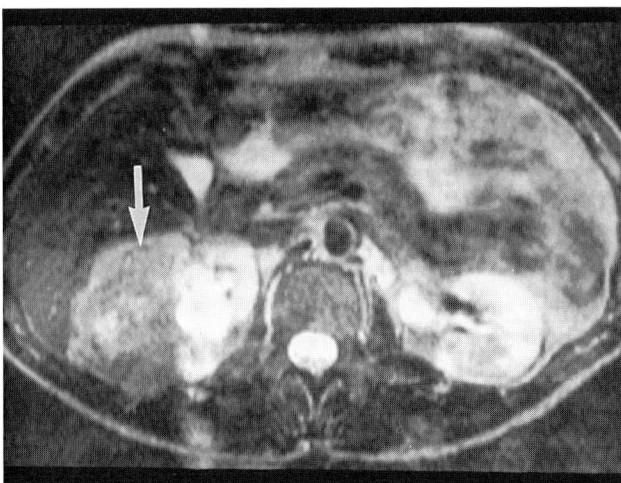

Figure 8–17. T2-weighted axial MRI of renal cell carcinoma (arrow). Water is bright. The accuracy of MRI in tumor staging has been reported as 96% and is especially useful in stage II, III, and IV.[20]

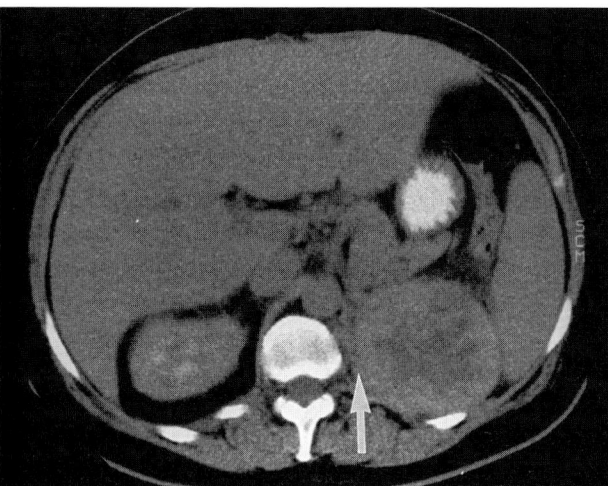

Figure 8–19. Renal cell carcinoma with extent to left iliopsoas muscle (arrow), placing it in the stage IV category. The left kidney is diffusely infiltrated and enlarged.

kidney is normal. Edema may mimic tumor in the perinephric fat. Nonspecific signs of extracapsular spread into the perinephric space are stranding/cobwebbing (which is seen in 50% of patients with stage I disease), collateral vessels, fat obliteration, fascial thickening, and soft-tissue mass (the most reliable sign). If the requisition explicity calls for staging, thin collimation with fast scanning following a rapid bolus of intravenous contrast may be obtained to enable the detection of tumor thrombosis, which appears as a low-density mass, in the renal vein or inferior vena cava with 95% accuracy (Fig. 8–20). Enlargement or displacement of the renal vein is not a reliable sign of invasion but may be associated. Rarely, neovascularity is present in the thrombus. If the injection is too rapid, the renal vein may fill prior to the IVC, mimicking a filling defect in the IVC. Because of its shorter and more oblique course, the right renal vein is more difficult to image than the left. Arm injection is preferable for renal vein assessment, but foot injection is better for IVC invasion. Ultrasound is sometimes superior in defining the superior extent of IVC thrombus (i.e., right atrial involvement).

Size of tumor and frequency of metastasis or renal vein involvement is directly proportional.[24] For lesions of less than 4 cm, 8.5% metastasize; for those of 4 to 8 cm (grade II), 17.9% metastasize; and for those of more than 8 cm (grade III), 50% metastasize. Hematogenous spread to lungs, bone, liver, adrenals, and opposite kidney is the most frequent. Using the appropriate windows and bolus contrast CT is excellent for overall detection. Lung and mediastinal metastasis is frequent enough to warrant routine chest CT. Unusual traits of RCC are that late metastasis can arise even 20 years after cure, and distant metastasis can disappear following nephrectomy. Nodes of greater than 2 cm are always abnormal; however those of 1 to 1.5 cm are nonspecific and sometimes equivocal. Renal hilum, pericaval, and periaortic nodes are most likely to be involved. Local adenopathy by metastasis and direct invasion into the psoas muscle or vertebrae are undoubtedly best detected by CT.

Problems encountered in staging include discriminating invasion of adjacent organs (liver, spleen, colon, pancreas) from indentation. A bulky right renal mass may obsure visualization of the venous structures.

Recurrent renal cell carcinoma occurs most often in the tumor bed, local nodes, liver, adrenal gland, contralateral kidney, and lumbar spine. Abdominal CT with adequate oral and intravenous contrast is important for routine postoperative surveillance. Renal sarcoma and adult Wilms' tumors are rare neoplasms that have no radiologic features that distinguish them from primary renal cell carcinoma. Thus, they are usually resected under the preoperative diagnosis of renal carcinoma.

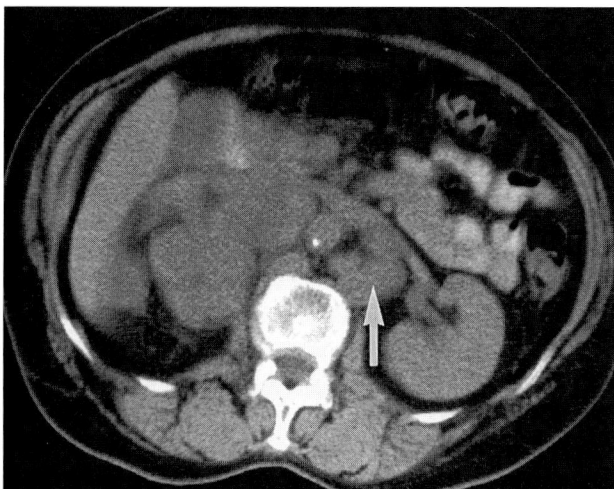

Figure 8–20. Right renal cell carcinoma with invasion of the inferior vena cava (stage III). The aorta has calcification in the walls and the vena cava is the dilated structure to the patient's right. Adenopathy (arrow) is present left of the aorta. Contrast bolus into the foot followed by rapid scanning at the level of the hilum would better delineate the findings, but this is sometimes avoided, to avoid damage to the normal kidney, when there is considerable uremia.

LYMPHOMA

Up to a third of lymphomas involve the kidney, particularly non-Hodgkin's, but the diagnosis is usually known prior to detection of renal involvement.[25] Multiple small focal masses are the most common presentation (Figs. 8–21, 8–22). Other patterns include a diffuse infiltration causing renal enlargement or a solitary mass, in which case CT-guided biopsy is useful to determine inoperative (lymphoma) from operative (carcinoma). Suggestive signs include bilaterality, homogeneity, splenomegaly, and extensive retroperitoneal adenopathy, which can displace the ureters. The lesions are often isodense with unenhanced parenchyma and are enhanced to a lesser degree than normal

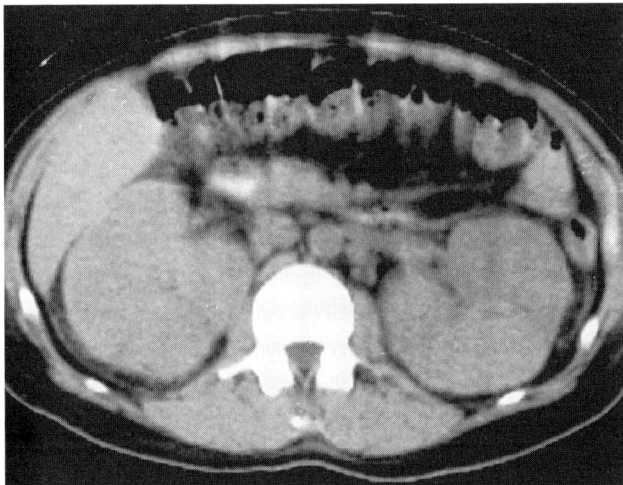

Figure 8–21. Renal lymphoma can give this unique picture of bilateral, homogeneous (on unenhanced studies), bulky renal enlargement. Extensive adenopathy (although not seen here) is highly suspicious for lymphoma.

renal tissue does. Biopsy is indicated if therapy does not produce a response.

The incidence of Kaposi's sarcoma in the AIDS population approximates 27%; 6 to 11% of AIDS lymphoma cases involve the kidneys.[11] Non-Hodgkin's is most common, but Hodgkin's and Burkitt's lymphoma also occur. AIDS-related lymphoma tends to be aggressive, advanced at presentation, and has a greater predilection for extranodal sites. Renal masses without adenopathy are more common than in the general population. CT is ideal for evaluation of multiple sites. Renal disease may appear as multiple masses, diffuse infiltration, or extensive adenopathy. Note there is increased risk for biopsy or invasive procedures on these patients

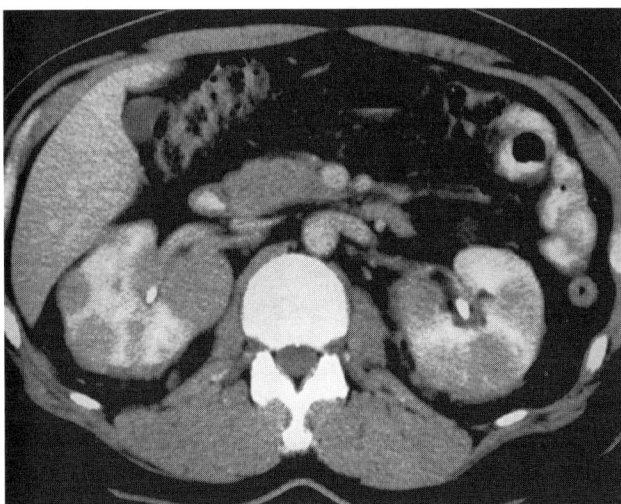

Figure 8–22. After treatment the same patient with renal lymphoma has decreased renal size. The heterogeneity of the kidneys can be visualized with contrast administration. Multiple low-density masses have infiltrated the parenchyma diffusely.

because DIC or pancytopenia can result in massive hemorrhage.

Lymphoma and Kaposi's sarcoma are increased in the AIDS population, and both can affect the kidneys and retroperitoneum. The kidney, adrenal glands, and bladder are not as frequently involved as lymph nodes, lung, liver, spleen, bowel, and skin.[11] Involvement of the kidneys tends to be microscopic and often not identifiable until autopsy. CT may, however, demonstrate bulky lymphadenopathy and infiltration of retroperitoneum by tumor, which can obstruct the collecting system and lead to renal failure.

Renal Metastasis

The most common renal malignancy in autopsy is metastatic disease; however, this tends to occur late in the course of neoplasia. Metastases also tend to enhance but less than normal parenchyma, and CT is considered the most sensitive modality for detection. Lung and melanoma are frequent primaries. Squamous cell carcinoma and metastatic breast carcinoma can give the picture of diffuse infiltration.

Benign Tumors

It is not always possible to differentiate benign from malignant on noninvasive studies. Benign fibromas or leiomyomas are strictly histologic diagnoses.

Adenomas fall in between categories and are considered remalignant, potentially malignant, or "carcinoma of low metastatic potential." The histology is well differentiated renal cortical glandular tissue. They are rarely seen below the age of 30. The incidence increases with age, male sex, and tobacco use.

Oncocytoma is a benign tumor often treated as renal carcinoma until pathologically proven otherwise. Oncocytic tissue may be present in carcinoma; therefore biopsy cannot exclude malignancy. The "characteristic" finding is a very homogeneous, well-circumscribed mass with a pseudocapsule when small, and a "central scar."[26] These findings are not reliable enough to exlcude malignancy. Calcification is rare. Renal vein or ureteral occlusion, metastasis, or renal nonfunction all exclude this diagnosis.

Multilocular cystic nephroma is a rare benign neoplasm of males under 3 years of age and females over 40 years.[26] They are virtually always resected. One-third occasionally contains malignant cells, which appear as complex masses or multiple cystic spaces with opacifying septae of variable thickness that may calcify. Herniation into the sinus can occur.

Reninomas or juxtaglomerular cell tumors are rare, small, mildly enhancing tumors. This diagnosis is suspected in the clinical setting of hypertension, hyperreninemia, and secondary aldosteronism.

Carcinoma, adenoma, and oncocytoma are potentially indistinguishable on CT and can even occur in the same kid-

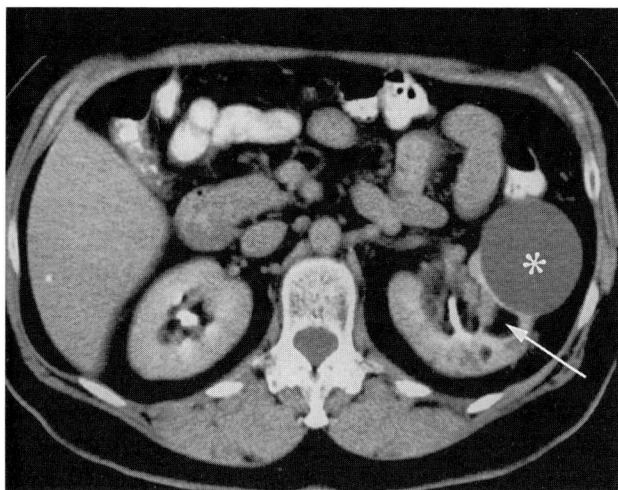

Figure 8–23. Angiomyolipoma. The pathognomonic feature is the fat (arrow) located well within the center of the lesion (very low density). Some malignancies can engulf small amounts of perinephric fat, but this usually occurs peripherally and is rare. A large simple cyst (asterisk) is also present.

ney. Thick, irregular walls; local invasion; blurring of perirenal fat; thickening of Gerota's fascia; necrosis; and hemorrhage can be present in either benign or malignant lesions.

Angiomyolipoma is also known as renal hamartoma, a benign tumor that ranges in size from 1 to 20 cm. The components are vessels (demonstrated enhancement); smooth muscle (appears as soft-tissue nodules, whorls, or strands in the perinephric fat); and fat, the pathognomonic feature (-80 to 120 HU) (Fig. 8–23). CT is confirmatory for this simple finding but complicated by the tendency of these tumors to bleed. Thin sections (3 to 5 mm) without contrast may be required to demonstrate a small amount of fat. Angiomyomas (total absence of fat) are rare. The fat must be located centrally to be reliably diagnostic because a large malignancy and/or the associated hemorrhage and edema can engulf a small region of perinephric fat. Eighty percent are solitary, are unilateral, and occur in young adult to middle-aged females. Twenty percent are multiple, bilateral, and associated with tuberous sclerosis.[26] This autosomal dominant disease is usually detected in infancy or childhood and is associated with multiple renal cysts and multiple bilateral renal, cutaneous, retinal, and cerebal hamartomas. (Fig. 8–24). Renal liposarcomas contain fat but are extremely rare, are usually located perirenally and can encase arteries.

THE COLLECTING SYSTEM

IVP and ultrasound may miss small pelvicalyceal filling defects, particularly in the setting of obesity or renal sinus lipomatosis. CT is excellent in detecting as well as differentiating these lesions. The differential diagnosis includes stone, urothelial tumor, hematoma, or sloughed renal tissue.[27] Usually the attenuation of stones is greater than that of hematoma and that of neoplasm. Liquefaction or calcification of thrombus alters this generalization, but administration of contrast to delineate tumor enhancement is useful. Dilatation of the collecting system from obstructing lesions is easily identified on CT. It is also useful to identify the level, location, and cause of obstruction. Excretion of contrast from the affected kidney may be delayed, and a fluid–fluid level of urine and contrast may be seen. With chronic obstruction, parenchymal thinning may occur.

STONES

The major function of CT in nephrolithiasis is to distinguish radiolucent calculi from other filling defects in the collecting system. Most stones are of mixed composition. Nonopaque stones are most often uric acid, but sometimes they are composed of cysteine, xanthine, and mucoid matrix.[14] Uric acid stones are the only type to cause an inflammatory response in the collecting system.[2] Even when they are radiolucent on x-ray, all stones are high attenuation on CT (193 to 540 HU). Tiny calcified stones may be better seen on plain film than on CT because of limited spatial resolution resulting from volume averaging. Contrast may obscure the stone; thus thin slices (<5 mm) without contrast are preferable for detection of stones. Oxalosis produces diffusely dense kidneys on unenhanced scans. Hematoma has an attenuation value of 58 to 60 HU, which overlaps with tumor; however, clots do not enhance, and they may change position or disappear in time.

TUMORS

Urothelial tumors have attenuation values of 20 to 46 HU on unenhanced scans and 64 to 84 HU with contrast enhancement. Urothelial malignancy represents 10 to 15% of

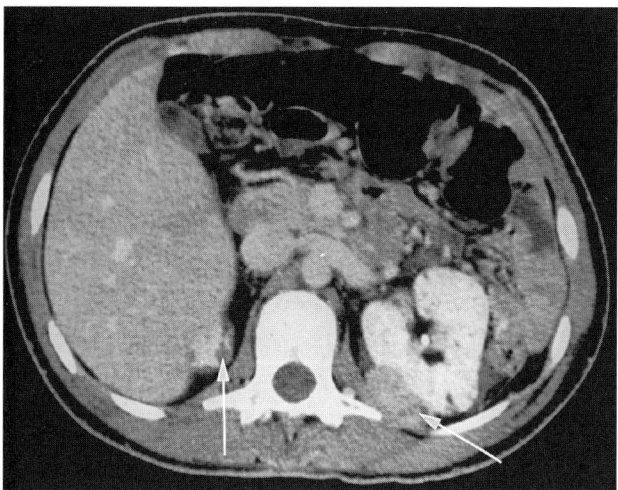

Figure 8–24. Tuberous sclerosis is associated with bilateral angiomyolipomas (arrows). Again fat is the telltale sign.

primary renal malignancy; 90% of these are transitional cell carcinomas. The remaining 10% are mainly squamous cell carcinoma, but occasionally adenocarcinoma can arise.[28] Renal cell carcinoma rarely distorts the collecting system, and when it does, the urothelial surface stays smooth and the collecting system is draped around the mass. On the other hand, urothelial malignancy can produce polypoid defects or mural irregularity of the collecting system or even amputate a minor or major calyx. Occasionally, transitional cell carcinoma can become as large as renal cell carcinoma. Either tumor can cause parenchymal destruction, venous occlusion, or ureteral obstruction and end renal function.

The typical presentation of transitional cell carcinoma is male (four times greater occurrence than in females) between the ages 40 and 70 (80%) with hematuria and flank pain.[29] Association with industrial carcinogens such as aniline dyes may be the reason for male predominance. Eighty-five percent is of the papillary variety, which is less malignant than other forms. The 5-year survival rate is 50%. The tumor grows by expansion when confined to the collecting system and can extend down the ureteral lumen. It becomes infiltrative when it invades the parenchyma. The kidney–tumor interface is often ill defined. The tumor is homogeneous and isodense to the parenchyma on unenhanced scans and hypodense after contrast. These tumors tend to be multicentric. Forty percent are associated with coexisting tumor in the ureter or bladder. A lobulated filling defect originating in the central collecting system without distorting the renal outline is expected, but occasionally they are round and exophytic (Fig. 8–25). The attenuation of the mass is greater than unopacified urine but less than any calculus, and enhancement is poor. Tumor necrosis is common, but calcification, hemorrhage, lymphadenopathy and venous invasion are rare. A prominent pelvic artery has been associated.[28] Seeding by needle biopsy can be avoided by retrograde ureteral brushing or urethroscopic biopsy.

Squamous cell carcinoma is an aggressive, infiltrative neoplasm that is strongly associated with chronic urinary tract infection and a high incidence of concurrent renal pelvic calculi. Prognosis is poor. The CT appearance may be similar to transitional cell carcinoma but these tumors tend to be more heterogeneous and lack calcification. Infiltrative squamous cell carcinoma is isodense with parenchyma before contrast and hypodense after. This tumor may be indistinguishable from xanthogranulomatous pyelonephritis on CT.

Adenocarcinomas are quite rare and may arise from metaplasia of the transitional epithelium. The findings are nonspecific, and association with stones and recurrent infections is noted.

EXTRARENAL LESIONS

Abnormality in the anterior pararenal fat is suspicious for pancreatic or bowel pathology. Inflammatory processes in this space can separate the posterior renal fascia into two layers.

Urinoma is a collection of fluid density that can occur from spontaneous calyceal rupture resulting from acute obstruction of iatrogenic traumatization. Resolution usually occurs in 3 to 4 days.

Retroperitoneal hematoma may occur with trauma, surgery, percutaneous intervention, shock wave lithotripsy, malignancy, or blood dyscrasia. The attenuation decreases as the clot matures because of decreased hemoglobin and water content. It may be isointense to contrast; therefore, a precontrast scan should be obtained (Fig. 8–26).

Retroperitoneal fibrosis is characteristically seen as a mantle of soft tissue encasing the ureters, distal aorta, and proximal iliac vessels (Fig. 8–27). The attenuation may be

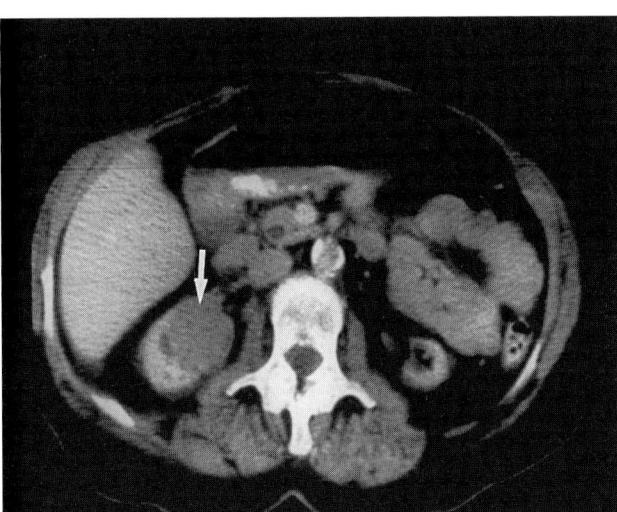

Figure 8–25. The mass (arrow) arising from the right collecting system is a transitional cell carcinoma, which in this patient was thought to be related to phenacetin use.

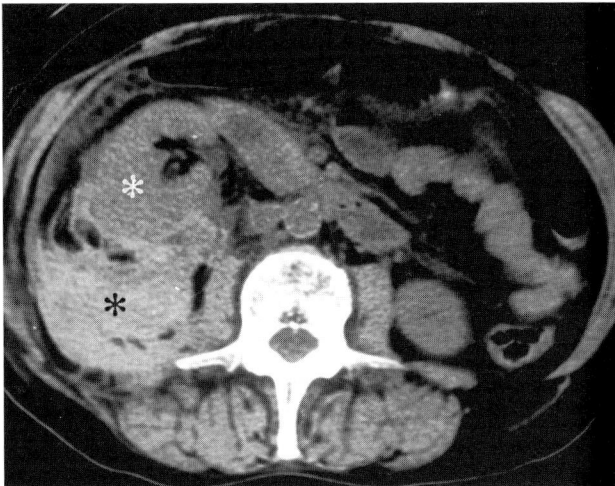

Figure 8–26. The right kidney (white asterisk) is significantly displaced anteriorly by a large collection of blood (black asterisk) in the posterior pararenal space that is higher in attenuation than unenhanced parenchyma. This is a well-known complication of renal biopsy.

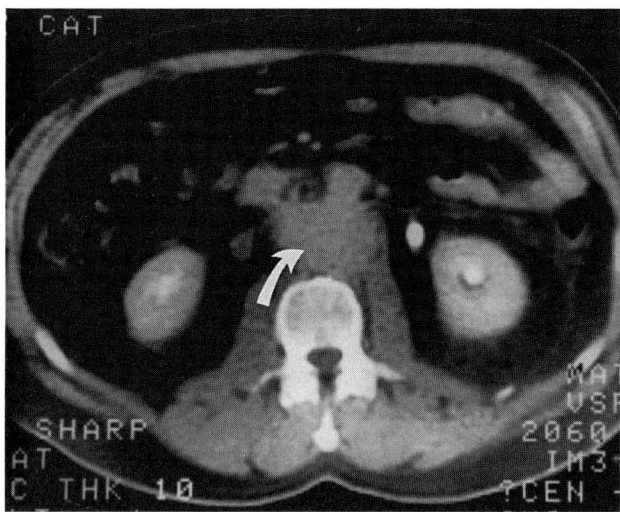

Figure 8–27. Retroperitoneal fibrosis is demonstrated as homogeneous, enhancing soft-tissue mass (arrow) enveloping the great vessels and extending to the psoas muscles. The ureters are often affected. Etiologies include methysergide ingestion, AAA, XRT, retroperitoneal hematoma, tumor, infection, urinoma and surgery. The differential diagnosis includes retroperitoneal tumor such as lymphoma and sometimes biopsy is required for definitive diagnosis.[15]

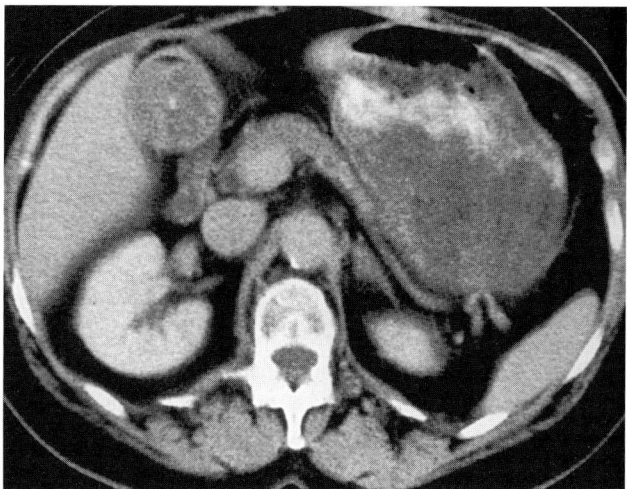

Figure 8–28. Left adrenal hyperplasia.

similar to tumor but the mass is located anterior and lateral to the aorta without displacing it anteriorly, as in lymphoma or metastatic disease.

Retroperitoneal sarcoma or extensive carcinoma from the pancreas, stomach, liver, and colon may involve the kidney. These may be indistinguishable from primary malignancy. Hricak et al found that MRI is more accurate in determining the origin of retroperitoneal tumors.[30] Selective arteriography can also suggest the origin.

ADRENAL GLAND

The normal gland is composed of anteromedial ridge and two asymmetric limbs that appear as a V or Y on cross-sectional imaging. Enlargement or focal lesion may distort the characteristic shape. Diffuse enlargement can be seen in hyperplasia, hemorrhage, infection, infiltrating neoplasm, or congenital metabolic deficiency.[31]

In bilateral adrenal hyperplasia the medulla may be seen as a high-density central linear band (Fig. 8–28). Tubercular adrenalitis often causes bilateral adrenal enlargement within 2 years of disease onset. Thereafter the glands may atrophy and calcify.[32] In idiopathic Addison's disease, the glands atrophy at the onset of disease.

Trauma

With routine use of CT for evaluation blunt thoracic or abdominal trauma, adrenal injury can also be detected. In a series by Burks et al most were unilateral, right-sided lesions, associated with thoracic or abdominal injuries on the same side.[33] Eighty-three percent of these injuries presented as discrete hematomas enlarging the gland. Other appearances include uniform swelling of the gland or diffuse irregular hemorrhage obliterating the gland. Blood in the surrounding fat can give it a "dirty" appearance or can mimic a thickened diaphragmatic crus. Complications of adrenal injury include delayed bleeding, infection, adrenal insufficiency, and caval thrombosis from compression of the inferior vena cava.

Masses

Small, well-defined smooth-rimmed, low-attenuation lesions involving part of the gland are characteristic of benignity. Greater than 2-cm lesions of low attenuation without a rim are more characteristic of malignancy;[34] however, appearances are variable, and biopsy or FNA is often necessary for distinction. Primary hyperaldosteronism or Conn's syndrome is most often the result of a small unilateral aldosterone-secreting cortical adenoma except in the pediatric population where bilateral nodular adrenocortical hyperplasia is more common. Not all adenomas are functional. Improved CT technique and high resolution has increased the detection of these lesions, which are often less than 2 cm and rarely more than 4 cm in size but have been seen up to 10 cm in diameter. A sensitivity of 82% and a positive predictive value of 100% has been reported by Dunnick et al.[35] The usual appearance on CT is a solid, encapsulated mass with attenuation values ranging from 30 to 50 HU. Some cortical adenomas have lower attenuation because of a high lipid component. Distinction of adrenal adenoma from a malignant lesion is not possible unless vascular invasion or metastasis is present to suggest malignancy (Fig. 8–29).

Bilateral micro- or macronodular hyperplasia of the adrenal cortex also causes idiopathic hyperaldosteronism. If a focal mass is seen in a patient with Conn's syndrome, ipsilateral adrenalectomy is often chosen because the false-pos-

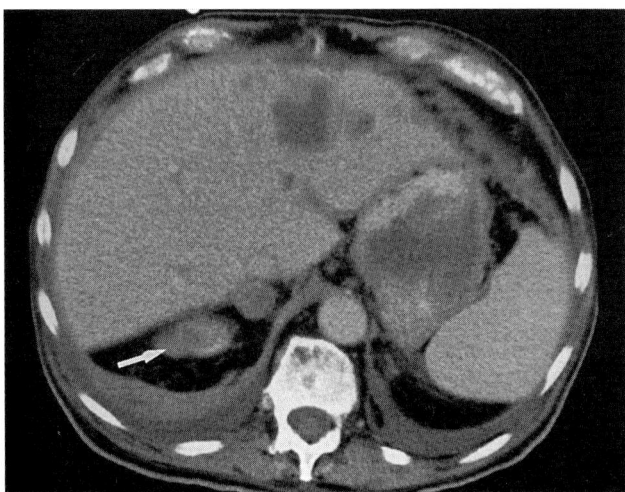

Figure 8–29. Adenocarcinoma of right adrenal gland seen as an ovoid, enhancing mass (arrow) on this postcontrast scan. The tumor may have originated in the stomach or prostate or may be a primary in this case.

itive rate for CT detection is almost nil.[35] If no mass is found, hormone sampling via the adrenal veins can be used to detect adenomas not visible on CT.

Other lesions of the adrenal cortex include myelolipomas, which are rare, well-circumscribed, benign tumors with fat and narrow elements. Cortical carcinomas present in women more often than in men and occur in those in their third to sixth decades, but they are also rare. They are often functional, causing masculinization, feminization, or Cushing's syndrome. These tumors are frequently large and aggressive with necrosis, hemorrhage, or calcification and metastasis to liver, nodes, or bone.

More commonly, adrenal tumors represent metastasis from other primary sites such as lung, breast, stomach, colon, pancreas, kidney, thyroid, melanoma, or lymphoma. These may be small circumscribed, unilateral, or bilateral. They may be isodense to normal tissue unless necrotic (Fig. 8–30).

The most common adrenal medullary tumor is the pheochromocytoma, which most commonly appears as a solitary, unilateral, encapsulated mass of 16 to 70 HU attenuation. They may be solid or cystic and are highly vascular, causing hemorrhage or necrosis; however, calcification is uncommon. They are usually greater than 2 cm in size except when associated with multiple endocrine adenoma syndromes, where they are often less than 1 cm in size. CT distinction from adenoma is difficult.

Neuroblastoma also arises in the adrenal medulla, appearing as a large, necrotic, hemorrhagic mass with calcification or a solid, noncalcific mass of soft tissue or fat density. Nodal, skeletal, liver, and pulmonary metastasis can occur.

BLADDER

Anatomy

The most anterior, rounded, fluid-filled structure in the pelvis is normally the bladder, which has a capacity of less than 400 to 500 mL. The ureters insert in the posterolateral surface and are approximately 2.5 cm apart in an empty bladder. When the bladder fills, the distance between ureters increases to 5 cm. At the entrance of the pelvis, the ureters cross anterior to the bifurcation of the common iliacs. This is a frequent site of obstruction by lithiasis.

Hernia

From 1 to 4% of inguinal hernias are associated with bladder herniation.[36] Urinary outlet obstruction (such as the prostatism) and loss of bladder tone secondary to aging (greater than 50 years) are felt to be contributing factors. Although most patients are asymptomatic, some may present with pain, hemospermia, and palpable mass. Because they can be unexpected during herniorrhaphy and can result in serious complications from intraoperative injury to the bladder, proper preoperative evaluation of high-risk patients (those over 50 and those with prostatism, recurrent inguinal or femoral hernias) is necessary. CT is superior to intravenous pyelography in visualizing the base of the bladder and in evaluation complications such as hydronephrosis, neoplasm, calculi, and strangulation.

Rupture

Patients sustaining abdominal or pelvic trauma are best evaluated with emergent CT with oral and intravenous contrast. CT has been shown to be as sensitive as conventional cystography for the detection of bladder injuries.[37] Rupture of

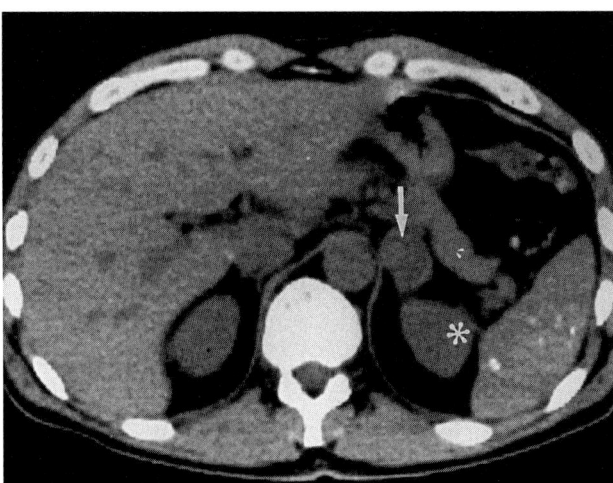

Figure 8–30. Malignant fibrous histiocytoma involving the left adrenal gland. This is a metastatic lesion from bone. The mass (arrow) is anteromedial to the superior pole of the left kidney (asterisk). Prognosis is poor.

the bladder wall may present with hematuria leakage of urine or contrast intra- or extraperitoneally. Note that a collection of contrast outside the bladder may be contained in another organ (i.e., the vagina), which usually can be differentiated from extravasation.

Hematomas can occur within the wall or lumen and have an attenuation pattern similar to hematomas occurring elsewhere.

Inflammation

Cystitis is a clinical laboratory diagnosis and commonly does not produce changes seen on CT. However, recurrent infection or evaluation for underlying pathology in atypical cases may lead to CT. Irregularity and/or thickening of the bladder wall is suspicious. Edema or inflammatory changes in surrounding fat or lymphadenopathy are secondary signs.

Tumors

The three major urothelial neoplasms are transitional, squamous cell, and adenocarcinoma, but transitional cell greatly outnumbers the others. Possibly related to environmental carcinogens, the incidence of bladder malignancies has increased 25% over the last decade. The male-to-female ratio is 3:1, with a peak incidence in the seventh decade of life. Over 20% of patients with bladder cancer die of the disease in any given year.[20] Most bladder tumors are noninvasive superficial carcinomas that do not become invasive. However, up to two-thirds recur; 25% of these recurrences are anaplastic to invasive. Staging directly affects prognosis and therapeutic choice. Since clinical staging is in error 66% of the time, CT is preferred. The goals of imaging include (1) accurate definition of bladder wall invasion (which is the single most important prognostic factor) (Fig. 8–31), (2) def-

inition of lymph node drainage areas and common sites for mets, and (3) follow-up of patients to detect recurrence. Two problems encountered in imaging are that tumor extent is often below spatial resolution and the postradiation fibrosis may look like active tumor.

Although calcification in bladder tumors is rare, detection is improved by CT (8%) as compared with radiographs (0.7 to 6.7%).[38] The location and pattern of calcification are fairly characteristic. Multiple fine punctate calcifications scattered within the mass are suggestive of mucin-producing adenocarcinoma, 50% of which calcify because of the presence of chondroitin sulfuric acid. Urachal carcinoma is predominantly mucinous adenocarcinoma, and calcification is usually in an arched or punctate pattern peripherally or a punctate pattern centrally (Fig. 8–32).[39]

Five percent of transitional cell carcinoma is associated with calcification.[38] The most common location is the surface of the tumor epithelium, which is thought to be related to infection. Central calcification secondary to necrosis, hemorrhage, or cystic degeneration has also been observed (Fig. 8–33).

Staging of pelvic malignancy is best achieved by a dynamic scanning technique, giving half of the intravenous contrast before and half during scanning. Therefore both vascular opacification and enhancement (to a lesser degree than the vessel) of the tumor are achieved. Minimal adenopathy is clinically relevent but difficult to distinguish from asymmetrical pelvic side wall vessels. This is seen in approximately 30% of normal male adults because of the more oblique course of the left common external iliac veins. Patterns of nodal enhancement are either uniform in small nodes, patchy in large nodes, or rim-enhancing with a low attenuation center.

Although clinical data and urography are more practical for detection, cross-sectional imaging is vital to staging. CT

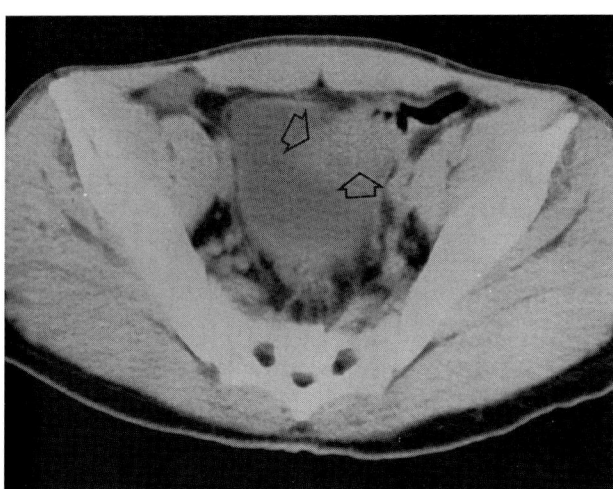

Figure 8–31. Colon cancer invading the bladder wall. The air in the left anterior pelvis is within the bowel. Adjacent to it is a soft-tissue mass (open arrows) that extends into the low-density, fluid-filled bladder.

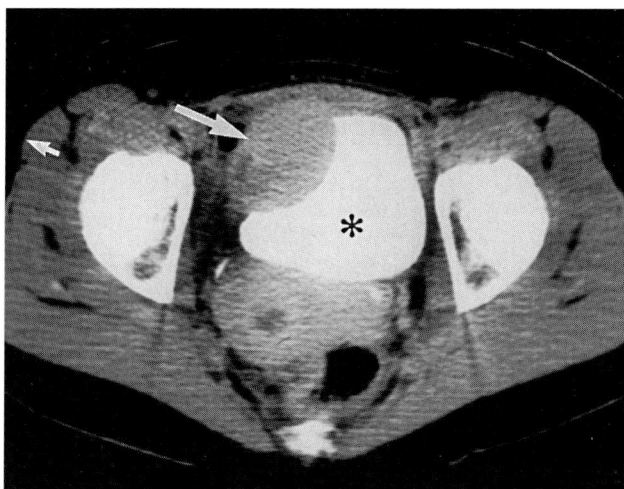

Figure 8–32. Urachal cyst. The round intermediate-density lesion (arrow) causing a defect on the contrast-filled bladder (asterisk) indicates cystic dilatation of the distal urachus proximal to the closed supravesical segment.

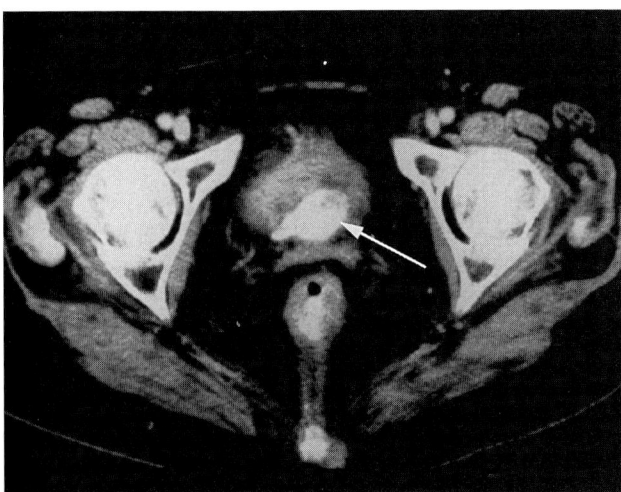

Figure 8–33. Carcinoma of the bladder seen as thickened, irregular walls with dense, plaquelike, massive calcification (arrow). According to Moon et al, calcification is seen in only about 8% of bladder tumors.[38] The most common location in transitional cell carcinoma is the surface of the tumor epithelium. This may be related to prior infection. Inguinal adenopathy is also present.

is best at assessing local extent but has limitations. Distinguishing stage A from stage B (extent to muscle) is not straightforward and may be better achieved by MRI or intravesical ultrasound (accuracy of 85 to 94%). Overall accuracy for detecting perivesical involvement ranges from 40 to 83%.

The paucity of fat in the pelvis limits CT's ability to evaluate invasion of neighboring structures. Adenopathy can only be detected when the involved nodes are enlarged (greater than 1 to 1.5 cm). MRI is more sensitive than CT in detecting perivesical invasion but requires lengthy imaging in multiple planes.

More than 50% of patients with invasive bladder carcinoma develop distant metastases. The most common sites are the bones, lungs, and liver; therefore screening CT of the chest and liver is often beneficial in candidates for curative therapy. CT is also the primary modality for follow-up of nodal or metastatic recurrence.

A NOTE ON CONTRAST NEPHROPATHY

Administration of intravenous contrast is not without risk. A rise in serum creatinine to one and a half times baseline administration is considered contrast-induced nephropathy.[40] The incidence approximates 0.15% but may reach 12% in certain clinical settings. With conservative management, the kidneys usually recover function within 7 to 12 days, but occasionally temporary or permanent dialysis is required. Established risk factors are renal disease, advanced age, dehydration, diabetes mellitus, multiple myeloma, hypertension, and heart disease. The volume and type of contrast also influence the risk for nephropathy. Persistent cortical attenuation (approximately 140 HU) 24 hours following contrast administration may indicate contrast nephropathy. IV contrast should be avoided in renal failure unless hemodialysis occurs within 24 hours.

REFERENCES

1. Engelstad BL, et al: the role of pre-contrast images in computed tomography of the kidney. *Radiology* 1980;136:153–155.
2. Haaga JR, Alfidi RJ, eds: *Computed Tomography of the Whole Body*, 2nd ed. St. Louis: CV Mosby, 1983.
3. Miles, MA, London NJ, Lavelle JM, et al: CT staging or renal carcinoma: a prospective comparison of threee dynamic computed tomography techniques. *Eur J Radiol* 1991;13(1):37–42.
4. Fanney DR, Casillas J, Murphy BJ: CT in the diagnosis of renal trauma. *Radiographics* 1990;10(1):29–40.
5. Lang EK: Intra-abdominal and retroperitoneal organ injuries diagnosed on dynamic computed tomograms obtained for assessment of renal trauma. *J Trauma* 1990;30(9):1161–1168.
6. Malmed AS, Love L, Jeffrey RB: Medullary CT enhancement in acute renal artery occlusion. *JCAT* 1992;16(1):107–109.
7. Gold RP, McClennan BL: Bacterial renal infection: role of CT (letter; comment). *Radiology* 1990;174(1):283–284.
8. Hoffman EP, Mindelzun RE, Anderson RU: Computed tomography in acute pyelonephritis associated with diabetes. *Radiology* 1980;135:691–695.
9. Kenney PJ: Imaging of chronic renal infections. *AJR* 1990;155(3):485–494.
10. Shah M, Haaga JR: Focal xanthogranulomatous pyelonephritis simulating a renal tumor: CT characteristics. *JCAT* 1989;13(4):712–713.
11. Kuhlman JE, Browne D, Shermak M, et al: Retroperitoneal and pelvic CT of patients with AIDS: primary and secondary involvement of the genitourinary tract. *Radiographics* 1991;11(3):473–483.
12. Kissane JM: Congenital malformations. In: Hepinstali RH, (ed) *Pathology of the Kidney*. Boston: Little, Brown, 1974, 69-119.
13. Glen DA, Gilbert FJ, Bayliss AP: Renal carcinomas missed by urography. *Br J Urol* 1989;63(5):457–459.
14. Dalla-Palma L, Pozzi-Mucelli R: Problematic renal masses in ultrasonography and computed tomography. *Clin Imag* 1990;14(2):83-98.
15. Dunnick NR, McCallum RW, Sandler CM: *Textbook of Uroradiology*. Baltimore: Williams & Wilkins, 1991;1–466.
16. Levine E, Grantham JJ: Calcified renal stones and cyst calcifications in autosomal dominant polycystic kidney disease: clinical and CT study in 84 patients. *AJR* 1992;159(1):77–81.
17. Cristallini EG, Paganelli C, Bolis GB: Role of fine-needle aspiration biopsy in the assessment of renal masses. *Diagn Cytopathol* 1991;7(1):32–35.
18. Bosniack MA: The small (less than or equal to 3.0 cm) renal parenchymal tumor: detection, diagnosis, and controversies. *Radiology* 1991;179(2):307–317.
19. Newhouse JH: The radiologic evaluation of the patient with renal cancer. *Urol Clin North Am* 1993;20(2):231–246.
20. Singer J, McClennan BL: The diagnosis, staging, and follow-up of carcinoma of the kidney, bladder, and prostate: the role of cross-sectional imaging. *Semin Ultrasound CT MR* 1989;10(6):481–497.
21. London NJM, Messios N, Kinder RB, et al: A propective study of the value of conventional CT, dynamic CT, ultrasonography

and arteriography for the staging of renal cell carcinoma. *Br J Urol* 1989;64:209–217.
22. Zagoria RJ, Dyer RB, Wolfman NT, et al: Radiology in the diagnosis and staging of renal cell carcinoma. *Crit Rev Diagn Imaging* 1990;31(1):81–115.
23. Amendola MA: Comparison of MR imaging and CT in the evaluation of renal masses. *Crit Rev Diagn Imaging* 1989;29(2):117–150.
24. Bosniack MA: Problems in the radiologic diagnosis of renal parenchymal tumors. *Urol Clin North Am* 1993;20(2):217–230.
25. Cohan RH, Dunnick NR, Leder RA, et al: Computed tomography of renal lymphoma. *JCAT* 1990;14(6):933–938.
26. Janus CL, Mendelson DS: Comparison of MRI and CT for study of renal and perirenal masses. *Crit Rev Diagn Imaging* 1991;32(2):69–118.
27. Netto NR, Claro JF: CT scanning in the diagnosis of pelvicalyceal filling defects. *Arch Esp Urol* 1990;43(6):683–685.
28. Gash JR, Zagoria RJ, Dyer RB, et al: Imaging features of infiltrating renal lesions. *Crit Rev Diagn Imaging* 1992;33(4):293–310.
29. Bree RL, Schultz SR, Hayes R: Large infiltrating renal transitional cell carcinomas: CT and ultrasound features. *JCAT* 1990;14(3):381–385.
30. Hricak H, Demas BE, Williams RD, et al: Magnetic resonance imaging in the diagnosis and staging of renal and perirenal neoplasms. *Radiology* 1985;154:709.
31. Yeh HC: US and CT evaluation of diffusely enlarged adrenal gland. [Review] *Crit Rev Diagn Imaging* 1992;33(5):437–460.
32. Buxi TB, et al: CT in adrenal enlargement due to tuberculosis: a review of literature with five new cases. [Review] *Clin Imaging* 1992;16(2):102–108.
33. Burks DW, Mirvis SE, Shanmuganathan K: Acute adrenal injury after blunt abdominal trauma: CT findings. *AJR* 1992;158(3):503–507.
34. Gillams A, Robert CM, Shaw P, et al: The value of CT scanning and percutaneous fine needle aspiration of adrenal masses in biopsy-proven lung cancer. *Clin Radiol* 1992;46(1)18–22.
35. Dunnick NR, Leight GS, Roubidoux MA, et al: CT in the diagnosis of primary aldosteronism: sensitivity in 29 patients. *AJR* 1993;160(2):321–324.
37. Horstman WG, McClennan BL, Heiken JP: Comparison of computed tomography and conventional cystography for detection of traumatic bladder rupture. *Urol Radiol* 1991;12(4):188–193.
36. Izes BA, Larsen CR, Izes JK, et al: Computerized tomographic appearance of hernias of the bladder. *J Urol* 1993;149(5):1002–1205.
38. Moon WK, Kim SH, Cho JM, et al: Calcified bladder tumors. CT features. *Acta Radiol* 1992;33(5):440–443.
39. Krysiewicz S: Diagnosis of urachal carcinoma by computed tomography and magnetic resonance imaging. *Clin Imaging* 1990;14(3):251–254.
40. Love L., Lind JA, Olson MC: Persistent CT nephrogram: significance in the diagnosis of contrast nephropathy. *Radiology* 1989;172(1):125–129.

9 Magnetic Resonance Imaging of the Urinary Tract

Elizabeth D. Brown, Richard C. Semelka

Magnetic resonance imaging (MRI) provides many benefits in the imaging of the urinary tract. Excellent soft-tissue contrast resolution and multiplanar imaging are possible without radiation exposure. Imaging with the use of intravenous gadolinium chelates is especially well suited to the study of the urinary tract, as the agent is eliminated exclusively by glomerular filtration. The purpose of this chapter is to introduce magnetic resonance principles and techniques used for imaging of the urinary tract. In addition, the normal and pathologic appearances are presented for each portion of the entire urinary tract.

PRINCIPLES OF MAGNETIC RESONANCE IMAGING

The primary strengths of magnetic resonance imaging (MRI) of the abdominal cavity include excellent soft-tissue contrast resolution and multiplanar imaging capabilities without radiation exposure. Recent improvements in sequences for abdominal imaging allow faster acquisition with better resolution and shorter scan times.

Physics of Magnetic Resonance Imaging

The physical principles of MRI are based on the fact that atomic nuclei with an odd number of protons or neutrons have an associated magnetic field surrounding them. The nuclei can act as tiny magnetic dipoles with a north and south pole. The magnetic field about each nucleus has a particular strength and direction. The hydrogen atom is the most convenient biologically active nucleus for study via magnetic resonance, as it is abundant and possesses strong magnetic properties. The protons are oriented randomly, and no net magnetization exists in the absence of an external magnetic field. However, if an external magnetic field is applied, the protons align themselves with and opposed to the direction of the field with a net positive direction, producing magnetization. When this external field is applied, it causes the proton's nuclear magnetic moment to precess around the magnetic field axis. If a radiofrequency energy is applied to a substance, the protons flip from the low-energy state to the high-energy state. This induction of transitions from one energy state to another is called resonance.[1] The field strength of the superconducting magnet is measured in Tesla (T). Field strengths are generally grouped into low field (0.1 to 0.35 T), midfield (0.5 T), and high field (1.0 to 2.0 T). The images presented in this chapter have been made on a high-field 1.5-T MR system.

Individual protons exchange a fixed amount of energy when they return to an equilibrium following the application of an external field. The time required for the magnetization in the z-axis to return to its equilibrium value is known as T1 relaxation or spin-lattice relaxation, as the value depends on the nuclei losing energy to their local environment or lattice. Because tissues show different T1 values, T1-weighted images provide intrinsic contrast between tissues, which can be accentuated with manipulation of the MR sequences[1,2] or by administration of T1-relaxing contrast agents.

On the other hand, T2 relaxation, or spin-spin relaxation time reflects the net loss of magnetization in the xy-plane due to dephasing. When a 180-degree radiofrequency pulse is applied, the protons align their precessional orientation and are temporarily "in phase." However, immediately following the pulse, they quickly lose phase coherence as a result of interactions with neighboring nuclei. Thus the precessional frequency of each proton differs slightly. The net transverse magnetization quickly decays to zero, and the time for this phenomenon to occur depends on the interactions between neighboring spinning nuclei. It is for this reason that the T2 relaxation is a collective phenomenon.[1]

The magnetization in the xy plane can be thought of as a magnet spinning at high speed. Thus a current is induced and can be amplified and measured (free induction decay). In a tissue in which all protons do not have the same resonance frequency, the signal will be the sum of the signals from the nuclei in these differing fields precessing at their own frequency and decaying with their own relaxation rate. This resulting signal is complex and is a function of time. However, it can be analyzed into its individual frequency components with a Fourier transform. Signal intensity is a measurement of the brightness of tissues displayed in an image. Tissue that is visually bright is described as high in signal intensity, whereas tissue that is dark is described as low in signal intensity.

T1 and T2 are independent of one another but occur simultaneously. T1 and T2 are intrinsic properties of a given tissue. In general, fluid appears dark on T1-weighted images and bright on T2-weighted images. Fat is bright on T1-weighted images and intermediate on T2-weighted images. Fat may however be attenuated and therefore low in signal intensity on T1- or T2-weighted images. Fibrous tissue and muscle are dark on T1- and T2-weighted images. Most disease processes result in increased fluid content of tissue and are therefore relatively dark on T1- and bright on T2-weighted images. In addition to T1 and T2, a third parameter, proton density, contributes to MRI. The manipulation of MR sequences is intended to emphasize different parameters to yield the desired information.[1]

The two critical parameters that are displayed on MR images are the repetition time (TR) and the echo time (TE). TR refers to the time between excitation radiofrequency pulses, and in general T2-weighted images possess a long TR (1500 to 3000 msec) whereas T1-weighted images possess a short TR (80 to 500 msec). TE refers to the time between the excitation pulses and data reception; in general, T2-weighted images have a long TE (70 to 150 msec) and T1-weighted images have a short TE (4 to 20 msec).

MR systems are equipped with three pairs of orthogonal gradient coils along the x, y, and z axes. Activation of a particular gradient coil produces a linear magnetic field gradient within the magnetic field along that orthogonal axis. The induced gradient selects a particular volume of tissue that resonates at the frequency of the transmitted radiofrequency pulses. Activation of two or three gradient coils simultaneously produces a linear gradient along an oblique direction. This concept allows multiplanar "slice selection" techniques.

The reduction of image artifacts is an important task in MR imaging of the abdomen and pelvis. The primary artifacts are: respiration-induced ghosting, bowel peristalsis, chemical shift, and blood flow artifacts. The most serious artifact, that resulting from respiratory-related motion of abdominal fat, is commonly compensated with the use of averaging of multiple acquisitions and reordering of the phase-encoding table based on the respiratory cycle. However, recently, other techniques have been used for the purpose of reducing this artifact: frequency fat suppression (fatsat); breath-hold imaging; snapshot imaging; and modified spin echo imaging called rapid acquisition with relaxation enhancement (RARE).

Techniques of Magnetic Resonance Imaging

FREQUENCY-SELECTIVE FAT SUPPRESSION

Frequency-selective fat suppression essentially removes the signal intensity (SI) of abdominal fat, thereby diminishing most of the ghosting artifacts.[3,4] This technique relies on the frequency shift of fat and water protons. The basic theory of this design is a frequency-selective excitation pulse that selectively excites protons at the frequency of fat. The resulting magnetization is immediately spoiled by a gradient pulse. A spin echo sequence then follows, which acquires data from water protons.

Advantages of this sequence include diminished ghosting artifact, removal of chemical shift artifact; improved dynamic range of signal intensities of soft tissues in the abdomen, and increased conspicuity of gadopentatate dimeglumine (gadolinium) enhancement. This latter advantage is achieved by removal of the high SI of fat, allowing better visualization of the high SI gadolinium.

The greatest limitation of fat suppression imaging is that the fat may be suppressed inhomogeneously because of variation of the uniformity of the main magnetic field within the imaging volume. Maximal uniformity of suppression may be possible with a good shim status of the magnetic field and adjustment of the chemically selective excitation pulse to the spectral frequency of lipids.[5] Currently, the latter method is used more commonly. However, the shim currents may be adjusted for each patient in order to optimize the homogeneity of the main magnetic field. The baseline shim currents can be selected from a menu of shim settings that are specific to the anatomic location and patient size.

Certain factors may limit the uniformity of fat suppression, such as the presence of ferromagnetic surgical implants, as they disturb the homogeneity of the magnetic field.

BREATH-HOLD IMAGING

Currently, three basic categories of fast imaging techniques are used clinically: spoiled gradient echo sequences [i.e., fast low-angle shot (FLASH) or spoiled GRASS][6–8]; rapid acquisition spin echo (RASE)[9]; and magnetization-prepared snapshot gradient echo (i.e., TurboFLASH).[6,10–12]

Fast Low-Angle Shot Technique. The breath-hold sequence known as FLASH has good inherent signal-to-noise ratio (SNR), spleen liver contrast, spatial resolution, and image quality. In addition, the FLASH sequence has the ability to acquire 14 to 22 images during a 19-second breath-hold. This provides imaging of the entire kidneys in one sequence. Thus the phases of gadolinium enhancement of the entire kidneys can be viewed in a serial fashion. The factors improving image quality include a high flip angle to maximize the SNR, T1 weighting, and a short TE.[6,8]

The spoiled gradient echo technique has the advantage of true T1 weighting, unlike other techniques, such as gradient recalled acquisition at steady state (GRASS), which gives information about T1 as well as T2. When information about T1 and T2 is given in a single image, the result can be confusing. For example, fluid in a cystic structure such as the bladder appears bright, whereas it appears dark with true T1 weighting.

Rapid Acquisition Spin Echo. The technique known as RASE is a spin echo sequence that shortens data acquisition to a breath-hold period by using a 128 × 256 matrix and half Fourier data reconstruction. The use of a short echo time (TE) provides an improved SNR and a larger number of images during the breath-hold. Currently, an echo time of 8 msec can be achieved.[6] However, the SNR for RASE is lower than that for FLASH. In addition, the number of images per breath-hold is less, and the spatial resolution is less for RASE images when compared with FLASH images. Despite these limitations, spin echo sequences are typically less sensitive to local magnetic field inhomogeneities. Thus for patients with ferromagnetic surgical clips that induce magnetic susceptibility and may compromise the quality of FLASH images, spin echo sequences may be advantageous.

Snapshot Gradient Echo. Magnetization-prepared snapshot gradient echo imaging (Turbo-FLASH) acquires the necessary data within 2 seconds or less, generating images that are independent of breathing.[6,10-13] Thus this sequence is ideal for uncooperative or very ill patients incapable of suspending breathing. The process consists of two steps. A preparation period determines the contrast in the resulting images, and the acquisition period follows, which is used to acquire the raw data of the image. In the clinical setting of Turbo-FLASH, the preparation period consists of an inversion pulse of 180 degrees followed by a variable wait time for recovery of the magnetization. The data acquisition period then consists of a series of gradient echoes. Pulse repetition time as short as 9 msec results in data acquisition time of about 1 second for a 128 × 356 image matrix. However, problems with Turbo-FLASH relate to the T1 relaxation during data acquisition. This may diminish the tissue contrast and spatial resolution.

RAPID ACQUISITION WITH RELAXATION ENHANCEMENT

The sequence known as rapid acquisition with relaxation enhancement (RARE) has demonstrated great potential for examining the pelvis.[14,15] Other eponyms used to describe this technique are fast spin echo and turbo spin echo. The sequence produces T2-weighted images with scan times up to 16 times faster than conventional spin echo (SE) sequences. Thus the T2-weighted SE images can be obtained in a single breath-hold, or a shorter scan time can be used to acquire high-resolution abdominal images with multiple averages in several minutes. The result is a T2-weighted sequence that decreases the imaging time fourfold compared with regular spin echo sequences. The principal advantages of RARE are the generation of images with higher spatial resolution (512 × 512 matrix), and the ability to acquire data in a breath-hold. High spatial resolution allows for better detection of smaller lesions. With the larger number of lines acquired per TR interval, the sequence can be completed in 21 seconds, which permits breath-hold data. The RARE technique may be modified to produce images which have an appearance analogous to an intravenous urogram. Resulting images have been described as MR urograms.

SATURATION PULSES

The quality of abdominal studies can be improved significantly with the use of spatially selective saturation pulses, which remove the flow artifact created by the pulsatile motion of blood. The targeted vessels are the inferior vena cava and the aorta. However, saturation pulses reduce the number of images that can be acquired per TR interval.

KIDNEYS

Magnetic Resonance Techniques

In most tissues the presence of gadolinium, a T1-relaxation enhancing agent, causes tissue brightening on T1-weighted images with an appearance similar to iodinated contrast on computed tomographic images. At higher concentration gadolinium causes blackening of the image due to local magnetic field inhomogeneity or T2-effects. In the kidneys, this effect can be used to evaluate the ability to concentrate urine in the medulla and produce concentrated urine. The intravenous agent gadolinium is freely filtered by renal glomeruli, undergoing no tubular reabsorption or secretion. For this reason, gadolinium is an ideal agent for study of the kidneys. In addition, the signal intensity of urine changes with the concentration of the agent. When dilute, gadolinium enhances T1 relaxation and creates a high signal intensity of urine; when concentrated, gadolinium induces magnetic susceptibility loss, and urine appears with a low SI.[16-18] Thus the concentrating ability of the kidneys can be studied using these properties. Four sequences are commonly used to examine the kidneys: (1) precontrast T1-weighted breath-hold FLASH; (2) precontrast fat-suppressed T1-weighted spin echo; (3) dynamic capillary phase T1-weighted FLASH; and (4) postcontrast fat-suppressed T1-weighted spin echo (Fig. 9-1).[19] MRI is more sensitive to the presence or absence of gadolinium than CT is to iodine. As such, viable tissue is shown to enhance, but regions with no blood flow (i.e., cysts) are very low in signal intensity.

Abnormalities of Position and Shape of Kidneys

Duplication of the collecting system may be difficult to detect on transaxial images. However, pelvic kidney and horseshoe kidney are easily recognized secondary to the intense uptake of gadolinium by the renal cortex and the resulting corticomedullary organization (Fig. 9-2). A prominent column of Bertin can be difficult to distinguish from a renal mass by many imaging methods. However, immediate and delayed postcontrast MR images show the column enhanc-

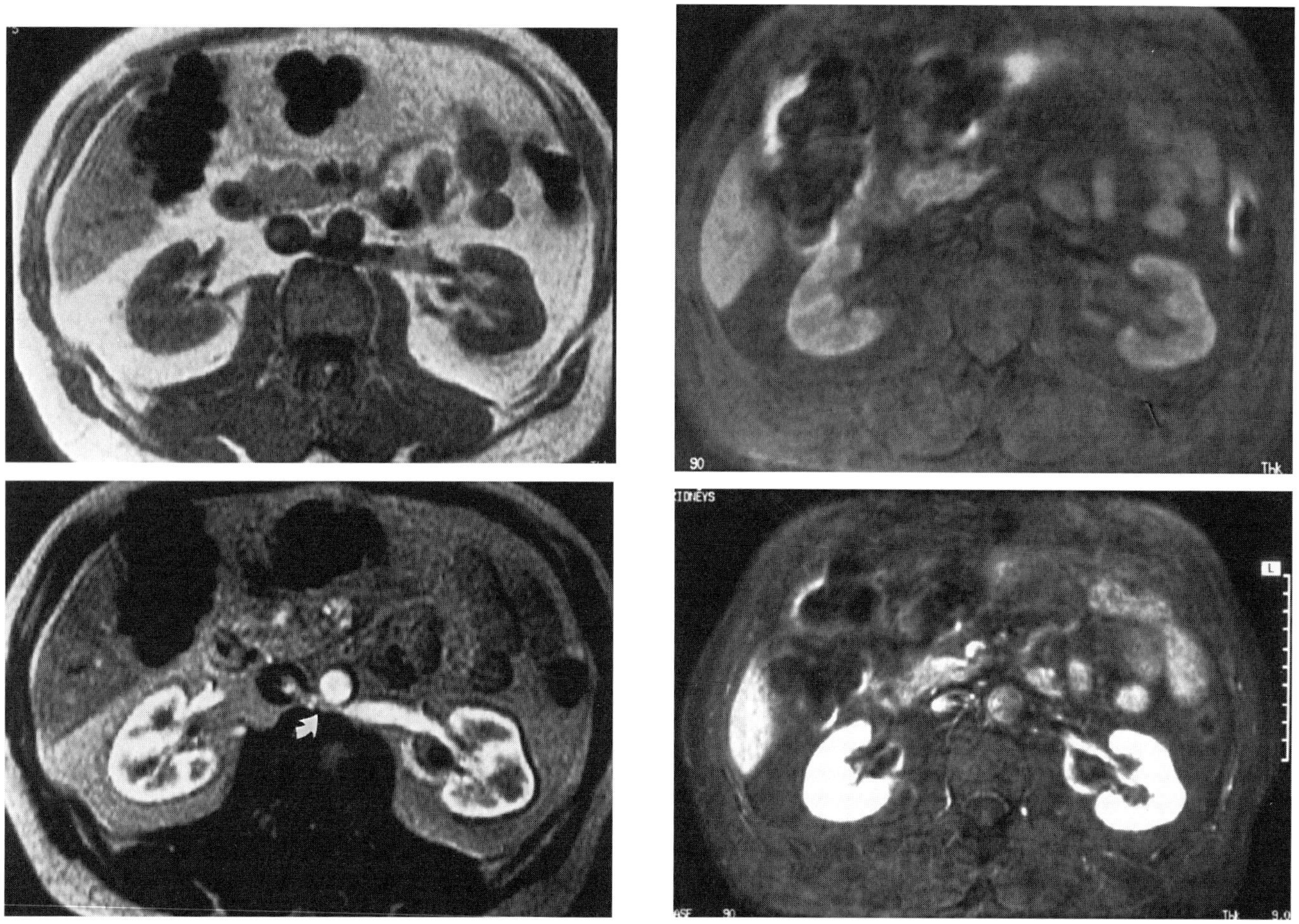

Figure 9–1. Normal kidneys. Precontrast FLASH (**A**), precontrast T1FS (**B**), 1-second postcontrast FLASH (**C**), and gadolinium-enhanced T1FS (**D**) images. Minimal corticomedullary (CM) differentiation is present on precontrast FLASH (**A**), whereas higher CM differentiation is apparent on precontrast T1FS (**B**). The highest CM differentiation on the immediate postcontrast FLASH image can be appreciated. Incidental note is made of a retroaortic left renal vein with high gadolinium-enhanced blood draining into the signal-void IVC (arrow). High spatial and contrast resolution, excellent image quality, and absence of phase or chemical shift artifact characterize gadolinium-enhanced T1FS (**D**) images. (Reprinted with permission from ref. 19.)

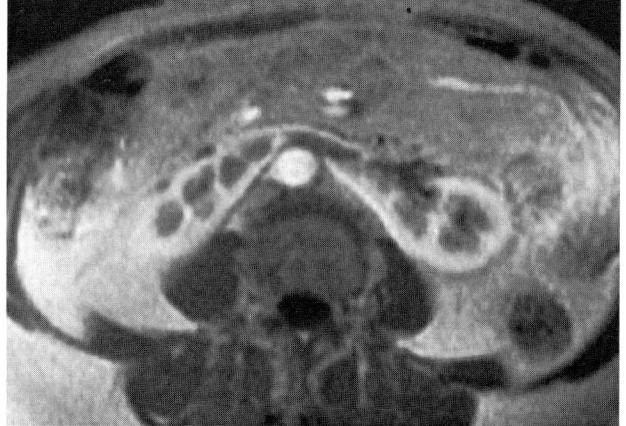

Figure 9–2. Horseshoe kidney. One-second postcontrast image. The corticomedullary differentiation demonstrates that the isthmus contains functional renal parenchyma. (Reprinted with permission from ref. 2.)

ing to the same extent as the renal cortex. Thus, the diagnosis is made without difficulty.

Diseases of the Parenchyma

BENIGN DISEASE

Cyst. Renal cysts are well shown on MR images as oval-shaped lesions that do not enhance with gadolinium. A cyst will typically possess sharp margins with renal parenchyma.[19,20] The fluid in a simple cyst should appear similar in composition to urine and show signal void on T1-weighted images. The cyst should have no definable wall when it extends beyond the renal cortex (Fig. 9–3). Complicated cysts contain blood, septations, or calcifications, and there should still be an absence of enhancement with gadolinium. MRI is particularly useful at evaluating calcified masses, as calcium is signal void on MR images (unlike CT in which it is very dense) and does not cause confusion with enhancing viable tissue.[20]

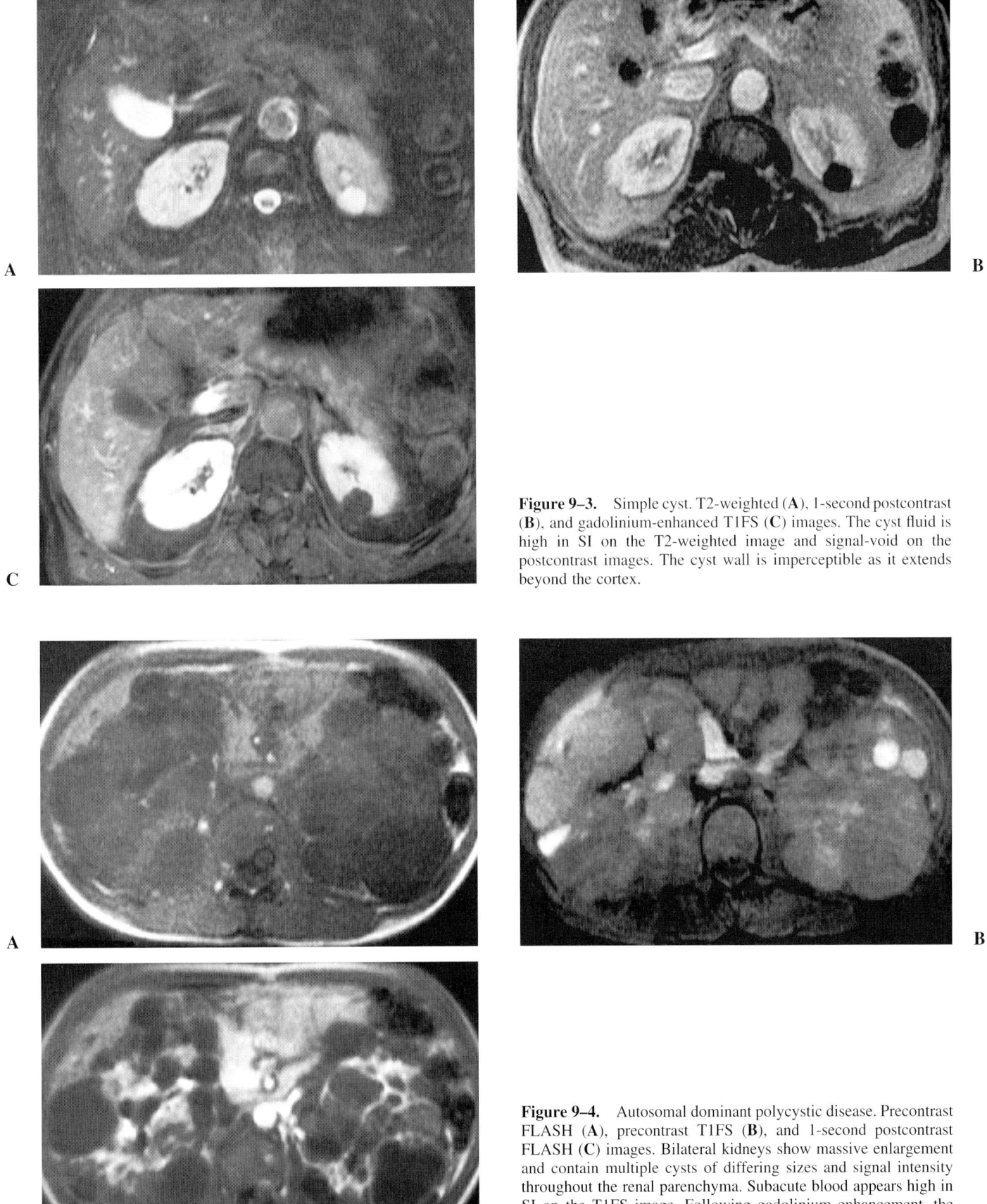

Figure 9–3. Simple cyst. T2-weighted (**A**), 1-second postcontrast (**B**), and gadolinium-enhanced T1FS (**C**) images. The cyst fluid is high in SI on the T2-weighted image and signal-void on the postcontrast images. The cyst wall is imperceptible as it extends beyond the cortex.

Figure 9–4. Autosomal dominant polycystic disease. Precontrast FLASH (**A**), precontrast T1FS (**B**), and 1-second postcontrast FLASH (**C**) images. Bilateral kidneys show massive enlargement and contain multiple cysts of differing sizes and signal intensity throughout the renal parenchyma. Subacute blood appears high in SI on the T1FS image. Following gadolinium enhancement, the remaining parenchyma enhances in a normal fashion, indicating some preservation of renal function. (Reprinted with permission from ref. 19.)

Parapelvic cysts may be difficult to distinguish from a dilated renal collecting system. Delayed postcontrast images may show that the high SI of dilute gadolinium contrasts well with the low SI of fluid in the parapelvic cysts.

Autosomal dominant polycystic kidney (ADPCK) disease typically appears as bilateral renal enlargement with numerous cysts of varying size that distort the renal architecture. The SI of the cysts usually varies because of the presence of blood products at different stages of degradation (Fig. 9-4). Because of the great sensitivity of MR to detect the presence of blood, this technique is well suited to evaluate patients with ADPCK who present with sudden abdominal pain or drop in hemoglobin to determine if hemorrhage into a cyst has occurred.

Long-term hemodialysis patients may develop multiple renal cysts of uncertain etiology.[21–23] The formation of such cysts may be related to ischemia or fibrosis and tends to follow atrophy of the kidneys. The location is usually superficial in the renal cortex, and hemorrhage is a common complication. As these patients have a 7% incidence of renal cancer,[23] MRI is important in that it provides excellent detection of renal cancer as a result of good parenchymal enhancement even in the setting of diminished renal function.

The neurocutaneous syndrome Von Hippel–Lindau disease is an autosomal dominant disorder. Patients are at increased risk of renal cysts, adenomas, and carcinomas.[24] Carcinomas tend to be multicentric and bilateral. The ability of MRI to distinguish cystic from solid tumors, even when small (1 cm) in diameter, renders it an effective method to evaluate patients with multiple bilateral tumors in whom multiple resections are contemplated.

Medullary sponge kidney may present with calculi, obstruction, infection, or hematuria. Findings are multiple cystic cavities in the papillae, frequently containing calculi. The findings may be segmental or unilateral but are usually bilateral.

Multilocular cystic nephroma is a benign lesion of noncommunicating cysts within a fibrous stroma. The typical appearance of the lesion is that of a multicystic renal mass with thick enhancing fibrous septations (Fig. 9–5). Cysts typically are mixed low to high in signal intensity on T1-weighted images. The multiplanar imaging capability of

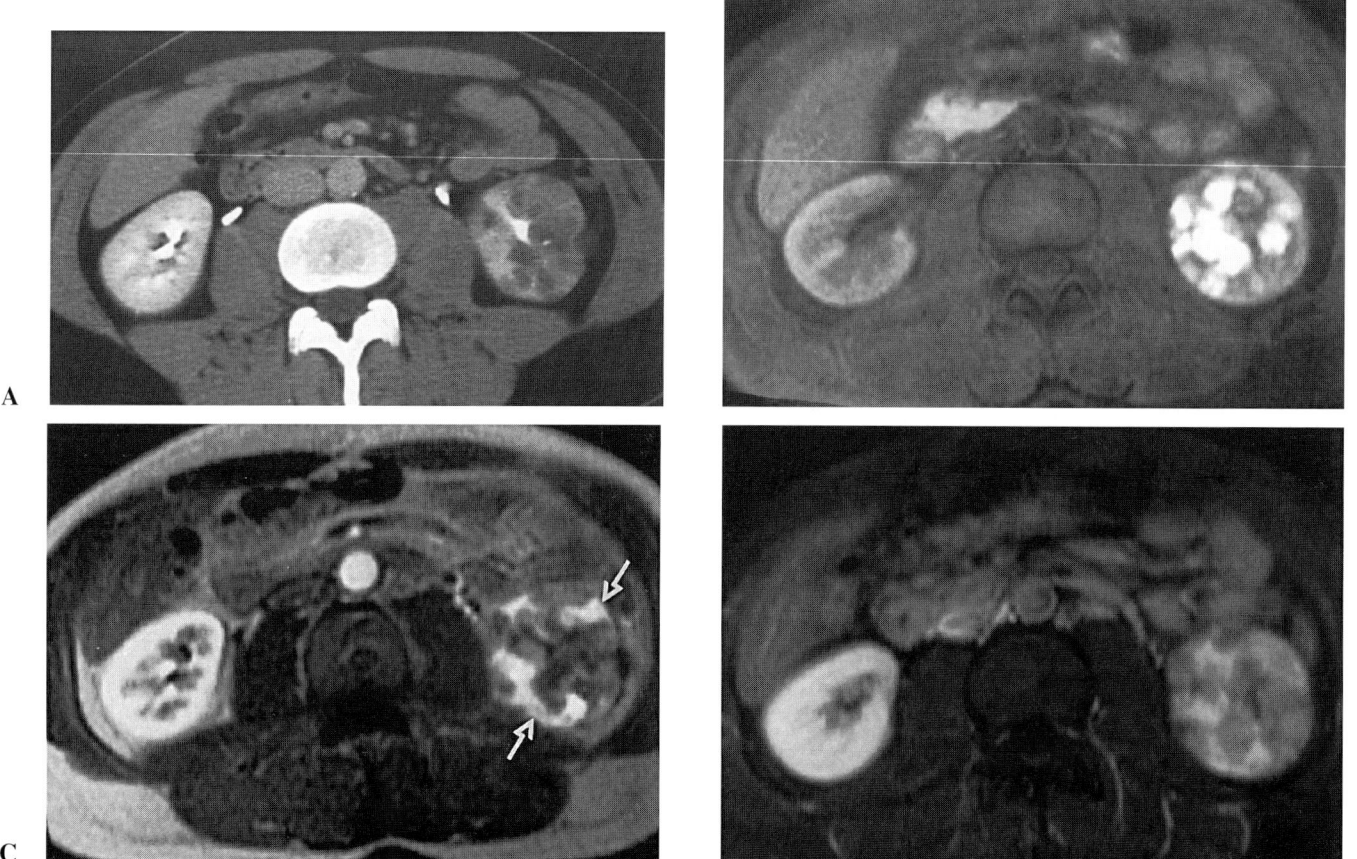

Figure 9–5. Multilocular cystic nephroma. Contrast-enhanced CT (**A**), T1FS (**B**), 1-second postcontrast FLASH (**C**), and gadolinium-enhanced T1FS (**D**) images. The CT demonstrates a multicystic mass arising from the lower pole of the left kidney. The T1FS image demonstrates that many of these cysts are high in SI, which is compatible with either subacute blood or protein. No SI increase of the cysts was identified on the 1-second postcontrast FLASH (**C**) or the gadolinium-enhanced T1FS (**D**) images. Fragments of renal cortex enhance in a normal fashion on the 1-second postcontrast image (arrows, **C**). (Reprinted with permission from ref. 2.)

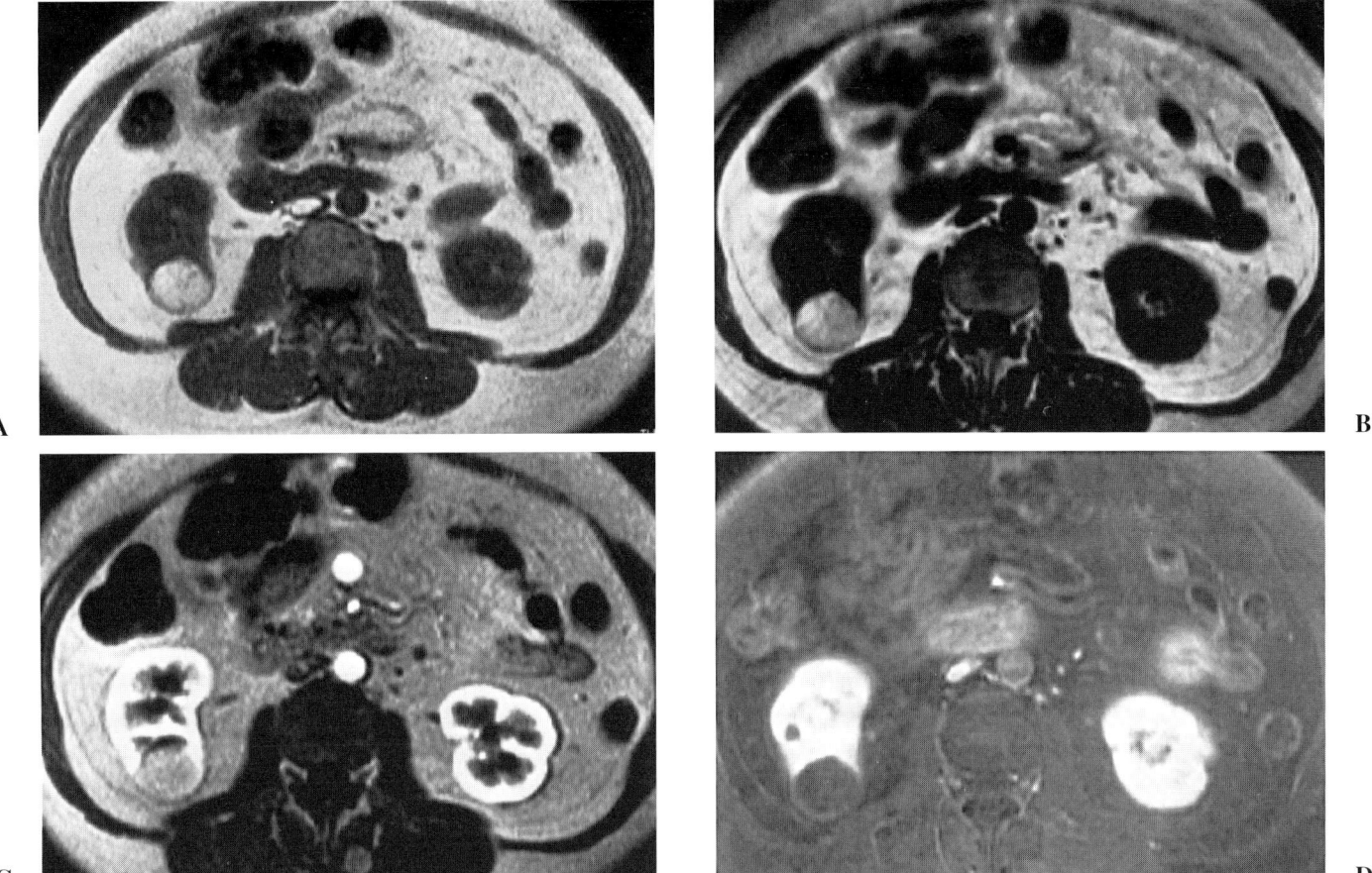

Figure 9–6. Angiomyolipoma. Precontrast FLASH (**A**), water-suppressed spin echo (**B**), and immediate postcontrast FLASH (**C**), and gadolinium-enhanced T1FS (**D**) images. A high-SI lesion on precontrast FLASH (**A**), which does not suppress with water suppression (**B**) but does suppress with fat suppression, is diagnostic for an angiomyolipoma. The lesion enhances poorly with gadolinium (**C**) and is a low-SI, sharply marginated lesion on T1FS (**D**). The appearance of the lesion on T1FS could be mistaken for a renal cyst without information from the precontrast FLASH image. (Reprinted with permission from ref. 19.)

MRI facilitates the demonstration that the cystic mass bulges into the renal pelvis, which is a characteristic feature of this entity.[25]

Angiomyolipoma. Angiomyolipomas contain blood vessels, smooth muscle, and fat, and are virtually always benign. Because of the large content of fat in most angiomyolipomas, characterization is possible on CT images and on combined T1-weighted regular and fat-suppressed images (Fig. 9–6).[26,27] If the lesions contain a large component of fat, tumors as small as 1 cm can be detected. This detection is a result of the high SI of fat on T1-weighted images that attenuates with fat suppression. However, if muscle or vascular components predominate in the angiomyolipoma, distinction from renal cell cancer may be difficult. Lesions less than 4 cm with a certain diagnosis of angiomyolipoma may be adequately managed with serial imaging studies.[28]

Adenoma. Renal adenoma is a benign tumor of renal cell origin that is typically a small, solid neoplasm.[29] This lesion is not distinguishable from papillary renal cell cancers on CT or MRI.[30] Small solid tumors may be adequately assessed with serial imaging to detect growth that would suggest malignancy.[31–34] Although there has not been an interval recommended for follow-up, a reasonable follow-up schedule would be an MRI at 3 months, 6 months, and annually thereafter.

MALIGNANT DISEASE

Renal Cell Carcinoma. Current generation CT and MR images are both able to detect renal cell carcinoma that measure 1 cm in diameter. Conventional MR sequences are useful in the characterization of renal tumors, assessment of extension of the tumors, and detection of tumor thrombus.[35] Spin echo images demonstrate a high contrast between tumor thrombus and signal-void blood.[35–40] Gadolinium-enhanced breath-hold and fat-suppressed techniques are superior to CT in differentiating cysts from solid tumors because of the increased sensitivity of MRI for gadolinium.[19,20,41]

Renal cell cancers typically appear as ill-defined masses

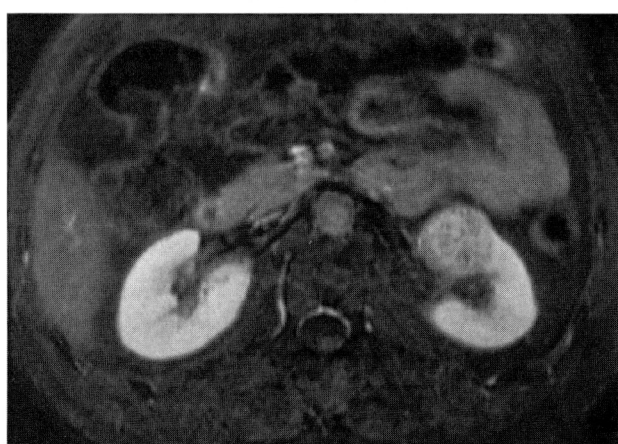

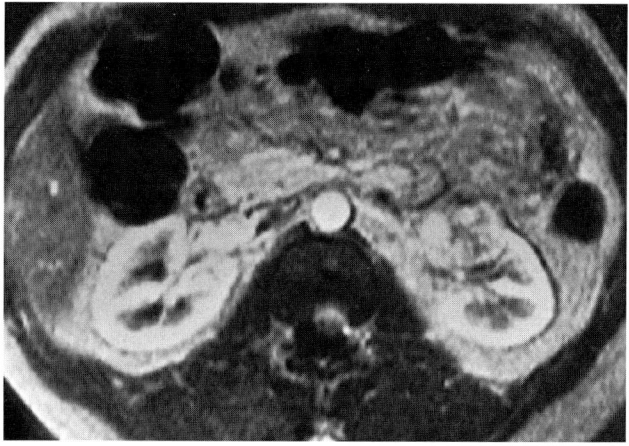

Figure 9–7. Stage I renal cell cancer. Precontrast FLASH (**A**), immediate postcontrast FLASH (**B**), and gadolinium-enhanced T1FS (**C**) images. A 3.5-cm tumor arises from the left kidney. The homogeneous, slightly hypointense mass on the precontrast image (**A**) enhances in a heterogeneous fashion after contrast enhancement (**B**) and is hypointense relative to renal cortex on gadolinium-enhanced T1FS (**C**). Although the tumor is well demonstrated on the postcontrast FLASH image, the tumor margins are not as well defined as on postcontrast T1FS. (Reprinted with permission from ref. 19.)

within the renal parenchyma. These tumors are often hypervascular and show heterogeneous enhancement on immediate postcontrast images, and diminished enhancement on more delayed postcontrast images. Tumor size is not a reliable criterion for diagnosing renal cancer or for distinguishing cancer from adenoma.[30–34] Therefore any nonfatty solid renal tumor should be considered a renal cell cancer until proven otherwise, and at the minimum should be followed closely on serial imaging. However, occasionally renal cell cancers show no change in size over intervals of more than 1 year.[32]

Completely intraparenchymal cancers are stage I cancers (Fig. 9–7). If the tumor extends beyond the cortical margins, the distinction between stage I and stage II cancers cannot be made based on imaging features. Large exophytic tumors can be stage I, and tumors with a small extrarenal component can be stage II.

Stage IIIa renal cancer is defined by extension into the renal vein, which frequently extends into the inferior vena cava (IVC). Although MRI has been recognized as superior to CT in the detection of thrombus, both modalities are acceptable in this use. However, MRI is better able to determine the extent of thrombus and to differentiate blood thrombus from tumor thrombus. Blood thrombus does not enhance with the use of gadolinium, but tumor thrombus does. Another technique to distinguish blood from tumor thrombus is to use a gradient echo technique. The presence of hemosiderin in blood clot renders blood thrombus a low signal intensity, whereas tumor thrombus is an intermediate signal intensity.

Stage IIIb renal cancer is defined by the presence of malignant nodes. Occasionally, MRI is able to demonstrate necrosis in lymph nodes (as shown by irregular low SI centers) that is not demonstrated on CT images.[26] In the presence of a necrotic primary tumor, necrotic lymph nodes may be specific for nodal involvement (Fig. 9–8). However, the presence of enlarged lymph nodes does not necessarily indicate stage IIIb or IIIc disease, as adenopathy may also be benign. In fact, in one study, 58% of patients with renal cell cancer had enlarged hyperplastic lymph nodes.[42] Stage IIIc renal cancer is defined by nodal involvement as well as by tumor extension into the renal vein.

Stage IV cancer involves extension to local or distant sites. Sites of metastases include lung (most common), adrenal glands, mediastinum, axial skeleton, and liver. Multiple bilateral renal tumors occur in fewer than 5% of patients with renal cancer. Cystic renal cell cancer may arise from tumor seeding of cysts. For this reason cysts in patients with multiple bilateral renal cancers should be viewed with suspicion.

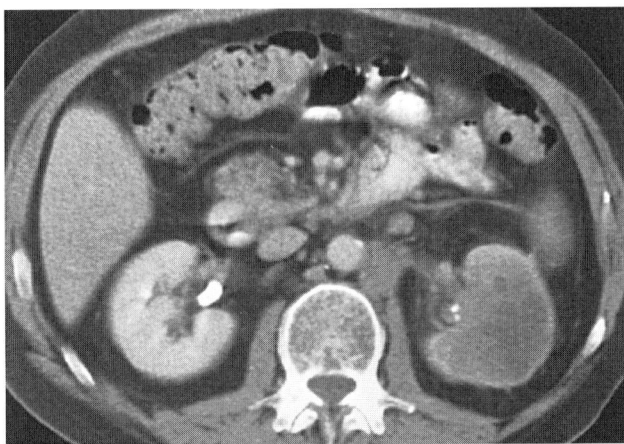
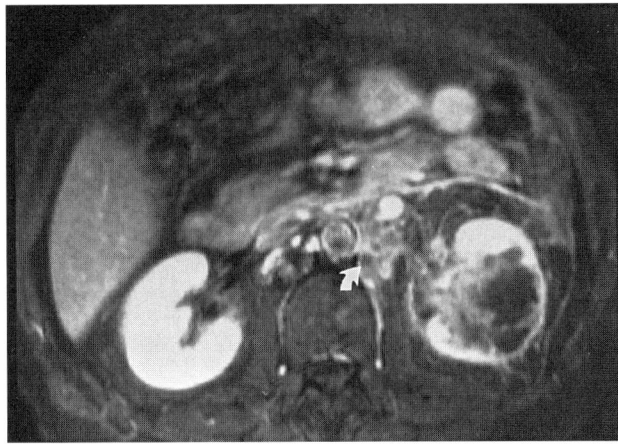

Figure 9–8. Stage IIIB renal cell cancer. Contrast-enhanced CT (**A**) and postcontrast T1FS (**B**) images. On the CT image, enlarged nodes are visible. However, on the postcontrast T1FS image, heterogeneous enhancement with a central low SI is apparent, which is similar to the primary tumor (arrow). (Reprinted with permission from ref. 19.)

Recent reports have shown MRI to be slightly superior to CT in the detection, characterization, and staging of renal cancer.[19,20] It has not yet been determined whether this superiority justifies the use of MRI of all renal masses. However, there are certain definite indications for the use of MRI, which include allergy to iodine contrast, indeterminate or calcified renal mass, and renal failure.[43–46] In patients with renal failure, the greater enhancement of renal parenchyma, the smaller volume of contrast needed, and the lesser renal toxicity provided by MRI justify the routine use of gadolinium-enhanced MRI in these patients (Fig. 9–9).[45]

MRI plays a considerable role in the detection and staging of renal cell cancers. As early detection leads to improved survival, the ability of MR to detect lesions as small as 1 cm in diameter may be important. As kidney-sparing surgery becomes more prevalent, accurate preoperative staging is increasingly critical.

Wilms' Tumor. Wilms' tumor is the most common renal malignant neoplasm in the pediatric patient and has a peak occurrence at the age of 2 years. Focal hemorrhage and necrosis are common findings. Although these tumors are usually solitary, they may be multiple in 5 to 10% of cases. At presentation, the tumor is usually a large mass that is calcified in only 5% of cases, whereas neuroblastomas calcify in 50% of cases. The appearance of Wilms' tumor is indistinguishable from renal cell cancer, appearing heterogeneous in signal intensity on contrast-enhanced images (Fig. 9–10). The patient's age alone constitutes the diagnosis in the patient less than the mid-teens, after which renal cell cancer is the most common renal tumor. Metastatic sites most common are the lungs, liver, and lymph nodes.

Lymphoma. Lymphomatous involvement of the kidneys is typically associated with widespread disease. However, isolated involvement of the kidney does occur.[47] The kid-

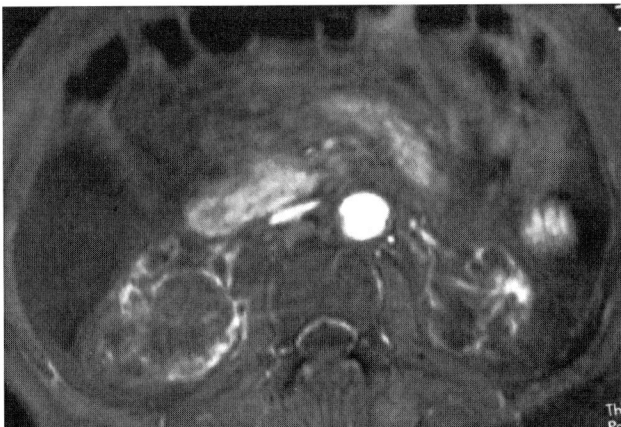

Figure 9–9. Renal cell cancer with chronic renal failure. Gadolinium-enhanced T1FS image. A 4-cm hypovascular renal cancer arises from the right kidney. Cortical enhancement persists despite chronic renal failure. (Reprinted with permission from ref. 2.)

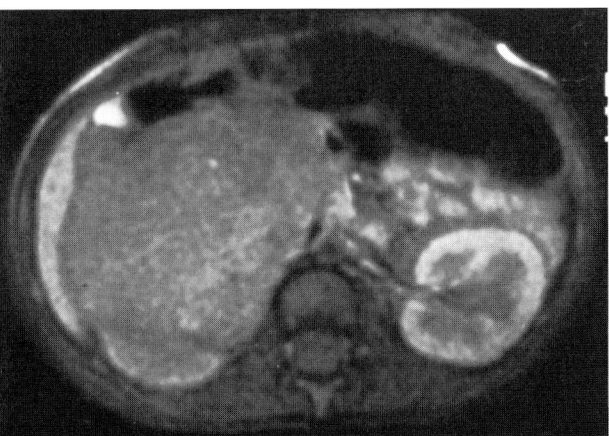

Figure 9–10. Wilms' tumor on a T1FS image. A large heterogeneous mass arises from the right kidney. (Reprinted with permission from ref. 2.)

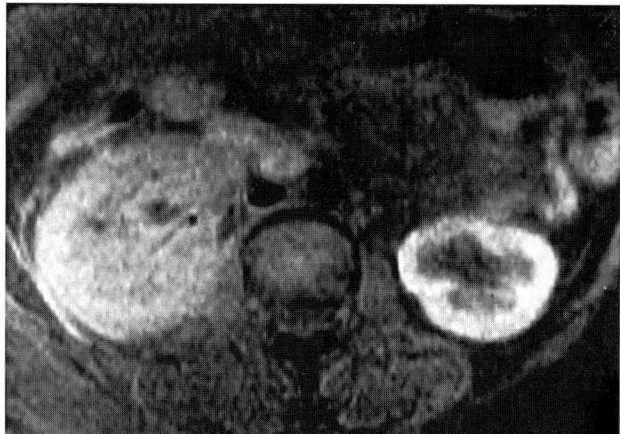
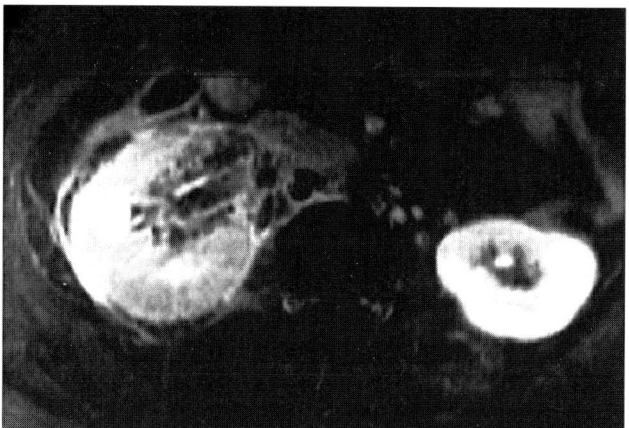

Figure 9–11. Lymphoma. T1FS (**A**), 1-second postcontrast FLASH (**B**), and gadolinium-enhanced T1FS (**C**) images. Diffuse renal enlargement and loss of corticomedullary differentiation on the T1FS image apparent in the right kidney (**A,B**). Low-SI lesions are noted in the medulla on the postcontrast images (**B,C**), most likely representing lymphomatous deposits. (Reprinted with permission from ref. 2.)

neys are more commonly affected by non-Hodgkin's lymphoma than by Hodgkin's lymphoma. The appearance of lymphomatous involvement varies and, includes: enlargement with maintenance of reniform shape, multiple bilateral nodules; direct invasion by retroperitoneal adenopathy; solitary renal mass; and perinephric involvement.[47] The most common pattern of involvement is direct invasion by retroperitoneal disease.

Lymphoma typically enhances minimally with gadolinium, which helps differentiate lymphoma from renal cell cancer, which usually contains regions of increased enhancement.[48] Typically, diffuse involvement appears as an increase in renal size with predominant involvement of the renal medulla (Fig. 9–11). Lymphomatous involvement of the kidney predelicts the renal medulla, which is a further distinction from renal cancer.[48] Large lymphatomatous masses can be differentiated from renal cell cancer as there is a greater tendency for lymphoma to encase the renal artery, which results in diminished enhancement of the entire kidney as a result of compromised renal blood flow.

Metastasis. Lung and breast cancer are the primary tumors to metastasize to the kidneys, and this usually occurs as a late manifestation of the disease. The usual appearance of metastases is that of multiple bilateral renal masses (Fig. 9-12).

OBSTRUCTION

Acute obstruction is recognized on MR images by the enlarged kidney size and persistence of contrast in the renal parenchyma, yielding a prolonged nephrogram phase. Diminished corticomedullary differentiation is present.[16] However, in chronic obstruction as in ischemia, the kidney has a smaller size, smooth contour, and decreased contrast enhancement. The collecting system remains dilated, which aids in differentiation from chronic ischemia (Fig. 9–13).

ISCHEMIA

The vascular diseases involving the kidney are usually thromboembolic in origin, as a result of underlying atherosclerotic disease. Acute and chronic renal ischemia is well shown with the use of MRI. The relative renal blood flow to the kidneys can be readily appreciated and compared on immediate post-gadolinium dynamic MR images to obtain a relative quantification of renal blood flow. Acute ischemia usually results in a normal or slightly enlarged kidney with diminished contrast enhancement. On the other hand, chronic ischemia usually results in a small kidney with a smooth boundary and diminished contrast enhancement, with persistence of the corticomedullary differentiation (Fig. 9–14).

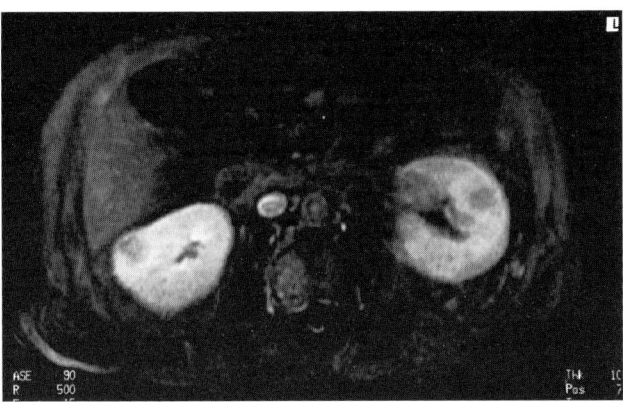

Figure 9-12. Metastases to the kidneys from adenocarcinoma of the lung. Gadolinium-enhanced T1FS image. Multiple bilateral metastases are demonstrated as poorly enhancing lesions. (Reprinted with permission from ref. 2.)

For patients with a source of emboli, renal emboli are a common complication, since the kidneys receive 20% of the cardiac output. The most common cause of renal emboli are mural thrombi in patients with a history of atrial arrhythmias or myocardial infarction.[49] Infarction tends to occur between calices and results in well-defined wedge-shaped defects in the renal outline (Fig. 9-15).[37]

HEMORRHAGE

MR images of hemorrhage typically show a high or mixed high SI fluid in the parenchyma or in the subcapsular region. In the setting of fluid collections, MR is more sensitive to detection of hemorrhage than is CT.

INFECTION

Acute Infection. Acute pyelonephritis is characterized by enlargement of the infected kidney. However, MRI is not commonly performed for the diagnosis of this entity, as it is usually based on clinical findings.

Reflux Nephropathy and Chronic Pyelonephritis. Renal scarring following reflux nephropathy is typically demonstrated in the polar regions adjacent to the renal calyces. Chronic pyelonephritis appears as calyceal dilatation and overlying cortical scarring. In the capillary phase of enhancement, cortical thinning is well demonstrated.

Abscess. The presentation of abscesses may be insidious, and its cause may be related to an ascending infection or hematogenous spread. Hematogenous infection may be found in patients with tuberculosis, intravenous drug use, or gram-positive cocci bacteremia. MR images of renal abscesses demonstrate irregular mass lesions with a signal-void

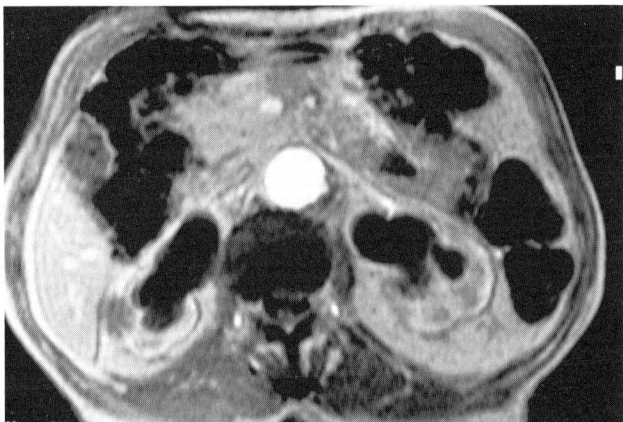

Figure 9-13. Chronic obstruction. One-second post-gadolinium FLASH image. Both kidneys are small and the cortex shows smooth contours and diminished enhancement. The collecting systems are markedly dilated.

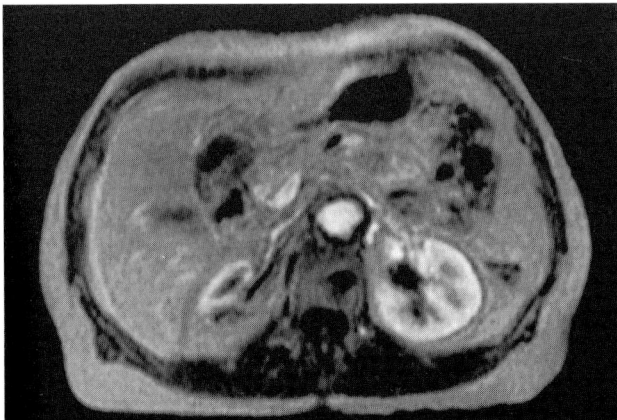

Figure 9-14. Chronic renal ischemia. One-second post-gadolinium FLASH image. The renal cortex is thin and smooth. Corticomedullary differentiation persists.

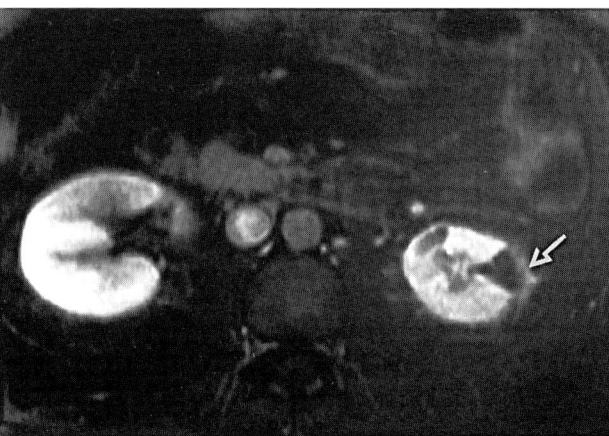

Figure 9-15. Embolic infarction. Gadolinium-enhanced T1FS image. A well-defined wedge-shaped defect is apparent in the lower pole of the left kidney. A thin rim of enhancement persists, consistent with a capsular vessel (arrow). (Reprinted with permission from ref. 2.)

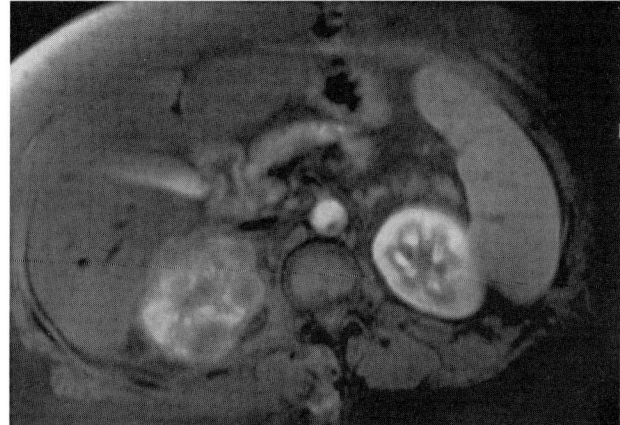

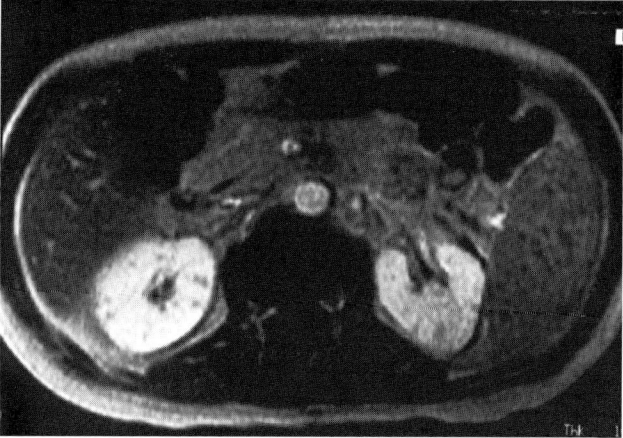

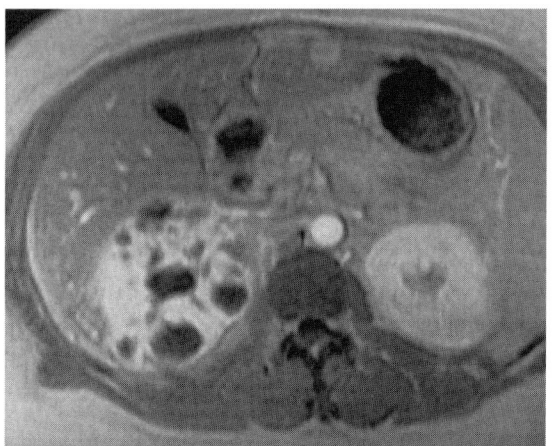

Figure 9–16. Abscesses. Precontrast T1FS (**A**) and 45-second post-gadolinium (**B**) images. Prominent renal abscesses distort the renal parenchyma of the right kidney. On the T1FS image (**B**), the left kidney contains high SI in the medulla, consistent with proteinaceous, purulent material in acute pyelonephritis.

Figure 9–17. Renal candidiasis. Ninety-second postcontrast FLASH image. Multiple 1- and 2-mm signal-void lesions are consistent with microabscesses of candidiasis. (Reprinted with permission from ref. 2.)

center (Fig. 9–16). The higher contrast resolution of MR over CT permits better distinction of focal bacterial nephritis and true bacterial abscess with a necrotic center. Perirenal inflammatory stranding is common with renal abscesses. In patients with elevated serum creatinine MRI is well suited to define abscesses and as follow-up imaging to observe resolution after treatment.[50]

Xanthogranulomatous Pyelonephritis. Xanthogranulomatous pyelonephritis (XGPN) is a chronic infection that develops in the presence of chronic obstruction.[50] *Proteus* species are involved with 60% of cases. Although the infection is usually a diffuse process, focal XGPN has been described.[51]

Candidiasis. The lesions of renal candidiasis in the context of systemic candidiasis are usually small (about 2 mm) and well defined. Fungus balls tend to occur in patients with diabetes mellitus and appear as nonenhancing masses in the collecting system (Fig. 9–17).

Disease of the Renal Collecting System

BENIGN DISEASE

Several benign masses may affect the renal collecting system. These include fibroepithelial polyp, pyelitis cystica, cholesteatoma, leukoplakia, and malakoplakia. The appearance of these lesions on MR images has not yet been defined.

MALIGNANT DISEASE

Transitional Cell Cancer. Transitional cell cancer is commonly multifocal (in 30 to 50% of cases) and bilateral (15 to 25%). Tumors appear as eccentric filling defects in the renal pelvis.[52,53] Concentric wall thickening may occur on occasion.[52,53] Tumors usually spread superficially, but rarely may be large focal masses. Invasion of the parenchyma may be difficult to detect. Despite the hypovascularity of these tumors, the SI may be high on gadolinium-enhanced T1 fat-suppressed (T1FS) MR images, presumably because of the abnormal clearance of contrast from the extracellular space (Fig. 9–18). The tumors tend to invade locally with regional lymphatic nodal involvement. Because of the tendency of transitional cell cancer to be multifocal and bilateral, evaluation of the entire urothelium with retrograde pyelography is necessary.

Metastasis. Renal metastases usually appear as multiple focal masses involving both kidneys. The SI of these masses is lower than adjacent parenchyma. The most common primary tumors to metastasize to the urothelium are melanoma, breast cancer, and ovarian cancer.

FILLING DEFECT

The most common filling defects in the renal collecting system are calculi. In North America, the most common

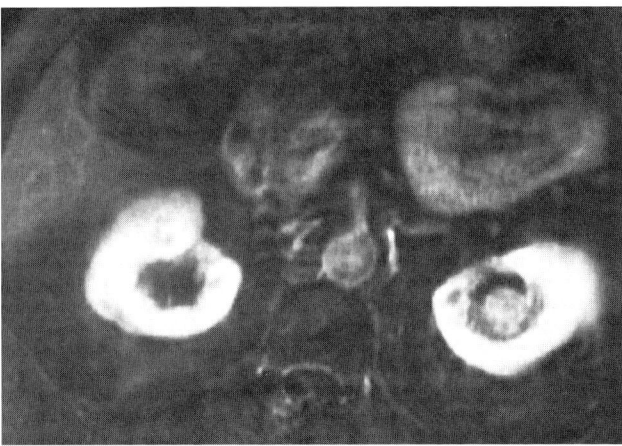

Figure 9–18. Transitional cell carcinoma. Gadolinium-enhanced T1FS image. The 2-cm tumor has diminished contrast enhancement and arises from a superior pole calyx in the left kidney. (Reprinted with permission from ref. 2.)

form of renal calculi are calcium oxalate stones, which account for approximately 65% of cases.[54] All renal calculi, despite calcium composition, are signal void on MR images. Classically, MRI has not been used for detection of renal calculi, as urine and calculi are both signal void on T1 images, which best demonstrate anatomy. However, in the well-hydrated patient, the use of gadolinium allows for high SI urine in the renal pelvis 2 to 30 minutes following contrast administration. Signal-void calculi as small as 1 to 2 mm in diameter can be detected when urine is high SI due to the presence of dilute gadolinium (Fig. 9–19). Obstruction of the collecting system causes alteration in the enhancement of renal parenchyma and in the transit of contrast material within the kidney. This is well shown on MR images. MR urography may hold future promise as a noninvasive, fast technique to demonstrate obstructing ureteric calculi.

Other filling defects, such as blood clots or fungus balls, are also well demonstrated with MRI. The typical appearance is a mass lesion seated in the contrast-filled collecting system.

Trauma

Abdominal trauma not infrequently leads to renal injury. Severity of the injury is best evaluated with tomographic imaging. Injury is usually classified as mild (contusion), moderate (laceration into the collecting system), or severe (disruption of the renal pedicle or complete crush).[55] Integrity of the vessels is well evaluated with the use of dynamic gadolinium imaging, which shows high SI in the vessels.

Renal Function

Serial imaging permits characterization of the distinct phases of gadolinium enhancement, which include cortical (or capillary), early tubular, ductal, and excretory phase.[16] The characteristics of gadolinium, which cause the SI of a fluid medium to change, depending on the concentration of gadolinium, allow evaluation of the concentrating ability of the kidneys. The assessment of the different phases of contrast enhancement allow distinction between normal collecting systems and nonobstructed dilated systems, as well as between acute and chronically obstructed systems. For optimal results, it is recommended that the patients be mildly dehydrated so as to provide physiologic renal concentration. This is adequately achieved with a 5-hour fast prior to the examination.

Because the renal transit time is not impaired in the condition of dilated nonobstructed kidneys, the signal intensity changes are similar to those of normal kidneys. Acutely obstructed kidneys are enlarged and have increased renal transit time. Therefore there is a prolonged, increasing SI nephrogram, and the appearance of contrast in the renal ducts and

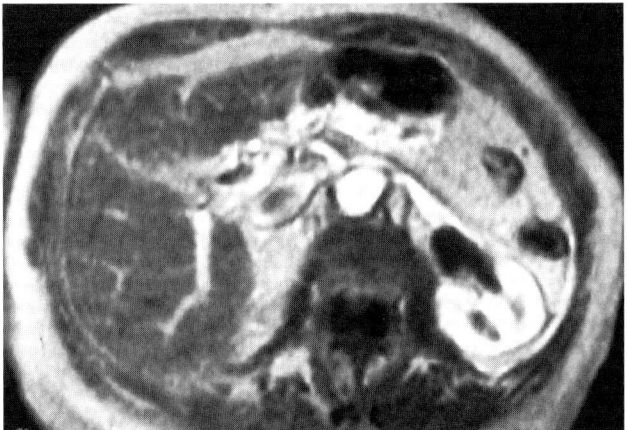 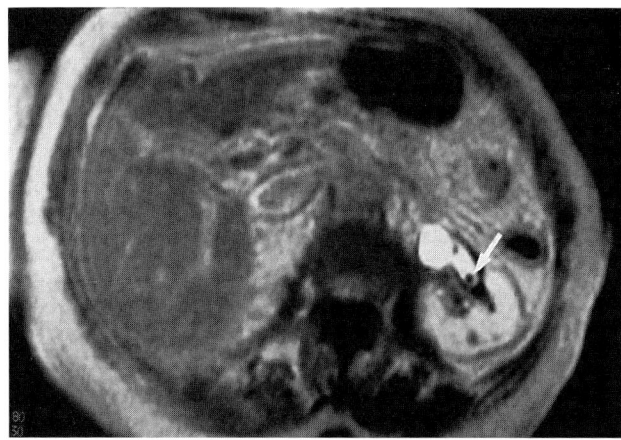

Figure 9–19. Renal calculi. One-second (**A**) and 10-minute post-gadolinium FLASH (**B**) images. The calculus is signal-void, and thus not detectable within the low-signal urine, which does not contain gadolinium. However, on the later image, urine is a high signal intensity, because of a low concentration of gadolinium, which permits visualization of the signal-void calculus (arrow). (Reprinted with permission from ref. 2.)

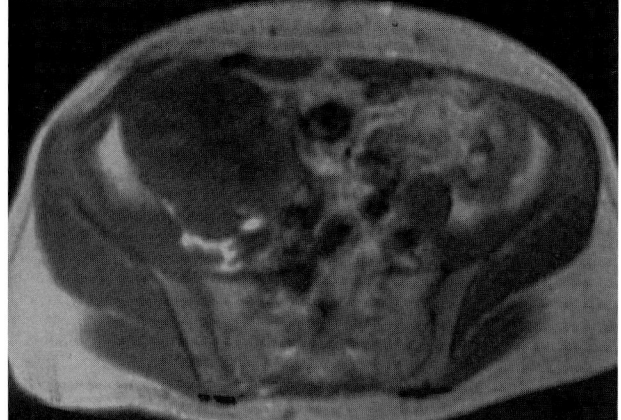
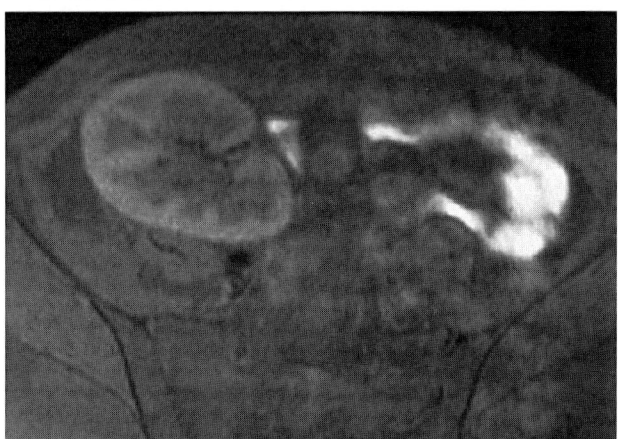
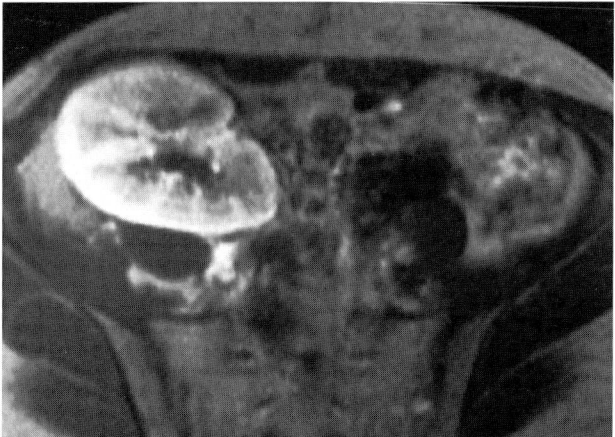

Figure 9–20. Functioning renal transplant. Precontrast FLASH (**A**), T1FS (**B**), and 1-second postcontrast FLASH (**C**) images. The corticomedullary differentiation is well demonstrated on the T1FS images, and the dynamic gadolinium-enhanced image shows a normal pattern of renal flow. (Reprinted with permission from ref. 2.)

collecting system is delayed. Chronic obstruction shows an increased transit time and diminished cortical enhancement.

Renal Transplants

The normally functioning renal transplant shows good corticomedullary differentiation on T1FS and dynamic gadolinium-enhanced images (Fig. 9–20). Conversely, a renal allograft undergoing rejection shows a loss of renal corticomedullary differentiation.[56] In fact, it appears that MR is more sensitive than quantitative scintigraphy or sonography in detection of renal transplant rejection.[57] However, the finding of loss of corticomedullary differentiation is a nonspecific one and is also seen with cyclosporine toxicity and other infiltrative renal diseases. Chronic rejection is demonstrated by loss of corticomedullary differentiation on T1FS images, and the degree of loss of corticomedullary differentiation on dynamic gadolinium-enhanced images may correlate with the severity of rejection.

The assessment of surgical complications such as urinoma and renal vascular patency is also possible with MRI. Additionally, MRI allows diagnosis of avascular necrosis of bone, which is a common occurrence in these patients.

Juxtarenal Processes

Juxtarenal processes include tumor, hemorrhage, abscesses, and urine leaks. Extravasation of urine may be the result of pyelosinus rupture caused by elevated intracollecting system pressure, which is most commonly caused by the presence of a calculus. Urine extravasation may also be the result of trauma.

URETER AND RETROPERITONEUM

Dilated ureters are well shown on MR images by the SI of the urine, which is dark on T1-weighted and bright on T2-weighted images. Coronal and sagittal views may provide better illustration of the extent of the dilated segment.

Retroperitoneal fibrosis, a sclerosing process centered over the lower lumbar spine, often leads to ureteral obstruction. MRI has certain advantages over CT in evaluation of retroperitoneal fibrosis. Multiplanar imaging characteristics allow full evaluation of the extent of the lesion as well as its relationship to neighboring structures. Typically, retroperitoneal fibrosis has a low to medium signal intensity on T1-weighted spin echo images,[58–60] and the T1 signal intensity may be lower than that seen with lymphoma.[61] The SI on T2-weighted images of inactive forms of retroperitoneal fibrosis tends to be low, secondary to decreased vascularity and dense collagen deposits, and this is generally observed in chronic benign retroperitoneal fibrosis after approximately one year of disease duration. Active forms, acute benign retroperitoneal fibrosis, show a higher SI because of edema and active inflammation.[60] Malignant retroperitoneal fibrosis is typically moderately high in SI on T2-weighted images. Both acute benign and malignant retroperitoneal fibrosis may enhance substantially with gadolinium, while chronic benign disease enhances minimally. MR may be useful in distinguishing chronic benign from malignant disease.[62] The distinction between acute benign and malignant retroperitoneal fibrosis may be more problematic, and clinical history is often important information to aid in establishing the correct diagnosis.

Retroperitoneal lymphadenopathy is well demonstrated with MRI.[63,64] Enlarged nodes are intermediate in SI on T1-weighted images and appear relatively bright on T2-weighted images. Lymph nodes also enhance with gadolinium. Using MR images obtained in multiple planes (i.e., transaxial, coronal, and sagittal), precise location of nodes of interest can be identified.[65]

BLADDER

Magnetic Resonance Techniques

A variety of MR techniques have been employed to study the bladder. Techniques that are particularly useful include T2-weighted spin echo, pre- and postintravenous gadolinium, T1-weighted fat-suppressed spin echo, and dynamic immediate postcontrast gradient echo sequences. T1-weighted images are effective at demonstrating morphology but are not as effective as the previously mentioned techniques at demonstrating depth of tumor invasion. As in other organ systems it is useful to combine imaging techniques that demonstrate different tissue contrasts. In the bladder it is useful to combine sequences that demonstrate high SI urine (i.e., T2-weighted imaging and delayed postgadolinium imaging) with techniques that demonstrate low SI urine (i.e., T1-weighted spin echo with or without fat suppression and immediate postcontrast dynamic gradient echo imaging). The acquisition of sequences that show different contrast between urine and bladder wall is important to effectively evaluate abnormalities in the bladder wall and lumen.

Another important feature of MRI is the multiplanar imaging capability that permits image acquisition in different planes to minimize partial volume effects when evaluating depth of penetration of bladder cancer (i.e., sagittal imaging for anterior and posterior wall and dome lesions, and coronal imaging for lateral wall and dome lesions).

The critical artifacts in MRI of the bladder involve motion, degree of bladder distention, and chemical shift. Involuntary motion artifacts include motion from respiration, intestinal peristalsis, and bladder motion. Respiratory movements can be reduced by the use of a tight abdominal band. Bladder distention is important. If the bladder is not distended, the detrusor muscle is thickened, mimicking thickening from disease states and making it difficult to recognize small tumors. If the bladder is too distended, the patient becomes uncomfortable and flat tumors can be missed secondary to overstretching of the muscle layer. Chemical shift artifact occurs at the water–fat interface, and appears as a dark band along the lateral wall on one side and a bright band along the lateral wall on the opposite side.[66] This appearance can mimic or mask an invasive bladder cancer. To correct for this, chemically selective fat suppression can be performed, or the frequency-encoding gradient can be rotated to select the direction that least interferes with examination of bladder wall adjacent to tumor.[66]

The use of surface coils can significantly improve the image quality of the pelvic structures. Double surface coils have been shown to improve pelvic MRI.[67–69] Even greater image improvements occur with the use of phased-array multicoils and endorectal coils.

The normal bladder wall appears as an intermediate signal intensity on T1-weighted images. The appearance of the bladder wall on T2-weighted images has previously been reported as a low-signal-intensity band that represents the entire muscular layer. More recently, this band has been divided into two bands of low SI (inner) and intermediate SI (outer). These have been characterized as the compact inner and looser outer arrangement of smooth muscle bundles.[70]

Benign Disease

DIFFUSE DISEASE

Bladder wall hypertrophy appears as an increased thickness of the bladder wall that is low in SI on T2-weighted images and does not enhance substantially with gadolinium. Signal intensity features are similar to those of a normal bladder wall (Fig. 9–21).

Inflammation of the bladder results in a thickened appearance of the bladder wall and may be focal. On T2-weighted images of inflamed bladder wall, four layers can be appreciated. An innermost low-signal-intensity band and inner high-signal-intensity band represent the thickened epithelium and lamina propria, respectively. An outer low-signal-intensity band and outermost intermediate-signal-intensity bands represent the inner compact muscle layer and outer loose muscle layer, respectively.[70] Increased enhancement following gadolinium administration is usually observed.

Hemorrhagic cystitis may demonstrate a complex appearance on MR images, as a result of the complexity of MR appearances of hemorrhage, based on the T1 and T2 characteristics of aging blood products. Active bleeding (oxyhemoglobin) has limited paramagnetic properties and behaves like simple fluid with a long T1 (low SI on T1-weighted images) and long T2 (high SI on T2-weighted images); acute blood (intracellular deoxyhemoglobin) has a long T1 (low signal intensity on T1-weighted images) and a short T2 (low signal intensity on T2-weighted images). Intracellular methemoglobin has a short T1 (high signal intensity on T1-weighted images) and a short T2 (low signal intensity on T2-weighted images). Extracellular

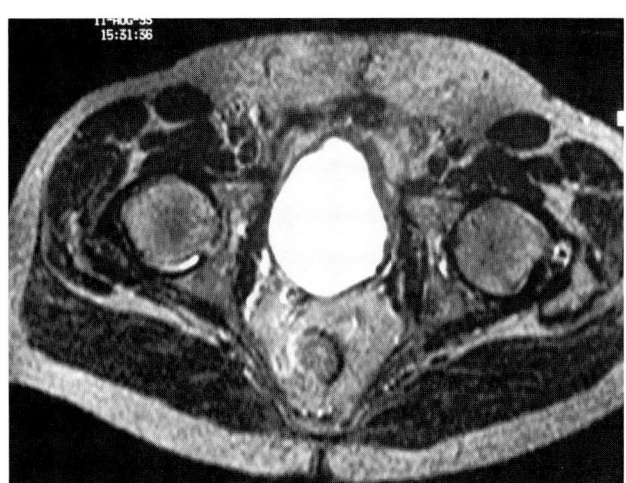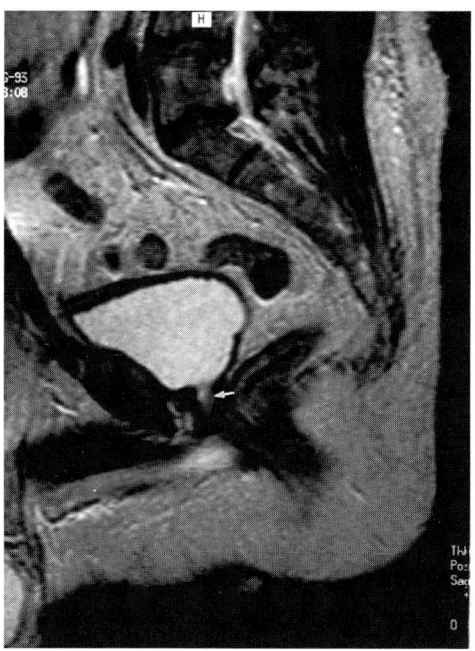

Figure 9–21. Bladder hypertrophy. Transverse (**A**) and sagittal T2SE (**B**) images. Bladder shows asymmetric hypertrophic changes. The bladder wall is low in SI, consistent with benign noninflammatory disease. A prostatic urethral defect is present as a result of transurethral resection of the prostate (arrow).

methemoglobin has a short T1 (high signal intensity on T1-weighted images) and a long T2 (high signal intensity on T2-weighted images), and this appearance is most typical for subacute hemorrhage. Intracellular hemosiderin in an old hematoma has a medium T1 (intermediate signal intensity on T1-weighted images) and a short T2 (low signal intensity on T2-weighted images).[71] Thus the appearance of hemorrhagic cystitis may demonstrate not only a thickened bladder wall, but also the complex signal characteristics of hemorrhage (Fig. 9–22).

Edema of the bladder wall as a result of acute bladder disease can be distinguished from bladder wall hypertrophy by its longer T2, which renders it high in SI on T2-weighted images.[72]

FOCAL DISEASE

Focal granulomatous reactions, either infectious or inflammatory (tuberculosis, bilharziosis), appear as intravesical lesions with high SI on T2-weighted images. They may behave similarly to bladder wall mass lesions.[65] Epithelioid granulomatous lesions, which can occur in patients undergoing immunotherapy (BCG) used for the treatment of malignant bladder lesions, may appear similar to malignant tumors on MRI. Although MRI accurately shows these lesions to be confined to the vesical wall, their presence can lead to false-positive findings.[65]

Calcifications of pathologic lesions (bilharziosis) shows a typical absence of signal on all sequences.[73] Bladder calculi are rare lesions that are well shown on T2-weighted images or late postgadolinium T1-weighted images. These sequences show good contrast between high SI urine and signal void calculi.[65]

Neurofibromatosis of the genitourinary tract, a rare entity, has distinct MR features that allow better characterization of the extent of the tumor within the bladder, pelvic side walls, and surrounding soft tissues than does CT. The described MR findings for type I neurofibromatosis (von Recklinghausen disease) are a T1-weighted SI slightly greater than that of skeletal muscle and a markedly increased SI relative to the surrounding tissues on the T2-weighted images. Most demonstrate enhancement with gadolinium administration. Obstructive hydronephrosis, a common complication, is presumably due to neurofibromas involving the trigone. Pelvic side wall tumors appear nodular and may extend into the obturator foramina.[74]

Bladder pheochromocytoma occurs most commonly in the trigone or near the ureteral orifices. Less often, it is found in the dome and lateral walls of the bladder. Characteristic MR features help distinguish this tumor from other tumors, including carcinoma.[75,76] Typically, these tumors show markedly increased, homogeneous SI on T2-weighted SE sequences.[77–79]

The diagnosis of pelvic lipomatosis can be supported with the use of MRI. The characteristic appearance is that of an extensive amount of fat surrounding the bladder (high SI on T1-weighted images).[80]

Bladder papillomas are most clearly shown on immediate postcontrast MR images as small enhancing masses arising from lesser enhancing wall. Dynamic postgadolinium enhanced MR images (15 to 45 seconds) may be most useful to demonstrate the superficial nature of these lesions.

Malignant Disease

PRIMARY DISEASE

Both T1- and T2-weighted images are useful in staging of bladder cancers.[81-88] The use of T1-weighted SE sequences is recommended to determine invasion of the perivesical fat and surrounding organs (except the prostate), and involvement of lymph node and bone marrow. T2-weighted images are recommended for assessment of the extent of tumor invasion into the muscle layer of the bladder wall and prostate.[66,81-85,88]

The use of intravenous gadolinium contrast agents has improved the imaging of bladder carcinomas. Gadolinium quickly distributes in the extracellular space without passing through intact cell membranes[89] and typically provides significant enhancement of urinary bladder carcinomas.[90-98] Bladder carcinomas tend to enhance greater than the surrounding bladder wall early after injection of contrast. Tumors are well seen approximately 5 to 15 sec after arterial enhancement.[97] This early phase of enhancement also demonstrates good conspicuity of bladder tumor against gadolinium-free urine in the bladder. Delayed postcontrast T1-weighted images show high signal intensity of urine, and the intraluminal portion of a bladder tumor is usually well delineated, although small tumors may be obscured.

Accuracy of MR in the staging of bladder carcinoma has been reported to range from 69 to 89%. Staging of small tumors particularly is improved with the use of gadolinium.[90,93,94,96,97] MRI offers several advantages over CT, which include higher contrast resolution and multiplanar imaging, which permits better imaging of the bladder dome, trigone, perivesical fat, prostate, and seminal vesicles. The higher contrast resolution is most useful in differentiation between muscular invasion (stage T3a) and invasion into the perivesical fat (stage T3b).[81-85,87,90] Bladder tumors at the base or dome are clearly better staged with MRI. For deeply infiltrative tumors (stages T3b, T4a, and T4b), MR is generally agreed to be the most accurate method of staging (Fig. 9–23). The most common cause of staging error in MR and CT studies is overstaging, and prior cystoscopic biopsy is likely a common cause of this overstaging.[98]

MR may be able to differentiate between superficial (stage T1) and deep invasion of the muscle layer of the bladder wall (stage T3a). This distinction is not possible with clinical staging, CT, or intravesical sonography.

MRI is particularly useful in the distinction between late fibrosis or granulation tissue and recurrence of carcinoma.

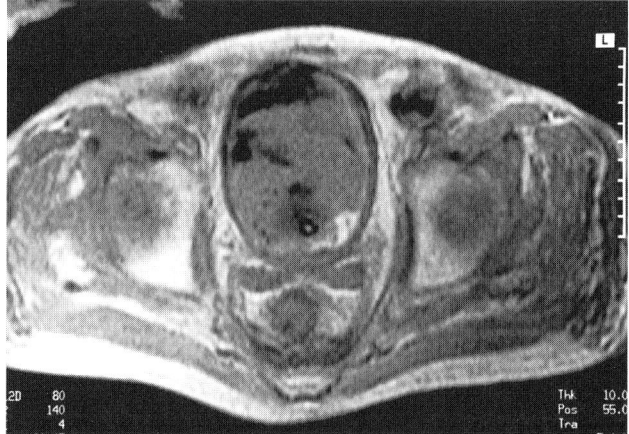
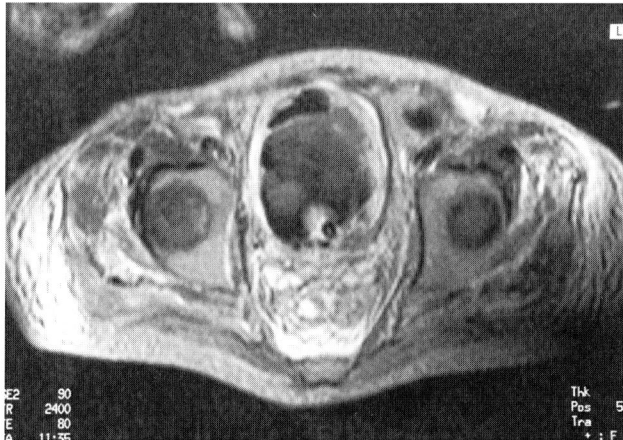
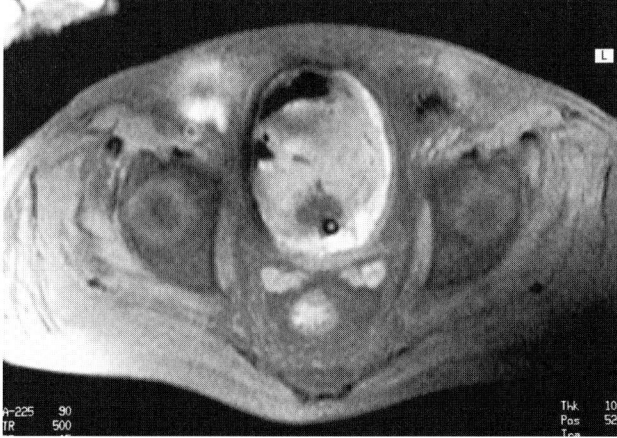

Figure 9–22. Bladder hemorrhage. FLASH (**A**), T2 (**B**), and T1FS (**C**) images. The bladder wall is thickened. Blood products of differing ages result in a range of signal intensities on the various sequences. A catheter lies within the bladder.

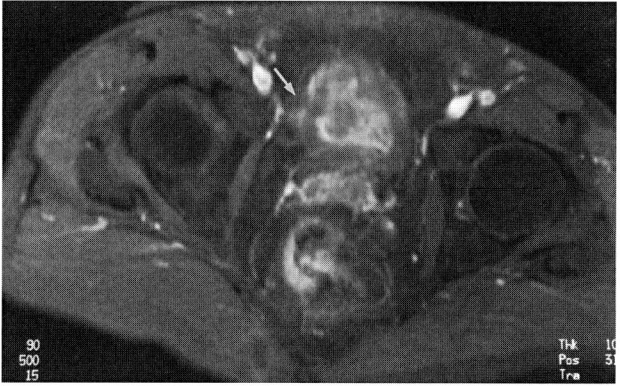

Figure 9–23. Stage T3b bladder cancer. Gadolinium-enhanced T1FS image. This tumor shows extension into the perivesical fat (arrow).

One year following transurethral resection, after most of the acute edema has resolved, residual scar can be distinguished from recurrence of tumor using T2-weighted images.[88,99] Recurrent tumor appears high SI, while scar appears low SI on T2-weighted images. However, prior to resolution of the edema, MR is not able to exclude recurrence.[88,90,93,94,96,97]

In the staging of lymph node metastases, MR and CT appear to be comparable. Accuracy for CT is 83 to 97%; that for MR, 73 to 98%. MR is, however, superior to CT in diagnosis of bone marrow metastases.[88,100]

MRI and clinical staging have complementary roles, and staging of urinary bladder tumors is best achieved with the use of both modalities. Because of the limitations in differentiating acute edema from tumor tissue, MR is most helpful if performed prior to the clinical staging.[101]

METASTATIC DISEASE

The most common metastases to the bladder arise from direct extension from pelvic neoplasms (Figs. 9–24, 9–25). The diagnostic accuracy of MRI in the detection of bladder mucosal invasion by pelvic tumors was reported to be 81% in one series.[102] The types of tumors studied in this series were cervical, colon, urethral, vaginal, vulvar, and lymphoid tissue. False-negative findings may arise from microscopic foci of invasion, whereas false-positive findings may stem from muscularis invasion without mucosal invasion. In this series, it was noted that postradiation changes and bullous edema are easily distinguished from tumor.[102]

Cervical carcinoma stage IVa involves bladder mucosa. This invasion is well shown with the use of gadolinium-enhanced T1-weighted images, which provides accurate diagnosis.[103,104]

URETHRA

Magnetic Resonance Techniques and Normal Anatomy

FEMALE ANATOMY

The normal female urethra demonstrates a characteristic targetlike appearance on T2-weighted or T1-weighted gadolinium-enhanced images.[105] The appearance of the MR image correlates with the histology of the female urethra.[105] The three layers that make up the urethra are the outer muscular layer, the middle submucosa, and the mucosa.[106–110]

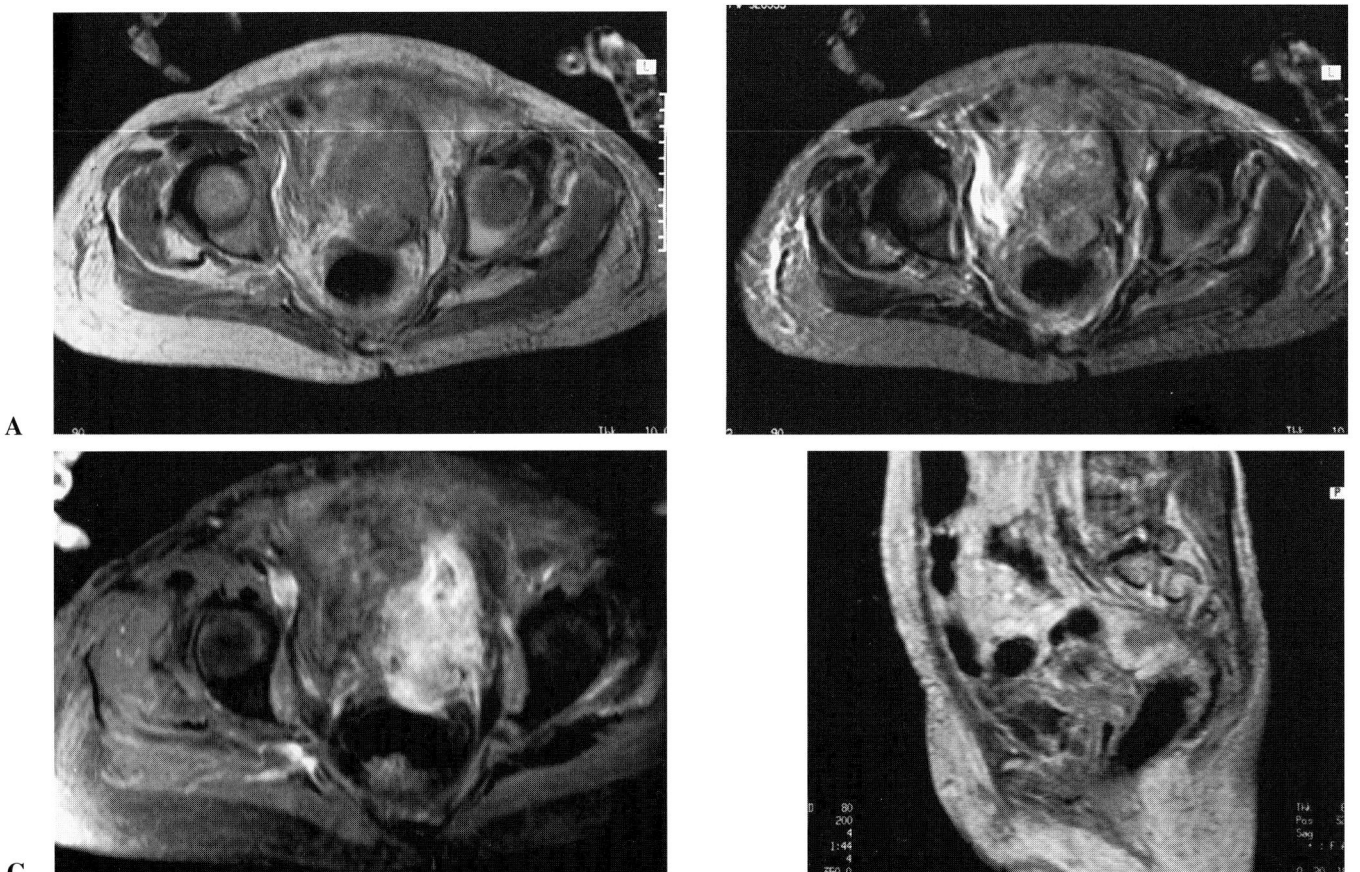

Figure 9–24. Invasion of bladder wall by vaginal adenocarcinoma. Proton density (**A**), T2 (**B**), gadolinium-enhanced T1FS (**C**), and sagittal gadolinium-enhanced FLASH (**D**) images. Extensive invasion of the bladder wall is noted. The tumor mass enhances heterogeneously with gadolinium (**C**). The extent of invasion is well appreciated on the sagittal image (**D**).

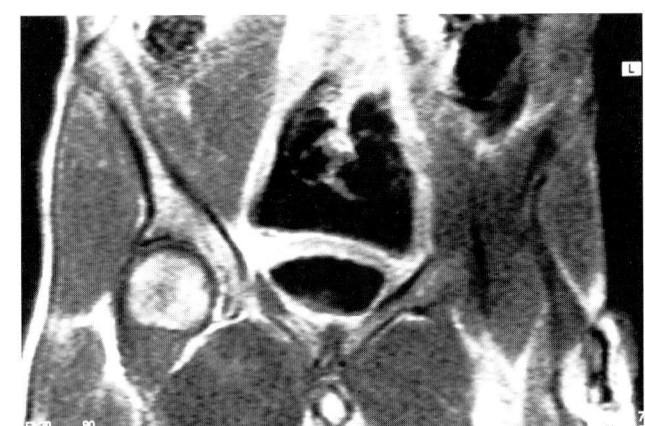
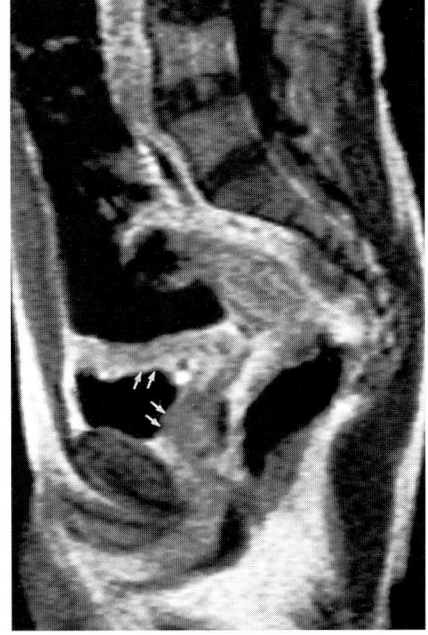

Figure 9–25. Invasion of bladder wall by rectal carcinoma. Coronal precontrast FLASH (**A**) and sagittal postcontrast FLASH (**B**) images. The bladder wall shows asymmetric thickening, especially along the posterior and superior portions of the bladder (arrows). On the coronal image (**A**), ascites surrounds a bowel loop above the bladder, which is suspended by its mesentery. Direct extension of rectal carcinoma onto the dome of the bladder is clearly shown on the sagittal and coronal images.

The outer, low-signal-intensity ring noted on MR images most likely represents the outer muscular layer, which consists of an inner layer of longitudinal and thin circular fibers of smooth muscle and an outer layer of striated muscle. The middle layer of the urethra, noted as a high-signal intensity on T2-weighted images, most likely represents the submucosa, containing a rich vascular plexus intermixed with smooth muscle bundles and loosely woven connective tissue. The innermost portion of the urethra appears on MR images as a low signal intensity, which probably represents the mucosa. The mucosa consists of folded stratified squamous, pseudostratified columnar, or transitional epithelium, depending on the portion of the urethra. A central dot of low SI is typically identified in the normal urethra but may not be seen in 20% of normal patients (Fig. 9–26).[105]

MALE ANATOMY

The male urethra is divided into three parts: the prostatic, membranous, and penile portions. The portion of the prostatic urethra at the base of the bladder neck is not usually visualized on MR images without the presence of a urinary catheter or history of previous transurethral resection. At the level of the verumontanum, which typically appears as a high-signal intensity on T2-weighted images, the urethra is located in the posterior portion of the prostate and takes on an anterior position at the apex of the prostate. The most distal portion of the prostatic urethra is surrounded by low-signal-intensity muscular ring.[105]

On T2-weighted transaxial images, the membranous urethra possesses a low-signal intensity ring, which represents the muscular external sphincter surrounding a higher-signal-intensity mucosa. In the sagittal plane, a high-signal-intensity stripe between the prostatic apex and the bulb of the penis is identified as the membranous urethra.[111–113]

The bulbous portion of the penile urethra is best demonstrated with coronal T2-weighted images and appears as a low-signal-intensity ring within the high-signal-intensity corpus spongiosum. However, the anterior penile urethra is rarely visualized on MR images.[112,113]

Congenital Anomalies

MR demonstrates well the complex anatomy associated with congenital anomalies and may aid in surgical planning. In one study of patients with epispadias, associated findings such as separated pubic bones, separation of the corpora cavernosa, and cephalad displacement of the corpus spongiosum were well demonstrated.[113]

Benign Disease

A recent study by Hricak and others has shown MRI to be more sensitive in the detection of urethral diverticula in female patients than urethroscopy or double-balloon urethrography.[105] On the T1-weighted axial images, diverticula usually appear as an enlargement in the urethra or adjacent to the urethra with a homogeneously low signal intensity. Im-

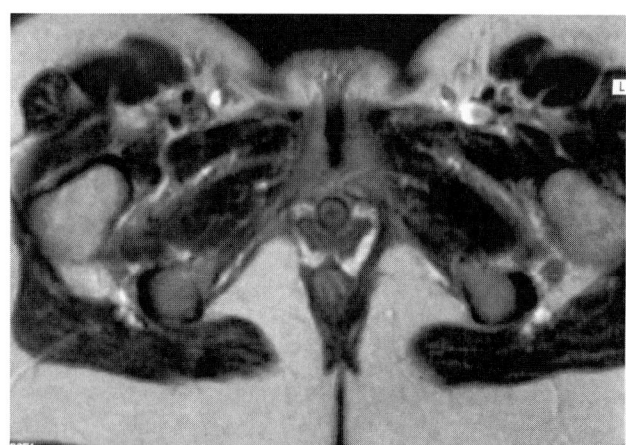 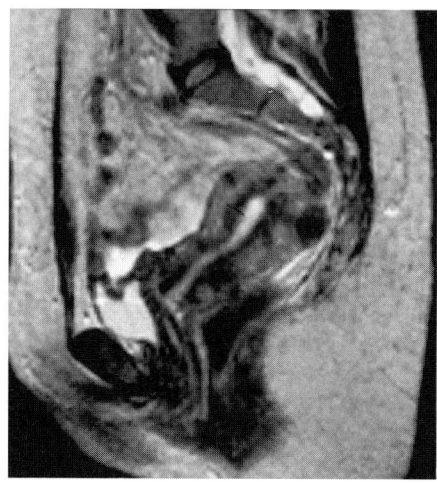

Figure 9-26. Normal urethra. Transaxial T2 turbo spin echo (**A**) and sagittal T2 spin echo (**B**) images. On the transaxial image (**A**), three rings are identified in the region of the urethra: The outer, low-SI ring surrounds a high-SI ring, which surrounds a central low SI. These layers most likely correlate with the muscularis, submucosa, and mucosa, respectively.

mediately following intravenous gadolinium administration, there is an increased contrast between urethral tissue, which enhances, and the low signal intensity of fluid in the diverticulum, which does not enhance.[105] On the T2-weighted images, diverticula appear as regions of higher SI than the urethra.[105]

MR has not commonly been used to diagnose stress urinary incontinence (SUI). However, it has been reported as a method to determine the precise anatomic changes responsible for stress urinary incontinence, and it may be a useful tool in surgical planning. In one study, patients showed weakening of the musculofascial extensions of the levator muscles. In the same study, the urethra of some patients was shown to have deficiencies of the smooth muscle coat.[114] Limitations of MRI for the diagnosis of SUI are that the patient cannot be examined in the erect position and that the static image may miss transient descent of the urethra. However, dynamic fast imaging may yield findings that correlate well with SUI symptoms.[115] With maximal straining, the bladder neck was found to descend not more than 1 cm below the pubococcygeal line in controls, whereas that distance was exceeded in 9 of 12 patients with SUI.[115]

Malignant Disease

FEMALE URETHRAL CARCINOMA

MRI appears to be limited in the detection of urethral tumors, because of the similar appearance of benign inflammation and malignant tumor on MR images. However, following the pathologic diagnosis of urethral carcinoma, MRI can be used to characterize tumor size, stage, and location (Fig. 9-27). MR has been shown to be very accurate in the demonstration of size and location. In addition, MR staging has been shown to be very sensitive in the evaluation of the extent of tumor, with a negative predictive value of 100%. However, because of the similar appearance of granulation tissue, edema, and tumor, overstaging may occur. Lymphadenopathy is best demonstrated with both T1 and T2 weighting and may be underestimated.[105]

MALE URETHRAL CARCINOMA

Squamous cell carcinoma and transitional cell carcinoma have similar appearances on MR images. On T1-weighted images, the signal intensities of the lesion were similar to or lower than that of the corpora spongiosum. On T2-weighted images, the signal intensity of the lesion has been noted to be equal to or lower than that of surrounding corpus spongiosum. MR accuracy in determination of the local extent of disease is good.[113]

Trauma

Urethral trauma is typically associated with extensive pelvic injury, including pelvic fractures, hemorrhage, and damage to other viscera.[116] MRI appears to be valuable in defining the pelvic anatomy, as well as soft-tissue and bony injuries, and may aid in surgical planning. Thin sections in each of the imaging planes are recommended. Images with T1 weighting are better for detection of displacement of abdominal organs. However, T2-weighted images are necessary to detect displacement of the membranous urethra. Dislocation of the urethra between the prostatic apex and membranous portions can occur in the lateral or anterior-posterior directions. This dislocation appears as misalignment of the apex of the prostate relative to the bulb of the penis.[112] Additionally, MR demonstrates organized hematoma and fibrosis that may be associated with urethral dislocation. Both will appear as a low signal intensity on T2-weighted images.[112]

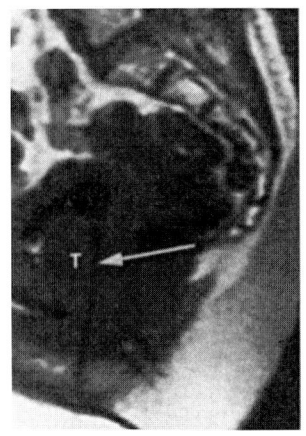 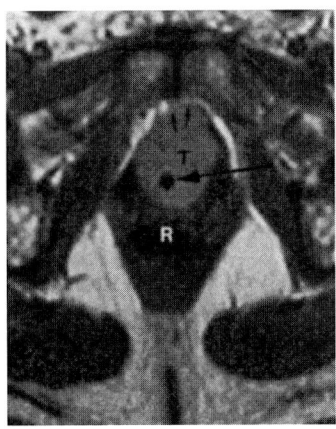 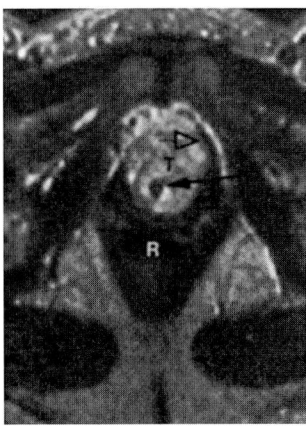

Figure 9–27. Squamous cell carcinoma of the female urethra on sagittal T1 (**A**), transaxial proton density (**B**), and T2 (**C**) images. A large tumor is apparent in the region of the urethra. The long arrows indicate a catheter in the urethra. The tumor extends into the retropubic adipose tissue (small arrows, **B**) and has completely invaded the outer muscle ring, especially along the anterior and right lateral portion. However, the left lateral muscular ring has not been invaded and remains low in signal intensity (open arrow). (Reprinted with permission from ref. 105.)

NEW DIRECTIONS OF MAGNETIC RESONANCE IMAGING

The future of abdominal MRI appears to hold three basic types of developments: imaging techniques that provide improved spatial or temporal resolution or selective imaging of a certain aspect of an organ system; specialized coils; and organ- or tissue-specific contrast agents.

Magnetic Resonance Imaging Techniques

Currently, T1-weighted images have good spatial and temporal resolution with the FLASH sequence. However, breath-hold T2-weighted sequences could benefit from considerable improvement in resolution. New sequences already hold promise for improvements in this area. A particularly promising technique is termed half fourier snapshot turbo spin echo (HASTE). In addition, modifications need to be made in magnetic field homogeneity and table incrementation facilitating the study of larger volumes of tissue along the z axis.

A technique known as rapid acquisition with relaxation enhancement (RARE-MR-urography) has been combined with T1-weighted imaging to rapidly and selectively depict fluid by heavy T2 weighting. This technique demonstrates fluid in cysts, calyces, renal pelvis, and other fluid-filled spaces without the use of contrast. In addition, this technique is independent of renal function and has been shown to be effective in the pediatric diagnosis of upper urinary tract abnormalities, including cysts in the pediatric patient.[117,118]

MR angiography has been used extensively in the diagnosis of carotid artery stenosis. Recently, similar techniques have been applied to imaging of the renal arteries with good results. Preliminary data show 100% sensitivity and 94% specificity in detection of proximal renal artery stenosis.[119] The detection of stenosis is independent of renal function and therefore may be complementary to scintigraphy. However, severe stenosis may be difficult to differentiate from occlusion, and diagnosis of stenosis in the mid and distal renal arteries appears to be less accurate.[120] In addition, projection arteriography and venography techniques are able to demonstrate direction of blood flow and differentiate arteries from veins.[121]

Specialized Coils

The use of body coils has been noted to improve the signal-to-noise ratio in imaging of the abdomen. Endorectal coils specifically improve imaging in the pelvis. However, endorectal coils alone tend to have limited spatial coverage. It appears that the use of an endorectal coil combined with an external anterior coil may increase the signal-to-noise ratio for larger spatial coverage.[80] Also, the use of high-resolution multicoils results in better signal-to-noise ratios for pelvic imaging, which improves imaging of the bladder and urethra.[122] Currently, many centers routinely employ multicoils for abdominal and pelvic MR studies. In addition to the preceding coils, which appear to have immediate clinical uses, implanted coils hold promise for MR microscopy research. These coils may be implanted about a kidney in an animal model to demonstrate microscopic changes resulting from chemically induced acute tubular necrosis or other renal diseases.[123]

Contrast Agents

Various new MR contrast agents have been developed that have applicability in the urinary tract. Gadolinium can be cross-linked with albumin to yield a macromolecule that remains largely confined to the intravascular space.[124–127] This molecule provides excellent enhancement of intravascular spaces, including the renal parenchyma and excluding the renal collecting system. Other intravascular gadolinium agents include albumin-(gadolinium)$_{35}$[128] and polysaccharide complexes of gadolinium.[129] Other agents that have been investigated include nonionic polyethylene glycol-ferrioxamine (PEG-ferrioxamine-B)[130] and dysprosium.

Lymph node–specific contrast agents have been investigated that may permit differentiation of lymph node involvement versus enlargement. Thus the staging of urinary tract carcinomas may be improved.

REFERENCES

1. Brown MA, Semelka RC: *MRI basic principles and applications.* New York: Wiley-Liss, 1995.
2. Semelka RC, Shoenut JP: *MRI of the Abdomen with CT Correlation.* New York: Raven Press, 1993.
3. Semelka RC, Chew W, Hricak H, Tomei E, Higgins CB: Fat saturation MR imaging of the abdomen. *AJR* 1990;155:1111–1116.
4. Mitchell DG, Vinitski S, Saponaro S, Tasciyan T, Burk DL Jr, Rifkin MD: Liver and pancreas: improved spin-echo T1 contrast by shorter echo time and fat suppression at 1.5T. *Radiology* 1991;178:67–71.
5. Semelka RC, Kroeker MA, Shoenut JP, Kroeker R, Yaffe CS, Micflikier AB: Pancreatic disease: prospective comparison of CT, ERCP, and 1.5T MR imaging with dynamic gadolinium enhancement and fat suppression. *Radiology* 1991;181:785–791.
6. Semelka RC, Simm FC, Recht M, Deimling M, Lenz G, Laub BA: T1-weighted sequences for MR imaging of the liver—comparison of three techniques for single breath hold volume acquisition at 1.0 and 1.5T. *Radiology* 1991;180:629–635.
7. Edelman RR, Siegel JB, Singer A, Dupuis K, Longmaid HE: Dynamic MR imaging of the liver with gadolinium: initial clinical results. *AJR* 1989;153:1213–1219.
8. Taupitz M, Hamm B, Speidel A, Deimling M, Branding G, Wolf K-J: Multisection FLASH: method for breath-hold MR imaging of the entire liver. *Radiology* 1992;182:73–79.
9. Mirowitz SA, Lee JKT, Brown JJ, Eilenberg SS, Heiken JP, Perman WH: Rapid acquisition spin-echo (RASE) MR imaging: a new technique for reduction of artifacts and acquisition time. *Radiology* 1990;175:131–135.
10. Haase A: Snapshot FLASH MRI: applications to T1, T2, and chemical-shift imaging. *Magn Reson Med* 1990;13:77–89.
11. Holsinger AE, Riederer SJ: The importance of phase encoding order in ultra-short TR snapshot gradient-echo MR imaging. *Magn Reson Med* 1990;16:481–488.
12. Holsinger-Bampton AE, Riederer SJ, Campeau NG, Ehman RL, Johnson CD: T1-weighted snapshot gradient-echo MR imaging of the abdomen. *Radiology* 1991;181:25–32.
13. Jakob PM, Haase A: Scan time reduction in snapshot FLASH MRI. *Magn Reson Med* 1992;24:392–396.
14. Smith RC, Reinhold C, Lange RC, McCauley TR, Kier R, McCarthy S: Comparison of conventional and fast spin-echo body coil MR imaging of the female pelvis. *Radiology* 1991;181(p):168.
15. Francis IR, Steiner RM, Herfkens RJ, Jain K, Glover GH: T2-weighted fast spin-echo MR imaging of the pelvis. *Radiology* 1991;181(p):169.
16. Semelka RC, Hricak H, Tomei E, Floth A, Stoller M: Obstructive nephropathy: evaluation with dynamic gadolinium enhanced MR imaging. *Radiology* 1990;175:797–803.
17. Choyke PL, Frank JA, Girton ME, et al: Dynamic gadolinium enhanced MR imaging of the kidney: experimental results. *Radiology* 1989;170:713–720.
18. Kikinis R, von Schulthess Gk, Jager P, et al: Normal and hydronephrotic kidney: evaluation of renal function with contrast enhanced MR imaging. *Radiology* 1987;165:837–842.
19. Semelka RC, Shoenut JP, Kroeker MA, MacMahon RG, Greenberg HM: Renal lesions: controlled comparison between CT and 1.5T MR imaging with nonenhanced and gadolinium-enhanced fat-suppressed spin-echo and breath-hold FLASH techniques. *Radiology* 1992;182:425–430.
20. Semelka RC, Hricak H, Stevens SK, Fingold R, Tomei E, Carroll PR: Combined gadolinium-enhanced and fat saturation MR imaging of renal masses. *Radiology* 1991;178:803–809.
21. Cho C, Friedland GW, Swenson RS: Acquired renal cystic disease and renal neoplasms in hemodialysis patients. *Urol Radiol* 1984;6:153–157.
22. Ishikawa I: Uremic acquired cystic disease of kidney. *Urology* 1985;26:101–107.
23. Levine E, Grantham JJ, Slucher SL, Greathouse JL, Krohn BP: CT of acquired cystic kidney disease and renal tumors in long term dialysis patients. *AJR* 1984;142:125–131.
24. Levine E, Collins DL, Horton WA, Schmenke RN: CT screening of the abdomen in von Hippel-Lindau disease. *AJR* 1982;139:505–510.
25. Kettritz U, Semelka RC, Siegelman ES, Shoenut JP, Mitchell DG: Multilocular cystic nephroma: MR imaging appearance with current techniques including gadolinium enhancement. *J Magn Reson Imaging* 1996;1:145–148.
26. Bosniak MA: Angiomyolipoma (hamartoma) of the kidney: a preoperative diagnosis is possible in virtually every case. *Urol Radiol* 1981;3:135–142.
27. Totty WG, McClennan Bl, Melson GL, Patel R: Relative value of computed tomography and ultrasonography in the assessment of renal angiomyolipoma. *J Comput Assist Tomogr* 1981;5:173–177.
28. Osterling JE, Fishman EK, Goldman SM, Marshall FF: The management of renal angiomyolipoma. *J Urol* 1986;135:1121–1124.
29. Quinn MJ, Hartman DS, Friedman AC, et al: Renal oncocytoma: new observations. *Radiology* 1984;153:49–53.
30. Press GA, McClennan BL, Melson GL, Weyman PJ, Mauro MA, Lee JKT: Papillary renal cell carcinoma: CT and sonographic evaluation. *AJR* 1984;143:1005–1010.
31. Bosniak MA: The small (<3.0 cm) renal parenchymal tumor detection, diagnosis and controversies. *Radiology* 1991;179:307–317.
32. Birnbaum BA Bosniak MA, Megibow AJ, Lubat E, Gordon RB: Observations on the growth of renal neoplasms. *Radiology* 1990;176:695–701.
33. Levine E, Huntrakoon M, Wetzel LH: Small renal neoplasms: clinical, pathologic, and imaging features. *AJR* 1989;153:69–73.
34. Curry NS, Schabel SI, Betsill WL Jr: Small renal neoplasms: diagnostic imaging, pathological features and clinical course. *Radiology* 1986;158:113–117.
35. Hricak H, Thoeni RF, Carroll PR, Demas BE, Marotti M, Tanagho EA: Detection and staging of renal neoplasms: a reassessment of MR imaging. *Radiology* 1988;166:643–649.
36. Hricak H, Amparo E, Fisher MR, Crooks L, Higgins CB: Abdominal venous system: assessment using MR. *Radiology* 1985;156:415–422.
37. Hricak H, Demas BE, Williams RD, et al: Magnetic resonance imaging in the diagnosis of renal and perirenal neoplasms. *Radiology* 1985;154:709–715.

38. Patel SK, Stack CM, Turner DA: Magnetic resonance imaging in the staging of renal cell carcinoma. *Radiographics* 1987;156:415–422.
39. Pritchett TR, Raval JK, Benson RC, et al: Diagnosis and staging of renal cell carcinoma: experience with five cases. *J Urol* 1987;138:1220–1222.
40. Fein AB, Lee JKT, Balfe DM, et al: Diagnosis and staging of renal cell carcinoma: a comparison of MR imaging and CT. *AJR* 1987;148:749–753.
41. Eilenberg SS, Lee JKT, Brown JJ, Mirowitz SA, Tartar VM: Renal masses: evaluation with gradient-echo gadolinium enhanced dynamic MR imaging. *Radiology* 1990;176:333–338.
42. Studer UE, Scherz S, Scheidegger J, et al: Enlargement of regional lymph nodes in renal cell carcinoma is often not due to metastases. *J Urol* 1990;144:243–245.
43. Semelka RC, Shoenut JP, Magro CM, Kroeker MA, MacMahon R, Greenberg HM: Renal cancer staging: Comparison of contrast-enhanced CT and gadolinium-enhanced fat suppressed spin echo and gradient echo MR imaging. *JMRI* 1993;3:597–602.
44. Goldstein HA, Kashanian FK, Blumetti RF, Holyoak WL, Hugo FP, Blumenfield DM: Safety assessment of gadopentatate dimeglumine in U.S. clinical trials. *Radiology* 1990;174:17–23.
45. Krestin GP, Schuhmann-Giamjsieri G, Haustein J, et al: Functional dynamic MRI, pharmacokinetics and safety of gadolinium in patients with impaired renal function. *Eur Radiol* 1992;16–23.
46. Rofsky NM, Weinreb JC, Bosniak MA, Lives RB, Birnbaum BA: Renal lesion characterization with gadolinium-enhanced MR imaging: efficacy and safety in patients with renal insufficiency. *Radiology* 1991;180;85–89.
47. Heiken JP, McClennan BL, Gold RP: Renal lymphoma. *Semin Ultrasound CT MR* 1986;7:58–66.
48. Semelka RC, Kelekis NL, Burdeny DA, Mitchell DG, Brown JJ, Siegelman ES. Renal lymphoma: demonstration by MR imaging. *Am J Roentgen* 1996; (in press).
49. Lessman RK, Johnson SF, Coburn JW, et al: Renal artery embolism: clinical features and long-term follow-up of 17 cases. *Ann Intern Med* 1978;89:477–481.
50. Brown ED, Brown JJ, Kettritz U, Shoenut JP, Semelka RC: Renal abscesses: appearance on gadolinium-enhanced magnetic resonance imaging. *Abdom Imaging* 1996; (in press).
51. Goldman SM, Hartman DS, Fishman EK, Finizio JP, Gatewood OM, Siegelman SS: CT of xanthogranulomatous pyelonephritis: radiologic-pathologic correlation. *AJR* 1984;142:963–969.
52. Cholankeril JV, Freundlich R, Ketyer S, Spirito AL, Napolitano J: Computed tomography in urothelial tumors of renal pelvis and related filling defects. *J Comput Assist Tomogr* 1986;10:263–272.
53. Weeks SM, Brown ED, Brown JJ, Adamis MK, Eisenberg LB, Semelka RC: Transitional cell carcinoma of the upper urinary tract: staging by MRI. *Abdom Imaging* 1995;20:365–367.
54. Elliot JS: Urinary calculus disease. *Surg Clin North Am* 1965;45:1393–1404.
55. Bretan PN, McAninch JW, Federle MP, Jeffrey RB: Computerized tomographic staging of renal trauma: 85 consecutive cases. *J Urol* 1986;61:113–118.
56. McCreath GT, McMillan N, Patterson J, et al: Magnetic resonance imaging of renal transplants: initial experience. *Br J Radiol* 1988;61:113–118.
57. Hricak H, Terrier F, Marotti M, et al: Post-transplant renal rejection: comparison of quantitative scintigraphy, ultrasonography and magnetic resonance imaging. *Radiology* 1987;162:685–688.
58. Amis ES: Retroperitoneal fibrosis. *AJR* 1991;157:321–329.
59. Arrive L, Hricak H, Tavares NJ, et al: Malignant versus non-malignant retroperitoneal fibrosis: differentiation with MR imaging. *Radiology* 1989;172:139–143.
60. Yuh WTC, Barloon TJ, Sickels WJ, et al: Magnetic resonance imaging in the diagnosis and follow-up of idiopathic retroperitoneal fibrosis. *J Urol* 1989;141:602–605.
61. Brooks AP, Rexnek RH, Webb JAW: Magnetic resonance imaging in idiopathic retroperitoneal fibrosis: measurement of T2 relaxation time. *Br J Radiol* 1990;63:842–844.
62. Newhouse JH: Clinical use of urinary tract magnetic resonance imaging. *Radiol Clin North Am* 1991;29:455–474.
63. Dooms GC, Hricak H, Crooks LE, et al: Magnetic resonance imaging of the lymph nodes: comparison with CT. *Radiology* 1984;153:719–728.
64. Lee JKT, Heiken JP, Ling D, et al: Magnetic resonance imaging of abdominal and pelvic lymphadenopathy. *Radiology* 1984;153:181–188.
65. Arrive L, Malbec L, Buy JN, Guinet C, Vadrot D: Male pelvis. In: Vanel D, McNamara MT, eds. *MRI of the Body*. New York: Springer-Verlag, 1989;242–255.
66. Lee JKT, Rholl KS: MRI of the bladder and prostate (review). *AJR* 1986;147:732–736.
67. Barentsz JO, Lemmens JAM, Ruijs SHJ, et al: Carcinoma of the urinary bladder: MR imaging using a double surface coil. *AJR* 1988;151:107–112.
68. Reiman TH, Heiken JP, Totty WG, Lee JKT: Clinical MR imaging with a Helmholtz-type surface coil. *Radiology* 1988;169:564–566.
69. Requardt H, Sauter R, Weber H: Helmholtzspulen in der Kernspintomographie. *Electromed* 1987;55:61–72.
70. Narumi Y, Kadota T, Inoue E, Kuriyama K, Horinouchi T, et al: Bladder wall morphology: in vitro MR imaging-histopathologic correlation. *Radiology* 1993;187:151–155.
71. Bradley WG Jr: Hemorrhage and brain iron. In: Stark DD, Bradley WG Jr, eds. *Magnetic Resonance Imaging, 1*. St. Louis: Mosby Year Book, 1992;721–728.
72. Rifkin MD, Piccoli CW: Male pelvis and bladder. In: Stark DD, Bradley WG, eds. *Magnetic Resonance Imaging, 2*. St. Louis: Mosby Year Book, 1992;2044–2057.
73. Bryan PJ, Butler HE, Nelson AD, Lipuma JP, Kopiwoda SY, et al: Magnetic resonance imaging of the prostate. *AJR* 1986;146:543–548.
74. Shonnard KM, Jelinek JS, Benedikt RA, Kransdorf MJ: CT and MR of neurofibromatosis of the bladder. *J Comput Assist Tomgr* 1992;16:433–438.
75. Warshawsky R, Bow SN, Waldbaum RS, Cintron J: Bladder pheochromocytoma with MR correlation. *J Comput Assist Tomogr* 1989;13:714–716.
76. Heyman J, Cheung Y, Ghali V, Leiter E: Bladder pheochromocytoma: evaluation with magnetic resonance imaging. *J Urol* 1989;141:1424–1426.
77. Fink JIJ, Reinig JW, Dwyer AJ, et al: MR imaging of pheochromocytoma. *J Comput Assist Tomogr* 1985;9:454–458.
78. Falke ThM, LeStrake L, Shaff MI, et al: MR imaging of the adrenals: correlated with computed tomography. *J Comput Assist Tomogr* 1986;10:242–253.
79. Quint LE, Glazer GM, Francis IR, Shapiro B, Chenevert TL: Pheochromocytoma and paraganglioma: comparison of MR imaging with CT and I-131 MIB6 scintigraphy. *Radiology* 1987;165:89–93.
80. Schnall MD, Connick T, Hayes CE, Lenkinski RE, Kressel HY: MR imaging of the pelvis with an endorectal-external multicoil array. *JMRI* 1992;2:229–232.
81. Fisher MR, Hricak H, Tanagho EA: Urinary bladder MR imaging. Part II. Neoplasm. *Radiology* 1985;157:471–477.
82. Amendola MA, Glaser GM, Grossman HB, et al: Staging of

bladder carcinoma: MRI-CT-surgical correlation. *AJR* 1986; 146:1179–1183.
83. Bryan PJ, Butler HE, LiPuma JP, et al: CT and MR imaging in staging bladder neoplasms. *J Comput Assist Tomogr* 1987; 11:96–101.
84. Rholl KS, Lee JKT, Heiken JP, et al: Primary bladder carcinoma: evaluation with MR imaging. *Radiology* 1987; 163:117–123.
85. Buy JN, Moss AA, Guinet C, et al: MR staging of bladder carcinoma: correlation with pathologic findings. *Radiology* 1988;169:695–700.
86. Koebel G, Schmeidl U, Griebel J, et al: MR imaging of urinary bladder neoplasms. *J Comput Assist Tomogr* 1988; 12:98–103.
87. Husband JE, Oliff JF, Williams MP, Heron CW, Cherryman GR: Bladder cancer: staging with CT and MR imaging. *Radiology* 1989;173:435–440.
88. Barentsz JO, Debruyne FMJ, Ruijs SHJ: *Magnetic Resonance Imaging of Carcinoma of the Urinary Bladder.* Norwell, MA: Kluwer, 1990.
89. Strich G, Hagan P, Gerber KH, et al: Tissue distribution and magnetic resonance spin lattice relaxation effects of gadolinium-DTPA. *Radiology* 1985;154:723–726.
90. Tachibana M, Baba S, Daguchi N, et al: Efficacy of gadolinium-diethylene-triaminepentaacetic acid-enhanced magnetic resonance imaging for differentiation between superficial and muscle-invasive tumor of the bladder: a comparative study with computerized tomography and transurethral ultrasonography. *J Urol* 1991;145:1169–1173.
91. Doringer E, Joos H, Forstner R, Schmoller H: MRI of bladder carcinoma: tumor staging and gadolinium contrast behaviors. *Fortschr Rontgenstr* 1991;154:357–363.
92. Neuerburg JM, Bohndorf K, Sohn M, et al: Urinary bladder neoplasms: evaluation with contrast-enhanced MR imaging. *Radiology* 1989;172:739–743.
93. Neuerburg JM, Bohndorf K, Sohn M, Teufl F, Gunther RW: Staging of urinary bladder neoplasms with MR imaging: is gadolinium helpful? *J Comput Assist Tomogr* 1991;15:780–786.
94. Sohn M, Neuerburg JM, Teufl F, Bohndorf K: Gadolinium-enhanced magnetic resonance imaging in the staging of urinary bladder neoplasms. *Urol Int* 1990;45:142–147.
95. Barentsz JO, van Erning LJThO, Ruijs JHJ, Bors WG, Jager G, Oosterhof G: Dynamic turbo-FLASH subtraction MR imaging: perfusion of pelvic tumors (abstr). *Radiology* 1992; 185(p):340.
96. Nicolas V, Spielmann R, Maas R, et al: The diagnostic value of MR tomography following gadolinium-DTPA compared to computed-tomography in bladder tumors. *Fortschr Rontgenstr* 1991;154:357–363.
97. Sparenberg A, Hamm B, Hammerer P, Samberger V, Wolf KJ: The diagnosis of bladder carcinomas by NMR tomography: any improvement with gadolinium? *Fortschr Rontgenstr* 1991;155:117–122.
98. Kim B, Semelka RC, Ascher SM, Chalpin D, Carroll P, Hricak H: Bladder tumor staging: comparison of contrast-enhanced CT, T1- and T2-weighted MR imaging, dynamic gadolinium-enhanced imaging, and late gadolinium-enhanced imaging. *Radiology* 1994;193:239–245.
99. Ebner F, Kressel HY, Mintz MC, et al: Tumor recurrence versus fibrosis in the female pelvis: differentiation with MR imaging at 1.5T. *Radiology* 1988;166:333–340.
100. Algra PR, Bloem JL, Tissing H, Falke ThHM, Arndt J-W, Verboom LJ: Detection of vertebral metastases: comparison between MR imaging and bone scintigraphy. *Radiographics* 1991;11:219–232.
101. Barentsz JO, Ruijs SHJ, Strijk SP: The role of MR imaging in carcinoma of the urinary bladder. *AJR* 1993;160:937–947.
102. Popovich MJ, Hricak H, Sugimura Kazuro, Stern JL: The role of MR imaging in determining surgical eligibility for pelvic exenteration. *AJR* 1993;160:525–531.
103. Hricak H, Hamm B, Semelka R, Cann CE, Nauert T, Secaf E, Stern JL, Wolf K-J: Carcinoma of the uterus: use of gadopentetate dimeglumine in MR imaging. *Radiology* 1991; 181:95–106.
104. Janus CL, Mendelson DS, Moore S, Gendal EL, Dottino P, Brodman M: Staging of cervical carcinoma: accuracy of magnetic resonance imaging and computed tomography. *Clinical Imaging* 1989;13;114–116.
105. Hricak H, Secaf E, Buckley DW, et al: Female urethra: MR imaging. *Radiology* 1991;178:527–535.
106. Gray H, Williams PL, Warwick R, Dyson M, Bannister LH, eds.: *Anatomy of the human body,* 37th ed. New York: Churchill Livingstone, 1989;1422–1423.
107. Krantz K: The anatomy of the urethra and anterior vaginal wall. *Am J Obstet Gynecol* 1951;62:374–386.
108. Huisman AB: Aspects on the anatomy of the female urethra with special relation to urinary continence. *Contrib Gyencol Obstet* 1983;10:1–31.
109. DeLancey JO: Correlative study of paraurethral anatomy. *Obstet Gynecol* 1986;68:91–97.
110. Carlile A, Davies I, Rigby A, Brocklehurst JC: Age changes in the human female urethra: a morphometric study. *J urol* 1988;139:532–535.
111. Popovich MJ, Hricak H: The prostate and seminal vesicles. In: *Magnetic Resonance Imaging of the Body,* 2nd ed. New York: Raven Press, 1992;915–916.
112. Popovich MJ, Hricak H: The penis/male urethra and scrotum. In: *Magnetic Resonance Imaging of the Body,* 2nd ed. New York: Raven Press, 1992;940–946.
113. Hricak H, Mariotti M, Gilbert TJ, Lue TF, Wetzel LH, McAninch JW, Tanagho EA: Normal penile anatomy and abnormal penile conditions: evaluation with MR imaging. *Radiology* 1988;169:683–690.
114. Klutke C, Golomg J, Barbaric Z, et al: The anatomy of stress incontinence: magnetic resonance imaging of the female bladder neck and urethra. *J Urol* 1990;143:563.
115. Yang A, Mostwin JL, Rosenshein NB, et al: Pelvic floor descent in women: dynamic evaluation with fast MRI imaging and cinematic display. *Radiology* 1991;179:25.
116. Palmer JK, Benson GS, Corriere JN Jr: Diagnosis and initial management of urological injuries associated with 200 consecutive pelvic fractures. *J Urol* 1983;130:712–714.
117. Sigmund G, Stoever B, Zimmerhackl LB, Laubenberger J, Nitzsche E, Frankenschmidt A, Hennig J: Cystic diseases of the kidney in children: MRI, including RARE-MR-urography. *Eur Radiol* 1991;1:27–32.
118. Sigmund G, Stoever B, Zimmerhackl LB, et al: RARE-MR-urography in the diagnosis of upper urinary tract abnormalities in children. *Pediatr Radiol* 1991;21:416–420.
119. Kent KC, Edelman RR, Kim D, et al: Magnetic resonance imaging: a reliable test for the evaluation of proximal atherosclerotic renal arterial stenosis. *J Vasc Surg* 1991;13:311–318.
120. Yucel EK: Magnetic resonance angiography of the lower extremity and renal arteries. *Semin US, CT, MRI* 1992;13:291–302.
121. Edelman RR, Wentz KU, Mattle H, Zhao B, Liu C, Kim D, Laub G: Projection arteriography and venography: initial clinical results with MR. *Radiology* 1989;172:351–357.
122. Smith RC, Reinhold C, McCauley TR, Lange RC, Constable RT, Kier R, McCarthy S: Multicoil high-resolution fast spin-

echo MR imaging of the female pelvis. *Radiology* 1992; 184:671–675.
123. Farmer THR, Johnson GA, Cofter GP, Maronpot RR, Dixon D, Hedlund LW: Implanted coil MR microscopy of renal pathology. *Magn Res Med* 1989;10:310–323.
124. Niemi P, Koskinen S, Reisto T: Tissue relaxation enhancement after intravenous administration of (ITCB-DTPA)-gadolinium conjugated albumin, an intravascular magnetic resonance imaging contrast agent. *Invest Radiol* 1991;25:674–680.
125. Schmiedl U, Ogan M, Paajanen H, et al: Albumin labeled with gadolinium as an intravascular, blood pool-enhancing agent for MR imaging: biodistribution and imaging studies. *Radiology* 1987;162:205–210.
126. Schmiedl U, Moseley ME, Sievers R, et al: Magnetic resonance imaging of myocardial infarction using albumin-Gd-DTPA, a macromolecular blood volume contrast agent in a rat model. *Invest Radiol* 1987;22:713–721.
127. Schmiedl U, Sievers RE, Brasch RC, et al: Acute myocardial ischemia and reperfusion: MR imaging with albumin-Gd-DTPA. *Radiology* 1989;170:351–356.
128. Vexler VS, Berthezene Y, Clement O, Muhler A, Rosenau W, Moseley M, Brasch R: Detection of zonal renal ischemia with contrast-enhanced MR imaging with a macromolecular blood pool contrast agent. *JMRI* 1992;2:311–319.
129. Gibby WA, Billings BS, Hall RP, Ovitt TW: Biodistribution and magnetic resonance imaging of cross-linked DTPA polysaccharides. *Invest Radiol* 1990;25:164–172.
130. Duewell St, Wuethrich R, von Schulthess GK, Jenny HB, Muller RN, Moerker T, Fuchs WA: Nonionic polyethylene glycol-ferrioxamine as a renal magnetic resonance contrast agent. *Invest Radiol* 1991;26:50–57.

10 Section 1: Endourology

Alan D. Jenkins

Thomas Edison's development of the incandescent light bulb revolutionized the way we live. It also led to the development of the profession of urology as we know it today. More than a century ago Nitze attached a light bulb to the end of a cystoscope and initiated endoscopy of the lower urinary tract.[1] The subsequent development of the rod lens system made cystoscopy an everyday occurrence and led to the development of transurethral resection of the prostate. The further development of rigid endoscopes and the adaptation of fiberoptics to provide images have permitted urologists to extend lower endoscopic procedures to the ureter and the kidney. Even the roots of modern laparoscopic procedures can be traced to the simple cystoscope.

This chapter covers the application of endourologic procedures to the lower and upper urinary tract. Although the emphasis of this discussion is on diagnostic aspects of endourology, many of these procedures are inherently therapeutic. A diagnostic endoscopic procedure often becomes a therapeutic endoscopic procedure.

LOWER TRACT ENDOSCOPY

Anatomy

Although the anatomy of the bladder and urethra is familiar to urologists, this information often is neglected when endoscopic procedures are performed. Anatomic relationships determine what can safely be performed endoscopically.

The adult bladder is surrounded by the bony pelvis and lies behind the symphysis pubis. In children, the bladder sits higher in the pelvis and can be palpated or percussed above the symphysis when it is full. The ureteral orifices—which, together with the bladder neck, form the trigone—are visible at either end of the interureteric ridge.

The adult female urethra is approximately 4 cm in length and travels along the posterior surface of the symphysis. The distal female urethra is lined with squamous epithelium, whereas the more proximal portion is lined with pseudostratified or transitional epithelium. Connective and elastic tissue make up the submucosa. Embedded within this are many periurethral glands.

In the male, the urethra travels through the prostate. Posteriorly, the prostatic urethra is perforated by the ejaculatory ducts at the verumontanum. As the urethra exits the prostate, it enters the genitourinary diaphragm, where it becomes the membranous urethra. The corpus spongiosum and the bulbospongiosus muscle surround the bulbous urethra. The penile urethra extends distally from the suspensory ligament of the penis and is surrounded by corpus spongiosum. The fossa navicularis is that portion of the urethra within the glans penis. The mucosa is squamous epithelium. Transitional epithelium lines the more proximal portions of the urethra.

The two corpora cavernosa and the corpus spongiosum are covered by Buck's fascia. Colles's fascia is found just beneath the skin of the penis and the scrotum. These fascial layers determine the route that irrigating fluid takes if a perforation occurs during a cystoscopic procedure.

Instrumentation

Although cystoscopy has been performed for many decades, the appearance of cystoscopes with a rod lens system and a fiberoptic light supply with a high-intensity light source greatly improved cystoscopic visualization. The further development of fiberoptic visualization permitted the development of flexible cystoscopes that are more comfortable for the patient and enable endoscopy of urinary diversions that would have been impossible with a rigid instrument. A criticism of all flexible endoscopes is that their visual field is granular. Manufacturers have been able to increase the fiber density so that this is not a significant problem in newer instruments.

Although the urethra will accommodate a 28 to 30 Fr instrument, such a large instrument is needed only if a large working channel is needed, as during a transurethral prostatectomy. A 19 or 21 Fr rigid instrument will suffice for the vast majority of diagnostic urethroscopic and cystoscopic procedures.

As a rule, flexible cystoscopes have a smaller diameter than rigid cystoscopes (Fig. 10–1). Instruments range in size from 14 to 16 Fr. The smaller size is more comfortable for patients and the working channel is large enough to pass grasping or biopsy instruments.

A flexible cystoscope is suitable for the vast majority of urethroscopic and cystoscopic procedures. Flexible cystoscopes, however, are inferior to rigid cystoscopes in two situations. The first is in a patient with acute bleeding and numerous clots in the bladder. Clots can be evacuated effectively only with a rigid instrument. A second criticism of

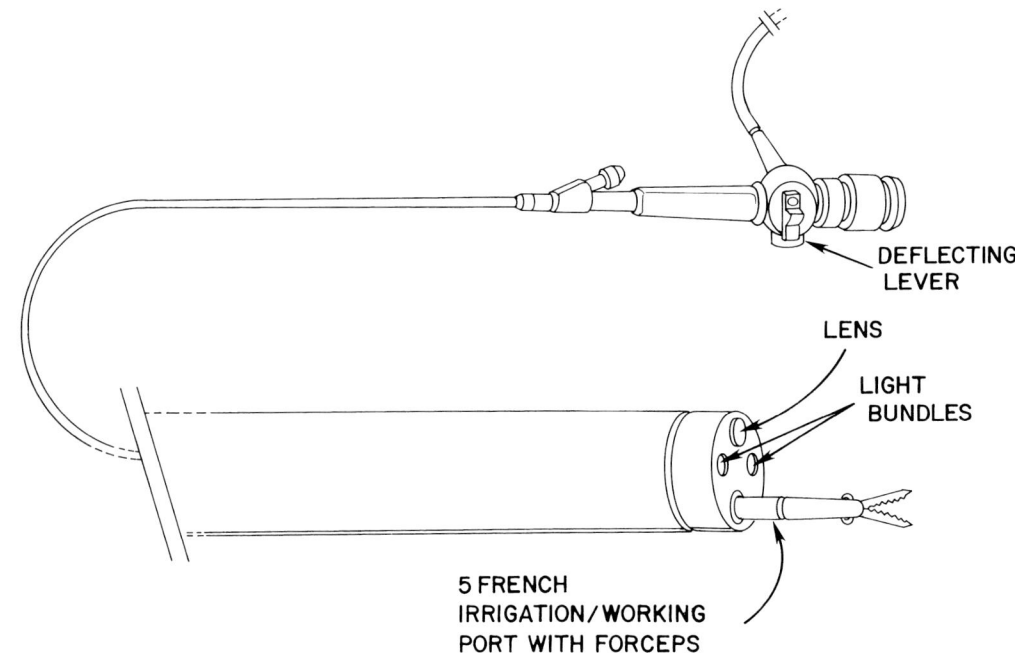

Figure 10–1. Basic design of a flexible endoscope. Flexible cystoscopes and nephroscopes are shorter and have a larger diameter than flexible ureteroscopes. The latter have a correspondingly smaller-diameter working channel. Instruments specifically designed for flexible nephroscopy have a shorter tip bending radius than flexible cystoscopes.

flexible cystoscopes is that retrograde ureterography is difficult to perform because cone tip ureteral catheters cannot be passed through the instrument. Although a guidewire can be passed easily through a flexible cystoscope and used to place a ureteral catheter, the performance of a retrograde pyelogram is much easier with a rigid cystoscope.

A last consideration with any endoscopic instrument is its care and maintenance.[2] All this equipment is very expensive. Although the rod lenses used with rigid instruments are fairly rugged, they can be damaged if they are dropped on the floor. Flexible cystoscopes are more delicate. They do not tolerate vigorous active deflection. Careful protocols must be followed when they are sterilized or instruments will be ruined. All personnel responsible for the care of these instruments should be very familiar with the manufacturers' recommendations.

Retrograde Urethrography and Cystography

The retrograde injection of water-soluble contrast agents into the urethra and bladder is a simple technique that is the cornerstone of the evaluation of urethral stricture disease and urethral or bladder trauma. Two basic techniques can be used to perform a retrograde urethrogram. A catheter tip syringe can be inserted in the urethral meatus while the physician holds the penis comfortably stretched. A radiograph is obtained when a sufficient amount of contrast has been injected to distend the urethra. Patients may complain of discomfort when the contrast reaches the external sphincter. Gentle but steady pressure usually will permit contrast to pass through the sphincter. Care should be taken to avoid excessive pressure; otherwise extravasation, usually into the venous system, will occur, and a very dramatic radiographic will be obtained. The major disadvantage of this technique is that much of the physician's hand is exposed to the x-ray beam. A preferred technique is the placement of the tip of a small Foley catheter (12 or 14 Fr) into the distal urethra and the gentle inflation of the balloon in the fossa navicularis. In this technique the physician's hands remain outside of the x-ray field.

If the urethrogram is normal during a lower tract evaluation for trauma, a Foley catheter is passed and a cystogram is performed. Contrast is instilled under gravity flow. No more than 200 mL should be instilled initially. A large quantity of contrast could be administered inadvertently if the patient has an intraperitoneal bladder rupture. Additional contrast can be instilled at a higher pressure if no extravasation is visible on the low-pressure cystogram. A final washout film should be taken to make sure that the patient does not have a small bladder tear posteriorly. As with all radiographic procedures, it is important that a preliminary radiograph be obtained.

Technique

Most cystourethroscopic procedures can be performed in an office setting after instillation of a topical anesthetic agent. A rare patient requires intravenous sedation. The need for anesthesia is reduced even further if a flexible instrument is used. The only situation in which a general anesthetic is needed is during the evaluation of a patient with a painful bladder disorder. Although these patients can undergo cystoscopy in the office, these usually are very painful and the examination is inadequate. The performance of cystoscopy under general anesthesia permits more adequate filling of the bladder. Concurrent hydraulic distention often provides symptomatic relief for some patients.

Rigid cystourethroscopy is performed with the patient in a dorsal lithotomy position. The patient is prepped and draped in a sterile fashion and the tip of the instrument is well lubricated. A viscous solution of lidocaine is injected in male patients 10 minutes before the procedure. Anesthetization of the female urethra is difficult, but the use of a 10% aerosol spray of lidocaine applied to the tip of the instrument often helps. The urethra should be examined under direct vision as the instrument is passed. The interior of the bladder should be examined in a systematic fashion. Most rigid cystoscopes are provided with 30- and 70-degree lenses. The former lens provides adequate visualization of the entire bladder in all but a few patients. Flexible cystoscopy[3] can be performed with the patient in a dorsal lithotomy position, in a frog-leg position for female patients, or in a supine position in male patients.

Care should be taken not to overdistend the bladder during the procedure and to empty the bladder at the end of the procedure. An ounce of antibiotic solution can be instilled at the end of the procedure, or the patient can take a single dose of an oral antimicrobial agent.

Indications

Cystoscopy is indicated for the evaluation of hematuria (gross or microscopic), urethral strictures undergoing an initial evaluation, filling defects revealed by urography, recurrent urinary tract infections, iatrogenic urethral injuries, and the evaluation of foreign bodies in the urethra or bladder. Urologists traditionally have cystoscoped patients with any type of voiding disorder, but routine cystoscopy in all patients is unnecessary. Cystoscopy in a woman with classic stress urinary incontinence or a man with classic prostatism probably has little benefit and provides little, if any, useful information. If there is any doubt, however, one should endoscope the patient.

Cystourethroscopy is an integral part of the evaluation of hematuria. Although most patients with microscopic hematuria have no visible lesions within the urethra or bladder, a thorough workup requires endoscopic visualization of the entire urethra and the bladder. Cystoscopy is mandatory in patients with gross hematuria. It is classic teaching that patients with gross hematuria should be endoscoped when they are bleeding actively. More often than not such patients are not bleeding when they are in the urologist's office. Whether or not to proceed with cystoscopy anyway depends on the clinical situation. A bladder lesion is more likely to be found in a 50-year-old woman with gross hematuria and a long smoking history than it is in a 20-year-old male with no smoking history. Immediate cystoscopy in the former patient is reasonable, but it may be more prudent to wait until the latter patient is bleeding actively before proceeding with endoscopy. If a patient is bleeding actively and no lesions can be seen in the urethra or the bladder, it is imperative that the urine effluxing from each ureteral orifice be examined in an attempt to lateralize the site of bleeding. The lateralization of the source of bleeding makes the subsequent evaluation and management far easier.

Cystoscopy also is an integral part of the evaluation of patients with recurrent urinary tract "infection." Patients often present with a history of episodes of irritative voiding and the finding of pyuria on a urinalysis. Recurrent urinary tract infections may never have been documented, but the presence of pyuria requires cystoendoscopy.

Cystoscopy also is required for the evaluation of filling defects within the urethra or bladder. Although calculi (radiolucent or radiopaque) can be detected with either plain film radiography or ultrasound examination, tumors can be proven only with an endoscopic procedure. Many filling defects in the bladder are transitional cell carcinomas or blood clots that have formed from such tumors bleeding. The papillary or sessile nature of a tumor can be ascertained during cystoscopy, and biopsies can be obtained. Cystoscopy also is an integral part of the workup of patients who have irritative voiding symptoms or positive urine cytologies that might be indicative of carcinoma in situ.

Urethroscopy of patients with urethral strictures usually is done just prior to a visual internal urethrotomy. Some strictures are caused by carcinoma, and biopsies should be taken if there is any doubt as to the nature of the stricture. A small guidewire can be passed during the urethroscopic procedure and used in a subsequent therapeutic procedure under anesthesia. The initial cystoscopy may offer the greatest chance of success at identifying a tiny lumen.

Foreign bodies in the urethra or bladder can be identified easily during cystoendoscopy. These objects may not be radiopaque and their nature cannot be ascertained with either plain radiography or ultrasound examination. Cystoscopy usually is the best approach for diagnosis and removal.

Lastly, the passage of a urethral catheter is not always a benign procedure. False passages can occur, and urethroscopy may be the only way to identify the true urethral lumen.[4] A guidewire can be placed once the lumen has been identified, and a Foley catheter with an end hole can be advanced over the guidewire.

Indwelling double pigtail catheters can be placed during flexible cystoscopy. A 0.035-in. or a 0.038-in. guidewire is passed under direct vision through the cystoscope. Once the guidewire has been advanced up the ureter and into the kidney, the cystoscope is removed. An 8 Fr exchange sheath is placed over this guidewire. When the obturator of this sheath is removed, the double pigtail catheter is inserted, and its final position is monitored under fluoroscopic control. A metal-tipped pusher is inserted so that the distal end of the double pigtail catheter protrudes from the ureteral orifice. A good rule of thumb is to place the metallic tip of the pusher at the top edge of the symphysis pubis in men and at the lower edge of the symphysis pubis in women.

Complications

Complications associated with cystourethroscopy are rare. Virtually all of them relate to an inability to ascertain where one is within the urethra. This can be a troublesome problem in patients with active bleeding. As long as the urethral lumen is identifiable within the center of the visual field of the endoscope, there is no danger of perforation. If, however, one does perforate the urethra, the procedure should be abandoned and a Foley catheter should be placed. Persistent attempts to continue endoscopic examination can lead to extravasation of irrigating fluid. Minimal fluid will extravasate as long as Buck's fascia is intact, but injury to this can allow irrigating fluid access to the subcutaneous penile tissue and the scrotum. If one does sustain a urethral perforation, it is best to identify the urethral lumen immediately and pass a guidewire. The guidewire can be used to pass an end hole Foley catheter to provide drainage of the bladder.

If the urethral lumen cannot be identified, a percutaneous bladder tube will have to be placed.[5] If the bladder is distended, this is a simple procedure. If the bladder is not easily palpable, then it can be allowed to fill with urine. Ultrasonographic guidance is very helpful if the full bladder cannot be palpated or percussed.

URETEROPYELOSCOPY

The ease of lower tract endoscopy was extended to the upper urinary tract with the development of thin rigid and flexible ureteroscopes. Virtually all procedures that are commonplace within the urethra or bladder can be done in the ureter and renal collecting system. The major differences between upper and lower tract endoscopy are the small caliber of the instruments, the delicate nature of the ureter, and the ample flow of blood through the kidney.

Anatomy

The ureter extends from the renal pelvis to the bladder and lies in the retroperitoneum (Fig. 10–2).[6] As the ureter exits the ureteropelvic junction, it passes anterior to the psoas muscle. Anteriorly, the right proximal ureter is adjacent to the descending portion of the duodenum while the jejunum is anterior to the upper portion of the left ureter. As the ureter passes distally, over the psoas muscle, it crosses the transverse processes of the 3rd, 4th, and 5th lumbar vertebrae. It then crosses the bifurcation of the common iliac artery. As it passes into the bony pelvis it crosses anterior to the hypo-

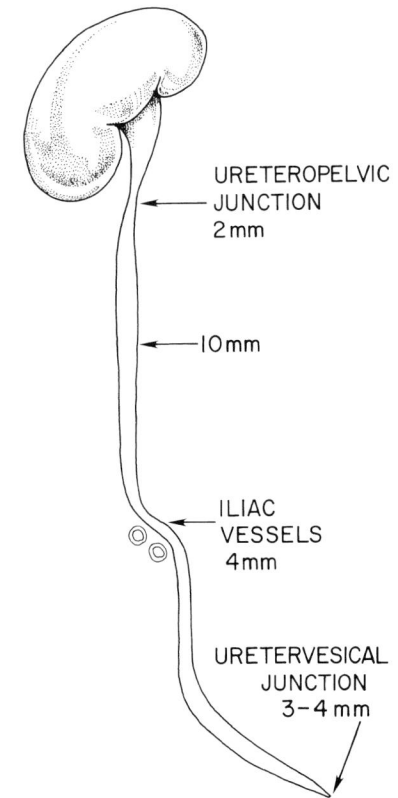

Figure 10–2. The ureter does not have a uniform diameter. The narrowest areas of the ureter are at the ureteropelvic junction, iliac vessels, and ureterovesical junction. Angulation of the ureter also occurs at the iliac vessels and ureteropelvic junction.

gastric artery and lies medial to the obturator nerve and artery. The ureter then passes through the ureterovesical junction that also is the narrowest portion of the ureter.

The upper ureter is supplied by the gonadal and renal arteries with occasional small aortic branches. The middle hemorrhoidal and superior vesicle arteries supply blood to the lower ureter.

The ureter is composed of three layers: an outer adventitia, a middle muscular layer, and the inner urothelium. The muscular layer in the lower ureter consists of three distinct layers: inner longitudinal, middle circular, and outer longitudinal fibers. The corresponding muscular layers in the upper ureter are less clearly defined. As the distal ureter passes through the bladder wall, the longitudinal fiber density decreases. This sparse muscular content in the distal ureter is thought to be the reason for the greater likelihood of perforation in the distal ureter.

Instrumentation

Ureteroscopes that were popular in the early 1980s were 11.5 Fr and between 39 and 45 cm in length (Fig. 10–3).[7] As with cystoscopes, the telescopes had a rod lens construction and were interchangeable. Also analogous with cystoscope design, original ureteroscopes had an offset working channel.

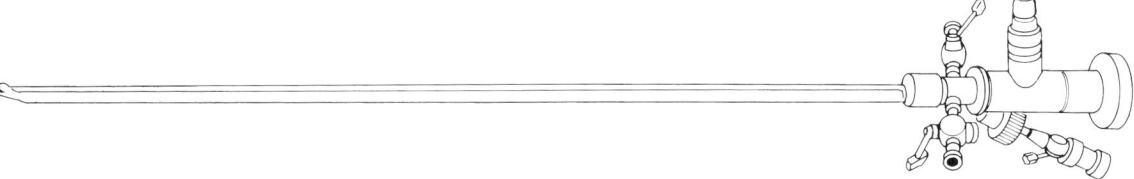

Figure 10–3. Rigid ureteroscope with an offset working channel. Such instruments with a rod lens telescopic system were popular in the 1980s, but all newer instruments have a fiberoptic telescopic system.

This permitted the passage of flexible accessories, but rigid accessories, such as an ultrasonic probe, could not be passed through this channel. The development of a ureteroscope with an offset lens allowed the passage of a rigid accessory such as an ultrasonic probe and continued visualization of the interior of the ureter during the procedure. The telescope had to be removed from early instruments during ultrasonic lithotripsy of a ureteral stone.

The 1980s also saw a shrinkage of the diameter of ureteroscopes. The limitations of rod lens construction held the reduction to about 9.5 Fr. Concurrently, flexible ureteroscopes were developed (see Fig. 10–1).[8] Flexible ureteroscopes as small as 7 Fr were manufactured, but these did not have a system for active tip deflection. Early flexible ureteroscopes with active deflection were no smaller than 10 Fr.

A compromise was achieved when the rod lens telescope was replaced with a fiberoptic telescope encased in a metal sheath. These instruments are smaller than the rod lens instruments and are more durable. Ureteroscopes with this design are commonly available today, and their sizes are as small as 7.5 or 6.5 Fr. This design has two disadvantages. One is the stippled visual field due to the optic fibers. As with all flexible instruments, this can be overcome by reducing the size of individual fibers and increasing the fiber density. Another disadvantage that is insurmountable is the small size of the working channel.[9] The working port size for smaller flexible ureteroscopes is approximately 3 Fr. Fortunately, instrument manufacturers have responded by making even smaller accessories. Actively deflectable flexible ureteroscopes with an adequate working channel and an 8.5 Fr size are readily available.

Retrograde Ureteropyelography

Although ureteroscopy can be performed without advance knowledge of a particular patient's ureteral anatomy, the procedure is easier and safer if a prior intravenous urogram or retrograde ureterogram is available. A contrast study of the ureter provides a road map and may identify kinks or narrow portions of the ureter that might be difficult to traverse with a ureteroscope. A retrograde ureterogram might not be performed if a patient has a history of a contrast allergy or if subsequent shock wave lithotripsy is to be done and the contrast would obscure a stone. Although the likelihood of a severe reaction to radiocontrast material is less with a retrograde than with an intravenous urogram, patients can still have severe reactions, even if the contrast is not injected directly into the vascular system.

Technique

Patients should have sterile urine before ureteroscopy. Most urologists also administer preoperative antibiotics, even though no studies support their use in this situation. As a general rule, general or regional anesthesia should be used. Although ureteroscopy can be performed with intravenous sedation, the lack of adequate anesthesia hinders one's ability to perform an adequate procedure. Patients undergoing ureteroscopy require an initial cystoscopic procedure to examine the urethra and bladder and identify the ureteral orifice. Although cystoscopy can be performed with relatively little discomfort, ureteral dilation, if performed, can be very painful, and the passage of the ureteroscope using a pressurized irrigation system can cause severe renal colic. A patient who is comfortable during the initial cystoscopy may develop severe pain as the ureteroscope is advanced up the ureter. Everyone will be happier and a more careful and thorough ureteroscopic examination can be performed if adequate anesthesia is used.

Patients should be placed in a dorsal lithotomy position. Ureteroscopic procedures are more easily done with fluoroscopic guidance, but this is not absolutely necessary. This can be accomplished with a specific endourology table or a portable C-arm and an operating room table with a radiolucent top.

The need for ureteral dilation is controversial.[10,11] Although a small rigid ureteroscope can be passed without formal dilation, the mere passage of a ureteroscope dilates the ureter. Most ureteroscopists prefer to dilate the ureter. Early ureteroscopists dilated only the ureterovesicle junction with metal bougies. These have been replaced with tapered, flexible ureteral dilators or dilating balloons. If so desired, a retrograde ureterogram is obtained and a guidewire is passed. A very safe guidewire is a 0.035- or 0.038-in. Bentson type of guidewire that has a long, flexible tip. It is virtually impossible to perforate the ureter with this guidewire. Another favorite guidewire for some urologists is one that has a hydrophilic coating. These guidewires become very slippery when wet and often can be slipped past an obstructing stone. Their slipperiness makes them treacherous to use because the irrigating fluid pressure can extrude them from the instrument and ureter. It probably is best to use these

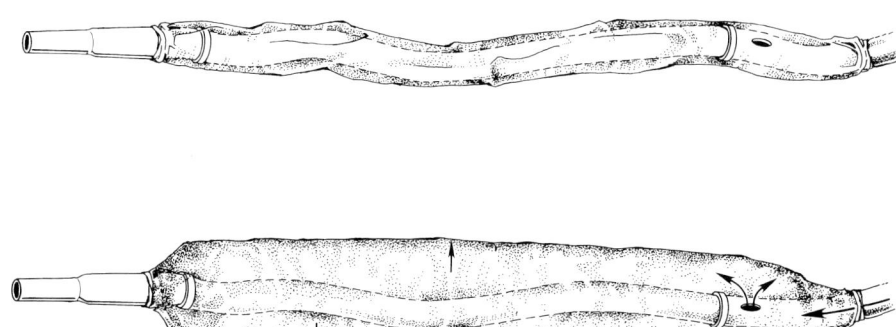

Figure 10–4. A typical balloon dilator has a 6 or 7 Fr shaft size, an inflated diameter of 5 mm, and a length of 4 cm; it will accommodate up to 15 atmospheres of pressure. The balloon is deflated in the upper diagram and inflated in the lower diagram. Radiopaque markers are placed where the maximum inflation diameter begins and ends.

wires only in a difficult situation. They should be exchanged for a more traditional wire once an obstructed area has been bypassed.

The guidewire is passed through the cystoscope and introduced into the ureteral orifice under direct vision. Fluoroscopic guidance is used to negotiate the wire up the ureter and into the renal pelvis. Once the tip of the guidewire has been placed in the renal pelvis, the remainder of the dilation can be performed under fluoroscopic control. The choice of dilation method is between a balloon catheter and tapered ureteral catheters. Most urologists favor the former, because balloon dilation is a one-step procedure. Inflated balloon diameters of 5 or 6 mm usually are used (Fig. 10–4). The length of balloons ranges between 2 and 10 cm. Although a 10-cm balloon is appealing because its longer length dilates a longer segment of ureter, there is a greater risk of balloon rupture. It is safer to use a balloon that has a length of only 4 cm.

Tapered ureteral dilators are somewhat more troublesome to use, but they provide the urologist with a measure of the compliance of the ureter. If it is increasingly difficult to advance the tapered ureteral catheters as the size increases from 6 to 8 to 10 Fr, then ureteral compliance is low. This should alert the urologist that this may be a very difficult ureteroscopic procedure. The most dangerous aspect of ureteroscopy is the temptation to use excessive force.

Dilation of the lower ureter proceeds readily in most patients, but not in all. Some patients, usually males, may have relatively narrow ureters that are not very compliant. Attempts can be made to balloon-dilate the entire length of the ureter, but resultant bleeding can impair visualization during ureteroscopy. If the ureteral dilation is a struggle, it may be prudent to place a temporizing double pigtail catheter for a week or two. This passively dilates the ureter and makes subsequent ureteroscopy much easier.

During ureteral dilation, a ringlike ureteral stricture may be encountered. These do not appear to be classic ureteral strictures but are weblike diaphragms. They do not cause clinical obstruction (unless a small stone becomes lodged proximal to them), but they are virtually impossible to dilate. Attempts to dilate these with a high-pressure balloon lead to the formation of a narrow waist in the balloon. The balloon may rupture if excessive force is applied. These tight diaphragms must be incised with a ureterotome or small electrocautery before the ureteroscope can be passed. They also may be soft-dilated with a temporizing double pigtail catheter.

Once the ureter has been dilated, the ureteroscope is passed under direct vision. Although it is not mandatory to place a second safety guidewire, the urologist should be certain that a solitary guidewire is not lost during the procedure. The ureteroscope can be advanced alongside the guidewire, but it usually is easier to advance the ureteroscope over the wire. The cystoscope can be removed during the ureteroscopic procedure, but it is often easier to leave the cystoscope sheath in place during the procedure. Irrigating fluid can drain out of the bladder, and bending of the ureteroscope is minimized in muscular men. Most ureteroscopes have a small beak like a cystoscope. The ureteroscope can be rotated 180 degrees to place the beak posterolateral (Fig. 10-5).

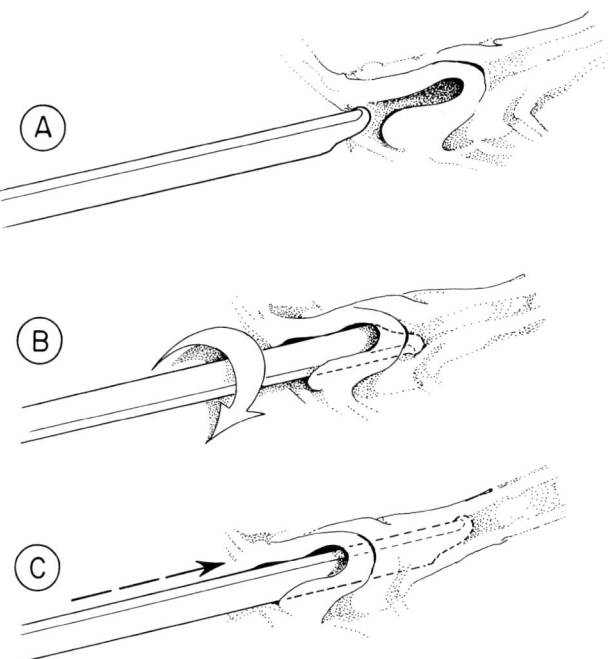

Figure 10–5. A 180-degree rotation of the instrument facilitates the introduction of a rigid ureteroscope with a beak. The urologist should remain cognizant of the location of the beak as the instrument is advanced up the ureter.

As the ureteroscope is advanced, the ureteral lumen should be kept in the central field of view of the instrument. This usually is easier if the ureteroscope is passed over a guidewire.

As with all endoscopic procedures, irrigation must be used during ureteroscopy. Given the potential for extraluminal extravasation, normal saline should be used as the primary irrigant. Water or glycine should be used only during ureteroscopic electrosurgical procedures. Even electrohydraulic lithotripsy can be performed with saline irrigation.

The small working channel of most ureteroscopes often requires a pressurized irrigation system. A simple approach is to use a pressurized cuff on a standard liter bag of normal saline.[12] Care must be taken to limit flow during the procedure, because a liter of irrigant will empty rapidly. Patients also may experience severe renal colic if attention is not paid to the pressure and flow of irrigant. An alternate approach to pressurization is a syringelike device that can intermittently flush the ureteroscope. Irrigant flow during most of the procedure is provided by gravity.

The entire ureteral wall is examined as the ureteroscope is advanced up the ureter. If balloon dilation has been used, there may be longitudinal tears in the mucosa. These small splits cause no permanent damage, but they offer the potential for extravasation, especially if irrigant pressure is kept high. The passage of the ureter over the common iliac artery is identified by posterolateral pulsations (see Fig. 10–2). The tip of the ureteroscope must be guided over this. As long as the ureteroscope advances smoothly up the ureter without bunching of the ureteral mucosa in front of the tip of the instrument, there is no danger of ureteral avulsion. If the mucosa forms folds in front of the instrument, advancement should be halted (Fig. 10–6). A smaller instrument should be used or this portion of the ureter should be dilated with a balloon.

Rigid ureteroscopes with a rod lens system tolerate minimal longitudinal bending. This is manifested by the formation of a small crescent in the visual field. These are very delicate instruments, and severe bending can break the instrument. Crescent formation will not be seen with a fiberoptic rigid ureteroscope. Nevertheless, the urologist must recognize that some bending can occur, especially when the ureteroscope passes over the iliac vessels.

A rigid ureteroscope often can be passed all the way into the renal pelvis. The ureteropelvic junction is seen as a dipping of the ureter posteriorly and the presence of a small mucosal fold posteriorly. Once the tip of the instrument has been advanced into the renal pelvis, irrigating fluid should be drained before proceeding. This relieves pressure in the renal pelvis and permits unhindered flow of irrigant during the remainder of the examination.

A duplicated collecting system offers no obstacle to ureteroscopy. Placement of the guidewire into the appropriate collecting system may require direct ureteroscopic visualization of the ureteral bifurcation. A guidewire can be placed initially in either collecting system so that the distal ureter can be dilated. Once the ureteroscope has been advanced into the lower ureter and the bifurcation identified, the appropriate lumen can be cannulated with another wire and the ureteroscopic procedure can proceed as with a single ureter.

Rarely, a ureterocele may be found, often containing a stone. The stone can be removed by making a small transverse incision in the distal-most portion of the ureterocele. This is therapeutic and permits one to enter the ureterocele with the ureteroscope and identify the ureteral lumen. A guidewire can be passed and ureteroscopy can be completed.

An ectopic or reimplanted ureter is a more difficult situation, because the angle of approach from the cystoscope may preclude direct passage of a guidewire. Deflectable guidewires often can be directed into the ureteral orifice and up the ureter. In this situation it is helpful if a radiographic road map of the distal ureter has been obtained before the ureteroscopy. The combination of a 6 Fr tapered ureteral dilator and a Bentson guidewire (Fig. 10–7) often can be used to place the tip of the wire into the ureteral orifice and rotate the distal 1 cm of wire so that it is aligned with the distal ureter. Submucosal perforation should be avoided, because it will become very difficult to identify and cannulate the true ureteral lumen.

Most urologists place a double pigtail catheter at the completion of ureteroscopy. If the distal ureter has not been dilated and there appears to be no injury to the intramural ureter, then it may be possible to leave the patient without a stent. In most situations, however, it is best to leave a stent. These stents can be left in place for 3 or 4 days. Options for removal include repeat cystoscopy or the use of a urethral suture that the patient can use to self-remove the stent (Fig. 10–8). Yet another option is to leave a 3- or 4-cm length of suture attached to the distal end of the double pigtail catheter in the bladder. This simplifies the removal of the stent with a flexible endoscope because the suture can be grasped with a pair of fine grasping forceps. Accessory forceps that can be passed through a flexible cystoscope often are too small to achieve adequate purchase on the stent itself. Most patients are placed on oral antibiotics for a few days after the procedure.

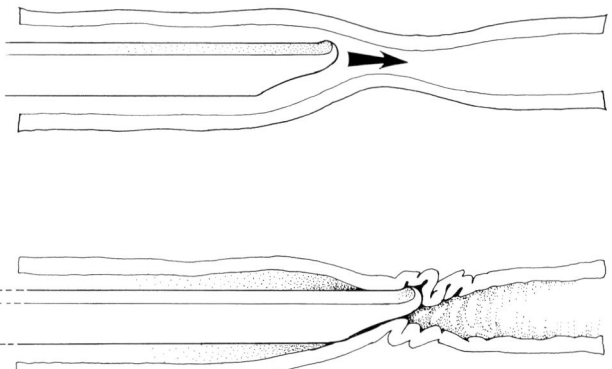

Figure 10–6. Advancement of a ureteroscope should be stopped if mucosal folds appear in front of the instrument. Persistent attempts to advance the instrument may avulse the ureter.

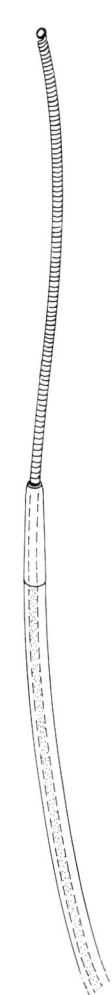

Figure 10–7. A 6 Fr tapered ureteral dilator and a 0.035-in. Bentson guidewire are a useful and safe combination to cannulate a difficult ureteral orifice or negotiate an obstructed or kinked ureter. The guidewire is advanced a short distance, followed by the dilator. The wire and catheter can be advanced in an inchwormlike fashion up the entire ureter.

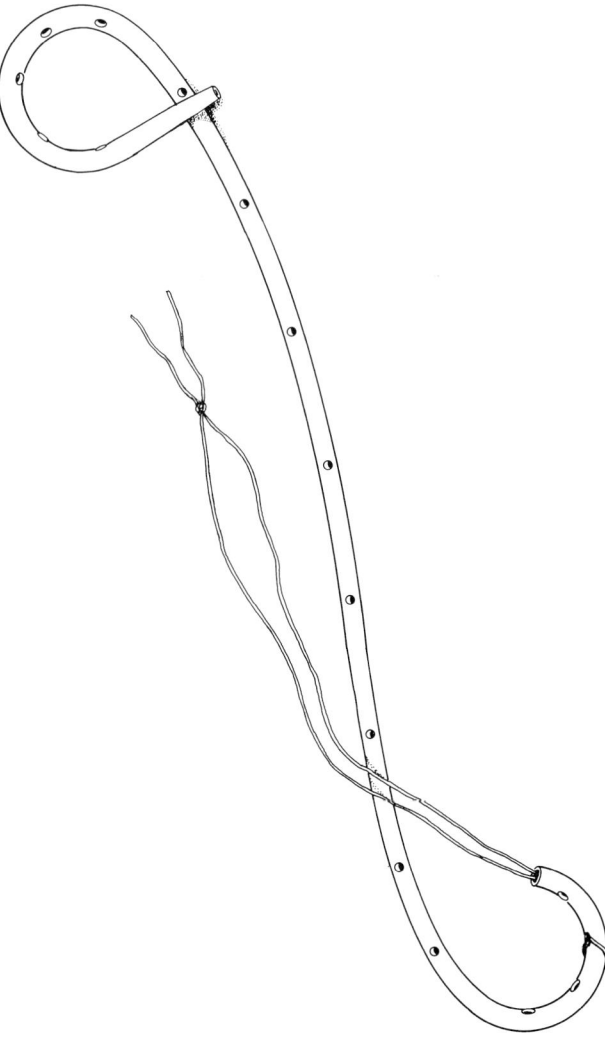

Figure 10–8. Double pigtail catheter with an attached suture. The suture can be left long to dangle out of the urethral meatus or short to permit easier removal with a flexible cystoscope.

Indications

The indications for ureteroscopy are the same as those for lower tract endoscopy, including evaluation of radiographic filling defects, obstruction,[13] gross hematuria, and a unilateral positive urinary cytology.[14] Ureteroscopy also can be used for upper tract surveillance after endoscopic treatment of a ureteral or renal pelvic tumor.

Ureteroscopy for evaluation of a positive urine cytology or a history of gross hematuria is aided by the preoperative lateralization of the hematuria or positive cytology.[15] This is why it is important that patients with gross hematuria undergo immediate cystoscopy. Likewise, urine cytologies can be obtained from each ureter to lateralize the source. Although bilateral diagnostic ureteroscopic procedures can be performed, they are twice as long and the patient is twice as uncomfortable postoperatively. Invariably, the time spent examining the second ureter and collecting system would have been better spent examining the ureter and collecting system that was the source of the bleeding or positive cytology.

Although ureteroscopy usually is used as a therapeutic procedure for ureteral calculi, it also can confirm that a midureteral filling defect is a uric acid calculus. Although ultrasound is an excellent means to accomplish this in the renal pelvis or bladder, it is difficult to examine the midureter sonographically. It also is possible to confirm the nature of a foreign body.

A ureteral stricture can be examined visually and biopsies obtained.[16] When ureteroscopy is performed for the examination of intraluminal lesions, vigorous manipulation with guidewires, catheters, and balloons should be avoided, because the associated trauma may obscure the nature of the filling defect. Although a guidewire can be placed adjacent to the lesion, it is wise not to pass dilators or inflate a balloon adjacent to such a filling defect. This can be done once the area has been seen.

In some situations it is not possible to advance the ureteroscope to the offending lesion for direct visualization. Fortunately, the acquisition of tissue samples with a brush biopsy device seems to be just as productive as direct visualization and a formal cup biopsy.

The nature and extent of a previous endoscopic ureteral injury can be determined ureteroscopically.[17] It may be possible to identify the true ureteral lumen and pass a guidewire and stenting catheter.

Complications

Complications associated with ureteroscopy range from a simple guidewire perforation to ureteral avulsion.[18] The former is of little significance, whereas the latter requires an open surgical repair.[19] The likelihood of a ureteroscopic injury seems to be related to the experience of the ureteroscopist, although the widespread availability of smaller ureteroscopes seems to have reduced the incidence of serious complications.

Since ureteroscopy is a retrograde procedure, the perforations create flaps of ureteral wall that tend to self-seal with the antegrade passage of urine. The placement of an indwelling double pigtail catheter avoids the development of high intraureteral pressures and allows the perforations to seal. A dwelling time of 2 to 3 days probably is sufficient for a small guidewire perforation, but a larger perforation may require that the stent be left in place for 2 or 3 weeks.

Submucosal perforations often occur just within the ureteral orifice along the lateral wall of the intramural ureter. If this happens, one often can place the tip of the ureteroscope in the orifice. The small mucosal perforation can be identified lateral to the true ureteral lumen. A guidewire can be advanced under direct vision into the true lumen and ureteroscopy can be completed.

Even balloon dilation of the ureter can cause longitudinal splitting of the ureteral mucosa or the entire ureteral wall.[20] These splits do not cause ureteral strictures and can be managed with a couple of weeks of internal stent drainage.

A theoretical criticism of double pigtail catheters is the potential to transmit voiding pressures to the upper urinary tract. Patients with double pigtail catheters often complain of flank pain, especially at the end of voiding.[21] Only rarely does extravasation worsen with a double pigtail stent. If this occurs, then a Foley catheter should be placed.

If it is not possible to pass a retrograde stent, then a percutaneous nephrostomy tube can be placed, followed by the antegrade passage of a double pigtail catheter. One should make sure that the ureter has not been avulsed, because this requires open surgical repair.

PERCUTANEOUS NEPHROSCOPY

The first percutaneous nephrostomy tube was placed 40 years ago by Goodwin and associates,[22] but another 25 years passed before the first renal calculi were removed percutaneously.[23] Percutaneous nephrostomy tube placement has since become a routine procedure. Endoscopic removal of renal pelvic tumors and correction of ureteropelvic junction obstruction have been added to percutaneous stone removal.

Anatomy

The kidneys are retroperitoneal organs located on either side of the vertebral column. The right kidney lies somewhat lower than the left. The descending portion of the duodenum lies anterior to the right renal pelvis. The hepatic flexure of the colon is anterior to the lower pole of the right kidney. Posteriorly, the twelfth rib and the diaphragm lie over the upper poles of each kidney. The left kidney is bounded anteriorly by the spleen, proximal jejunum, and splenic flexure of the colon. The tail of the pancreas also extends across the renal hilum anteriorly on the left. Immediately anterior to the intrarenal pelvis is the renal vein and the renal artery.

The renal artery divides into anterior and posterior branches before entering each kidney (Fig. 10–9).[24] Within the renal parenchyma, the branch arteries form the interlobar arteries that ascend between the renal pyramids. These arch along the base of the pyramids to form the arcuate arteries. The interlobular arteries branch from the arcuate arteries and then form the afferent arterioles, glomeruli, and efferent arterioles. The location of the relatively large interlobar arter-

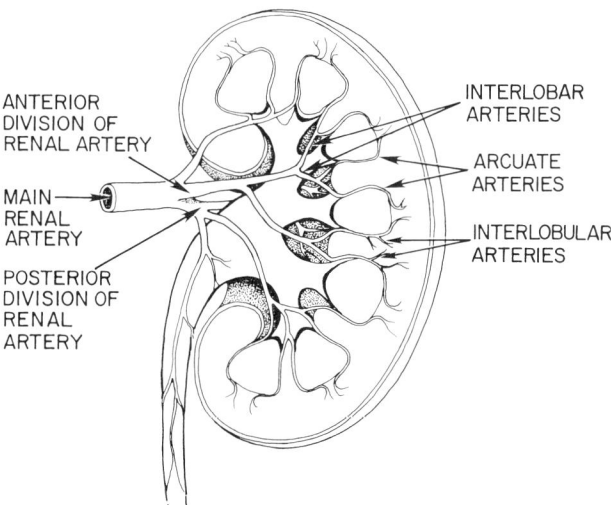

Figure 10–9. Anterior view of the arterial vasculature of the kidney and its relationship to the renal parenchyma and collecting system. The percutaneous renal endoscopist should remember that the relatively large interlobar arteries lie adjacent to the infundibula.

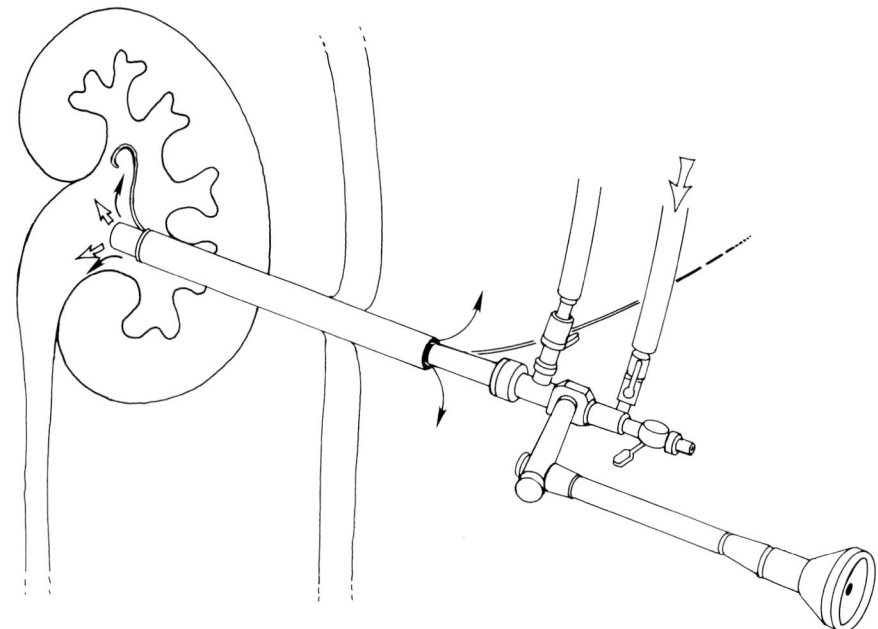

Figure 10–10. A working sheath has been placed with its distal tip in the renal collecting system, which is then examined with a rigid nephroscope. This arrangement maintains a low intrapelvic pressure, because irrigating fluid drains back out of the sheath around the nephroscope. The rigid nephroscope can easily be replaced with other instruments such as a flexible nephroscope or ureteroscope.

ies adjacent to the infundibula should be kept in mind when performing percutaneous endoscopic procedures.

Within the renal collecting system, the papillae form the apex of the renal pyramids.[25] Endoscopically, a papilla appears as a cone-shaped structure with radial striations. It has a pink color and is more friable than the surrounding urothelium. The circular fornix at the base of the papilla also is subject to injury during endoscopic procedures, because its attachment to the papilla is rather delicate. Further evidence of the delicate attachment of the fornix to the papilla is provided by the occasional forniceal tear with urinary extravasation that can occur in a patient with an acutely obstructing ureteral calculus. Care should be taken when endoscopically probing either the papilla or fornix. Urine formed in the calyces passes through the infundibula and then into the renal pelvis. The ureteropelvic junction usually can be identified during antegrade endoscopy as a funnel-shaped narrowing of the renal pelvis.

Instrumentation

The equipment used for percutaneous nephrostomy can be divided into two categories: that needed for placement and dilation of the nephrostomy tract and that needed for visual examination of the intrarenal collecting system. Although retrograde percutaneous access to the collecting system has been described,[26] it has never gained popularity. The rationale for this technique had been to enable a urologist to place a percutaneous nephrostomy tube using familiar retrograde endoscopic techniques. Urologists who were interested in placing their own percutaneous nephrostomy tubes found that it was much easier simply to place them percutaneously in an antegrade fashion using the same techniques that had been developed by interventional radiologists.

The initial percutaneous nephrostomy tract can be placed under ultrasonic or fluoroscopic guidance.[27] The collecting system must be opacified if the latter is chosen. This can be

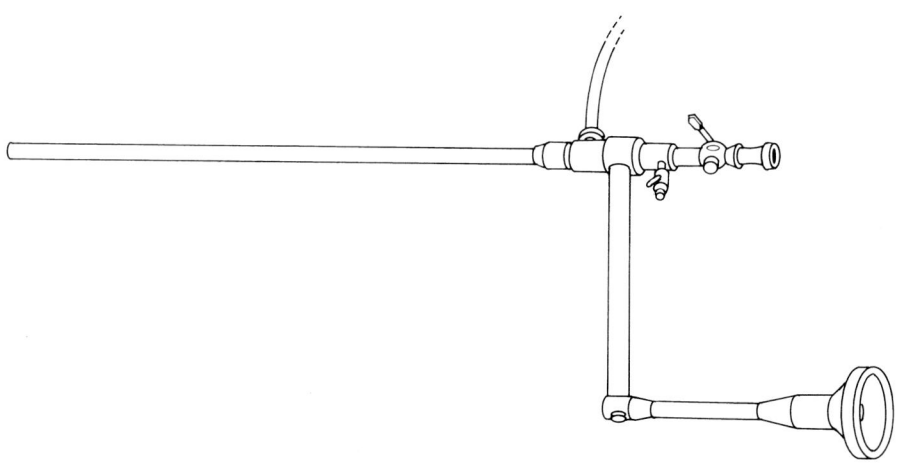

Figure 10–11. Rigid nephroscopes have an offset lens. This provides a straight working channel through which an ultrasonic lithotrite can be inserted.

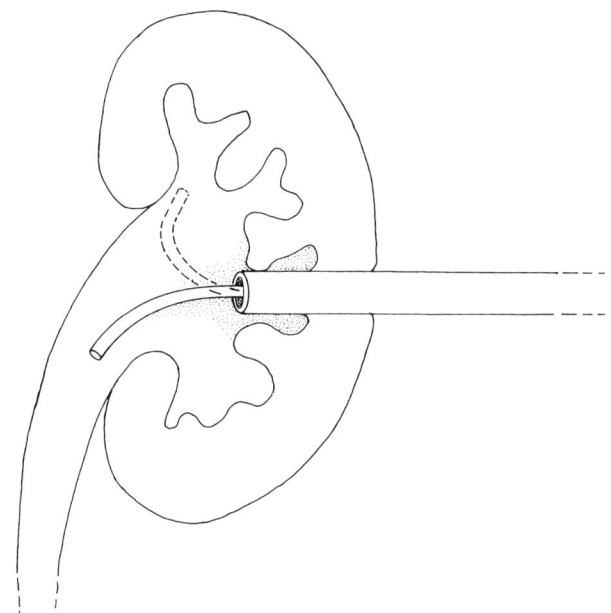

Figure 10–12. If the entire renal collecting cannot be seen with a rigid instrument, a flexible nephroscope can be inserted via the working sheath. Care should be taken not to induce intrarenal bleeding during rigid nephroscopy, because subsequent examination with a flexible instrument may be rendered difficult, if not impossible. The tip of a flexible instrument should be straightened before removal, because the edge of the sheath can tear the plastic covering of a flexible instrument.

accomplished with the intravenous or retrograde injection of radiocontrast material, or the fluoroscopic placement of a skinny needle into the renal collecting system. Aspiration of urine confirms that the skinny needle is in the collecting system.

Once percutaneous access has been achieved, the tract is dilated up to 1 cm in diameter. Dilation techniques include the sequential passage of tapered plastic or telescopic metal dilators,[28] or inflation of a high-pressure balloon. Most percutaneous nephroscopists prefer to use a working sheath (Amplatz) instead of the integral metal sheath that is supplied by the nephroscope manufacturer (Fig. 10–10).

Although a standard cystoscope can be used to examine the interior of the kidney, all nephroscopes have an offset lens (Fig. 10–11). Percutaneous nephroscopy was developed primarily for the removal of renal calculi. Ultrasonic fragmentation is the most common means to fragment larger calculi, and its use requires a straight working channel.

Usually it is impossible to examine the entire intrarenal collecting system with a rigid nephroscope. A flexible cystoscope can be passed through the working sheath and can be used to examine portions of the intrarenal collecting system not seen with a rigid instrument (Fig. 10–12). The only caveat is that the renal collecting system is not as capacious as the bladder and the flexible endoscope must have a small radius of deflection. Fortunately, all modern flexible cystoscopes can be used to examine the interior of the kidney.

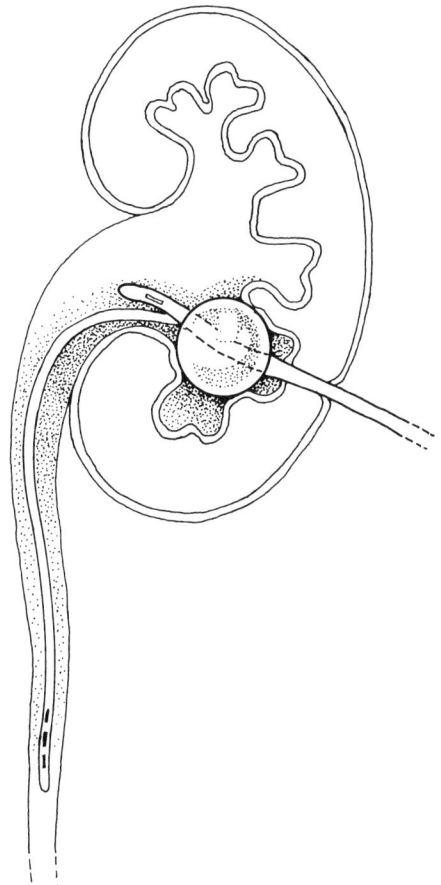

Figure 10–13. A Foley catheter is left in the renal pelvis, and a 5 Fr end hole catheter is left two-thirds of the way down the ureter as a safety catheter. The latter provides access to the renal collecting system if the nephrostomy tube falls out. A double pigtail catheter can be used instead of a ureteral catheter if temporary internal drainage is desired after the nephrostomy tube is removed.

Most renal infundibulae will accommodate a 16 Fr flexible endoscope, and it may even be possible to pass such an instrument down a dilated ureter. A flexible ureteroscope can be used to examine calyces attached to more narrow infundibulae and to examine a normal-caliber ureter. The antegrade passage of a flexible ureteroscope is particularly helpful in the examination of the ureter in a patient who has had a cystectomy and urinary diversion.

A nephrostomy tube should be placed when the procedure is completed. Numerous specialty percutaneous nephrostomy tubes have been developed for this purpose, but a standard Foley catheter suffices (Fig. 10–13).

Antegrade Pyeloureterography

An antegrade radiographic contrast study of the renal pelvis and ureter is almost always obtained, because the vast majority of percutaneous endoscopic procedures are performed under fluoroscopic control. This confirms the position of a stone within the renal pelvis or one of the calyces or the presence of a suspected or known filling defect. An antegrade pyelogram is especially useful for the evaluation of ureteral obstruction. The passage of contrast is monitored fluoroscopically as it is injected into the renal pelvis. A formal Whittaker test also can be performed to evaluate the presence and severity of obstruction. Fortunately, the need for Whittaker tests has declined with an increase in quality of Lasix renal scans. The presence of clinically significant obstruction already has been confirmed in the vast majority of patients before the placement of a percutaneous nephrostomy tube. The interventional procedure usually is intended to be therapeutic (endoscopic incision of a narrow ureteropelvic junction or ureterointestinal anastomotic stricture) rather than diagnostic. Nevertheless, it is comforting to confirm that a patient with an elevated $T_{1/2}$ on a Lasix renal scan does have an anatomically narrow ureteropelvic junction.

Technique

Although percutaneous nephrostomy tubes are almost always placed with local anesthesia and percutaneous nephroscopy can be performed with local anesthesia, vigorous manipulation of the interior of the kidney and performance of any therapeutic procedure are easier if a general or regional anesthetic is administered. Vigorous intravenous sedation should be avoided, because the prone position of these patients makes respiratory depression a more serious anesthetic complication if it should occur.

Patients are placed in a prone position and the kidney is punctured from a posterolateral direction. The goal is to puncture the kidney through the parenchyma, which prevents urinary leakage after the nephrostomy tube is removed. A more direct puncture through the posterior portion of the kidney also is more likely to injure one of the larger segmental arteries. The location of the puncture site along the longitudinal axis of the kidney is determined by the specific indication for percutaneous nephroscopy. A direct calyceal puncture should be made for an isolated calyceal stone. The tract for removal of a large staghorn calculus should be made in the upper or lower pole. A midpole puncture provides direct access to the ureteropelvic junction for an endopyelotomy. Tube placement for the examination of a filling defect should be such that visualization is optimized and local resection of a transitional cell tumor can be accomplished safely and completely.

The location of the ascending colon on the right and the descending colon on the left should be recognized when the initial puncture is made. If there is any doubt as to the lateral and posterior location of the colon, a preoperative CT scan can be obtained to delineate the anatomy. When an upper pole tract is selected, the adjacent spleen on the left should be recognized, and the location of the diaphragm and overlying pleura should be recognized for both kidneys. Nephrostomy tract placement above the twelfth or even eleventh rib is necessary in some patients.[29] Although the likelihood of developing a pneumothorax or a hemothorax is greater with a supracostal puncture, these complications are relatively infrequent, especially when a working sheath is used. The puncture should be lateral to the paraspinous muscles.

The initial tract can be placed under sonographic guidance or after opacification of the collecting system. A blind initial puncture can be made with a 22-gauge thin-wall needle. The approximate location is ascertained from previous radiographs. Once urine is aspirated, contrast is injected to opacify the collecting system. Identification of the renal collecting system usually is not a problem, because many patients undergoing percutaneous nephrostomy tube placement have radiopaque calculi that can be used as a guide. Patients with UPJ obstruction have a dilated renal collecting system that simplifies direct puncture.

A second puncture usually is made with an 18-gauge needle that will accommodate a 0.035- or 0.038-in. guidewire. Once this guidewire has been advanced into the kidney, it should be negotiated through the ureteropelvic junction, down the ureter, and into the bladder. This is not always possible in patients with a large staghorn calculus or an obstructed ureteropelvic junction. Nevertheless, placement of the guidewire in the ureter minimizes the likelihood that it will become dislodged during the subsequent dilation. Initial tract dilation is accomplished with tapered dilators up to approximately 10 Fr. A 10 Fr exchange sheath is placed, followed by a second or safety guidewire. Subsequent tract dilation is done with larger tapered dilators or a high-pressure balloon, which is preferred by most physicians. The tract need not be dilated greater than 30 Fr. The tract should be dilated from the skin to the renal parenchyma. An Amplatz working sheath is placed after dilation, and the rigid nephroscope is inserted. As with ureteroscopic procedures, the irrigating solution should be normal saline. Glycine or water are needed only when electrosurgical resection of a renal pelvic tumor is undertaken. Even electrohydraulic lithotripsy of a renal pelvic calculus can be done with normal saline irrigation.

Examination of the intrarenal collecting system with a rigid nephroscope is a simple procedure. Most of the intrarenal collecting system can be examined with careful manipulation. Perirenal scarring from a previous open surgical procedure limits mobility of the kidney. Care must be taken not to split any infundibula with overzealous manipulation. Likewise, the renal pelvic wall is thinner than the bladder wall and can be easily perforated. The renal vessels lie anterior to the renal pelvis, along with the jejunum on the left and the descending portion of the duodenum on the right. The peritoneal cavity can be entered with vigorous advancement of the nephroscope. The procedure should be abandoned if this occurs, because virtually all the irrigant will leak out of the kidney and into the abdomen.

Flexible nephroscopy and flexible antegrade ureteroscopy can be done, but acute bleeding from tract placement will limit visualization. Flexible nephroscopy may have to be postponed for 2 or 3 days. If a nephrostomy tube is left in place, it can be replaced with a working sheath and flexible nephroscopy can be done with only mild intravenous sedation. Care should be taken that the covering of a flexible instrument is not torn by the lip of the working sheath. The tip of the nephroscope should be straightened before the instrument is withdrawn from the sheath.

Examination of a duplicated collecting system requires that more attention be paid to exact placement of the nephrostomy tract. The tube should be placed in that portion of the collecting system that contains the presumed lesion. Examination of the entire collecting system may require placement of two separate tracts. An alternative would be flexible retrograde ureteroscopy.

The approach to a horseshoe kidney is complicated by its more anterior position. Although a horseshoe kidney has numerous aberrant vessels, these vessels enter the kidney anteromedially. Inadvertent vascular injury does not seem to be a significant risk. These kidneys also must be approached from a more medial skin puncture. Access through the paraspinous muscles and the more anterior location of a horseshoe kidney results in a longer nephrostomy tract. Although standard nephroscopes usually are long enough to reach the collecting system, the entire length of the instrument must be used. The mobility of a horseshoe kidney is less than that of a normal kidney. Consequently, the puncture site must be chosen even more carefully. Targeted stones and filling defects should be punctured directly.

Indications

As with other endoscopic procedures, the indications can be divided into diagnostic or therapeutic. Most diagnostic procedures rapidly become therapeutic, because placement of a percutaneous nephrostomy tube, dilation of the tract, and examination of the intrarenal collecting system constitute an invasive procedure. Examination of the upper collecting system during the workup of a positive cytology or recurrent gross hematuria is best accomplished with retrograde ureteroscopy. Although the intrarenal collecting system can be examined through a percutaneous antegrade tract, it is likely that the placement of the tract and its subsequent dilation may obscure the offending lesion. In those situations where it is not possible to advance a ureteroscope into the renal collecting system, it probably is more prudent to leave a double pigtail catheter in place for 1 or 2 weeks.[30] This dilates the ureter and expedites repeat ureteroscopy.

Primary percutaneous nephroscopy should be limited to examination and resection of known filling defects, endoscopic removal of calculi or endoscopic incision of an intrarenal stricture, congenital UPJ obstruction, or stricture of a ureterointestinal anastomosis. Percutaneous nephrostomy tube placement with antegrade pyelography, however, is an accepted method to opacify a collecting system (and provide drainage) when little contrast is excreted by the kidney after intravenous injection.

Complications

The largest experience with percutaneous nephroscopy is in patients who have had stones removed.[31] Loss of percutaneous access is the most frustrating and avoidable complication of percutaneous renal surgery. This can be minimized by placing a safety guidewire and remaining cognizant of the location of both guidewires during the entire procedure.

Extravasation of irrigation fluid can occur during the procedure. A large volume can fill the intrapleural or intraperitoneal space. The former can be minimized with a working sheath, whereas the latter can be minimized by avoiding perforation of the collecting system anteriorly. If the latter does occur, the procedure should be terminated and a nephrostomy tube placed. Use of an Amplatz sheath also minimizes perinephric extravasation, because intrapelvic pressure is kept low. Extravasation of massive amounts of fluid can be avoided if the surgeon remains aware of how much irrigation fluid is being used and how much is being removed from suction attached to the ultrasonic probe or leakage through the working sheath. The procedure should be terminated and a nephrostomy tube placed if there is any doubt. A renal pelvic perforation will close within a couple of days and the proedure can be completed safely at that time. Extravasation of contrast media can occur during initial tract placement. Patients with a history of a contrast reaction should be premedicated with steroids.

Bleeding during percutaneous nephroscopic surgery is not unusual,[32] particularly when a transitional cell tumor is resected, a large stone is removed, or an endopyelotomy is performed. It is not uncommon for patients to lose one or two units of blood. The quantity lost seems to be proportional to the duration of the procedure. Fortunately, vigorous hemorrhage limits visualization and forces one to halt the procedure. Veins usually are the source of bleeding, and placement and clamping of a nephrostomy tube provide intrarenal tamponade. Such bleeding usually resolves within half an hour. The intrarenal clot will lyse within a day. Special balloon catheters provide more active tamponade, but their use is not mandatory.[33]

Arterial bleeding is a more serious problem. This is more likely to occur during an endopyelotomy. Tamponade may help, but an arteriogram should be performed and the transected vessel embolized if the bleeding continues and the patient becomes hemodynamically unstable.

Late bleeding may occur when the nephrostomy tube is removed. This usually is self-limited, but acute distention of the renal collecting system causes severe colic. Fewer than 10% of patients require perioperative transfusion.

Development of an arteriovenous fissure is a potential complication of percutaneous renal surgery.[34] This should be suspected if the patient has recurrent episodes of severe gross hematuria and renal colic secondary to clot passage. An arteriovenous fistula is diagnosed and treated with arteriography and selective embolization.

A low-grade fever may occur in up to 20% of patients after percutaneous nephrostolithotomy.[35] Patients with septic upper tract obstruction require decompression. Even though placement of a percutaneous nephrostomy tube is therapeutic, such patients may become even more unstable for several hours after tube placement. Although these patients may become hypotensive, they usually respond to intravascular volume replacement and stabilize within 12 to 24 hours.

As with all invasive endoscopic procedures, an attempt should be made to sterilize the urine, but this is not possible in every patient. Prophylactic antibiotics usually are used, in spite of the lack of careful studies to support such a practice.

ENDOSCOPY OF URINARY DIVERSION

Flexible endoscopes permit the urologist to examine lower tract urinary diversions visually. Rigid endoscopy of ileal conduits can be done, but examination of the entire length of the conduit is rarely possible. Flexible instruments overcome this limitation.

A mainstay of the evaluation of patients with ileal conduits has been the retrograde injection of contrast through the conduit with the hope that it would reflux up the ureters and into the kidneys. This is an efficient means to introduce contrast into the upper collecting system, but many new diversionary procedures use antirefluxing anastomoses of the ureters to the bowel segment. Retrograde injection of contrast still can be used to evaluate the conduit or pouch, but the capacious nature of many continent urinary diversions makes it difficult to interpret these studies accurately.

Indications

The indications for endoscopic examination of a urinary diversion are the same as those for the examination of the bladder or upper urinary tract, including the presence of a filling defect or stricture, usually at the anastomosis. Sonography is very helpful in differentiating a transitional cell tumor from a calculus, but visual examination can be used if there is any doubt as to the exact etiology of the filling defect.

Strictures of a ureteroileal anastomosis usually are diagnosed with an intravenous urogram or sonogram. Accurate delineation of such a stricture usually requires that contrast be introduced into the upper collecting system through an intravenous or percutaneous antegrade injection. If the latter is necessary, subsequent endoscopy is facilitated if a nephrostomy tube is placed and a guidewire is advanced down the ureter and through the anastomosis.[36,37] This simplifies identification and examination of the anastomosis during retrograde endoscopy.

Technique

Endoscopy of a conduit or a continent diversion should be done with a flexible instrument. A rigid instrument can be used, but it may not be possible to advance it to the end of a conduit or see the entire interior surface of a continent pouch. The patulous nature of a conduit can make endoscopy frustrating, but usually it is possible to negotiate the endoscope to the end of the loop. The anastomoses of the ureters to the conduit are identifiable as pale or dimpled areas. If the anastomosis is strictured, it will be very difficult, if not impossible, to identify the actual lumen. In other instances the flexible instrument will pass through the anastomosis and up the ureter.

If the anastomosis is refluxing, identification is aided by the pre-endoscopic injection of saline that has been mixed with methylene blue or indigo carmine. The blue liquid refluxes into the upper tracts and will efflux from the anastomotic sites during endoscopy. Another option is the intravenous injection of indigo carmine. This is beneficial only if some urine can pass through the anastomosis.

Another complicating factor with continent urinary diversions is the presence of mucus. The mucus can be irrigated from the pouch if a pre-endoscopic catheter is passed. It also may be difficult to pass a flexible instrument through an abdominal wall stoma with a continent diversion. As with all endoscopic procedures, the lumen should be kept in the center of the field of the endoscope. This minimizes the likelihood of perforation. No catheters or drains need to be left in place after the procedure, but the continent pouch should be drained.

REFERENCES

1. Carson CC III: Endourology. In: Glenn JF, ed.: *Urologic Surgery*, 2nd ed. New York: Harper & Row, 1975;287–305.
2. Gregory E, Simmons D, Weinberg J: Care and sterilization of endourologic instruments. *Urol Clin North Am* 1988; 15(3):541–546.
3. Kennedy TJ, Preminger GM: Flexible cystoscopy. *Urol Clin North Am* 1988;15(3):525–528.
4. Badlani GH, Smith AD: Intraoperative endourologic urethral manipulation. *Urol Clin North Am* 1990;17(1):25–29.
5. O'Brien WM: Percutaneous placement of a suprapubic tube with peel away sheath introducer. *J Urol* 1991;145:1015–1016.
6. Huffman JL, Bagley DH: Upper urinary tract anatomy for the ureteroscopist in Huffman JL, Bagley DH, Lyon ES, eds.: *Ureteroscopy*. Philadelphia: WB Saunders, 1988;31–40.
7. Lyon ES, Huffman JL, Bagley DH: Ureteroscopy and ureteropyeloscopy. *Urology* 1984;23(5):29–36.
8. Kavoussi L, Clayman R, Basler J: Flexible, actively deflectable fiberoptic ureteronephroscopy. *J Urol* 1989;142:949–954.
9. Wilson WT, Eberhart RC, Preminger GM: Flow, pressure, and deflection characteristics of flexible deflectable ureterorenoscopes. *J Endourol* 1990;4(3):283–289.
10. Huffman JL, Bagley DH: Balloon dilation of the ureter for ureteroscopy. *J Urol* 1988;140:954–956.
11. Stoller ML, Wolf JS, Hofmann R, et al: Ureteroscopy without routine balloon dilation: an outcome assessment. *J Urol* 1992; 147:1238–1242.
12. Harrison SCW, George VK, Sibley GN: Simple method of hydrostatic dilation of the ureter for ureteroscopy. *Br J Urol* 1990;65:218.

13. Bagley DH, Huffman JL, Lyon ES: Flexible ureteropyeloscopy: diagnosis and treatment in the upper urinary tract. *J Urol* 1987;138:280–285.
14. Huffman JL, Morse MJ, Herr HW, et al: Ureteropyeloscopy: the diagnostic and therapeutic approach to upper tract urothelial tumors. *World J Urol* 1985;3:58–63.
15. Bagley DH, Allen J: Flexible ureteropyeloscopy in the diagnosis of benign essential hematuria. *J Urol* 1990;143:549–553.
16. Netto Jr NR, Ferreira U, Lemos GC, et al: Endourological management of ureteral strictures. *J Urol* 1990;144:631–634.
17. Cormio L, Battaglia M, Traficante A, et al: Endourological treatment of ureteric injuries. *Br J Urol* 1993;72:165–168.
18. Kramolowsky EV: Ureteral perforation during ureterorenoscopy: treatment and management. *J Urol* 1987;138:36–38.
19. Lytton B, Weiss RM, Green DF: Complications of ureteral endoscopy. *J Urol* 1987;137:649–653.
20. Clayman RV, Elbers J, Palmer JO, et al: Experimental extensive balloon dilation of the distal ureter: immediate and long-term effects. *J Endourol* 1987;1(1):19–22.
21. Pryor JL, Langley MJ, Jenkins AD: Comparison of symptom characteristics of indwelling ureteral catheters. *J Urol* 1991;145:719–722.
22. Goodwin WE, Casey WC, Woolf W: Percutaneous trocar (needle) nephrostomy in hydronephrosis. *JAMA* 1955;157(11):891–894.
23. Fernström I, Johnson B: Percutaneous pyelolithotomy: a new extraction technique. *Scand J Urol Nephrol* 1976(10):257.
24. Sampaio FJB: Review: anatomic background for intrarenal endourologic surgery. *J Endourol* 1992;6(5):301–304.
25. Sampaio FJB, Mandarim-De-Lacerda, CA: 3-Dimensional and radiological pelviocaliceal anatomy for endourology. *J Urol* 1988;140:1352–1355.
26. Hunter PT, Newman RC, Finlayson B, et al: Retrograde nephrostomy in 100 patients. *World J Urol* 1985;3:2–6.
27. Stables DP: Percutaneous nephrostomy. techniques, indications, and results. *Urol Clin North Am* 1982;9(1):15–29.
28. Alken P: The telescope dilators. *World J Urol* 1985;3:7–10.
29. Karlin GS and Smith AD: Approaches to the superior calix: renal displacement technique and review of options. *J Urol* 1989;142:774–777.
30. Pang KK, Fuchs GJ: Ureteral stents and flexible ureterorenoscopy. *J Endourol* 1993;7(2):145–149.
31. Lang EK: Percutaneous nephrostolithotomy and lithotripsy: a multi-institutional survey of complications. *Radiology* 1987;162:25–30.
32. Stoller ML, Wolf Jr JS, St. Lezin MA: Estimated blood loss and transfusion rates associated with percutaneous nephrolithotomy. *J Urol* 1994;152:1977–1981.
33. Babayan RK: Stents and catheters in percutaneous renal surgery. *J Endourol* 1993;7(2): 163–168.
34. Patterson DE, Segura JW, Leroy AJ, et al: The etiology and treatment of delayed bleeding following percutaneous lithotripsy. *J Urol* 1985;133:447–451.
35. Lee WJ, Smith AD, Cubelli V, et al: Complications of percutaneous nephrolithotomy. *AJR* 1987;148:177–180.
36. Kramolowsky EV and Clayman RV: Advances in endosurgery. *Urol Clin North Am* 1988;15(3):413–418.
37. Meretyk S, Clayman RV, Kavoussi LR, et al: Endourological treatment of ureteroenteric anastomotic strictures: long-term followup. *J Urol* 1991;145:723–727.

10 Section 2: Renal Angiography

John F. Angle, Charles J. Tegtmeyer, Alan H. Matsumoto

Despite advances in noninvasive imaging, renal angiography continues to be an important tool in the evaluation and treatment of renal and perirenal masses, hematuria, retroperitoneal hemorrhage, and renovascular hypertension. The role of diagnostic renal angiography and percutaneous transcatheter vascular therapy will be reviewed.

PREOPERATIVE EVALUATION

Renal angiography is helpful in the preoperative evaluation of patients with renal neoplasms. More than 30% of patients have multiple renal arteries, and an angiogram will accurately depict the number, size, and location of the renal arteries.[1] An angiogram will also identify nonrenal collateral arteries that have been parasitized by a renal tumor (Fig. 10-14). The overall vascularity, the amount of arteriovenous shunting, and the exact blood supply to the neoplasm can be defined. During the angiographic evaluation, the contralateral kidney is routinely evaluated for a synchronous tumor, renal artery stenosis, or other significant disease process that might drastically alter the surgical approach.

Patients undergoing renal arteriography to evaluate a renal tumor may have already had noninvasive studies that suggest a liver mass. If these examinations do not clearly define whether the hepatic mass is benign or malignant, a hepatic arteriogram can frequently define the nature of the liver mass. Renal neoplasms metastatic to the liver have a vascular pattern similar to that of the primary tumor from which they arise.[2] Therefore if a hepatic angiogram performed on a patient with a renal carcinoma demonstrates a liver mass with a vascular pattern similar to that of the renal mass, the study is diagnostic of renal carcinoma metastatic to the liver. Incidental hepatic masses, such as hemangiomas, also have characteristic angiographic findings.[3]

In the same setting as the arteriogram, a venogram of the inferior vena cava (IVC) and the renal veins of the affected kidney can be performed. This information is important in tumor staging and operative planning (Fig. 10–15).[4] In 21 to 55% of patients with renal cell carcinomas, venous invasion is present at the time of diagnosis. Tumor extends into the IVC in up to 70% of patients with venous extension.[5] The venogram will define the extent of venous extension relative to the hepatic veins and right atrium. Tumor growth up to or beyond the level of the hepatic veins greatly alters the surgical approach to nephrectomy.[6]

Patients with bilateral renal tumors, renal insufficiency, or one kidney and a renal mass may be considered for localized resection of the renal mass. Because of significant variability in arterial anatomy, it can be difficult to plan segmental resection from cross-sectional images. Angiography provides important information about the segmental vascular anatomy.

Preoperative embolization of hypervascular renal cell carcinomas has been shown to significantly reduce intraoperative blood loss.[7] The agent most frequently used for preoperative embolization is absolute alcohol (American Regent Laboratories, Shirley, NY). It is delivered through a balloon occlusion catheter in the main renal artery.[8] This agent induces vascular thrombosis at the arteriolar or capillary level, reducing the venous flow and the inflow from collateral vessels. The main renal artery can still be easily clamped in the operating room. Renal tumor embolization must be complete to be most effective, so it is important to embolize aberrant renal and parasitized nonrenal collateral arteries.[7] Particulate embolic material (Polyvinyl alcohol, Interventional Therapeutics Co., San Diego, CA) is used to occlude parasitized lumbar arteries in order to minimize the chance of causing spinal infarction. The embolization procedure is usually performed within 24 hours of the planned surgery in order to minimize the duration of postembolization symptoms that the patient experiences.

Nonresectable renal carcinomas can lead to gross hematuria, spontaneous retroperitoneal hemorrhage, or intractable pain. Transcatheter embolization can be used for palliation in these cases. These patients will usually develop the postembolization syndrome, which includes fever, pain, nausea, and vomiting for 3 to 4 days following the embolization.[8]

INDETERMINATE MASSES

With the widespread use of ultrasound (US), computed tomography (CT), and magnetic resonance imaging (MRI) in the evaluation of renal masses, angiography is often overlooked. In situations where the origin of a retroperitoneal or intra-abdominal mass is unclear by cross-sectional imaging, an angiogram can often localize the organ of origin of the mass.[9] Selective contrast injections of renal, adrenal, lumbar, hepatic, and mesenteric vessels facilitate delineation of the exact arterial supply to an abdominal or retroperitoneal mass. The origin of blood supply is a good indicator of the organ

Renal Angiography   221

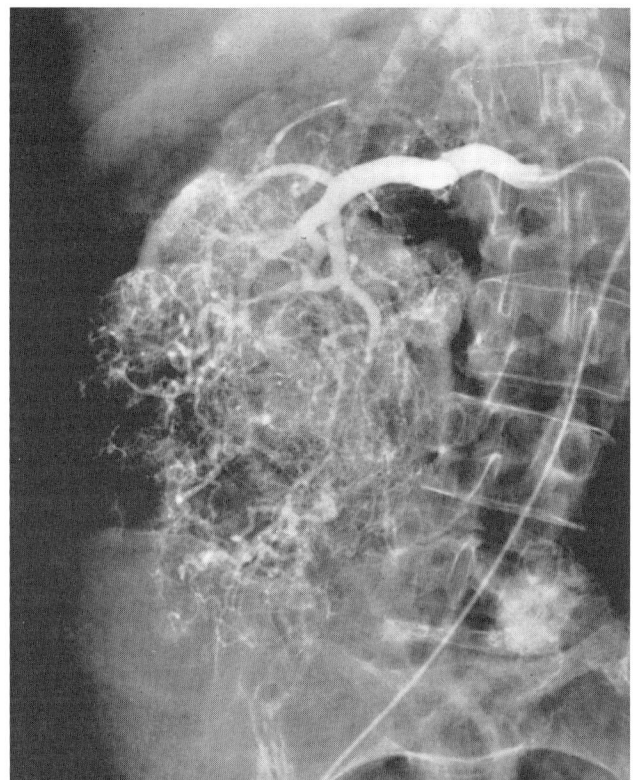

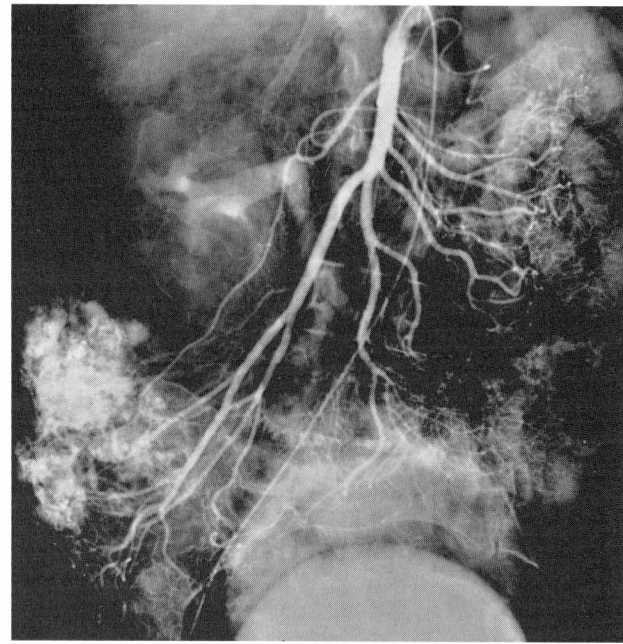

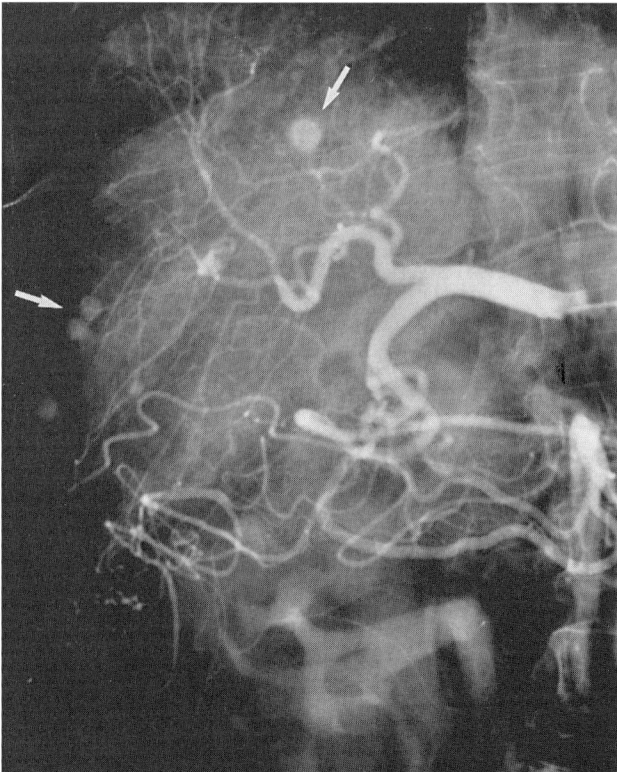

Figure 10–14. (**A**) Selective angiogram demonstrates the vascular changes of renal cell carcinoma. (**B**) Extensive parasitization from the superior mesenteric artery is seen. (**C**) Multiple liver metastases are demonstrated on hepatic arteriography (arrows).

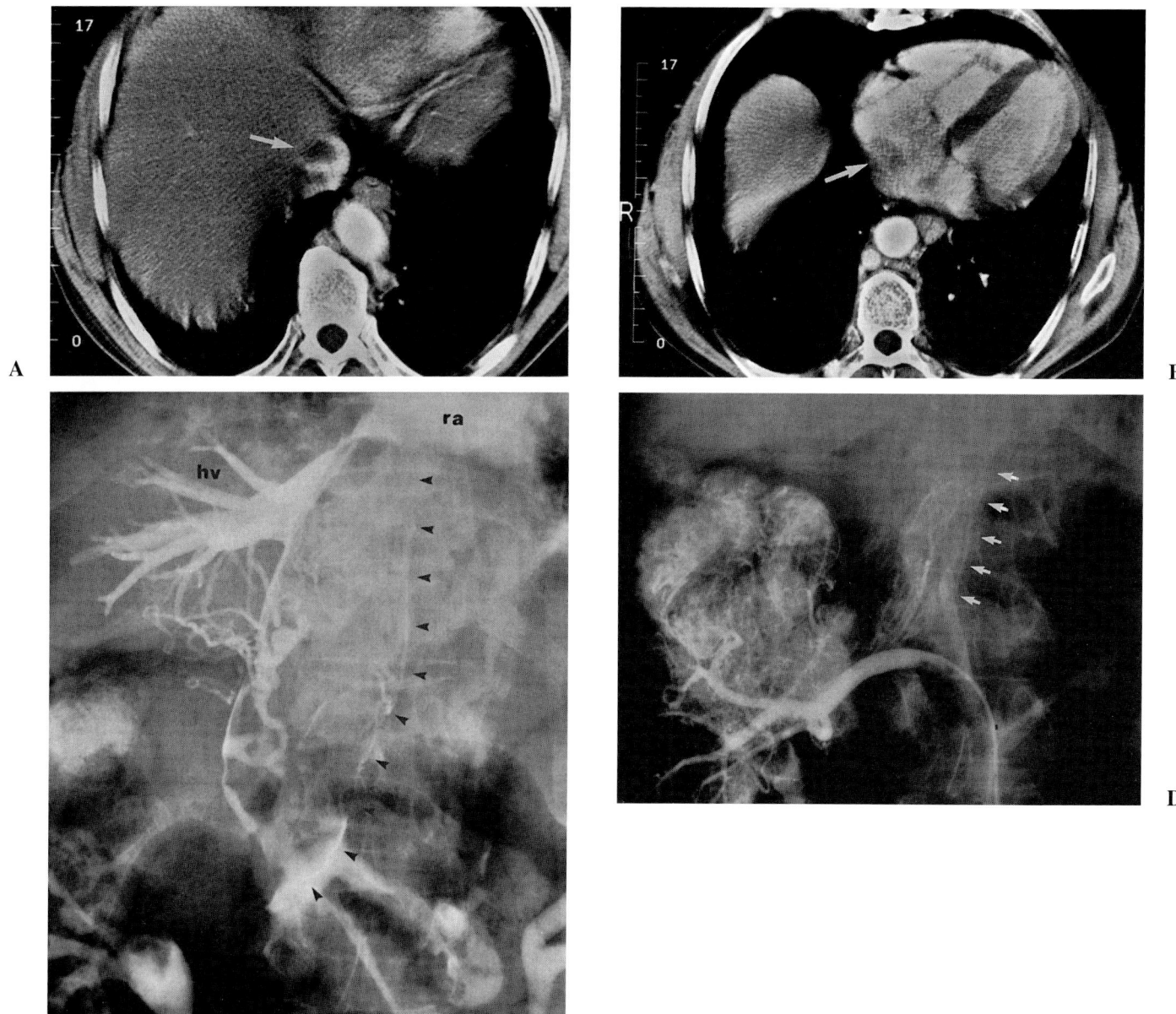

Figure 10–15. (**A,B**) CT scan demonstrates tumor thrombus near the floor of right atrium. (**C**) Venogram clearly shows the relation of the tumor thrombus to the right atrium (arrowheads). HV, hepatic veins; RA, right atrium. (**D**) Selective renal arteriogram reveals a renal tumor with tumor vascularity extending into the inferior vena cava (arrows). In a combined procedure with cardiothoracic surgeons, this renal cell carcinoma was resected.

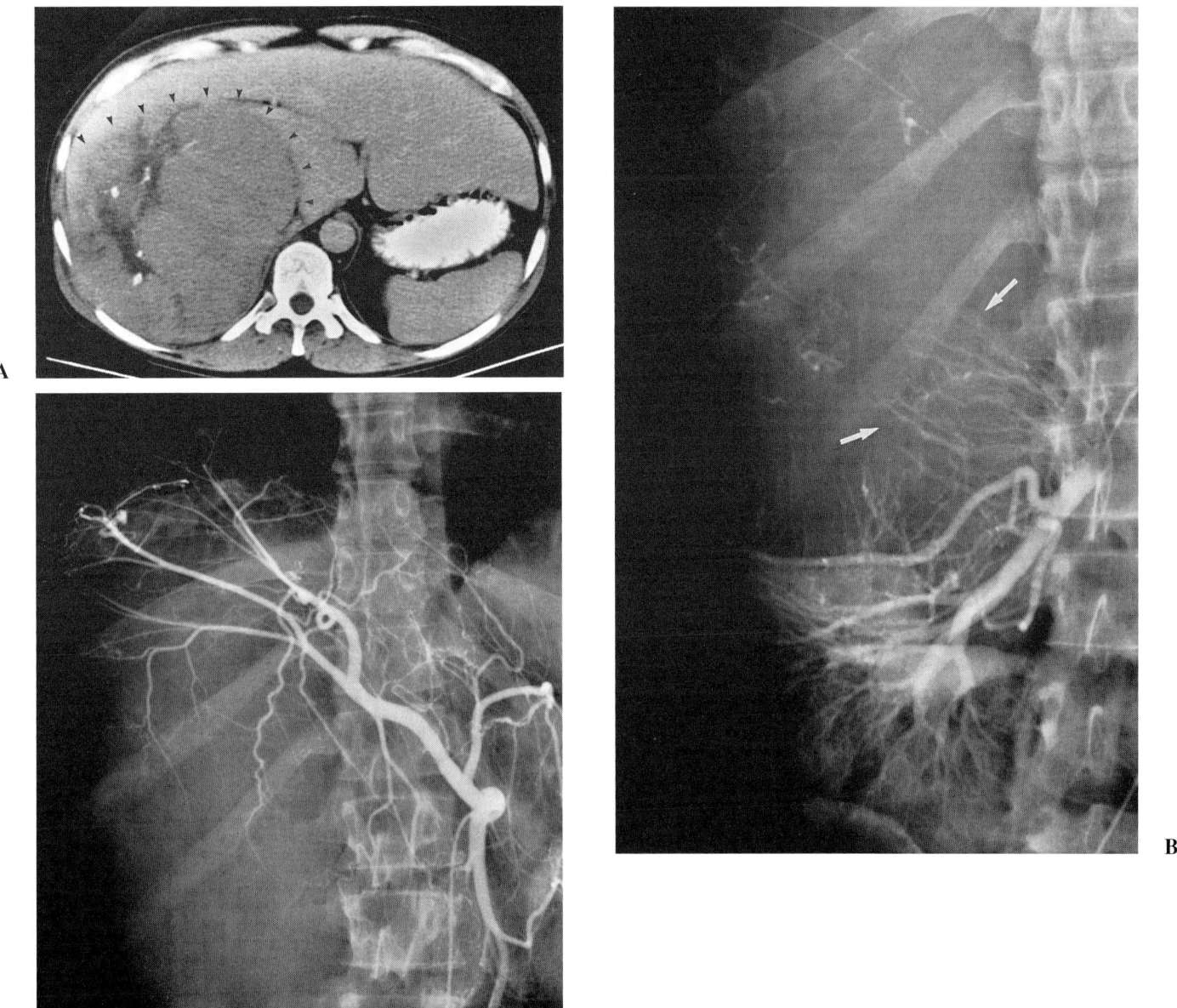

Figure 10–16. (**A**) CT scan shows a large retroperitoneal mass arising from either the kidney, adrenal, or liver (arrowheads). (**B**) The angiogram localized the mass to the adrenal gland. Selective injection of the renal artery reveals abnormal inferior adrenal arteries (arrows). (**C**) Celiac arteriogram shows marked cephalad displacement of the liver.

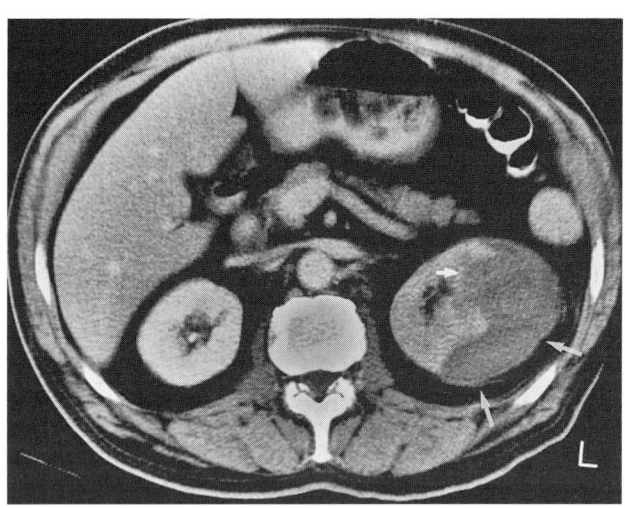 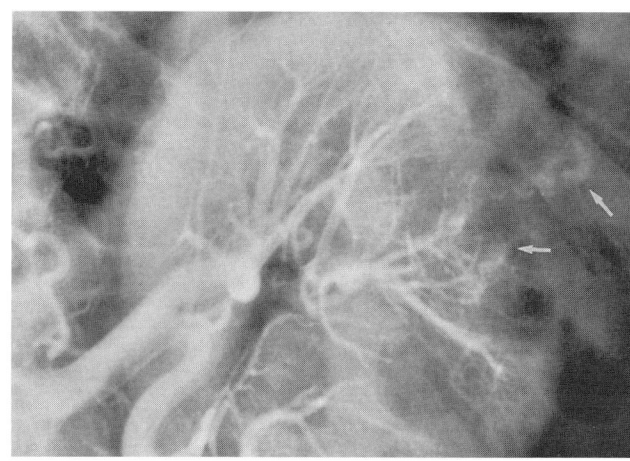

Figure 10–17. (A) CT reveals a subcapsular hematoma (arrows) and suggestion of an underlying renal mass (small arrow). (B) Magnification view of a selective left renal arteriogram reveals vascular encasement, and venous pooling. These angiographic findings are markers for malignancy, which was confirmed at surgery.

from which a neoplasm arises. One of the most common examples is the differentiation between an adrenal and an upper pole renal mass (Fig. 10–16).

Once the angiogram demonstrates the origin of a mass, evaluation of the angiogram can often provide a diagnosis. At a minimum, angiography can usually differentiate benign- from malignant-appearing vascularity (Fig. 10–17). The vessels feeding a renal cell carcinoma characteristically have an irregular appearance with abnormal tapering and unusual branching. Most renal cell carcinomas are hypervascular. An intense capillary blush and the presence of early-filling veins or abnormal venous lakes are additional angiographic signs of malignancy.[10] Renal angiography has been reported to have a 97% diagnostic accuracy for renal cell carcinoma.[11] Renal angiography can be most helpful when a renal mass is complicated by renal hemorrhage or when multiple renal cysts are present (Fig. 10–18).[12]

The widespread use of CT and US has led to the detection of many small or unsuspected renal masses. Angiography is being increasingly used to evaluate these small indeterminate renal masses. In patients with Von Hippel–Lindau disease and small renal tumors, angiography has been shown to have a 35% sensitivity in detecting renal neoplasms and a 100% specificity for determining which masses are malignant.[13] The high specificity confirms the reliability of the angiographic signs of malignancy.

The sensitivity of renal angiography can be enhanced by performing selective magnification angiography in multiple projections. Renal arteriography followed by selective intra-arterial epinephrine (Wyeth Laboratories, Philadelphia, PA) injections further improves the sensitivity of angiography.[14] Epinephrine (1:1000) is diluted to 1 μg/mL. Two to 4 μg of epinephrine is injected into the renal artery immediately prior to the angiogram. Epinephrine decreases flow in normal renal artery branches and tumor vessels fail to constrict. This differential response of the renal arteries to the epinephrine allows a subtle hypovascular renal cell carcinoma to become apparent during angiography. The actual accuracy of renal angiography for detecting renal carcinomas varies with each patient population studied, but overall it remains a fairly sensitive and highly specific examination.[11]

Renal venograms are an essential part of the workup for any indeterminate or small renal mass. The presence of venous tumor thrombus differentiates a benign from a malignant tumor. Selective venograms of the renal or adrenal veins can demonstrate subtle venous extension of tumor that might not be detected by CT, US, or MRI (Fig. 10–19).

The angiogram can also identify previously undetected metastases. Careful evaluation of the abdominal aortogram and selective celiac, hepatic, and lumbar angiograms may demonstrate metastases not seen on CT or US.[15] Lymph node involvement by metastatic tumor is identified on CT by size criteria. A hypervascular lymph node on angiography in a patient with renal cell carcinoma is highly specific for tumor spread, even if it is normal in size on CT. Spread into the mesentery can be easily missed by cross-sectional imaging studies but can be detected by angiography.

Renal carcinoma may present with symptoms suggestive of a bone metastasis. A screening bone scan obtained in a patient with a renal mass may also raise concern of a bone metastasis. Selective angiography of the affected area may reveal a vascular pattern similar to that seen in the primary renal mass, confirming spread of renal carcinoma to bone metastasis.[16]

Angiography is not a replacement for CT or US, but it is an important adjunct in the evaluation of renal tumors and for preoperative planning of kidney-sparing surgery.

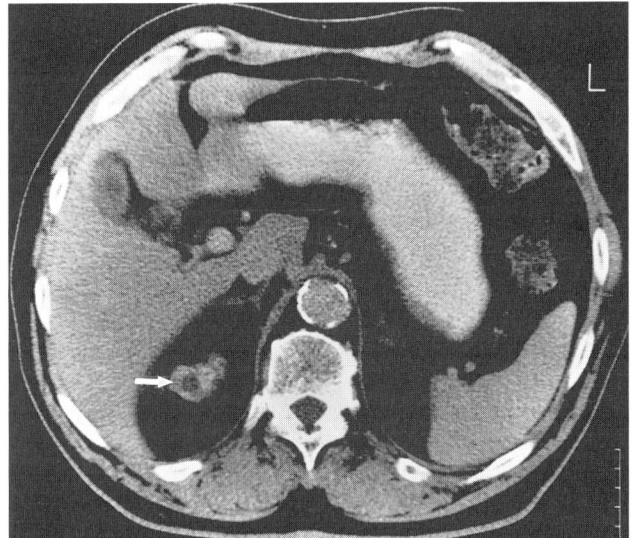
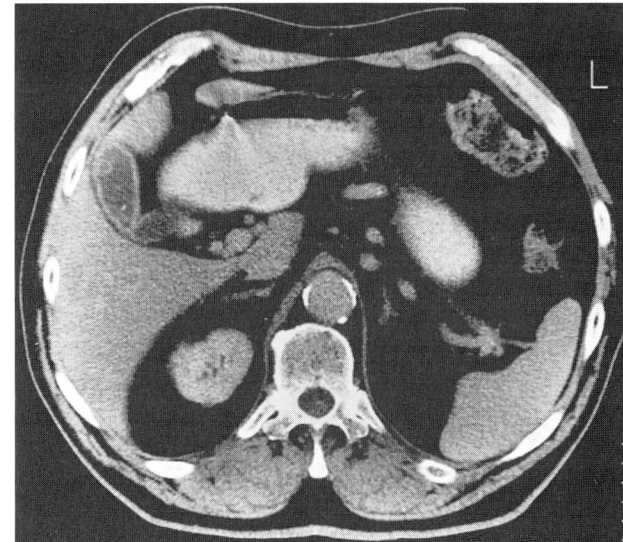
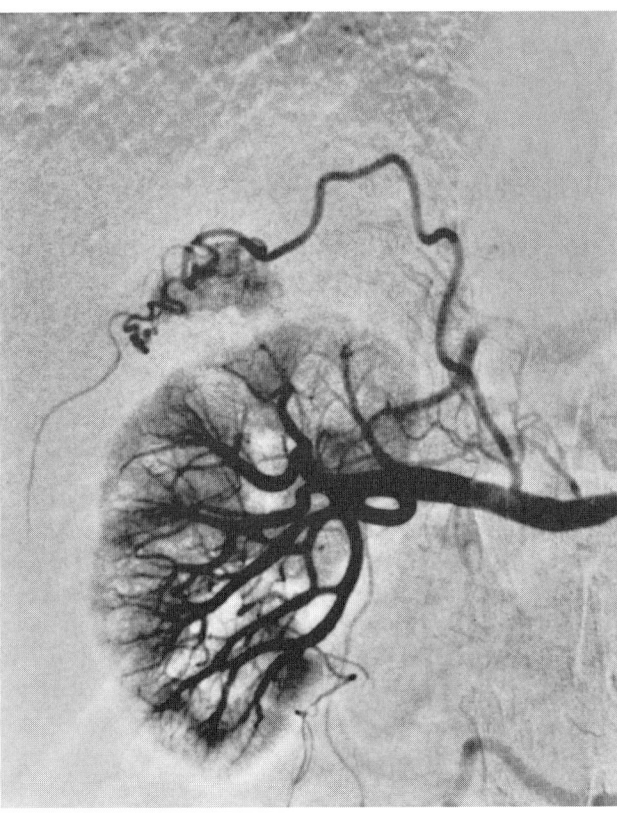

Figure 10–18. (A,B) CT examination shows a suspcious appearing cyst in the upper pole of the right kidney (arrow). (C) Selective right renal arteriogram demonstrates obvious tumor vascularity. Note the supply is predominantly from a capsular artery.

HEMATURIA

In the management of patients with hematuria, angiography can often localize the site and etiology of bleeding. Patients with no medical renal disease or urinary tract infection who present with painless hematuria are often evaluated with an intravenous urogram and CT. If these studies are normal, cystoscopy and retrograde pyelography are performed. If these examinations reveal a unilateral upper urinary tract source of bleeding, angiography should be performed to exclude an arteriovenous malformation (AVM), arterial aneurysm, or other vascular abnormality.

Patients with an AVM or aneurysm as the cause of hematuria can often be embolized using percutaneous transcatheter techniques. The abnormal artery is occluded superselectively to preserve as much renal function as possible. The technique is effective in occluding arteriovenous fistulas in more than 90% of patients (Fig. 10–20).[17,18] Following embolization, transient hypertension occurs in 5% of patients.[17] Patients with injury to intrarenal artery branch from

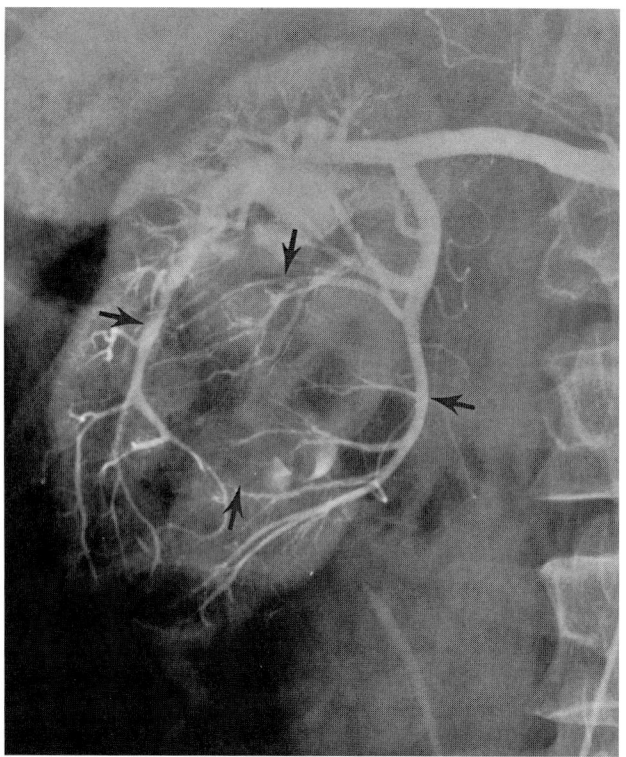
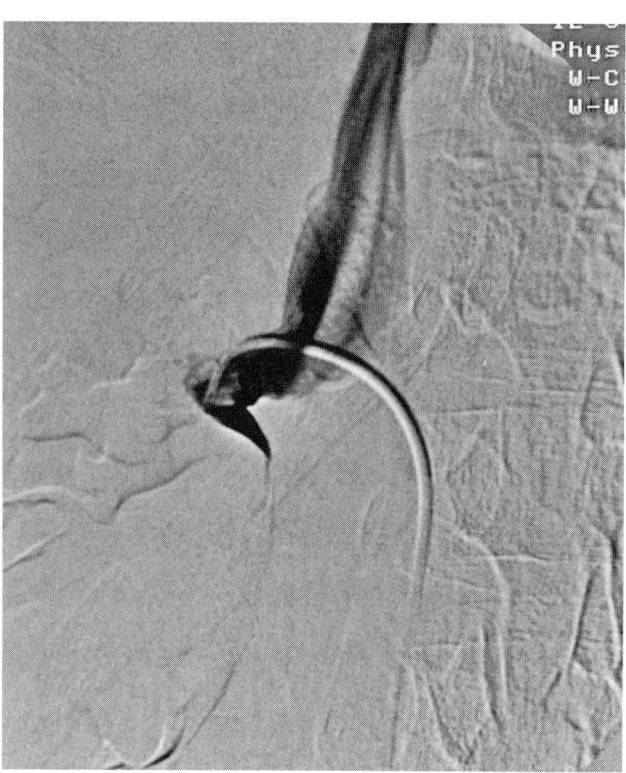

Figure 10–19. (A) Selective right renal angiogram reveals a nonspecific hypovascular mass (arrows). (B) Selective right renal venogram demonstrates venous occlusion secondary to tumor in the right renal vein, confirming the suspected diagnosis of renal cell carcinoma.

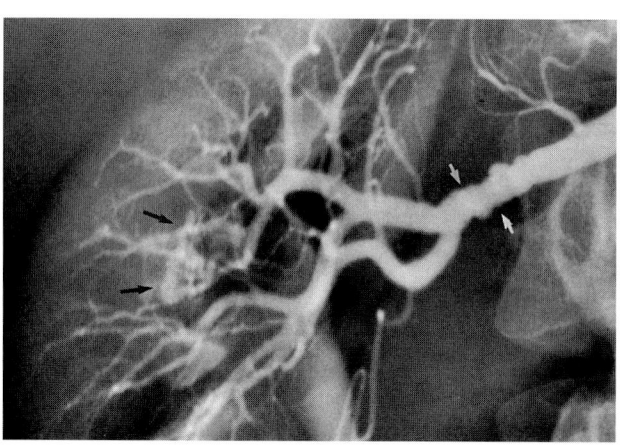
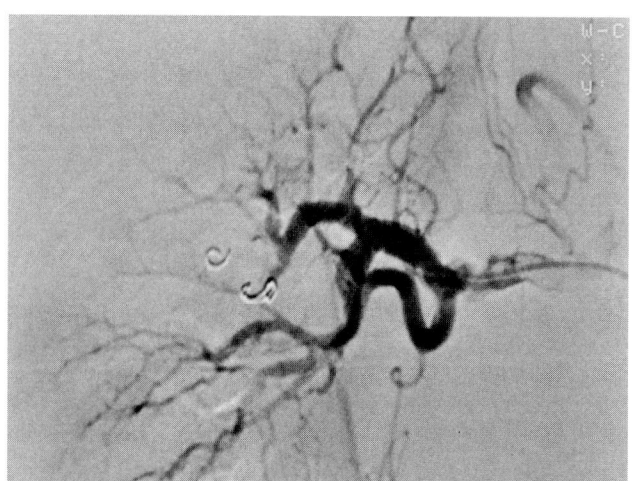

Figure 10–20. (A) Selective right renal arteriogram in a patient with persistent hematuria demonstrates an AVM (arrows). Incidental note is made of FMD in the distal renal artery (small arrows). (B) After superselective transcatheter embolization of the feeding renal artery branch, the vascular malformation has been occluded. The kidney has nearly normal perfusion postembolization.

TRAUMA

Patients with blunt or penetrating renal trauma may require angiography. The evaluation of trauma patients remains controversial, but patients with persistent hematuria arising from the kidney or ureter should have angiography. Trauma patients with an intravenous urogram demonstrating an asymmetric nephrogram should be further evaluated with CT or angiography (Fig. 10–21). Any patient being considered for operation to treat traumatic injury to the kidney should first have an angiogram. If the angiogram is not performed, then percutaneous embolization is excluded as a treatment option.

a biopsy, percutaneous nephrostomy, or other causes of hematuria can also be treated with percutaneous transcatheter embolization.

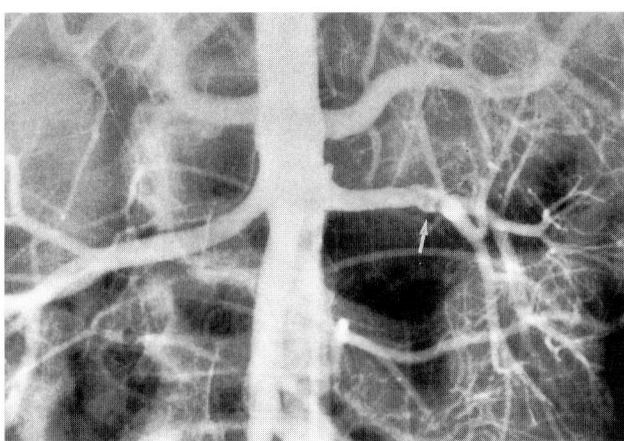

Figure 10–21. Ten-year-old girl with blunt trauma. She had hypoperfusion of the left kidney on intravenous urogram and CT. A nonselective injection of the abdominal aorta demonstrates intimal injury in the left renal artery (arrow).

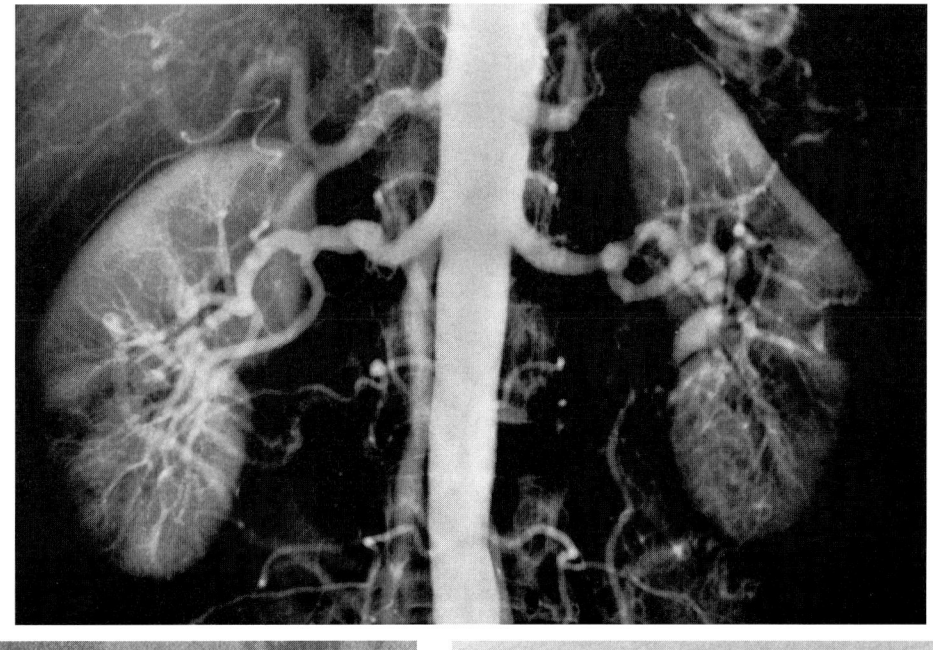

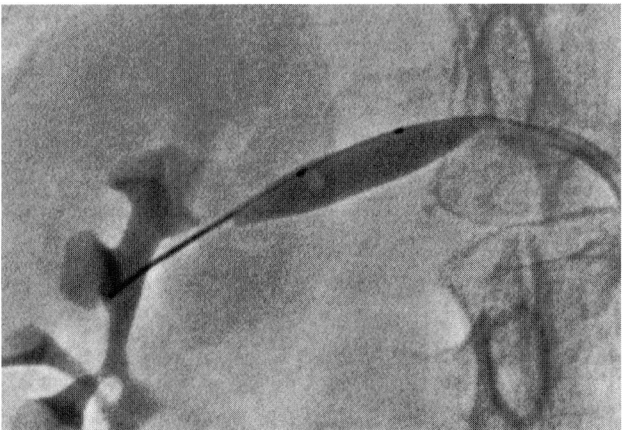

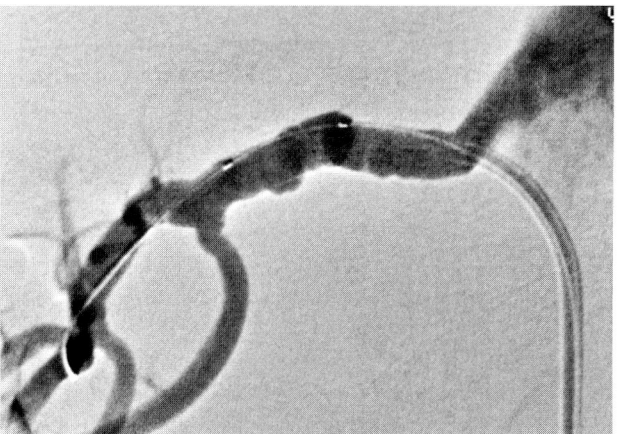

Figure 10–22. (A) Renal arteriogram with narrowing on the right due to fibromuscular dysplasia (arrow). (B) The lesion has been crossed using a 5-mm Tegtwire (Meditech, Boston, MA). (C) After renal PTA the vessel is widely patent.

RENOVASCULAR HYPERTENSION

Renal artery stenosis accounts for about 5% of cases of hypertension.[19] The etiology is usually atherosclerosis or fibromuscular disease (FMD). Clinical signs and symptoms include the sudden acceleration of hypertension, hypertension that is difficult to control even with multiple medications, a sudden decrease in renal function when treated with captopril, and/or a flank bruit.[20] Peripheral and selective renal vein renin samples, captopril nuclear medicine scans, duplex ultrasound, intravenous digital subtraction angiography, magnetic resonance angiography, and CT have been used to screen for renovascular hypertension.[21–23] As yet none of these screening tests has been shown to be reliable or cost effective. Renal angiography remains the gold standard for defining renal artery stenoses, and it provides access for definitive therapy with percutaneous transluminal angioplasty (PTA).

Patients with a clinical picture suggestive of renovascular hypertension or patients with a positive screening test should have a renal angiogram. At our institution, patients with angiographically significant renal artery stenosis and an appropriate clinical history for renovascular hypertension are treated with PTA immediately following the diagnostic angiogram. Those that have equivocal stenoses have selective renal vein renin sampling done at the same time as the angiogram and are treated according to the results either medically or with PTA.

The results of renal PTA vary with the etiology of the arterial stenosis. In patients with FMD the initial technical success rate is greater than 95%. The clinical cure rate is 25 to 85%, with 85 to 100% demonstrating clinical benefit (Fig. 10–22).[24,25] PTA is the treatment of choice for symptomatic FMD of the renal arteries.[24,26] In patients with atherosclerotic renal artery stenosis, the initial technical success rate of renal PTA is 75 to 97%. Approximately 25% of patients are cured and another 55% show clinical improvement in follow-up of 1 to 2 years.[26–28] The addition of newer techniques involving atherectomy devices and vascular stents further improves the initial technical success rate, but long-term results with these devices are not yet available.[29]

RENAL TRANSPLANTS

Hypertension is common in renal transplant patients. This is often due to rejection, but transplant renal artery stenosis can also cause hypertension or renal insufficiency. Evaluation of renal transplants with angiography can provide important information on the patency of the iliac artery providing inflow to the transplanted renal artery, the transplant renal artery, the intrarenal arterial branches, and the renal vein. Many transplant renal artery stenoses are amenable to PTA (Fig. 10–23). The technical success rate for angioplasty of transplant renal arteries is 76%; clinical improvement is demonstrated in 81% of patients at 1 year.[30]

RENAL DONORS

Renal angiography is performed routinely in prospective kidney donors. Although more than one-third of patients

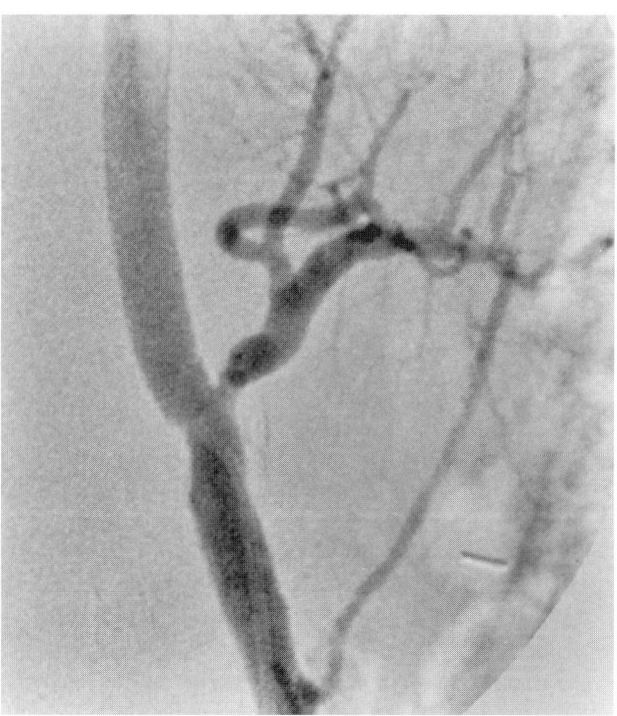
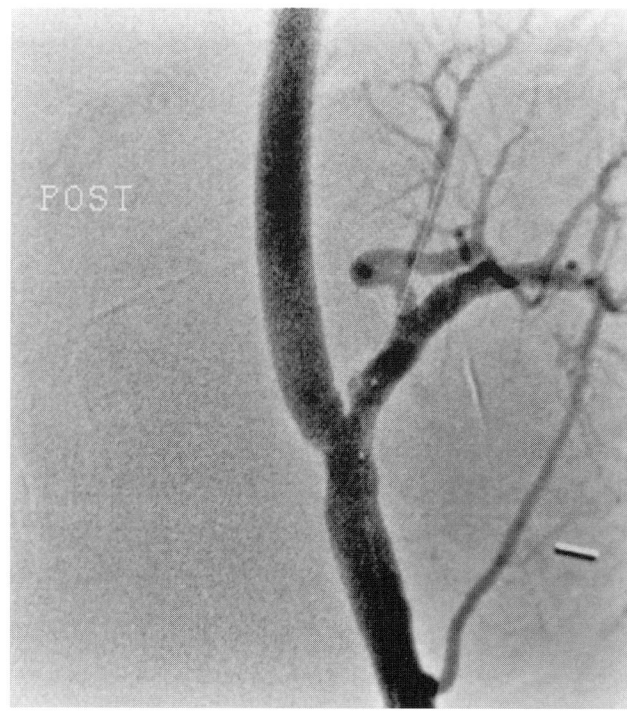

Figure 10–23. (A) Proximal renal transplant artery narrowing. (B) After balloon dilatation there is no significant residual narrowing.

have multiple renal arteries, only 12% have multiple renal arteries bilaterally.[31] Thus angiography is an essential prerequisite to choosing the correct kidney to harvest. Angiography will also demonstrate significant renovascular disease in 6% of potential renal donors.[31]

SUMMARY

Renal angiography remains an important diagnostic and therapeutic tool. In the evaluation of renal masses, angiography provides an accurate evaluation of tumor origin, vascularity, and location for surgical planning, and provides an opportunity for preoperative embolization. Although many patients with renal masses have an extensive cross-sectional imaging evaluation, renal angiography continues to provide the sole method to accurately delineate the arterial and venous anatomy. In many cases, angiography can localize a retroperitoneal tumor that is of uncertain origin by other studies.

In the workup of hematuria or spontaneous retroperitoneal hemorrhage, angiography is invaluable in localizing the site of bleeding, and in many centers arterial embolization provides a safe and effective treatment.

Despite advances in cross-sectional imaging, arteriography remains the standard for evaluation of renovascular hypertension. The success of renal artery PTA for the treatment of renovascular hypertension has also been well demonstrated.

REFERENCES

1. Merklin RJ, Michels NA: The variant renal and suprarenal blood supply with data on the inferior phrenic, ureteral and gonadal arteries. *J Int Coll Surg* 1958;29:41–76.
2. Abrams HL: Renal tumor versus renal cyst. In: Abrams HL, ed. *Abrams Angiography Vascular and International Radiology 2*, 3rd ed. Boston: Little, Brown, 1983;1123–1174.
3. Hellekant C, Nyman U: Routine celiac angiography in patients with renal cell carcinoma. *J Urol* 1979;122:17–19.
4. Simpson A, Murray GB, Mitty HA: Angiographic patterns of venous extension of hypernephroma. *J Urol* 1974;111:441–444.
5. Goncharenko V, Gerlock AJ Jr, Kadir S, Turner B: Incidence and distribution of venous extension in 70 hypernephromas. *Am J Roentgenol* 1979;133:263–265.
6. Henriksson C, Aldenborg F, Haljamae H, et al: Renal cell carcinoma with vena cava extension: diagnostic and surgical features of 41 cases. *Scand J Urol Nephrol* 1987;21:291–296.
7. Bakal CW, Cynamon J, Lakritz PS, Sprayregen S: Value of preoperative renal artery embolization in reducing blood transfusion requirements during nephrectomy for renal cell carcinoma. *J Vasc Interv Radiol* 1993;4:727–731.
8. Rabe FE, Yune HY, Richmond BD, et al: Renal tumor infarction with absolute ethanol. *Am J Roentgenol* 1982;139:1139–1144.
9. Kolmannkog F, Kolbenstuedt A, Brekke IB: Computed tomography and angiography in adrenocortical carcinoma. *Acta Radiol* 1992;3:45–49.
10. Levine E: Renal cell carcinoma: radiological diagnosis and staging. *Semin Roentgenol* 1987;22:248–259.
11. Watson RC, Fleming RJ, Evans JA: Arteriography in the diagnosis of renal carcinoma. *Radiology* 1968;91:888–897.
12. Tegtmeyer CJ, Cail W, Wyker AW, Jr, et al: Angiographic diagnosis of renal tumors associated with polycystic disease. *Radiology* 1978;126:105–109.
13. Miller DL, Choyke PL, Walther MM, et al: Von Hippel-Lindau disease: inadequacy of angiography for identification of renal cancer. *Radiology* 191;179:833–836.
14. Kahn PC, Wise HM Jr: The use of epinephrine in selective angiography of renal masses. *J Urol* 1968;99:133–138.
15. Nakamura M, Vozumi J, Veda T, Kumazawa J: Renal cell carcinoma with unusual metastases detected by angiography. *Urol Int* 1992;48:446–449.
16. Bosniak MA, O'Connor JF, Caplan LH: Renal arteriography in patients with metastatic renal cell carcinoma: its use as a substitute for histopathologic biopsy. *JAMA* 1968;203:249–254.
17. Benett JB, Kadir S: Embolization for the management of aneurysms, fistulas and AVMs of the renal artery. In: Kadir S, ed. *Current Practice of Interventional Radiology*. Philadelphia: BC Becker, 1991;631–637.
18. Tarkington MA, Matsumoto AH, Dejter SW, Regan JB: Spectrum of renal vascular malformation. *Urology* 1991;38:297–300.
19. Danielson M, Dammstrom BG: The prevalence of secondary and curable hypertension. *Acta med Scand* 1981;209:451–455.
20. Simon N, Franklin SS, Bleifer KH, et al: Clinical characteristics of renovascular hypertension. *JAMA* 1972;220:1209–1217.
21. Galanksi M, Prokop M, Chavan A, et al: Renal artery stenosis: spiral CT angiography. *Radiology* 1993;189:185–192.
22. Dunnick NR, Svetkey LP, Cohan RH, et al: Intravenous digital subtraction renal angiography: use in screening for renovascular hypertension. *Radiology* 1989;171:219–222.
23. Debtain JF, Spritzer CE, Grist TM, et al: Imaging of the renal arteries: value of MR angiography. *Am J Roentgenol* 1991;157:981–990.
24. Tegtmeyer CJ, Selby JB, Hartwell GD, Ayers C, Tegtmeyer V: Results and complications of angioplasty in fibromuscular disease. *Circulation* 1991;83(suppl):155–161.
25. Wise KL, McCann RL, Dunnick NR, Paulson DF: Renovascular hypertension. *J Urol* 1988;140:911–924.
26. Lüscher TF, Lie JT, Stanson AW, et al: Arterial Fibromuscular Dysplasia. *Mayo Clin Proc* 1987;62:931–952.
27. Tegtmeyer CJ, Kellum CD, Ayers C: Percutaneous transluminal angioplasty of the renal artery. *Radiology* 1984;153:77–84.
28. Sos TA: Angioplasty for the treatment of azotemia and renovascular hypertension in atherosclerotic renal artery disease. *Circulation* 1991;83(suppl 1):162–166.
29. Hennequin LM, Joffre FG, Rousseau HP, et al: Renal artery stent placement: long-term results with the Wallstent endoprosthesis. *Radiology* 1994;191:713–719.
30. Rodriguez-Perez JC, Plaza C, Reyers R, Pulido-Duque JM, et al: Treatment of renovascular hypertension with percutaneous transluminal angioplasty: experience in Spain. *J Vasc Interv Radiol* 1994;5:101–109.
31. Spring DB, Salvatierra O Jr, Palubinskas AJ, et al: Results and significance of angiography in potential kidney donors. *Radiology* 1979;133:45–47.

11 Pediatric Uroradiology

Thomas E. Sumner, Sam T. Auringer

Evaluation of the abnormal urinary tract in children has changed as new and improved imaging techniques have been developed. During the last decade, the intravenous urogram (IVU) has generally been replaced by ultrasonography for depiction of anatomy and for assessment of renal function by nuclear imaging. Infant IVUs are frequently suboptimal because a full bladder impedes upper tract emptying and because newborn kidneys have low concentrating ability. Tomographic sections may facilitate visualization of renal outlines and collecting systems when IVUs are obtained. We prefer ultrasonography for initial evaluation of the upper and lower pediatric urinary tract; this technique alone may be diagnostic, or it may be supplemented by voiding cystourethrography (VCUG) and radionuclide imaging. The IVU remains useful for evaluation of stone disease and diagnosis of ectopic ureter in the incontinent young female patient.

Prenatal ultrasound screening for urinary tract abnormalities is frequently performed. Oligohydramnios is a common indication for ultrasound evaluation of the fetal urinary tract since fetal urine is the major contributor to the formation of amniotic fluid. In utero detection of reflux, obstruction, and tumors has been reported. Parents with a history of genetic renal diseases, such as polycystic kidney disease, or congenital disorders, such as renal dysplasia, may request prenatal screening. Postnatal imaging is required to confirm abnormalities suggested by prenatal ultrasonography. Equivocal prenatal and postnatal sonograms may require further evaluation with a VCUG, renal scintigraphy, or both.

This chapter discusses indications for and major findings observed during postnatal imaging of pediatric urinary tract abnormalities. Specific genitourinary tract abnormalities to be discussed are listed in Table 11–1.

RENAL AGENESIS AND ECTOPIA

Renal agenesis results from failure of formation or atresia of one or both metanephric diverticula or ureteric buds. Bilateral agenesis occurs with a frequency of 1 in 4000; boys are affected approximately three times more commonly than girls.[1] Bilateral renal agenesis is associated with fetal compression and severe bilateral pulmonary hypoplasia caused by oligohydramnios from fetal anuria.

Postnatal sonography reveals discoid or "pancake" adrenals that occupy the renal fossa and mimic kidneys (Figs. 11–1, 11–2).[1] Unilateral renal agenesis, much more common than the bilateral form, occurs in 0.1 to 0.2% of live births; it affects the left kidney more often than the right and is also more common in boys than in girls.[2] Coexistent genitourinary tract anomalies are common.[2] Approximately 66% of girls with unilateral renal agenesis have an ipsilateral müllerian duct anomaly.[2] With absence of the uterus and upper two-thirds of the vagina (Mayer–Rokitansky–Küster–Hauser syndrome), there is a 12 to 16% incidence of renal agenesis. The adrenal glands remain present in renal agenesis and ectopia; they occupy the renal fossae and are elongated and discoid. Since the normal newborn adrenal is large and easily seen, one must be careful not to mistake the adrenal for a small kidney; this error may be avoided by searching for the large medullary pyramids that typify neonatal kidneys (Fig. 11–3). A kidney in an ectopic position, usually in the pelvis, is common and should not be evaluated with ultrasound alone. It likely results from anomalous migration of the ureteric bud and is usually associated with failure of ascent, unusual orientation, and abnormal number of pelves and calyces. As a result, ectopic kidneys are susceptible to hydronephrosis, infection, and calculi formation. Furthermore, ectopic kidneys are predisposed to additional anomalies such as multicystic dysplasia and obstruction, and full evaluation may require other imaging studies such as IVU or nuclear scintigraphy (Fig. 11–4). Other variations of renal ectopia include crossed renal ectopia, crossed-fused renal ectopia, and horseshoe kidney.

Horseshoe kidney, with an incidence of 1 in 400 births, is the most common renal fusion anomaly. It results from the partial failure of renal ascent and the fusion of the lower

Table 11–1. Pediatric Urinary Tract Abnormalities

Renal agenesis and ectopia
Ureteropelvic junction obstruction
Ureterovesical junction obstruction
Duplication anomalies/ureterocele complex
Posterior urethral valves
Prune-belly syndrome
Vesicoureteral reflux
Urinary tract infection
Renal cystic disease
Renal vein thrombosis
Adrenal hemorrhage

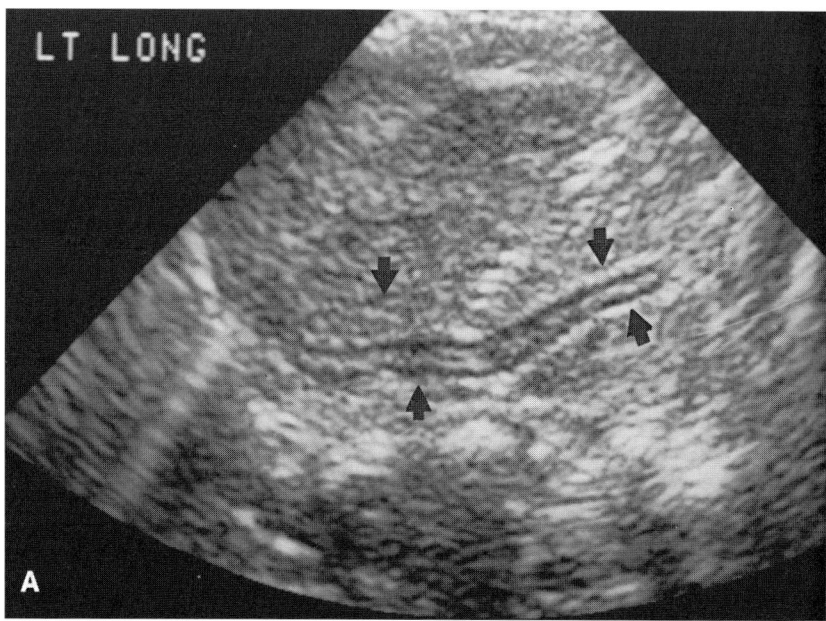
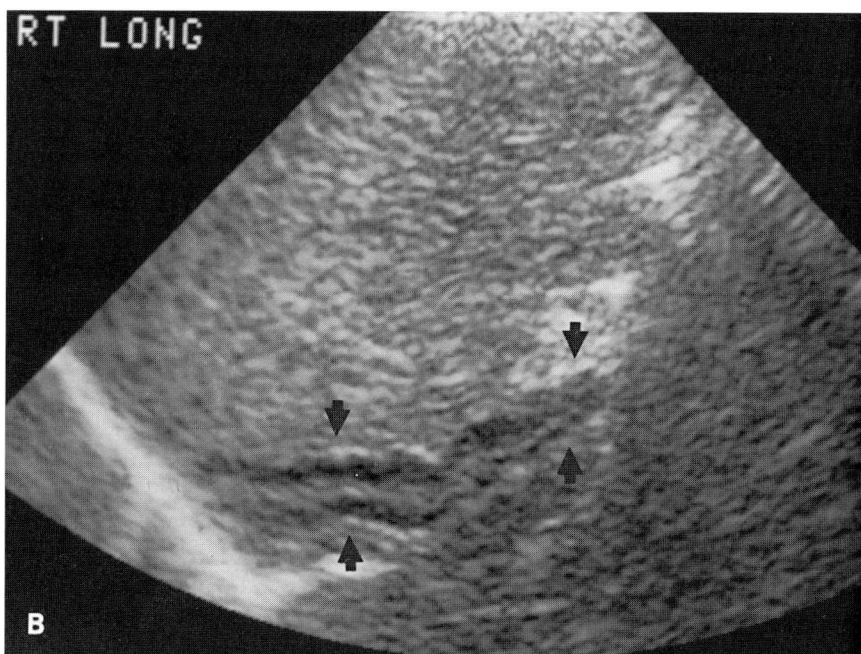

Figure 11–1. Bilateral renal agenesis. **(A)** Longitudinal sonogram through the left flank shows an elongated adrenal gland (arrows) and no demonstrable kidney. **(B)** Longitudinal scan through the right flank shows a discoid ("pancake") adrenal (arrows) occupying the renal fossa.

poles of the kidneys, producing a parenchymal or fibrous isthmus that crosses the midline. Approximately one-third of patients have associated genitourinary, cardiovascular, or skeletal anomalies. Similar to other ectopic kidneys, horseshoe kidneys are more susceptible to hydronephrosis, calculi, and infection. Typical sonographic findings are medially oriented inferior poles and an isthmus of tissue crossing the midline (Fig. 11–5).

OBSTRUCTION AND REFLUX

Although obstruction and reflux are physiologically separate entities, they may coexist. Both produce dilated upper tracts, and the widespread use of prenatal ultrasonography has led to frequent in utero detection of hydronephrosis. When intrauterine hydronephrosis is detected, postpartum sonography is indicated for confirmation, and additional imaging with VCUG, scintigraphy, or both may be warranted to exclude reflux. Postpartum sonography is best performed several days to 1 week after delivery so that patient rehydration and improved glomerular filtration rate will optimize detection of obstructing lesions.

The most common obstructive uropathies, accounting for 87% of cases of neonatal hydronephrosis, are ureteropelvic junction (UPJ) obstruction, ureterovesical junction (UVJ) obstruction, duplication anomalies and ureterocele, and posterior urethral valves (PUV).[3] Less common conditions pro-

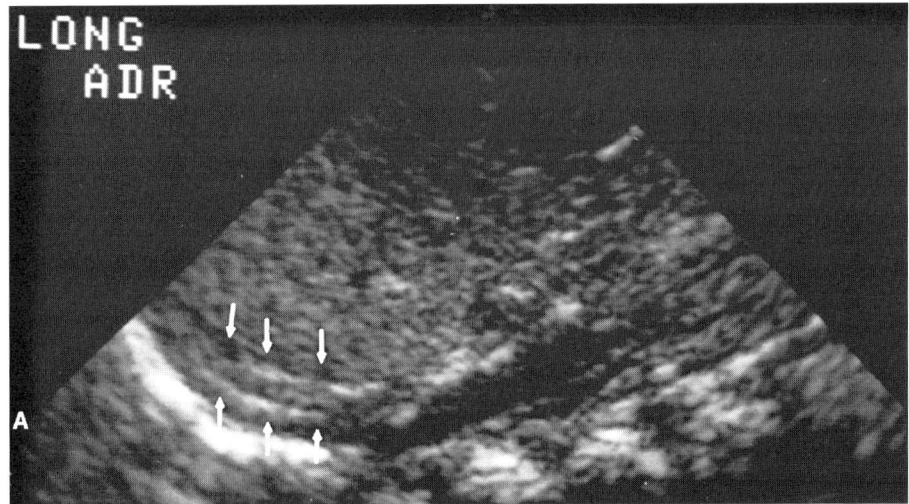

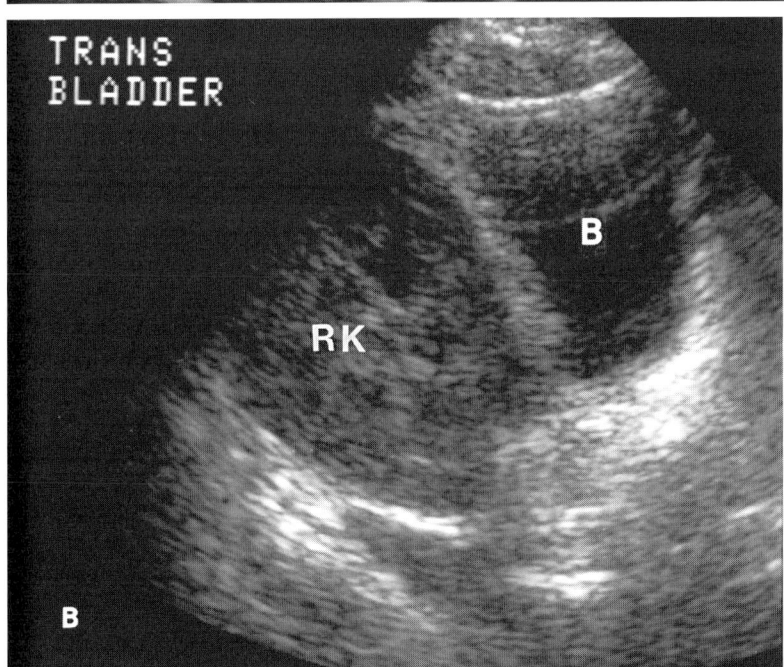

Figure 11–2. Mayer–Rokitansky–Küster–Hauser syndrome. **(A)** Longitudinal sonogram reveals elongated right adrenal (white arrows). **(B)** Transverse view shows solitary abdominopelvic right kidney (RK), bladder (B).

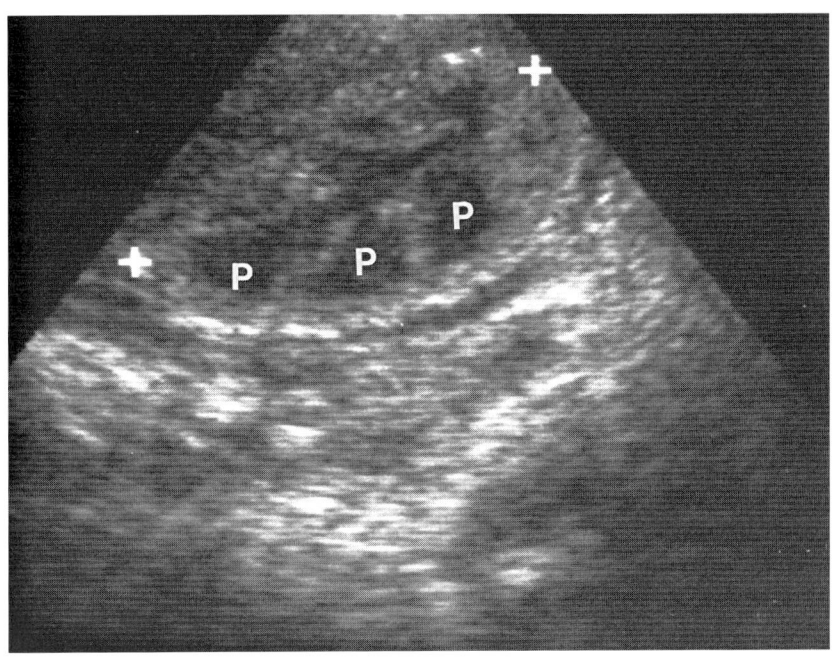

Figure 11–3. Normal infant kidney. Longitudinal sonogram shows the typical prominent hypoechoic renal pyramids (P).

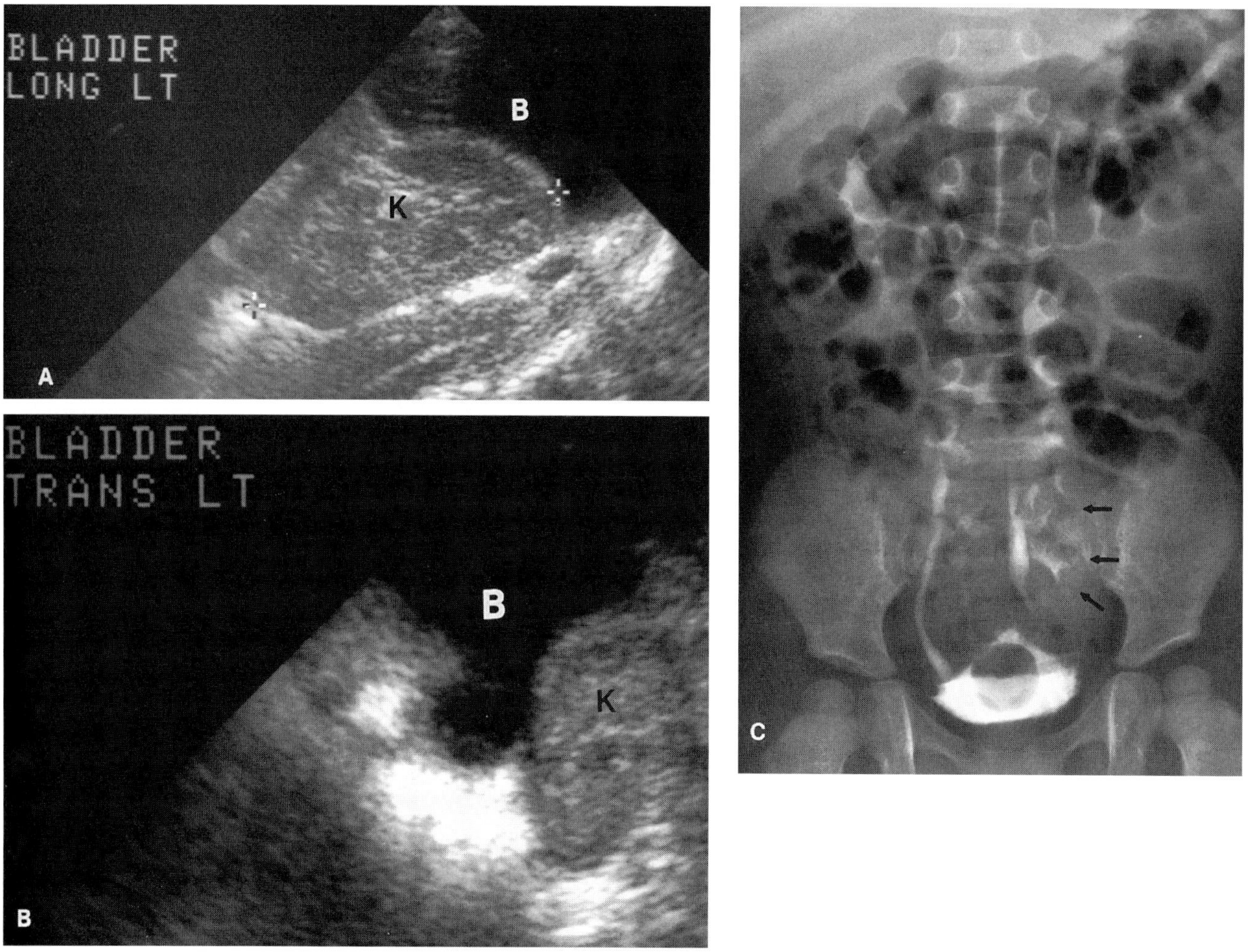

Figure 11–4. Pelvic kidney. **(A)** Longitudinal and **(B)** transverse sonograms show the left pelvic kidney (K), (B) bladder. **(C)** Excretory urography confirms pelvic location of left kidney (arrows).

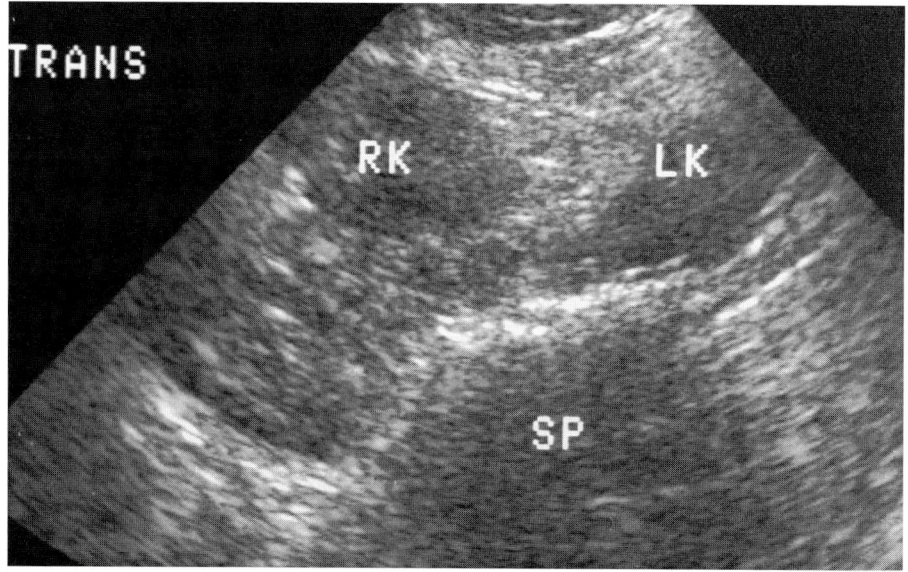

Figure 11–5. Horseshoe kidney. Transverse sonogram shows medially oriented lower poles of the kidneys (RK, LK) crossing anteriorly to the spine (SP).

ducing hydronephrosis are prune-belly syndrome, vesicoureteral reflux (VUR), megacystis–microcolon–intestinal hypoperistalsis syndrome, and cloacal anomalies.

Ureteropelvic Junction Obstruction

The most common obstructive lesion of the urinary tract in children is UPJ obstruction, which accounts for approximately 40% of all cases of significant hydronephrosis.[3] UPJ obstruction is more common on the left and boys are affected five times more frequently than girls.[4] UPJ obstruction is bilateral in approximately 30% of cases.[5] UPJ obstruction is suggested by abnormal in utero ultrasound results; a palpable mass; or, in older children, abdominal pain, hematuria, or urinary tract infection. Flank pain associated with increased fluid intake is another classic presentation. The etiology of UPJ obstruction remains controversial, but a congenital etiology is favored, and intrinsic stenosis or extrinsic compression from muscle fibers, adhesions, or aberrant vessels may be the culprit. Regardless of its origin, the result is hydronephrosis, which may cause renal dysplasia if it is severe.

Sonography is the initial imaging modality regardless of the patient's age. A typical image shows multiple interconnecting cystic structures converging on a dilated pelvis (Fig. 11–6). Additional sonographic features are visible renal parenchyma and lack of visualization of a distal ureter. The renal parenchyma is usually thin, with normal or increased echogenicity, or contains cysts corresponding to histologic areas of renal dysplasia (Fig. 11–7).[6] Severe obstruction may result in urinoma formation or urinary ascites secondary to rupture of the collecting system. As mentioned, the ureter is typically normal and not visualized. If ipsilateral ureteral dilatation is detected, coexisting VUR or distal ureteral obstruction should be suspected and VCUG performed to evaluate for reflux.

The degree and level of obstruction can be assessed with IVU or renal scintigraphy. We prefer diuretic renal scintigraphy to differentiate urinary tract obstruction from urinary tract dilatation without significant obstruction. Diuretic renal scintigraphy is generally performed with 99m Tc-labeled DTPA or 99m Tc-labeled MAG 3 as the tracer; a diuretic (generally furosemide) is administered intravenously after the tracer has collected in the hydronephrotic collecting system. Renal washout is then assessed with a computer-generated time activity curve (Fig. 11–8).

Ureterovesical Junction Obstruction

Megaureter is the term used to describe a dilated and tortuous ureter that can be the result of obstruction, reflux, atony, or maldevelopment. Usage of this term, however, is inconsistent in the urologic and radiologic literature. When the etiology is known, *megaureter* should be preceded by the terms *primary, secondary, obstructive, nonobstructive, refluxing, nonrefluxing,* or a combination. In this discussion, the term *primary megaureter* will be used to refer to a subcategory of obstructed megaureter, hence the term *primary obstructive megaureter* (POM). POM results from a normal-caliber aperistaltic 0.5- to 4-cm distal (juxtavesical) ureteral segment, which causes a functional obstruction.[7]

Primary obstructive megaureter is the most common cause of distal ureteral obstruction in children.[8] Prenatal ultrasound detection of hydronephrosis is the most frequent clinical pre-

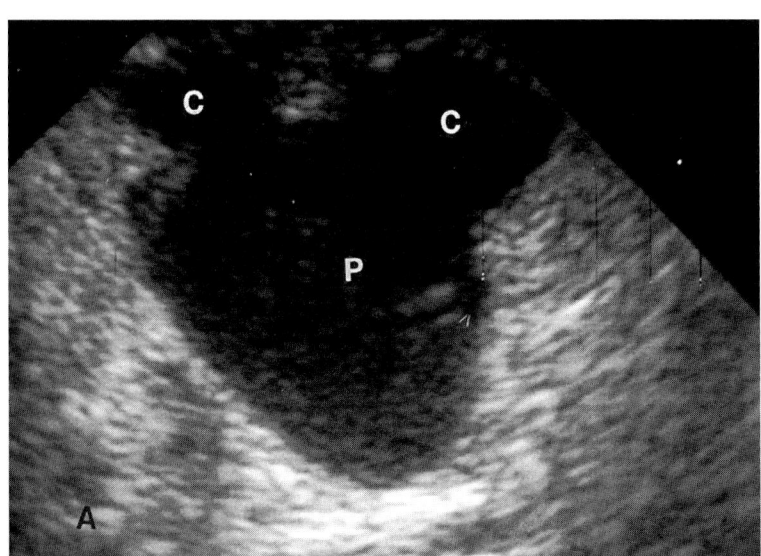
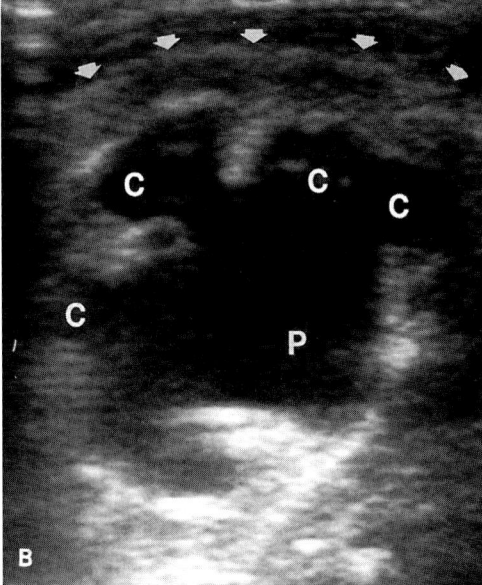

Figure 11–6. Ureteropelvic junction (UPJ) obstruction. **(A)** Longitudinal and **(B)** transverse sonograms show dilated calyces (C) communicating with a markedly dilated pelvis (P). Note the thin rim of parenchyma (arrowheads) surrounding the dilated collecting system. No distal ureter was visualized.

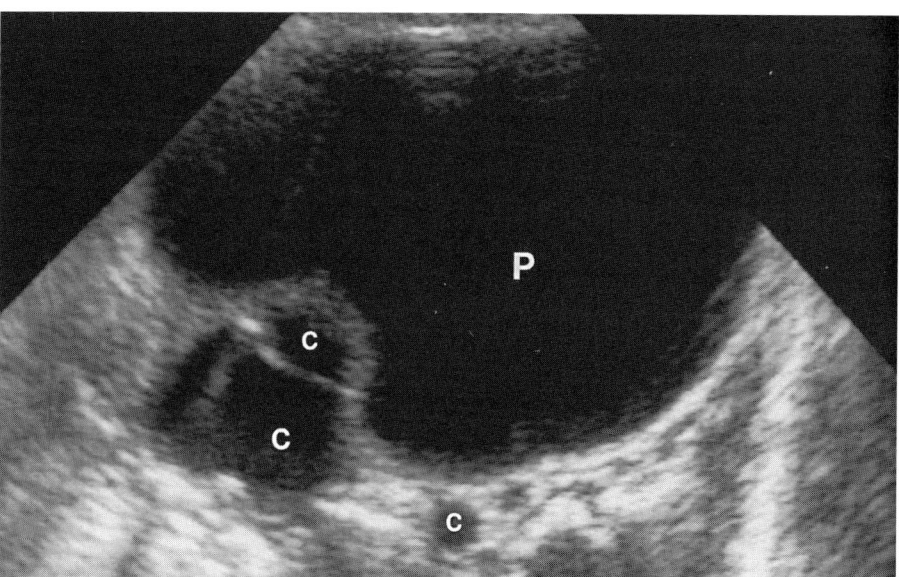

Figure 11–7. UPJ obstruction with dysplasia. Transverse scan demonstrates markedly dilated pelvis (P) with peripheral cystic dysplastic parenchyma (C).

sentation; urinary tract infection, often with urosepsis and flank mass, is common in infancy and childhood.[9] Most patients are male (67%), the POM is usually unilateral (85%), and when it is unilateral, it occurs usually on the left side (78%).[9] POM is more often bilateral in patients less than 1 year old; contralateral renal agenesis occurs in about 10% of cases.

Sonography of POM reveals ureteral dilatation, which may terminate in a narrow distal segment, lower ureteral hyperperistalsis with an adynamic narrowed termination, and disproportionate lower ureteral dilatation as compared with upper ureteral and pelvocalyceal dilatation (Fig. 11–9).[10] Differentiating between an obstructed collecting system and a nonobstructed renal collecting system that is dilated because of reflux is difficult. Since routine ultrasonography cannot rule out significant VUR, evaluation should include a VCUG to exclude reflux and distal obstruction. A functional assessment, usually with a nuclear renal scan (99m Tc-labeled DTPA), is suggested for split renal function quantitation and to establish a baseline for follow-up studies (Fig. 11–9). Significant spontaneous regression or complete resolution of POM may occur in infancy.[11] Patients with a mildly dilated and mildly obstructed primary megaureter are treated nonoperatively with long-term antibiotics; patients with intermediate dilatation and obstruction require surgery if dilatation worsens. Surgical treatment for severe POM consists of excision of the obstruction and antireflux reimplantation with or without limited ureteral tailoring.[12] Severe ureteral decompensation, advanced hydronephrosis, repeated infections, stone formation, and less than 10% function are indications for nephroureterectomy.[13]

Primary refluxing megaureter is due to a short or absent intravesical ureter. This disorder may be familial and associated with other urinary tract anomalies, such as prune-belly syndrome, duplication anomalies with ureteroceles, and megacystis–microcolon–intestinal hypoperistalsis syndrome. Another consideration is the megacystis–megaureter association with hydroureteronephrosis; a large, thin-walled bladder; and high-grade reflux. The cause of the megaureter and enlarged bladder is the constant recycling of massive amounts of refluxed urine. Prenatal ultrasonographic diagnosis of hydronephrosis has identified a select group of neonates with this condition: male predominance (80%), grade IV to grade V reflux (80%), and bilateral reflux with renal functional impairment (50 to 60%) based upon differential renal scintigraphy.[14] *Secondary refluxing megaureter* is due to a neurogenic bladder or to bladder outlet obstruction such as posterior urethral valves or ureteroceles. *Primary nonobstructive, nonrefluxing* megaureter has neither juxtavesical/bladder outlet obstruction nor reflux. Dilatation may be

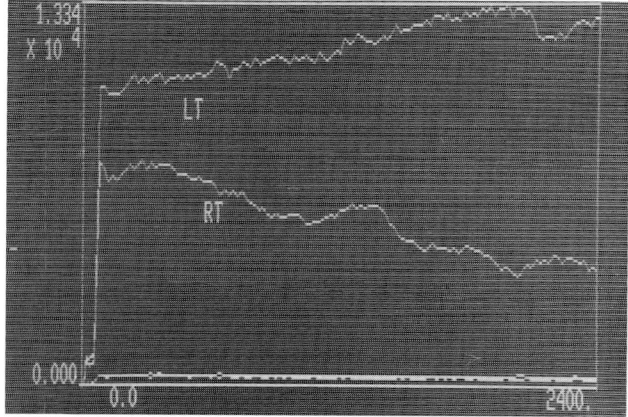

Figure 11–8. Left UPJ obstruction. Diuretic ^{99m}Tc DTPA renogram after Lasix administration demonstrates normal washout on right and lack of washout on left, consistent with obstruction.

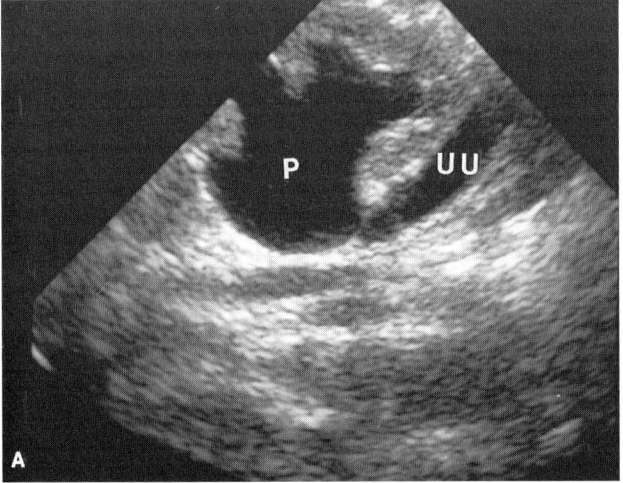
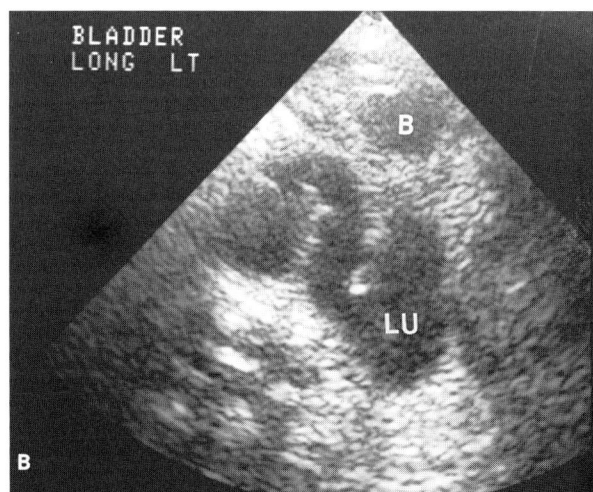
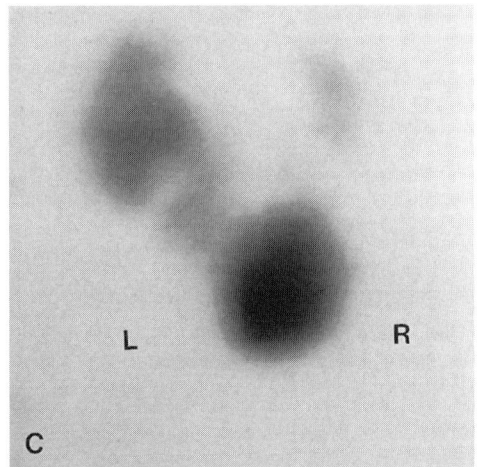
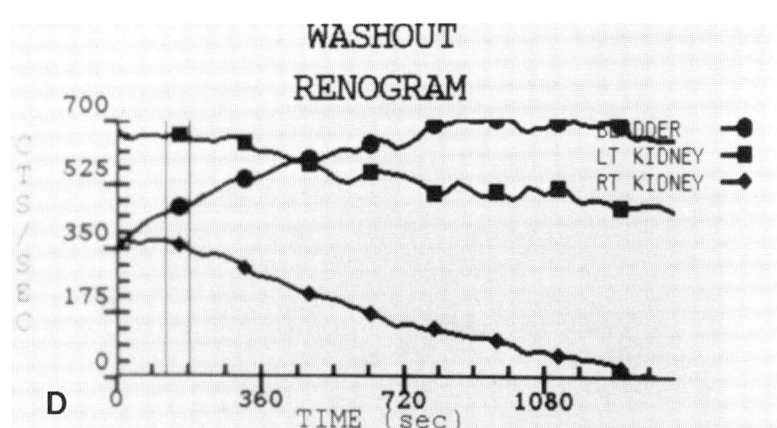

Figure 11–9. Primary megaureter. **(A)** Longitudinal sonogram shows the left renal pelvis (P) and upper ureter (UU). **(B)** Longitudinal sonogram shows tortuous lower ureter (LU) and bladder (B). Note disproportionate dilatation of the LU with respect to the UU and kidney. **(C)** ^{99m}Tc renogram reveals left megaureter. **(D)** Diuretic renogram demonstrates primary obstructed left megaureter.

segmental or may involve the entire ureter, and upper tract drainage usually is not significantly abnormal. *Secondary nonrefluxing, nonobstructive megaureter* may be due to atony from urinary tract infection or to high urine flow and volume.[15] As with primary obstructive megaureter, evaluation of these entities frequently requires both VCUG and nuclear renal function studies; the final diagnosis is one of exclusion.

Duplication Anomalies/Ureterocele Complex

As a group, duplication anomalies are common; approximately 10% of the population has partial duplication of the collecting system. The spectrum ranges from complete duplication with a supernumerary kidney to complete separation of the collecting system in a single kidney. Bilateral duplication occurs in 40% of patients; unilateral duplication has an equal right and left incidence.

Partial duplication of the collecting system results from proximal branching of the ureteric bud. After this branched bud contacts the metanephric blastema, metanephric nephrogenesis ensues. Incomplete duplication occurs as a result and ranges from a bifid renal pelvis to Y-shaped ureters with a common ureter distal to the point of initial branching. Ultrasound reveals a nonobstructed duplex kidney larger than the normal single-system kidney, with an interruption of the echogenic central pelvic fat (Fig. 11–10). This entity is an asymptomatic normal variant unless a coexistent anomaly is present.

Complete duplication of the collecting system occurs when two distinct ureteric buds develop from the ipsilateral wolffian duct. These two buds usually course together and contact the metanephric blastema in proximity to each other, resulting in two separate collecting systems and two ureters with separate insertions. The upper pole ureter has an anomalous insertion. As the mesonephric duct is incorporated into

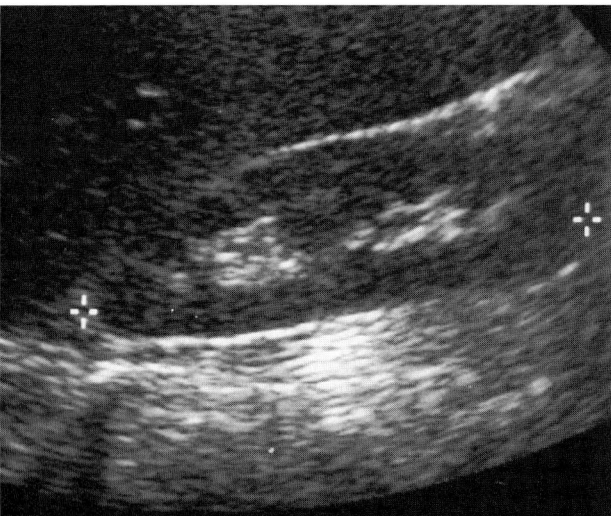

Figure 11–10. Nonobstructed duplex kidney. Longitudinal renal sonogram shows separation of superior and inferior pelvic echoes.

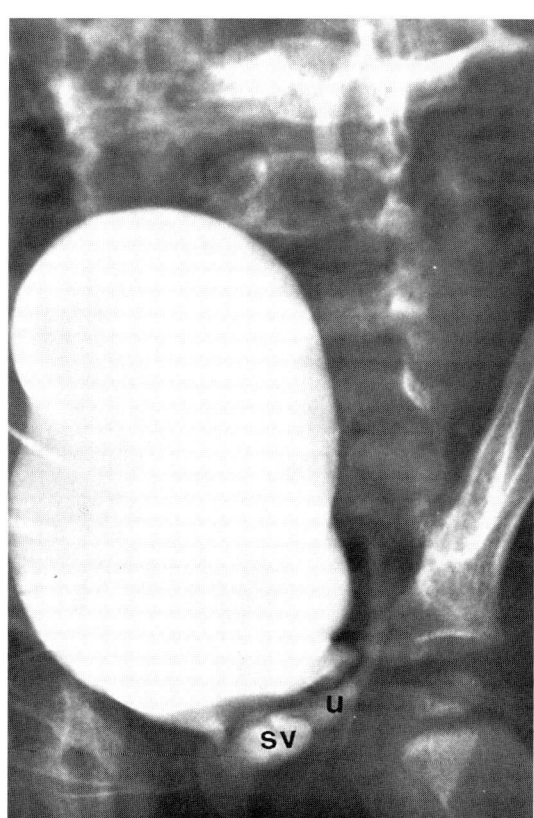

Figure 11–12. Ureteral duplication with an ectopic ureter in a male patient. Voiding cystourethrogram demonstrating upper moiety ureter (U) ectopically inserting into seminal vesicle (SV).

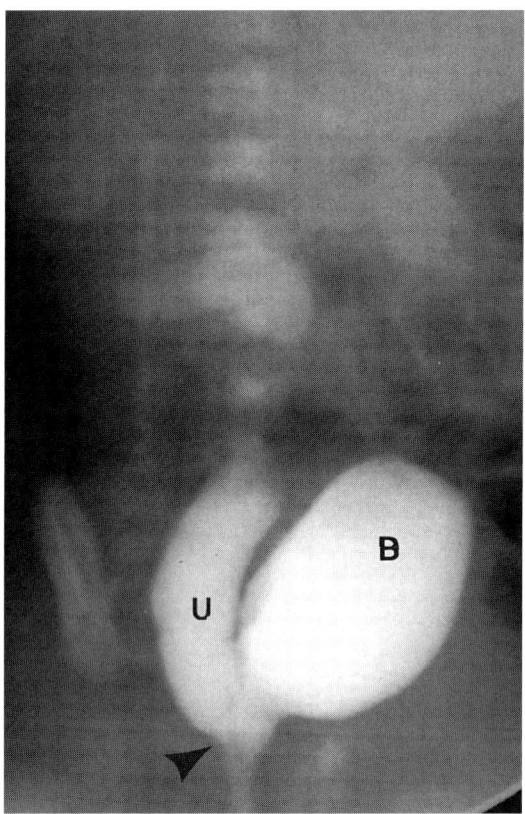

Figure 11–11. Ureteral duplication with an ectopic ureter in a female patient. Voiding cystourethrogram demonstrates upper moiety ureter (U) ectopically inserting into urethra (arrowhead), bladder (B).

the urogenital sinus, it carries the upper pole ureter to an insertion distal and medial to its normal trigonal location (Weigert–Meyer rule). As a result, the upper pole moiety inserts ectopically into the bladder neck, urethra, vagina, uterus, or vestibule in girls (Fig. 11–11) and into the bladder neck, posterior urethra, epididymis, seminal vesicle, or vas deferens in boys (Fig. 11–12). Approximately 30% of ectopic ureters terminate either in the bladder neck or slightly more distally in the urethra at the level of the external sphincter. Infection is the common presentation when the ectopic ureter enters above the external sphincter, whereas incontinence results from ectopic insertion below the external sphincter. The classic duplication anomaly has an ectopic ureterocele associated with the upper pole ureter, causing hydroureteronephrosis of the upper pole moiety (Fig. 11–13). The lower pole ureter inserts laterally and superiorly to its normal trigonal position, predisposing it to vesicoureteral reflux.

Sonography of a duplicated system with an ectopic ureter usually reveals a dilated upper pole collecting system surrounded by a thin rim of parenchyma of normal echogenicity (Fig. 11–14A). The ectatic dilated upper pole ureter usually can be imaged distally where it either terminates outside the bladder or enters into an ectopic ureterocele, which may be

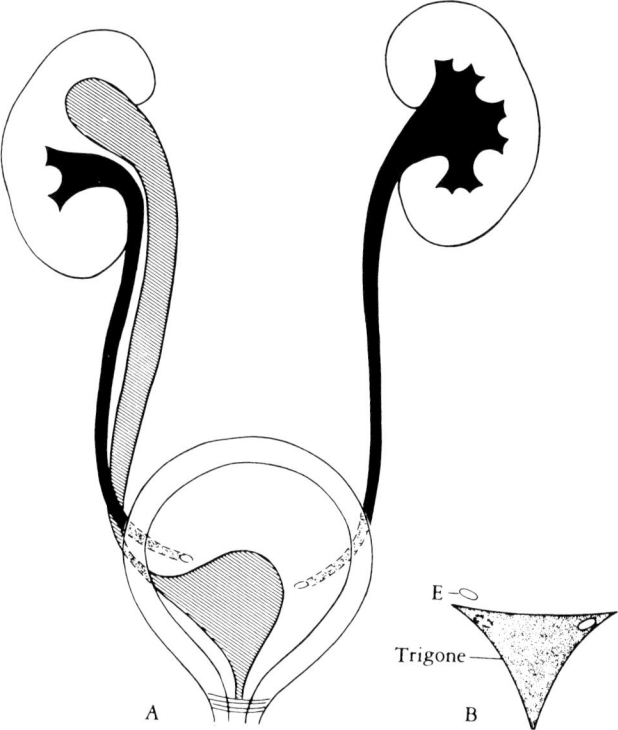

Figure 11–13. Weigert–Meyer rule. (A) Typical features of ectopic ureterocele. There is usually obstruction of the upper urinary tract. Flattening of the lower-pole calyces produces a "drooping lily" appearance. The ureter of the lower-pole moiety is displaced laterally on the side of the ureterocele. The mass in the bladder is due to a ureterocele of the distal ureter of the upper-pole moiety. The Weigert–Meyer rule states that the ectopic ureteral orifice of the upper-pole moiety is medial and caudal to its normal trigonal location. (B) Frequently, the ureteral orifice for the lower-pole moiety is slightly ectopic (E). It lies lateral and cephalad to its normal trigonal location. There may be vesicoureteral reflux into the ureter draining the lower-pole moiety.

intravesical at the bladder neck or prolapsed into the urethra (Fig. 11–14B–D). However, upper pole moiety anomalies with duplication cover a wide spectrum. They may be atrophic, may or may not contain a central fluid collection, and may be difficult to detect. Sometimes the upper pole is highly echogenic with small cysts due to dysplasia; if hypoplastic, the subtended ureter may be diminutive.[16] Lower pole ureteral dilatation may be due to reflux or to obstruction by an ectopic ureterocele.

Ureteroceles are approximately four to seven times more common in girls than in boys. Ureteral duplication is present in 75% of children with ureteroceles; single-system ectopic ureteroceles are rare and are usually seen in boys. A simple ureterocele arises from a normally positioned ureteral orifice near the corner of the trigone. Theories of origin include persistence of the Chwalla membrane, leading to an obstruction where the mesonephric duct joins the primitive urogenital canal, or possibly obstruction at a higher level resulting from incomplete canalization of the ureteral bud at its orifice.

Simple ureteroceles are seldom seen in children and rarely prolapse or become large enough to cause vesical neck obstruction.[17] However, when present, the severity of associated ureterectasis and hydronephrosis is greater in children than in adults, and urinary tract infection is the usual presentation.[18] Simple ureteroceles typically have the classic cobra head or spring onion appearance on intravenous urography (Fig. 11–15A). Sonography reveals an intravesical sonolucent mass with a thin wall (Fig. 11–15B). Reflux can occur but is rare with this type of ureterocele.[19]

Posterior Urethral Valves

Posterior urethral valves are the most common form of congenital urethral obstruction in boys.[20] PUVs are the second leading cause of neonatal hydronephrosis, and in utero they are the most common cause of urethral obstruction. This condition may present in utero, in children, and occasionally in adults. Macpherson et al.[21] reported that approximately 8% of occurrences were discovered in utero, 34% in neonates, and 32% within the first year of life; significantly, 25% were diagnosed in patients over 1 year of age.

Young et al.[22] in 1919 originally proposed three types of PUVs. This classification, shown next, is still in use today (Fig. 11–16).

Type 1 (90%): Thickened mucosal folds from the caudal verumontanum fused anteriorly at a lower level
Type 2 (5%): Mucosal folds, extending cranially from the verumontanum to the bladder neck
Type 3 (5%): Disclike membrane or diaphragm located below the verumontanum

Prenatal sonography demonstrating severe hydroureteronephrosis in a male fetus should suggest the possibility of posterior urethral valves. Varying degrees of renal dysplasia, resulting from VUR secondary to urethral obstruction, occur before the twentieth gestational week. Therefore intrauterine intervention after week 20 is not successful in preventing renal damage.[23]

Neonates typically present with bilateral flank masses and bladder distention secondary to urethral obstruction. The bladder compensates by developing intramural muscular hypertrophy and trabeculation (Fig. 11–17A). The ureters may be compressed along their intravesical portion, thus producing UVJ obstruction; conversely, they may be dilated and ectatic as a result of massive VUR (Fig. 11–17B,C). Both mechanisms may produce severe hydroureteronephrosis. Interestingly, 40% of cases have no associated ureteral dilatation; in 10 to 20% of these cases, hydroureteronephrosis results in spontaneous periureteric rupture, which allows escape of urine and subsequent decompression of the urinary tract.[24] More frequently, however, the kidney decompresses

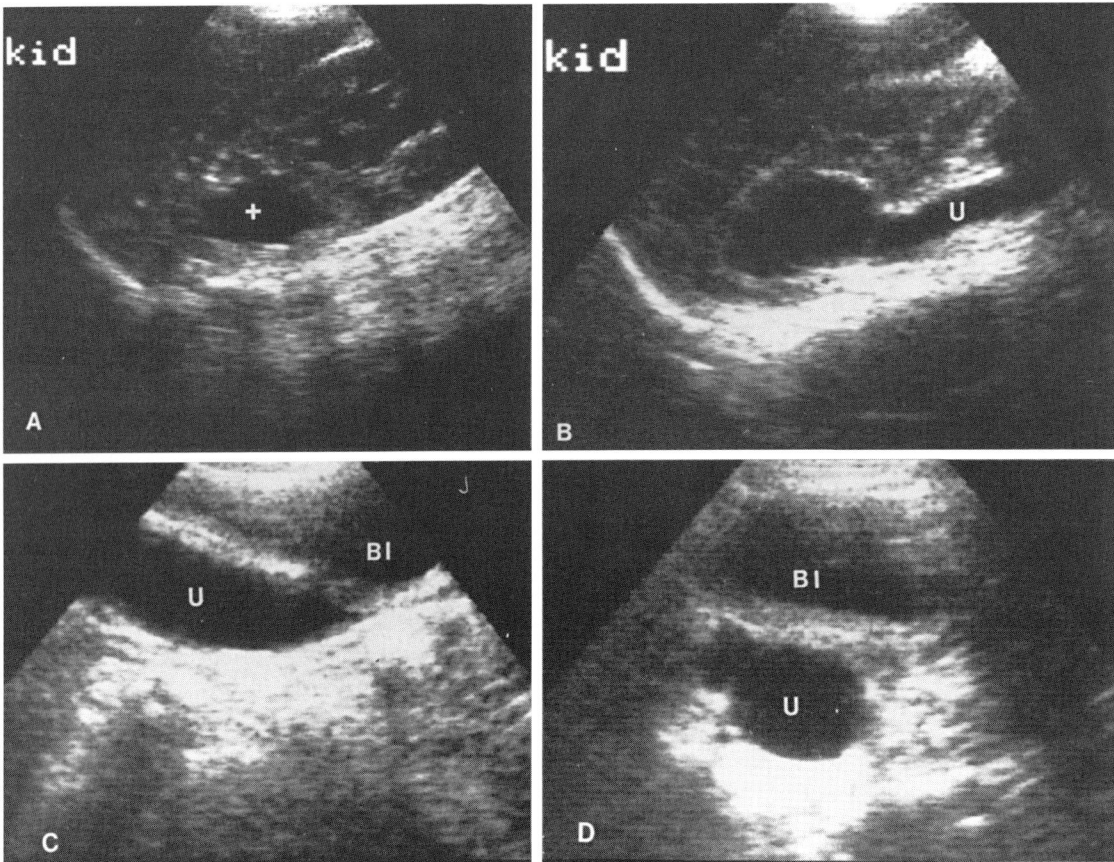

Figure 11-14. Ectopic ureterocele. **(A–C)** Sequential longitudinal renal sonograms demonstrate the hydronephrotic upper moiety (+) in A, its dilated ureter (U) in B, and distal upper-moiety ureteral (U) dilatation to the level of the bladder (Bl) in C; **(D)** Transverse bladder sonogram demonstrates the right ectopic ureterocele (U) in the bladder (Bl).

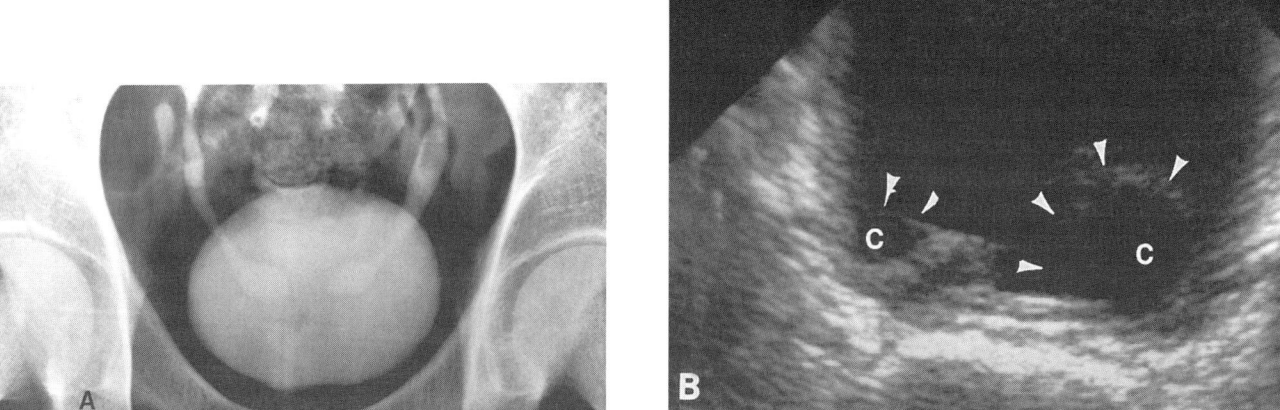

Figure 11-15. Simple ureterocele. **(A)** Bilateral "cobra head" appearance is seen during excretory urography. **(B)** Transverse bladder sonogram reveals cysts (C) with echogenic walls (arrows) representing ureteroceles at the bladder base.

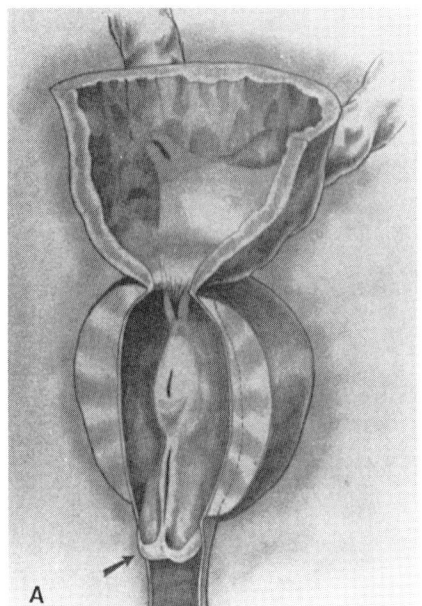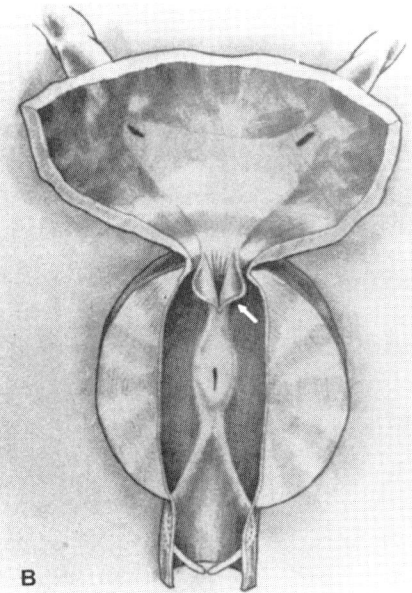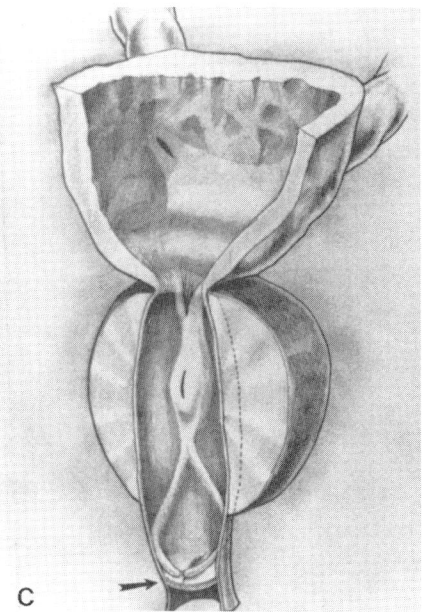

Figure 11–16. Types of posterior urethral valves. The original classification proposed by Young[22] in 1919 is still in use today. **(A)** Type 1 posterior urethral valves (arrow) are mucosal folds extending anteroinferiorly from the caudal aspect of the verumontanum, often fusing anteriorly at a lower level. They are derived from the plicae colliculi and constitute the majority of valves. **(B)** Type 2 posterior urethral valves (arrow) are mucosal folds extending anterosuperiorly from the verumontanum toward the bladder neck. A rare occurrence, they are probably an effect rather than a cause of bladder obstruction. **(C)** Type 3 posterior urethral valves (arrow) are disclike membranes located below the verumontanum and unrelated to it. They constitute a small percentage of posterior urethral valves.

itself by rupturing at the area of least resistance—the calyceal fornix—with resultant urine extravasation into the perirenal space (urinoma) or peritoneal cavity (ascites) (Fig. 11–18).

Fluid occasionally accumulates in the pleural space (urothorax). Severe bladder outlet obstruction will cause oligohydramnios, and the classic Potter syndrome may be seen with pulmonary insufficiency (hypoplasia), air leak (pneumothorax), and severe renal dysplasia. Hydronephrotic type IV multicystic dysplastic kidney may result from massive in utero bladder and ureteric distention.[21,24] Thinning and stretching of abdominal-wall musculature as a result of chronic severe bladder distention may produce an appearance mimicking the prune-belly syndrome. Infants and children with lesser degrees of obstruction commonly present with voiding abnormalities (inability to void or voiding with a poor, intermittent stream) or an abdominal mass (hydronephrosis); less commonly, the patients present with failure to thrive and chronic urinary retention.

The VCUG is the "gold standard" for diagnosis of posterior urethral valves (Fig. 11–19).[25] The bladder is usually thick-walled, with sacculations and trabeculations; reflux (unilateral or bilateral) occurs in 50% and is accompanied by varying degrees of hydroureteronephrosis. Reflux is typically unilateral and left-sided in neonates with PUVs; because the contralateral kidney is usually spared, the prognosis is favorable. Bilateral reflux is common in severely affected infants with posterior urethral valves detected in utero (Fig. 11–20). The major diagnostic findings are

1. A dilated posterior urethra
2. Marked discrepancy in size between the normal anterior and dilated posterior urethra
3. A posteriorly located orifice between the anterior and posterior urethra, not a central lumen
4. Visualization of the valves

Prognosis depends upon the degree of renal damage and dysplasia. Evaluation of renal function is by serum creatinine and renal scintigraphy (usually Tc 99m-labeled DTPA). Treatment of posterior urethral valves can be controversial.[26] Distal temporary diversion, vesicostomy, or cystostomy has been used primarily in infants whose urethras are too small to accept available resectoscopes and in larger infants who have significant renal failure. Proximal temporary diversions, ureterostomies or pyelostomies, have been used for diversion of urine flow in small infants or larger children with renal failure. Proximal diversions have also been used as treatment for markedly dilated and tortuous ureters that have not responded to valve ablation and vesicostomy. Primary valve ablation is most often performed in older children with normal renal function. After ablation endoscopy, there may be persistent though reduced dilatation of the pos-

242 Diagnosis of Genitourinary Disease

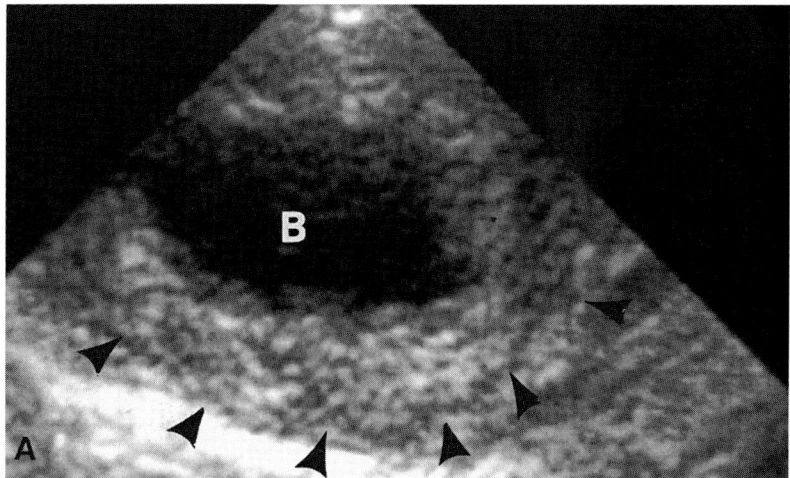

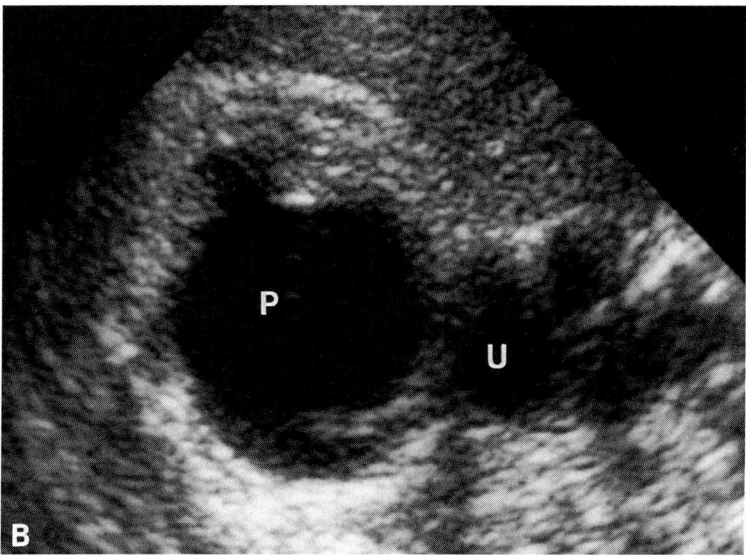

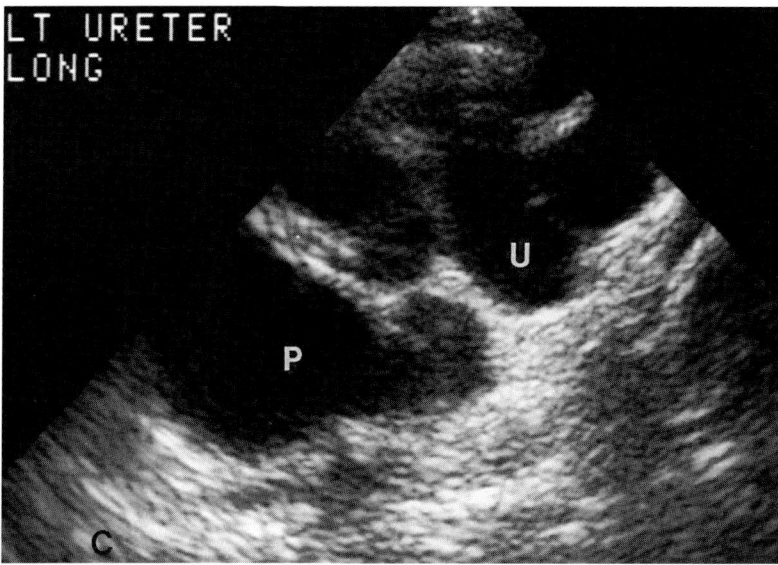

Figure 11–17. Posterior urethral valves. **(A)** Transverse pelvic sonogram reveals thick-walled bladder (B); arrowheads delineate bladder wall. **(B)** Longitudinal sonogram of the right kidney shows dilated pelvis (P) and ectatic ureter (U). **(C)** Longitudinal sonogram of the left kidney shows dilated pelvis (P) and ectatic ureter (U).

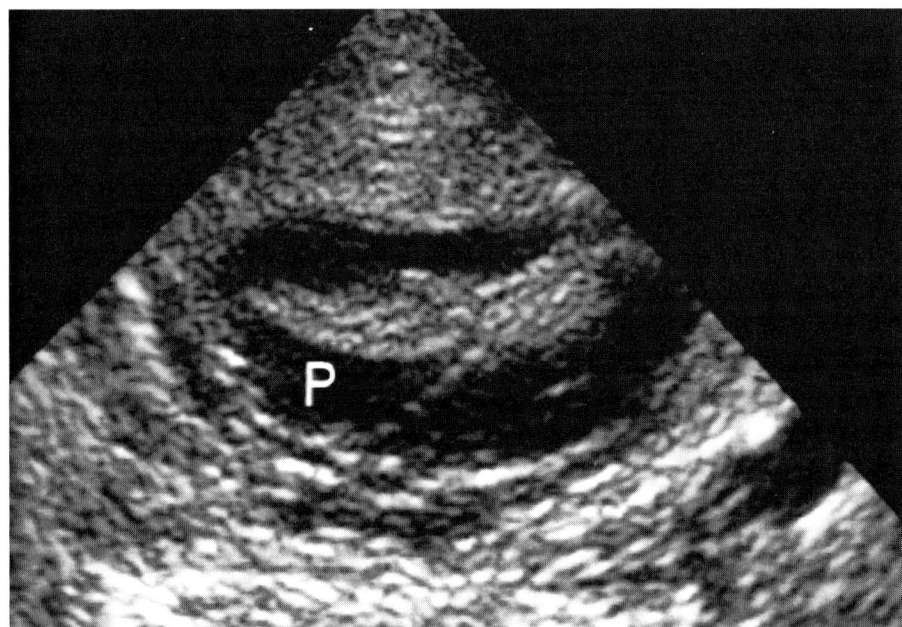

Figure 11–18. Urinoma. Longitudinal renal sonogram reveals fluid in the perirenal space (P) in an infant with posterior urethral valves.

terior urethra (Fig. 11–21). This dilatation persists for years in 20% of patients.[27] Urethral dilatation 2 to 3 years after the ablation is likely permanent but does not necessarily indicate persistent urethral obstruction. Therefore periodic renal function evaluation (usually Tc 99m-labeled DTPA) is recommended. As expected, the degree to which hydroureteronephrosis returns to normal is proportional to its preoperative severity. Overall poor prognosis is directly related to delay in diagnosis (older than 2 years) and associated persistent vesicoureteral reflux. A 9-year follow-up of 25 posterior urethral valve patients revealed that 40% had growth retardation and 44% had end-stage renal disease.[28]

Prune-Belly Syndrome (Eagle-Barrett)

Prune-belly syndrome is the triad of deficient abdominal musculature, urinary tract anomalies, and cryptorchidism.[29] Urinary tract findings include large hypotonic, dilated, tor-

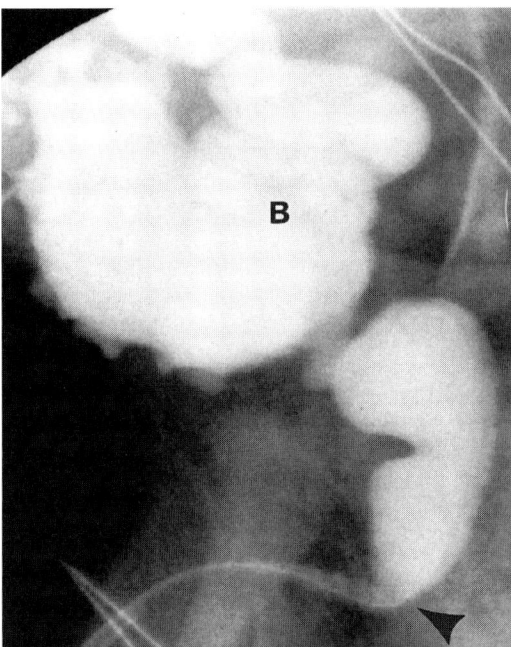

Figure 11–19. Posterior urethral valves. Voiding cystourethrogram shows posterior urethral valves (arrowhead), dilated posterior urethra, and trabeculated bladder (B).

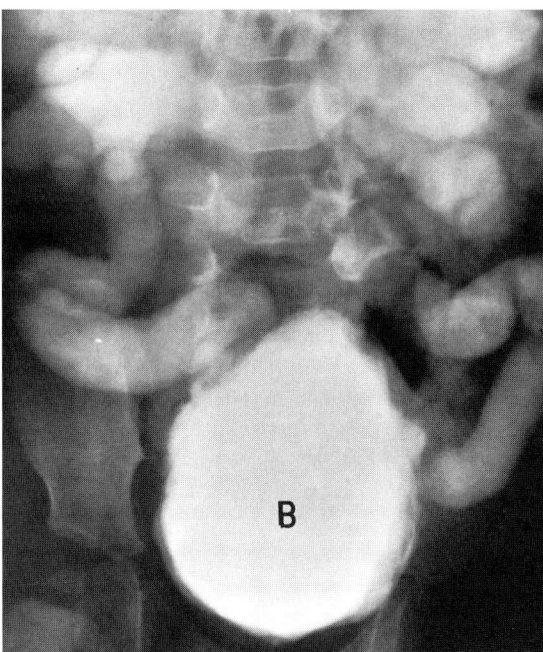

Figure 11–20. Posterior urethral valves. Voiding cystourethrogram demonstrates trabeculated bladder (B) with massive bilateral reflux.

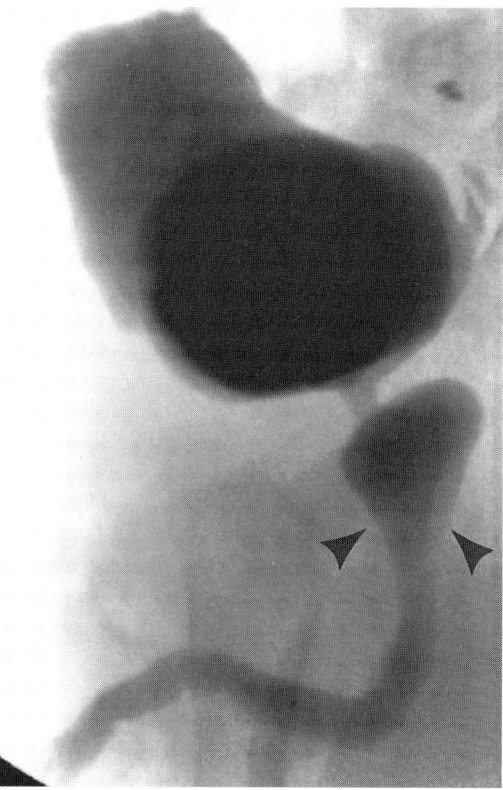

Figure 11–21. Posterior urethral valves. Postoperative voiding cystourethrogram shows persistent dilatation of the posterior urethra (arrowheads).

without visible normal renal parenchyma. Group 2 patients have marked ureteral dilatation with mild to moderate pelvocalyceal dilatation. Group 3 patients have either minimal dilatation or normal urinary tracts.[31]

VCUG in these patients demonstrates the large bladder, often with a urachal remnant, and a dilated posterior urethra (Fig. 11–22); actual obstructing valves have not been demonstrated in surviving patients with prune-belly syndrome. Functional imaging may be performed with IVU or scintigraphy.

Vesicoureteral Reflux

Reflux is an important cause of urinary tract dilatation. An increasing number of neonates whose prenatal screening sonograms revealed intermittent or persistent hydronephrosis with and without large bladders are referred for postnatal evaluation. In utero reflux with subsequent neonatal reflux without obstruction has been reported.[32,33] However, the fact that other neonates are normal at birth suggests that their in utero reflux was exclusively an intrauterine condition.[34]

Detection of VUR in early childhood is of paramount importance. Since reflux affects renal growth, early detection may prevent atrophy and scarring. Both excretory urography and ultrasound may be normal in the presence of reflux; hence the best initial imaging study for detection of reflux is radiographic VCUG. Radionuclide cystography is often recommended for follow-up studies to decrease patient ra-

tuous ureters; dilatation and muscular hypertrophy of the bladder (with urachus); dilated proximal prostatic urethra; and mild to severe multicystic dysplastic kidneys. Berdon and coworkers[30] described three groups based upon radiologic and clinical findings:

Group 1: Most severe involvement; stillborn or die soon after birth with urethral obstruction from valves or even atresia and show bilateral cystic renal dysplasia; pulmonary hypoplasia and oligohydramnios.
Group 2: Moderate severity without pulmonary hypoplasia; dilated bladder without urethral obstruction; VCUG may reveal large bladder with patulous bladder neck and dilated posterior urethra; dilated ureters and renal pelves and dysmorphic calyces.
Group 3: Mild involvement with features ranging between those of group 2 and a normal urinary tract.

This syndrome occurs in from 1 in 35,000 to 1 in 50,000 live births and almost exclusively affects males (96%). The anterior abdominal wall musculature is wrinkled, although all three muscle layers are present.

Sonography in prune-belly syndrome parallels the clinical manifestations. Group 1 patients have dysplastic kidneys

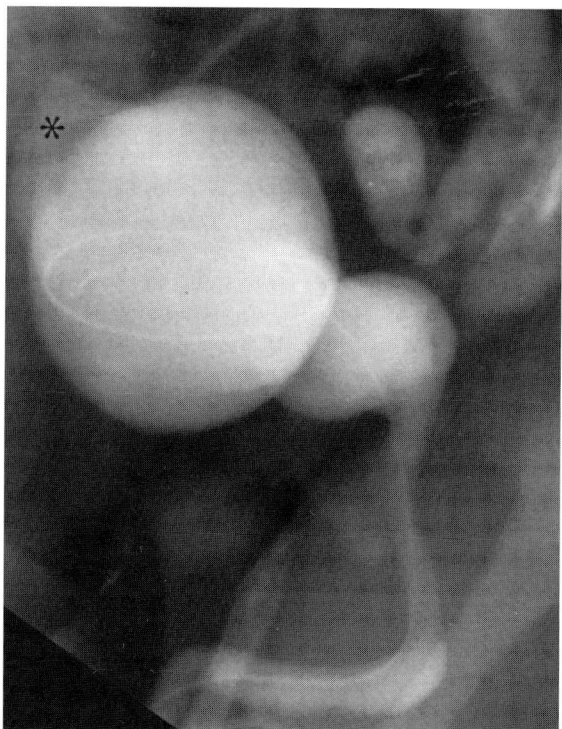

Figure 11–22. Prune-belly syndrome. Voiding cystourethrogram shows a large bladder with a urachal remnant (*) and a dilated posterior urethra without obstructing valves.

diation dose. The VCUG is also sensitive for identifying intrarenal reflux (IRR). The importance of IRR, its detection, and possible sequela (reflux nephropathy) was described by Hodson.[35] Some patients with IRR may progress to scarred kidneys without any known infection (Fig. 11–23A–C). Vesicoureteral reflux occurs in less than 0.5% of asymptomatic children[36]; however, it occurs in 8.26% of siblings of children with VUR.[36,37] Therefore many believe that VUR is a primary abnormality. The sibling population is reportedly at substantial risk for renal damage, even in the absence of a history of urinary tract infection, and even if the reflux is of only moderate severity.[38] Therefore it has been recommended that these siblings be screened for reflux. If reflux is present, further evaluation of their renal parenchyma with cortical scintigraphy is urged.[38]

The relationship between VUR and urinary tract infection remains controversial. Previously, VUR was considered secondary to distal obstruction, infection, or both. Now most investigators favor a primary abnormality incompetence of the ureterovesical junction.[39,40] Both the increased incidence of reflux in siblings and a 20-fold greater incidence of reflux in white versus black children tend to support the conclusion that reflux is a primary phenomenon.[39] Gross and Lebowitz[39] have also reported that 88% of children with reflux have sterile urine and that there is no significant difference in the incidence of sterile (88 to 90%) and infected (10 to 12%) urine in nonrefluxing versus refluxing children. It has also been suggested that some children have transient mild reflux as a result of urinary tract infections with inflammation of the bladder wall and the intravesical ureteral segment; this mechanism may explain the reversible hydronephrosis occasionally observed in the neonate with urinary sepsis.[41] VUR is present in 30 to 50% of children with urinary tract infection.[42-44] The frequency of VUR associated with urinary tract infection is inversely proportional to patient age.

Urinary Tract Infection

Urinary tract infection (UTI) is the most common abnormality of the urinary tract in children. Symptomatic UTI

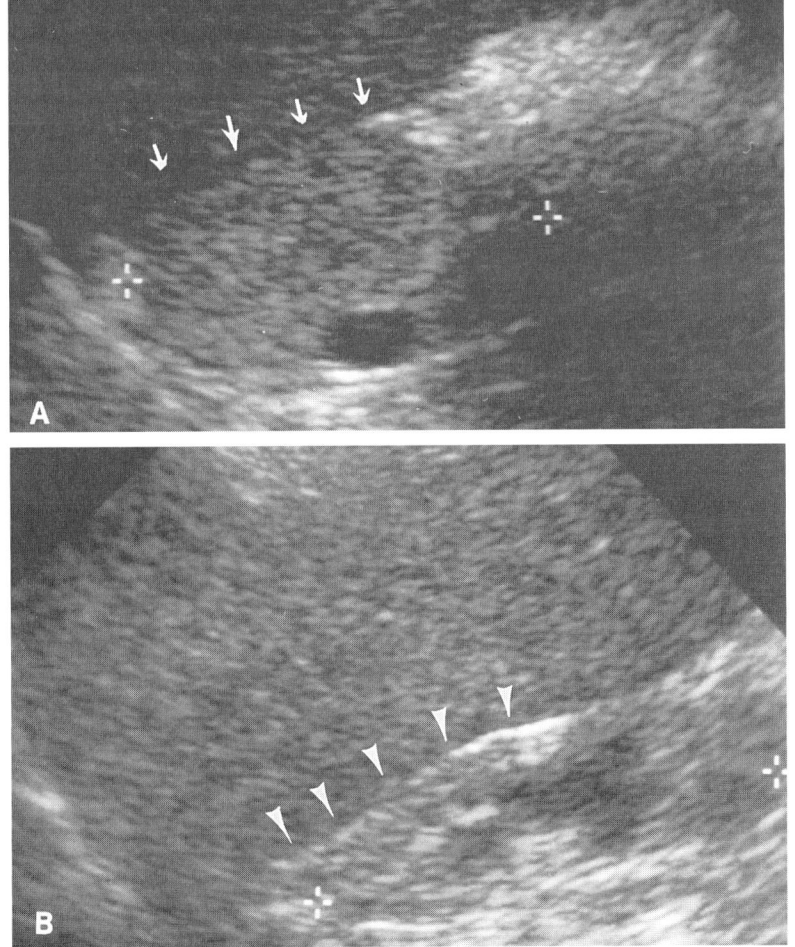

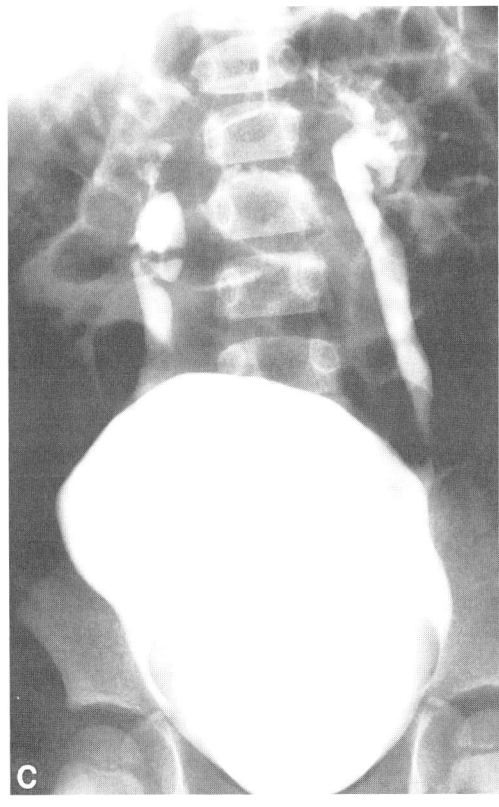

Figure 11–23. Reflux nephropathy. Longitudinal sonograms of (**A**) left and (**B**) right kidneys (arrows) demonstrate small echogenic atrophic kidneys (+ delineates renal borders). (**C**) Voiding cystourethrogram shows bilateral reflux.

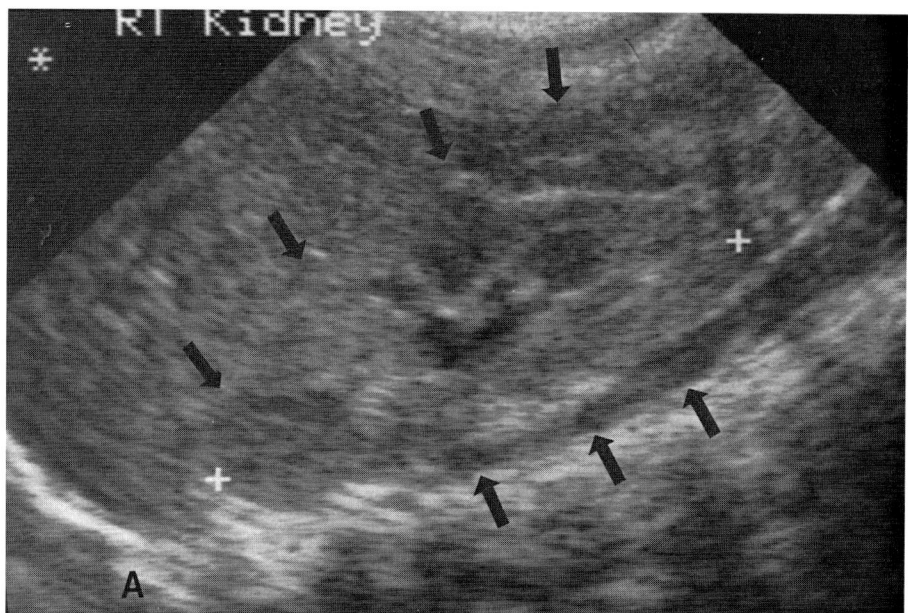

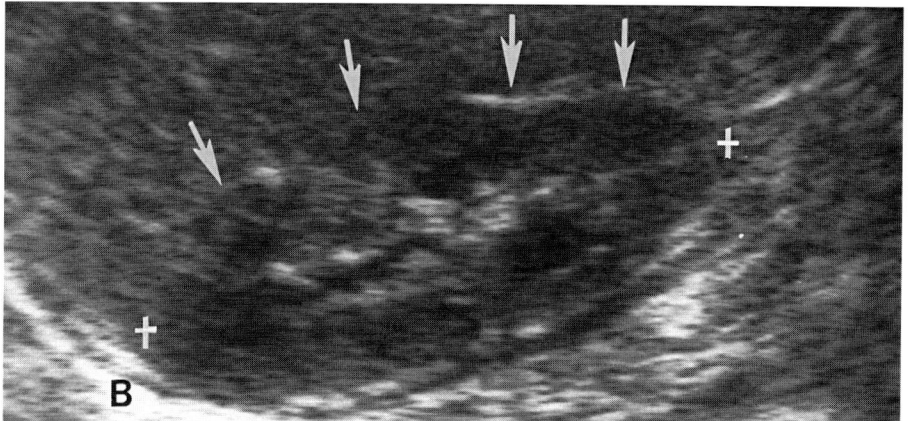

Figure 11-24. Acute pyelonephritis. (**A**) Initial longitudinal renal sonogram demonstrates nephromegaly with increased echogenicity and indistinct corticomedullary junction. (**B**) Follow-up longitudinal sonogram demonstrates normal renal size and echogenicity. Arrows and + symbols delineate renal borders.

affects 1 to 3% of children under 11 years of age, and asymptomatic bacteriuria is even more prevalent.[45] Although lower tract infection usually resolves without sequelae, delay in treatment or inappropriate treatment of upper tract infection can lead to renal scarring. Sequelae of renal scarring include hypertension, growth failure, and in severe cases affecting both kidneys, chronic renal failure.

The imaging evaluation of the initial UTI in children has changed. Previously, the standard screening tests were radiographic VCUG to detect vesicoureteral reflux and intravenous urography (IVU) to evaluate the upper tracts and kidneys for scarring, pyelonephritis, and decreased function. We now first investigate the lower urinary tract with either the radiographic or nuclear VCUG in girls and the radiographic VCUG in boys. The upper urinary tract is now imaged with sonography and nuclear medicine rather than the IVU. Ultrasound surpasses urography in evaluation of congenital anomalies, pyonephrosis, and perinephric collections; acute pyelonephritis and renal abscesses are also seen.[46,47] Invasive procedures, such as diagnostic and therapeutic aspirations, can be performed under sonographic guidance.

As the modalities of nuclear medicine and computed tomography (CT) have developed, they have been used with increasing frequency in the evaluation of UTI. Renal nuclear scintigraphy with cortical agents such as 99m glucoheptonate (GH) or dimercaptosuccinic acid (DMSA) has supplanted IVU for detection of acute pyelonephritis and renal scarring; acute pyelonephritis can also be imaged with gallium-67 (^{67}Ga) citrate- or indium-111 (^{111}In)-labeled white blood cells. For children, the increased radiation exposure associated with gallium imaging limits its usage, and the blood volume required for white cell labeling with indium-111 is prohibitive in children. Although mild renal scarring may be more likely missed with ultrasound than with radionuclide scintigraphy, mild focal scarring is probably of little practical importance. CT is extremely sensitive for identifying renal, perinephric, and retroperitoneal abnormalities, such as abscesses, which may not be easily detected with sonography, particularly in patients with excess bowel gas.

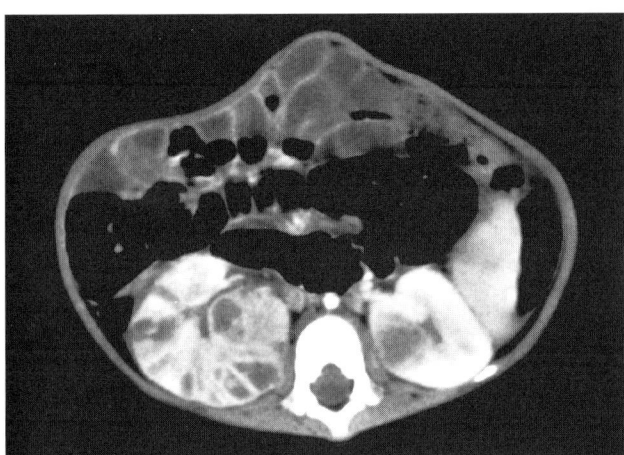

Figure 11–25. Acute pyelonephritis. CT scan shows bilateral multifocal low-attenuation areas.

ages are obtained.[49] Recent studies employing single-photon-emission computed tomography (SPECT) for renal cortical imaging of pyelonephritis in children have not shown a statistically significant advantage over pinhole imaging with DMSA and GH.[50]

Acute lobar nephronia is a focal area of pyelonephritis without frank suppuration.[51] On sonography, the focal area of infection appears as a relatively anechoic or echogenic mass with loss of corticomedullary differentiation. Rapidity of change on serial sonograms helps to differentiate lobar nephronia from other processes such as tumors or abscesses (Fig. 11–26A). Nuclear scintigraphy may also be helpful in differentiation (Fig. 11–26B). CT may show inhomogeneous areas or a normal appearance on precontrast scans with a patchy inhomogeneous appearance observed after contrast enhancement.[52] Scarring may develop in children after a documented episode of acute lobar nephronia.[48]

Urographic and sonographic findings in acute pyelonephritis may be minimal to absent. Diffuse enlargement is the earliest common sign. Generalized decreased echogenicity resulting from edema has been described, as has a diffuse increase in renal echogenicity (Fig. 11–24). All patients with a normal sonogram also have a normal urogram, but the reverse is not necessarily true.[48] CT is more sensitive than urography in detecting tissue attenuation differences caused by inflammatory edema and microabscesses (Fig. 11–25). Perirenal and retroperitoneal spaces are best evaluated by CT. Renal cortical imaging can identify acute parenchymal inflammation, as well as the scars of reflux nephropathy. Both technetium 99m DMSA and technetium 99m GH are used; the dose of radiation is similar for both agents, but DMSA is preferred at some institutions as better-quality im-

Renal Cystic Disease

Classifications of renal cystic disease range from simple to complex. Based upon microdissection techniques, most discussions use the Osathanondh and Potter[53] classification based upon developmental abnormalities of the collecting ducts, as follows:

Type I: autosomal recessive (infantile) polycystic kidney disease (ARPKD)

Type II: multicystic dysplastic kidney (MCDK)

Type III: autosomal dominant (adult) polycystic kidney disease (ADPKD), medullary sponge kidney, and cysts associated with syndromes

Type IV: hydronephrotic multicystic kidney

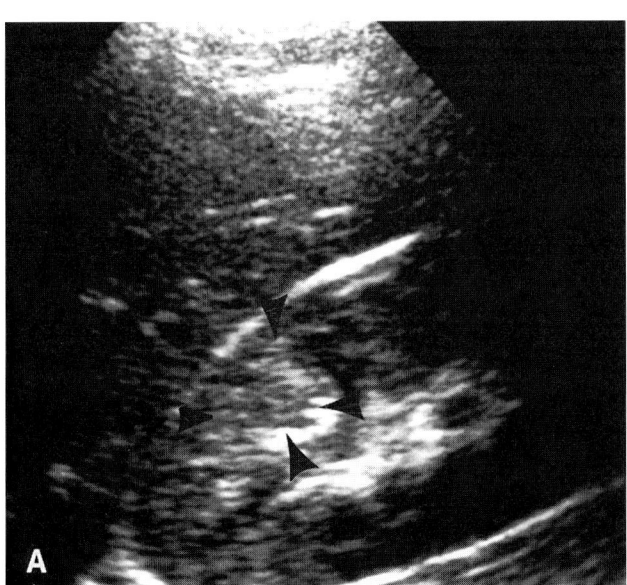 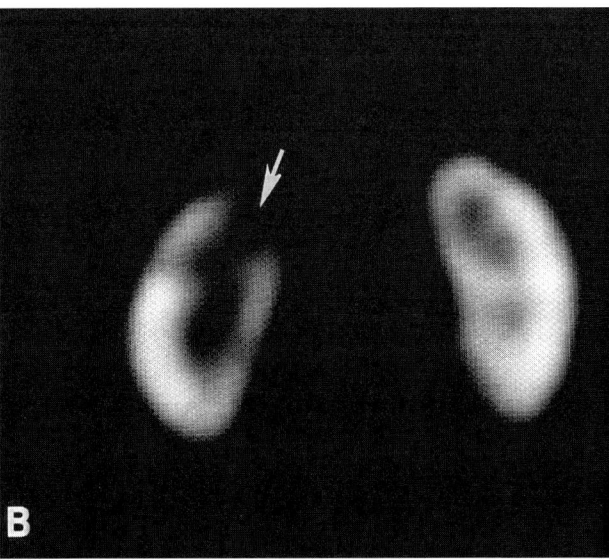

Figure 11–26. Lobar nephronia. (A) Longitudinal right renal sonogram shows focal increased echogenicity in upper pole (arrows). (B) Nuclear scintigraphy reveals lack of tracer uptake in the right upper pole (arrow).

Table 11–2. Cystic Diseases of the Kidney

Bilateral Cysts

Autosomal recessive polycystic kidney disease (ARPKD)
Autosomal dominant polycystic kidney disease (ADPKD)
Glomerulocystic disease
Cystic disease of renal medulla
Cysts associated with multiple malformation syndromes
Acquired cystic disease with chronic hemodialysis

Unilateral Cysts

Multicystic dysplastic kidney (MCDK)
Simple cysts

Source: Modified from Siegel MJ: Urinary tract. In: Siegel MJ, ed. *Pediatric Sonography*. New York: Raven Press, 1991.

The inclusion of multiple cystic entities into type III has not been universally accepted.[54] Bernstein[55] in 1976 proposed a classification dividing renal dysplasia into four groups:

1. Multicystic dysplasia resulting from ureteropelvic dysplasia
2. Focal and segmental cystic dysplasia resulting from obstruction of one of the ureters of a duplex kidney
3. Cystic dysplasia associated with nonatretic urinary tract obstruction (e.g., posterior urethral valves)
4. Heredofamilial cystic dysplasia

Although this schema has been supported by more recent research, it is of interest that it proposed a common mechanism of obstruction for all but the heredofamilial dysplasias.[56]

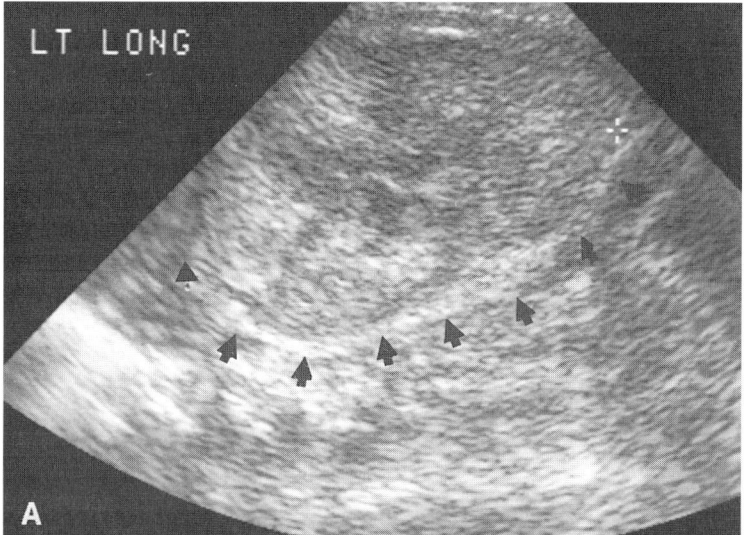

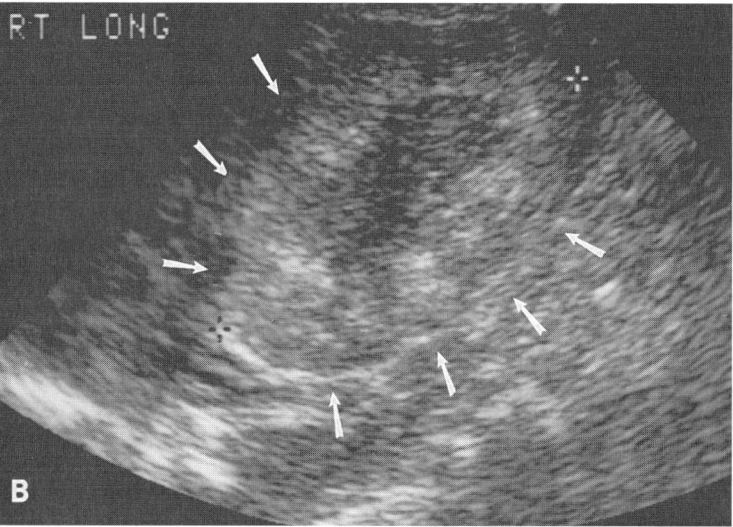

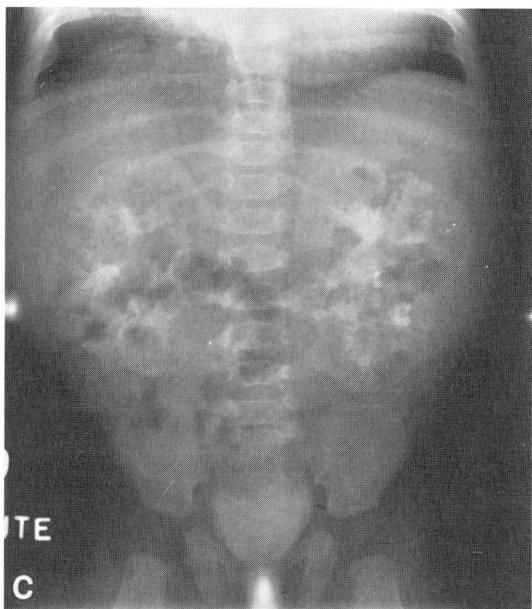

Figure 11–27. Neonatal autosomal recessive polycystic kidney disease. Longitudinal sonograms of (**A**) left and (**B**) right kidneys (arrows) reveal bilateral nephromegaly with loss of normal architecture. (**C**) Excretory urogram shows spoke–wheel appearance of contrast material in dilated collecting tubules.

Ultrasonography is now the usual initial imaging modality, but a specific diagnosis of the type of cystic disease may be impossible from ultrasonography alone, as morphologic criteria in themselves are inadequate for diagnosis. For example, "polycystic" kidneys may actually appear echogenic rather than echo-free because multiple acoustic interfaces within the involved parenchyma result in hyperechogenicity. As suggested by Teele and Share,[57] geneticists using chromosomal markers are becoming recognized as the final arbiter between the different types of renal cystic disease. Recently, Siegel[15] has provided a very practical and usable sonographic differential approach based upon bilateral versus unilateral disease (Table 11–2), which will serve as a framework for the following discussion of renal cystic disease. Neoplasms are discussed in Chapter 20.

Autosomal Recessive Polycystic Kidney Disease

Although autosomal recessive polycystic kidney disease (ARPKD) was previously termed "infantile" polycystic kidney disease, this is a misnomer in that ARPKD can occur initially in toddlers and older children. Family history of the disease frequently is lacking because of the recessive inheritance pattern. The most common presentation is a neonate with bilateral flank masses. A history of oligohydramnios indicates severe renal dysplasia and variable degrees of pulmonary hypoplasia. The "cysts" are actually dilated collecting tubules creating multiple interfaces that result in large echogenic kidneys in the newborn (Fig. 11–27A,B). Although rarely performed today, IVU reveals nephromegaly with radiating streaks of contrast material in dilated collecting tubules in the typical neonatal form of ARPKD (Fig. 11–27C). If the baby survives, macroscopic cysts may develop, but they are not as large or as numerous as those encountered in autosomal dominant polycystic kidney disease (ADPKD). Children with ARPKD can be divided into four types based upon age at presentation and degree of renal involvement: perinatal, neonatal, infantile, and juvenile (Table 11–3). In addition, ARPKD is a spectrum with an inverse relationship between renal disease and hepatic fibrosis. Neonates have minimal liver dysfunction, whereas adolescents may present with hemoptysis resulting from esophageal varices and portal hypertension. This form of ARPKD is called "juvenile polycystic disease" or tubular ectasia with congenital hepatic fibrosis. Renal sonography usually reveals increased medullary echogenicity (Fig. 11–28),[58] and results of hepatic sonography may vary from normal to increased parenchymal echogenicity with biliary ductal ectasia.

Autosomal Dominant Polycystic Kidney Disease

ADPKD is also known as adult polycystic renal disease. Most patients have a strong family history; the estimated frequency of disease is one per 1000 children. Less than 10% of patients present within the first decade of life. Neonates with ADPKD generally have enlarged, diffusely echogenic kidneys on sonography.[58] Occasionally, cysts of varying sizes are seen. Since ARPKD and ADPKD have similar sonographic features, diagnosis usually depends upon family history, tissue sampling, and occasionally, prenatal chromosomal studies.[59] When diagnosed in utero, ADPKD usually appears as multiple cysts within slightly mildly enlarged kidneys. Although the appearance is similar to ARPKD, the degree of oligohydramnios is not as severe in ADPKD as in ARPKD.[60] Interestingly, infants with ADPKD differ from older children with ADPKD and from infants with ARPKD in that the disease may be unilateral or asymmetric at presentation in older children.

Glomerulocystic Disease

Glomerulocystic disease is rare and sporadic. The pathologic hallmark is cystic dilatation of Bowman's space around the glomeruli.[61] Usually, renal cysts of varying size are seen,

Table 11–3. Autosomal Recessive Polycystic Kidney Disease in Childhood

	DISEASE TYPE			
Feature	Perinatal	Neonatal	Infantile	Juvenile
Age of presentation	Birth	First month	3–6 months	1–5 years
Mode of presentation	Massive renal enlargement, normal liver	Large kidneys and liver	Large kidneys, hepatosplenomegaly	1–5 years Variable renal enlargement, hepatosplenomegaly
Kidney: proportion of dilated tubules	>90%	60%	25%	<10%
Liver: proportion of dilated, infolded bile ducts	All	All	All	All
Periportal fibrosis	Minimal	Mild	Moderate	Marked
Typical course	Early death from uremia	Progressive renal failure	Chronic renal failure, systemic and portal hypertension	Severe portal hypertension

Source: Adapted with permission from Blyth H, Ockenden BG: Polycystic disease of kidneys and liver presenting in childhood. *J Med Genet* 1971;8:257–284.

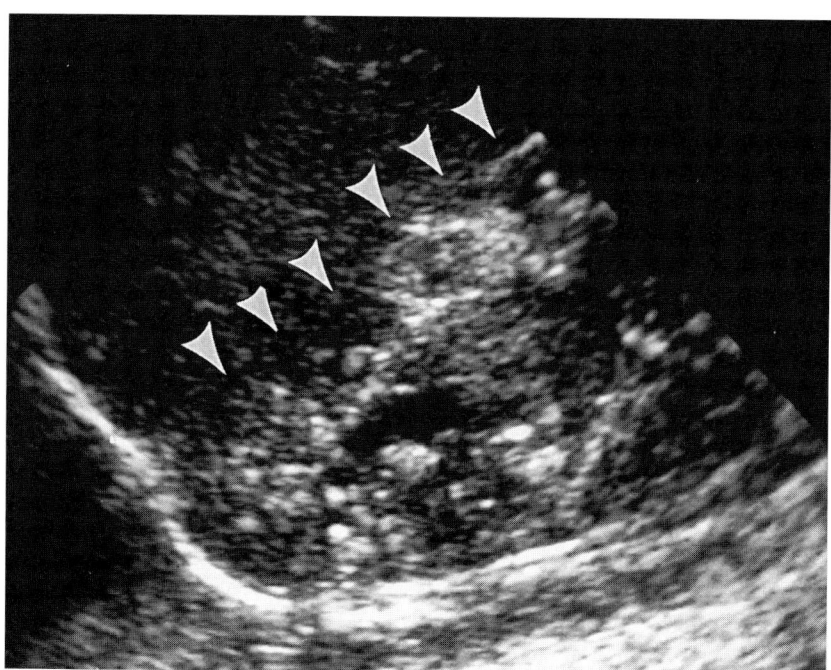

Figure 11–28. Juvenile autosomal recessive polycystic kidney disease. Longitudinal sonogram of kidney (arrows) demonstrates increased echogenicity, mainly in the medullary region.

but the condition may be indistinguishable from either ARPKD or ADPKD.[62] Palpable abdominal masses with renal failure early in life are the most common presentation.

CYSTIC DISEASE OF RENAL MEDULLA

Juvenile nephronophthisis and medullary sponge kidney (MSK) are the two forms of medullary cystic disease encountered in pediatric patients. The terms *juvenile nephronophthisis* and *renal medullary cystic disease* refer to the same renal abnormality; however, juvenile nephronophthisis is inherited as an autosomal recessive condition, and renal medullary cystic disease is inherited as an autosomal dominant condition. Both conditions may be associated with other anomalies. Renal sonography reveals small echogenic kidneys with variable cysts.[58] MSK, also called renal collecting tubular ectasia, is not an inherited disease and is not associated with other anomalies. Ultrasonography may reveal hyperechogenicity of the renal pyramids resulting from calcium deposition.[63] Although MSK is usually diagnosed after childhood, children with MSK may present with urinary tract infection, calculi, or hematuria.

Miscellaneous Cysts

Renal cysts may be associated with chromosomal and malformation syndromes; the most common are listed in Table 11–4. Most patients have multiple cysts in the cortex, in the medulla, or throughout both kidneys. Tuberous sclerosis, an autosomal dominant syndrome, may present in the neonate with macroscopic cystic disease resembling ADPKD or, more commonly, in an older child with several cysts, angiomyolipomas, or both.

Many patients undergoing long-term intermittent hemodialysis acquire renal cysts. The incidence is proportional to dialysis time; there is a marked increase in cystic disease after the third year.[64] Cysts vary in size and number. Complications include intrarenal or perirenal hemorrhage and an increased incidence of renal adenomas and carcinomas.[64]

Multicystic Dysplasia

Multicystic dysplastic kidney (MCDK), the second most common abdominal mass in the newborn following hydronephrosis, is usually unilateral. Boys and girls are equally

Table 11–4. Renal Cysts Associated with Malformation Syndromes

CHROMOSOMAL DISORDERS	GENETIC DISORDERS
Trisomy D	Autosomal dominant
Trisomy E	Tuberous sclerosis
Trisomy 21	von Hippel–Lindau disease
Turner syndrome	Autosomal recessive
	Meckel syndrome
	Asphyxiating thoracic dystrophy (Jeune syndrome)
	Cerebrohepatorenal syndrome (Zellweger syndrome)
	X-linked dominant
	Orofacial-digital syndrome type 1

Source: Sty JR, Wells RG, Starshak RJ, Gregg DC: The genitourinary system. In: *Diagnostic Imaging of Infants and Children, 1*. Gaithersburg, MD: Aspen Publishers, 1992.

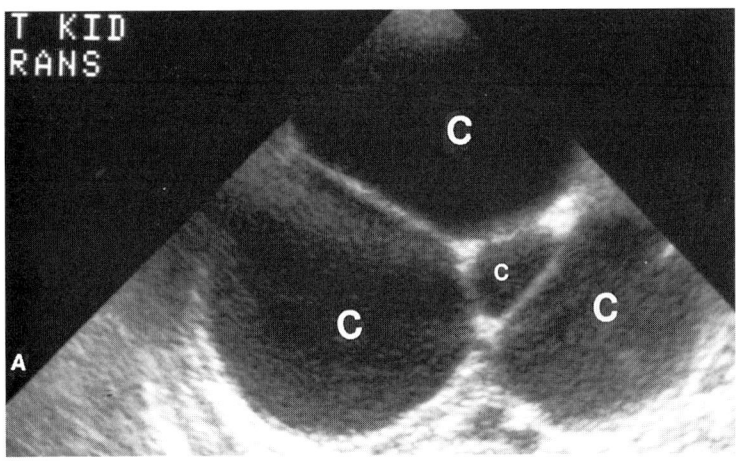
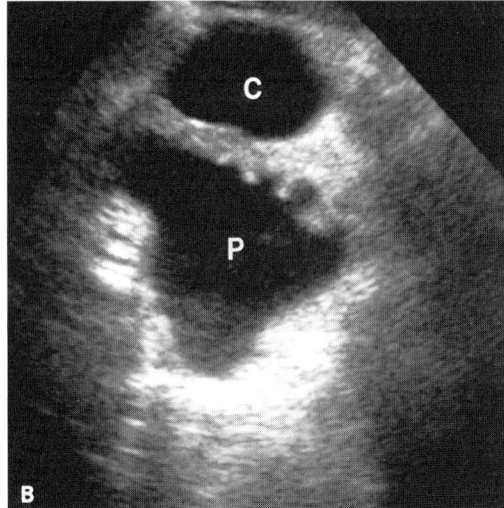

Figure 11–29. Multicystic dysplastic kidney. **(A)** Transverse renal sonogram reveals multiple noncommunicating cysts of varying sizes without a central renal pelvis or normal parenchyma. **(B)** Transverse sonogram reveals renal pelvis (P) and large eccentric cyst (C).

affected, and MCDK is more common on the left. However, contralateral urinary tract anomalies occur in up to 40% of these patients.[65] The most common associated anomaly is UPJ obstruction; ectopic ureteroceles are also frequently seen. The pelvoinfundibular (classic) type of MCDK is caused by atresia of the ureter and renal pelvis, leading to failure of proper induction of the metanephric blastema. If only the upper ureter is atretic, the less common hydronephrotic type of MCDK develops.[66] In both types of MCDK the ureters and renal vessels may be small or atretic. Sonography of MCDK typically reveals multiple noncommunicating cysts of varying sizes, eccentric location of the largest cysts, absence of an identifiable renal pelvis, and dysplastic or absent renal parenchyma (Fig. 11–29A). In the less common hydronephrotic form of MCDK, a renal pelvis can be seen (Fig. 11–29B). Differentiating mild to moderate hydronephrosis from MCDK may require radionuclide renal scanning; however, severe hdyronephrosis with nearly absent renal function may be indistinguishable from MCDK. If clinically indicated, a percutaneous needle puncture of the collecting system may be performed for fluid analysis, and contrast material may be injected for radiographic imaging. A patent connection between calyces and the renal pelvis is present with UPJ obstruction but is absent with MCDK. VCUG may be performed to identify reflux on the abnormal side and to evaluate the contralateral side. As ureteral atresia commonly accompanies MCDK, ipsilateral reflux is rare and, when present, occurs into a small distal ureter. However, VCUG may reveal reflux into a hydronephrotic MCDK with a patent ureter. The management of unilateral MCDK in babies remains controversial. Some pediatric urologists prefer nonoperative management after diagnosis by ultrasound and renal scintigraphy, whereas others prefer nephrectomy and cite possible infection, hypertension, and rare malignant transformation of the multicystic kidney.[67,68]

Simple Cysts

The incidence of simple cysts in children is difficult to establish; autopsy studies cite a 5% incidence.[69] Reports in the urologic and radiologic literature usually lack pathologic proof or follow-up studies. The most common clinical presentation is a palpable abdominal mass, but hematuria and incidental detection during urography or sonography are reported presentations.[70] Ultrasound demonstrates one or more thin-walled anechoic masses with good through-transmission of sound (Fig. 11–30). The presence of internal echoes suggests that a simple cyst may have been complicated by hemorrhage, infection, or calcification; if cystic neoplasm is a consideration, percutaneous aspiration with sonographic guidance may be diagnostic and therapeutic.

Differential considerations for a cyst include pyelocalyceal diverticulum, localized obstructive hydronephrosis (particularly in the upper pole and related to a duplication anomaly with ureterocele), an ectatic calyx, a liquefied hematoma, or rarely, a renal artery aneurysm or venous malformation.[57] Doppler sonography should be included in the sonographic evaluation to exclude a vascular lesion.

Renal Vein Thrombosis

Another cause of a unilateral or (less commonly) bilateral renal mass is renal vein thrombosis (RVT). Usually occurring in the neonate, RVT is associated with dehydration and hemoconcentration, and with decreased renal perfusion and oxygenation; occasionally, it occurs in association with the nephrotic syndrome. Blood loss, sepsis, and diarrhea are additional commonly associated conditions; furthermore, RVT is more prevalent in infants of diabetic mothers. Sexes are equally affected, but in boys there is equal frequency on either side, whereas in girls the left side is affected three

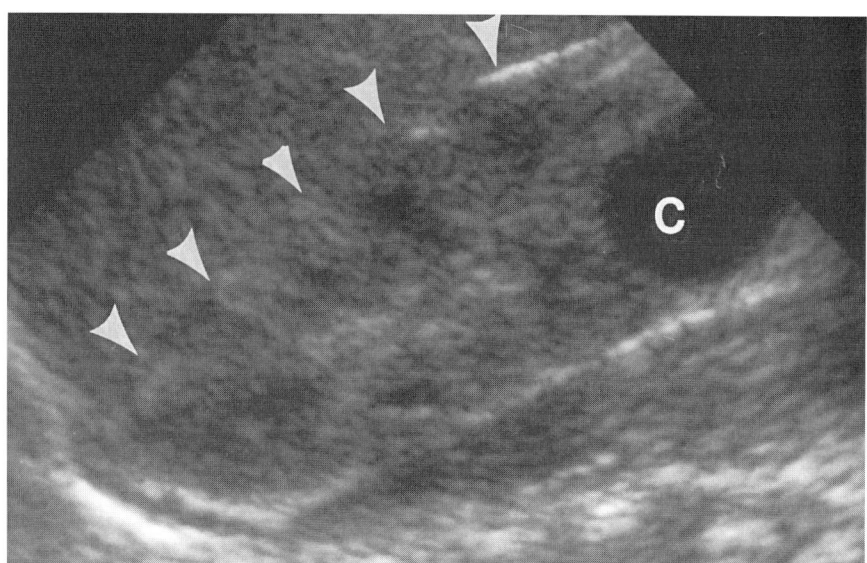

Figure 11–30. Solitary cyst. Longitudinal sonogram shows single cyst (C) in lower pole of kidney (arrowheads).

times more often than the right. Flank mass, hematuria, and transient hypertension are common presenting signs; other findings include proteinuria and coagulopathy with thrombocytopenia. The diagnosis of RVT is usually confirmed with ultrasonography (including Doppler). Renal sonography demonstrates an enlarged echogenic kidney with loss of corticomedullary differentiation secondary to edema and hemorrhage (Fig. 11–31A). Hyperechoic streaks within the perilobular and interlobar regions have been associated with RVT. Doppler signs of RVT are a higher-resistance index and absent, steady, or less pulsatile venous flow on the affected side.[71] Propagation of thrombus into the inferior vena cava can be delineated (Fig. 11–31B). If further confirmatory imaging is needed, renal scintigraphy will show decreased to absent perfusion and function. The outcome depends upon the degree of venous occlusion or infarction and relative venous recanalization and collateral venous flow; complete recovery may occur, or severe atrophy may develop within weeks to months. Reticular calcification within the intrarenal veins of the resultant small end-stage kidney is reported in 30% of cases.[72]

Adrenal Hemorrhage

Adrenal hemorrhage is primarily a neonatal condition. In fact, it is the most common neonatal adrenal lesion; the estimated incidence is 1.7 to 5.8 cases per 1000 live births. Involvement is more frequent in male infants and is bilateral in 5 to 10% and right-sided in 70% of cases.[73] The etiology of adrenal hemorrhage remains unknown, but associated conditions include birth trauma (especially in infants of diabetic mothers), perinatal stress, hypoxia, coagulation disorders, septicemia, and shock. In older children, adrenal hemorrhage can occur as a result of trauma or as a complication of adrenocorticotropic hormone or anticoagulant therapy, severe stress, or overwhelming sepsis.[74] Clinical presentation of the neonate is usually prompted by a palpable mass or complications, such as uncontrollable bleeding or jaundice. RVT (almost always left-sided) commonly causes decreased ipsilateral renal function.[75]

Sonography is the primary imaging study in the diagnosis of neonatal adrenal hemorrhage. The findings depend on the time of the bleed relative to imaging. Initially, the hemorrhagic adrenal is anechoic, and as a clot forms the mass becomes more complex and echogenic (Fig. 11–32A,B). The clot then usually becomes smaller over a 3- to 6-week period, and characteristic calcification occurs within several months (Fig. 11–32C). However, because adrenal hemorrhage may appear as an echogenic or mixed-echogenicity suprarenal mass on initial sonograms, depending upon the age and extent of hemorrhage, it is important to obtain serial sonograms to confirm decreasing size, as expected with adrenal hemorrhage, and to exclude the differential diagnoses of neuroblastoma, adrenal abscess, and Wolman's disease. Adrenal neuroblastoma typically appears echogenic, although it may have hypoechoic necrotic areas and fluid–fluid levels. Purely cystic neuroblastoma is extremely rare. The most important differentiating feature between adrenal hemorrhage and neuroblastoma is that the latter does not change in shape or character over time. Doppler evaluation may be helpful in demonstrating the avascularity of neonatal adrenal hemorrhage versus the vascularity of neuroblastoma. Urinary catecholamine levels, elevated in 85 to 90% of patients with neuroblastoma, should be obtained in all cases of presumed neonatal adrenal hemorrhage. Magnetic resonance imaging (MRI) has also been utilized to increase diagnostic specificity.[76] Adrenal hemorrhage has intense signal on both T1- and T2-weighted MR images; adrenal neuroblastoma typically produces low or intermediate signal intensity on

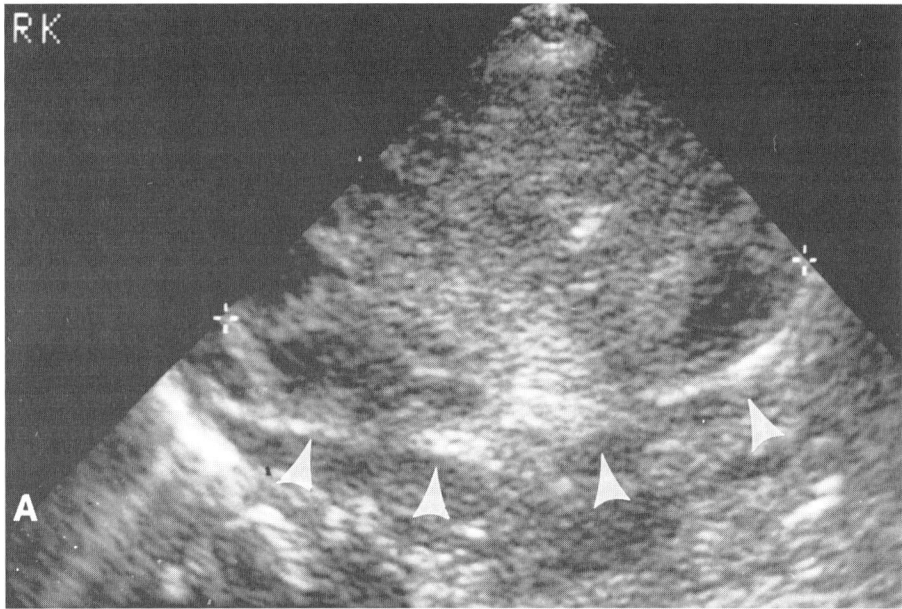

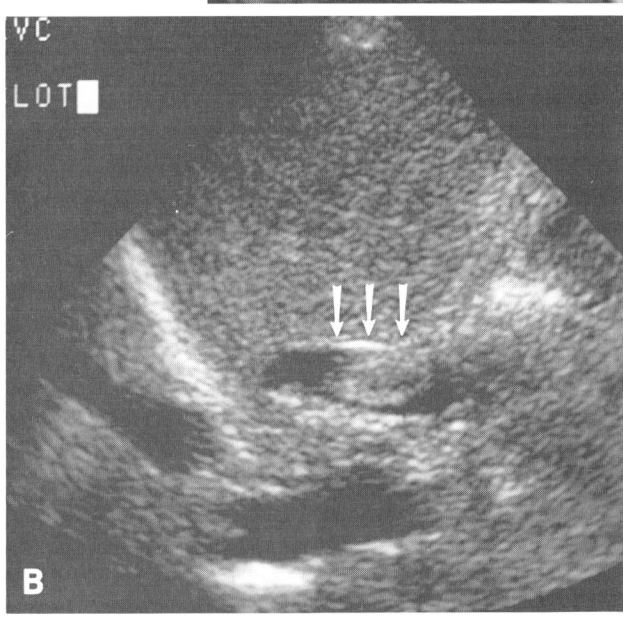

Figure 11–31. Renal vein thrombosis in an infant of a diabetic mother. (**A**) Longitudinal sonogram shows an enlarged echogenic right kidney (+ delineates borders). (**B**) Longitudinal sonogram demonstrates thrombus within the lumen of the inferior vena cava (white arrows).

T1-weighted images and moderate or high signal intensity on T2-weighted images. An adrenal abscess is a rare lesion found in infants (usually not neonates) with sepsis, and its sonographic appearance, though often hypoechoic with scattered internal echoes, may vary with serial sonograms.[77] Tc-99m glucoheptonate renal imaging has been used to differentiate adrenal abscess from adrenal hemorrhage and neuroblastoma.[78] Wolman's disease (familial xanthomatosis with massive adrenal calcification) is usually seen in older infants and is an autosomal recessive disease marked by severe failure to thrive, diarrhea, vomiting, and abdominal distention with hepatomegaly. Adrenal gland calcification and enlargement can be documented by plain radiographs, sonography, or CT.

SUMMARY

Pediatric uroradiology is an ever-changing subspecialty. Although the pediatric urinary tract abnormalities discussed in this chapter have been recognized for many years, their radiologic evaluation continues to evolve. Ultrasonography has replaced the IVU for anatomy depiction, and nuclear scintigraphy provides qualitative and quantitative assessment of renal function. Recent technological developments such as pulsed and color Doppler have enhanced noninvasive ultrasound imaging of particular entities, such as RVT and renal vascular hypertension. CT and MRI currently have limited application in pediatric uroradiology and are mainly useful in abdominal abscess and neoplasia detection; how-

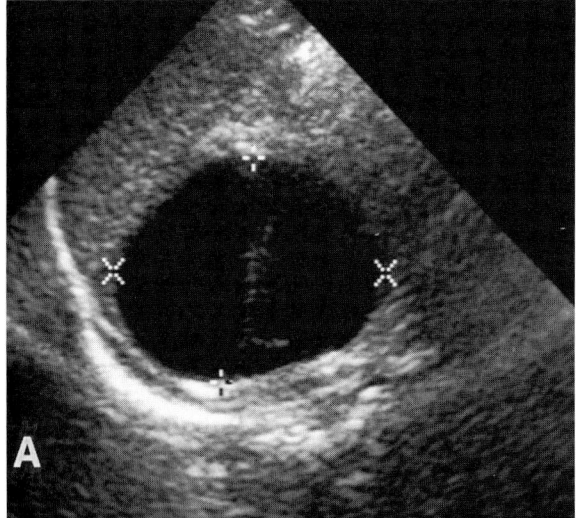
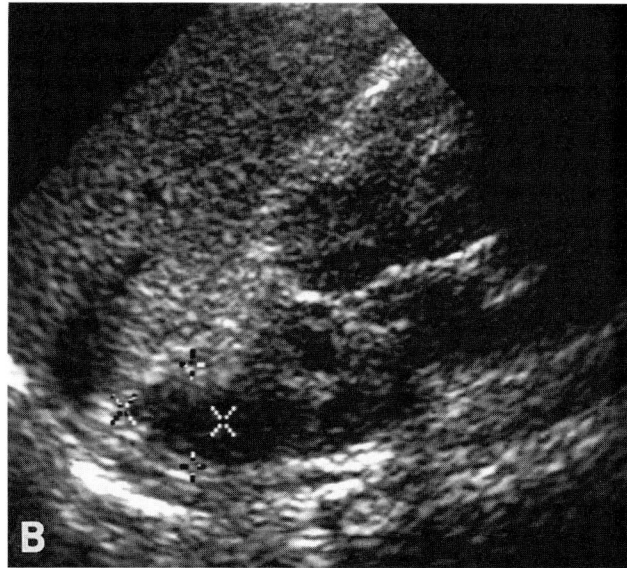
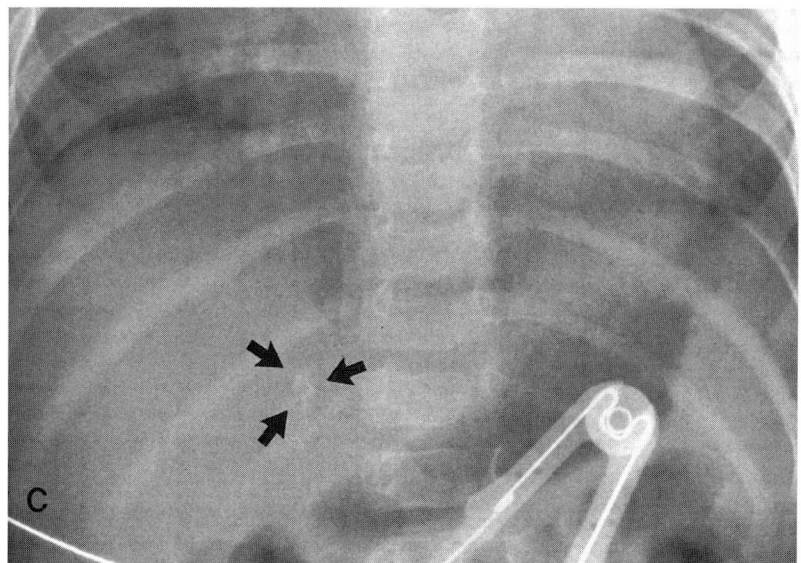

Figure 11–32. Adrenal hemorrhage. (**A**) Initial longitudinal sonogram shows a relatively anechoic mass superior to the kidney. (**B**) Follow-up longitudinal scan shows an echogenic, contracted adrenal gland (+). (**C**) Abdominal radiograph reveals triangular coarse calcifications in the suprarenal region (arrows).

ever, future developments may increase utilization of both techniques. Because pediatric uroradiologic imaging varies somewhat, we have attempted to discuss current concepts within the framework of our own experience and that of authors cited in the references. In this manner we hope to have provided a logical and efficient imaging approach to relatively frequently encountered pediatric urologic problems.

REFERENCES

1. Dubbins PA, Kurtz AB, Wapner RJ, Goldberg BB: Renal agenesis: spectrum of in utero findings. *J Clin Ultrasound* 1981;9:189–193.
2. Kissane J: Congenital malformations. In: Heptinstall RH, ed. *Pathology of the Kidney*, 2nd ed. Boston: Little, Brown, 1974; 69–119.
3. Brown T, Mandell J, Lebowitz RL: Neonatal hydronephrosis in the era of sonography. *AJR* 1987;148:959–963.
4. Romero R, Pilu G, Jeanty P, Ghidini A, Hobbins JC: The urinary tract and adrenal glands. In: *Prenatal Diagnosis of Congenital Anomalies*. Norwalk, CT: Appleton & Lange, 1988; 255–299.
5. Young DW, Lebowitz RL: Congenital abnormalities of the ureter. *Semin Roentgenol* 1986;21:172–187.
6. Sanders RC, Hartman DS: The sonographic distinction between neonatal multicystic kidney and hydronephrosis. *Radiology* 1984;151:621–625.
7. Pfister RC, Hendren WH: Primary megaureter in children and adults: clinical and pathophysiologic features of 150 ureters. *Urology* 1978;12:160–176.
8. Aaronson IA, Cremin BJ: *Clinical Pediatric Uroradiology*. Edinburgh: Churchill Livingstone, 1984;203–208.
9. Meyer JS, Lebowitz RL: Primary megaureter in infants and children: a review. *Urol Radiol* 1992;14:296–305.
10. Wood BP, Ben-Ami T, Teele RL, Rabinowitz R: Ureterovesical obstruction and megaloureter: diagnosis by real-time US. *Radiology* 1985;156:79–81.

11. Babut JM, Fremond B, Sameh A, Vidal V: Primary megaureter in the neonate with prenatal or postnatal diagnosis. *Z Kinderchir* 1988;43:150–153.
12. Hanna MK, Jeffs RD: Primary obstructive megaureter in children. *Urology* 1975;6:419–427.
13. Sripathi V, King PA, Thomson MR, Bogle MS: Primary obstructive megaureter. *J Pediatr Surg* 1991;26:826–829.
14. Mandell J, Lebowitz RL, Peters CA, Estroff JA, Retik AB, Benacerraf BB: Prenatal diagnosis of the megacystis–megaureter association. *J Urol* 1992;148:1487–1489.
15. Siegel MJ: Urinary tract. In: Siegel MJ, ed. *Pediatric Sonography*. New York: Raven Press, 1991;257–309.
16. Share JC, Lebowitz RL: Ectopic ureterocele without ureteral and calyceal dilatation (ureterocele disproportion): findings on urography and sonography. *AJR* 1989;152:567–571.
17. Diard F, Eklöf O, Lebowitz R, Maurseth K: Urethral obstruction in boys caused by prolapse of simple ureterocele. *Pediatr Radiol* 1981;11:139–142.
18. Rabinowitz R, Barkin M, Schillinger JF, Jeffs RD, Cook GT: Bilateral orthotopic ureteroceles causing massive ureteral dilatation in children. *J Urol* 1978;119:839–840.
19. Borden TA, Martinez A: Vesicoureteral reflux associated with intact orthotopic ureterocele. *Urology* 1977;9:182–183.
20. Cremin BJ: A review of the ultrasonic appearances of posterior urethral valve and ureteroceles. *Pediatr Radiol* 1986;16:357–364.
21. Macpherson RI, Leithiser RE, Gordon L, Turner WR: Posterior urethral valves: an update and review. *Radiographics* 1986;6:753–791.
22. Young HH, Frontz WA, Baldwin JC: Congenital obstruction of the posterior urethra. *J Urol* 1919;3:289–365.
23. Turner RJ: Early antenatal diagnosis and natural progression of untreated posterior urethral valve syndrome. *Tex Med* 1985;81:51–54.
24. Angtuaco TL, Miller SF, Ferris EJ: Congenital urinary tract abnormalities: prenatal and neonatal diagnosis. *Curr Probl Diagn Radiol* 1990;19:165–198.
25. Griesbach WA, Waterhouse RK, Mellins HZ: Voiding cystourethrography in the diagnosis of congenital posterior urethral valves. *AJR* 1959;82:521–529.
26. Glassberg KI: Current issues regarding posterior urethral valves. *Urol Clin North Am* 1985;12:175–185.
27. King LR: Posterior urethra, In: Kelalis PP, King LR, Belman AB, eds: *Clinical Pediatric Urology, 1*, 2nd ed. Philadelphia: WB Saunders, 1985;527–558.
28. Tejani A, Butt K, Glassberg K, Price A, Gurumurthy K: Predictors of eventual end stage renal disease in children with posterior urethral valves. *J Urol* 1986;136:857–860.
29. Williams DI: *Urology in Childhood*. New York: Springer-Verlag, 1974;195–229.
30. Berdon WE, Baker DH, Wigger HJ, Blanc WA: The radiologic and pathologic spectrum of the prune belly syndrome: the importance of urethral obstruction in prognosis. *Radiol Clin North Am* 1977;15:83–92.
31. Garris J, Kangarloo H, Sarti D, Sample WF, Smith LE: The ultrasound spectrum of prune-belly syndrome. *J Clin Ultrasound* 1980;8:117–120.
32. Blane CE, Koff SA, Bowerman RA, Barr M Jr: Nonobstructive fetal hydronephrosis: sonographic recognition and therapeutic implications. *Radiology* 1983;147:95–99.
33. Scott JES: Fetal ureteric reflux. *Br J Urol* 1987;59:291–296.
34. Broyer M, Guest G, Lestage F, Gacoin FB: Prenatal diagnosis of urinary tract malformations. *Adv Nephrol Necker Hosp* 1985;14:21–38.
35. Hodson CJ: Neuhauser lecture. Reflux nephropathy: a personal historical review. *AJR* 1981;137:451–462.
36. Levitt SB, Duckett J, Spitzer A, et al: Medical versus surgical treatment of primary vesicoureteral reflux: report of the International Reflux Study Committee. *Pediatrics* 1981;67:392–400.
37. Van den Abbeele AD, Treves ST, Lebowitz RL, et al: Vesicoureteral reflux in asymptomatic siblings of patients with known reflux: radionuclide cystography. *Pediatrics* 1987;79:147–153.
38. Buonomo C, Treves ST, Jones B, Summerville D, Bauer S, Retik A: Silent renal damage in symptom-free siblings of children with vesicoureteral reflux: assessment with technetium Tc 99m dimercaptosuccinic acid scintigraphy. *J Pediatr* 1993;122:721–723.
39. Gross GW, Lebowitz RL: Infection does not cause reflux. *AJR* 1981;137:929–932.
40. Lebowitz RL, Mandell J: Urinary tract infection in children: putting radiology in its place. *Radiology* 1987;165:1–9.
41. Pais VM, Retik AB: Reversible hydronephrosis in the neonate with urinary sepsis. *N Engl J Med* 1975;292:465–467.
42. Rolleston GL, Shannon FT, Utley WLF: Relationship of infantile vesicoureteral reflux to renal damage. *BMJ* 1970;1:460–463.
43. Blickman JG, Taylor GA, Lebowitz RL: Voiding cystourethrography: the initial radiologic study in children with urinary tract infection. *Radiology* 1985;156:659–662.
44. Strife JL, Bisset GS III, Kirks DR, et al: Nuclear cystography and renal sonography: findings in girls with urinary tract infection. *AJR* 1989;153:115–119.
45. Cardiff-Oxford Bacteriuria Study Group: Sequelae of covert bacteriuria in school girls: a four-year follow-up study. *Lancet* 1978;1:889–893.
46. Kangarloo H, Gold RH, Fine RN, Diament MJ, Boechat MI: Urinary tract infection in infants and children evaluated by ultrasound. *Radiology* 1985;154:367–373.
47. Leonidas JC, McCauley RGK, Klauber GC, Fretzayas AM: Sonography as a substitute for excretory urography in children with urinary tract infection. *AJR* 1985;144:815–819.
48. Slovis TL, Sty JR, Haller JO: *Imaging of the Pediatric Urinary Tract*. Philadelphia: WB Saunders, 1989.
49. Andrich MP, Majd M: Diagnostic imaging in the evaluation of the first urinary tract infection in infants and young children. *Pediatrics* 1992;90:436–441.
50. Eggli DF, Tulchinsky M: Scintigraphic evaluation of pediatric urinary tract infection. *Semin Nucl Med* 1993;23:199–218.
51. Rosenfield AT, Glickman MG, Taylor KJW, Crade M, Hodson J: Acute focal bacterial nephritis (acute lobar nephronia). *Radiology* 1979;132:553–561.
52. Lee JKT, McClennan BL, Melson GL, Stanley RJ: Acute focal bacterial nephritis: emphasis on gray scale sonography and computed tomography. *AJR* 1980;135:87–92.
53. Osathanondh V, Potter EL: Pathogenesis of polycystic kidneys. *Arch Pathol* 1964;77:459–512.
54. Hartman DS: *Renal Cystic Disease*. Philadelphia: WB Saunders, 1989;1–154.
55. Bernstein J: A classification of renal cysts, in Gardner KD, ed. *Cystic Disease of the Kidney*. New York: John Wiley, 1976;7–30.
56. Mahony BS: The genitourinary system. In: Callen PW, ed. *Ultrasonography in Obstetrics and Gynecology*, 2nd ed. Philadelphia: WB Saunders, 1988;254–276.
57. Teele RL, Share JC: *Ultrasonography of Infants and Children*. Philadelphia: WB Saunders, 1991.
58. Hayden CK Jr, Swischuk LE, Smith TH, Armstrong EA: Renal cystic disease in childhood. *Radiographics* 1986;6:97–116.
59. Reeders ST, Breuning MH, Corney G, et al: Two genetic markers closely linked to adult polycystic kidney disease on chromosome 16. *BMJ* 1986;292:851–853.
60. Pretorius DH, Lee ME, Manco-Johnson ML, Weingast GR,

Sedman AB, Gabow PA: Diagnosis of autosomal dominant polycystic kidney disease in utero and in the young infant. *J Ultrasound Med* 1987;6:249–255.

61. McAlister WH, Siegel MJ, Shackelford GD, Askin F, Kissane JM: Glomerulocystic kidney. *AJR* 1979;133:536–538.
62. Worthington JL, Shackelford GD, Cole BR, Tack ED, Kissane JM: Sonographically detectable cysts in polycystic kidney disease in newborn and young infants. *Pediatr Radiol* 1988;18:287–293.
63. Patriquin HB, O'Regan S: Medullary sponge kidney in childhood. *AJR* 1985;145:315–319.
64. Glassberg KI, Filmer RB: Renal dysplasia, renal hypoplasia, and cystic disease of the kidney. In: Kelalis PP, King LR, Belman AB, eds. *Clinical Pediatric Urology, 2*, 2nd ed. Philadelphia: WB Saunders, 1985;922–971.
65. Kleiner B, Filly RA, Mack L, Callen PW: Multicystic dysplastic kidney: observations of contralateral disease in the fetal population. *Radiology* 1986;161:27–29.
66. Felson B, Cussen LJ: The hydronephrotic type of unilateral congenital multicystic disease of the kidney. *Semin Roentgenol* 1975;10:113–123.
67. Hartman GE, Smolik LM, Shochat SJ: The dilemma of the multicystic dysplastic kidney. *Am J Dis Child* 1986;140:925–928.
68. Gordon AC, Thomas DFM, Arthur RJ, Irving HC: Multicystic dysplastic kidney: is nephrectomy still appropriate? *J Urol* 1988;140:1231–1234.
69. Mir S, Rapola J, Koskimies O: Renal cysts in pediatric autopsy material. *Nephron* 1983;33:189–195.
70. Siegel MJ, McAlister WH: Simple cysts of the kidney in children. *J Urol* 1980;123:75–78.
71. Laplante S, Patriquin HB, Robitaille P, Filiatrault D, Grignon A, Décarie J-C: Renal vein thrombosis in children: evidence of early flow recovery with Doppler US. *Radiology* 1993;189:37–42.
72. Sutton TJ, Leblanc A, Gauthier N, Hassan M: Radiological manifestations of neonatal renal vein thrombosis on follow-up examinations. *Radiology* 1977;122:435–438.
73. Kuhn J, Jewett T, Munschauer R: The clinical and radiographic features of massive neonatal adrenal hemorrhage. *Radiology* 1971;99:647–652.
74. Levin TL, Morton E: Adrenal hemorrhage complicating ACTH therapy in Crohn's disease. *Pediatr Radiol* 1993;23:457–458.
75. Lebowitz JM, Belman AB: Simultaneous idiopathic adrenal hemorrhage and renal vein thrombosis in the newborn. *J Urol* 1983;129:574–576.
76. Willemse APP, Coppes MJ, Feldberg MAM, Kramer PPG, Witkamp TD: Magnetic resonance appearance of adrenal hemorrhage in a neonate. *Pediatr Radiol* 1989;19:210–211.
77. Atkinson GO Jr, Kodroff MB, Gay BB Jr, Ricketts RR: Adrenal abscess in the neonate. *Radiology* 1985;155:101–104.
78. Wells RG, Sty JR, Hodgson NB: Suprarenal abscess in the neonate: technetium-99m glucoheptonate imaging. *Clin Nucl Med* 1986;11:32–34.

12 Urinary Tract Infections

Michael P. Donovan, Culley C. Carson III

Urinary tract infections are a major source of morbidity and health care costs in the United States. In 1992 urinary tract infections accounted for 286,000 hospital admissions and were involved in another 1.547 million hospitalizations.[1] These infections are also the leading cause of gram-negative bacteremia and death due to sepsis in hospitals. The occurrence of nosocomial bacteremia and sepsis is commonly associated with urinary tract instrumentation, usually indwelling catheters, and urinary infections with gram-negative organisms.[2] The urinary tract is second only to the upper respiratory tract in the occurrence of infections seen by physicians. Almost half the patients seen in the urologist's office and hospital practice involve the diagnosis and treatment of urinary tract infection.

Urinary tract infections occur in all ages of both sexes but are more common in women, 10 to 20% of whom will have a urinary infection at some time during their lives. Although many of these infections are of low morbidity, the incidence of renal scarring as a sequela of urinary infections in autopsy series is reported as high as 15% of patients studied.[2,3] These autopsy findings imply that many asymptomatic urinary infections gradually lead to chronic pyelonephritis with renal scarring. Severe renal damage, even to the point of renal failure, can begin as a single episode of lower urinary tract infection and progress inexorably to renal failure.

Urinary tract infections, both acute and chronic, are challenging diagnostic and management problems. It is of extreme importance to both patient and physician to separate urinary tract infections into those that require vigorous and continued therapy and follow-up, and those that are of lesser import. The use of localization techniques, cultures, radiography, and imaging modalities such as ultrasound, radionucleotide studies, computerized tomography, and magnetic resonance imaging allows for such a segregation.

INFECTIONS OF THE LOWER URINARY TRACT

Bacterial Cystitis

The urinary bladder is the most common site of infection in the urinary tract. Infections of the bladder in females frequently coexist with urethral infections, and in males they often coexist with infections of the prostate. The importance of these infections lies in their common occurrence and economic impact as well as in the knowledge that most upper urinary tract infections begin with bacterial cystitis. This cystitis may subsequently ascend to involve the kidneys. The discovery of a lower urinary tract infection, therefore, draws attention to the urinary tract, and an attempt to prevent a serious future pyelonephritis must be considered despite the apparently benign nature of the infection.

For purposes of evaluation and treatment urinary tract infections are often classified by Stamey's original description as either first infections, unresolved bacteriuria, bacterial persistence, or reinfection.[4] It is also helpful to differentiate asymptomatic bacteriuria from acute uncomplicated urinary tract infection or complicated urinary tract infection. Asymptomatic bacteriuria implies urinary colonization, whereas urinary tract infection implies clinical, histologic, or immunologic evidence of host injury by bacterial replication.[5] Complicated urinary tract infections are those that occur in a patient who has a functionally, metabolically, or anatomically abnormal urinary tract that makes it possible for bacteria that are usually not pathogenic to cause infections, or infections by pathogens resistant to antibiotics.[6] Nephrolithiasis, bladder outlet obstruction, urethral strictures, reflux, and double collecting systems all interfere with the free flow of urine and create a complicated setting in which these infections are more likely to occur.[6,7]

Human urine is normally sterile as it enters and leaves the urinary bladder. It is remarkably resistant to infection by ordinary bacteria. The chemical makeup of the urine and the ability of the bladder to empty completely with each voiding combine to form the host resistance to colonization and infection from bacteria of the lower urinary tract.

Bacteriuria is defined as bacterial colonization of the urine and the urinary tract. It can occur in patients with or without symptoms.[8] Significant bacteriuria has been defined as greater than 100,000 organisms of a single species per milliliter (mL) of voided urine. Quantitative urine cultures have been used to discriminate contamination from infection and between infected and noninfected asymptomatic bacteriuria. Kass's pioneering work clearly showed that patients with enterobacteriaceae greater than 100,000 colonies/mL in their urine on three successive voided specimens have infected urine in 95% of cases. The sensitivity of one such specimen is 80%.[8] Studies of acutely symptomatic young women with bladder bacteriuria on suprapubic aspirate, however, have shown that only one-half of the patients had greater than

100,000 colony-forming units (CFU)/mL on culture of the midstream specimen.[9] Midstream urine cultures of only 100 to 10,000 gram-negative bacteria are found in approximately a third of ambulatory women with acute dysuric episodes.[10] In correctly collected urine samples in symptomatic female patients, therefore, counts as low as 100 bacteria/mL may indicate significant infection.[4,9–11] In symptomatic men, urine cultures of 1000 CFU/mL of a uropathogen are considered significant bacteriuria.[12] In catheterized patients even lower levels of bacteriuria may be significant. Bacterial counts of 100 CFU/mL of a single species have been shown to progress to counts of 100,000 CFU/mL within 24 to 48 hours and reflect actual infections.[13]

Bacteriuria is most commonly due to *Escherichia coli*, followed in incidence by *Klebsiella*, *Enterobacter*, *Serratia*, *Proteus*, and *Pseudomonas*. In nonhospitalized ambulatory patients *Staphylococcus saprophyticus* is an important uropathogen and accounts for a significant number of infections in young women.[14] Along with gram-negative organisms, enterococci and other staphylococcal species are more common in nosocomial and complicated urinary infections. In debilitated and bedridden patients gram-positive organisms have been increasingly identified as urinary tract pathogens.[15] Urinary tract infection with more than one organism is rare and raises suspicion for underlying urogenital pathology.

The diagnosis of urosepsis can best be made by urine culture. Leukocyte esterase nitrite dipstick urinalysis, microscopic analysis of spun urine, Gram staining of urinary sediment, and hemocytometric cell counting have all been used to screen for lower urinary tract infection with fairly good results. Leukocyte esterase is released by white blood cells in the urine and is a very sensitive test for detecting pyuria associated with urinary infections. A positive nitrite test indicates the presence of bacteria that can convert nitrate to nitrite and is more specific for bacteriuria. One caveat, however, is that not all bacteria have this capacity. In symptomatic patients the leukocyte esterase-nitrite dipstick test is sensitive for detecting infections that will correlate with 10,000 CFU/mL of cultured urine 88% of the time.[16] The diagnostic accuracy of this screening test is increased when combined with a standard urinalysis and Gram staining of the urine sediment. Appropriate Gram staining of the urine sediment results in the identification of significant numbers of gram-negative organisms and can be correlated with midstream urine cultures of more than 100,000 CFU/mL.[10,16] Any bacteria seen with light microscopy on high power in an unspun urine specimen generally correlate with urine cultures of greater than 100,000 CFU/mL. Patients with compromised host resistance, urologic instrumentation, or presence of a foreign body within the urinary tract may have unreliable urine dipstick or Gram stain findings, and only urine culture may reliably diagnose urosepsis.

Pyuria is often used to diagnose urinary tract infection and to differentiate urinary colonization from true urinary tract infection. Nonpathologic limits for pyuria have been established as less than 10 leukocytes/mm^3 in uncentrifuged urine. Using this definition, pyuria is present in less than 1% of asymptomatic nonbacteriuric patients versus 96% of symptomatic men and women with significant bacteriuria.[5] Microscopic analysis of centrifuged urine is less reliable and does not always correlate with the number of cells per cubic millimeter. Generally, 5 to 10 leukocytes per high-powered field (HPF) in centrifuged urine are considered significant, although as few as 2 leukocytes/HPF have been shown to correlate with 10 leukocytes/mm^3 in uncentrifuged urine.[17] Although significant bacteriuria in symptomatic patients is usually associated with pyuria, the association is not invariable in all patients. In one study of pregnant women with asymptomatic bacteriuria only 49% had pathologically significant pyuria.[18] Pyuria without bacteriuria can also occur in patients with chlamydial infection, tuberculosis, polycystic renal disease, hypertension, or diabetes mellitus. Microscopic hematuria is present in approximately 50% of urinary tract infection and helps differentiate infection from colonization.

The importance of careful, midstream urine collection cannot be overemphasized. Appropriate meatal, labial, and glanular cleansing with antiseptic solutions, such as iodophor, prior to midsteam collection is of great importance. In patients in whom this technique is impossible, urethral catheterization or suprapubic needle aspiration of the bladder may be necessary to provide an adequate urine specimen. Immediate refrigeration of the specimen and culture inoculation within 12 hours of collection further add to the reliability of the bacteriologic determination. Cultures can be carried out on disposable blood agar and eosin-methylene blue (EMB) agar plates. A simple and accurate technique for office cultures using dip-slides has given even the smallest physician's office the availability of rapid, reliable culture methods.

There is little doubt that microorganisms are frequently introduced into the bladder in a retrograde fashion.[19] The ability of host defenses to eradicate these microorganisms prior to the onset of frank infection requires active host resistance as well as normal voiding flow dynamics. The balance between these host defenses and the infective ability of the microorganism is critical. Trauma, obstruction, foreign bodies, and many other factors increase the facility with which organisms colonize and infect the lower urinary tract.

The incidence of urinary tract infections varies according to the different patient populations and their host defenses. In females there is a progressive increase in incidence of bacteriuria from 1 to 2% of preschool and schoolgirls to 2 to 3% by young adulthood and then an additional increase of 1 to 2% for each decade of life.[11,20] Urinary tract infection is uncommon in young or middle-aged men with a reported incidence of less than 1%, but it begins to rise after the fifth decade until it approaches the frequency in females.[12] Interesting differences in the incidence of urinary infections have been noted with regard to patients and their host defenses. Kunin showed that significant caliectasis, hydronephrosis, unilateral small kidney, reflux, vesical trabeculation, and the megacystis syndrome were frequently associated with asymptomatic bacteriuria in a general population of school girls.[21] Uncomplicated maternity patients have a reported incidence of 4.74 to 5.9% of asymptomatic bacteriuria.[20] In diabetic pregnant patients this figure approaches 12.5% with the highest incidence of asymptomatic bacteriuria noted in pregnant women who have a history of previous urinary tract infection.[22] Aging and hospitalization can further compromise host resistance to urinary tract infection. Stamey reported a 10 to 20% incidence of urinary tract infections on hospital medical wards.[19] The incidence of facility-acquired infections in the elderly has been reported in as many as one-third of nursing home patients followed for 4 months.[23] Of these, 47% were urinary tract infections. Chronic indwelling Foley catheters were implicated in approximately half of these infections.

The problem of frank urinary tract infection in children is far more serious. Frequently, these infections begin in infancy or even in the neonatal period. In the first few months of life, males are more commonly affected; females are the most commonly affected group in later childhood. It is this group that is most susceptible to progression to chronic pyelonephritis.[24]

There is no universal study capable of differentiating lower urinary tract infection from acute uncomplicated upper urinary tract infection. Localization techniques such as bladder washout studies, ureteral catheterization for collection of urine, and percutaneous renal collection of urine are needed only in selected complicated cases and are unecessarily invasive for the majority of patients with acute bacteriuria. Although noninvasive techniques, like the antibody-coated bacteria studies, have shown promise, their widespread clinical usefulness has not been confirmed. Most patients without clinical symptoms or signs of upper urinary tract involvement are, therefore, treated as though they have cystitis only.

Adult patients with lower urinary tract infections, even of the recurrent variety, require few diagnostic procedures in addition to urine studies. The classic manifestations of cystitis; dysuria, urgency, and frequency are caused by inflammation of the urethra and bladder outlet and may be present without infection. Patients may complain of gross hematuria, pyuria, malodorous urine, and abdominal pain if their urines are heavily infected. Few findings are present on physical examination. The only findings present are urethral infection and, occasionally, suprapubic tenderness.

Patients with upper urinary tract infections frequently require radiographic procedures to guide management and to detect anatomic or obstructive abnormalities. Congenital abnormalities, renal calculi, and obstructive pathology are best evaluated by excretory urography. Urography should be obtained in all patients with urinary infections who are at high risk for surgically treatable urinary tract abnormalities.

This high-risk group includes all children with urinary infections, males with urinary infections not confined to the prostate, patients with relapsing infections, and those patients in whom urinary infections have progressed to bacteremia. These patients should be studied with an excretory urogram and postvoiding bladder film to evaluate upper tracts and residual urine. All excretory urograms should include nephrotomography. Voiding cystourethrograms should be obtained in all children with urinary tract infections to diagnose vesicoureteral reflux. Since vesicoureteral reflux may be related to progressive renal scarring, especially in school-age children, these studies should be done in any child with bacteriuria.

Urologic evaluation with excretory urography is indicated when the patient presents with upper urinary tract symptoms, such as flank pain and high fever, or when the patient has had these symptoms in a past episode.[25] Other indications are persistent microscopic hematuria, a history of obstruction, or stone disease. Cystoscopy is indicated in populations at high risk for a bladder tumor or when hematuria is persistent. Clinical suspicion of a urethral diverticulum can be confirmed using a voiding cystourethrogram or double balloon urethrogram. Urodynamic evaluation is useful only in patients whose history is consistent with abnormal voiding pattern.[25]

Urologic evaluation using excretory urography and cystography has been uniformly nonproductive in lower tract infections. Several studies have shown that women with lower urinary tract infections or the urethral syndrome, which rarely have upper tract pathology, are frequently evaluated with multiple radiographic studies with low yield.[26,27] Patients with the urethral syndrome—frequency, urgency, dysuria in the absence of "significant bacteriuria"—rarely have urographic abnormalities.[26] Incidental findings may be detected on excretory urography, but these are usually clinically insignificant.[27] Cystourethroscopy is usually not necessary and will be normal in 86% of patients.[26]

Full evaluation of patients with lower urinary tract infections is necessary if significant voiding dysfunction, symptoms associated with upper tract infections, or bacteriuria unresponsive to appropriate antibiotic therapy are present. In those patients excretory urography and cystoscopy may reveal anatomic abnormalities, foreign bodies, obstructive uropathy, of neurogenic vesical dysfunction.

Cystitis Emphysematosa

Cystitis emphysematosa is a rare manifestation of urinary tract infection in which bacteria produce gas in the bladder wall and lumen. These infections are usually found in patients with severe diabetes mellitus and gas-forming urinary bacteria. More commonly, however, gas in the bladder and, indeed, the upper urinary tract is iatrogenic. Infections of cystitis emphysematosa are usually caused by common aerobic pathogens such as *Escherichia coli*, *Enterobacter*, *Proteus*, *Pseudomonas*, and less commonly, staphylococcal and streptococcal species.[28] Rarely, *Clostridia* may produce the gas, especially in association with an enteric or perineal infection.[29]

More than half the cases of gas-producing infection in the urinary tract occur in diabetic patients.[28] It has been suggested that the presence of hyperglycemia will allow

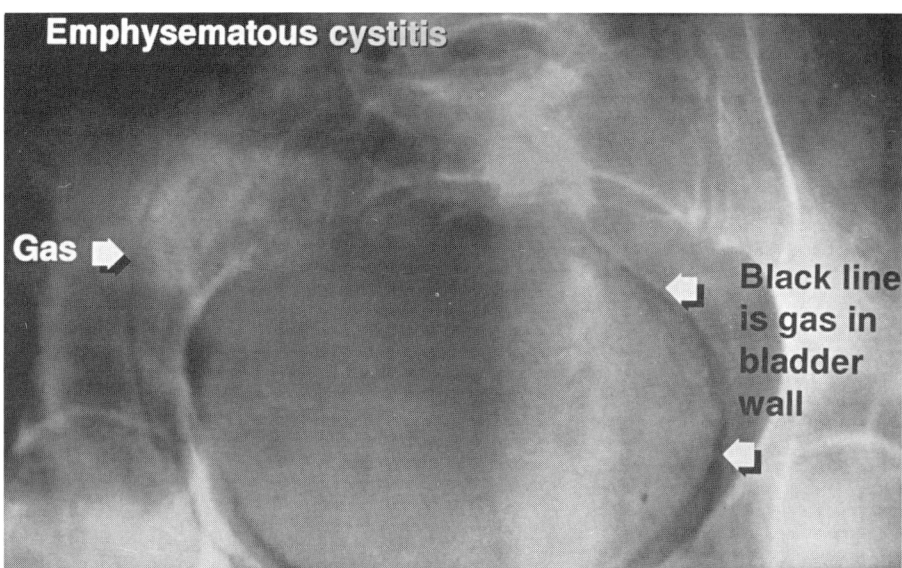

Figure 12–1. Emphysematous cystitis in a diabetic patient. Notice the gas shadow (dark line) outlining the fluid-filled bladder. (Courtesy of Dr. R. Older.)

fermentation by certain strains of bacteria with the production of gas. The gas is then deposited within the tissues of the bladder wall. The gas present usually collects within the wall of the bladder but may also accumulate in the bladder lumen.

The differentiation of gas collections caused by emphysematous cystitis from gas present after instrumentation or caused by vesicoenteric or other fistulas is best done by cystogram and cystoscopy. Urographically, collections of gas are seen to overlie the bladder region on kidney and urinary bladder (KUB), and pelvic film. Excretory urography confirms that the gas lies within the bladder. Films at various degrees of bladder emptying and oblique views will further add to localization. Sonographic findings are nonspecific but may show echogenic diffuse wall thickening associated with posterior acoustic shadowing.[28] CT scans will also demonstrate gas within the bladder wall and are more precise at defining the extent and location of the gas collections. Cystoscopy is the most reliable diagnostic procedure and can help differentiate between intravesical gas accumulations, gas present after instrumentation, and vesical fistulas.[30] Typical findings of emphysematous cystitis on cystoscopy include marked acute cystitis with vesicles of various size and interspersed areas of hemorrhage (Figs. 12–1, 12–2).

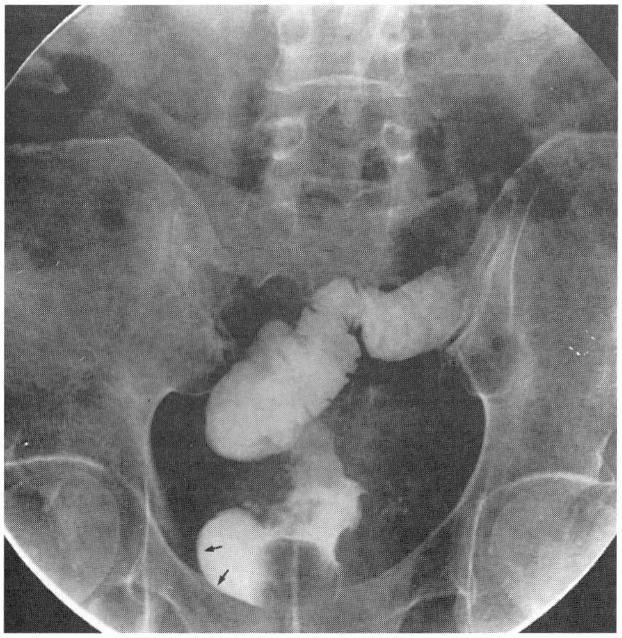

INFLAMMATORY BLADDER LESIONS: CYSTITIS CYSTICA, CYSTITIS GLANDULARIS, MALAKOPLAKIA, INTERSTITIAL CYSTITIS, AND EOSINOPHILIC CYSTITIS

Inflammatory bladder lesions arise occasionally in the evaluation of urinary tract infection and in some cases may actually represent reactions to chronic infection. These lesions include cystitis cystica, cystitis glandularis, malakoplakia, interstitial cystitis, and eosinophilic cystitis. Of these, interstitial cystitis and eosinophilic cystitis are not associated with known infections and will only be covered briefly.

Cystitis Cystica

Cystitis cystica is a benign bladder condition of unclear etiology. Evidence suggests that the lesions of cystitis cystica are a manifestation of an immunologic mediated reaction by which the urinary tract attempts to deal with an infection or irritation within the bladder. Pathologically, there is a gen-

Figure 12–2. Vesicocolic fistula cystogram. Arrows identify the bladder. There is massive efflux of contrast media into a segment of small bowel.

Urinary Tract Infections 261

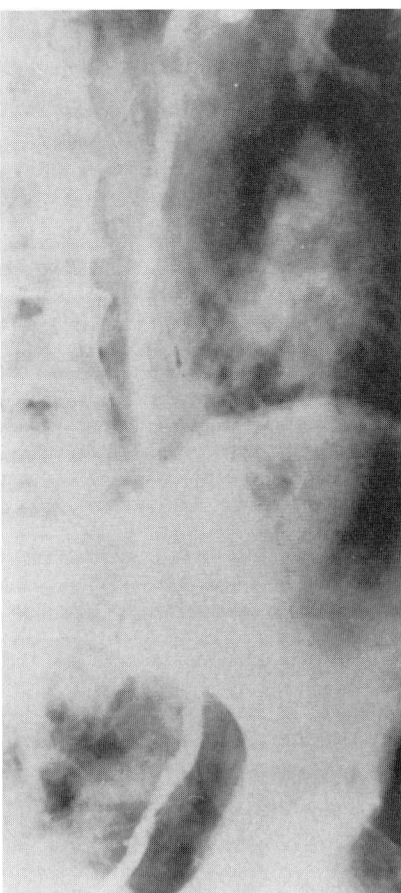

Figure 12–3. Ureteritis cystica. Multiple cystic structures and cobblestoning of the ureter are seen throughout the course of the ureter in this patient with chronic upper tract urinary tract infections.

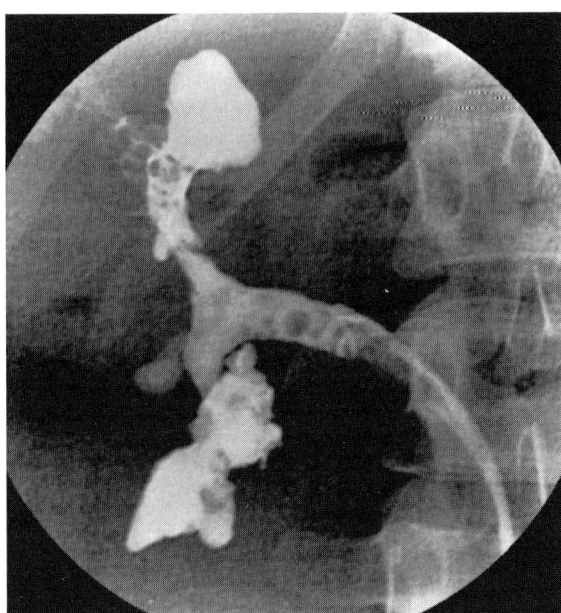

Figure 12–4. Pyelitis cystica retrograde pyelogram. Diffuse pyelitis cystica is seen in this patient with chronic urinary infections and hydronephrosis.

eral disorganized urothelial architecture with lymphocyte infiltration, occasional von Brunn's nests, and multiple cysts.[31] Increased immunoglobulin production has been described in the epithelial cells but their role in the development of inflammatory crypts or von Brunn's cell nest into mature cysts is unclear.[32]

Cystoscopically, small rounded cysts are present, usually in the trigone and at the bladder outlet. The cysts are colorless or slightly yellow in appearance. They are usually less than 1 cm in size, are multiple, and are pathologically benign. Urographically, findings are typical of multiple small cystic structures. Whether present only in the bladder or extending to ureter and renal pelves, small, smooth-walled, radiolucent filling defects are seen, causing a scalloped appearance of the bladder wall and upper urinary tracts. These lesions are nonobstructive and can be differentiated from other types of lucent filling defects. Because of their resemblance to urothelial malignancy, however, urine cytology, brush biopsy, and retrograde pyelography may be necessary to confirm the diagnosis. The introduction of air bubbles during retrograde pyelography may frequently cause some confusion, as small, localized areas of cystic change in the upper tracts may mimic these bubbles. Bubble evacuation, additional contrast media instillation, and delayed films will usually reveal a change in position of air bubbles while the lesions of cystitis cystica remain static. These lesions may remain for long periods, despite eradication of infection and relief of obstruction. For this reason differentiation from transitional cell carcinoma is essential. Cystitis cystica is an important diagnostic finding and when present only in the bladder can easily be confirmed by cystoscopic examination. These cysts are most common in women with chronic urinary infection and usually resolve with adequate control of bacteriuria. One study found that 97 of 439 girls evaluated with recurrent urinary tract infection had cystoscopic findings of cystitis cystica.[33] These chronic infections associated with cystitis cystica are often difficult to treat and eradicate (Figs. 12–3, 12–4).

Cystitis Glandularis

Cystitis glandularis is a rare manifestation of mucosal metaplasia resulting from chronic infection or foreign-body irritation. Like cystitis cystica, cystitis glandularis is thought to arise from gland formation of von Brunn's nests and may represent a continuum of metaplasia within the urothelium.[34,35] Cystitis glandularis, however, is associated with primary adenocarcinoma of the bladder and is considered a premalignant lesion similar to metaplastic intestinal mucosa.[34] These lesions have been reported frequently in patients with extrophy of the bladder and pelvic lipomatosis.[35,36] It has been suggested that pelvic lymphedema and venous stasis lead to the histologic changes seen in cystitis glandularis. Closure of extrophic bladders in infancy decreases the metaplastic changes seen in the bladder mucosa of children with extrophy.[36]

Evaluation with excretory urography reveals only nonspecific lucent filling defects on cystography. Imaging studies with CT, sonography, and MRI will demonstrate bladder wall thickening and frequently well-defined lesions in the bladder but are nonspecific. Diagnosis must be made by biopsy of the lesion and histologic examination. Cystitis glandularis is treated by removal of chronic vesical irritation with excision and fulguration of the lesion. Close cystoscopic follow-up of these patients is required to eliminate the possibility that cystitis glandularis will progress to adenocarcinoma of the bladder.

Malakoplakia

Malakoplakia is a disease of impaired macrophage response to infection that can involve any organ system but is most commonly found in the urinary tract.[34] Although most cases involve the bladder, these lesions have also been found in the kidneys, ureters, prostate, and testes.[37] Patients usually present with lower urinary tract irritative symptoms and hematuria. Most have a history of recurrent urinary tract infections treated with various antibiotics, usually without an adequate course of therapy. Malakoplakia is more common in women, with a peak incidence in the fifth decade. An association between host altered immune response caused by systemic disease and the development of malakoplakia has been noted.[38]

Cystoscopy is frequently diagnostic in these cases, revealing yellowish lesions, 2 to 3 cm in diameter with a velvety, raised appearance. Many patients pass large amounts of debris while voiding. The lesions can be found on any part of the bladder but are most common on the posterior wall and bladder base.

In as many as 25% of patients with malakoplakia of the bladder, the upper tract structures are also involved.[39] The definitive diagnosis of this condition, however, rests on a biopsy that reveals a sheetlike histiocytic inflammatory reaction that contains numerous Michaelis-Gutmann bodies. These Michaelis-Gutmann bodies are easily identified as concentrically laminated calcospherules, which are deeply basophilic staining with PAS stain. They are thought to be the remnants of partially digested bacteria.[37]

Malakoplakia is a difficult radiographic diagnosis. Excretory urography is frequently normal, especially if only the lower tract is involved. Lesions of the ureter and renal pelvis include ureteropelvic junction obstruction, lucent filling defects of the ureter or calyces, and a generalized dilation and scalloped appearance of the ureters.[37,39] If lucent lesions are seen in the upper tracts, retrograde pyelography with selective ureteral cytology collections and brush biopsy may be necessary to differentiate malakoplakia and transitional cell carcinoma. Sonography, MRI, and CT have been useful in determining the extent of disease and monitoring response to treatment but are unable to differentiate malakoplakia lesions from other pelvic masses.[38]

Interstitial Cystitis

Interstitial cystitis is an enigmatic inflammatory disease of the urinary bladder most commonly found in middle-aged women. Patients with this condition complain of severe bladder pain on filling that is relieved by frequent voiding. Bladder capacity is usually limited and progressively decreasing as the process continues. Urinalysis may reveal microscopic hematuria but the urine is sterile. Pathologically, there are varying degrees of inflammatory infiltrate in the submucosa and muscularis with edema, and in cases of longer duration, fibrosis. Although multiple pathogenetic mechanisms have been suggested there is no evidence for a bacterial, fungal, or viral etiology.[34] There have been several reports of transitional cell carcinoma in situ associated with symptoms similar to interstitial cystitis, especially when symptoms are present in men.[40]

Cystoscopy is usually diagnostic and reveals petechial bleeding and mucosal glomerulations with bladder distention. The classic cystoscopic findings of Hunner's ulcers are only rarely seen.

Eosinophilic Cystitis

Eosinophilic cystitis is an uncommon inflammatory disorder of the urinary bladder that causes irritative voiding symptoms. Clinically, the disease is characterized by striking episodes of dysuria, frequency, urgency, and gross hematuria.[41] The majority of cases have been reported in women and children, frequently with an associated history of allergy and peripheral eosinophilia. The condition is also seen in older men and may be related to the presence of bladder injury secondary to other urinary tract disease, or chronic urinary obstruction. Peripheral eosinophilia may or may not be present. Urinalysis frequently shows numerous eosinophils, and biopsy specimens have severe eosinophilic infiltration of all layers of the vesical wall.[34,41] Cystoscopy is diagnostic with severe mucosal injection and polypoid lesions seen in the bladder. Excretory urography is nonspecific in these cases but occasionally reveals dilation of the upper tracts, vesicoureteric reflux, and bladder contraction. Treatment of these patients with antihistamines, antibiotics, and corticosteroids is frequently beneficial.

PROSTATITIS

The diagnosis and treatment of prostatitis requires diligence and persistence on the part of both the physician and the patient. Although the diagnosis of acute bacterial prostatitis is made with ease and its treatment is straightforward, chronic bacterial prostatitis and other forms of prostatic disease are more difficult. The documentation of infection is often elusive despite careful evaluation.

Prostatitis can best be discussed by separating into four groups: acute bacterial prostatitis, chronic bacterial prostatitis, nonbacterial prostatitis, and prostatodynia. These categories allow for improved diagnosis and treatment.

Acute Bacterial Prostatitis

In most cases the diagnosis of acute bacterial prostatitis is straightforward and readily apparent on physical examination. The patient is frequently febrile and toxic with severe rigors, back pain, perineal pain, dysuria, urgency, frequency, and mild to moderate obstructive symptoms. Approximately one-third of patients will present in acute urinary retention secondary to prostatic inflammation in an already enlarged and partially obstructing gland.[42] Rectal examination supports the diagnosis with a severely swollen tender prostate that causes exquisite discomfort on palpation of the gland. Urine culture and prostatic fluid have many polymorphonuclear leukocytes, and the infecting organisms are frequently seen on Gram stain of these fluids. Massage of an acutely infected prostate, however, should be proscribed, because bacteremia and septicemia may result. Overwhelming prostatic infections allow the bacteria to enter the bladder, and the infecting organism can often be cultured from midstream urine collection.

The most common offending pathogens include *E. coli*, *Proteus*, members of the *Klebsiella-Enterobacter* group, and the enterococci. Once the Gram stain of the urine has established acute urinary infection and urine and blood cultures are sent, therapy with bedrest, analgesics, and broad-spectrum parenteral antibiotics should be instituted with appropriate bladder drainage if necessary by suprapubic diversion. Unlike the infections of chronic bacterial prostatitis, numerous antibiotics penetrate the acutely inflamed prostate. Antibiotic therapy can be tailored to the offending organism based on definitive blood and urine culture and sensitivity reports.

As a result of acute bacterial prostatitis, prostatic abscesses may ensue. In patients in whom systemic signs and symptoms continue unabated while on appropriate antibiotic treatment, bedrest, and fluids, the possibility of a prostatic abscess should be entertained. Prostatic abscesses may be multiple and are often associated with painful prostatic enlargement and fluctuance on digital rectal examination.[42] Drainage in these cases must be performed either transrectally, perineally, or by transurethral resection or incision of the prostate. Only when combined with drainage will antibiotic treatment, as for acute prostatitis, resolve the infection (Fig. 12–5).

Radiographically, acute prostatitis has few specific findings. Voiding studies during the acute episode may reveal narrowing of the prostatic urethra, large residual urines, and findings of bladder outlet obstruction. Likewise, an intact prostatic abscess is unlikely to be diagnosed radiographically by plain radiographs or IVP. Occasionally, abscesses will obtain large enough sizes to produce a filling defect at the bladder base to be seen on IVP.[42] Once a prostatic abscess has drained either spontaneously or surgically, filling of the resultant cavity on retrograde urethrogram or voiding cystourethrogram can be expected. These cavities are frequently epithelialized and remain as open diverticuli indefinitely. These cavities may be a nidus for chronic prostatitis or chronic urinary infections. Cystoscopy is usually not helpful and often reveals nonspecific elongation of the prostatic urethra and trigonal elongation. Transrectal ultrasound and CT scan have been used to diagnose prostatic abscesses with a high degree of accuracy.[42,43] Transrectal ultrasound of prostatic abscesses often reveals heterogeneous areas or irregular hypoechoic areas within the gland.[43] CT will show focal areas of low attenuation and can be used to determine the extent of the prostatic abscess better than ultrasound. These studies can then be used to guide percutaneous drainage (Fig. 12–6).

Chronic Bacterial Prostatitis, Nonbacterial Prostatitis, and Prostatodynia

Prostatitis is one of the most common genitourinary tract complaints of men. It is estimated that about half of all men experience prostatic symptoms at some time during their adult life.[4] Chronic bacterial prostatitis accounts for a relatively small number of these patients, with more than 90% of men eventually diagnosed with nonbacterial prostatitis or prostatodynia.[44,45] The usual causes of chronic bacterial prostatitis are the same gram-negative organisms that cause urinary tract infections and acute bacterial prostatitis. Gram-positive organisms, mostly enterococci, may also cause

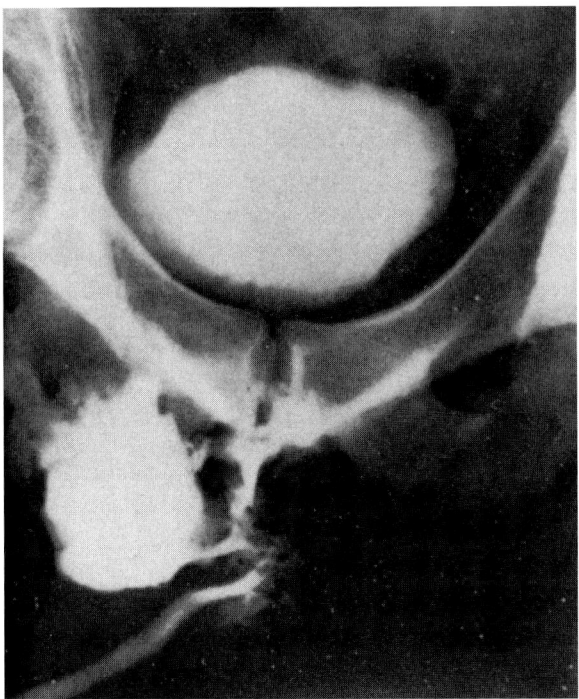

Figure 12–5. Periurethral abscess. This retrograde cystourethrogram shows massive extravasation of contrast into a periurethral abscess in a patient who has had multiple urethral strictures following gonorrhea.

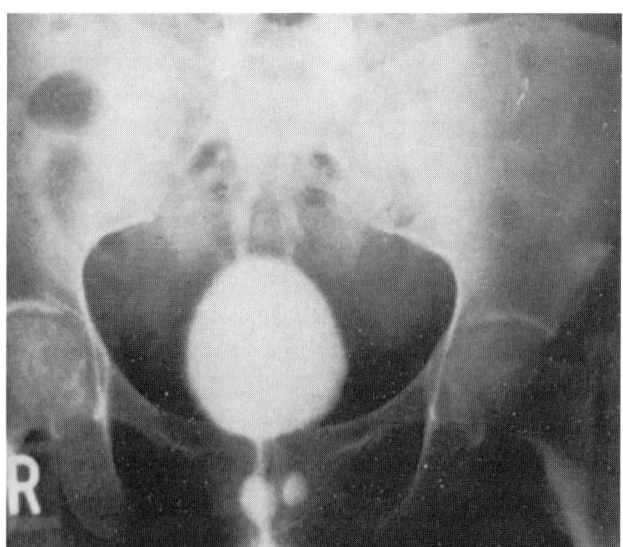

Figure 12–6. Chronic prostatic abscess cavity. Cystourethrogram shows prostatic abscess cavity to the left of the dilated prostatic urethra.

chronic infections of the prostate. Unusual bacteria such as *Mycobacterium tuberculosis* and *Neisseria gonorrhea* or fungi may occasionally cause prostatic infections. *Ureaplasma urealyticum* (T-strain mucoplasma) and *Chlamydia trachomatis* have been studied extensively using antigen-specific immunoglobulins and immunofluorescent stains in patients with nonbacterial prostatitis.[46] The results so far have been inconclusive, and these organisms are generally considered unproven pathogens in chronic prostatic inflammation.

Most patients with chronic bacterial prostatitis present with symptoms of bladder inflammation, and a small number have asymptomatic bacteriuria. The typical symptomatology of chronic bacterial prostatitis includes perineal pain, scrotalgia, dysuria, frequency, urgency, and postejaculatory discomfort. These symptoms may be accompanied by obstructive symptoms in patients with coexistent prostatic hyperplasia. The signs and symptoms of chronic bacterial prostatitis may be indistinguishable from nonbacterial prostatitis and prostatodynia. The diagnosis of nonbacterial prostatitis is based on the findings of significant prostatic inflammation, defined as 10 or more WBCs per HPF on examined expressed prostatic secretions, with lipid-laden macrophages and negative cultures. Prostatodynia patients will show no inflammation upon microscopic examination of prostatic fluid and will have negative cultures. Routine culturing of prostatic secretions in patients with symptoms of chronic prostatitis are often inadequate and may be confusing because these expressed secretions may be contaminated by urethral bacteria. The use of needle biopsy and culture of prostatic tissue is often unreliable because of the focal nature of the disease and the likelihood of contamination.

The diagnosis of chronic bacterial prostatitis rests on quantitative localization techniques as described by Meares and Stamey.[47] Cultures are obtained of urethral urine (VB-1), midstream urine (VB-2), expressed prostatic secretions selected after prostatic massage (EPS), and urine voided after prostatic massage (VB-3). Occasionally, expressed prostatic secretions cannot be collected and a semen collection and culture must be obtained to culture the prostatic fluid accurately.

The technique for collecting these specimens is quite simple and can be undertaken in any clinic or private office. Patients are instructed to come to the clinic with a full bladder and void the first 10 mL of urine into a sterile container. This specimen is the voided bladder number 1 (VB-1) specimen. The patient then continues to void 100 mL of urine, which is discarded. A second 10-mL aliquote is collected in a sterile container and labelled VB-2. The patient is instructed to cease voiding and prostatic massage is undertaken. Prostatic secretions are then collected in a sterile container and labeled EPS (expressed prostatic secretions). The patient then voids his remaining urine and a fourth aliquote, labeled VB-3, is collected. These specimens are immediately innoculated into culture media. If significant bacteriuria is present in the VB-2 and VB-3 specimens, a short 2- to 3-day course of antibiotics that concentrate in the urine is given to sterilize the urine. In this short time period these agents will not affect bacterial counts in the prostate in patients with chronic bacterial prostatitis. Chronic bacterial prostatitis is diagnosed by the number of bacteria in the EPS or VB-3 specimens. Colony counts in these specimens must be at least 10 times greater than those in the VB-1 or VB-2 specimens to document chronic bacterial prostatitis.

The radiographic examination of patients with chronic bacterial prostatitis is usually unnecessary and findings are nondiagnostic. Patients in whom tuberculosis prostatitis is diagnosed should, however, undergo radiographic evaluation as described in the tuberculosis section. Occasionally, prostatic calculi are seen on plain abdominal films or transrectal ultrasounds done for other indications. These calculi have also been found in as many as 75% of middle-aged men and are present in 100% of elderly men with chronic prostatitis on transrectal ultrasound.[46] Prostatic calculi may account for the high treatment failure in chronic bacterial prostatitis (Fig. 12–7).

The treatment of chronic bacterial prostatitis is difficult and often requires long courses of antibiotics. Alterations in prostatic secretions in bacterial prostatitis are important in the pathogenesis of bacterial prostatitis and account for the poor perfusion of certain drugs into prostatic fluid. In both acute and chronic bacterial prostatitis the prostatic fluid becomes less viscous and more alkaline than normal, containing significantly depressed levels of zinc, spermine, and prostatic antibacterial factor. Prolonged administration of antibiotics is usually desirable and a 12- to 14-week course may be necessary for eradicating chronic bacterial infections. Drugs such as trimethoprim-sulfamethoxazole or trimethoprim alone are able to achieve therapeutic levels in chronic bacterial infections in a significant number of pa-

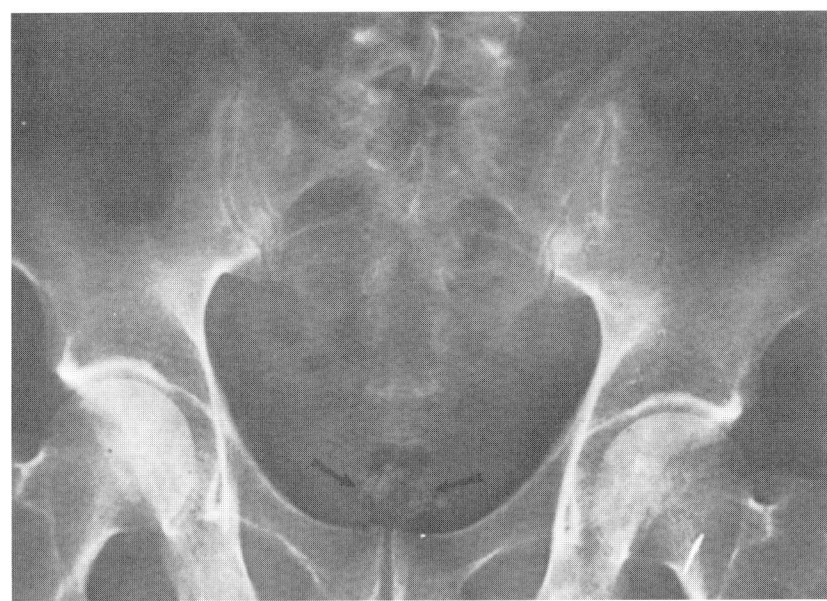

Figure 12–7. Prostatic calculi. Arrows define multiple prostatic calculi in patient with chronic bacterial prostatitis.

tients. Other agents—including doxycycline, minocycline, geocillin, ampicillin, indanyl carbenicillin, and cephalexin—have been used with variable success but do not concentrate well in prostatic fluid. The newer fluoroquinolones are highly lipid soluble and concentrate well in prostatic fluid and tissues. These antimicrobials have good activity against the Enterobacteraceae, *Pseudomonas*, and staphylococcal species. Preliminary studies are encouraging, with significantly higher cure rates than standard antimicrobial therapy. The usual treatment period is 4 weeks, with no additional benefit demonstrated with longer courses of therapy.[48] Despite adequate therapy directed at the specific organisms involved a cure of bacterial prostatitis remains very difficult. For those patients who fail to respond completely to a full course of appropriate antimicrobial therapy, continuous low-dose suppression may be an option. Extended transurethral resection of the prostate and even complete excision of the prostate, seminal vesicles, and vas deferens have been advocated in selected symptomatic refractory cases of chronic bacterial prostatitis.[46] In cases of relapsing disease a more limited transurethral resection of the prostate using real-time sonography has been proposed by Meares to remove infected prostatic calculi.[46] Most prostatic calculi, however, are not colonized by bacteria and cause no harm.

Nonbacterial prostatitis and prostatodynia have symptoms similar to those with chronic bacterial prostatitis but no infecting organisms are identified by routine cultures. Perineal pain, low back discomfort, postejaculatory pain, and dysuria are frequently present and resistant to treatment with antibiotics. Patients are afebrile and repeated differential urine cultures fail to reveal causative organisms. Cultures, including those for *Ureaplasma urealyticum*, *Chlamydia trachomatis*, and viruses have also been negative.[49] Elevated levels of prostatic antigen-specific antibodies have been reported in prostatic fluid of men with nonbacterial prostatitis, but these are nonspecific for infections with *Chlamydia*, *Ureaplasma*, or other less common pathogens.[48]

Prostatodynia patients are typically young to middle-aged men, usually with no previous history of urinary tract infections. Symptoms are similar to those of men with nonbacterial prostatitis. Microscopic examination of expressed prostatic secretions do not contain increased numbers of WBCs (greater than 10 per HPF) or large numbers of lecithin bodies. Cultures, including those for nonbacterial pathogens, have been negative. Musculoskeletal abnormalities are thought to be responsible for symptoms more often than prostatic ones. Often there is discomfort during palpation of the anal and paraprostatic muscles, despite a normal prostate examination, which may reflect tension myalgia of the pelvic floor.[46]

Therapy for nonbacterial prostatitis and prostatodynia is even more difficult than that for chronic bacterial prostatitis. No specific, effective treatment is known. Some patients improve with periodic prostatic massage, anticholinergic drugs, warm sitz baths, anti-inflammatory drugs, and other supportive therapy. Patients with prostatodynia may have symptomatic improvement with alpha blocking agents such as phenoxybenzamine and prozosin aimed at relaxing urethral and bladder neck muscle spasms. Pelvic floor tension myalgia is a less frequent cause of prostatodynia but may respond to oral diazepam alone or in combination with a selective alpha-one antagonist.[46] Unnecessary urethral instrumentation and excessive diagnostic testing should be avoided in these patients. Transurethral resection also is usually ineffective in these individuals.

Granulomatous Prostatitis

Granulomatous prostatitis is an uncommon chronic inflammatory condition of the prostate first described more than 50 years ago. Physical examination of these patients reveals a rock hard indurated prostate, or prostate nodule, indistinguishable from carcinoma of the prostate on rectal examination. Epstein and Hutchins classified granulomatous prostatitis into four categories: specific, nonspecific, post-transurethral resection, and allergic granulomatous prostatitis.[50] This condition has been associated with tuberculosis, syphilis, brucellosis, viruses, fungi, eosinophilic granulomatosis, and Wegener's granulomatosis.[51] Intravesical bacillus Calmette-Guerrin therapy for superficial transitional cell carcinoma of the bladder has also been associated with granulomatous prostatitis and is suggested by the history of prior therapy for bladder cancer.[52,53] The nonspecific forms of the disease often follow a recent urinary tract infection and are associated with recurrent febrile episodes, chills, and irritative voiding symptoms.[52] The prostate specific antigen (PSA) values may be slightly elevated or normal.[54] Since prostatic induration is always present the previously described triad of recurring febrile episodes, dysuria, and prostatic induration can be used only in retrospect. The diagnosis in these cases is made only by needle biopsy and microscopic examination of the prostatic tissue. Radiographically, many of these patients have prostatic calculi. Excretory urography is usually nonproductive, although occasional incidence of urethral obstruction has been seen in patients with severe allergic granulomatous prostatitis. Transrectal ultrasound findings are variable with multiple large and small hypoechoic areas found throughout the peripheral, transitional, and central zones. These areas are indistinguishable from those of diffuse prostatic carcinoma.[54] Once the diagnosis is confirmed, resolution of the process is frequently spontaneous and no therapy may be needed.

SEMINAL VESICULITIS

Documented bacterial infections of the seminal vesicles are quite uncommon. These infections often occur in patients with established infections of the prostate gland or epididymis, with associated seminal vesicle infections. Abnormal vesiculography is common in these cases, occurring in 21 of 24 vesiculograms in one series of patients with chronic bacterial prostatitis. Segmental stenosis or complete shrinking of the seminal vesicles is frequently found, often on the same side as previous episodes of epididymo-orchitis.[55] Isolated infections of the seminal vesicles probably occur after adequate therapy for prostatic infections has eliminated bacteria from the prostatic secretions. A nidus of infection can then remain within the seminal vesicle to produce symptoms of seminal vesiculitis. Symptoms most commonly encountered are those of perineal pain, postejaculatory pain, diminution of ejaculate volume, hematospermia, and ill-defined stress in the scrotum, testes, buttocks, and coccygeal area.[56] Since many of these symptoms also occur in patients with bacterial prostatitis and prostatodynia, seminal vesiculitis cannot be diagnosed by history alone.

Evaluation of seminal vesicular infections is done by a combination of semen cultures and differential prostatic cultures, as previously described. If semen cultures are positive and differential prostatic cultures are negative, it can be concluded that significant bacteria are present within the seminal vesicle. This is a rare occurrence, and usually the diagnosis of seminal vesiculitis rests on radiographic evaluation of seminal vesicle morphology. Traditionally, visualization of the seminal vesicles has been accomplished with vesiculography. This is a complex and invasive procedure requiring considerable experience in technique and interpretation.

The technique of seminal vesiculography is best performed by the vasoseminal route with injection of contrast media into the vas deferens. Patients are evaluated by identifying the vas transscrotally and exposing the vas deferens through a small scrotal incision. This can be done using local anesthesia in a manner similar to that of routine bilateral vasectomy. Once the vas is identified and isolated, a 25-gauge needle is used to cannulate the lumen of the vas in a proximal direction. Using a 15-mL syringe, urographic contrast media is injected slowly into each vas deferens. Films are obtained during each injection.

Chronic infection and inflammatory changes may result in distortion or partial obstruction of the seminal vesicles. Radiographically, seminal vesiculography in patients with seminal vesiculitis reveals dilated seminal vesicles that fill poorly and are quite irregular in appearance. The ampullae of the vas deferens are usually poorly visualized and only partially patent. Although no radiographic findings are pathognomonic for seminal vesiculitis Dunnick and coworkers described an abnormal feathery appearance of the ampullae of the vas deferens, presumably due to multiple small ducts or diverticulae, in the majority of patients examined with seminal vesiculography for presumed seminal vesiculitis.[53] The ejaculatory ducts may be partially or totally occluded. This occlusion usually impedes the free efflux of contrast into the posterior urethra during seminal vesiculogram. The vas deferens itself is usually normal proximal to the ampulla (Figs. 12–8, 12–9).

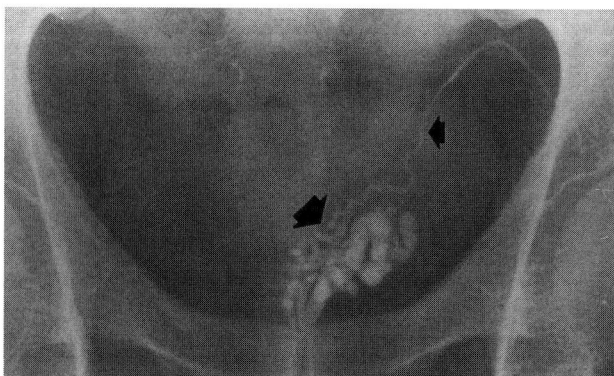

Figure 12–8. Seminal vesiculogram. Normal-appearing seminal vesical in a patient with oligospermia. Vas deferens (small black arrow) and ampulla (larger black arrow). (Photograph courtesy of Dr. R. Older.)

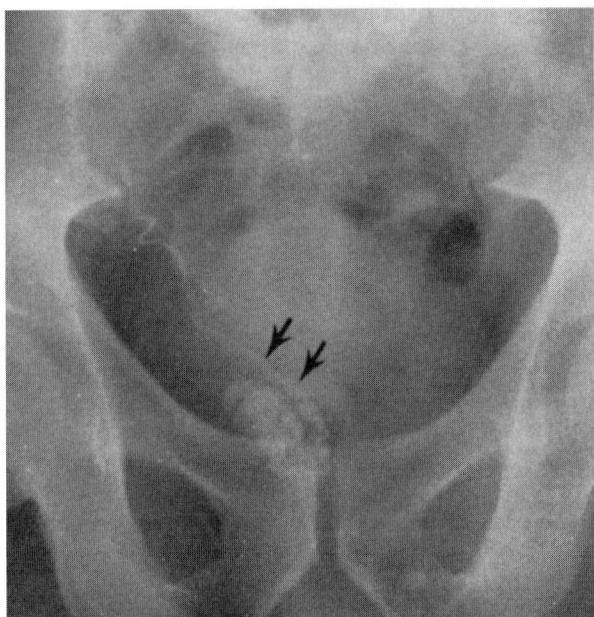

Figure 12–9. Seminal vesiculogram in a patient with seminal vesiculitis. Note globular appearance of vesicle with poor filling and poor visualization of the ampulla with small diverticula of the distal vas deferens (arrows).

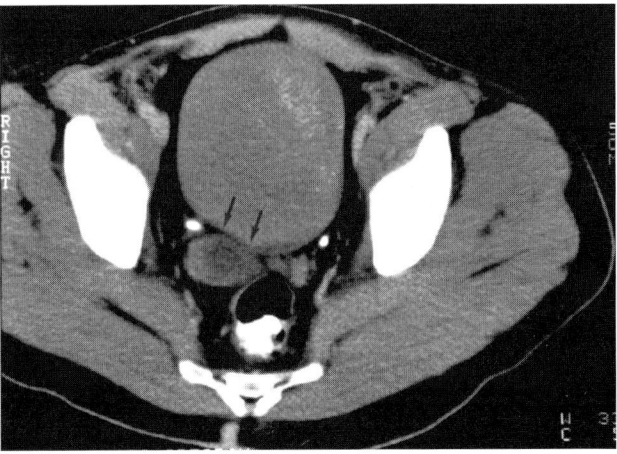

Figure 12–10. CT of a seminal vesical abscess in a patient with genitourinary tuberculosis. Arrows in bladder point to a right seminal vesical abscess. (Photograph courtesy of Dr. D. M. Warshauer.)

In contrast, the normal seminal vesicle is differentiated from that of seminal vesiculitis in being sharply delineated with a smooth, even convolution and regular, round saccules. Free efflux on contrast into the posterior urethra with frequent outlining of the verumontanum is also seen in these normal studies. All components of the vasoseminal system, including the seminal vesicles, ejaculatory ducts, and ampullae of the vas deferens are symmetrical in position and filling by contrast media.

After the seminal vesiculogram has been completed, further assurance of the diagnosis can be added by the injection of 50 mg of doxycycline per vas. Frequently, this injection will produce symptomatic improvement. Since this pain relief is frequently short-lived, definitive treatment of persistent, recalcitrant seminal vesiculitis may be accomplished by extirpation of the seminal vesicles transvesically.[53]

In recent years transrectal ultrasound, CT, and magnetic resonance imaging (MRI) have been used in the evaluation of ejaculatory dysfunction with excellent results. These imaging modalities have the advantage of being noninvasive and often provide superior anatomic detail of the seminal vesicles architecture. Although the seminal vesicles may vary in size when measured at different times, transrectal ultrasound is capable of determining symmetry and excluding other pathologic abnormalities such as tumor, cysts, abscess, or obstruction.[57] Recently, newer MRI with endorectal surface coils have been used in evaluating ejaculatory dysfunction with even greater detail. Changes in signal enhancement and diffuse thickening of the seminal vesical walls are characteristic of the chronic inflammatory changes seen in seminal vesiculitis.[58] These special coils are not routinely available but hold promise as future diagnostic tools in the evaluation of patients suspected of having seminal vesiculitis (Fig. 12–10).

UPPER URINARY TRACT INFECTION

Pyelonephritis is an inflammation of the renal parenchyma and its collecting system. This process is usually caused by an acute bacterial infection but may be caused by fungi, viruses, or parasites. The degree of bacterial infection can progress from acute uncomplicated bacterial pyelonephritis to worsening stages of interstitial inflammation to frank abscess formation. Permanent renal injury from bacterial invasion with residual renal scarring is frequently seen. Bacterial pyelonephritis can be divided into acute and chronic forms with specific differences in diagnosis, treatment, and prognosis.

Acute Bacterial Pyelonephritis

Acute pyelonephritis is caused by bacterial invasion of the renal parenchyma and is manifested by high fever, rigors, flank pain, malaise, and frequently lower urinary tract infection. Microscopically, pyuria, urine leukocyte casts, and bacteriuria are found on urinalysis. This acute renal parenchymal infection can lead to severe renal impairment, loss of renal function, and bacteremia. Many cases of acute pyelonephritis are not diagnosed, and residual effects are found only at autopsy. As many as 50% of infections can be asymptomatic and resolve spontaneously.[59] Gross or microscopic hematuria may be present, and oliguria may be associated with acute pyelonephritis.

Physical examination usually reveals abdominal pain with severe flank pain to flank percussion. Flank pain is usually unilateral but may be bilateral. Tenderness is predominantly localized to the ipsilateral costovertebral angle. Abdominal tenderness and pain may cause confusion on physical examination. Pain may be upper quadrant or diffuse and may mimic other intra-abdominal processes. Bowel sounds may be diminished and the abdomen distended. Many patients exhibit marked hypertensive episodes along with acute prelonephritis and may present with severely elevated blood pressure.

Children frequently present with high fever of unknown origins, vomiting, diarrhea, and failure to thrive. In children who are toilet trained, urinary urgency, frequency, and enuresis may be observed. Frequently, a recent history of foul-smelling urine may be volunteered by parents.

The diagnosis of acute pyelonephritis rests on the microscopic and bacteriologic examination of the urine. Careful midstream or catheterized urine specimens must be obtained and examined microscopically to determine the presence or absence of bacteria. Urinalysis will frequently reveal leukocyte casts, significant pyuria, bacteria, and microscopic hematuria. Urine Gram stains will commonly reveal the gram-negative pathogens. Urine culture should be obtained immediately and will usually grow significant cultures of *E. coli*, *Proteus*, *Pseudomonas*, *Enterococcus*, or *Klebsiella*. Blood cultures should be obtained before antibiotic therapy is begun. The presence of P-fimbriae on *E. coli* strains has been shown to be an important virulence marker for the development of pyelonephritis. Commercially available agglutination screening tests for P-fimbriae have been used to identify these pathogens and show a high correlation with documented pyelonephritis.[60]

Kidneys affected by acute pyelonephritis appear grossly enlarged and bulging on cut surface with the appearance of massive edema. Multiple microscopic abscesses and microhemorrhages are seen, especially in the subcapsular renal surface. Most of these changes appear in the renal cortex with infected areas interspersed with grossly normal-appearing tissue. If only a small renal segment is affected, a wedge-shaped area may stand out from the remainder of the kidney as an isolated infected segment. This is often referred to as acute focal bacterial nephritis or lobar nephronia as the extent of the infection may be determined by the renal lobes. This acute inflammatory process proceeds to cortical parenchymal destruction around the abscesses. Large numbers of polymorphonuclear leukocytes are present in the stroma surrounding the renal tubules.[3,61]

Clinical findings—including urine studies, physical examination, and history—are most important in diagnosing upper urinary tract infections and determining appropriate treatment. In acute uncomplicated pyelonephritis imaging studies are unnecessary. Failure to respond to appropriate therapy within 24 to 48 hours, however, is an indication that further evaluation is needed.

The most sensitive study to detect the presence of acute bacterial pyelonephritis is a radionuclide scan using a cortical agent like DMSA or glucoheptonate. Findings of nonspecific diminution or absence of activity in the involved area suggest renal involvement and have a reported sensitivity of 86% and specificity of 81%.[62] These studies are especially useful in children and may identify those kidneys at risk for subsequent cortical scarring.[63] Gallium-67 and Indium-111 nuclear studies have also been reported to localize in acutely infected kidneys in as many as 86% of patients with upper tract infections.[64] However, these scans require at least 24 hours after injection for interpretation, and this lengthy time period may be prohibitive in an acutely ill patient. These studies, although sensitive at detecting renal infection, provide little information about the severity or extent of the infection. Similar findings may be seen in both lobar nephronia and abscess formation.

Excretory urography, renal ultrasound, and CT scans provide little additional information in uncomplicated pyelonephritis. Excretory urography is abnormal in 25% of patients with acute bacterial pyelonephritis symptoms.[65] Patients who have excretory urography during an episode of acute pyelonephritis usually show renal architectural distortions caused by severe renal parenchymal swelling within a rigid capsule.[61] These alterations are primarily seen in the nephrogram phase of the study. A prolonged nephrogram and delayed definition of the calyceal architecture resulting from diminished contrast collection are characteristic of acute pyelonephritis. There is frequently narrowing and distortion of the calyces and infundibula. The involved kidneys appear enlarged with an apparent increased parenchymal thickness from severe edema (Fig. 12–11).[61,66]

If renal involvement is unilateral, delayed visualization of the involved kidney may be evident on IVP. Occasionally, only a small segment of the kidney may be involved. This is usually referred to as focal bacterial nephritis and may lead to the radiographic appearance of the so-called acute lobar nephronia. These areas present as a usually polar renal mass and must be differentiated from tumor or abscess.

Ultrasound is a quick and sensitive study capable of differentiating these areas from abscesses. Typically, these areas will reveal a solid hypoechoic mass or wedge-shaped segment of parenchyma that is poorly marginated from adjacent parenchyma but lacks a definable wall. The normally sharp corticomedullary definition is lost.[67,68] Unlike abscesses, there is no evidence of liquefication. When abnormalities are small, less than 2 cm, pre- and postcontrast enhanced CT defines the type and location of the infection better than does ultrasound.[67,68] Because of the high water content of these edematous areas, they appear as areas of low attenuation on nonenhanced CT images. With contrast administration there is delayed enhancement, often seen as patchy or striated streaks of contrast, typical of slow flow through functioning renal parenchyma. These areas lack a definable wall differentiating them from a renal abscess. When severe infection is present perinephric extension can be identified by thickening or "whiskering" of the normal perinephric septa, obliteration of the normal perinephric fat, and thickening of Gerota's fascia.[69] Gallium scanning may also be used to evaluate indeterminate masses on IVP and will usually reveal a positive gallium image in the region of the acute lobar nephronia mass (Figs. 12–12, 12–13).

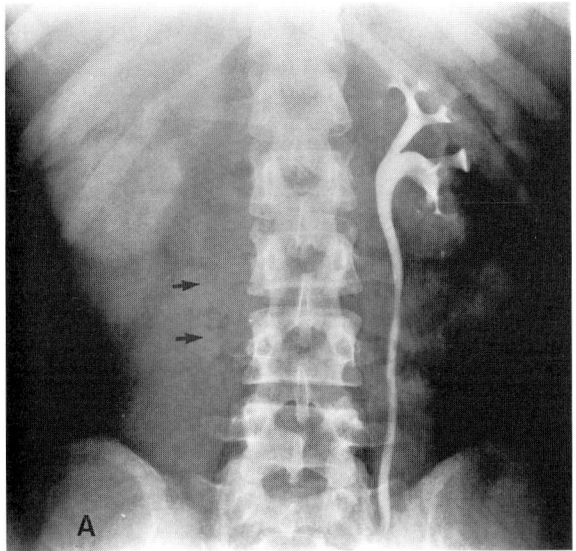
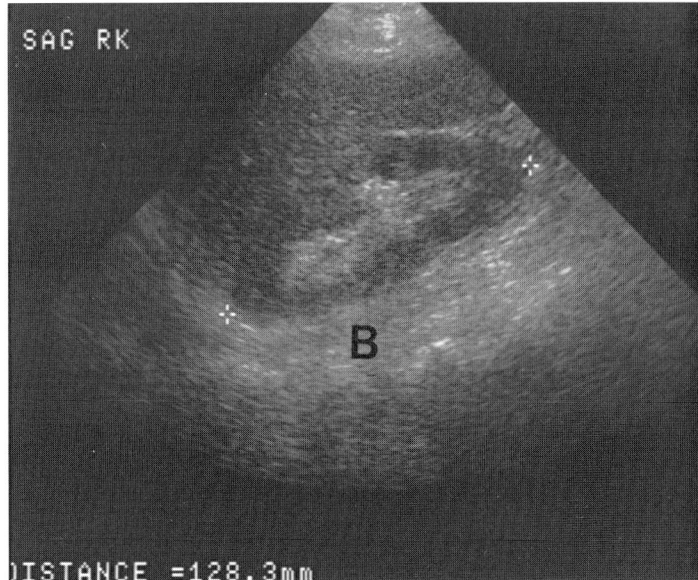
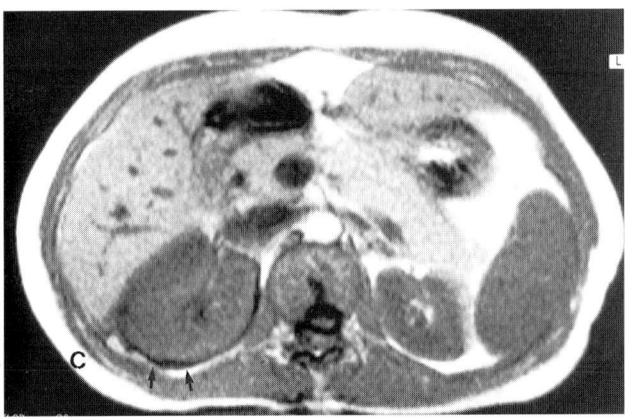

Figure 12–11. Acute right pyelonephritis: IVP, ULS, and MRI. (**A**) Excretory urogram in acute right pyelonephritis showing enlarged kidney with delayed function. Arrows point to contrast in ureter. (**B**) Ultrasound in same patient showing renal parenchyma edema (contralateral kidney measured 102.5 mm). (**C**) T1-weighted MRI of same patient showing perinephric fluid collection (arrows).

When used as the primary imaging modality in acute pyelonephritis, ultrasound will demonstrate abnormalities in approximately 50% of patients.[66] Ultrasonography in acute pyelonephritis reveals a small pyelocalyceal system without hydronephrosis or obstruction. The renal parenchyma is thickened and swollen with an increased anechoic pattern and multiple low-level scattered echoes. There will be increased ultrasonic shadowing because of the high fluid content of the infected kidney. These findings are consistent with the pathologic changes of acute pyelonephritis, that is, marked inflammatory edema of the renal parenchyma.[67,68] The most characteristic sonographic finding, acute renal swelling from marked inflammatory edema of the renal parenchyma, is present in 81% of patients but may only be apparent in retrospect.[67]

MRI has not been used routinely in the evaluation of acute renal infection because of cost constraints and the length of time required for scanning. On T1-weighted images there is an overall decrease in signal intensity and corticomedullary differentiation. On T2-weighted images the cortex and medulla are of high intensity and may be heterogeneous, again reflecting the high water content from inflammation and edema. Thickening of renal fascia and inflammatory changes

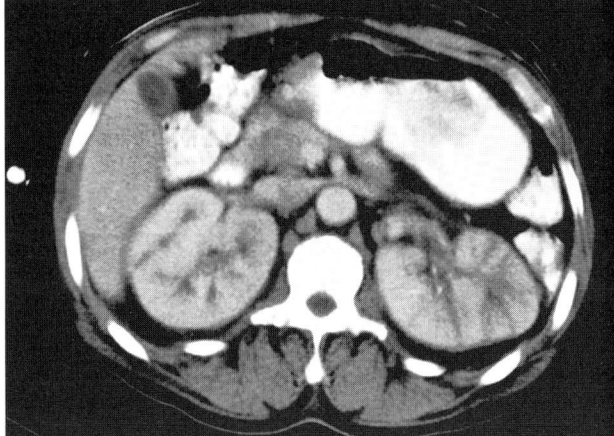

Figure 12–12. Acute pyelonephritis. CT scan in a patient with bilateral acute pyelonephritis showing marked edema and striation of the renal parenchyma. (Photograph courtesy of Dr. D. M. Warshauer.)

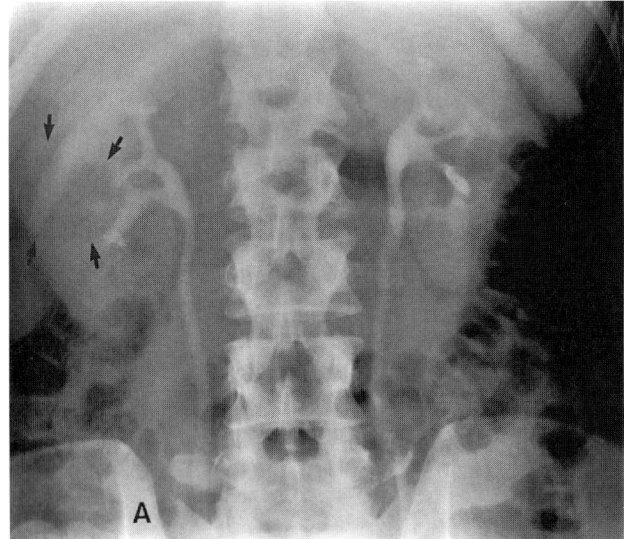
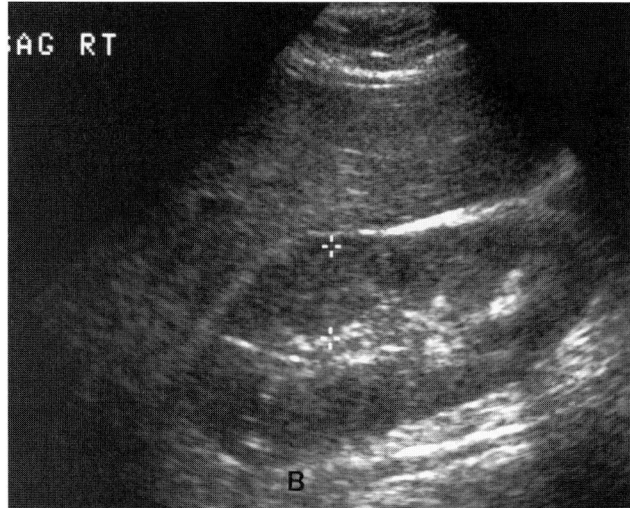
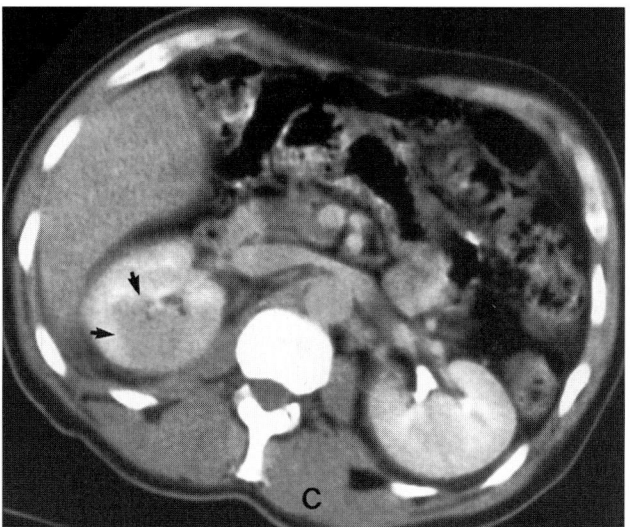

Figure 12–13. Focal bacterial nephritis (lobar nephronia): IVP, ULS, and CT. (**A**) Excretory urogram showing focal renal mass and diminution of nephrogram density in right lateral aspect of kidney (arrows). (**B**) Ultrasound in same patient showing poorly defined mass (markers). (**C**) Arrows point to area of patchy inhomogeneous enhancement on contrast CT of focal bacterial nephritis. (Photographs courtesy of Dr. R. L. Clark.)

of the perinephric fat are best appreciated on T1-weighted images.[69]

Renal angiography in patients with acutely infected kidneys is rarely necessary, and frequently these angiograms will be normal. Findings in the renal arteriography of acute pyelonephritis include renal cortical striation in the nephrogram phase with multiple, diffuse parenchymal lucencies.[70] There may also be a decrease in size and number of interlobar arterial branches with corticovascular stretching.

After a single episode of renal infection, many patients will have normal follow-up urograms.[61] The abnormalities seen during the acute phase will usually resolve during the healing phase. Follow-up CT scans after symptoms resolve demonstrate disappearance of the lesions by 10 to 16 weeks.[71,72] There is, however, a significant incidence of cortical scarring and even atrophy resulting from acute pyelonephritis. Soulen and associates reported new cortical scars on follow-up CT scans in 6 of 12 patients with an initially normal renal contour.[72]

COMPLICATED CASES OF ACUTE PYELONEPHRITIS: EMPHYSEMATOUS PYELONEPHRITIS AND RENAL ABSCESS

Emphysematous Pyelonephritis. Emphysematous pyelonephritis is a rare, life-threatening complication of severe pyelonephritis characterized by intraparenchymal gas formation. All the documented cases have been in adults and are usually associated with impaired host defenses.[73] These infections are more common in women and have left-sided predominance. Most cases are unilateral, but bilateral cases are present 12% of the time.[73] Patients are almost always diabetic, with obstruction documented in approximately one-third of cases. Like emphysematous cystitis these severe parenchymal infections create an environment of low oxygen tension that allows the infecting organisms to ferment glucose to lactate and carbon dioxide, accounting for the gas in the tissue. As the infection progresses, gas will extend to the perinephric space and retroperitoneum. This should be differentiated from emphysematous pyelitis, where air is confined to the renal pelvis and calyces.

The offending organisms are facultative anaerobes, most commonly *E. coli*; *Klebsiella*, *Proteus*, and *Aerobacter* account for the remainder of cases. Patients with emphysematous pyelonephritis are usually quite ill, with most displaying the classic triad of fever, vomiting, and flank pain. Frequently there is bacteriuria, bacteremia, leukocytosis, hyperglycemia, lethargy, confusion, and variable degrees of azotemia. Physical examination findings are similar to those of pyelonephritis. A crepitant mass may occasionally be palpable on examination of the flank and suggests the diagnosis.

Emphysematous pyelonephritis is a surgical emergency, with mortality rates as high as 50% despite appropriate intervention. Nephrectomy has been the traditional therapy, although with prompt diagnosis some cases have been treated successfully with percutaneous drainage.[66,73]

On plain radiography gas within the parenchyma of the kidney appears as mottled gas shadows over the involved kidney or less commonly as a cresenteric collection over the upper pole. These findings are identified in one-third of cases and usually signify a later stage when there is a relatively large collection of gas.[74] Excretory urography is rarely helpful in making the diagnosis. Most involved kidneys are poorly functioning or nonfunctioning, especially if obstruction is present. Nephrotomograms may, however, increase

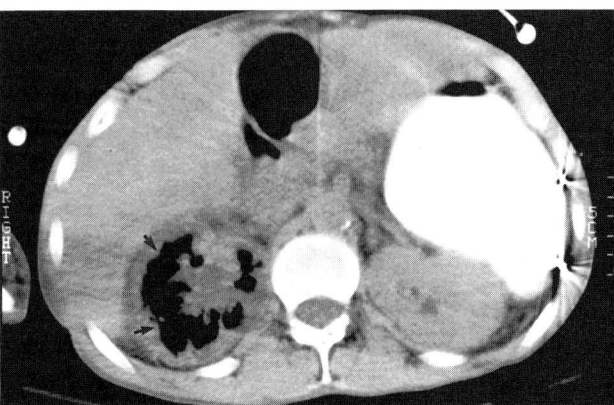

Figure 12–15. Emphysematous pyelonephritis. Noncontrast CT scan with intraparenchymal gas collections (arrows) in a patient with right emphysematous pylonephritis.

the radiographic yield for identifying gas within the renal parenchyma. Ultrasonography will demonstrate shadowing with internal echoes, the so-called dirty shadowing, in contradistinction to the clean shadowing associated with calculi.[68] This finding is characteristic of air interfaces and suggests the diagnosis of emphysematous pyelonephritis. Gas shadowing may obscure large portions of the infected kidney, and exact sonographic localization of the air is usually difficult. CT scan is the most sensitive test to detect emphysematous pyelonephritis. Since contrast administration may be contraindicated in azotemic diabetic patients, unenhanced CT images can be used to demonstrate intraparenchymal gas (Figs. 12–14, 12–15, 12–16).

Although most patients require nephrectomy, medical therapy with or without percutaneous drainage has been recommended in selected cases where there is still good kidney function. Often this allows time for the patient to be medically stabilized, during which time broad-spectrum antibi-

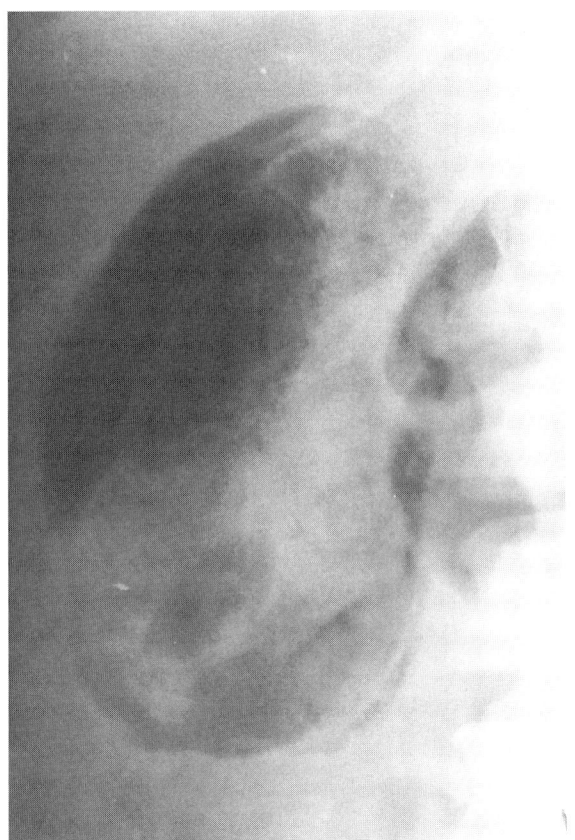

Figure 12–14. Emphysematous pyelonephritis. Gas dissects the renal parenchyma and extends to the subcapsular space. (Photograph courtesy of Dr. R. Older.)

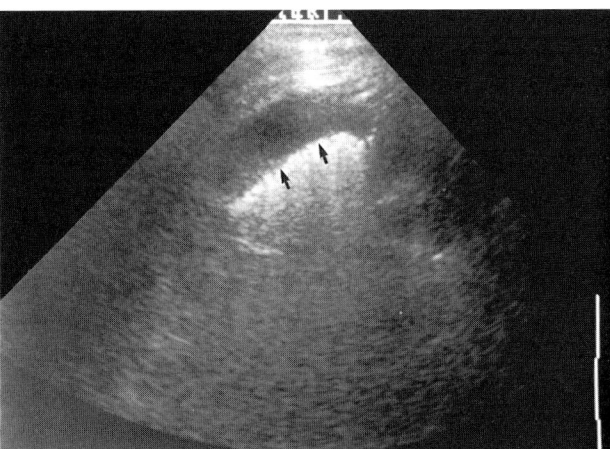

Figure 12–16. Emphysematous pyelonephritis. Arrows point to gas interface producing "dirty shadowing" in patient with intraparenchymal gas due to emphysematous pyelonephritis. (Photograph courtesy of Dr. D. M. Warshauer.)

otics are administered. If the kidney is extensively destroyed or if the patient fails to improve after several days open surgical drainge or delayed nephrectomy can be performed.

Renal Abscess. Renal and perinephric abscesses are rare complications of urinary tract infections secondary to renal obstruction, especially in an infected kidney or renal segment. Bacteria usually ascend from a bladder colonized by pathogenic organisms. Renal abscess formation may result from progression of acute lobar nephronia with coalition of microabscesses or from hematogenous spread of infection from remote infection foci or during episodes of bacteremia. Perinephric abscess formation is usually the result of rupture of a renal abscess into the perirenal space. In general, Gerota's fascia serves as a relative barrier to further contiguous spread. The responsible pathogenic organisms are usually gram-negative enteric pathogens. Abscesses caused by gram-positive cocci are usually spread hematogenously. Abscesses frequently pose a diagnostic dilemma that may only be resolved by exploratory surgery. With improved diagnostic techniques, however, more renal abscesses can be diagnosed and managed without open surgery.

Predisposing factors in patients with renal abscesses include previous urologic surgery, previous urinary tract infections, nephrolithiasis, immunosuppression, diabetes mellitus, vesicoureteral reflux, obstructive uropathy, and bacteremia.[75] Less commonly, polycystic renal disease with infected cyst, obstruction caused by renal tumors, renal papillary necrosis, tuberculosis with severe scarring, intravenous drug abuse, steroid abuse, alcoholism, and hemodialysis may be implicated.[75,76] Hematogenous origin from remote sites such as dental abscesses, acute prostatitis, furuncles, and other localized infections may lead to perirenal or renal abscess. Gram-positive abscesses usually begin as cortical abscesses and were the most common types of perinephric infections in the era before broad-spectrum antibiotics.[75] This type of abscess still occurs in intravenous drug users and in those patients with dermatologic conditions or secondary skin infection. In one recent series, gram-positive abscesses accounted for 11% of all cases of renal abscess.[76]

The clinical course of perinephric abscess is one of insidious onset and delayed diagnosis. Patients frequently present with several weeks of malaise, fever, and diffuse, poorly localized abdominal pain with or without an abdominal mass.[75,76] Patients with fever, pain, and a bulging flank with palpable mass constitute the classic presenting feature of this condition. Fever is usually low grade, and patients are rarely toxic. Although the flank and costovertebral angle are the most common sites for abdominal pain, the location may be variable. When overlying the psoas muscle, abscesses may produce ipsilateral hip, thigh, or knee pain. This pain is exacerbated by walking and weight bearing and is diminished by hip flexion. In as many as 10% of cases the pain may be entirely abdominal, confusing the diagnosis.[74] Occasionally, these abscesses will present as spontaneously draining flank infections. Urinary symptoms may be minimal or absent. Hematuria, pyuria, or urinary retention may occur. Most patients, however, do not have frequency, urgency, or irritative symptoms (Fig. 12–17).

Urinalysis may be completely normal or may have protienuria, microscopic hematuria, or pyuria. Urine cultures may be sterile in more than 20% of patients. Polymicrobial cultures are found in almost one-third of cases, with *E. coli* and *Proteus* most commonly isolated. In one series correct preoperative cultures were found in only 28% of cases.[77] Leukocytosis and anemia are common findings. The most useful clinical observation as reported by Thorley and associates is the failure of resolution of fever within 3 to 4 days of antibiotic treatment, despite culture-proven sensitivity to the therapeutic agent.[78] Complete blood count and radiographic studies, therefore, are absolutely necessary to make the diagnosis of perinephric abscesses.

Plain abdominal films obtained prior to excretory urography or as a definitive study aid perinephric abscess diagnosis only in advanced stages of infection. Hazy shadows in the retroperitoneum with obliteration of the psoas muscle shadow and a mass effect overlying the renal fossa may suggest perinephric abscess. Likewise, the presence of renal calculi has been noted in association with perinephric abscess in as many as 30% of patients.[79] These findings may be associated with significant lumbar scoliosis with scoliotic concavity toward the side of the abscess.[75] Large upper pole abscesses, especially those in contact with the ipsilateral diaphragm, may produce atelectasis, flattening of the posterior segment of the diaphragm, or free fluid in the ipsilat-

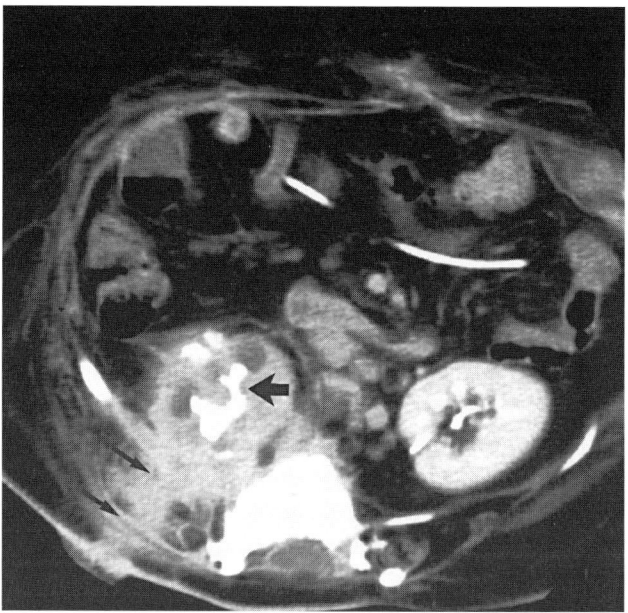

Figure 12–17. Nephrocutaneous fistula. Contrast-enhanced CT scan in a patient with staghorn calculus (wide arrow) who presented with spontaneously draining staphylococcal abscess of the right flank. Smaller arrows point to fistula from kidney.

eral chest. Plain film of the abdomen may also show dilation of loops of small bowel consistent with paralytic ileus (Fig. 12–18).

Gas collection may frequently be seen in perirenal infections, especially in association with diabetes mellitus or obstruction. These gas collections can be seen in the renal parenchyma, as air–fluid levels within the abscess cavity itself, or in renal collecting system. Vesicoenteric fistula must be ruled out in these cases. Most commonly, however, these gas collections occur in diabetics with obstructive uropathy in the presence of gas-forming organisms.[73]

Once contrast media have been administered, further information regarding the renal deformity or chronic infection can be obtained. Stretching of calyceal or infundibular outlines may be early evidence of the mass effect of renal abscess. Incomplete filling of various segments of the kidney when displaced by the pressure of the abscess collection may also be seen. If the process is long-standing, incomplete calyceal visualization or even complete obliteration or enlargement of the segment of renal tissue may be seen on intravenous urogram. In these cases, retrograde pyelogram may be necessary to further define this area of the infected kidney.

Normal kidneys are freely mobile in the retroperitoneal space and can descend as much as two to three vertebral widths on standing. Supine and upright films may be helpful in making the diagnosis of perirenal abscess. Since fixation of the kidneys is well known with severe retroperitoneal inflammatory processes, the failure of the kidney to descend on upright film adds further evidence for retroperitoneal infection and renal abscess.

Abscesses that form within the parenchyma, especially in close proximity to the calyces, are referred to as cortical abscesses. These abscesses frequently enlarge and spontaneously drain into the collecting system of the kidney. Patients will frequently notice immediate pain relief and defervescence after these erosions. Excretory urograms obtained after this spontaneous drainage reveal cavitation that appears quite similar to that seen in renal tuberculosis. These abscesses may also rupture toward the periphery of the kidney, allowing fistulization between the renal calyces and renal capsule. A collection of contrast media beneath the renal capsule with connections to the collecting system is frequently seen on the retrograde pyelogram or excretory urogram in these cases. Occasionally, with severe, prolonged infection, pyonephrosis or complete filling of the renal parenchyma and calyces with purulent material can be seen. Accumulation of pus in the renal pelvis may also occur proximal to an obstruction such as calculi, strictures, congenital anomalies, or malignancy. CT, sonography, and MRI will usually demonstrate a hydronephrotic-appearing kidney. The diagnosis is suggested by internal echoes on sonography or by debris within the fluid collections with CT or MRI. These images can be useful if diagnostic aspiration is considered. More commonly, retrograde drainage with a ureteral catheter or stent is performed. Contrast dispersed around purulent debris can be well appreciated on retrograde pyelography (Fig. 12–19).

Renal angiography in the evaluation of suspected intrarenal or perirenal abscess has largely been supplanted by CT

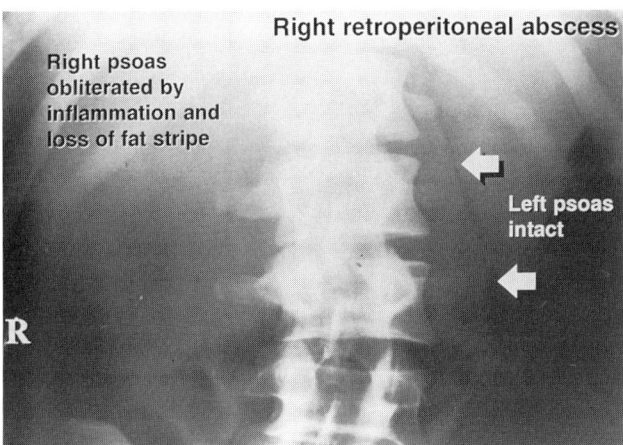

Figure 12–18. Perinephric abscess. Plain abdominal film shows obliteration of the right psoas muscle shadow and convexity of the lumbar spine away from the right perinephric abscess. (Photograph courtesy of Dr. R. Older.)

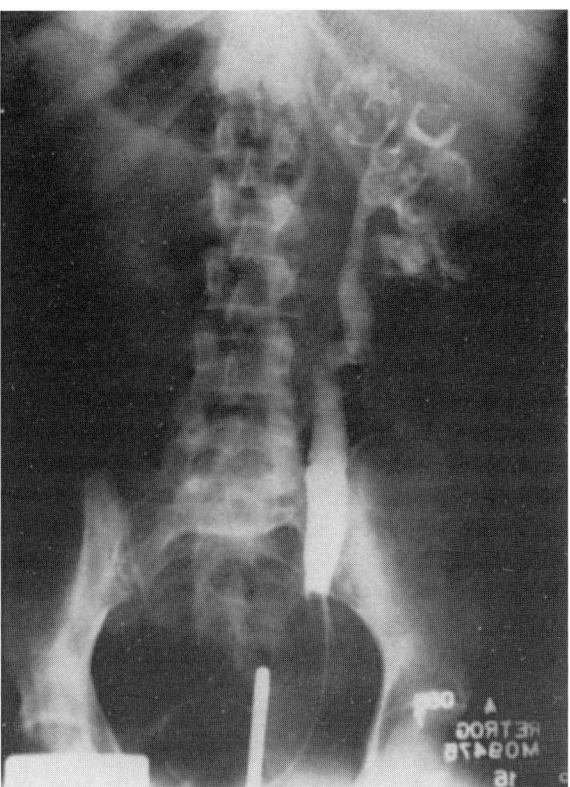

Figure 12–19. Pyonephrosis retrograde ureteropylogram. Severe renal infection and pyonephrosis behind a distal ureteral obstruction. Contrast outlines dilated, pus-filled calyces and extravasates into renal tissue.

and sonography. Angiographically these lesions are typical for those of inflammatory lesions. Arteries are frequently spread apart and the intralobar arteries are attenuated in appearance. There is prolonged nephrogram phase with delay in arteriocapulary drainage. Linear densities are seen radiating from the renal periphery during the nephrogram. There is an increase in the number and size of capsular vessels.[70] When perinephric extension is involved, evidence of neovascularity originating from intrarenal vessels may be seen.[80] In later stages, when pyonephrosis ensues, small vessels surround large pus-filled calyces, forming multiple hazy bordered hypovascular areas. Epinephrine infusion may be employed and has been reported to produce a vasoconstrictive response in patients with abscesses but no vasoconstriction in patients with neoplasia. The use of epinephrine may be valuable in differentiating infection and malignancy in some cases (Fig. 12–20).

Ultrasound evaluation of these abscesses may also contribute to the diagnosis and differentiation of mass lesions. Enhanced through-transmission of the ultrasound beam and refraction of the beam at the junction of the fluid collection and adjacent soft tissue differentiate renal abscesses from other solid masses. Frequently, however, complex masses with internal echoes are seen in many studies. Because of these internal echoes, ultrasound is frequently confusing and nondiagnostic in renal abscesses, especially in early stages. False-negatives may occur in as many as one-third of cases.[68] CT scan is the most sensitive and specific imaging modality for the diagnosis of renal abscesses. These studies provide a more detailed image of the kidneys and adjacent mass lesions. Abscesses appear as either a well-defined area of low attenuation or decreased enhancement.[65] Frequently there is a surrounding inflammatory wall of slightly higher attenuation seen on unenhanced images, the so-called rind sign.[75] When gas is present within the lesion this is pathognomonic for renal abscess. Unless gas is seen within the lesion, CT cannot differentiate hematoma, necrotic malignancy, or urinoma from inflammatory lesions. Both CT and sonography have also provided additional modalities for imaging renal or perirenal infections in patients with nonfunctioning kidneys. CT scan is more sensitive when lesions are small, the patient has a large body habitus, or there is perinephric extension. In one recent series CT was able to detect 7 of 15 intrarenal and extrarenal abscesses not seen on ultrasound.[81] Ultrasound is valuable, therefore, only in correlation with other imaging techniques. MRI is an additional imaging modality for identifying abscesses but with limited experience.[69] On T1-weighted images, the abscess signal intensity is low and may be inhomogeneous. On T2-weighted images there is increased signal, but here too the signal may be inhomogeneous (Figs. 12–21, 12–22, 12–23).

Gallium citrate (67Ga) was first described for use in localizing highly malignant tumors.[82] Because of its ability to selectively label leukocytes and macrophages, 67Ga is also useful in localizing deep-seated abscesses. Unfortunately, however, gallium scanning is diagnostic only 48 to 72 hours after administration of the isotope. Collection of this isotope within the abscess, therefore, requires significant time between its administration and diagnosis. In a patient in whom confusing diagnostic signals are obtained and in whom long-term workup is in progress, gallium scanning may add invaluable information of differentiating renal abscesses from other renal masses. A necessary caution, however, must be inserted, because gallium accumulation can also be seen in malignant neoplasms, acute tubular necrosis, and vasculitis.[82] Radionucleotide scanning with pertechnetate, glucoheptonate, and DMSA has been used, but these are nonspecific and will reveal only a "cold" area or area of diminished isotope uptake (Fig. 12–24).

Percutaneous fine-needle aspiration of renal mass lesions under ultrasound or CT guidance can be performed for both diagnosis and therapy. Fine-needle aspiration of pus or Gram stain of collected fluid can be used to confirm an abscess. Additional material collected can then be sent for culture and a larger catheter can be placed for drainage. Lambiase and coworkers reported eventual cures in 55% of intrarenal and 68% of perirenal abscesses treated with percutaneous drainage alone.[83] An additional 16 to 18% of patients had temporization with percutaneous drainage prior to definitive nephrectomy. The complications from percutaneous drain-

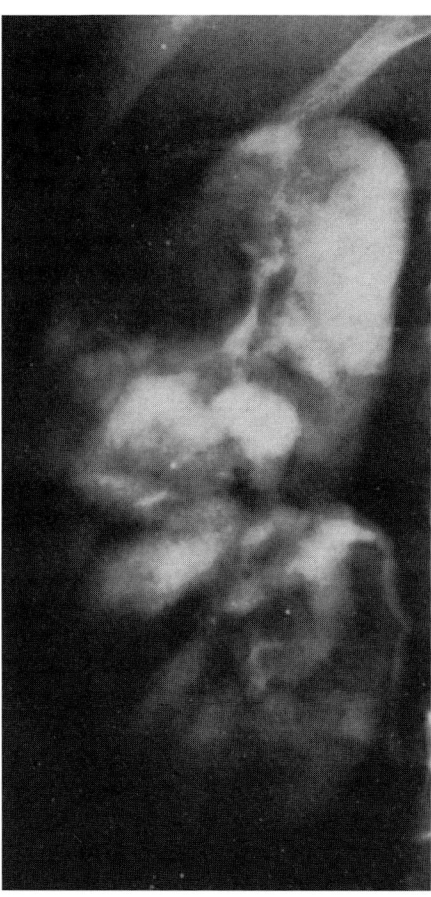

Figure 12–20. Renal carbuncle. Right calyceal stretching and mass effect confirmed by arteriogram in renal carbuncle.

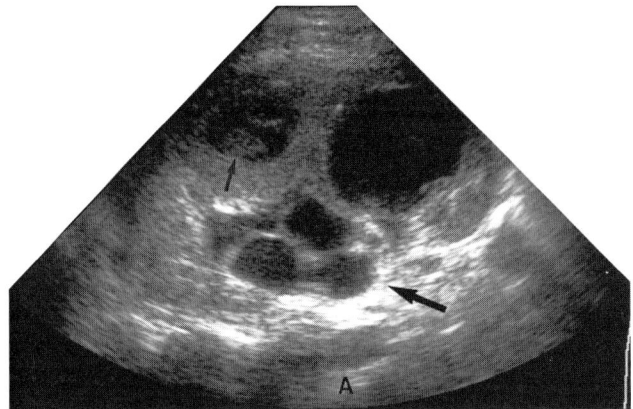
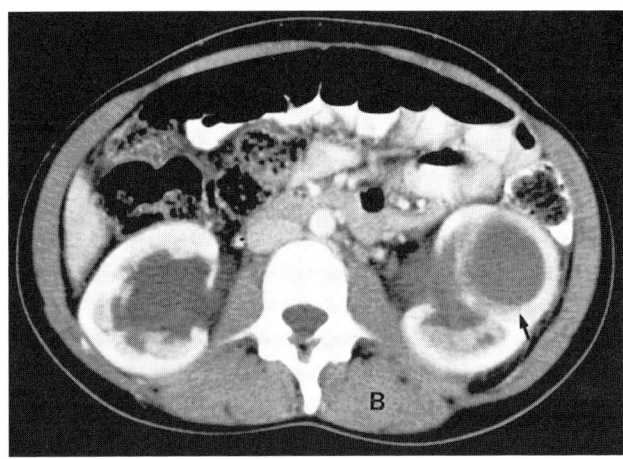
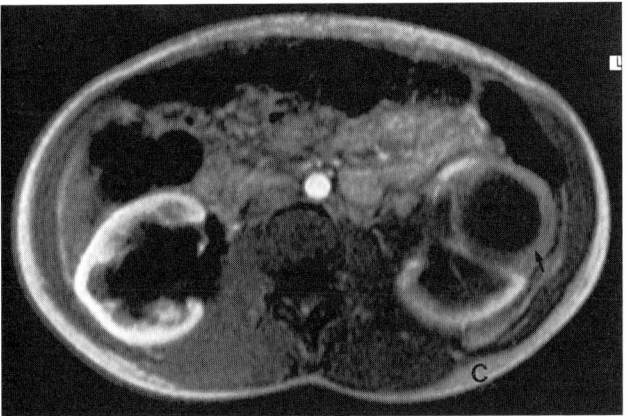

Figure 12–21. Case of a young female patient with several-month history of recurrent pyelonephritis unresponsive to antibiotics: ULS, CT, MRI. **(A)** Ultrasound with two large abscesses. Small arrow points to echogenic foci within the smaller abscess representing debris. Large arrow points to cluster of incidental peripelvic cysts. **(B)** Contrast-enhanced CT scan with arrow pointing to the larger abscess. **(C)** Gadolinium-enhanced T1-weighted MRI of the same patient.

age are few and often far outweighed when the patient is critically ill and unable to tolerate major surgery safely. The frequent occurrence of multiple and multilocular abscesses, however, makes surgical drainage for definitive diagnosis and treatment necessary in many cases.

Chronic Bacterial Pyelonephritis

Chronic pyelonephritis refers to a long-standing, bacterial infection producing progressive destruction of the renal parenchyma. The infection may be active or inactive as determined by symptoms and bacteriuria.

Although these recurrent infections lead to renal damage, not all patients with recurrent urinary infections progress to end-stage renal failure. For this reason it is important to evaluate patients for site of infection and localize bacteria to kidney or bladder. Bacterial growth in urine collected by direct ureteral catheterization and the bladder washout test have both been used successfully to localize upper urinary tract infections.[84,85] These tests, however, are invasive and in the case of ureteral catheterization require a surgical procedure. Over the years numerous noninvasive tests have been developed for infection localization. Techniques such as antibody-coated bacteria in the urine, the urinary lactic dehydrogenase isoenzyme technique, urinary beta-2 microglobulin, measurement of antibodies to Tamm–Horsfall pro-

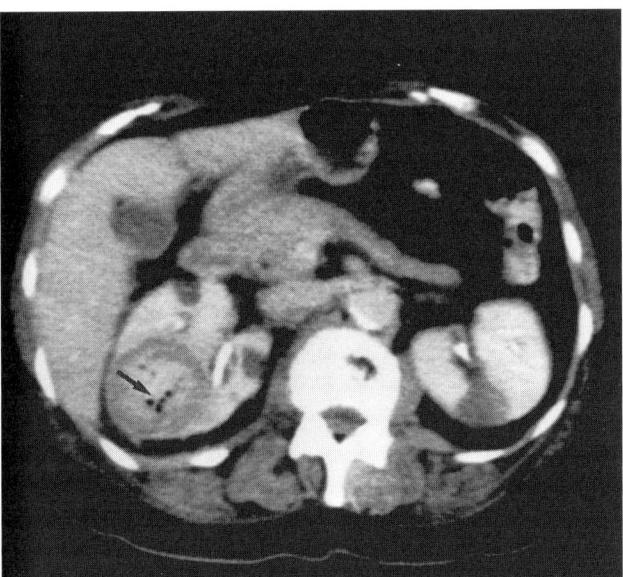

Figure 12–22. Renal abscess. Contrast-enhanced CT showing gas in right renal abscess (arrow). Note bilateral incidental cysts. (Photograph courtesy of Dr. D. M. Warshauer.)

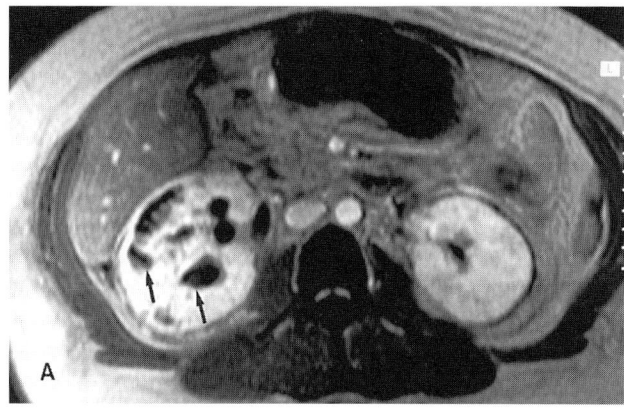
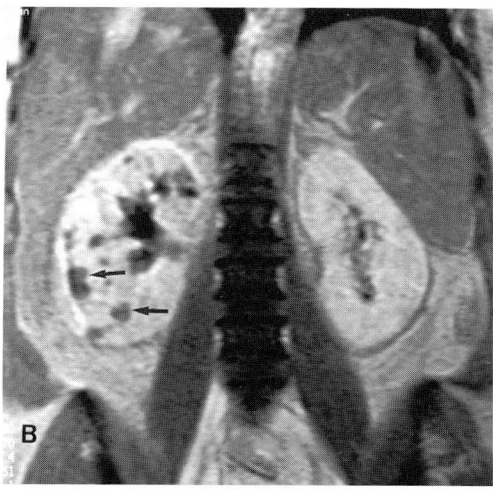

Figure 12–23. Renal abscess. (**A**) Transaxial gadolinium-enhanced T1-weighted MRI of patient with multiple right renal abscesses (arrows). (**B**) Coronal T1-weighted images of same patient.

tein, serum c-reactive protein, urinary beta-glucuronidase, and determinations of maximal urinary concentrating ability have all been used in an attempt to localize bacterial infections. Most of these studies are nonspecific and have not gained widespread use because of technical reasons or cost.

In 1974 Thomas and associates reported a technique of detecting antibody coating of bacteria in the urine.[86] The principle behind this technique is that bacteria infecting the renal parenchyma respond to serum immunoglobulins to which bladder bacteria are not exposed. These renal antibodies respond to bacterial presence by coating the offending organisms. Bacteria found in the urine collections are incubated with a flourescein-conjugated anti-human globulin and examined with a fluorescent microscope for fluorescein labeling. In Thomas's original report 34 of 35 patients with upper tract infections showed a positive antibody-coated bacteria test. On the other hand, only one of 20 patients with lower tract infection had a positive test. The results of this test were compared with ureteral catheterization studies in several subsequent evaluations of this technique.[87] Antibody coating has failed to be as reliable as first reported, but few false-positives can be anticipated in carefully done studies. False-positives can, however, be found in children and in patients with bacterial prostatitis, chronic cystitis, or ileal conduit. Because of these mixed results, the widespread use of this procedure as a reliable localization technique cannot be recommended.

Localization of urinary infections by the use of lactic dehydrogenase (LDH) isoenzyme has been reported in children.[88] Lactate dehydrogenase is present in the body in several isoenzymatic forms. Of these, only isoenzymes 4 and 5 are present in large concentrations in the renal medulla and are shed in the urine during episodes of renal infection. Electrophoresis of aliquots of urine collected from the bladder

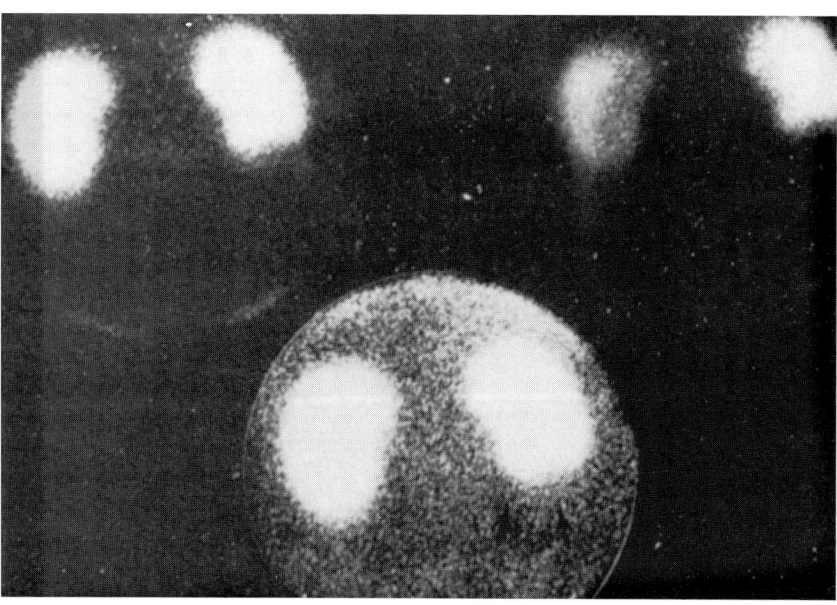

Figure 12–24. Right renal abscess. Radionucleotide scan shows right renal abscess that appears as an area of decreased uptake of isotope in the lower pole of the kidney.

are carried out to define the five isoenzymes of LDH. A markedly elevated level of LDH isoenzyme 5 is the most sensitive indicator of active pyelonephritis. In comparison with the antibody-coated bacteria test, the LDH measurement has been shown to be more sensitive at differentiating upper and lower urinary tract infections, but considerable overlap can exist between LDH levels for the two groups.[89]

The urinary beta-2 microglobulin is another indirect localization method used to differentiate upper and lower urinary tract infections. The beta-2 microglobulin is a small protein synthesized by most nucleated cells that is filtered by the kidney and then reabsorbed almost completely in the renal tubules in undamaged kidneys. In pyelonephritis there is tubular damage to the kidney with a decreased ability for reabsorption. Elevated urinary concentration of beta-2 microglobulin and a decreased urinary concentrating ability are thus found. In a study by Schaijn and associates the beta-2 microglobulin test was elevated in 19 patients with radiographic evidence of pyelonephritis but in none of the 15 patients with cystitis or the 44 control patients.[90] This test, however, requires a 24-hour urine collection, and urinary alkalinization is necessary because the protein is destroyed at a pH greater than 6.

The Tamm–Horsfall protein has been studied in a number of urologic disorders. This protein is produced exclusively by cells in the ascending loop of Henle and is normally found in the urine. In obstructive renal disease or severe vesicoureteral reflux this large protein can be deposited in renal interstitium and Bowman's space, where it stimulates antibody formation. An enzyme-linked immunosorbent assay can then be used in these cases to measure for antibodies to Tamm–Horsfall protein. Studies that have used this technique to localize bacteriuria, however, have not proved specific, and antibodies are often elevated in cases without infection. Other indirect measures of renal infection such as the c-reactive protein, urinary beta glucuronidase test, and determinations of maximum urinary concentrating ability are more nonspecific and have not been found useful in the majority of cases.

Experimental models of renal infections have shown that even with ureteral catheterization techniques, often considered the gold standard for diagnosing upper urinary tract infection, the accuracy of diagnosing chronic bacterial infections is 50%.[91] Even when these studies are accurate radiographic evaluation is usually necessary as they provide little pathologic information about the involved kidney.

The initial changes in the renal collecting system in chronic pyelonephritis were best described by Hodson and associates in both animal models and human studies.[3] The major anatomic changes of these scarred kidneys include a deep, focal, cortical renal scar with the renal calyx below it showing marked clubbing. These classic scars may be unilateral or bilateral and usually involve the renal poles. Histologic examination of the renal parenchyma in these areas reveals marked parenchymal atrophy, scarring, and fibrosis. As the involved areas of the kidney increase in size, parenchymal thickness diminishes and calyceal clubbing continues. In severely affected kidneys with progressive scarring, the entire kidney may diminish in size and atrophy with diminished function on excretory urography (Fig. 12–25).

Radiographically, kidneys with chronic pyelonephritis are often smaller and are easily detected using excretory urography, ultrasound, or CT scan. Good-quality excretory urography with nephrotomography is usually adequate in making the diagnosis. The associated calyceal scarring with retraction of the papillae are demonstrated on excretory urography as thinning of the renal cortex and calyceal clubbing. Retrograde studies are rarely necessary in these patients. Ultrasound will detect cortical scars as linear hypoechoic areas perpendicular to the surface of the kidney.[69] CT scan is not routinely used to diagnose chronic pyelonephritis, but it will demonstrate focal and diffuse loss of renal parenchyma, replacement of renal pelvic fat, and cortical scars.[69]

With segmental scarring, normal areas of the kidney may develop compensatory hypertrophy, resulting in segmental enlargement and the formation of a pseudo-tumor.[92] These lesions may be indeterminate on excretory urography and further diagnostic studies may be necessary to differentiate this hypertrophied segment from renal cell carcinoma or renal abscess. Both CT scan and ultrasound are capable of differentiating pseudo-tumor from other renal lesions. Angiography is less frequently used today but can also differentiate areas of pseudo-tumor. These areas characteristically have no neovascularity, arteriovenous shunting, or puddling of contrast media.[93] Radionuclide scanning may also differentiate renal cell carcinoma from pseudo-tumor. The latter characteristically has normal isotopic uptake in comparison to the contralateral kidney or normal areas in the affected kidney. Renal neoplasms are seen as areas of decreased isotopic activity (Figs. 12–26, 12–27).

Although associated hypertension has been found in approximately one-third of chronic pyelonephritis cases, angiography is seldom helpful.[94] Thinned, irregular cortex is

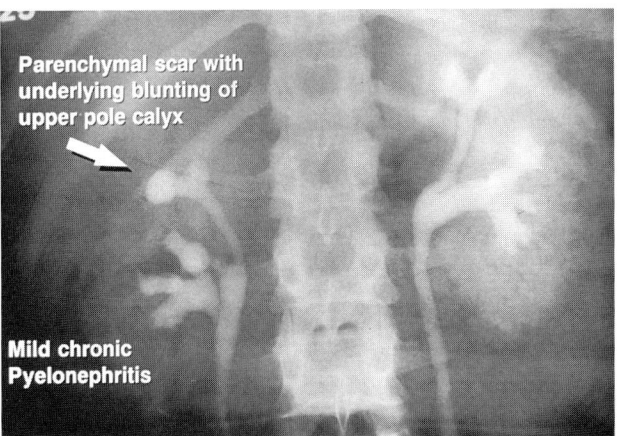

Figure 12–25. Mild chronic pyelonephritis. Arrows outline polar parenchymal scar with underlying blunting of the upper pole calyx. This configuration appeared after an episode of severe acute pyelonephritis. (Photograph courtesy of Dr. R. Older.)

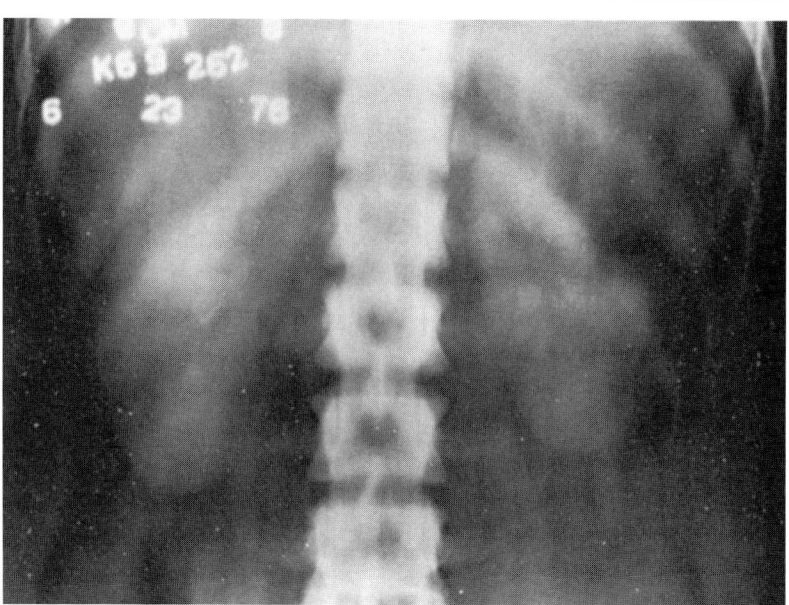

Figure 12–26. Chronic pyelonephritis, pseudotumors. Renal tissue regeneration between cortical scarring produces a pseudo-tumor effect.

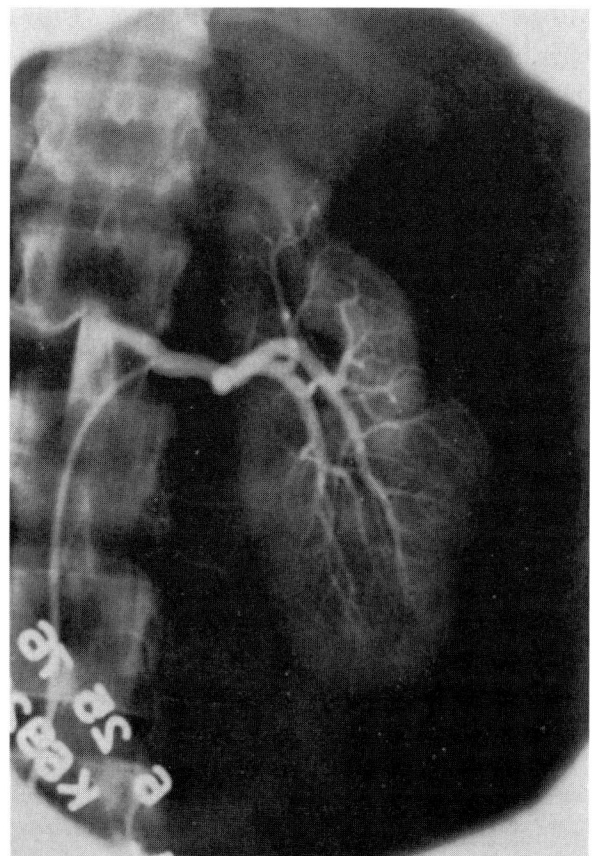

Figure 12–27. Chronic pyelonephritis. Arteriogram emphasizes parenchymal scarring and pseudo-tumor formation with regeneration.

readily apparent. The renal artery may be narrowed, especially in its distal two-thirds. The interlobar arteries may be absent in a vascular area or may show pruning. Arcuate arteries, likewise, are diminished in number and size, and capsular arteries may be dilated.[70] The renal venous tree also shows widespread obliteration and may contribute to the tissue damage in the pyelonephritic kidney.[94]

Chronic atrophic pyelonephritis, also known as reflux nephropathy, was first described by Kleeman and has several specific features that differentiate it from other forms of chronic pyelonephritis.[59] These features include its frequent association with vesicoureteral reflux and common onset of symptoms before the age of 5 years. It is usually rapidly progressive and, if bilateral, frequently progresses to chronic renal failure during the third decade of life.[95] Renal growth during childhood is greatly diminished in these patients, and the overall kidney size, as measured on IVP, is more than 1.5 cm less that its normal mate. These kidneys may be followed by radionuclide studies and renal ultrasound to determine progression of scarring and renal growth. If functional information is desired nuclear medicine is the study of choice. These kidneys do maintain renal function and may resume renal growth potential if urine is maintained sterile and if vesicoureteral reflux is eliminated.[96] The majority of these patients will demonstrate similar renal morphology on follow-up IVP and stable renal function after a long period of observation.[95]

Xanthogranulomatous Pyelonephritis

Xanthogranulomatous pyelonephritis is a rare and atypical form of chronic renal parenchymal infection. The infection results in a chronic granulomatous inflammatory disease characterized by parenchymal destruction and replacement by lipid-laden macrophages, the so-called foamy or xanthoma cells. On cut surface, accumulation of these foamy histiocytes appears as yellow nodules within the renal parenchyma. Renal involvement may be diffuse or segmental. Unlike chronic pyelonephritis, perinephric extension is common. Perinephric abscesses and fistulas to the bowel or flank have been reported.[66,97] Associated focal squamous metaplasia of the urothelium and transitional cell carcinoma of the renal pelvis have also been reported. These tumors are thought to arise from chronic inflammation of the renal pelvis from the disease process.[98] Xanthogranulomatous pyelonephritis can mimic renal neoplasm and other inflammatory renal parenchymal diseases and is frequently misdiagnosed.

This unusual reaction to chronic infection is usually found in adults in the fourth through the sixth decades and is more common in females.[98] Several cases have been reported in infants and in children.[99] The disease is universally one-sided and only one case of bilateral xanthogranulomatous pyelonephritis has been reported. Similar to other chronic renal infections, symptoms are frequently nonspecific, multiple, and chronic in nature. Patients often appear chronically ill with common presenting symptoms of flank pain, low-grade fevers, chills, persistent urosepsis, malaise, weight loss, and constipation.[100] Urinary symptoms are minimal, although recurrent urinary tract infections and frequently a history of sporadic and incomplete antibiotic treatment may be elicited. Symptoms usually have been present for more than 6 weeks, and a history of previous calculus disease, diabetes mellitus, or obstructive uropathy is common.

Many bacteria seem to share the ability to cause this uncommon reaction to chronic infection. The most common causative organisms are *E. Coli* and *Proteus*. In some patients more than one organism and even gram-positive cocci have been isolated.[98] Urine and blood cultures are not very reliable and are frequently sterile, sometimes because of previous antibiotic treatment. The presence of sterile urine cultures and the presence of chronic parenchymal infections suggests calyceal obstruction preventing contaminated urine from reaching the bladder. Significant pyuria may be present in as many as 40% of patients despite sterile urine cultures.[101] Xanthoma or foam cells occasionally may be found in the urine.[2] The inability to retrieve causative organisms from urine culture makes early, correct diagnosis of these infections difficult. Bacterial cultures of the renal tissue at the time of surgery identify the responsible organisms. Bacteria removed from the kidney, however, may be different from those recovered from the urine.

Other laboratory results include frequent chronic microcytic anemia, elevated erythrocyte sedimentation rate, and the syndrome of reversible hepatic dysfunction similar to that seen in patients with renal cell carcinoma.[98] Stouffer's syndrome associated with reversible hepatic dysfunction is based on findings of elevations in SGOT, SGPT, bilirubin, and alkaline phosphatase that, after nephrectomy, return to normal levels. This syndrome occurs in approximately 17% of patients with xanthogranulomatous pyelonephritis.[98]

Radiographic diagnosis is quite difficult, as radiographic signs are highly variable. The kidney can be affected locally or diffusely, and frequently, perinephric extension of the disease process in association with perinephric abscess formation produces ill-defined renal margins and a nondescript renal mass. Branched renal calculi or calcifications are present in more than 80% of cases.[100,102] Eighty-five percent of patients have a nonfunctioning kidney, often with ureteropelvic obstruction. Renal mass lesions are present in 75% of cases composing the so-called tumefactive form. Retrograde pyelography usually demonstrates an abnormal pelvocalyceal system owing to diffuse parenchymal enlargement and involvement of the collecting system from the disease process. Nephrotomography reveals a solid renal mass, indistinguishable from renal cell carcinoma. Similarly, ultrasonography is nonspecific and usually reveals only a solid mass, which is indistinguishable from a renal tumor. CT findings are more specific and can demonstrate the extent of perirenal involvement as well as the details of intrarenal lesions. Typically, there is renal enlargement with multiple low-attenuation areas, representing dilated calyces or abscesses, with little parenchymal function. Associated renal calculi are common and can be appreciated best on nonenhanced images. CT scan findings, however, suggest the specific diagnosis in only a few cases.[103] MRI has also been used to evaluate xanthogranulomatous pyelonephritis but offers little additional information.[69] Because of better fat enhancement these images are sensitive for detecting extrarenal spread, which produces high-intensity signal on T2-weighted images (Figs. 12–28, 12–29).

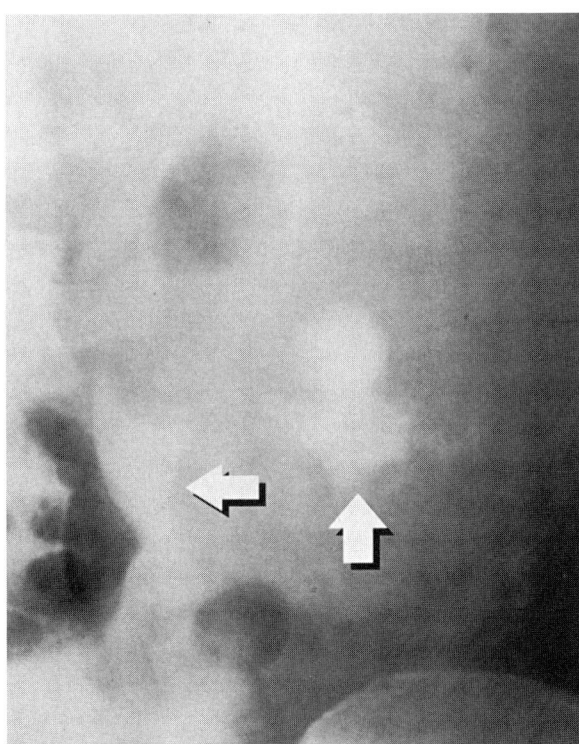

Figure 12–28. Xanthogranulomatous pyelonephritis. Multiple calcifications (arrows) in left kidney of patient with proven xanthogranulomatous pyelonephritis. Note mass lesion of lateral renal border consistent with tumefactive xanthogranulomatous pyelonephritis. (Photograph courtesy of Dr. R. Older.)

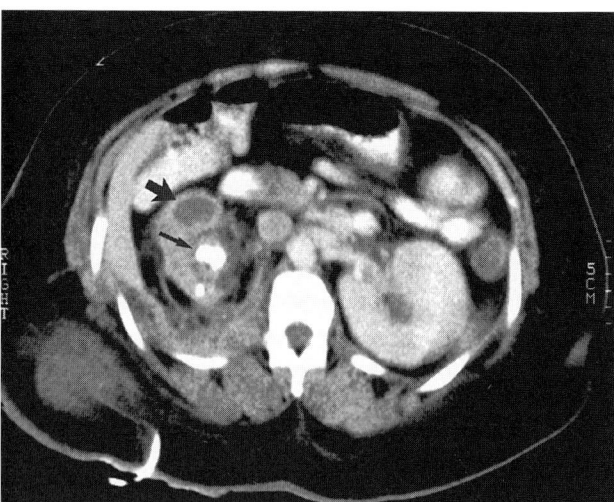

Figure 12–29. Xanthogranulomatous pyelonephritis. Contrast-enhanced CT in diabetic patient with xanthogranulomatous pyelonephritis and perinephric inflammation. Smaller arrow points to calculi in renal pelvis. Note area of spherical low attenuation (wide arrow) often seen with xanthogranulomatous pyelonephritis. A right flank percutaneous drain is also present.

Angiography is usually not indicated in the evaluation of xanthogranulomatous pyelonephritis but has been used in the past to help differentiate these lesions from carcinoma. The angiographic appearance of xanthogranulomatous pyelonephritis, however, is quite variable, frequently being confused with hypovascular or necrotic forms of renal cell carcinoma. The suggestion of abnormal vascularity is also present in many cases.

Despite the correct preoperative diagnosis, radical nephrectomy is still required. Correct preoperative diagnosis, however, provides assurance that the disease is not malignant and provides the surgeon with the knowledge that this is a chronic infective process. This is especially important in children where nephron-sparing surgery may be considered. Vigorous preoperative antibiotic treatment should be undertaken once the diagnosis is made. The presence of a patient who is chronically ill and whose excretory urograms reveal a nonfunctioning kidney or renal mass in association with renal calcifications should suggest the diagnosis of xanthogranulomatous pyelonephritis.

Pyelonephritis of Pregnancy

Bacteriuria and urinary tract infections are the most common medical complication of pregnancy. The overall prevalence of bacteriuria is 4 to 7% of all pregnancies.[21,22] Screening for asymptomatic bacteriuria is usually done in the first trimester. Identification and treatment of infections can reduce progression to symptomatic infections and the concomitant risk to maternal and fetal health by 80 to 90%.[104] Physiologic changes of the urinary tract during pregnancy are well documented. Ureteral dilation has been reported during pregnancy for many years. The exact etiology of this ureterectasis remains elusive, but its right-sided predominance is well known. Ureteral dilation usually begins as early as the seventh week of gestation and progresses until term. The cause has been attributed to hypertrophy of Waldeyer's sheath resulting from hormonal changes, to reduced peristalsis as a result of progesterone, and to physical obstruction caused by an enlarging uterus. Ureteral volume can also increase up to 25-fold during pregnancy, and bladder tone decreases markedly by the third trimester. Postpartum, ureteral dilation and bladder tone rapidly return to normal, in the absence of infection, usually by the second month.[104]

The incidence of infection increases as pregnancy progresses. The clinical findings of fever, flank tenderness, chills, nausea, and vomiting are similar to those in nonpregnant patients. The increased ureteral volume and decreased peristalsis during pregnancy seem to enhance the ability of urinary infective organisms to progress to pyelonephritis. Clinical pyelonephritis, also more common on the right side, occurs in 1 to 2% of all pregnancies.[104] The association of asymptomatic bacteriuria and the subsequent development of acute symptomatic urinary tract infections have been previously documented.[104,105] If left untreated almost one-third of women with bacteriuria will develop pyelonephritis at some time during their pregnancy.[106] This is especially true in women with diabetes or with a history of previous urinary tract infections. The association of vesicoureteric reflux with pregnancy is unusual. Cystourethroscopic findings may show chronic inflammatory changes of the bladder but rarely demonstrate significant lower urinary tract pathology.[106] It seems, therefore, that cystography and cystourethroscopy are not necessary for evaluation of urinary infections during pregnancy.

Excretory urography should usually be deferred until after delivery. In those cases with the possibility of obstruction or in whom multiple severe recurrences of infection occur despite adequate antibiotic therapy, excretory urography should be carried out to exclude complicating, obstructive lesions. If excretory urography is carried out, the technique must be modified in order to diminish radiation dosage to which the fetus is exposed. In most cases, an abbreviated excretory urogram will provide the necessary information for diagnosis and treatment of urinary obstruction. Usually, a preliminary film followed by a single tomographic film and 10-minute postinjection view are adequate to eliminate obstruction from the differential diagnosis. Rare earth screens also reduce radiation in these cases.

The ideal management of pyelonephritis of pregnancy is prevention. Identification of patients with bacteriuria during the first trimester and sterilization of the urine with continued follow-up and repeat urinary evaluation will prevent many cases of pyelonephritis during pregnancy. In patients with acute upper tract infections during pregnancy, administration of appropriate antibiotic is guided by culture and in vitro antibiotic sensitivity studies. Sterilization of infected urine is absolutely necessary in patients with bacteriuria of pregnancy. Pregnant women who develop symptomatic urinary tract infections or pyelonephritis have associated prematurity in 20 to 50% of cases.[104] The contribution of treated asymptomatic bacteriuria to prematurity or maternal-fetal complications is unclear.[21]

In the series by Dempsey and coworkers almost 10% of treated patients went on to develop recurrence of urinary tract infection.[21] Screening during the first trimester may, therefore, help identify high-risk women who will need closer follow-up. Failure to eliminate bacteriuria with repeated therapy or recurrence of the same organism may indicate underlying structural abnormality or renal parenchymal infection. These women should have follow-up cultures and a complete urologic evaluation after delivery.

REFERENCES

1. National Hospital Discharge Survey: annual summary. National Center for Health Statistics. Vital Stat, 1992.
2. Kunin CM: *Detection, Prevention, and Management of Urinary Tract Infections*. Philadelphia: Lea & Febiger, 1987.
3. Hodgson CJ, Wilson S: Natural history of chronic pyelonephritis scarring. *Br Med J* 1965;2:191.
4. Stamey TA: *Pathogenesis and Treatment of Urinary Tract Infection*. Baltimore: Williams & Wilkins, 1980.
5. Stamm WE: Measurement of pyuria and its relation to bacteriuria. *Am J Med* 1983;75:53.
6. Stamm WE, Hooton TM: Management of urinary tract infections in adults. *N Engl J Med* 1993;329:1328.
7. Brettman LR: Pathogenesis of urinary tract infections: host susceptibility and bacterial virulence factors. *Urology* 1988; 32(Suppl):21.
8. Kass EH: The diagnosis of infections of the urinary tract. *Arch Int Med* 1957;100:709.
9. Stamm WE, et al: Diagnosis of coliform infection in acutely dysuric women. *N Engl J Med* 1982;307:463.
10. Latham RH, Wong ES, Larson A, Coyle M, Stamm WE: Laboratory diagnosis of urinary tract infection in ambulatory women. *JAMA* 1985;254:3333.
11. Kunin CM, White LV, Hua TH: A reassessment of the importance of "low-count" bacteriuria in young women with acute urinary symptoms. *Ann Intern Med* 1993;119:454.
12. Lipsky BA: Urinary tract infections in men: epidemiology, pathophysiology, diagnosis, and treatment. *Ann Intern Med* 1989;110:138.
13. Stark RP, Maki DG: Bacteriuria in the catheterized patient. What quantitative level of bacteriuria is relevant? *N Engl J Med* 1984;311:560.
14. Hedman P, Ringertz O: Urinary tract infections caused by *Staphylococcus saprophiticus*: a matched case control study. *J Infect* 1991;23:145.
15. Boscia JA, et al: Epidemiology of bacteriuria in an elderly ambulatory population. *Am J Med* 1986;80:208.
16. Blum RN, Wright RA: Detection of pyuria and bacteriuria in symptomatic ambulatory women. *J Gen Inter Med* 1992; 7:140.
17. Baerheim A, Albrektsen G, Eriksen AG, Laerum E, Sandberg S: Quantification of pyuria by two methods: correlation and interobserver agreement. *Scand J Prim Health Care* 1989; 7:83.
18. Williams JD, Leigh DA, Rosser E, Brumfitt W: The organization and results of a screening program for the detection of bacteriuria of pregnancy. *J Obstet Gynaecol Br Emp* 1965; 72:327.
19. Stamey TA: A clinical classification of urinary tract infections based upon origin. *South Med J* 1975;68:934.
20. Dempsey C, Harrison RF, Moloney A, Darling M, Walshe J: Characteristics of bacteriuria in a homogeneous maternity hospital population. *Eur J Obstet Gynecol Reprod Biol* 1992; 44:189.
21. Kunin CM, Zacha E, Paquin AJ: Urinary infections in school children. In: Prevalence of bacteriuria and associated urologic findings. *N Engl J Med* 1962;266:1289.
22. Golan A, Wexler S, Amit A, Gordon D, David MP: Asymptomatic bacteriuria in normal and high-risk pregnancy. *Eur J Obstet Gynecol Reprod Biol* 1989;33:101.
23. Lee YL, Thrupp LD, Friis RH, Fine M, Maleki P, Cesario TC: Nosocomial infection and antibiotic utilization in geriatric patients: a pilot prospective surveillance program in skilled nursing facilities. *Gerontology* 1992; 38:223.
24. Spencer JR, Schaeffer AJ: Pediatric urinary tract infection. *Urol Clin North Am* 1986;13:661.
25. Corriere JN Jr: Avoiding "overkill" in diagnosis and treatment of lower urinary tract infection. *Urology* 1988; 32(suppl):17.
26. Carson CC, Osbourne DW, Segura JW: Evaluation and treatment of the urethral syndrome. *J Urol* 1980;124:609.
27. Fowler JE, Pulaski TE: Excretory urography, cystography, and cystoscopy in the evaluation of women with urinary tract infection. *N Engl J Med* 1981;304:462.
28. Quint HJ, Drach GW, Rappaport WD, Hoffman CJ: Emphysematous cystitis: a review of the spectrum of disease. *J Urol* 1992;147:134.
29. Carson CC, Malek RS, ReMine WH: Urologic aspects of vesicoenteric fistulas. *J Urol* 1978;119:774.
30. Katz DS, Aksoy E, Cunha BA: *Clostridium perfringens* emphysematous cystitis. *Urology* 1993;41:458.
31. Jost SP, Dixon JS, Gosling JA: Ultrastructural observations on cystitis cystica in human bladder urothelium. *Br J Urol* 1993;71:28.
32. Walther MM, Campbell WG Jr, O'Brien DP 3d, Wheatley JK, Graham SD Jr: Cystitis cystica: an electron and immunofluorescence microscopic study. *J Urol* 1987;137:764.
33. Aabech HS, Lien EN: Cystitis cystica in childhood: clinical findings and treatment procedures. *Acta Paediatr Scand* 1982;71:247.
34. Tomaszewski JE: Cystitis. In: Hill GS, ed. *Uropathology*. New York: Churchill, Livingstone, 1989.
35. Heyns CF, De Kock MLS, Kirsten PH, van Velden DJJ: Pelvic lipomatosis associated with cystitis glandularis and adenocarcinoma of the bladder. *J Urol* 1991;145:364.
36. Rudin L, Tannenbaum M, Lattimer JK: Histologic analysis of the extrophied bladder after anatomical closure. *J Urol* 1972;108:802.
37. Stanton MJ, Maxted W: Malakoplakia: a study of the literature and current concepts of pathogenesis, diagnosis, and treatment. *J Urol* 1981;125:139.
38. Baumgartner BR, Alagappian R: Malakoplakia of the ureter and bladder. *Urol Radiol* 1990;12:157.
39. Schneiderman C, Simon MA: Malakoplakia of the urinary tract. *J Urol* 1968;100:694.
40. Lamm DL, Gittes RF: Inflammatory carcinoma of the bladder and interstitial cystitis. *J Urol* 1977;117:49.
41. Castillo J Jr, Cartagena R, Montes M: Eosinophilic cystitis: a therapeutic challenge. *Urology* 1988;32:535.
42. Granados EA, Riley G, Salvador J, Vincente J: Prostatic abscess: diagnosis and treatment. *J Urol* 1992;148:80.
43. Cytron S, Weinberger M, Pitlik SD, Servadio C: Value of transrectal ultrasonography for diagnosis and treatment of prostatic abscess. *Urology* 1988;32(suppl):454.

44. Brunner H, Weidner W, Schiefer H-G: Studies on the role of Ureaplasma urealyticum and *Mycoplasma hominis* in prostatitis. *J Infect Dis* 1983;147:807.
45. Kreiger JN, Egan KJ: Comprehensive evaluation and treatment of 75 men referred to chronic prostatitis clinic. *Urology* 1991;38:11.
46. Meares EM Jr: Prostatitis. *Med Clin North Am* 1991;75:405.
47. Meares EM, Stamey TA: Bacteriologic localization patterns in bacterial prostatitis and urethritis. *Invest Urol* 1968;5:492.
48. Schaeffer AJ, Darras FS: The efficacy of norfloxacin in the treatment of chronic bacterial prostatitis refractory to trimethoprim-sulfamethoxazole and/or carbenicillin. *J Urol* 1990;144:690.
49. Shortliffe LM, Sellers RG, Schachter J: The characterization of nonbacterial prostatitis: search for an etiology. *J Urol* 1992;148:146.
50. Epstein JI, Hutchin GM: Granulomatous prostatitis: distinction among allergic, non-specific, and post-transurethral resection lesions. *Hum Pathol* 1984;15:818.
51. Stillwell TJ, Engen DE, Farrow GM: The clinical spectrum of granulomatous prostatitis: a report of 200 cases. *J Urol* 1987;138:320.
52. Miyashita H, Trancoso P, Babaian RJ: BCG-induced granulomatous prostatitis: a comparative ultrasound and pathologic study. *Urology* 1992;39:364.
53. Dunnick NR, Ford K, Osborne D, Carson CC, Paulson DF: Seminal vesiculography: limited value in vesiculitis. *Urology* 1982;20:454.
54. Clements R, Thomas KG, Griffiths GJ, Peeling WB: Transrectal ultrasound appearances of granulomatous prostatitis. *Clin Radiol* 1993;47:174.
55. Baert L, Leonard A, D'Hoedt M, Vandeursen R: Seminal vesiculography in chronic bacterial prostatitis. *J Urol* 1986;126:844.
56. Hatcher PA, Carson CC: Pain in seminal vesiculitis: diagnosis and treatment. *Probl Urol* 1989;3:256.
57. Littrup PJ, et al: Transrectal ultrasound of the seminal vesicles and ejaculatory ducts: clinical correlation. *Radiology* 1988;168:625.
58. Schnall MD, Pollack HM, Van Arsdalen K, Kressel HY: The seminal tract in patients with ejaculatory dysfunction: MR imaging with an endorectal coil. *Am J Roentgenol* 1992;159:337.
59. Kleeman CR, Huwitt WL, Guze LB: Pyelonephritis. *Medicine* (Baltimore) 1960;39:3.
60. Ryberg J, Helin I: A simple agglutination test for screening P-fimbriated *Escherichia coli* in children with urinary tract infections gives valuable clinical information. *Scand J Infect Dis* 1991;23:573.
61. Cameron DD, Azimi F: The value of excretory urography in the diagnosis of acute pyelonephritis. *J Urol* 1974;112:546.
62. Conway J: The role of scintigraphy in urinary tract infection. *Semin Nucl Med* 1988;18:308.
63. Stoller ML, Kogan BA: Sensitivity of 99m technetium-dimercaptosuccinic acid for the diagnosis of chronic pyelonephritis: clinical and theoretical considerations. *J Urol* 1986;135:977.
64. Hurwitz SR, et al: Gallium-67 imaging to localize urinary tract infections. *Br J Radiol* 1976;49:156.
65. Thornbury JR: Acute renal infections. *Urol Radiol* 1991;12:209.
66. Merenech WM, Popky GL: Radiology of renal infection. *Med Clin North Am* 1991;75:425.
67. Piccirillo M, Rigsby CM, Rosenfield AT: Sonography of renal inflammatory disease. *Urol Radiol* 1987;9:66.
68. Johnson JR, Vincent LM, Wang K, Roberts PL, Stamm WE: Renal ultrasonographic correlates of acute pyelonephritis. *Clin Infect Dis* 1992;14:15.
69. Goldman SM, Fishman EK: Upper urinary tract infection: the current role of CT, ultrasound, and MR. *Semin Ultrasound CT MR* 1991;12:335.
70. Frimann-Dahl J: Angiography in renal inflammatory disease. In: Kincaid OW, ed. *Renal Angiography*. Chicago: Year Book Medical Publisher, 1966.
71. Tsugaya M, et al: Computerized tomography in acute pyelonephritis: the clinical correlations. *J Urol* 1990;144:611.
72. Soulen MC, Fishman EK, Goldman SM: Sequelae of acute renal infections: CT evaluation. *Radiology* 1989;173:423.
73. Michaeli J, Mogle P, Perlberg S, Heiman S, Caine M: Emphysematous pyelonephritis. *J Urol* 1984;131:203.
74. Bohlman ME, et al: Emphysematous pyelitis and emphysematous pyelonephritis characterized by computerized tomography. *South Med J* 1991;84:1438.
75. Morgan WR, Nyberg LM Jr: Perinephric and intrarenal abscesses. *Urology* 1985;26:529.
76. Edelstein H, McCabe RE: Perinephric abscess. Modern diagnosis and treatment in 47 cases. *Medicine* (Baltimore) 1988;67:118.
77. Raghavaihh NV: The diagnosis of renal cortical abscess. *J Urol* 1978;120:237.
78. Thorley JD, Jones SR, Sanford JP: Perinephric abscesses. *Medicine* 1974;53:441.
79. Altemier WA, Culbertson WR, Fullen WD: Intraabdominal sepsis. *Adv Surg* 1971;5:281.
80. Koehler PR: The roentgen diagnosis of renal inflammatory masses: special emphasis on angiographic changes. *Radiology* 1974;112:257.
81. Soulen MC, Fishman EK, Goldman SM, Gatewood OMB: Bacterial renal infection: role of CT. *Radiology* 1989;171:703.
82. Lavender JP, et al: Gallium-67 citrate scanning in neoplastic and inflammatory lesions. *Br J Radiol* 1971;44:361.
83. Lambiase RE, Deyoe L, Cronan JJ, Dorfman GS: Percutaneous drainage of 335 consecutive abscesses: results of primary drainage with 1-year follow-up. *Radiology* 1992;184:167.
84. Stamey TA, Govan DE, Palmer JM: The localization and treatment of urinary tract infections: the role of bactericidal urine levels as opposed to serum levels. *Medicine* 1965;44:276.
85. Fairley KF, Bond AG, Brown RB, Habersberger P: Simple test to determine the site of urinary-tract infection. *Lancet* 1967;2:7513.
86. Thomas V, Shelokov A, Forland M: Antibody-coated bacteria in the urine and the site of urinary tract infection. *N Engl J Med* 1974;290:558.
87. Hawthorne NJ, et al: Accuracy of antibody-coated bacteria tests in recurrent urinary tract infections. *Mayo Clin Proc* 1978;53:651.
88. Carvajal HF, Passey RB, Burger M: Urinary lactic dehydrogenase isoenzyme 5 in the differential diagnosis of kidney and bladder infection. *Kidney Int* 1975;8:176.
89. Lorentz WB Jr, Resnick MI: Comparison of urinary lactic dehydrogenase with antibody-coated bacteria in the urine sediment as a means of localizing the site of urinary tract infection. *Pediatrics* 1979;64:672.
90. Schardijn GHC, Statius van Eps LW, Pauw W, Hoefnagel C, Noogen WJ: Comparison of reliability of tests to distinguish upper from lower urinary tract infection. *Br Med J* 1984;289:284.
91. Miller TE, Findon G, Lecamwasam JP, Yap P: Ureteric catheterization in the diagnosis of pyelonephritis: an experimental evaluation. *Kidney Int* 1990;38:835.

92. King MC, Friedenberg RM, Tina LB: Normal renal parenchyma simulating tumor. *Radiology* 1968;91:217.
93. Hodson CJ: The radiological contribution toward the diagnosis of chronic pyelonephritis. *Radiology* 1967;88:857.
94. Suat CP, Lindop GBM: Chronic pyelonephritis: the significance of renal renin and the vascular changes in the human kidney. *J Pathol* 1991;163:343.
95. Filly R, et al: Development and progression of clubbing and scarring in children with recurrent urinary tract infection. *Radiology* 1974;113:145.
96. Carson CC, Kelalis PP, Hoffman AD: Renal growth in small kidneys after ureteroneocystotomy. *J Urol* 1982;127:1146.
97. Sussman SK, Gallman WH, Cohan EH, et al: CT findings in xanthogranulomatous pyelonephritis with co-existent renocolic fisula. *J Comput Assist Tomogr* 1987;11:1088.
98. Chuang C-K, et al: Xanthogranulomatous pyelonephritis: experience in 36 cases. *J Urol* 1992;147:333.
99. Kierce F, Caroll R, Guiney EJ: Xanthogranulomatous pyelonephritis in childhood. *Br J Urol* 1985;57:261.
100. Petronic V, Buturovic J, Isvaneski M: Xanthogranulomatous pyelonephritis. *Br J Urol* 1989;64:336.
101. Goldman SM, Gatewood OMB: Inflammatory renal disease. *Prob Urol* 1989;3:607.
102. Malek RS, Elder JS: Xanthogranulomatous pyelonephritis: a critical analysis of 26 cases and of the literature. *J Urol* 1978;119:589.
103. Claes H, Vereecken R, Oyen R, Van Damme B: Xanthogranulomatous pyelonephritis with emphasis on computerized tomography scan. Retrospective study of 20 cases and literature review. *Urology* 1987;29:389.
104. Andriole VT, Patterson TF: Epidemiology, natural history, and management of urinary tract infections in pregnancy. *Med Clin North Am* 1991;75:359.
105. Williams SD, et al: The treatment of bacteriuria in pregnancy. In: O'Grady F, Brumfitt W, eds. *Urinary Tract Infection*. London: Oxford University Press, 1968.
106. Diokno AC, Compton A, Seski J, Vinson R: Urologic evaluation of urinary tract infection in pregnancy. *J Reprod Med* 1986;31:23.

13 Tuberculosis, Fungal Diseases, and Parasitic Diseases of the Urinary Tract

Durwood E. Neal, Jr., Eric Walser

FUNGAL, MYCOBACTERIAL, AND PARASITIC INFECTIONS

Until recently, fungal, mycobacterial, and parasitic infections remained somewhat uncommon. These infections occur sporadically, and few series could be generated in any one institution or region. A dramatic upswing has been seen in each of these infections in the last decade, however.[1,2] These infections not only are occurring more commonly in the genitourinary tract, but are found more frequently in other organ systems as well. The relative increase in the numbers of infected persons is undoubtedly due in part to the fact that there is an increase in the immunosuppressed population. Certainly these patients are far more susceptible to the unusual infections and they tend to be followed very closely from an overall medical perspective, leading to a possible increase in the reporting of these diseases. Despite the relative stabilization or decrease in the availability of organs for transplant, the absolute number of patients surviving long term with a transplanted organ is higher than ever. With improvement in immunosuppressive therapy and antirejection treatment, these patients and their organs are surviving longer. This has increased both the population at risk for unusual infections and the pool of patients in the general population with whom these infections tend to be associated.

Perhaps the fastest-growing at-risk population is that which is infected with the human immunodeficiency virus (HIV). It is estimated that there are approximately 300,000 new cases every year, and despite a great deal of public awareness and education, the numbers of infected patients continue to rise.[2] By the fact that there is a specific immunodeficiency in the T-cell population in this group, which is the hallmark of this disease, infections that are primarily handled by the cell-mediated immune system would be most affected. Each of these three disease entities is more common in patients who have cell-mediated immunity defects, because it is this component of the body's defense mechanism that must be intact to eradicate these pathogens.

By necessity, an increase in all these diseases has been seen along with the rise of immunocompromised individuals. Also, the therapy has greatly improved and the current antifungal, antimycobacterial, and antihelminthic drugs are better than ever. Diagnostic modalities such as serologic techniques and imaging studies have also progressed. Establishment of the diagnosis of these diseases within the urinary tract is problematic, and each carries its own set of caveats.

MYCOBACTERIAL INFECTIONS

Genitourinary tuberculosis (TB) has been a recognized entity for many years. The effects of this infection on the urinary tract are well understood and, until about 10 years ago, the incidence of infection was stable or decreasing.[1] In an age of immunosuppression, these infections are becoming more common and unfortunately more difficult to eradicate with the standard antituberculosis chemotherapeutic regimens. In addition to *Mycobacterium tuberculosis*, other species have been recognized as well. *M. avium-intracellulare* (MAI), *M. bovis*, and others are recognized more frequently now, especially in the patients with acquired immunodeficiency syndrome (AIDS).[3]

The pathogenesis involves an initial pulmonary infection that may or may not be clinically recognizable. Much less commonly, the organisms are spread by other means. After infection, there is hematogenous spread to the renal parenchyma. Unlike most other urinary tract infections, this is the primary mode of spread. Ascending infection is probably extremely rare. The organisms ultimately cause the development of caseating granulomas, which may be found in the renal parenchyma or anywhere along the urothelial tract. The granulomatous infectious process results in two forms of damage to the urinary system. First, the renal parenchyma may be destroyed by the enlarging granuloma (Fig. 13–1). Second, the infection may involve the urothelium, with the granulomas causing scarring and stricture formation with subsequent obstruction (Fig. 13–2). In the most severe cases, autonephrectomy occurs with diffuse renal calcification (Fig. 13–3).

DIAGNOSIS

Presentation is often associated with recurrent bacterial urinary tract infection (UTI).[4] A high index of suspension should occur in the patient with recurrent bacterial UTIs in

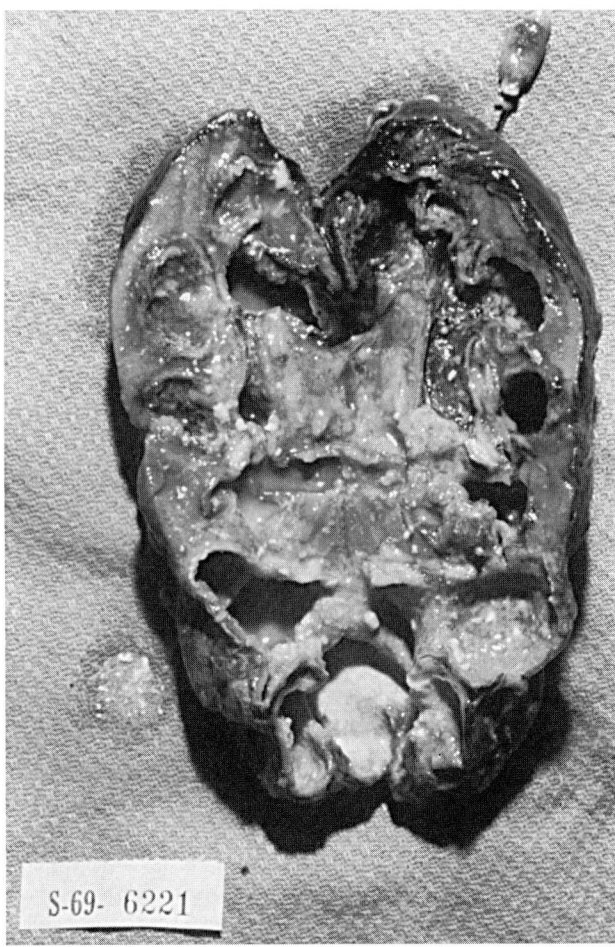

Figure 13–1. Renal parenchyma destroyed by tuberculous granulomata.

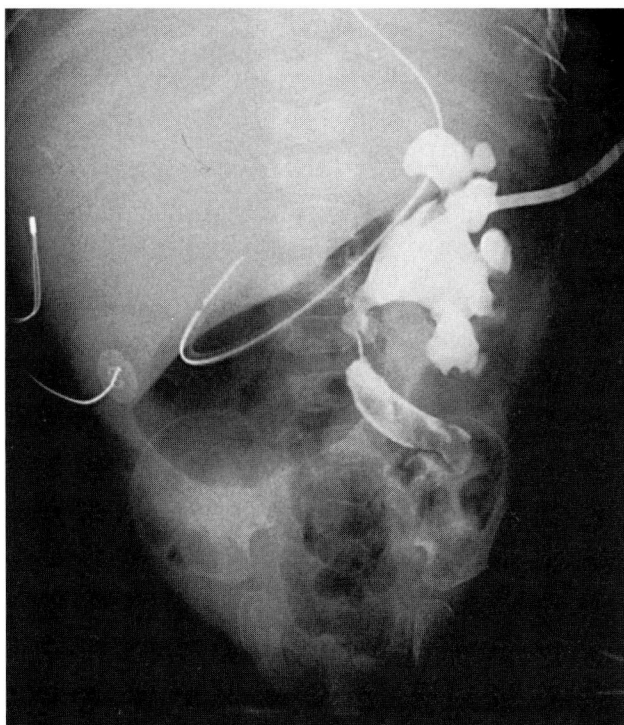

Figure 13–2. Nephrostogram showing multiple ureteral strictures in tuberculous prelonephritis.

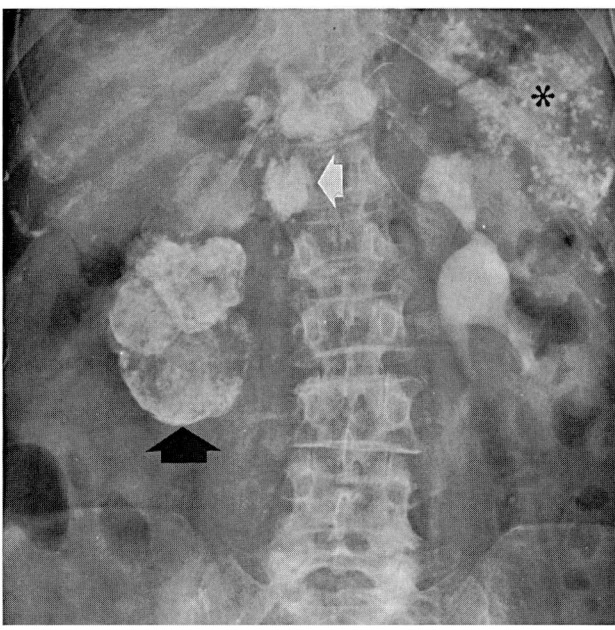

Figure 13–3. Autonephrectomy ("Putty" kidney) (black arrow) on right. Calcified lymph nodes and multiple splenic granulomas (asterisk) are also manifestations of tuberculosis.

whom other sources of infection cannot be demonstrated. Another hallmark of the diagnosis is culture-negative leukocyturia and persistent microscopic hematuria. In fact, in the setting of sterile pyuria, it is incumbent upon the physician to rule out the presence of mycobacterial infection. On occasion, patients will present with an indurated, tender testis and epididymis. One physical finding that may suggest this disease is an indurated, beaded vas deferens. Suspicion of mycobacterial infection should be high when this sign is present.

The diagnosis may be made by a number of methods; however, the most reliable is culture of the urine for mycobacteria.[4] Because these organisms are slow-growing and somewhat fastidious, patience is required with establishment of a culture-positive diagnosis. Most authors recommend at least three first morning urine specimens and others recommend as many as five. The first morning urine is best because the urine tends to be more concentrated and has a greater chance of containing the tubercle bacillus. It is common for the cultures to take from 4 to 8 weeks to grow. Special growth medium is typically used that has numerous enrichments to improve the isolation of these organisms. In the past, the urine or other body fluids were injected into guinea pigs to allow better growth of the organisms; however, this is no longer necessary.

Skin testing for cutaneous hypersensitivity with purified protein derivative (PPD) remains a valuable diagnostic tool. When used with the proper controls, such as mumps antigen, *Candida* antigen, *Trichophyton*, and others, the test may be very accurate. The change from a previously negative skin test to a positive should lead one to intensive investigation for the presence of tuberculosis. Often patients may be anergic to tuberculosis as well as the other skin test antigens. In this circumstance, it may be difficult to tell if a patient has been exposed to mycobacteria. Other diagnostic modalities such as urine, sputum cultures, and radiographs must be utilized in this instance.

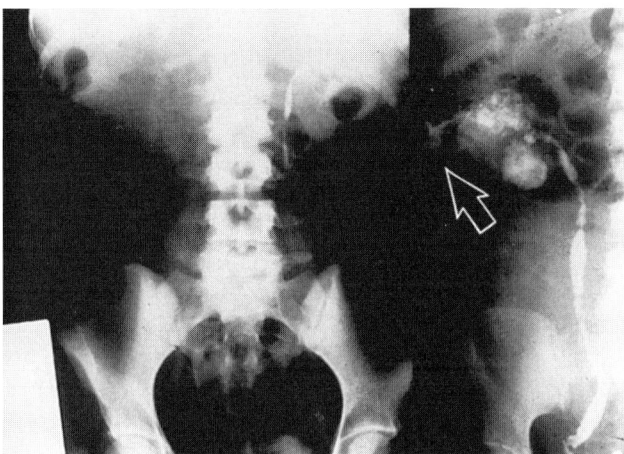

Figure 13–4. Intravenous pyelogram and retrograde pyelogram showing loss of function and perinephric extravasation (arrow). Multiple ureteric strictures are also present.

RADIOLOGY

The goals of modern imaging in renal TB are three. First, although "classic" renal TB has characteristic urographic findings, computerized axial tomographic scanning (CT) and ultrasonography (US) are frequently used in the initial evaluation of these patients. Accordingly, radiologists must be familiar with the cross-sectional appearance of renal TB. Second, current imaging techniques must detect the atypical appearance of renal TB as well as the manifestations of atypical TB (MAI) in the immunocompromised patient (ICP). The third goal of imaging is to provide radiologic guidance for biopsy and drainage procedures.

The urographic appearance of renal TB reflects the pathologic process of chronic granulomatous infection. Although TB involves the kidney after primary pulmonary infection, less than one-half of patients with renal TB have abnormal chest radiographs, and only 10% have clinical signs of active pulmonary TB.[5,6] After inhalation, the organisms hematogenously seed the periglomerular capillaries where cortical granulomatosus form and may stabilize for years, or even calcify. Upon reactivation, the infection spreads to the medulla. The ensuing papillitis can extend to the collecting system, causing destruction, stricture formation, and loss of function (Fig. 13–4). End-stage renal TB is autonephrectomy or "putty kidney," which is an atrophic, calcified, nonfunctioning renal remnant (Figs. 13–5 to 13–7). A single kidney is involved in more than 70% of patients.[7]

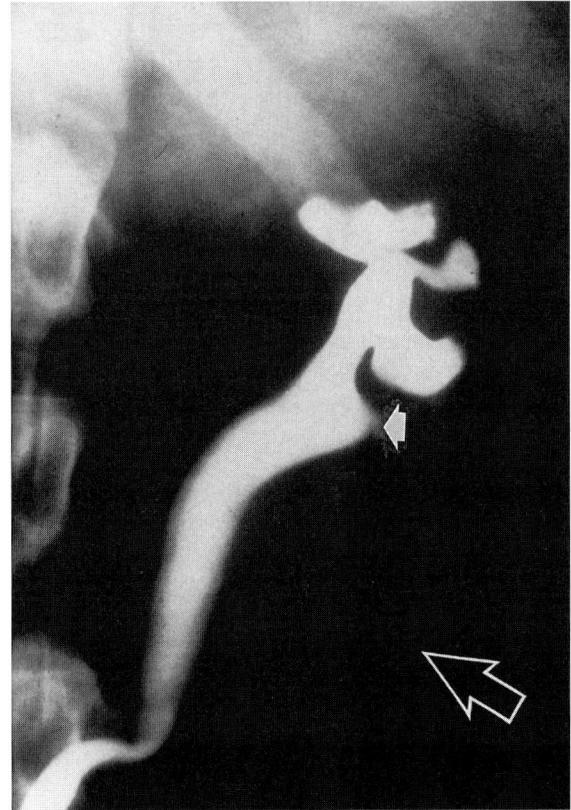
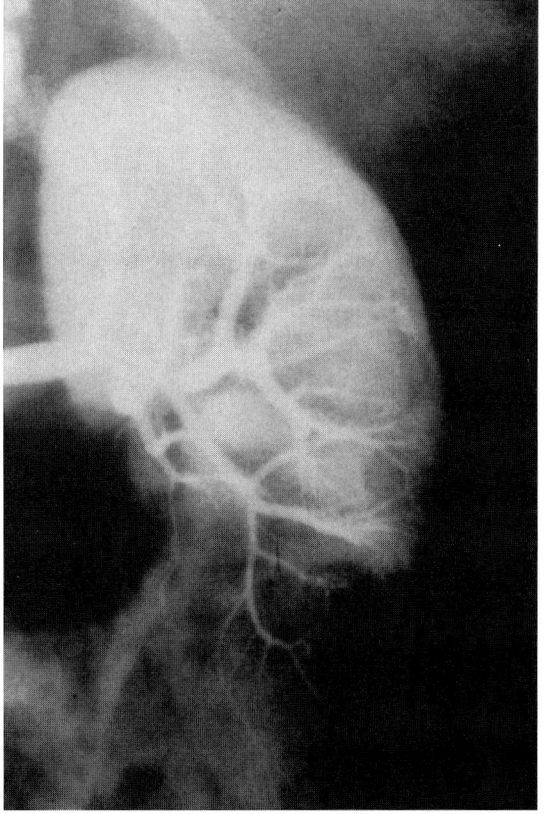

Figure 13–5. (**A**) Retrograde pyelogram showing loss of lower pole (open arrow) and amputated calyx (solid white arrow). (**B**) Arteriogram of same kidney with hypovascular lower pole.

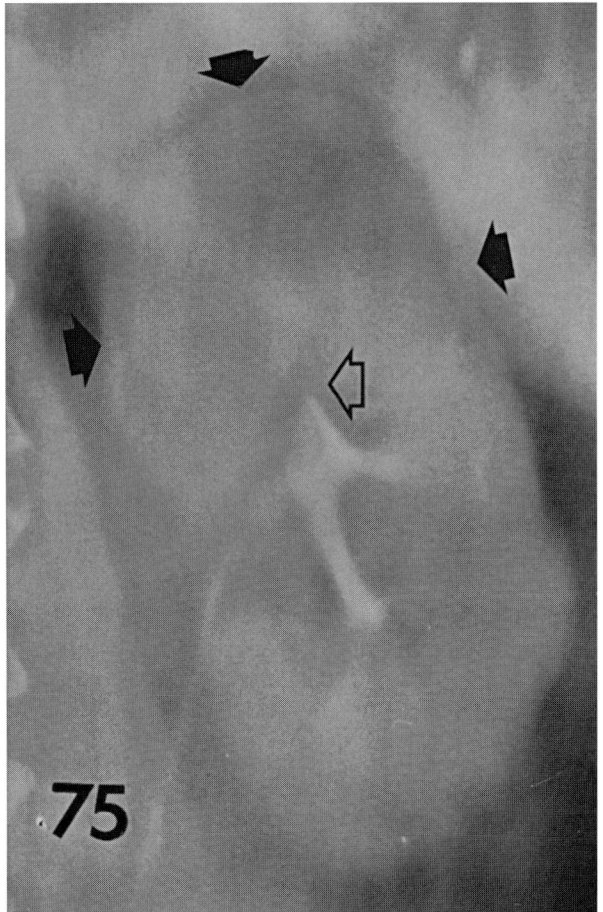

Figure 13-6. Typical amputated left upper pole calyx (open arrow) and granulomatous mass (black arrows) proximal to amputated calyx.

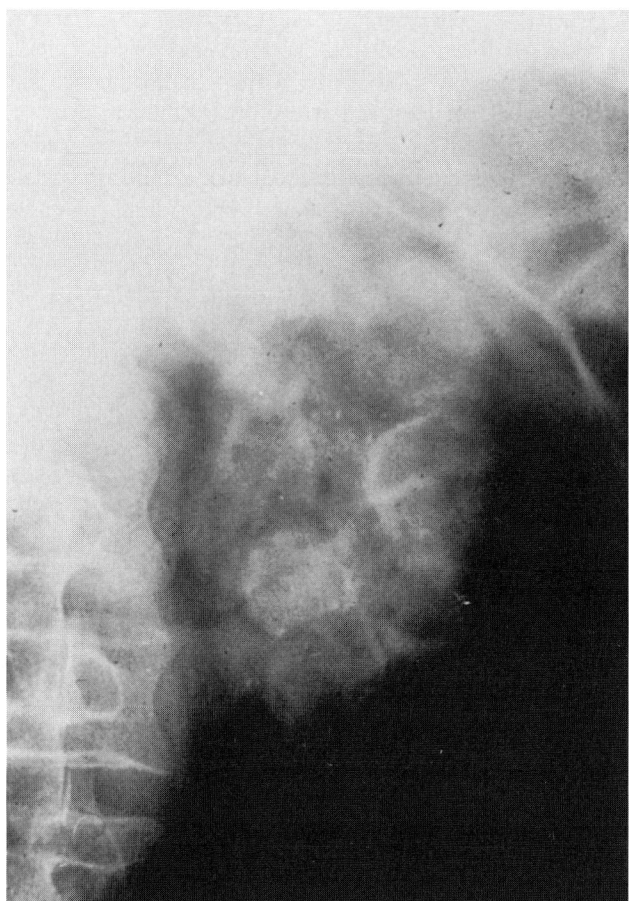

Figure 13-7. Lower pole tuberculous calcifications.

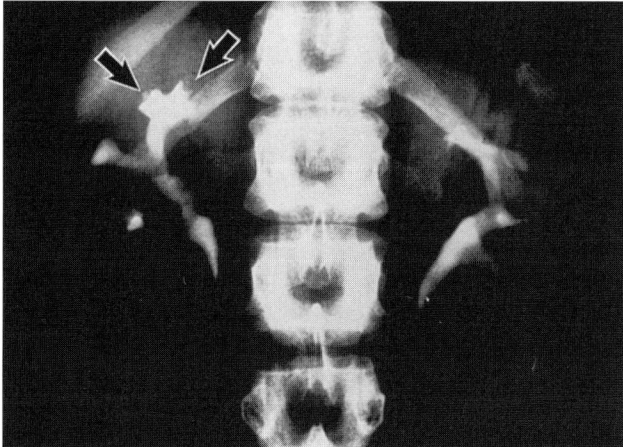

Figure 13-8. Papillitis (upper pole) forms early TB (arrows).

UROGRAPHY

The hallmark of renal TB infection is "destructive obstruction," referring to the processes of necrotizing papillitis and stricture formation. The earliest urographic finding in renal TB is "fuzzy" or irregular calyceal contours, which are consequences of papillitis (Fig. 13-8). However, approximately 15% of patients with renal TB have a normal excretory urogram.[6] The progressive papillitis leads to pericalyceal cavity formation. Strictures form in the infundibulum, pelvis, or ureter and can progress to obstruction of all or a segment of the kidney (Fig. 13-9). A characteristic finding in renal TB is the "phantom calyx," which is an obstructed, nonfunctioning calyx proximal to an infundibular stricture (see Figs. 13-5 and 13-6). Parenchymal inflammatory masses may develop, especially in these obstructed systems, and eventually calcify. Chemotherapy may halt active inflammation and salvage renal function. However, scarring usually continues despite adequate pharmacologic therapy; subsequently, cortical scars, calyceal clubbing, and ureteral strictures may develop (Fig. 13-10). Patients undergoing treatment for renal TB must be monitored frequently for signs of renal obstruction. Ureteral or ureteropelvic junction strictures must be stented or a nephrostomy tube placed to prevent obstructive damage to the remaining renal tissue.

Early signs of ureteral TB include dilation, ulceration, and mucosal irregularity.[5] Ureteral calcification in TB is uncommon and occurs late in the disease. Late ureteral TB presents with strictures and ureteral shortening. The typical urographic image is multiple strictures in the distal ureter, which

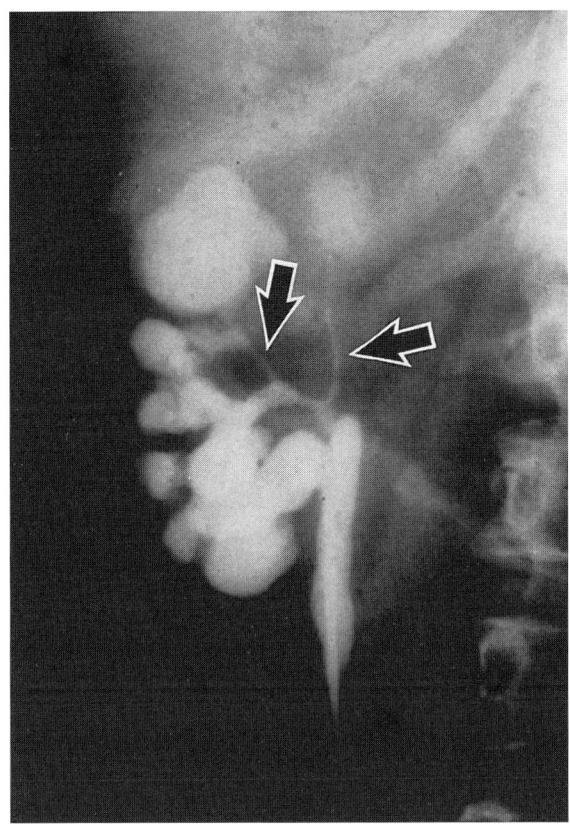

Figure 13–9. Upper pole infundibular strictures secondary to TB (arrows).

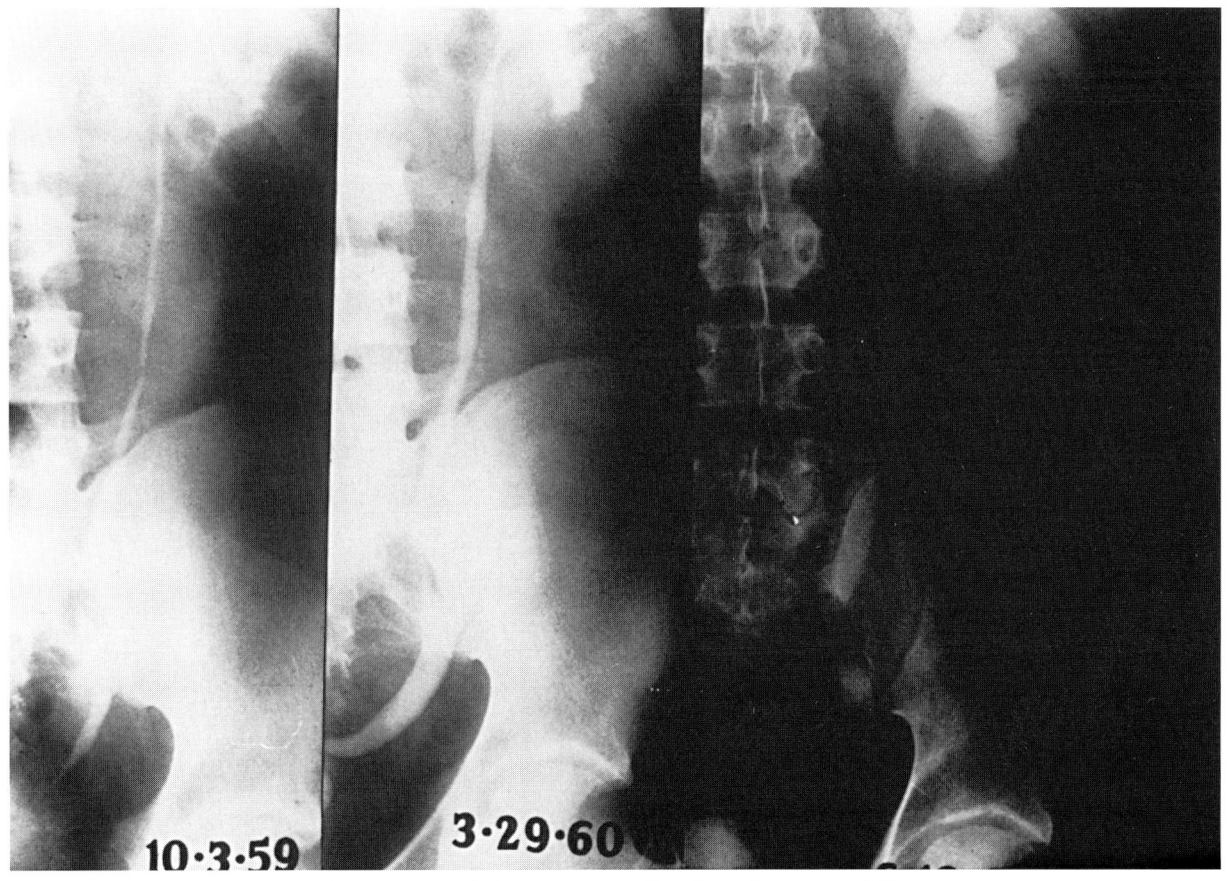

Figure 13–10. Gradual obstruction over time from distal ureteral TB stricture.

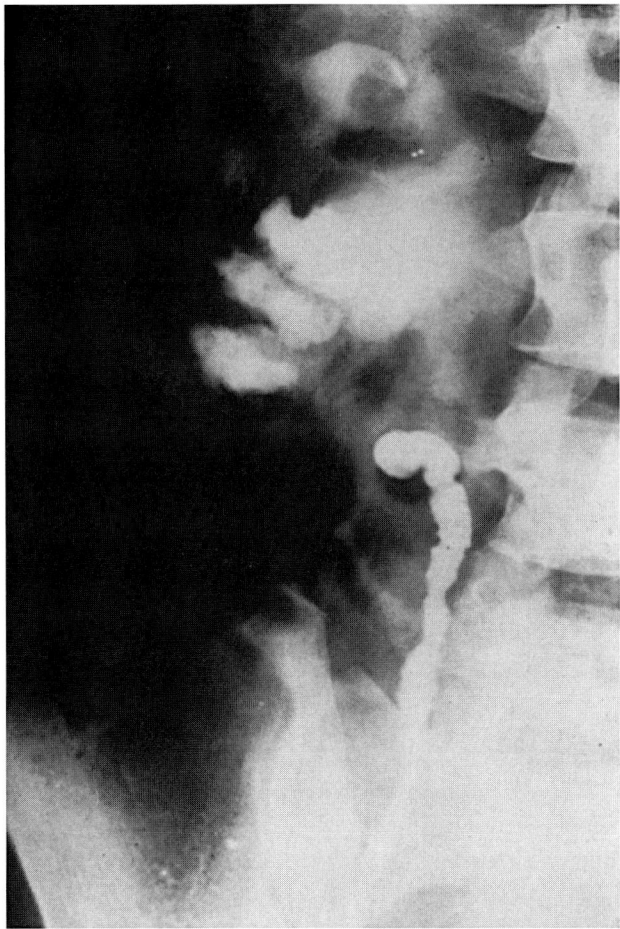

Figure 13–11. Beaded ureter from TB.

appears beaded and tortuous because of fibrotic contractions (Fig. 13–11). Later in the disease, a diffusely stenotic, shortened ureter develops ("pipestem ureter"), which is usually coexistent with advanced ipsilateral renal damage (Fig. 13–12). Extremely dilated ureters with mural calcification confined to the distal portion are usually found as a consequence of schistosomiasis, not TB, although progressive renal calcification occurs (Fig. 13–13).

Bladder TB involvement mirrors ureteral infection with progressive irregular contraction. Diverticula or inflammatory masses may develop in the distorted shrunken bladder. As the ureters and bladder become fibrotic, vesicoureteral reflex can occur, causing further damage to the kidneys. Calcification of the bladder wall rarely occurs, but it differs from schistosomal calcification in that it is usually more coarse and patchy.

CT/US FINDINGS

Ultrasound is relatively insensitive in distinguishing renal TB from other lesions. Because isoechoic inflammatory masses and calcification are poorly seen, renal function cannot be properly evaluated (Fig. 13–14). Ultrasound is most useful in monitoring patients undergoing treatment for renal TB, because frequent screening for obstructive complications (i.e., hydronephrosis) can be performed without radiation or intravenous contrast administration. CT effectively images renal TB and is a better modality than excretory urography for several reasons. CT is more sensitive for identifying calcifications and demonstrates nonfunctioning renal tissue (Fig. 13–15). In addition, perinephric extension of TB, as well as involvement of other organs (e.g., Potts disease), is best visualized by CT. Typical CT findings in renal TB are caliectasis and focal cortical scarring (>80%). Calcification is seen in 37 to 71% of cases. Low-density parenchymal inflammatory masses are present in 37% of patients with tuberculosis pyelonephritis (Fig. 13–16).[8,9]

Regardless of the imaging modality, the diagnosis of renal tuberculosis hinges on the recognition of the characteristic association of destruction and obstruction—namely, necrosis/calcification and strictures, all resulting in the loss of functioning renal tissue (Fig. 13–17).

In the immunocompromised patient, abdominal mycobacterial infections probably originate in mesenteric lymph nodes after invasion of the small bowel mucosa. Bulky, mesenteric adenopathy with extensive central necrosis is identified on CT images.[9] Enlarged lymph nodes with central areas of low density are suggestive of TB or other mycobacterial infection, because Kaposi's sarcoma or AIDS-related lymphoma rarely demonstrates central necrosis. Visceral involvement follows mesenteric TB and appears as hepatic, splenic, and renal microabscesses, which may calcify. Calcified visceral abscesses may also be seen in disseminated CMV or *Pneumocystis* infections.[10] Needle biopsy and cultures can identify the offending organisms. On fine-needle aspiration, mycobacterial infections yield macrophages filled with AFB. Granulomas are not seen in aspirates from ICPs (immunocompromised individuals) because of immunosuppression.

PHARMACOTHERAPY

The most common of the antituberculosis drugs in use today is isoniazid, in combination with ethambutol, streptomycin, pyrazinamide, and rifampicin. For many years the treatment of this disease required long-term therapy with combinations of antimicrobials. This has changed in the last few years because of the efficacy of a short-course regimen.[11] J. G. Gow has demonstrated the effectiveness of short-course chemotherapy with a variety of combinations.[12] This has been fortuitous, in that one of the primary concerns with therapy has been compliance. He recommends a treatment course of pyrazinamide, isoniazid, and rifampicin for 2 months followed by a 2-month course of isoniazid and rifampicin. All these drugs are highly excreted in the urine and have been demonstrated to penetrate into renal parenchyma and tuberculosis cavities with great efficacy. The regimen uses pyrazinamide at 25 mg/kg body weight per day (with a maximum of 2 g). Isoniazid is given at 300 mg daily and rifampicin at 450 mg daily. The latter two drugs are

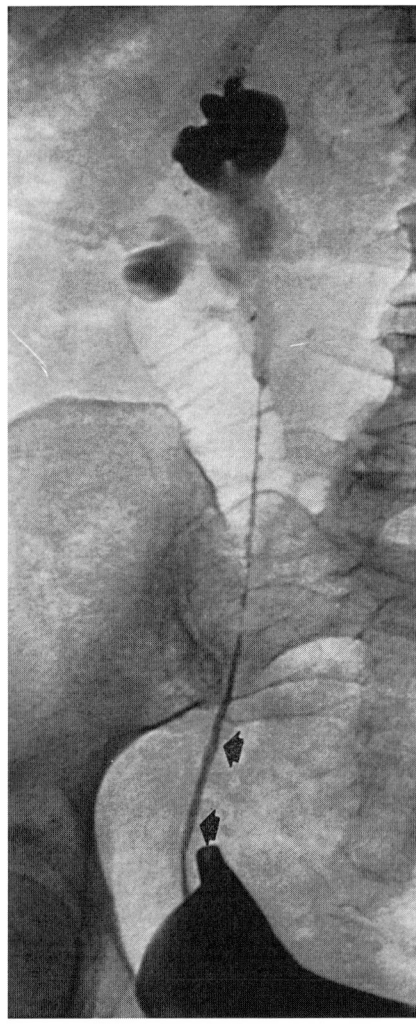
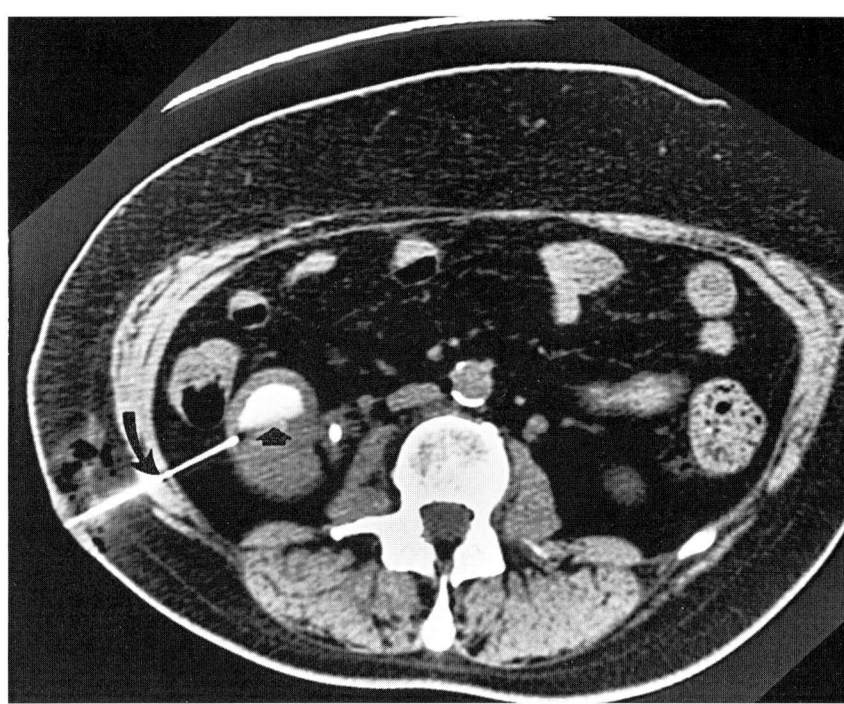

Figure 13–12. (A) Distal "pipestem" ureter (arrows). More proximally, the ureter is narrowed and beaded. (B) Diagnosis of TB in this patient was made from CT-guided needle (curved arrow) aspiration of a cavitary lesion (arrow).

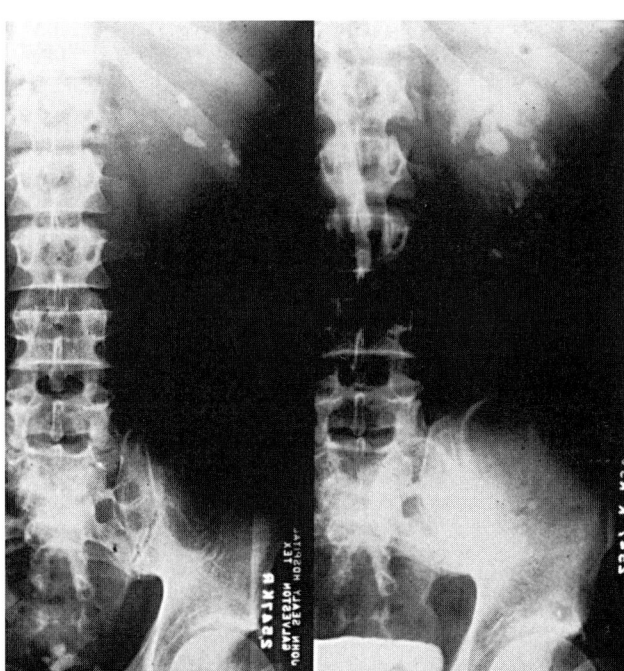

Figure 13–13. Progressive renal TB calcification.

given as a single dose to prevent subtherapeutic levels occurring in the tissues and serum. After the first 2 months, isoniazid is given at 600 mg as a single dose three times a week with rifampicin at 900 mg per dose three times per week. At the end of this 4 months of therapy, most patients will be cured of their infection. He also comments that streptomycin should be used for symptomatic relief, especially if there is a dominant component of tuberculous cystitis with the attendant severe voiding symptomatology.

Other drugs have been used as well for the management of these patients. When there is stricture formation or other scar tissue within the urinary tract, steroids may have some benefit.[12] Also, in cases of acute tuberculous cystitis, patients may obtain symptomatic relief with a short course of prednisone. Additionally, patients have been treated locally with isoniazid and rifampicin as an intravesical installation for the treatment of severe cystitis. If necessary, the renal pelvis may be irrigated through a percutaneous nephrostomy tube for local treatment. These should perhaps be reserved for the most severe cases or in circumstances where oral drugs are difficult to administer secondary to toxicity. Certainly if toxicity or hypersensitivity occurs to any of the drugs that are

292　Diagnosis of Genitourinary Disease

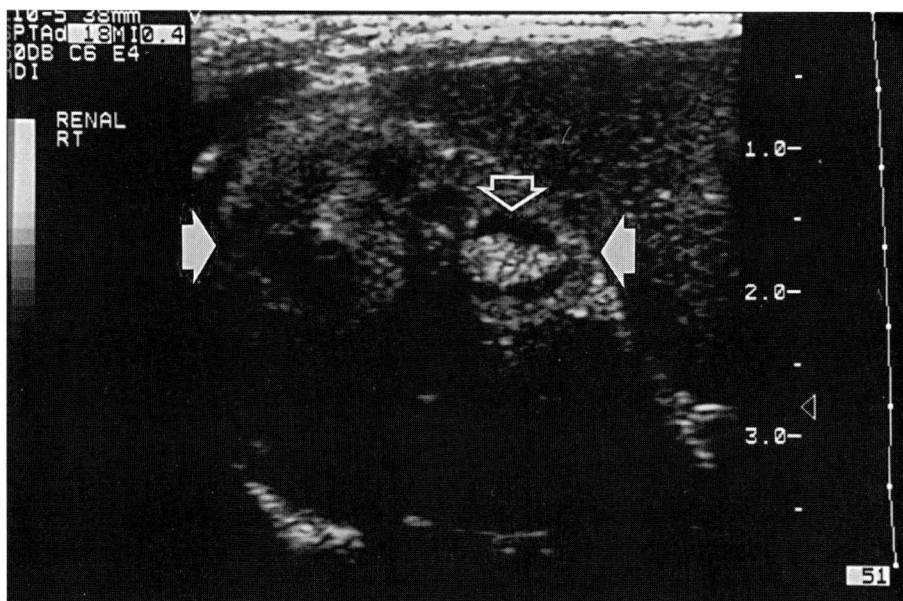

Figure 13–14. Ultrasound showing progressive destruction of the right kidney (white arrow) with cavity formation (open white arrow).

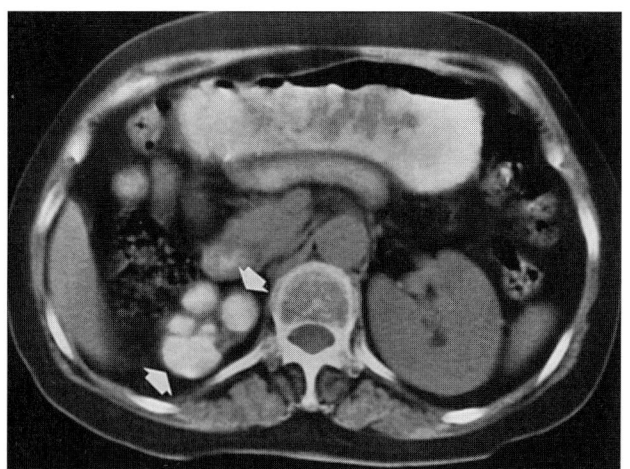

Figure 13–15. Nonfunctioning calcified kidney (arrows).

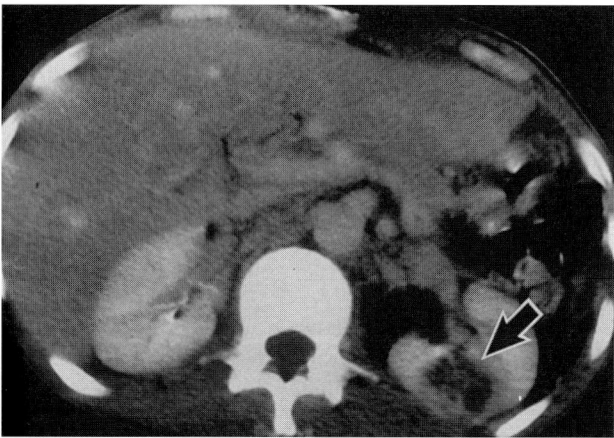

Figure 13–16. Parenchymal tuberculous inflammatory mass (arrow).

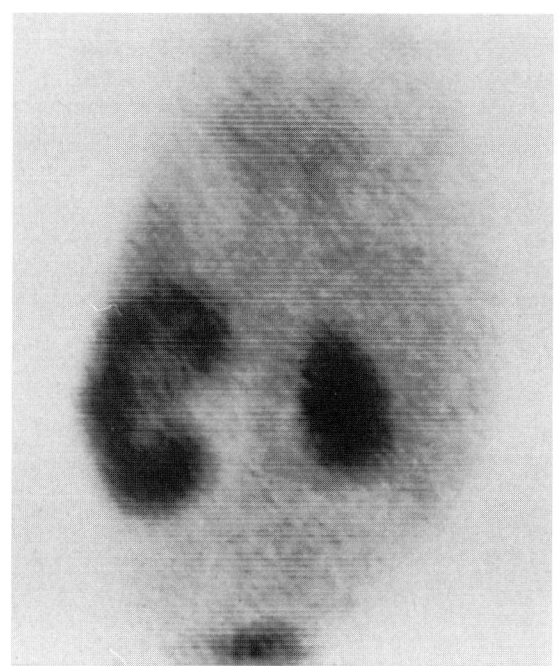

Figure 13–17. Nuclear scan showing decrease in renal function on the right.

administered in the recommended regimen, drugs such as cycloserine, ethionamide, and others may be used as substitutes. In more recent times, these organisms have become more and more resistant to traditional antituberculosis chemotherapy.[13–16] It has been shown that the fluoroquinolones, specifically ciprofloxacin and others, in high doses may exert an antimycobacterial effect as well.[17–19] The newest-generation macrolide, clarithromycin, has also shown efficacy and is considered by some to be the treatment of choice for an atypical mycobacteria.[20] This particular regimen, however, awaits approval from the Food and Drug Administration.

Overall, approximately 10% of all tuberculosis cases are infected with drug-resistant organisms, exhibiting resistance to either isoniazid, rifampicin, or both.[16] The incidence of resistance to both drugs is approximately 3.5%. It is for this reason that new drugs are constantly being tested against mycobacteria, and when these standard drugs are employed, three or four drug combinations are highly recommended.

INTERVENTIONAL RADIOLOGY

Although the radiographic findings in renal TB are usually characteristic, needle-aspiration biopsy is occasionally useful to clarify indeterminate renal masses, particularly in the ICP, because multifocal lymphoma can simulate visceral infections. In addition, needle-aspiration biopsy and culture can differentiate calcified renal cell carcinomas from tuberculosis and other inflammatory masses. The different diagnoses of renal TB include congenital multicystic kidney disease, renal papillary necrosis, pyogenic abscess, and calyceal diverticulum. Radiographically, brucellosis often resembles renal TB.

Percutaneous nephrostomy and renal pressure-flow testing (Whittaker) can be used to diagnose and treat patients who develop uretheral strictures. Metallic ureteral stents (spirals) could be used in these instances, although they are a new modality and little experience with them has been reported. Perinephric or psoas abscesses respond well to percutaneous catheter drainage, similar to those caused by the usual uropathogens.

SURGERY

Nephrectomy is indicated in only the worst cases of tuberculous nephritis. The most obvious reason for ablative surgery is nonfunction along with chronic infection. A relative indication includes extensive disease that is not amenable to surgical correction. The most common operative reconstruction is in the ureter. The ureterovesical junction is the most commonly involved segment; however, strictures at the ureteropelvic junction and at the middle and lower third of the ureter also occur. The strictures more commonly occur during the course of therapy as the granulomas begin to heal, causing fibrosis and calcifications. Most authors recommend treatment with corticosteroids during chemotherapy to reduce the degree of stricture formation. After 4 to 8 weeks of this type of pharmacotherapy, surgical correction is indicated if there is no improvement. Other surgical alternatives include dilation of the ureter, ureteral reimplantation, ureteroureterostomy, and others. For those patients who have extreme cystitis symptoms after therapy as a result of a contracted, severely damaged bladder, augmentation cystoplasty or supravesical diversion may be indicated with a continent pouch or ileal conduit.

In the future, with technology advancing rapidly, there certainly will be antituberculous chemotherapy. In addition, with the elimination of some of the immunosuppressive diseases with vaccines and other treatments, the population at risk will be reduced. Finally, there has been an increased interest in vaccinations against tuberculosis. Worldwide, Bacille Calmette Guerin (BCG) has been used as an antituberculosis vaccine. Numerous published reports discuss its efficacy for the prevention of tuberculosis.[21-24] It has been available throughout the world since 1921, and approximately 3 billion people have been vaccinated with it.[25] A recent article in the *Journal of the American Medical Association* analyzed all the prospective and case-controlled trials in the literature and found that the BCG vaccine reduced the risk of tuberculosis overall by approximately one-half.[25] Furthermore, there was even greater protection against tuberculous meningitis, disseminated tuberculosis, and disease-related death. Clearly, an evaluation of BCG vaccination in the United States needs to be considered with the increase in numbers of cases and the increasing difficulty with treatment. One must also consider compliance with therapy when deciding on a vaccination program because even the short-course regimens are 4 months in duration.

FUNGAL DISEASES

Numerous fungal organisms commonly inhabit the genitourinary tract. These organisms are frequently isolated as commensals or saprophytes and may not cause disease. In certain individuals, however, many yeasts and other fungi may cause invasive disease. This is far more common in the immunosuppressed population, but it can occur in any patient with a debilitating condition or even in normal, healthy people.

Almost all hospitalized patients are at risk of developing a fungal infection involving some organ system. The urinary tract is somewhat less commonly involved than the gastrointestinal or integumentary system; however, genitourinary fungal infections are still rather common.

The most common fungal organism to be isolated from the urinary tract is *Candida albicans*.[26] This organism is isolated with great regularity from the urine of patients who are catheterized, on antibiotic therapy, or both. In addition, central venous catheters are a significant risk factor. In these scenarios, selective pressure is given to the growth of *Candida*, which may be present as a commensal organism on the urethral meatus, in the groin, or in the perineal/vaginal area. With destruction of the normal flora by the action of antibacterials, overgrowth with these organisms is commonly seen. It is in these that the differentiation between colonization and invasive disease becomes difficult to distinguish. In the case of the former, discontinuation of the antibiotics and/or removal of the urinary tract foreign body (e.g., urethral catheter) may be all that is necessary to allow natural defense mechanisms to eradicate the organism. In the case of a true infection, potentially highly toxic medications may be needed to eliminate the disease. As the fungi grow, they develop fungal accretions in which the organisms live, multiply, and are protected against not only the body defense mechanisms but also antimicrobial chemotherapy.[27]

Numerous other fungal organisms have also been isolated from the urinary tract. A variety of other molds and yeasts may be found in the kidneys, bladder, or prostate, but they typically have a different point of origin—namely, the lungs. *Histoplasma capsulatum*, *Coccidioides immitis*, *Blastomyces dermatitidis*, and *Cryptococcus neoformans* have all been isolated from the urinary tract. The most clinically significant disease in each of these cases is usually not in the urinary system, because most of these diseases are far more severe and life-threatening as pulmonary or meningeal infections. Interestingly, the urinary system may often offer a safe haven for these organisms, where they lie relatively protected from antifungal chemotherapy.[28] On occasion the systemic disease caused by any of these agents may initially manifest itself to the patient and physician with genitourinary complaints. This, however, is undoubtedly the exception and not the rule. A few other fungal organisms have been sporadically isolated from the urine, including *Aspergillus* species, *Sporothrix*, *Mucor*, and others. These occur almost exclusively in immunosuppressed individuals, but when they are detected, the disease is usually life-threatening and difficult to treat.

These organisms often present as a result of their primary infection and may be incidentally isolated from the urinary tract. In the case of *Candida*, the urinary tract is often the primary source of the infectious process, and the symptoms are those of cystitis or pyelonephritis, with dysuria, frequency, urgency, and suprapubic pain, along with fever, chills, and flank pain, in the cases of upper tract infection. For patients with systemic fungal disease, urinalysis, along with a urinary fungal culture to determine the extent of the infection, should be routine. Conversely, for patients who have *Candida* or other yeasts isolated from their urine, investigation with blood cultures and other tests may be necessary to ascertain whether systemic disease exists. The presence of greater than 10,000 colonies per milliliter of urine should be considered significant, especially in the patient population that is at risk. The difficulty has often been that one cannot differentiate between a diagnosis of upper tract versus lower tract *Candida* infection. Systemic signs and symptoms are a fairly reliable indicator; however, they are not always present. Colony counts have been used, but they are generally inadequate. When patients have less than 10,000 colonies per milliliter, there may be a systemic infection, whereas patients with greater than 100,000 colonies per milliliter may only be colonized. Several investigators have used serologic studies to measure candidal antigens; however, the results may be variable and difficult to interpret.[26,29,30] *Candida* enolase, an enzyme unique to this yeast, has been investigated as being a marker of systemic disease, but it has not been found to be 100% sensitive.[31]

The treatment for either local or systemic infection is certainly very different and ranges from no treatment to toxic systemic therapy. With the addition of fluconazole, an imidazole that is highly excreted in the urine, this distinction has become less important.[32] Prior to this drug's availability, bladder infection was treated effectively with local amphotericin B irrigation. Because the only systemic agent for candiduria was amphotericin B, it was not often administered unless there was convincing evidence of systemic or upper tract infection. Again, it must be remembered that *Candida* in the urine could merely be colonizing the bladder and not actually infecting it; thus the elimination of risk factors may resolve the condition.

RADIOLOGY

In the immunocompromised or debilitated patient, urinary tract fungal colonization can lead to disseminated disease with visceral microabscess formation and high morbidity. This situation contrasts with immunocompetent individuals who can harbor urinary fungi without systemic involvement. Urinary involvement may be due to systemic disease and hematogenous seeding, although ascending infection from the bladder can occur. The acute form of candidal pyelonephritis causes renal enlargement, results in microabscess formation, and is radiographically similar to acute pyelonephritis with a delayed, irregular nephrogram on IVP or CT (Fig. 13–18).[33] Small abscesses can extend into the peri-

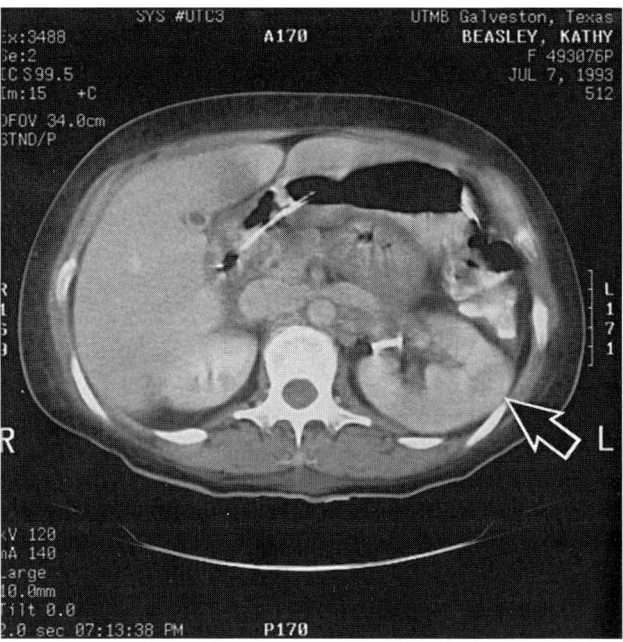

Figure 13–18. Parenchymal abscess due to *Torulopsis glabrata* (arrow).

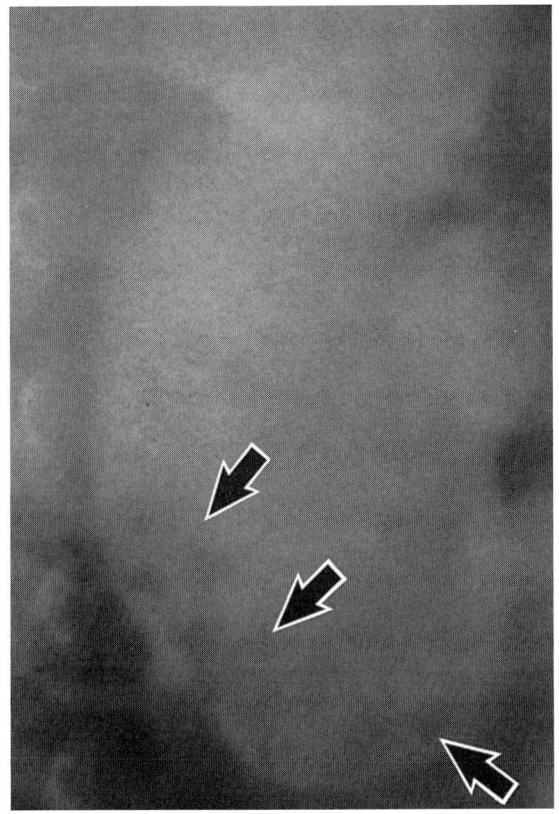

Figure 13–19. Multiple fungus balls in renal pelvis (arrows).

nephric space if the infection remains untreated. Chronic candidal infections resemble chronic pyelonephritis with cortical scarring and calyceal clubbing, which may be visualized on US, CT or IVP.[34] Papillary necrosis can occur, especially in premature infants and diabetics.[35] Of diagnostic importance is the formation of fungal accretions ("fungus ball") in chronic *Candida* infections.[27] A fungus ball, composed of mycelia and necrotic debris, produces a filling defect at urography, which conforms to the renal pelvis and calyces, although it may have an irregular, shaggy border (Figs. 13–19, 13–20). Because *Candida albicans* is gas-forming, CT or plain films show a bladder or renal pelvic mass containing a lacy network of air lucencies—a pathognomonic finding.[36] *Torulopsis glabrata* urinary infections are less common but produce similar radiographic findings, except that they do not form pseudohyphae and therefore do not make fungus balls. Renal involvement may occur with disseminated *Coccidioides* and other fungi, which radiographically resemble TB, although the ureter is infrequently affected.[37]

Treatment

PHARMACOTHERAPY

As was mentioned, no pharmacotherapy may be necessary for patients with localized candidiasis of the bladder except discontinuation of drugs causing selective pressure (e.g., antibiotics) or removal of the intravesical foreign body (e.g., Foley catheter). Localized bladder irrigation is undertaken with amphotericin B in a dosage of 50 mg/L of distilled water, per day. Some clinicians have also used miconazole in a dosage of 50 mg/L of saline per day. Most of these are

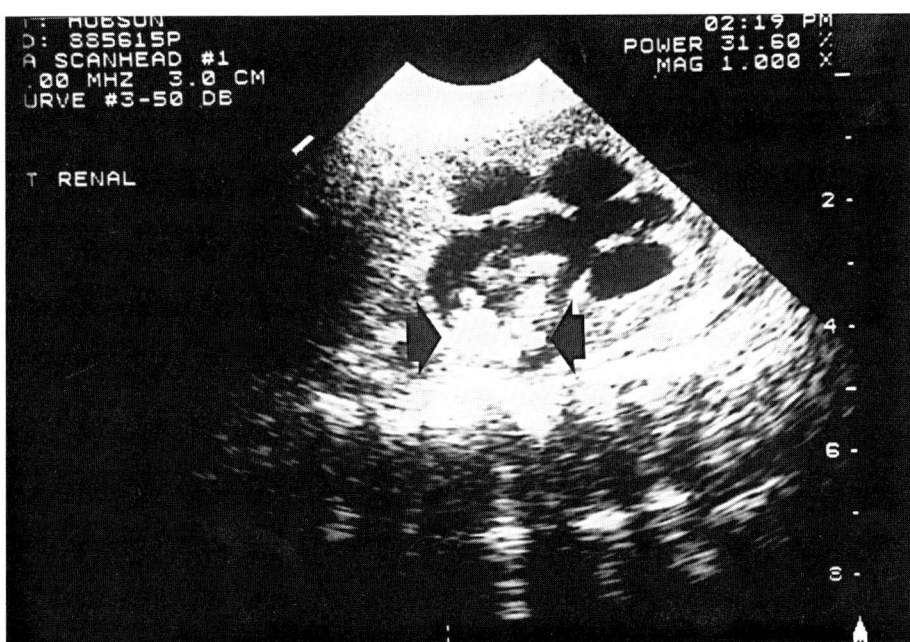

Figure 13–20. Ultrasound showing fungus (arrows) ball in renal pelvis of hydronephrotic kidney. The absence of distal shadowing in a lesion this large excludes calculi as the etiology.

continued for 7 days, and the treatment may be repeated. Oral fluconazole is also efficacious for treating this condition. With this agent's long half-life, it can be given once a day as 100 or 200 mg.

Systemic infection is usually treated with amphotericin B. This drug is given intravenously for a total dose of approximately 1 g over several days, with a total dosage of 6 mg/kg of body weight. Most clinicians do not give more than a total dose of a gram.[26] Fluconazole has also been used both intravenously and orally for the treatment of both localized and systemic infection. It has a special advantage in the urinary tract, because the drug is excreted approximately 90% unchanged in the urine.[34] In addition, excellent tissue levels are achieved, and the drug is well absorbed via the oral route, with few side effects. Flucytosine has also been used to treat candiduria. It is usually given in a dosage of 50 to 200 mg/kg per cay for several weeks.[26] This drug has the unwanted side effect of bone marrow toxicity when given over a long period of time. In addition, drug resistance to this agent occurs fairly rapidly, which limits its long-term usage. The dosage must be reduced when renal failure is present. Ketoconazole and miconazole have also been used for systemic candidiasis, but their excretion in the urine is relatively low; therefore, they have not been as efficacious. In any case, amphotericin B still remains the gold standard against which all other treatment regimens must be compared.

INTERVENTIONAL RADIOLOGY

To reduce systemic toxicity, renal fungal accretions are often treated with topical therapy through ureteral catheters. Alternatively, if the fungus ball obstructs the ureter, percutaneous nephrostomy can be performed for antegrade administration of antifungal drugs. In addition, the fungus burden can be reduced by percutaneous extraction of the fungal ball.[38] The access is obtained in the usual fashion and extraction is accomplished in a manner similar to percutaneous nephrostolithotomy, using a stone basket, grasping forceps, or the ultrasound probe with aspirator capability.

Surgery is rarely indicated for these diseases except as mentioned in the previous section. Occasionally, nephrectomy may be necessary if renal function is poor by isotope renal scan, but open surgical drainage is rarely, if ever, indicated. Surgical correction of any underlying anatomic defects is definitely indicated, especially those that cause stasis and obstruction.

Accessory Gland Infection

Prostate infections may be difficult to treat because amphotericin B does not achieve adequate therapeutic levels in the prostate gland.[39] Consequently, prostatic abscesses caused by such agents as *Candida albicans*, *Histoplasma capsulata*, and *Cryptococcosis neoformans* have been difficult to treat.[28] These can also spread to the ejaculatory ducts and ultimately to the epididymis, causing granulomatous disease and epidymal abscesses. A new drug, itraconazole, has been utilized for treatment of numerous fungal infections, and it has the theoretical benefit of a high lipid solubility and therefore may concentrate more in the prostate gland.[40,41] Little urologic information is available on this drug; however, its spectrum of action is greater than the other imidazoles and may be beneficial for the long-term therapy of some of the unusual fungal infections.

Localized infection to the genitalia and glans penis is usually adequately treated with local agents. Establishment of the diagnosis is critical in these incidences, especially in patients who are immunosuppressed, because local manifestations may indicate systemic disease. Miconazole, clotrimazole, ketoconazole, amphotericin B, and others are available topically and have shown efficacy in the treatment of cutaneous mycoses when no underlying systemic infection exists.

PARASITIC DISEASES

Schistosomiasis

Schistosomes are by far the most common urinary parasites.[42] It is estimated that they infect 200 million people in the world, primarily in Africa and the Middle East. In all, approximately 75 countries throughout the world are reservoirs for schistosomiasis.[43] Of all the species of *Schistosoma*, the genus, *hematobium* has the only predilection for the urinary tract. It is estimated that there are 400,000 cases in the United States currently, and this may be due to an increase in tourists and other visitors from endemic areas.[42,23] In terms of world health consequences, schistosomiasis is the most common cause of hematuria worldwide; without a doubt it causes more genitourinary tract pathology than any other microorganism.[42-44]

As may be inferred, schistosomiasis is more prevalent in areas where there are limited sanitary conditions. Agricultural economies have all shown an increase in the incidence of this disease. The organism's natural host is the *Bulinus* species of snail, and they tend to live and multiply in areas of stagnant water that result from irrigation of crops. In East Africa, wherever there is large usage of irrigation and damming of rivers, more cases of schistosomiasis are seen. Perhaps the most obvious increased prevalence occurred in Egypt after the construction of the Aswan dam in 1970. This had been preceded by a decrease in the prevalence of the disease.[45]

This parasite originates with the snail. Sporocysts are formed in the snail after it is infected with the aquatic miracidium, formed from the egg. Ultimately, it is excreted as cercaria, which are free-swimming ineffective larvae. They infect humans by penetrating the skin, at which time the tail and glycocalyx of the free-swimming stage is lost. The organism penetrates into the circulation and matures in the hepatic venous system. The female lives inside the male;

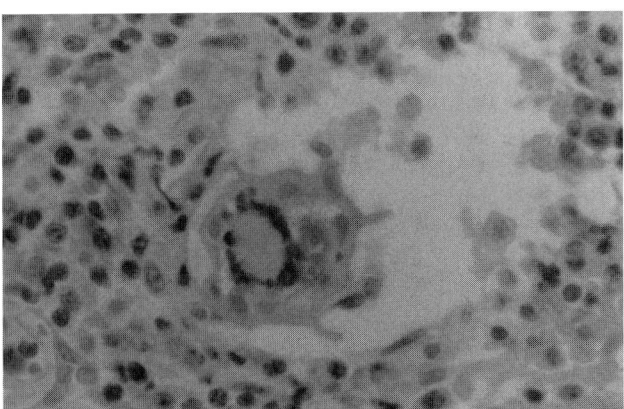

Figure 13–21. Granuloma and inflammation due to schistosomiasis.

when it is mature, the female is deposited in the pelvic venules, where it can lay up to 3000 eggs a day, for as long as 10 years. These ova, having been deposited in the tiny venules, may migrate through the endothelium, into the perivascular tissues, and through other tissue planes; ultimately, they may be excreted in the urine or other body fluids. Most notably, the migration into the bladder causes excretion of egg clusters, which may be identified in the urine.[44,45] The mechanism by which this occurs is still under investigation. The mature adult is seen within men, and these worms may be identified in the blood vessels and other tissues. After the eggs are excreted in waste matter, they develop into the miracidium form in water, which ultimately penetrates into the snail again.

Granuloma formation takes place in the tissues where the worms deposit ova (Fig. 13–21).[45] This results from an intense, cell-mediated immune response to *Schistosoma* antigens. Some of the eggs are destroyed by this inflammatory process, and their by-products and other eggs typically calcify, which gives the characteristic picture radiographically (Fig. 13–22).[44]

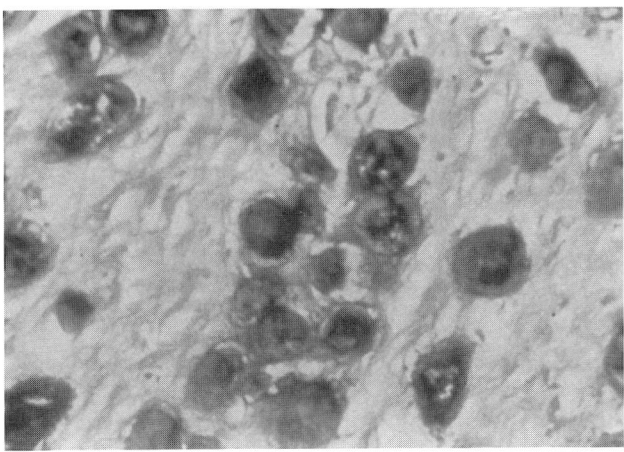

Figure 13–22. Calcified ova in tissue.

SYMPTOMS AND SIGNS

Where the cercaria enter the skin, there is a macular rash, which is referred to as "swimmer's itch" because of the fact that it is common to find it among people who have been swimming in infected water.[44] This pruritic rash lasts approximately 3 days. In patients who have had multiple exposures, immediate-type hypersensitivity reactions can be seen. There is usually a 4- to 6-week period after this time, which allows the schistosome to mature and form adult worms. The onset of egg production usually brings on the diffuse symptom complex associated with the disease. Most patients exhibit fever, nausea, vomiting, and a variety of voiding complaints. The most notable of these include hematuria, dysuria, and diffuse irritative voiding symptoms, all of which are nonspecific.[46] The physical examination will normally reveal hepatosplenomegaly, lymphadenopathy, and more important, dependent lymphedema, resulting from obstruction of the small veins and ultimately the lymphatics, because of invading ova. When the organism is located within a venule, the blood vessel typically collapses around it, effectively eliminating circulation. Laboratory studies usually show anemia with eosinophilia. Other elements of chronic infection, such as abnormal liver function tests, decreased lymphocyte count, hypoalbuminemia, and other findings may be noted. Elevations in the erythrocyte sedimentation rate and C-reactive protein will be seen as well.[44]

Most patients will have antibodies against the ova, but they may not always be detected, especially in patients who have become anergic. Because a positive serology is both sensitive and specific, it is helpful; however, these levels may remain high even after eradication of the organism. Because antibody levels may be too low to detect early in the infection, the test has limited value.[47]

Within the genitourinary system, the eggs may be identified in the urine. It is also important to note that recurrent bacterial urinary tract infections are commonly associated with this infection. These can even be noted as bacteremia as a result of the chronic infection of the blood vessels. When the urine is negative for ova, an occasional 24-hour urine collection may be necessary to increase the diagnostic accuracy of this test. The eggs are typically excreted in a circadian rhythm, making a single urine specimen less sensitive.[48]

RADIOLOGY

Unlike TB, schistosomiasis infections begin in the bladder and only secondarily involve the upper urinary tract. Cercaria, the infective form, are produced in the snail and enter the skin of humans exposed to infected water. After development in the portal vein, the parasites move to the pelvic veins and the female burrows into the mucosa of the bladder and lower ureters, where she deposits eggs. The deposition of eggs incites considerable inflammation and scarring, and calcium impregnates the dead ova in the bladder wall, caus-

298 Diagnosis of Genitourinary Disease

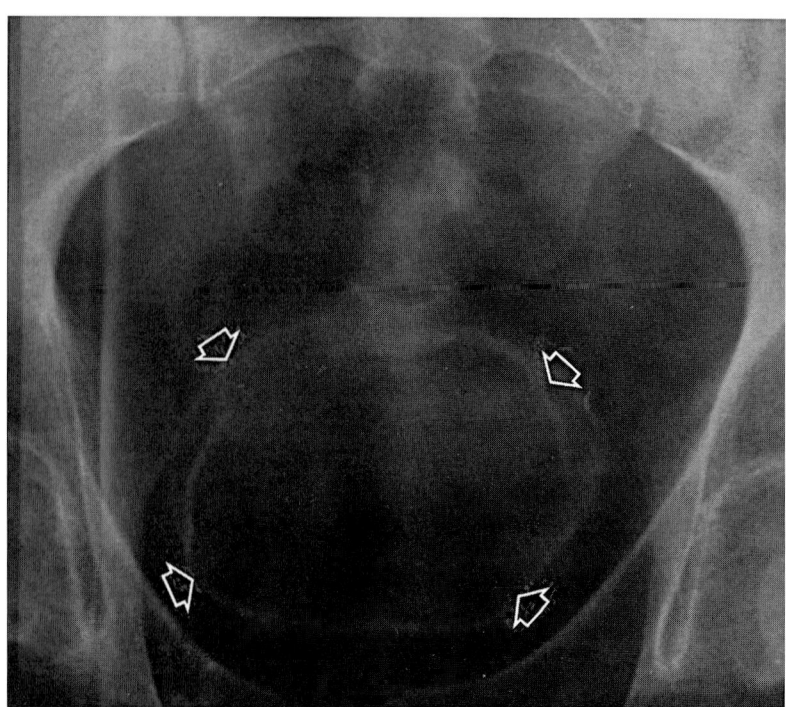

Figure 13–23. Calcified bladder (arrows) wall secondary to schistosomiasis.

ing the characteristic calcification of the bladder and lower ureters. On plain films, the earliest finding is a faint line of calcification above the symphysis pubis. With progressive disease, the entire bladder may calcify, and 34% of patients exhibit lower ureteral calcifications (Figs. 13–23, 13–24).[49] Approximately 40% of patients with schistosomal cystitis have associated calculi.[50]

Urographic and cystographic studies show a contracted bladder with an irregular shape. Filling defects may represent inflammatory polyps, calculi, or tumors. A cobblestone appearance on cystogram often indicates cystitis cystica. Squamous metaplasia is a frequent finding in chronic bilharziasis and predisposes to squamous cell carcinoma. Any interruption or asymmetry of the concentric bladder calcification is suggestive of neoplasm because carcinoma destroys

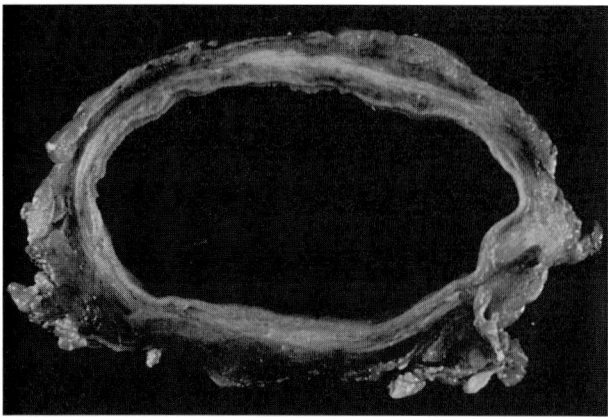

Figure 13–24. Calcified bladder with "sandy"-appearing mucosa.

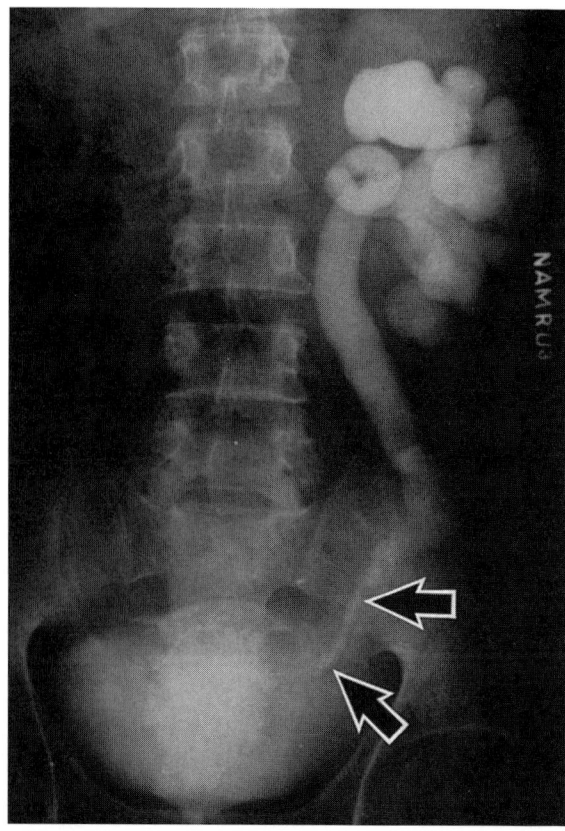

Figure 13–25. Distal ureteral stricture due to schistosomiasis.

the mural calcification, which may be identified on plain abdominal radiographs.

Ureteral strictures frequently develop and most commonly occur in the intramural portion of the distal ureter or at the level of the third lumbar vertebrae, where there are extensive venous anastomoses between the periureteral and portal veins. Ureteral dilation implies stricture or reflex but may also occur as a result of destruction of the periureteral nerve plexus by ova deposition (Fig. 13–25).[51] The kidney is rarely involved in schistosomal infections, but obstructive or reflux uropathy can complicate ureteral or bladder involvement. The prostate and seminal vesicles are involved in men with schistosomal infection revealing seminal vesicles that are often calcified. Urethral involvement leads to stricture formation and perineal fistulas.

CT evaluation of bladder schistosomiasis infections adds little to the urographic findings, although bladder masses with perivesicular extension are better evaluated with CT. Extensive shadowing from the bladder on sonography indicates bladder wall calcification, large calculi, or air.[52] A pelvic radiograph will establish the cause in these cases.

regimen combines an organophosphate, a pyrazinoisoquinoline. The former drug is given at 7.5 to 10 mg/kg per day divided into three doses, given at 2-week intervals. Because this drug is an organophosphate and therefore inhibits acetylcholinesterase at the neuromuscular junction, this is the source of the primary toxic effect, but these are rare. In general, it is recommended that people who are chronically exposed to organophosphate should not take this drug because of the risk of cumulative effects. The latter drug is a specific antischistosomal drug that has shown limited, if any, toxic effects. Tetravalent antimony, which was a mainstay of treatment for many years, has been abandoned.

Interventional Radiology. Bladder fibrosis in schistosomal cystitis is extensive in the region of the trigone, causing bladder neck contraction and close apposition of the ureteral orifices. This percutaneous nephrostomy or antegrade stenting is indicated in obstructed ureters that fail retrograde cystoscopic stent placement. Bladder tumors are best biopsied cystoscopically, but CT-guided biopsy can be performed in patients with urethral strictures or fistulas.

PHARMACOLOGY

The chemotherapy of schistosomiasis is usually effective when the acute disease is being treated. Most authors recommend two agents: metriphonate and pyraziquantel.[53] This

SURGERY

Only with chronic infestation is surgical intervention necessary. Strictures and calculi are encountered most often in this disease process (Fig. 13–26). Open resection is often

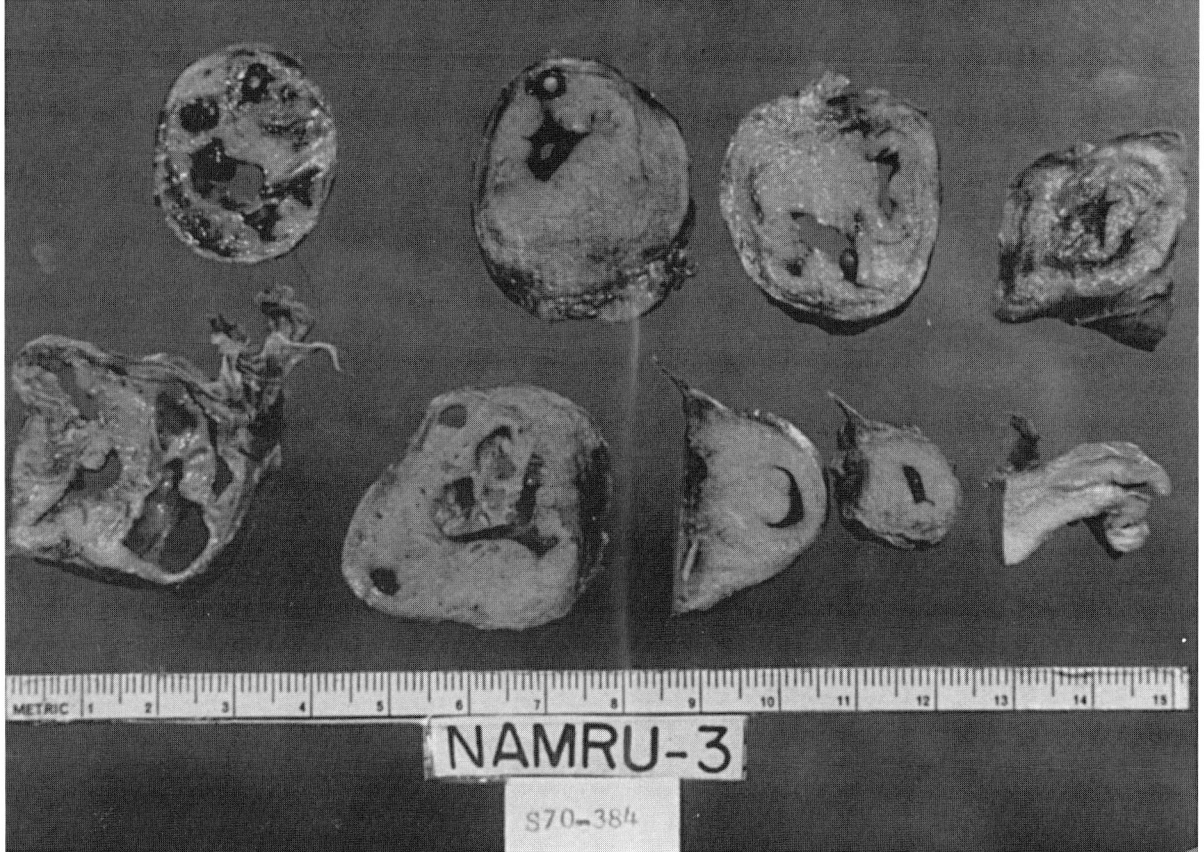

Figure 13–26. Gross specimen showing ureteritis due to *Schistosoma hematobium*.

necessary for this disease. On rare occasions a kidney will need to be removed, secondary to chronic obstruction and nonfunction.

SEQUELAE OF DISEASE

Bladder Cancer. The most disturbing and difficult to manage side effect of schistosomiasis is a dramatic increase in the incidence of bladder cancer. Both squamous cell carcinoma and adenocarcinoma have been reported with increasing frequency. They are both far more common in the dysfunctional bladder and may ultimately result from chronic bladder infection (Fig. 13–27). Because these bladders are commonly chronically infected with bacteria, large amounts of nitrosamines are produced, which are known carcinogens that may cause bladder tumors.[54] Many different treatment regimens have been recommended for the patient with bilharzial bladder cancer, but survival is poor. Roughly 75% of the patients are dead within 10 years of diagnosis. Of all patients, 18.5% have lymph node metastasis at the time of surgery.[55] In all, this disease is difficult to treat and long-term survival is unusual.

Filariasis

The involvement of the genitourinary system with filarial diseases is primarily limited to the manifestations of elephantiasis of the penis and scrotum, epididymitis, hydrocele, and chyluria. The primary infecting organism is *Wuchereria bancrofti*; *Brugia malayi* and *Brugia timori* are also implicated.[56,57] All these organisms infect the human lymphatic system and are spread primarily by mosquito bites, the most common of which is *Culex pipiens*. Other mosquitoes have been implicated as well. A number of these parasites have been described in humans but are nonlymphatic and are not commonly found in the genitourinary system. These include *Loa loa*, *Onchocerca volvulus*, and *Dirofilaria* species.

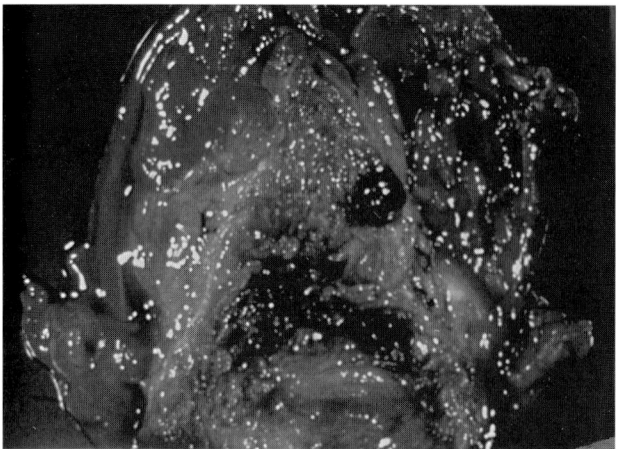

Figure 13–27. Squamous cell carcinoma in defunctionalized bladder.

These organisms are transmitted by mosquito bites where the infective larvae are injected into the skin along with saliva and other enzymes of the mosquito. There is a long incubation period, which may be as long as 4 months, where the larvae multiply within the lungs. After this, the organisms are transmitted to the larger lymphatic vessels, specifically in the periaortic iliac and inguinal lymph channels.[58] Many of these organisms have a particular predilection for certain areas.

HOST RESPONSE

Patients usually develop both a humoral and cell-mediated immune response to infection with these organisms.[57] The humoral response is primarily an IgE-mediated response, and hypersensitivity may occur. The cell-mediated response is primarily due to T cell activation. This immunostimulation does not confer immunity to the infection. Most of the patients will exhibit peripheral eosinophilia, granulomatous reactions, and deposition of antigen–antibody complexes. Lymphedema occurs during the period prior to established infection, referred to as the prepatent period. Patients have lymphadenopathy and lymphangitis during this time. As the infection progresses, the manifestations of epididymitis, abscesses, hydroceles, and anemia may result. As the infection progresses, more distal lymphatics tend to become involved, and a worsening of the previously described lesions occurs, along with chyluria, which results from rupture of intrapelvic lymph channels in the urinary system, specifically the kidney.[59]

DIAGNOSIS

Ideally, detection of the specific parasite in the blood, urine, or other body fluids would establish the diagnosis. Pathologic identification by histology is confirmatory. Several serologic tests measure antibodies to these organisms but are not as specific for current infection. Rarely, lymphangiography may be needed to determine the cause of lymphatic obstruction and to differentiate it from other possible diagnoses. In addition, plain film x-rays may show calcifications and calcified granulomas, but these are not always diagnostic.

TREATMENT

The treatment of filariasis involves both the destruction of the adult filariae and the interruption of microfilaremia. Diethylcarbamazine will disrupt the microfilaremia, thereby decreasing the vector-born transmissions; however, it is unclear whether this may actually kill the adult worm. The total dose should be 72 mg/kg divided as 6 mg/kg per day.[60,61] This drug may cause side effects that are usually allergic in nature. Headache and other constitutional symptoms may also be seen. The drug must be used for 2 or more weeks, and frequently it must be repeated. One of the more effective antifilarial drugs is ivermectin, given as a single dose of 25 μg/kg.[61] Often this drug must be repeated to prevent recurrent disease. Local care of the lymphedema with support hosiery and other measures may be necessary.

Rarely is surgery necessary except in the cases of genital elephantiasis. Reduction scrotoplasty is frequently helpful in conjunction with pharmacologic therapy.

Rare Parasitic Diseases

A number of other human parasites have been described in the genitourinary system. The most common of these perhaps are the other species of *Schistosoma* such as *mansoni* and *japonica*. In addition, *Echinococcus granulosus* has been reported in humans, causing hydatid cysts of the kidney and other organs.[62] These may appear to be tumors of the kidney, chiefly being their differential diagnosis. *Enterobius vermicularis*[63] and *Entamoeba histolytica*[64] have also been sporadically reported in the genitourinary system. The former may cause epididymitis and peritonitis, whereas the latter may form intrarenal or perinephric abscesses that may be difficult to distinguish from other forms of renal inflammatory disease. Most antihelminthic drugs are curative in these situations. Occasionally, surgical intervention with drainage of an abscess or even nephrectomy may be necessary to eradicate the infection.

REFERENCES

1. Rieder HL, Cauthen GM, Comstock GW, Snider DE: Epidemiology of tuberculosis in the United States. *Epidemiol Rev* 1989;11:79–98.
2. Centers for Disease Control and Prevention. Tuberculosis mortality—United States, 1992. *MMWR Morb Mortal Wkly Rep* 1992;42:696–697, 703–704.
3. Masur H: The Public Health Service Task Force on Prophylaxis and Therapy for *Mycobacterium avium* Complex. Recommendations on prophylaxis and therapy for *Mycobacterium avium* complex disease in patients infected with the human immunodeficiency virus. *N Engl J Med* 1993;329:898–904.
4. Gow JG, Barbosa S: Genitourinary tuberculosis: a study of 1117 cases over a period of 34 years. *Br J Urol* 1984;56:449–455.
5. Elkin M. Urogenital tuberculosis. In: Pollack HM, McClennan B, eds. *Clinical Urography*. Philadelphia: WB Saunders, 1990; 1020–1052.
6. Hartman DS: Radiologic-pathologic correlation of the granulomatous lesions of the kidney. In: Stamey TA, ed. *Monographs in Urology, 1, 2*. Philadelphia: WB Saunders, 1985; 403–417.
7. Davidson AJ: *Radiology of the Kidney*. Philadelphia: WB Saunders, 1985;403–417.
8. Okazawa N, Sekiya T, Tada S: Computed tomographic features of renal tuberculosis. *Radiat Med* 1985;9:209–213.
9. Goldman SM, Fishman EK, Hartman DS, Siegelman SS: Computed tomography of renal tuberculosis and its pathological correlates. *J Comput Assist Tomogr* 1985;9:771–776.
10. Jeffrey RB Jr: Abdominal imaging in the immunocompromised patients. *Radio Clin North Am* 1985;9:30:579–595.
11. Mitchinson DA: Treatment of tuberculosis. *J R Coll Physicians Lond* 1980;14:91.
12. Gow JG, Liverpool GB: The current management of patients with genitourinary tuberculosis. *AUA Update Series*, Vol. 11, lesson 26, AUA Office of Education, 1992.
13. Frieden TR, Sterling T, Pablos-Mendez A, Kilburn JD, Cauthen GM, Dooley SM: The emergence of drug-resistant tuberculosis in New York City. *N Engl J Med* 1993;328:521–526.
14. Edlin BR, Tokars JI, Grieco MH, et al: An outbreak of multidrug resistant tuberculosis among hospitalized patients with the acquired immunodeficiency syndrome. *N Engl J Med* 1992; 326:1514–1521.
15. Fischl MA, Uttamchandani RB, Daikos GL, et al: An outbreak of tuberculosis caused by multiple drug-resistant tubercle bacilli among patients with HIV infection. *Ann Intern Med* 1992; 117:177–183.
16. Bloch AB, Cauthen GM, Onorato IM, et al: Nationwide survey of drug-resistant tuberculosis in the United States. *JAMA* 1994; 271:665.
17. Collins CH, Uttley HC: In vitro susceptibility of mycobacteria to ciprofloxacin. *J Antimicrob Chemother* 1985;16:575–580.
18. Fenlon CH, Cynamon MH. Comparative in vitro activities of ciprofloxacin and other 4-quinolones against *Mycobacterium tuberculosis* and *Mycobacterium interacellulare*. *Antimicrob Agents Chemother* 1986;29:386–388.
19. Gorzynski EA, Gutman SI, Allen W: Comparative antimycobacterial activities of Difloxacin, temafloxacin, enoxacin, pefloxacin, reference fluoroquinolones, and a new macrolide, clarithromycin. *Antimicrob Agents Chemother* 1989;33:591–592.
20. Barradell LB, Plosker GL, McTavish D: Clarithromycin: a review of its pharmacological properties and therapeutic use in *Mycobacterium avium–intracellulare* complex infection in patients with acquired immune deficiency syndrome. *Drugs* 1993;46(2):289–312.
21. Centers for Disease Control: Nosocomial transmission of multidrug-resistant tuberculosis among HIV-infected persons—Florida and New York, 1988–1991. *MMWR Morb Mortal Wkly Rep* 1991;40:585–591.
22. Tuberculosis Prevention Trial, Madras: Trial of BCG vaccines in South India for tuberculosis prevention. *Indian J Med Res* 1980;72(suppl):1–74.
23. ten Dam HG, Toman K, Hitze KL, Guld J: Present knowledge of immunization against tuberculosis. *Bull World Health Organ* 1976;54:225–269.
24. Fine PEM, Rodrigues LC: Modern vaccines: mycobacterial diseases. *Lancet* 1990;335:1016–1020.
25. Colditz GA, Brewer TF, Berkey CS, Wilson ME, Burdick E, Fineberg HV, Mosteller F: Efficacy of BCG vaccine in the prevention of tuberculosis. *JAMA* 1994;271:698–702.
26. Wise GJ, Silver DA: Fungal infections of the genitourinary system. *J Urol* 1993;149:1377–1388.
27. Chisholm ER, Hutch JA: Fungal ball (*Candida albicans*) formation in the bladder. *J Urol* 1961;86:559.
28. Neal Jr, DE, Rodriguez G: Fungal prostatitis. *Cliniguide Fund Inf* 1993;4:1–5.
29. Suits T, Wise GJ, Walters B: Candidal antigenemia: a prognostic determinant. *J Urol* 1989;141:1381.
30. Ness MJ, Vaughan WP, Woods GL: Candida antigen latex test for detection of invasive candidiasis in immunocompromised patients. *J Infect Dis* 1989;159:495.
31. Walsh TJ, Hathorn JW, Sobel JD, Merz WG, Sanchez V, Maret SM, Buckley HR, Pfaller MA, Schaufele R, Silva C: Detection

of circulating *Candida* enolase by immunoassay in patients with cancer and invasive candidiasis. *N Engl J Med* 1991; 324:1026.
32. Neal Jr DE: Use of fluconazole in Candidal infections of the genitourinary tract. *Cliniguide Fund Infec* 1993;2:1–5.
33. Kenney PJ: Imaging of chronic renal infections. *AJR* 1990; 155:485–494.
34. Elkin M: *Radiology of the Urinary System.* Boston: Little, Brown, 1980;232–233.
35. Spring DB: Fungal diseases of the urinary tract. In: Pollack HM, McClennan B, eds. *Clinical Urography.* Philadelphia: WB Saunders, 1990;987–994.
36. Davidson AJ: *Radiology of the Kidney.* Philadelphia: WB Saunders, 1985;443–447, 450.
37. Berkow R, Fletcher AJ, eds: *The Merck Manual of Diagnosis and Therapy.* New Jersey: Merck & Co., 1987;1621.
38. Doemeny JM, Banner MP, Shapiro MJ, Amendola MA, Pollack HM: Percutaneous extraction of renal fungus ball. *AJR* 1988;150:1331–1332.
39. Staib F, Seibold M, L'age M, et al: Cryptococcus neoformans in the seminal fluid of an AIDS patient. A contribution to the clinical course of cryptococcosis. *Mycoses* 1989;32:171–180.
40. Saag MS, Dismukes WE: Azole antifungal agents: emphasis on new triazoles. *Antimicrob Agents Chemother* 1988;32:1.
41. Wheat LJ: Effect of successful treatment with amphotericin B on *Histoplasma capsulatum* variety *capsulatum* polysaccharide antigen levels in patients with AIDS and histoplasmosis. *Am J Med* 1992;92:153.
42. Mahoud AAF: Schistosomiasis: current concepts. *N Engl J Med* 1977;297:1329–1331.
43. WHO Expert Committee: The control of schistosomiasis. *Technical Report Series* 728, World Health Organization, Geneva, 1985.
44. Grasso M, Bagley D, Kelada AS, Shalaby MA: Genitourinary schistosomiasis. *Infect Urol* 1990;3:5:132–139.
45. Mobarak AB: The schistosomiasis problem in Egypt. *Am J Trop Med Hyg* 1982;31:87–91.
46. Doehring E, Vester U, Ehrich JHH, et al: Circadian variation of oval excretion, proteinuria, hematuria, and leukocyturia in urinary schistosomiasis. *Kidney Int* 1985;27:667–671.
47. Fleck SL, Moody AH: Serological diagnosis. In: *Diagnostic Techniques in Medical Parasitology.* London: Wright Publishing, 1988;113–119.
48. Doehring E: Schistosomiasis in childhood. *Eur J Pediatr* 1988; 147:2–9.
49. Hanafy BM, Youssef TK: Radiological aspects of bilharzial ureter. *Urology* 1975;6:118.
50. Afif MA: Roentgenographic manifestations of urinary bilharziasis and calculus formation in Egypt and intravenous pyelography. *AJR* 1934;31:208.
51. Ghoneum MA, Ashamallah A: Role of perineuritis in atonic dilated bilharzial ureter. *Int Surg* 1976;61:411.
52. Abdel-Wahab MF, Ramzy I, Esmat G, Kafass HE, Strickland GT: Ultrasound for detecting *Schistosoma haematobium* urinary tract complications: comparison with radiographic procedures. *J Urol* 1992;148:346–350.
53. Webbe G: Treatment of schistosomiasis. *Eur J Clin Pharmacol* 1987;32:433–436.
54. Smith JH, Christie JD: The pathobiology of *Schistosoma hematobium* infection in humans. *Hum Pathol* 1986;17:333–345.
55. Ghoneim MA, Ashmalla AK, Awaad HK, et al: Randomized trial of cystectomy with or without preoperative radiotherapy for carcinoma of the Bilharzial bladder. *J Urol* 1985;134:266–268.
56. Ottesen EA: Filariasis now. *Am J Trop Med Hyg* 1989; 41(suppl):8.
57. Ottesen EA: Infection and disease in lymphatic filariasis: an immunological perspective. *Parasitology* 1992;104:S71–S79.
58. Grenfell BT, Michael E: Infection and disease in lymphatic filariasis: an epidemiological approach. *Parasitology* 1992; 104:S81–S90.
59. Tani S, Akisada M: Lymphographical findings of the lymphaticopelvic fistulization in filarial chyluria. *Jpn J Trop Med* 1970;11:55.
60. Partono F, Purnomo, Oemijati S, Soewarta A: The long-term effects of repeated diethylcarbamazine administration with special reference to microfilaremia and elephantiasis. *Acta Trop* 1981;38:217.
61. Ottesen EA, Vijayasekaran V, Kumaraswami V, et al: A controlled trial of ivermectin and diethylacarbamazine in lymphatic filariasis. *N Engl J Med* 1990;322:1113.
62. Borrell JH, Barnes JM: Renal manifestations of hydatid diseases. *NY State J Med* 1933;33:1390.
63. Symmers W St C: Pathology of enterobiasis, AMA. *Arch Pathol Lab Med* 1950;50:475.
64. Brandt H, Perez Tamayo R: Pathology of human amoebiasis. *Hum Pathol* 1970;1:351.

ACKNOWLEDGMENTS

This chapter is dedicated to Katie and Caleb Neal, without whom it would have been impossible.

The authors are extremely grateful to Donna Ayala for preparation of the manuscript.

14 Urinary Stone Disease

Bruce I. Carlin, Martin I. Resnick

Although much of the pathophysiology of stone formation has been elucidated, clinical investigators are becoming increasingly aware of the multitude of factors responsible for the development of urinary calculi. No one factor has been identified that is common to all stone formers, and it is evident that patients with stones of similar composition have varying identifiable causes of their disease. Increased understanding of the medical abnormalities associated with the development of urolithiasis has led to a more effective delivery of medical and preventive therapy, thereby decreasing the recurrence rate of stone formation.[1] However, much is still unknown, and further work is warranted to deliver more effective care.

This chapter serves as both an overview of the pathophysiology of the formation of urinary calculi and a summary of their clinical presentation.

THEORIES OF STONE FORMATION

Four basic theories are proposed to explain the formation of urinary stones: precipitation–crystallization, matrix, epitaxy, and urinary inhibitors. Although these processes have been studied separately, it is generally accepted that more than one takes place during stone formation. In addition, it is proposed that the importance of each theory varies when stones of different etiologies are concerned.

Precipitation–Crystallization. It has long been recognized that for urinary crystals to form, urine must be supersaturated with respect to the specific ions comprising the crystal[2] and that once a nucleus of crystal forms, the crystals aggregate by chemical and electrical forces. Increasing the saturation of urine with respect to the ions leads to an increased rate of nucleation, crystal growth, and aggregation, and thus to an increased likelihod of stone growth.

According to this theory, the development of clinical disease relies entirely on the concentrations of the ions within the urine. Three zones of urinary saturation are thought to be involved with stone precipitation. The stable zone of undersaturation is a state in which the product of the ion concentrations does not exceed the solubility product and therefore no nucleation or growth of the crystal can occur, and dissolution may occur. In the oversaturated zone, the product of the ion concentration exceeds the formation product and there is spontaneous nucleation, with rapid growth and no dissolution. The metastable zone of supersaturation is a condition in which the product of the ion concentration is less than the formation product but greater than the solubility prouct; thus the stone grows from previously formed crystals, no new nuclei form, and stone dissolution can occur.[2-4]

This theory has some inconsistencies and does not completely account for the etiology of stone formation. It does not explain why some patients form urinary stones at a lower degree of urine supersaturation while others have no clinical disease at higher degrees. In addition, it does not propose a mechanism for the formation of heterogeneous stones. Therefore other theories must be explored.

Matrix. The composition of most urinary stones involves not only a crystalline phase, but also an organic phase, which is composed of protein, nonamino sugars, glucosamine, water, and organic ash. The role of this substance, matrix, must be considered in discussing stone formation because it makes up 2.0 to 9.0% (dry weight/weight basis) of urinary stones and 42 to 84% of true matrix stones and is arranged within the stones in organized concentric laminations.[5,6] Much work has suggested that some of the components of matrix—such as matrix substance A, uromucoid, and glycosaminoglycans—have an active role in lithogenesis in that their concentrations in the urine of stone formers greatly exceed those of non–stone formers.[6-8] There is evidence, however, that these constituents of matrix may inhibit stone formation.[6] Confirmatory evidence involving the role of these factors in the pathogenesis of urinary calculi is not currently available.

Epitaxy. This theory proposes that crystals of similar lattice structure will aggregate, thus forming stones of a heterogeneous nature. For example, the lattice structure of calcium oxalate and monosodium urate have similar structures, and therefore crystals of calcium oxalate can aggregate when a nucleus of monosodium urate crystals has formed previously.[3,9] In contrast, if the lattice structure of two crystals is incompatible, as is the case with calcium oxalate and struvite, the crystals will not aggregate.

Inhibitors. The consistent observation that many non–stone formers excrete urine in the metastable region of the supersaturation curve has prompted investigators to search for inhibitors of stone formation within the urine. Clinically, the three most important inhibitors at this time are urinary citrate,[10] diphosphonate,[11] and magnesium ion[12] in that treatment can be directed at these three variables; preparations such as UroCit K, magnesium supplements, and ethane-1-hydroxy-1,1-diphosphonate (EHDP)[11] have been found to be efficacious in decreasing the recurrence rate of urinary stones. Other substances that have been found to inhibit calculus formation include Nephrocalcin,[13] a glycoprotein that has been found to be deficient in the urine of patients who form calcium oxalate stones, and Uropontin,[14] an aspartate-rich protein that has been shown to directly inhibit calcium oxalate crystal aggregation. In addition, phosphates, mucoploysaccharides, and amino acids (specifically alanine) have been shown to exhibit significant inhibitory activity. Questions remain about the role of these substances in clinical stone disease and their exact mechanism of action.

PATHOPHYSIOLOGY

Calcium Stones

Calcium stones account for approximately 80% of all urinary calculi and usually contain a mixture of calcium oxalate and calcium phosphate, although pure calcium oxalate or calcium phosphate stones are not infrequent. Calcium oxalate stones occur in the monohydrate and the dihydrate forms, whereas calcium phosphate occurs in the apatite ($Ca_{10}[PO_4]_6[OH]_2$) or the brushite ($CaHPO_4 \cdot 2H_2O$) forms.

The most common metabolic abnormality in patients who form calcium stones is hypercalciuria. Between 30 and 60% of all patients with calcium stones will be hypercalciuric in the absence of hypercalcemia.[15] The primary abnormalities in these patients have been divided into absorptive hypercalciuria, renal hypercalciuria, and resorptive hypercalciuria. Other metabolic aberrations in the urine that predispose to increased stone formation include hyperoxaluria, hyperuricosuria, hypocitraturia, heterozygous cystinuria, and hypomagnesuria. In addition, many other disease states also contribute to the propensity for formation of urinary calculi.

Differentiation of these metabolic abnormalities is achieved by a metabolic evaluation that can be performed on an inpatient or ambulatory basis. Many types of protocols have been developed[1,16–18]; what is important is that the protocol be uniform. In this way, comparison of one patient to another is possible, and patients can be followed over a period of time after therapy is instituted. More than 90% of calcium stone formers can be stratified in this way.[19] Unless a situation exists requiring surgical intervention, it is preferable to proceed with metabolic evaluation prior to effecting stone removal. In the event that surgical intervention is necessary, it has been demonstrated that only a 2- to 3-week postoperative period is needed before full evaluation can be undertaken.[20]

For the initial part of this evaluation, the patient is maintained on his regular diet, and two 24-hour urine specimens are collected. Quantitative assays of the urine for calcium, phosphorus, uric acid, magnesium, citrate, oxalate, and creatinine, and a qualitative screening assay for the presence of cystine using the nitroprusside test are performed. Following these two collections, the patient is placed on a restricted-sodium–calcium diet (400 mg calcium; 100 meq sodium) for 1 week. After this period of stabilization, another 24-hour urine specimen is analyzed in the same fashion. The pH of the urine is measured serially, and if it is consistently above 5.3, an ammonium chloride loading test is performed. Serum calcium, phosphorus, uric acid, and creatinine levels are determined on the regular diet and on the restricted diet. If the patient is found to be hypercalcemic, a serum immunoreactive assay for parathormone is performed.

Subsequently, fasting and calcium load tests should be performed as follows. After the patient has fasted from 9 P.M. to 7 A.M. (distilled water only), he is instructed to void at 7 A.M. and discard the overnight sample. The patient then collects a 2-hour sample (7 A.M. to 9 A.M.), which is labeled the fasting sample. At 9 A.M. the patient is administered 1 g of calcium gluconate orally, and a urine sample is collected from 9 A.M. to 1 P.M., representing the calcium load sample. The volume of these two specimens is recorded and both are analyzed for calcium and creatinine. All precalcium load urine specimens should have a ratio of milligrams of calcium to milligrams of creatinine that is less than 0.11. Urine calcium is considered to be elevated on the postcalcium load specimen if this ratio exceeds 0.2.

Absorptive Hypercalciuria. The primary disturbance in absorptive hypercalciuria is intestinal hyperabsorption of calcium. It is unclear at this time whether this represents an increased response to 1,25-$(OH)_2$ vitamin D_3 stimulation or a process independent of vitamin D. As more calcium is absorbed, the patient becomes transiently hypercalcemic, and this suppresses parathormone secretion. Renal filtration of calcium is increased and less is reabsorbed by the kidney, primarily because of the decreased parathormone secretion. The result is hypercalciuria, which can be suppressed by decreasing the calcium intake in the diet and worsened with a calcium load. Thus with preceding evaluation, patients with absorptive hypercalciuria will have a normal fasting urine calcium/creatinine ratio but will demonstrate an abnormally high response to calcium load.

Renal Hypercalciuria. The aberration in renal hypercalciuria relates to an impairment of the renal tubular resorption of calcium or calcium leak. Many studies of this phenomenon suggest etiologies of infection, tubular ectasia, and a functional tubular defect. Renal leak of calcium causes mild hypocalcemia, and this triggers a response by the parathyroid glands and causes increased intestinal absorption of calcium and increased mobilization of calcium stores. Patients with renal hypercalciuria therefore will have elevated fasting and calcium load urine calcium/creatinine ratios.

Resorptive Hypercalciuria. Resorptive hypercalciuria is a relatively unusual form of hypercalciuria that is found in patients with primary hyperparathyroidism. Excess parathormone secretion stimulates the intestinal absorption by increasing the synthesis of $1,25\text{-}(OH)_2$ vitamin D_3 and increased mobilization of calcium stores. As in renal hypercalciuria, the urine calcium/creatinine fasting and calcium load ratios are elevated. The serum parathormone level, however, will distinguish these two entities (Table 14–1).

Hyperoxaluria. Hyperoxaluria is defined as an excretion of oxalate above the normal range of 10 to 50 mg/day. Changes in the oxalate concentration in the urine are 15 times as potent as similar changes in the calcium concentration in altering the saturation of calcium oxalate,[21] and therefore hyperoxaluria leads to a significant increase in the precipitation of calcium oxalate. Oxalate is found in high concentrations in tea, coffee, spinach, and rhubarb, and the daily dietary intake of oxalate in the typical Western diet varies from 70 to 920 mg/day.

Clinical hyperoxaluria is divided into primary and secondary hyperoxaluria. Primary hyperoxaluria is a rare autosomal recessive disorder that is subclassified into glycolic aciduria and L-glyceric aciduria that predisposes patients to produce increased endogenous oxalate and to form urinary calculi. Patients with primary hyperoxaluria typically develop renal failure and die by age 20.

Secondary or acquired hyperoxaluria is a more common entity and can occur in patients with pyridoxine deficiency, enteric hyperoxaluria, and increased intake of oxalate and oxalate precursors such as vitamin C. The pathogenesis of enteric hyperoxaluria involves gastrointestinal malabsorption of fatty acids, which bind intraluminal calcium and form salts that are excreted in the feces. This leads to the increased intestinal absorption of unbound oxalate. Diseases associated with enteric hyperoxaluria include biliary tract disease, pancreatic insufficiency, inflammatory bowel disease, and jejunoileal bypass for morbid obesity.[21]

Hyperuricosuria. Hyperuricosuria has been reported in approximately 20% of patients forming calcium oxalate stones[22,23] and is defined as the excretion of greater than 800 mg/day of uric acid for men and 750 mg/day for women. The mechanism of action of uric acid in predisposing to the formation of calcium oxalate stones has yet to be clearly established. It may be related to the epitactic growth of calcium oxalate crystals around a nucleus of uric acid crystals[4,15,22] or to the action of uric acid as a counterinhibitor of the urinary mucopolysaccharides, which inhibit calcium oxalate crystallization.[4,24] Recent studies suggest that the action of uric acid may simply be a "salting-out" phenomenon that involves the precipitation of a nonelectrolyte, calcium oxalate, from solution after the addition of an electrolyte, uric acid.[25–27]

Hypocitraturia. The incidence of hypocitraturia in calcium stone formers is 15 to 50%[28] and is defined as the excretion of less than 320 mg of citrate per day.[10] Citrate acts as an inhibitor of calcium urolithiasis by forming complexes with calcium, thereby increasing the solubility of calcium in the urine, and by inhibiting the aggregation of calcium phosphate and calcium oxalate crystals.[10] Disease states such as chronic diarrhea, intestinal malabsorption, and renal tubular acidosis promote hypocitraturia and thus increase the incidence of calcium urolithiasis.

Heterozygous Cystinuria. An unexpectedly high incidence of heterozygous cystinuria has been found in calcium stone formers.[24] The incidence of this metabolic abnormality in males and females is 11.8% and 17.1%, respectively. The true mechanism of action of cystine is unknown, but it is possible that cystine has a role in calcium urolithiasis that is similar to uric acid.

Hypomagnesuria. Magnesium ion has been shown to form complexes with oxalate in the urine and to decrease tubular resorption of citrate. It has been proposed therefore that magnesium acts as a urinary inhibitor of calcium stone formation and that hypomagnesuria may predispose to calcium urolithiasis.[12]

Sarcoidosis. In patients with sarcoidosis, there is an increased sensitivity of the intestinal epithelium to vitamin D_3 and thus an increased absorption of calcium from the gastrointestinal tract. This results in an elevated level of urinary calcium excretion and urinary stone formation. Patients with sarcoidosis characteristically have a chest radiograph that demonstrates bilateral enlarged lymph nodes and a reticulonodular infiltrative pattern. Physical examination often reveals the presence of cervical adenopathy and hepatosplenomegaly. Serum B-globulins are increased and biopsy of

Table 14–1. Summary of the Metabolic Evaluation of Patients with Hypercalciuria

METABOLIC DISORDER	SERUM CA	RESTRICTED CA (URINE)	FASTING CA (URINE)	CA LOAD (URINE)	PTH (SERUM)
Absorptive	N	N or I	N	I	N
Renal	N	I	I	I	N
Resorptive	I	I	I	I	I

lymph nodes or an intradrenal injection of sarcoid homogenate, coupled with subsequent biopsy of the resultant nodule (Kveim Test), confirms the diagnosis.

Renal Tubular Acidosis. Three types of renal tubular acidosis exist, but only type I predisposes to the formation of calcium urolithiasis. Type I renal tubular acidosis is characterized by an inability of the distal nephron to secrete hydrogen ion. Patients are thus unable to excrete urine of a pH of less than 5.8 and present with hyperchloremic acidosis and hypokalemia, with wasting of calcium and phosphorus. Besides calcium urolithiasis and nephrocalcinosis, patients also develop muscle weakness and osteomalacia.[29]

Struvite Stones

Struvite or infectious stones account for 15 to 20% of all renal calculi. The stones are composed of both magnesium ammonium phosphate ($MgNH_46H_2O$) and carbonate apatite ($Ca_{10}[PO_4]_6CO_3$), and they usually assume a staghorn configuration, filling the collecting system of the kidney (Figure 14–1). These stones are always associated with urinary tract infections with urea-splitting bacteria such as *Proteus* species, *Klebsiella*, *Pseudomonas*, and *Staphylococcus aureus*. With this type of infection, urinary ammonium concentration rises and the urine becomes alkaline, thus inducing the precipitation of magnesium ammonium phosphate and carbonate apatite. Patients at risk for the development of struvite stones are those with chronic or recurrent pyelonephritis, indwelling Foley catheters, spinal cord injury, and ileal conduit diversion.[30] Preferably, the diagnosis should be established preoperatively so that appropriate antibiotic therapy can be instituted during the postoperative period to reduce the incidence of recurrent stone formation.

Uric Acid Stones

In the United States approximately 5% of all renal stones are composed primarily of uric acid. Conditions that lead to the formation of uric acid stones include medullary sponge kidney, distal small bowel disease (regional enteritis), jejunoileal bowel resection, and ileostomy placement. In addition, a highly acidic urine, a highly concentrated urine, and the excess excretion of uric acid as in systemic gout or myeloproliferative disorders will lead to increased uric acid stone formation. However, less than 50% of patients with uric acid stones have an elevated serum level of uric acid.[22]

Cystine Stones

Cystine stones account for only about 1% of all urinary calculi. Cystinuria is a rare autosomal recessive disorder of the epithelial cells of the renal tubule that prevents renal absorption of the dibasic amino acids cystine, lysine, ornithine, and arginine.[31] Because of the poor solubility, cystine crystalluria and stone formation result. These patients usually have acidic urine, which leads to a higher rate of precipitation. In the homozygous patient, the daily excretion of cystine usually exceeds 500 mg, and stone formation occurs at an early age. Heterozygotes excrete 100 to 300 mg/day of cystine and usually do not have clinical urolithiasis; as already mentioned, this abnormality is present in patients who form calcium stones.

CLINICAL PRESENTATION

Epidemiology. The highest incidence of urolithiasis is in the interval between 30 and 60 years of age, and the esti-

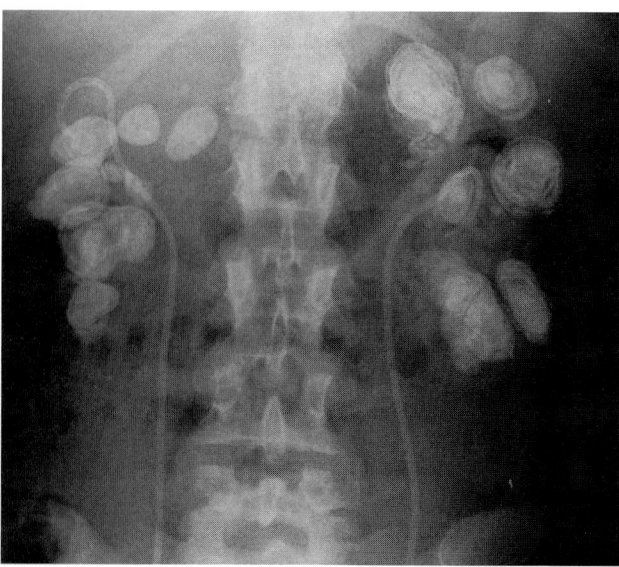

Figure 14–1. (A) A branched, radiopaque mass in the left kidney that is consistent with a staghorn renal calculus. (B) Another example of staghorn calculi. Note the characteristic concentric laminations.

mated annual incidence for males and females is 109.5 per 100,000 population and 36.0 per 100,000 population, respectively.[32] Recurrence rates at 5 years vary between 25 and 50%,[33] and are highest in the first year after presentation with the initial stone. Caucasians develop clinical urolithiasis three to four times as frequently as blacks; 61% of black stone formers are females as compared to whites, in which approximately 65% are male.[34]

The direct correlation between increased environmental temperature and the incidence of urinary stones has been demonstrated in that the incidence rates in the Northern Hemisphere are 1.5 to 2.0 times greater in the months between April and October, with a peak incidence in August.[35] In addition, there is a significant difference in the mean rate of hospital discharges for urinary stone disease in the states in the southeastern United States as compared to the rest of the country.[36]

Presenting Signs and Symptoms. The mode of presentation of patients with stone disease has been recognized since the earliest times. The ancient Hindu physician Sysruta stated[37]: ''The tortured patient grinds his teeth, presses on his abdomen, and rubs his penis. Urine, flatus, and feces are passed with severe pain. In such a case, the stone is black, rough, irregular, and covered with spikes like the maneleaceadanba flower....'' The symptoms that patients with urolithiasis experience depend on the anatomic location of the stone.[38] Pain is the most common symptom. Patients with renal calculi experience dull aching pain in the flank and usually have costovertebral angle tenderness. As the stone passes into the ureter and causes obstruction of urinary flow, patients suffer from colicky pain that frequently is referred to the testes in males and the labia and groin in females. Three areas of the upper urinary system where the stone is most likely to become lodged are the ureteropelvic junction, the point where the ureter passes over the iliac vessels, and the ureterovesical junction.

Many associated symptoms are encountered. Patients often complain of nausea and vomiting; the afferent autonomic sensory nerve fibers that innervate the genitourinary system synapse in the celiac ganglion in common with those from the gastrointestinal tract. Gross hematuria is often present in patients with stone disease and sometimes can be the chief complaint in the absence of any pain. If the stone is struvite in composition or if it is associated with a urinary tract infection, the patient can present with complaints of dysuria and fever.

A detailed history of other medical conditions, such as hypertension, diabetes mellitus, sarcoidosis, hyperparathyroidism, inflammatory bowel disease, and gout, should be sought because the treatment plan will change accordingly. A detailed family history for urolithiasis and other related diseases is essential. The use of habitual medications such as vitamin D preparations, antacids, or alkylating agents should be documented. Finally, a dietary history including intake of dairy products, tea, soda, and fluids can be helpful, especially in repeat stone formers.

Physical Examination. Physical examination should be thorough and an assessment made, not only to evaluate the general well-being of the patient but also to identify any specific diseases that may be associated with stone formation. Upon presentation in the emergency room, most patients will be experiencing ureteral colic and will be in obvious distress; typically, the patient will be tossing about, unable to find comfort in any one position. During this period of severe agitation, the patient's pulse rate will be elevated and the patient will be hypertensive. Diaphoresis and tachypnea are often present. Fever is usually absent unless there is an associated urinary tract infection.

Abdominal examination generally reveals tenderness on palpation over the kidney or midureter where the stone is impacted. Particular attention should be directed to palpation of the flank for the presence of a mass, indicative of a chronically obstructed kidney. Abdominal examination should also be made to assess bladder emptying because urinary retention is occasionally associated with stone passage. Auscultation of the abdomen in the patient experiencing acute colic often reveals decreased bowel sounds associated with a reflex paralytic ileus.

The presentation of urinary calculous disease can mimic other abdominal processes; thus a general abdominal examination is always necessary to help differentiate urinary stone disease from gastroenteritis, cholecystitis, appendicitis, and pelvic inflammatory disease.

Laboratory Evaluation. At the time of presentation all patients should have a urinanalysis and, if indicated, a urine culture. The examining physician should perform the urinalysis, looking for the presence of microscopic hematuria, pyuria, and bacilluria. The presence of crystals within the urine can be diagnostic of stone disease and can be helpful in initiating treatment.[39-41] The physician should pay particular attention to the pH of the urine specimen; the pH is elevated in the presence of struvite stones and is depressed in the presence of uric acid stones and thus can contribute to individualizing therapy.

A serum chemistry survey and a complete blood count (CBC) should be obtained as adjuncts to the other tests in order to screen for infection, renal disease, malignancy, or other associated metabolic disorders.

Another essential aspect of the workup is the stone analysis. All patients should be instructed to strain their urine and collect the sediment. With the ready availability of commercial laboratories performing reliable crystallographic analyses, quantitative data regarding stone composition and qualitative information regarding the center (nidus) and outer rim of the stone can be obtained. Patients undergoing extracorporeal lithotripsy should also be instructed to strain

308 Diagnosis of Genitourinary Disease

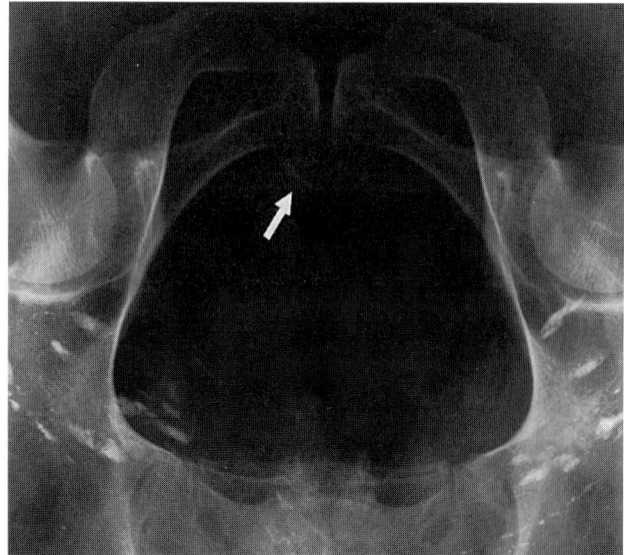

Figure 14–2. Prostatic calcifications identified on scout abdominal film (arrows).

RADIOLOGIC EVALUATION

Plain Films and Tomograms. Many radiologic modalities are available to aid in the characterization of urinary stones. The information most useful for the urologist planning treatment is the composition of the stone, the location of the stone, and the stone burden.

It is important that the clinician begin this investigation with plain films of the abdomen that rule out other causes of abdominal pain and include the area above the diaphragm to just below the symphysis pubis. In addition, it is necessary to obtain these studies before administering intravenous contrast media because occasionally urinary stones can be obscured and subsequently missed after the contrast is injected. Thus two preliminary films that are routinely obtained are one 14- × 17-in. film that includes the symphysis pubis inferiorly and a second, smaller film of 10 × 12 in. that centers on the kidneys; occasionally, more than two films are needed to cover the entire urinary tract.

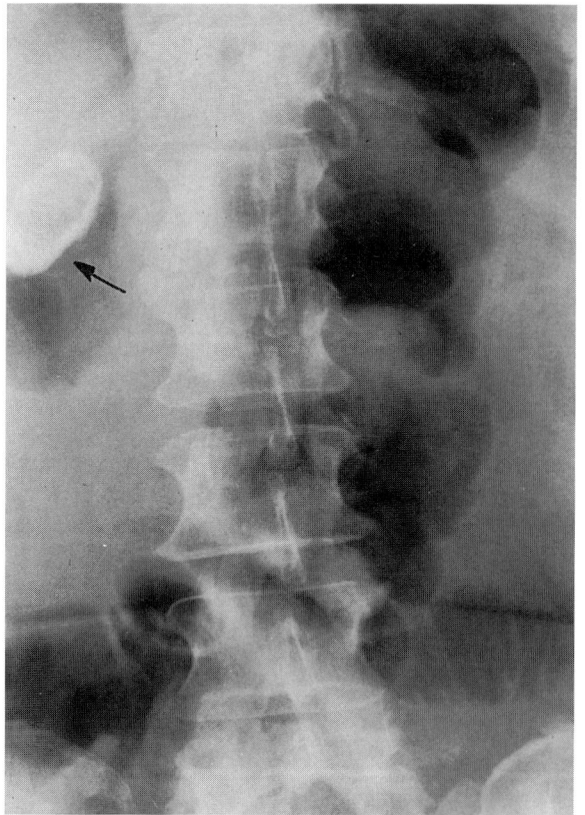
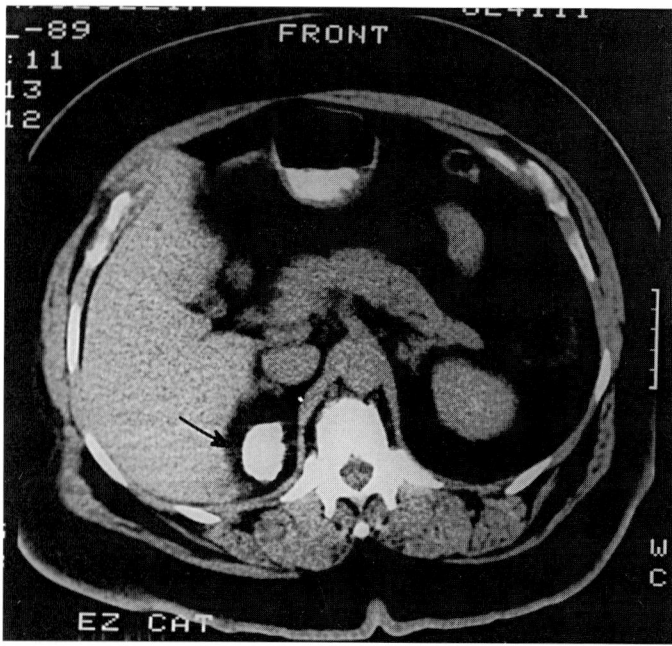

A
B

Figure 14–3. A 63-year-old with back pain. (A) A plain abdominal radiograph reveals a rounded density with a calcified rim in the right upper quandrant. Differential diagnosis includes a calcified adrenal mass versus a calcified renal mass. (B) CT scan of the abdomen of the same patient identifies a 3- × 3-cm calcified round retroperitoneal lesion that is consistent with calcified adrenal mass. Upon exploratory laparotomy, a benign calcified adrenal cyst was removed.

More than 90% of urinary stones can be detected by plain film.[42-45] The composition of the stone is suggested by plain film, as the different types of stones vary in radiopacity.[44] Calcium oxalate monohydrate stones are the most opaque stones and often present as round or oval with smooth, distinct borders. Calcium oxalate dihydrate stones, in contrast, tend to be less dense and demonstrate an irregular or brushite border. Struvite stones are somewhat less dense and have characteristic laminations that may be appreciated by plain films (see Fig. 14–1). In addition, struvite stones are often found in a staghorn configuration, but this is not specific to struvite calculi. Cystine stones are faintly opaque and usually are homogeneous in appearance. Infrequently, these stones may assume a staghorn appearance. Uric acid and xanthine stones are radiolucent at the KV_p used in typical abdominal films; however, if the stone contains any calcium, they can appear faintly opaque with laminations of calcified material.

Extraurinary calcifications that mimic urinary stones include costal cartilage; gallstones; calcified mesenteric lymph nodes; vascular, pancreatic, or adrenal calcifications (Fig. 14–3), phleboliths, prostatic calculi (see Fig. 14–2); and bone islands in the sacroiliac area.[45] In these cases when the diagnosis of urolithiasis is uncertain, further workup is necessary. Plain film tomograms have been shown to identify increased numbers of urinary calculi and differentiate urinary calculi from extraurinary calcifications.[46] If a patient presents with an unclear plain film where overlying feces, gas, or bony structures are obscuring the kidneys or if there is a question of extraurinary calcification, plain film tomograms are indicated.

Intrarenal calcifications that may mimic urinary stones include calcified renal papillae, calcified neoplasm, cholesteatomas, granulomas, and arterial calcifications.[45] These entities cannot be differentiated by plain films or tomograms; thus more invasive studies are indicated.

Intravenous Urography. The intravenous urogram is relatively inexpensive and simple to perform and remains the most valuable study in the initial evaluation of the patient with suspected urolithiasis. In this test, a water-soluble contrast media consisting of an iodinated benzene compound is injected intravenously and serial films are obtained. This test is generally well tolerated by patients, though common side effects include nausea, vomiting, flushing, warmth, or a metallic taste in the mouth. Adverse reactions to contrast media are uncommon and include mild to severe allergic reactions and nephrotoxicity. Prevention of these reactions involves premedicating patients with a history of contrast material reaction with a regimen of antihistamines and corticosteroids, and hydrating patients with known renal insufficiency, vascular disease, and diabetes mellitus with intravenous fluids to prevent acute renal failure. The use of nonionic contrast media has been shown to decrease the incidence of contrast media reactions significantly, but its use may be limited by its high cost. The most effective preventive measure, however, is the identification of risk for reaction and monitoring patients appropriately during the study.

The protocol for intravenous urography is universal, but deviation from this protocol is sometimes necessary in individualizing the evaluation based on the anatomy of the patient. Typically, the first film obtained after a bolus of contrast material is a coned-down 1-minute kidney film. In the nonobstructed kidney, a dense nephrogram will be visualized, whereas in the obstructed kidney, the nephrogram phase is delayed and the renal outline is not well visualized. A 3- to 5-minute coned-down film is then obtained to demonstrate the collecting system and renal pelvis in the normal kidney and to await the presence of the nephrogram phase in the obstructed kidney.

Serial films are taken until the collecting system of the obstructed kidney is visualized and the point of obstruction is identified. Routine findings in this film showing the pyelogram phase of the obstructed kidney are swelling and enlargement of the kidney, blunting of the calyceal architecture, and dilation of the ureter until the point of obstruction. Occasionally, extravasation of contrast material is seen representing a forniceal tear resulting from passage of the stone (Figs. 14–4, 14–5, 14–6).

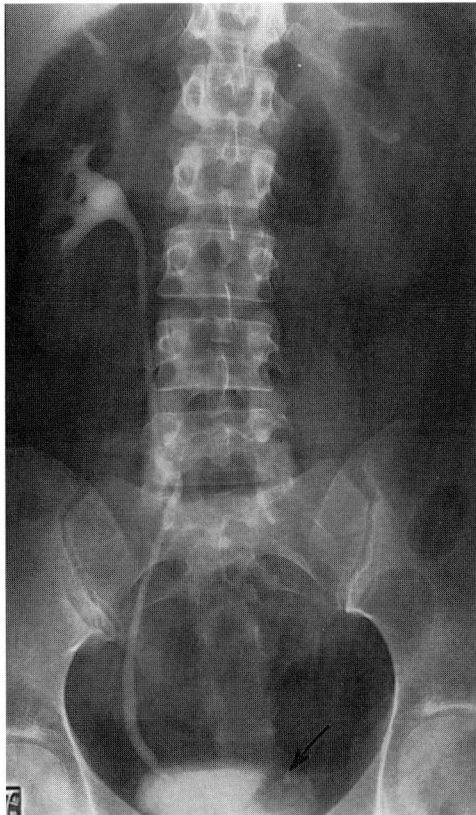

Figure 14–4. A 35-year-old patient with left ureteral colic. Intravenous pyelogram demonstrating a delayed nephrogram on the left side with a calcification in the area of the ureterovesical junction that is consistent with an obstructing calculus.

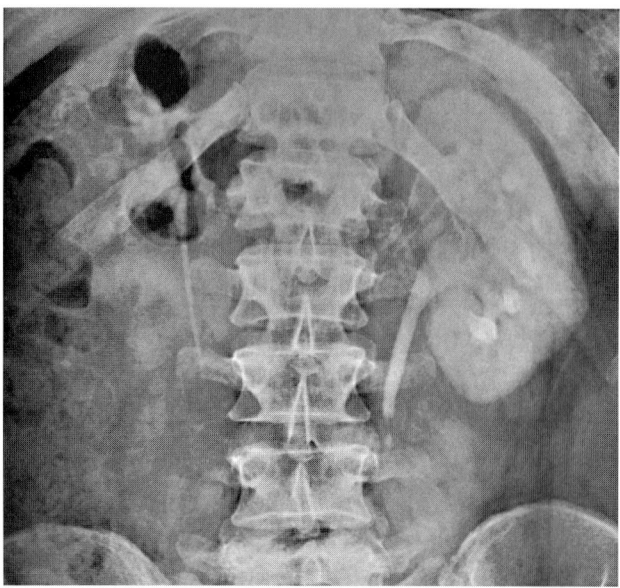

Figure 14–5. Left midureteral calculus. Acute left ureteral colic. Ten-minute film. Dense nephrogram on left as well as mildly dilated calyces and proximal ureter. Note pyelolymphatic extravasation.

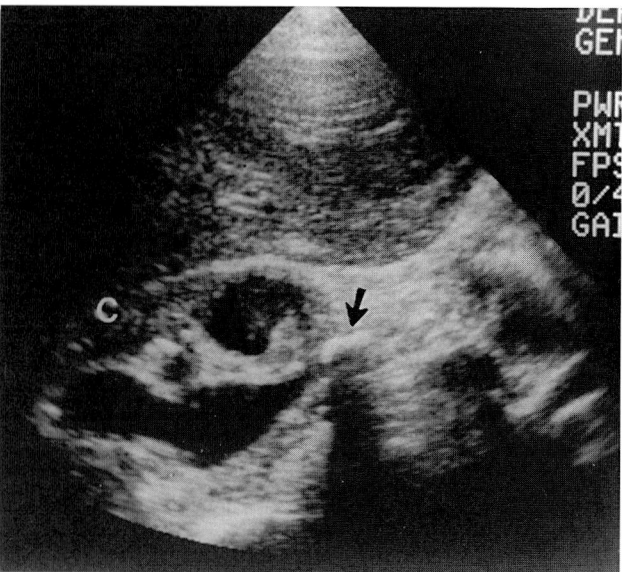

Figure 14–7. Transverse sonogram of the right kidney. Cortical atrophy (**C**) and pelvicalyceal dilatation due to an impacted stone (arrow) at the ureteropelvic junction.

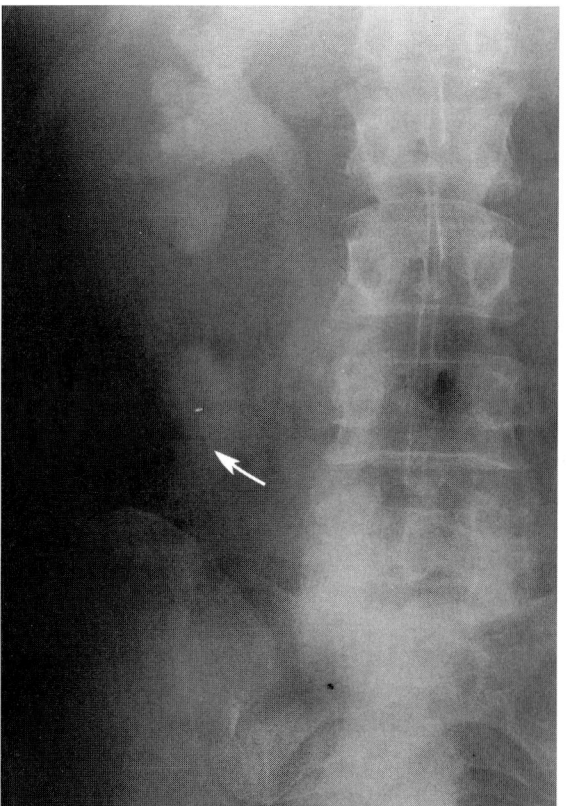

Figure 14–6. A 75-year-old with acute onset of right flank pain. Intravenous pyelogram demonstrates clubbing of the renal calyces and uniform dilatation of the right ureter on the 20-minute film. In the region of the midureter, there is extravasation of contrast media outside the ureter consistent with a ureteral tear due to passage of a stone (arrow).

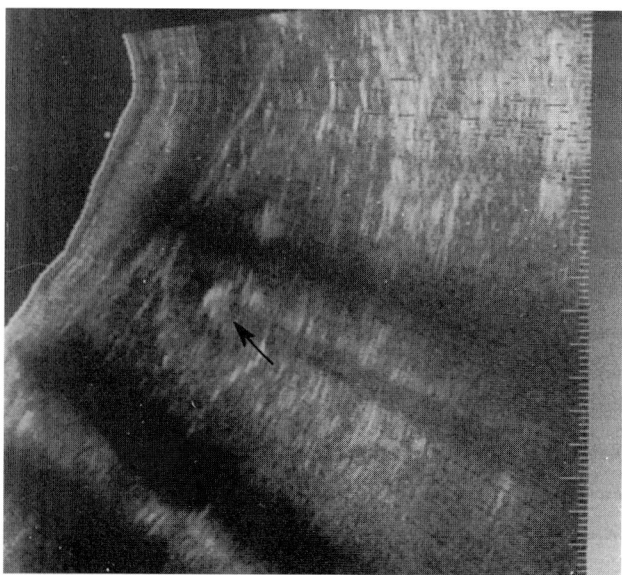

Figure 14–8. Ultrasound examination of the abdomen reveals an echogenic structure within the renal pelvis of the left kidney of a patient with left flank pain. No hydronephrosis is identified, but there is increased parenchymal echogenicity of the kidney consistent with diffuse parenchymal disease.

Many other films can be obtained to aid in the characterization of the pathology present. The patient can be placed in the Trendelenburg position to encourage filling and visualization of the collecting system, and thus can be moved into the reverse Trendelenburg position to visualize filling of the lower ureter and bladder. Oblique films are used to evaluate the distal ureter and ureterovesical junction and occasionally may visualize the obstructing stone with better ability than the AP view. Postvoid films are always performed to assure good emptying of the bladder and to rule out bladder and urethral calculi.

The overall diagnostic accuracy of excretory urography has ranged from 81.5 to 85% in patients with acute flank pain. However, detection of stones in the lower ureter and ureterovesical junction has been found to be less accurate, with rates of 68 to 74%.[47,48]

Ultrasound. The use of ultrasound for the diagnosis of urinary stones is controversial. Most clinicians agree that ultrasound is helpful in assessing the degree of hydronephrosis in obstruction and in measuring the thickness of the renal parenchyma in patients with urolithiasis and chronic renal failure. However, the difficulty in using ultrasound reliably to detect urinary calculi lies in the fact that there is minimal acoustic contrast between the stone and the surrounding tissues; this is in contrast to the detection of biliary stones, where the bile serves to increase the acoustic contrast.[43] Reported in the literature is the inability of ultrasound to detect stones in the midureter and its identification of false-positives from echogenic foci such as calcified arteries and other hilar structures.[43,45,47] In addition, ultrasound does not provide any information as to the functional status of the examined kidney (Figs. 14–7, 14–8, 14–9).

Although some investigators support the use of ultrasound to evaluate patients with acute renal colic and purport that there is a sensitivity of 96.8% for the identification of urinary

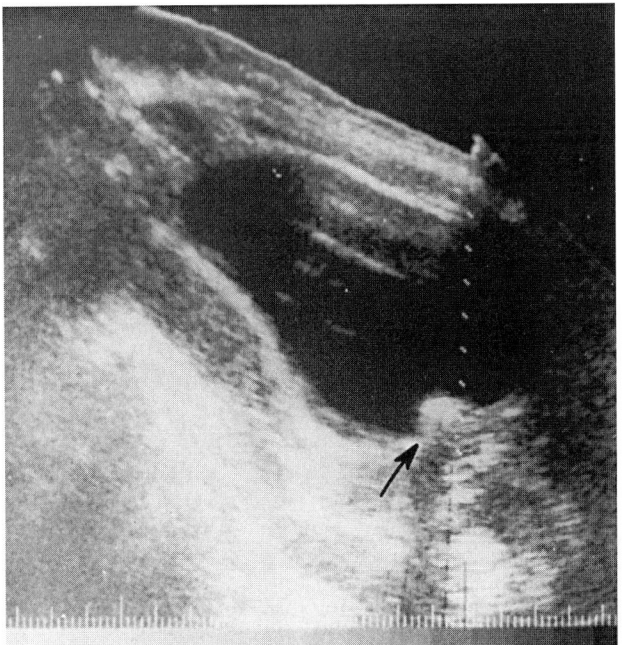

Figure 14–9. Ultrasound examination of the pelvis reveals an echogenic structure within the bladder that casts acoustic shadowing consistent with a bladder calculus.

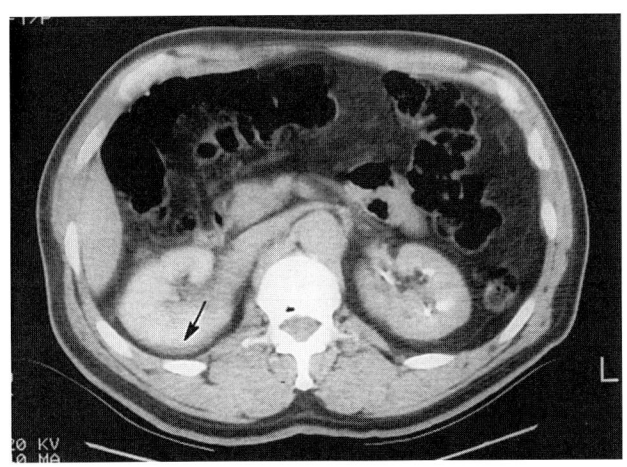
A

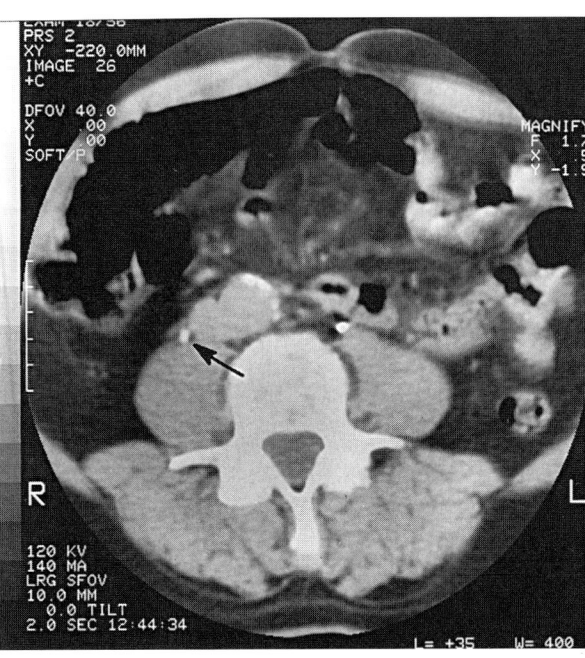
B

Figure 14–10. CT scan of the abdomen and pelvis. A 74-year-old with sudden onset of abdominal and back pain. **(A)** A postcontrast image identifying a dense nephrogram in the right kidney without contrast within the right collecting system. Dilation of the right renal pelvis and ureter is evident. There is a small, low-density fluid collection around the right kidney that is consistent with extravasated urine (arrows). **(B)** A small density is visualized in the region of the distal right ureter that represents a ureteral calculus (arrow).

stones when used in conjunction with excretory urography,[48] others have demonstrated the far greater superiority of excretory urography and have shown that ultrasound fails to detect 30 to 50% of urinary calculi.[43,47]

Computed Tomography. Computed tomography is rarely used in the initial evaluation of a patient with acute renal colic because it is expensive and subjects the patient to a relatively high radiation dosage. This technique is particularly useful, however, in differentiating urinary stones from other pathologic entities within the urinary tract. Computed tomography is particularly effective in the evaluation of radiolucent filling defects found on excretory urography. In addition, computed tomography is much more sensitive in detecting small stones and evaluating the relation of the kidney to extrarenal structures (Figures 14–3, 14–10).[44,49,50]

The differential diagnosis of a radiolucent filling defect on excretory urography includes uric acid or xanthine calculous disease, transitional cell neoplasm, sloughed papilla, blood clot, cholesteatoma, or papilloma. Many investigators have demonstrated that urinary calculi are identified in vivo by computed tomography with very high attenuation values in the range of 75 to 586 Hounsfield units, HU (Table 14–2). Except for cholesteatoma, the other pathologic entities are associated with much lower attenuation values (Table 14–3). In vitro computed tomographic analysis has been used to characterize and stratify calculi of various chemical composition[51]; at this time this stratification has not been possible in vivo, although calcium-containing stones have been shown to demonstrate higher attenuation values.[45,49] It should also be noted that computed tomography should be performed initially without intravenous contrast because many of the mentioned pathologic entities have been shown to enhance with contrast material.[42,52]

Retrograde Pyelography. With the development of ultrasound and computed tomography, retrograde pyelography is utilized less often because it is relatively invasive and requires the insertion of a cystoscope. This study, however, allows a controlled opacification of the renal pelvis and ureter and thus has many applications in the diagnosis and treatment of urinary calculi. It is particularly effective when in-

Table 14–2. Evaluation of Urinary Stones by Computed Tomography

CHEMICAL COMPOSITION	ATTENUATION VALUES (HU)
Calcium[42,45,49]	278–510
Cystine[42]	586
Uric acid[42,44,49,50]	75–402
Xanthine[42]	391
Triamterene[55]	132
Matrix[52]	16

Table 14–3. Differential Diagnosis of a Filling Defect on Intravenous Pyelography*

PATHOLOGY	ATTENUATION VALUES (HU)
Urinary stone	70–586
Transitional cell tumor[44,45,50]	15–45
Blood clot[44,45,50]	50–75
Fungus ball[50]	25
Normal renal parenchyma[45]	35–45

*Note the significant difference in attenuation values found on computed tomography between urinary stones and the other pathologic entities.

complete visualization of the collecting system occurs after intravenous pyelography and may be helpful in the evaluation of filling defects found on intravenous pyelography. It is essential when manipulation of a ureteral calculus is necessary or if placement of a ureteral stent is warranted.

Retrograde pyelography may be difficult or technically unsuccessful in a number of circumstances. Insertion of the ureteral catheter into the ureteral orifice may be impossible if an enlarged prostate blocks the orifice, if the ureter is ectopic, or if the ureter has been reimplanted previously. In addition, if the catheter has been introduced into the ureteral

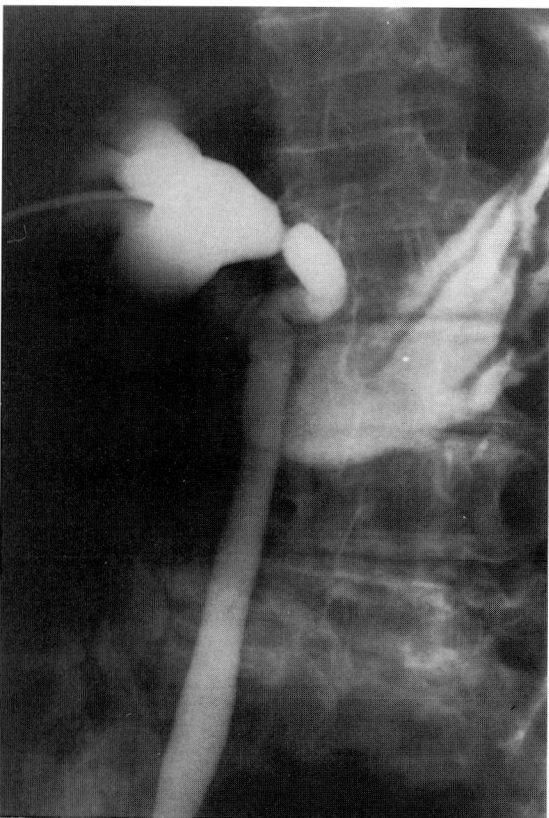

Figure 14–11. Complication of antegrade pyelography. Catheter passed through renal pelvis into duodenal bulb. Renal pelvis and ureter are opacified and hydronephrosis is readily identified. Contrast is also visualized in the stomach.

orifice successfully, bypassing a more proximal obstruction may be impossible.

Complications of retrograde pyelography include perforation of the ureter or renal pelvis, infection, and acute renal failure caused by ureteral obstruction resulting from edema after manipulation of the ureter.[53] In addition, although the incidence of minor and severe reactions to contrast media injected during retrograde pyelography is much lower than during intravenous pyelography, reactions have been reported and patients need to be monitored appropriately.

Antegrade Pyelography. Antegrade pyelography involves the placement of a percutaneous nephrostomy and is useful diagnostically when opacification of the urinary collecting system after intravenous pyelography and retrograde pyelography has been unsuccessful. This technique also has many therapeutic applications, which include nephrostomy drainage of the kidney, antegrade ureteral stenting, percutaneous nephrolithotomy, and perfusion chemolysis of renal stones.

The complications encountered when placing a percutaneous nephrostomy include bleeding, pseudoaneurysm formation, arteriovenous fistula formation, hematuria, catheter dislodgement, urinoma formation, infection, and visceral perforation (Fig. 14–11).[54]

REFERENCES

1. Pak C, Peters P, et al: Is selective therapy of recurrent nephrolithiasis possible? *Am J Med* 1981;71:615–622.
2. Finlayson B: Physiochemical aspects of urolithiasis. *Kidney Int* 1978;13:344–360.
3. Drach GW: Urinary lithiasis: etiology, diagnosis, and medical management. In: Walsh PC, et al, eds. *Campbell's Urology*, 6th ed. Philadelphia: WB Saunders, 1992;2085–2156.
4. Resnick MI, Pak C: *Urolithiasis: A Medical and Surgical Reference*. Philadelphia: WB Saunders, 1990.
5. Boyce WH: Organic matrix of human urinary concretions. *Am J Med* 1968;45:673–683.
6. Morse R, Resnick M: Urinary stone matrix. *J Urol* 1988;139:602–606.
7. Nishio S, Abe Y, Wakatsuki A, et al: Matrix glycosaminoglycan in urinary stones. *J Urol* 1985;134:503–505.
8. Roberts S, Resnick MI: Glycosaminoglycans content of stone matrix. *J Urol* 1986;135:1078–1083.
9. Fleisch H: Inhibitors and promoters of stone formation. *Kidney Int* 1978;13:361–371.
10. Nicar MJ, Skurla C, Sakahee K, Pak C: Low urinary citrate excretion in nephrolithiasis. *Urology* 1983;21:8–14.
11. Bone H, Zerwekh J, Britton F, Pak C: Treatment of calcium urolithiasis with diphosphonate: efficacy and hazards. *J Urol* 1979;121:568–571.
12. Rushton HG, Spector M: Effects of magnesium deficiency on intratubular calcium oxalate formation and crystalluria in hyperoxaluric rats. *J Urol* 1982;127:598–604.
13. Asplin J, DeGanello S, Nakagawa N, Coe F: Evidence that nephrocalcin and urine inhibit nucleation of calcium oxalate monohydrate crystals. *Am J Physiol* 1991;30:F824–F830.
14. Shiraga H, Min W, VanDusen WJ, et al: Inhibition of calcium oxalate crystal growth in vitro by uropontin: another member of the aspartic acid–rich protein superfamily. *Proc Natl Acad Sci USA* 1992;89:426–430.
15. Menon M, Krishnan CS: Evaluation and medical management of the patient with calcium stone disease. *Urol Clin North Am* 1983;10:595–615.
16. Drach GW, Perin R, Jacobs S: Outpatient evaluation of patients with calcium urolithiasis. *J Urol* 1979;121:564–567.
17. Pak C, Kaplan R, Bone H, Townsend J, Waters O: A simple test for the diagnosis of absorptive, resorptive, and renal hypercalciurias. *N Engl J Med* 1975;292:497–500.
18. Pak C, Fetner C, et al: Evaluation of calcium urolithiasis in ambulatory patients. *Am J Med* 1978;64:979–987.
19. Pak C: Should patients with single renal stone occurrence undergo diagnostic evaluation? *J Urol* 1982;127:855–858.
20. Urivetzky M, Ravalli R, Weinberg J, Smith AD: Biochemical evaluation of calcium stone patients: how soon can it be done after stone surgery/passage? *Urology* 1990;36:410–414.
21. Menon M, Mahle CJ: Oxalate metabolism and renal calculi. *J Urol* 1982;127:148–150.
22. Coe FL: Uric acid and calcium oxalate nephrolithiasis. *Kidney Int* 1983;24:392–403.
23. Coe FL, Kavalach AG: Hypercalciuria and hyperuricosuria in patients with calcium nephrolithiasis. *N Engl J Med* 1974;291:1344–1350.
24. Resnick MI, Goodman HO, Boyce WH: Heterozygous cystinuria and calcium oxalate urolithiasis. *J Urol* 1979;122:52–54.
25. Grover PK, Ryall RL, Potezny N, Marshall VR: The effect of decreasing the concentration of urinary urate on the crystallization of calcium oxalate in undiluted human urine. *J Urol* 1990;143:1057–1061.
26. Grover PK, Ryall RL, Marshall VR: Calcium oxalate crystallization in urine: role of urate and glycosaminoglycans. *Kidney Int* 1992;41:149–154.
27. Ryall RL, Grover PK, Marshall VR: Urate and calcium stones—picking up a drop of mercury with one's fingers? *Am J Kidney Dis* 1991;17:426–430.
28. Seftel A, Resnick MI: Metabolic evaluation of urolithiasis. *Urol Clin North Am* 1990;17:159–169.
29. Smith LH: Calcium-containing renal stones. *Kidney Int* 1978;13:383–389.
30. Griffith DP: Struvite stones. *Kidney Int* 1978;13:372–382.
31. Evans WP, Resnick MI, Boyce WH: Homozygous cystinuria: evaluation of 35 patients. *J Urol* 1982;127:707–709.
32. Johnson C, Wilson D, O'Fallon W, Malek R, Kurland L: Renal stone epidemiology: a 25-year study in Rochester, Minnesota. *Kidney Int* 1979;16:624–631.
33. Uribarri J, Oh MS, Carroll HJ: The first kidney stone. *Ann Int Med* 1989;111:1006–1009.
34. Sarmina I, Spirak JP, Resnick MI: Urinary lithiasis in the black population: an epidemiological study and review of the literature. *J Urol* 1987;138:14–17.
35. Prince CL, Scardino PL, Wolan CT: The effect of temperature, humidity, and dehydration on the formation of renal calculi. *J Urol* 1956;75:209–215.
36. Sierakowski R, Finlayson B, Landes RR, Finlayson CD, Sierakowski N: The frequency of urolithiasis in hospital discharge diagnoses in the United States. *Invest Urol* 1978;15:438–441.
37. Resnick MI, Boyce WH: Aetiological theories of renal lithiasis: a historical review. In: Wickham, JEA, ed. *Urinary Calculous Disease*. New York: Churchill Livingstone, 1979;1–20.
38. Spirnak JP, Resnick MI: Urinary stones. In: Tanagho E, McAninch JW, eds. *Smith's General Urology*, 12th ed. Stamford, CT: Appleton and Lange, 1988.
39. Daudon M, Marfisi C, Lacour B, Bader C: Investigation of urinary crystals by Fourier transform infrared microscopy. *Clin Chem* 1991;37:83–87.
40. Schumann GB, Schweitzer SC: Examination of the urine. In:

Henry JB, ed. *Clinical Diagnosis and Management by Laboratory Methods.* Philadelphia: WB Saunders, 1991;428–430.
41. Strasinger SK: *Urinalysis and Body Fluids: A Self-instructional Text.* Philadelphia: FA Davis, 1985;98–102.
42. Federle MP, McAninch JW, Kaiser JA, Goodman PC, Roberts J, Mall JC: Computed tomography of urinary calculi. *AJR* 1981;136:255–258.
43. Laing FC, Jeffrey RB, Wing VW: Ultrasound versus excretory urography in evaluating acute flank pain. *Radiology* 1985;154:613–616.
44. Segal AJ, Spataro RF, Linke CA, Frank IN, Rabinowitz R: Diagnosis of nonopaque calculi by computed tomography. *Radiology* 1978;129:447–450.
45. Van Arsdalen KN, Banner MP, Pollack HM: Radiographic imaging and urologic decision making in the management of renal and ureteral calculi. *Urol Clin North Am* 1990;17:171–190.
46. Schwartz G, Lipschitz S, Becker JA: Detection of renal calculi: the value of tomography. *AJR* 1984;143:143–145.
47. Hill MC, Rich JI, Mardiat JG, Finder CA: Sonography vs. excretory urography in acute flank pain. *AJR* 1985;144:1235–1238.
48. Saita H, Masao M, Fukushima H, Ohyama C, Nagata Y: Ultrasound diagnosis of ureteral stones: its usefulness with subsequent excretory urography. *J Urol* 1988;140:28–31.
49. Parienty RA, Ducellier R, Pradel J, Lubrano JM, Coquille F, Richard F: Diagnostic value of CT numbers in pelvocalyceal filling defects. *Radiology* 1982;145:743–747.
50. Pollack HM, Arger PH, Banner MP, Mulhern CB, Coleman BG: Computed tomography of renal pelvic filling defects. *Radiology* 1981;138:645–651.
51. Newhouse J, Prien E, Amis E, Dretler S, Pfister R: Computed tomographic analysis of urinary calculi. *AJR* 1984;142:545–548.
52. Sheppard PW, White FE: Demonstration of a matrix calculus using computed tomography. *Br J Radiol* 1987;60:1028–1029.
53. Imray TJ, Lieberman RP: Retrograde pyelography. In: Pollack HM, ed. *Clinical Urography: An Atlas and Textbook of Urological Imaging.* Philadelphia: WB Saunders, 1990;244–255.
54. Elyaderani MK, Kandzari SJ: Percutaneous nephrostomy. In: Elyaderani MK et al, eds. *Invasive Uroradiology,* The Collamore Press, 1984.
55. Guervara A, Springman K, Drach G, Hillman B: Triamterent stones and computerized axial tomography. *Urology* 1986;27:104–106.
56. Angell A, Resnick M: Surface interaction between glycosamines and calcium oxalate. *J Urol* 1989;141:1255–1258.
57. Barney JD: Lithiasis. In: Ballenger EG, ed. *History of Urology.* Baltimore: Williams & Wilkins, 1939, 1–25.
58. Boyce WH: Calculous disease (editorial). *J Urol* 1982;127:859.
59. Boyce WH, Resnick MI: Biochemical profiles of stone-forming patients: a guide to treatment. *J Urol* 1979;121:706–710.
60. Dean TE, Harrison NW, Bishop NL: CT scanning in the diagnosis and management of radiolucent urinary calculi. *Br J Urol* 1988;62:405–408.
61. Geterud K, Henriksson C, Pettersson S, Zachrisson BF: Computed tomography after percutaneous renal stone extraction. *Acta Radiol* 1987;28:55–58.
62. Goldman IL, Resnick MI: The diagnosis and management of uric acid lithiasis: a retrospective epidemiologic study *J Lithotripsy Stone Dis* 1989;1:107–112.
63. Hillman B, Drach G, Tracey P, Gaines J: Computed tomographic analysis of renal calculi. *AJR* 1984;142:549–552.
64. Jenkins A: Calculus formation. In: *Adult and Pediatric Urology,* 2nd ed. Gillenwater J, et al (eds). St Louis: Mosby-Year Book, 1991;403–443.
65. Kuwahara M, Kageyama S, Kurosu S, Orikasa S: Computed tomography and composition of renal calculi. *Urol Res* 1984;12:111–113.
66. Morse R, Resnick MI: A study of the incorporation of urinary macromolecules onto crystals of different mineral compositions. *J Urol* 1989;141:641–644.
67. Morse R, Resnick MI: Ureteral calculi: natural history and treatment in an era of advanced technology. *J Urol* 1991;145:263–265.
68. Morse R, Resnick MI: A new approach to the study of urinary macromolecules as a participant in calcium oxalate crystallization. *J Urol* 1988;139:869–873.
69. Murphy LJ: *The History of Urology.* Springfield, IL: Charles C Thomas, 1972.
70. Newhouse JH, Pfister RC: Antegrade pyelography. In: Pollack HM, ed. *Clinical Urography, An Atlas and Textbook of Urological Imaging.* Philadelphia: WB Saunders. 1990;2704–2714.
71. Pollack HM, Arger PH, Goldberg BB, Mulholland SG: Ultrasonic detection of nonopaque renal calculi. *Radiology* 1978;127:233–237.
72. Rao BK, Bryan PJ: Sonography of acute and chronic renal failure. In: Resnick MI, et al, eds. *Ultrasonography of the Urinary Tract.* Baltimore: Williams & Wilkins, 1991;204–235.
73. Resnick MI, Kursh ED, Cohen AM: Use of computerized tomography in the delineation of uric acid calculi. *J Urol* 1984;131:9–10.
74. Rodman JS, Williams JJ, Peterson CM: Dissolution of uric acid calculi. *J Urol* 1984;131:1039–1044.
75. Saksouk F, Tipton-Donovan A, Amis E, Goldman S: Computed tomography of perirenal and pararenal inflammatory disease complicating renal calculi. *Urology* 1984;24:200–204.

15 Section 1: Urinary Tract Obstruction and Dilatation: Upper Urinary Tract

Robert L. Waterhouse, Jr.

Urinary tract obstruction can be defined as a condition in which there is a structural and physiologic impediment to urinary outflow. Structural impediment is often implied by dilatation of urinary tract structures. However, the correlation between anatomic findings and their physiologic significance is less than perfect in defining obstruction. To compound the problem further, several factors contribute to the appearance of the urinary tract in any given individual at any given time. There is a wide variability in the manner in which the normal urinary tract will appear on various imaging studies based on the conditions that may be present (e.g., dehydrated versus hydrated state).

Obstruction is a dynamic process that may be more or less obvious, depending on the time it is investigated (e.g., ureteral pelvic junction obstruction may only be manifested during diuresis). Also, there are technical limitations to all imaging techniques and artifacts that may provide images that lead to misinterpretations of the actual clinical circumstance. These considerations amplify the importance of having a thorough understanding of the physiology of obstruction and knowledge of the capabilities and pitfalls of the various imaging modalities currently available.

ULTRASOUND

Ultrasound or sonography is a noninvasive imaging technique that has applications in the diagnosis and evaluation of upper urinary tract obstruction. Real-time gray-scale imaging should be performed in transverse and longitudinal planes.[1] The renal sinus and central portion of the kidney must be carefully and deliberately examined to discern if there is any evidence of pyelocaliectasis. Modest separation of the normally compact renal sinus echoes can be suspicious for mild hydronephrosis in the patient being screened for obstruction (Fig. 15–1). Besides these morphologic changes, more objective and reproducible quantification of obstruction may be obtained from morphometric measurements, including renal volume and the anteroposterior diameter of the renal pelvis. Such biometric studies are useful in the preoperative diagnosis and postoperative monitoring of children with obstructive uropathy.[2] However, these morphometric measurements are not widely used in clinical practice today.

As noted, the renal sinus is a very important area to examine when performing sonography to identify renal obstruction. It is composed of the collecting system, blood vessels, lymphatics, and fibrofatty tissue.[3] In the nonobstructed kidney, this region is oval-shaped on longitudinal imaging and is termed the "echodense central renal complex" or "central echo complex" (Fig. 15–2). On transverse scans, the complex is more rounded and centrally located. Although a narrow, sonolucent area can occasionally be seen within the central complex without obstruction, the diagnosis of hydronephrosis depends on detection of a defined central sonolucency or "splitting" of this complex.[4] The degree of hydronephrosis corresponds to the extent of splitting of the complex.[5,6] Using the most subtle criteria for sonographic detection of obstruction, ultrasound has excellent performance with false-negative rates reported as low as less than 1%.[7] In more recent studies, false-negative rates of 2 to 3% are reported.[8,9] However, a few rare conditions lead to the inability to diagnose hydronephrosis by sonography (Table 15–1).

Retroperitoneal fibrosis is particularly worrisome in this regard because renal obstruction in certain instances can be both severe and long-standing without demonstrable hydronephrosis on ultrasound.[10] Retroperitoneal malignancy and/or metastases as cause of renal obstruction may present a similar problem. Of the cases in which the obstructed kidney was not deemed hydronephrotic, the majority had hydronephrosis evident in the contralateral kidney.[8,9] Therefore the patient with unilateral hydronephrosis and renal failure warrants particularly careful inspection and suspicion. It is postulated that an inherent inability of the renal pelvis to distend may be secondary to either intrinsic poor compliance or tumor infiltration into the walls of the ureter and renal pelvis, producing a noncompliant system. Antegrade or retrograde contrast studies may be useful in these situations.

Although the degree of separation or dilatation of the collecting system is used to grade the severity of the hydronephrosis, it does not necessarily correlate with the amount of

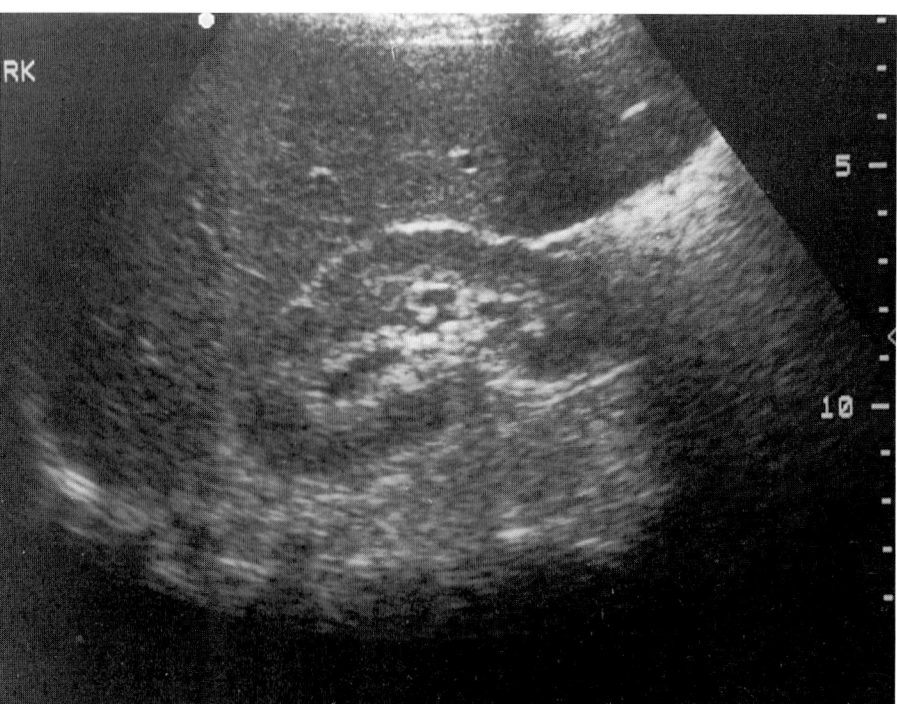

Figure 15–1. Mild hydronephrosis. The right kidney has modest separation of the renal sinus (appears white) with prominence of the collecting system (black).

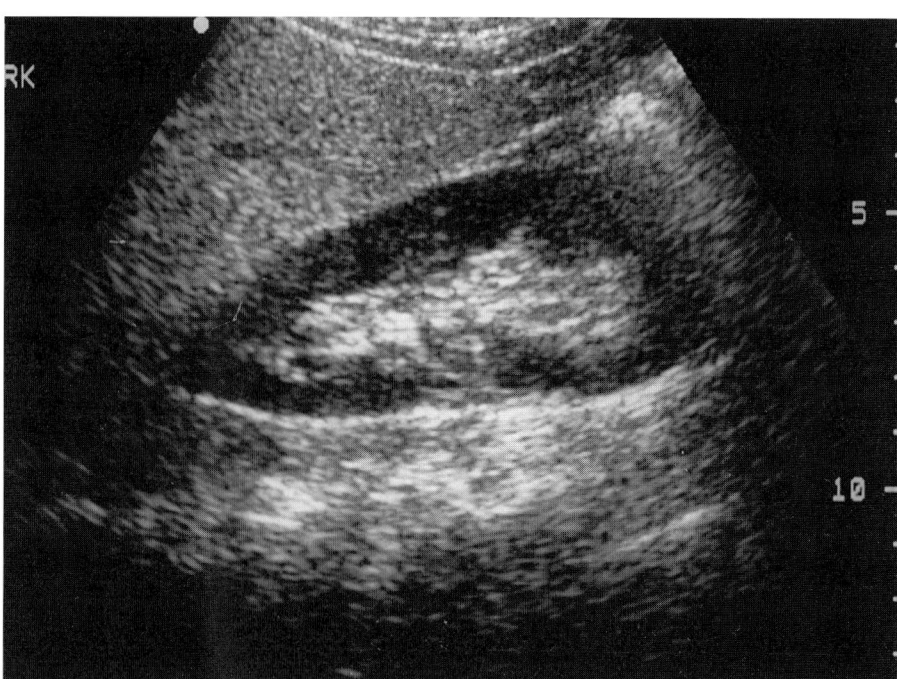

Figure 15–2. Normal kidney sonogram.

obstruction. Whether the hydronephrosis is mild, moderate, or severe, parenchymal thickness should be assessed and is of additional benefit in attempting to determine the degree of obstruction.

Once dilatation of the renal collecting system is identified during sonography, it should be followed to the ureter and as far distally as possible, in an attempt to identify the level of obstruction. In the nondilated state, the ureter is not readily imaged on ultrasound; therefore the actual visualization of the ureter may be considered significant. It may also be appropriate in these situations to scan the bladder for intravesicle sources of upper urinary tract obstruction. Here the potential etiology may derive from pathology in or around the distal ureter or bladder outlet. In the situation of a distended bladder, the kidneys should be rescanned after bladder emptying.[11] Subsequent improvement in hydronephrosis indicates the problem may involve the bladder outlet.

On the contrary, there are several situations in which non-

Table 15–1. Conditions Associated with Obstruction that May Not Be Detected on Sonography

Staghorn calculus with acoustic shadowing obscuring dilatation
A recent acute renal obstruction
Spontaneous decompression of obstructed system through backflow of extravasation
Numerous cysts or cystis disease
Retroperitoneal fibrosis
Misinterpretation of caliectasis as large renal pyramids
Dehydrated state with partial obstruction
Retroperitoneal metastases
Neonates with low glomerular filtration rate

obstructed upper urinary tracts may simulate hydronephrosis (Table 15–2). False-positive diagnoses of hydronephrosis range from 8 to 26%.[12] Although almost half the patients clinically suspected of obstruction with mild hydronephrosis on sonography will prove to be obstructed,[13] when mild hydronephrosis is discovered incidentally, only about 5% of those patients will prove to have obstruction.[14] In addition to the usual findings of a dilated collecting system on sonography, the demonstration of a dilated ureter aids in confirming the diagnosis of mild hydronephrosis as truly representative of obstruction.

INTRAVENOUS UROGRAPHY

Intravenous urography (IVU), also termed *intravenous pyelography* (IVP), is the traditional, classic method to view the urinary tract for evaluation of obstruction and other entities. Compared with sonography, it offers the benefit of both anatomic and functional information about the urinary system. Intravenous urography is also more invasive than sonography, for it involves both radiation exposure and the potential risks and morbidity that accompany the use of in-

Table 15–2. Conditions that Simulate Hydronephrosis on Sonography

Extrarenal pelvis
Simple cyst
Polycystic kidney disease
Medullary cystic disease
Lymphoma
Fluid-filled bowel loops
Renal artery aneurysm
Neonatal renal pyramids
Pyelonephritis
Vesicoureteral reflux
High flow
Congenital megacalycosis

travenous iodinated contrast. However, minor degrees of ureteral dilatation apparent on intravenous pyelography may not be delineated on sonography. Furthermore, ultrasound is more operator dependent, for there is much individual variability in how the examination is conducted in addition to the difference in interpretation of the entire live real-time study versus the static "spot" images kept as records. IVU is performed in a standard fashion with minor modification as needed by a radiologist who monitors the examination.

The three most prominent established features of obstruction on urography are the obstructive nephrogram, delayed-contrast excretion, and dilatation.[1] The degree to which any or all of these features are present provides information regarding the acuity of the obstruction (Fig. 15–3). The patterns of these features also vary according to the completeness of the obstruction. In an acute blockage of the upper urinary tract, contrast enters the nephron, but its transit through the tubules is delayed, creating a pattern of increasing nephrogenic density.[15–17] Nephrogenic density in an obstructed system maximizes in 3 to 6 hours but may last for 24 or more hours.[1] It is important to note that a hyperdense nephrogram may not develop in a case of acute obstruction if there is significant underlying renal disease or infection. In chronic obstruction, the nephrogram is often faint and not hyperdense, as renal function and renal blood flow are reduced (Fig. 15–4).[18] However, in long-standing urinary tract blockage, the nephrogram provides useful information about renal deterioration by measuring parenchymal thickness.

A delay in contrast opacification of the collecting system is a prominent finding in both acute and chronic obstruction. The degree of delayed excretion corresponds with the severity of the obstruction. Prolonged contrast transit and hypoactive peristalsis contribute to a slow mixing of contrast

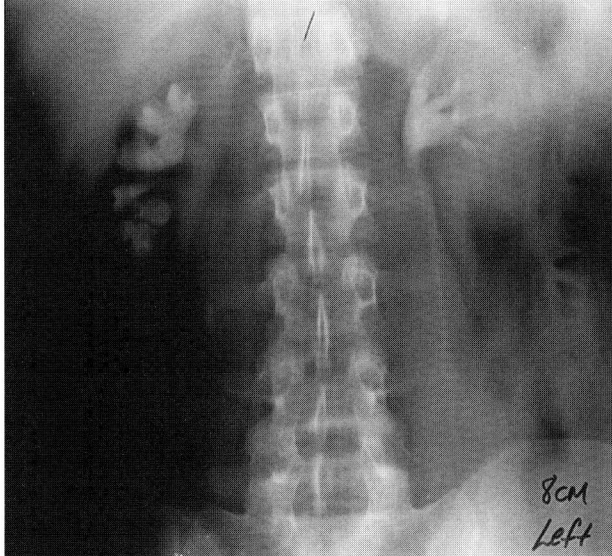

Figure 15–3. Patient with acute partial obstruction secondary to ureteral calculus illustrating hyperdense nephrogram, delayed excretion, and dilatation.

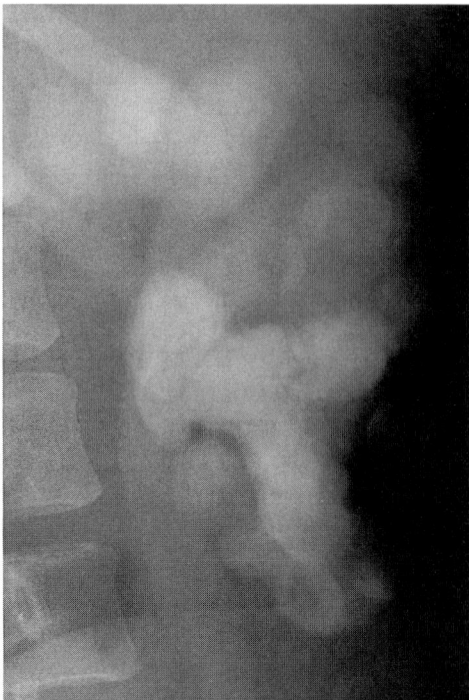

Figure 15–4. Patient with chronic high-grade partial obstruction showing absence of hyperdense nephrogram with marked dilatation secondary to ureteral stricture and partial staghorn calculus.

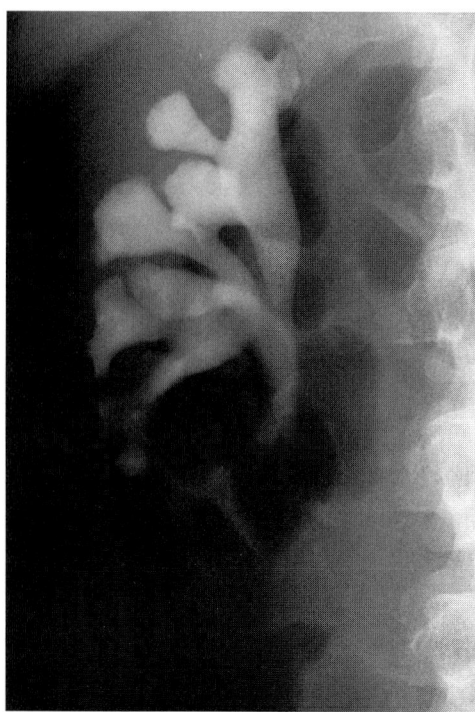

Figure 15–5. Patient with chronically dilated collecting system secondary to residual calyectasis after a stone that was obstructing for more than 3 years was removed.

into a static system. The delay can take from a few minutes to several hours. It is both important and helpful to take delayed images to follow the contrast over time as it columnizes down to the point of obstruction. On occasion the level of blockage is not well delineated because of poor concentrating ability of the impaired kidney or loss of contrast from the collecting system through extravasation via forniceal rupture.[19,20]

Similar to delayed excretion, the degree of dilatation sometimes corresponds to the severity of obstruction. This tendency is stronger for long-standing obstruction because features of hyperdense nephrogram and delayed-contrast excretion may overshadow dilatation in the acute situation.[21] However, directly correlating dilatation to the amount of obstruction should never become an assumption because each can exist independent of the other (Fig. 15–5). With chronic ureteral obstruction, the natural progression of dilatation is to develop ureteral tortuosity. Unfortunately, this finding can be overinterpreted because of physiologic variants. Overall, intravenous urography provides a wealth of information about upper urinary tract obstruction when the study is interpreted carefully and extensively in the context of the clinical scenario.

COMPUTED TOMOGRAPHY

Computed tomography (CT) has specific applicability in identifying the etiology of ureteral obstruction when intravenous urography has not been definitive and/or more invasive testing is undesirable or not helpful (e.g., retrograde pyelography). Both nonintravenous contrast-enhanced CT and intravenous contrast-enhanced CT are useful in this situation. Also, many patients with abdominal or pelvic pathology have a CT scan as part of the evaluation for their primary disease process, and obstruction of the upper urinary tract is detected incidentally.

Noncontrast-enhanced CT studies are often done when patients have decreased renal function or allergic reactions to intravenous contrast. The near water CT attenuation of the collecting system differs sharply with the renal parenchyma and the surrounding perinephric fat (Fig. 15–6). The three-dimensional capability of CT imaging also adds to understanding the source of obstruction, as the dilatation of the collecting system can be followed to its transition zone and the responsible etiology is often obvious at that point. However, noncontrast scanning does have its limitations and artifactual findings. Cysts and nonobstructed dilated calyces can be confused with true obstruction. Because this type of scanning is not a functional study, it cannot always delineate between inconsequential dilatation and significant obstruction.[12,22]

The addition of intravenous contrast enhancement to CT scanning helps to obviate this limitation because functional information can be retrieved (see Fig. 15–6). In acute obstruction, a progressively dense nephrogram develops from cortex to medulla (Fig. 15–7). There is a delay in opacification of the collecting system corresponding to the degree

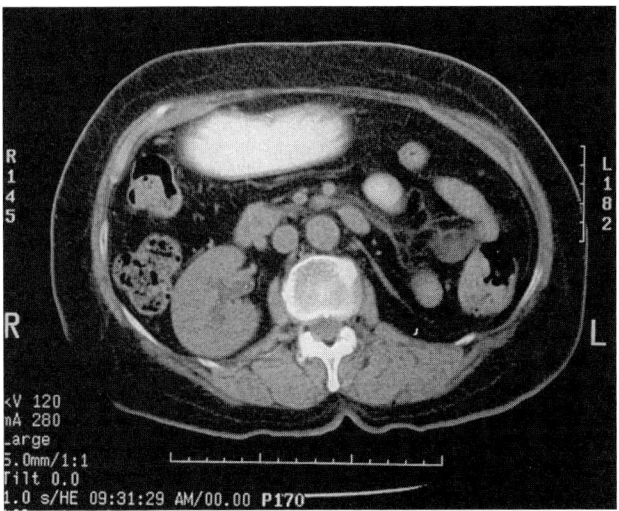 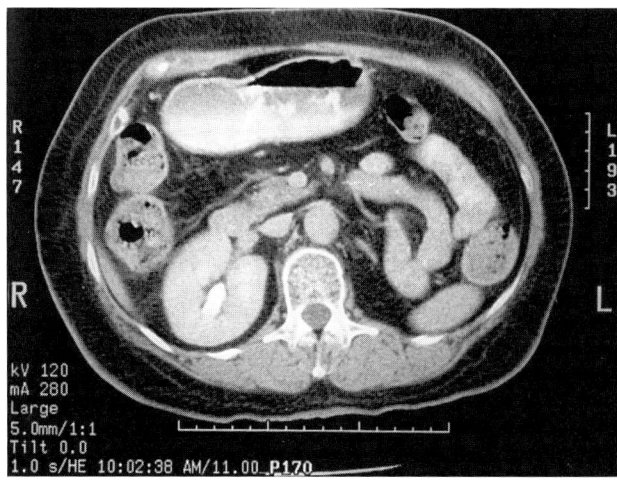

Figure 15–6. Computed tomography of kidney (**A**) without intravenous contrast, (**B**) with intravenous contrast.

of obstruction.[1] Urine contrast layering in the dependent portion of the collecting system is common. Parenchymal thickness is easily assessed to determine the acute or chronic nature of obstruction.[23,24] In chronic ureteral obstruction the dilated ureter is readily followed to the responsible etiology (Fig. 15–8). In this way CT scanning is likely the procedure of choice for evaluating extrinsic sources of ureteral obstruction.

RADIOISOTOPE SCANNING

Diuretic renography with radioisotopes is used to evaluate renal obstruction in a more quantitative fashion than either CT scanning or intravenous urography will allow. Assessing the upper urinary tract for obstruction using renography involves excretion and retention of a radionuclide, sufficient renal function to produce a subsequent diuresis, and a technique to quantitate this clearance.[25] Technetium-99m DTPA, magnesium-3, and iodine-123 hippuran are suitable radioisotopes because of their rapid clearance.[26,27] Furosemide is the standard diuretic, with diuresis beginning within 5 minutes, peaking at 30 minutes, and lasting for up to 3 hours. The diuretic effect is dose dependent, and a standardized dose between 0.5 mg/kg and 1.0 mg/kg is recommended. The timing of diuretic injection is also critical; ideally, diuretics should not be injected until radioactivity in the collecting system has plateaued. However, 15 to 20 minutes is commonly used as a compromise, because of delays in radioisotopes clearing the blood.[1]

There are several other factors to address in order to optimize renography. Patient position becomes important because of the existence of gravity-dependent obstruction.[27]

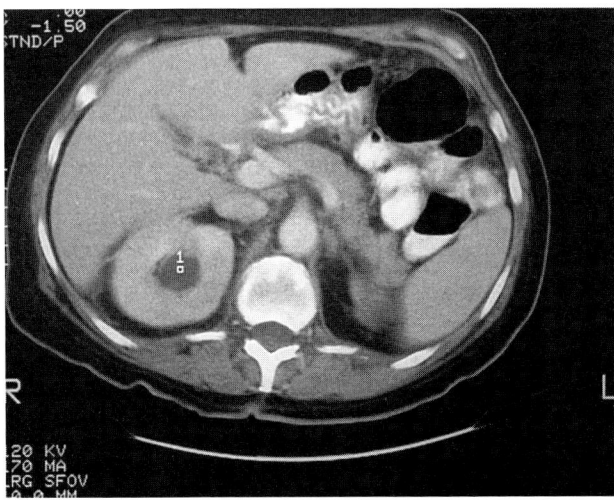 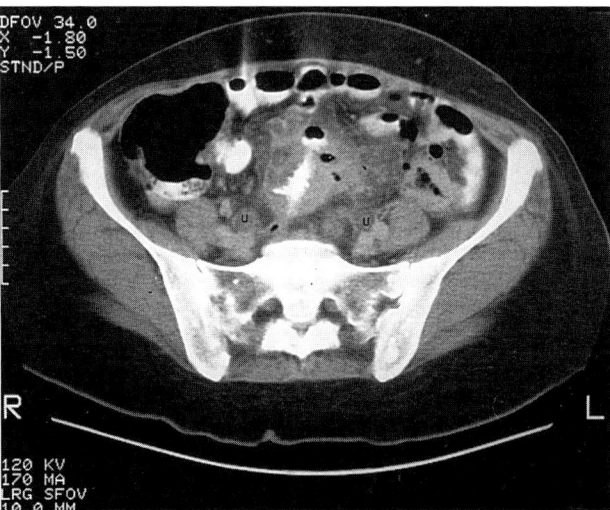

Figure 15–7. Computed tomography of kidney with intravenous contrast in patient with acute obstruction.

Figure 15–8. Computed tomography of chronically obstructed upper urinary tract with dilated ureters followed down to a pelvic mass from ovarian malignancy.

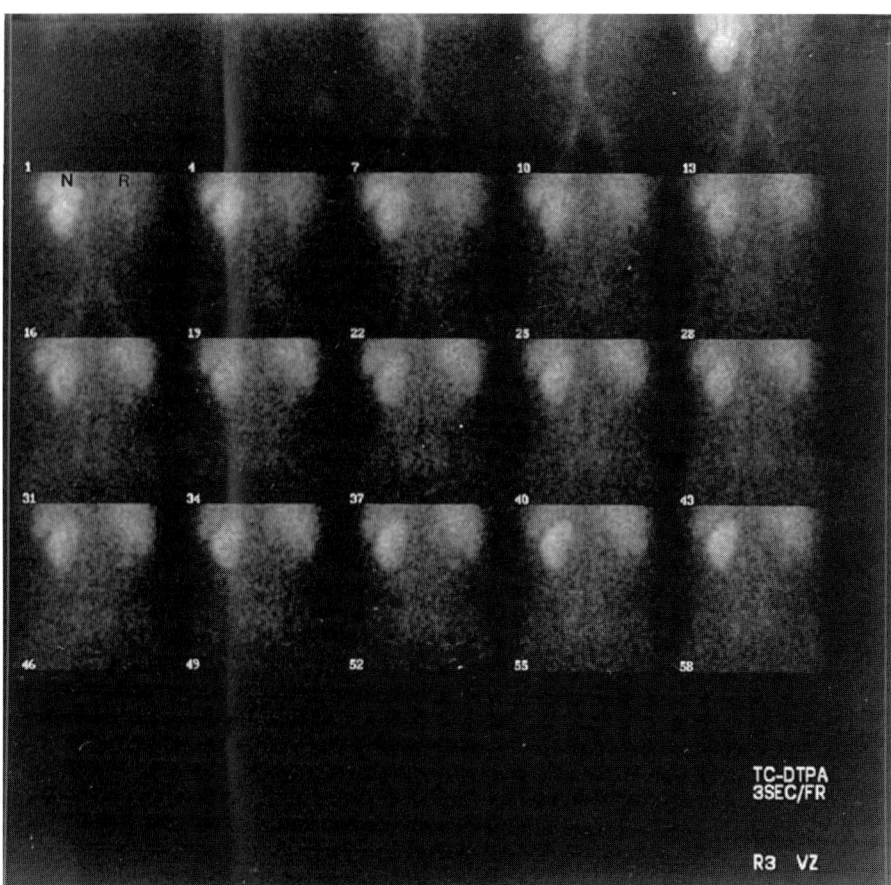

Figure 15–9. Renogram with TC-DTPA showing the typical posterior view of a patient with normal (N) left renal blood flow and reduced (R) right renal blood flow secondary to chronic right ureteral obstruction.

Sitting erect allows gravity to encourage drainage. Impaired bladder emptying or elevated bladder pressure can create an impediment to upper urinary flow in the absence of upper urinary tract obstruction.[28] Ideally, the bladder should be empty at the beginning of the procedure. If concerns exist about elevated bladder pressure as in neurogenic bladder dysfunction or dysfunctional voiding, bladder catheterization during the study is useful. Similarly, concerning vesicoureteral reflux, bladder drainage prevents spurious findings. "J-hooking" of the ureter, which occurs occasionally after ureteroneocystostomy, is also eliminated by bladder catheterization during the procedure.[29] Moreover, adequate hydration and sufficient renal function are absolutely critical to the quality of the study.

Once the renogram is started, renal blood flow is assessed during the first minute after injection. Images are taken at 3- to 4-second intervals (Fig. 15–9). Renal uptake and function are then assessed. A static image is taken to determine the area of interest where the cursor will detect function and excretion. The critical outline of the area of interest defines how accurately the kidney is scanned in total versus its background.

The excretory phase is performed by taking static images at 2- to 3-minute intervals, continuing for 30 minutes or more after Lasix is injected, if necessary. A computer mathematically calculates washout graphs of the excretion and $T\frac{1}{2}$ values that represent the time it takes for half of the radionuclide to clear the kidney. A normal system will have prompt washout with a $T\frac{1}{2}$ of less than 10 minutes (Fig. 15–10). An obstructed system has a marked delay in excretion, with a $T\frac{1}{2}$ of greater than 20 minutes (see Fig. 15–10). Unfortunately, there is an interval of $T\frac{1}{2}$ values between 10 and 20 minutes in which studies show delayed excretion, but enough to permit a definitive diagnosis of obstruction (Fig. 15–11). In these situations, repeating the study later or comparing the results to those of other dynamic tests such as a Whitaker test may yield a diagnosis. Although renograms are extremely helpful, they must be considered as part of the armamentarium and should not be considered the sole universal gold standard of obstruction.[26]

RETROGRADE PYELOGRAPHY

Retrograde pyelography has little utility in defining the presence or absence of obstruction. However, it is helpful when trying to decide if the cause is intraluminal or extraluminal. A retrograde study also defined the level of obstruction when the ureter is not visualized on antegrade procedures. Retrograde pyelography is more invasive but remains an informative procedure when necessary (Fig. 15–12).[1]

Urinary Tract Obstruction and Dilatation   321

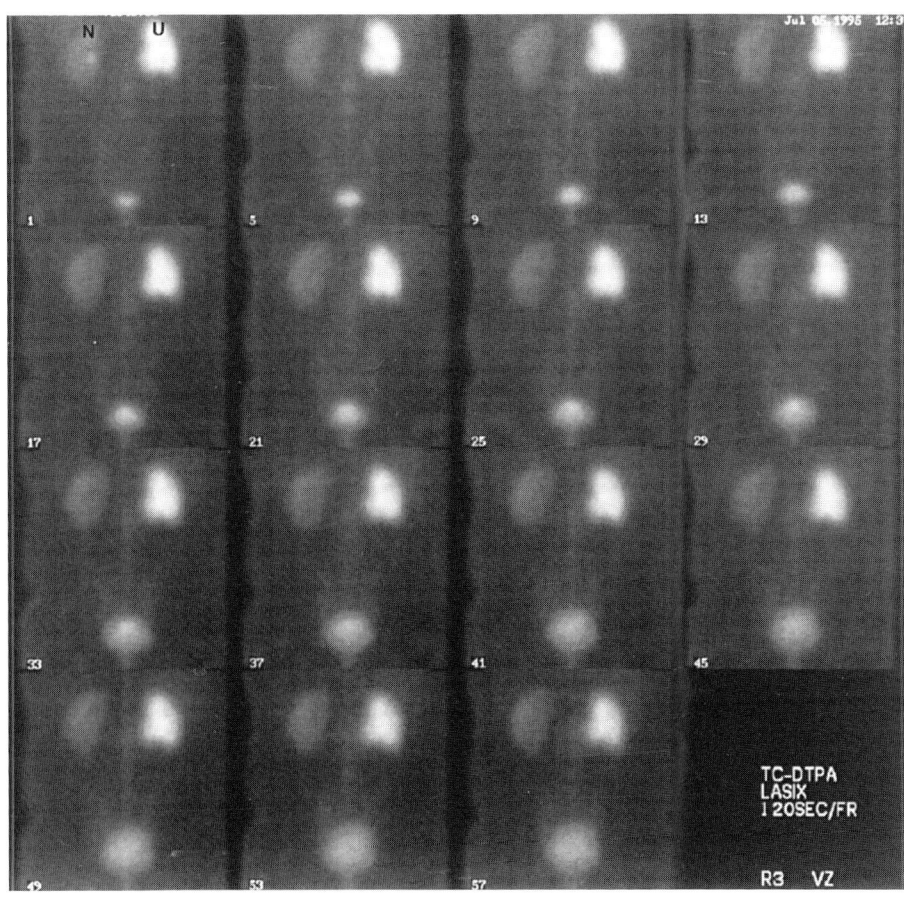

Figure 15–10. Renogram of a patient with a normal (N) left kidney showing prompt uptake and excretion with a marked delay in excretion of the left kidney after Lasix at greater than 57 minutes. The patient has right ureteropelvic junction obstruction (U).

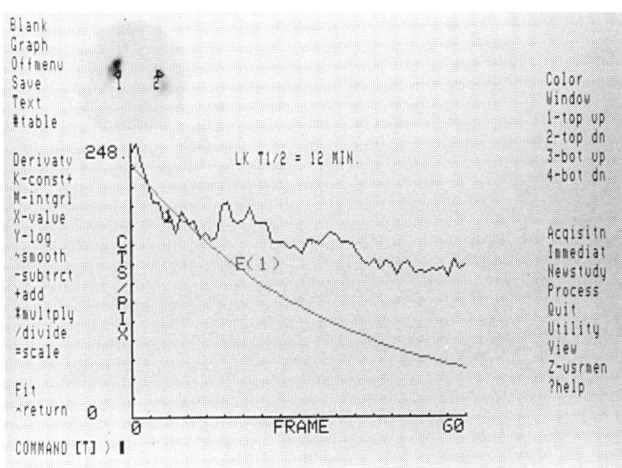

Figure 15–11. Renogram of patient that is indeterminate for obstruction with curve showing mild delay in excretion but borderline $T\frac{1}{2}$.

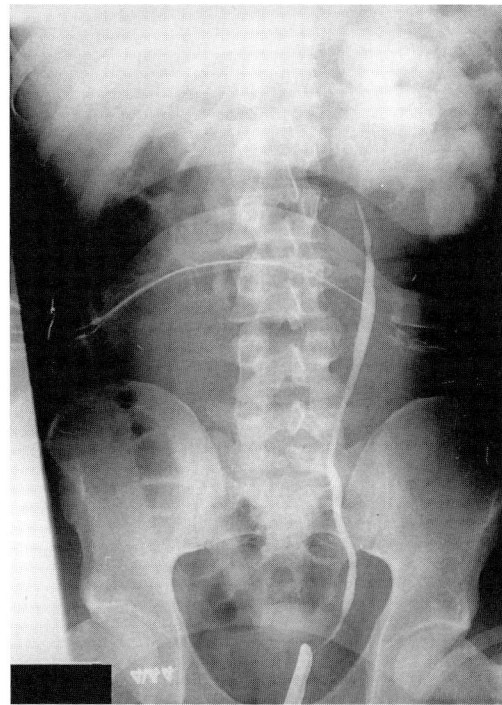

Figure 15–12. Patient with ureteropelvic junction obstruction who underwent retrograde pyelogram to delineate the ureter because it was never visualized on intravenous urogram.

CONCLUSION

All the imaging modalities discussed in this chapter have a role in evaluating upper urinary tract obstruction. It is important that the person ordering these tests have knowledge not only of the imaging techniques but also of urinary tract anatomy and the pathophysiology of obstruction. Similarly, it is critical that the individual interpreting these studies have this understanding and apply it to the specific clinical scenario of the patient being studied.

REFERENCES

1. Talner LB: Urinary obstruction. In: Pollack, HM, ed. *Clinical Urography*. Philadelphia: WB Saunders, 1990;1535–1628.
2. Dinkel E, Dittvech M, Peters H, et al: Sonographic biometry in obstructive uropathy of children: preoperative diagnosis and postoperative monitoring. *Urol Rad* 1985;7:1.
3. Amis ES, Cronan JJ, Pfister RC, Yoder IC: Ultrasonic recurrences in diagnosing renal obstruction. *Urology* 1982;19:101.
4. Sanders RC, Coward MR: The ultrasonic characteristics of the renal pelvic calyceal echo complex. *JCU* 1977;5:372.
5. Cunningham JT: Nonobstructive fragmentation of central renal pyelocalyceal echo complex. *Urology* 1979;13:94.
6. Scheible W, Tulner LB: Grayscale ultrasound and the genitourinary tract: a review of clinical applications. *Radiol Clin North Am* 1979;17:281.
7. Lee JKT, Balon RL, Melson GL, et al: Can real time ultrasonography replace static B-scanning in the diagnosis of renal obstruction? *Radiology* 1981;139:161.
8. Maillet PS, Pelle-Franco DP, Lavile M, et al: Nondilated obstructive acute renal failure: diagnostic procedures and therapeutic management. *Radiology* 1986;160:659.
9. Naidich JB: Nondilated obstructive uropathy: Percutaneous nephrostomy performed to reverse renal failure. *Radiology* 1986;160:653.
10. Lulli AF: Retroperitoneal fibrosis and inapparent obstructive uropathy. *Radiology* 1977;122:339.
11. Morin ME, Baker DA: The influence of hydration and bladder distention on the sonographic diagnosis of hydronephrosis. *JCU* 1979;7:192.
12. McClennan BL: Current approaches to the azotemic patient. *Radiol Clin North Am* 1979;17:197.
13. Curatola G, Mazzitelli R, Monzoni G, et al: The value of ultrasound as a screening procedure for urological disorders and renal failure. *J Urol* 1983;130:8.
14. Kamholtz RG, Cronan JJ, Dorfman GS: Obstruction in the minimally dilated renal collecting system: US evaluation. *Radiology* 1989;170:51.
15. Fry IK, Cattell WR: The nephrographic pattern during excretion urography. *Br Med Bull* 1972;28:227.
16. Newhouse JH, Pfister RC: The nephrogram. *Radiol Clin North Am* 1979;17:213.
17. Wesson MB, Fulmer CC: Influence of ureteral stones on intravenous urograms. *AJR* 1931;28:27.
18. Davies P, Price H: The urographic signs of acute on chronic obstruction of the kidney. *Clin Radiol* 1980;31:205.
19. Korobkin M, Jacobs RP, Clark RE, Minagi H: Diminished radiopacity of contrast material: a urographic sign of ureteral calculus. *AJR* 1978;131:847.
20. Theander G, Wehlin L: Retention of water-soluble contrast medium in the urinary and genital tracts. *Acta Radiol* 1977;18:187.
21. Pollack HM: Some limitations and pitfalls of excretory urography. *J Urol* 1976;116:537.
22. Amis ES Jr, Cronan JJ, Pfister RC: Pseudohydronephrosis on noncontrast computed tomography. *J Comput Assist Tomogr* 1982;6:511.
23. Bosniak MA, Megibow AJ, Ambos MA, et al: Computed tomography of ureteral obstruction. *AJR* 1982;138:1107.
24. Megibow AJ, Mitnick JS, Bosniak MA: The contribution of computed tomography to the evaluation of the obstructed ureter. *Urol Radiol* 1982;4:95.
25. Maizels M, Firlit CF, Conway JJ, King LR: Troubleshooting the diuretic renogram. *Urology* 1986;28:355.
26. Jewkes RF, Jeyasingh K: Comparisons of 123 I-hippuran and 99m Tc-DTPA. *Nucl Med Comm* 1982;2:278.
27. Shore RM, Uehling DT, Basskewitz R, Polyn RE: Evaluation of obstructive uropathy with diuretic renography. *Am J Dis Child* 1983;137:236.
28. Koff SA, Thrall JH, Keyes, JW Jr: Assessment of hydroureternephrosis in children using diuretic radionuclide urography. *J Urol* 1980;123:531.
29. Hensle TW, Berdon WE, Baker DH, Goldstein HR: The ureteral "J" sign: radiographic demonstration of iatrogenic distal ureteral obstruction after ureteral reimplantation. *J Urol* 1982;127:766.

15 Section 2: Bladder Outlet Obstruction

David R. Couillard, Steve W. Waxman, George D. Webster

The mechanisms by which we are able to store and expel urine involve the integrated function of the bladder, the bladder outlet, and urethra. Obstruction of the lower urinary tract is characterized by its location, and it may be structural, functional, or both (Table 15.3). Structural factors causing obstruction include vesical neck contracture, prostatic hypertrophy, prostate carcinoma, urethral valves, and urethral stricture disease. These conditions connote mechanical blockage to urinary flow and, except for benign prostatic hyperplasia (BPH), may be diagnosed by visually identifying the impediment endoscopically or radiologically. Functional conditions include dyssynergic function of the bladder neck or distal sphincter mechanisms and may result from neurogenic, myogenic, pharmacologic, or psychogenic causes and require more sophisticated diagnostic techniques to elucidate the abnormality accurately.

Bladder outlet obstruction may not be accurately defined by patient symptomatology and ideally requires urodynamic study for diagnosis. By definition, outflow obstruction is urodynamically characterized by a high detrusor pressure associated with a low voiding flow rate. The urologic evaluation of the bladder outlet necessitates a thorough and systematic history and physical examination and appropriate laboratory, radiographic, and endoscopic studies. Although not required in all patients, urodynamic study is optimal and may include simultaneous fluoroscopy (videourodynamics) and neurophysiologic techniques. With this added sophistication one can assure an accurate diagnosis of both functional and anatomic etiologies for obstructive uropathy.

SYMPTOMS

The patient interview should obtain a history that includes the chief complaint, onset and duration of all symptoms, and the chronology of events. The past surgical and medical history, review of systems, family history, social history, and a list of medications and allergies are all important. History taking may be facilitated by printed ''workup sheets,'' which may be completed by the patient prior to actual consultation.

A 3-day voiding diary is an invaluable adjunct to the diagnosis and treatment of patients with urinary incontinence or voiding problems. The log should document voiding times and volumes, and ideally should also note incontinent eqisodes, incontinence pad changes, activity status, and so on. Patients with lower urinary tract symptoms are notoriously inaccurate in their description of symptoms, and the frequency–volume chart provides significantly more credible data than information obtained by history alone.[1] The voiding diary also provides a baseline for comparison review following treatment and, by identifying customary functional capacity, acts as a guide to direct the filling volume when cystometry is later performed. It is not unusual for patients complaining of marked urinary frequency to be shown to have excessively large 24-hour urine outputs as the cause, and for the elderly patient with nocturia to be shown to be having a normal physiologic diuresis (Figure 15–13). Neither of these events requires further urologic investigation. The voiding diary is also invaluable for the establishment of a behavioral therapy program for those patients with symptoms of bladder overactivity.

Obstructive Symptoms

Obstructive symptoms are represented by hesitancy, poor flow, terminal dribbling, and ultimately retention. Such symptoms may be due not only to structural impediments to flow or functional bladder outlet obstruction, but also to poor detrusor contractility. This is particularly the case in women, in whom bladder outlet obstruction is uncommon; however, even in men with these symptoms, urodynamics finds detrusor dysfunction, not obstruction, to be the cause in 25 to 30%.[2–4] The relative importance of individual symptoms is questionable, although hesitancy and weak stream have been nonspecifically correlated with urodynamic evidence of outlet obstruction.[5–6] It is also not possible to predict reliably the outcome of treatment based on the presence or degree of any one symptom.

Hesitancy is the delay in initiating micturition. According to several authors it correlates with the presence of BPH.[7–9] It may be due to the increased opening time resulting from the outlet obstruction or to a decrease in bladder contractility. This symptom is often more prominent when the patient rises to void during the night or first thing in the morning, at which time it may represent poor activation of the micturition reflex or slight decompensation caused by overdistention. Urethral stricture disease can also produce hesitancy.

Table 15–3. Etiologies of Lower Urinary Tract Obstruction

Structural
Bladder neck contracture
Prostate carcinoma
Urethral valves
Urethral strictures
Fistulas, diverticula
Foreign body
Functional
Nonneurogenic
Bladder neck dysfunction
Dysfunctional voider (Hinman's)
Neurogenic
Proximal smooth muscle (BN) dyssynergia
Detrusor–sphincter dyssynergia
Benign Prostatic Hypertrophy

Poor force of urinary stream can be objectively quantified by uroflowmetry and can be due to either outlet obstruction or detrusor dysfunction. Like hesitancy, some consider this a cardinal symptom of BPH.[7–9] Unlike BPH, the urinary stream has less tendency to diurnal variation in urethral stricture disease.

Terminal dribbling results from continued drainage at the end of micturition, which is a result of either urine trapped in the bulbar urethra or a weak detrusor, demonstrating fatigue.[10]

Straining to void by the use of abdominal Valsalva is a nonspecific symptom caused by a variety of urologic disorders that result in a failure to empty. In the neurologically impaired patient with an acontractile bladder, an external force (the credé maneuver) may be applied to facilitate emptying. Typically, the man with bladder outlet obstruction from BPH does not strain to void because this could reduce flow by forcing the enlarged prostatic lobes together, further obstructing the outlet. These patients usually find relaxation more effective. However, patients with stricture disease find straining improves flow, and the turbulence created by the nonlaminar flow across the stricture may cause spraying of the stream. In women, urethral distortion can result from surgery, vaginal prolapse, or pelvic floor relaxation; here too straining can increase obstruction. Such patients often find that flow is improved by changing position on the commode, relaxation, and even manual replacement of the vaginal prolapse.

Two other symptoms include *intermittency* (stopping and starting during voiding) and *incomplete emptying* (the sensation of significant residual urine after micturition). Both can represent obstruction or detrusor dysfunction.

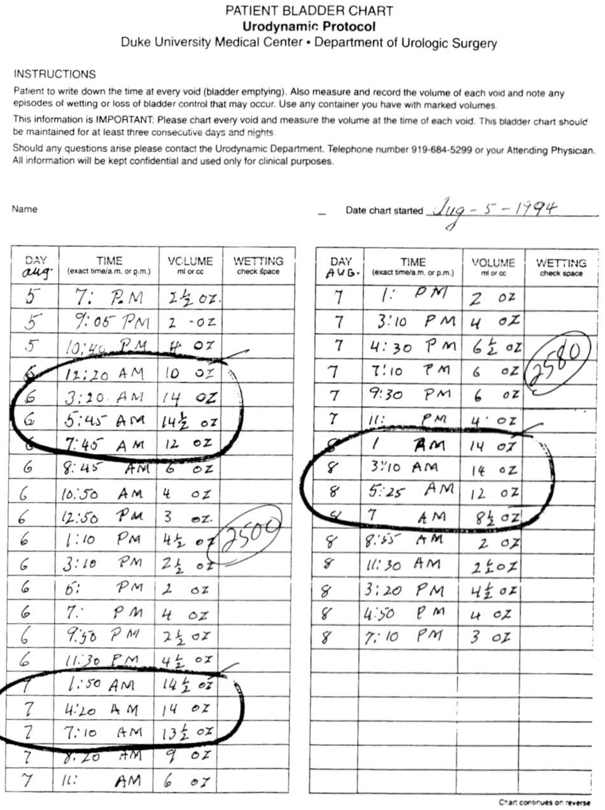

PATIENT BLADDER CHART

Urodynamic Protocol

Duke University Medical Center • Department of Urologic Surgery

INSTRUCTIONS

Patient to write down the time at every void (bladder emptying). Also measure and record the volume of each void and note any episodes of wetting or loss of bladder control that may occur. Use any container you have with marked volumes.

This information is IMPORTANT: Please chart every void and measure the volume at the time of each void. This bladder chart should be maintained for at least three consecutive days and nights.

Should any questions arise please contact the Urodynamic Department. Telephone number 919-684-5299 or your Attending Physician. All information will be kept confidential and used only for clinical purposes.

Name ____ Date chart started Aug-5-1994

DAY aug.	TIME (exact time/a.m. or p.m.)	VOLUME ml or cc	WETTING check space	DAY AUG.	TIME (exact time/a.m. or p.m.)	VOLUME ml or cc	WETTING check space
5	7: P.M	2½ oz.		7	1: PM	2 oz	
5	9:05 PM	2 -oz		7	3:10 PM	4 oz	
5	10:40 PM	4 oz		7	4:30 PM	6½ oz	2580
6	12:20 AM	10 oz		7	7:10 PM	6 oz	
6	3:20 AM	14 oz		7	9:30 PM	6 oz	
6	5:45 AM	14½ oz		7	11: PM	4 oz	
6	7:45 AM	12 oz		8	1 AM	14 oz	
6	8:45 AM	6 oz		8	3:10 AM	14 oz	
6	10:50 AM	4 oz		8	5:25 AM	12 oz	
6	12:50 PM	3 oz.		8	7 AM	8½ oz	
6	1:10 PM	4½ oz	2500	8	8:55 AM	2 oz	
6	3:10 PM	2½ oz		8	11:30 AM	2½ oz	
6	6: PM	2 oz		8	3:20 PM	4½ oz	
6	7: PM	4 oz		8	4:50 PM	4 oz	
6	9:50 PM	2½ oz		8	7:10 PM	3 oz	
6	11:30 PM	4½ oz					
7	1:50 AM	14½ oz					
7	4:20 AM	14 oz					
7	7:10 AM	13½ oz					
7	8:20 AM	9 oz					
7	11: AM	6 oz					

Chart continues on reverse

Figure 15–13. A voided volume chart (bladder diary) in an elderly woman with nocturia. The study confirms nocturnal diuresis.

Irritative Symptoms

Irritative symptoms comprise urinary frequency, nocturia, urgency, and urge incontinence. These symptoms often represent the presence of detrusor hyperactivity and are more accurately termed *instability symptoms*. Normal daytime voiding frequency is approximately every 2 hours or longer throughout the day but obviously will vary widely, depending on fluid intake. *Frequency* is best considered by analyzing the frequency/volume chart (voiding diary). Increased frequency of voiding can occur as a result of many processes other than fluid intake, and the most common are bladder hypersensitivity states of a variety of etiologies and bladder hyperactivity (Table 15–4). *Nocturia* is the interruption of sleep by the urge to void. It has the same causes as diurnal frequency, but as noted earlier, some patients mobilize fluid at night with a resulting physiologic nocturnal diuresis. *Urgency* is the extreme desire to void, which if not heeded, may result in incontinence. Frequency, urgency, and especially nocturia can be the most bothersome symptoms of the lower urinary tract that prompt the patient to seek medical attention.

As noted earlier, these symptoms are commonly attributed to detrusor instability that occurs as a consequence of outflow obstruction. Filling cystometry in men with prostatism demonstrates detrusor instability in 55 to 80% of patients, and the incidence decreases approximately 60% following transurethral prostatectomy (TURP).[2] In some men undergoing TURP the preoperative irritative symptoms may not be of obstructive etiology, in which event it is unlikely that

Table 15–4. Clinical Events Influencing Frequency

Fluid intake
Diuretic therapy
Bladder capacity
Habit
Infiltrating or ulcerative bladder neoplasmata, carcinoma in situ
Dyssynergic bladder neck
Urethral stricture
Local bladder disease
    Interstitial cystitis
    Calculus
    Tumor
    Postirradiation
Systemic disease (diabetes mellitus, diabetes insipidus, renal failure)
Chronic retention of urine
Neurologic bladder disorders
Detrusor instability
Prostatitis
Perivesical inflammatory conditions

From Rollema H: Clinical significance of symptoms, signs and urodynamic parameters in benign prostatic hypertrophy. In: Krane RJ, Siroky MB, Fitzpatrick JM, eds. Philadelphia: JB Lippincott, 1994; Table 61–1.

their surgery will improve that aspect of their symptomatology (Table 15–5). It is essential that in men whose predominant symptoms are irritative that pressure-flow urodynamic study be performed to ensure that obstruction really exists and that TURP is really necessary. In this population the detrusor overactivity may be due to aging (see later). Interestingly, when the incidence of detrusor instability in healthy elderly male volunteers is compared with that in patients with documented BPH, no significant difference is noted (53 to 52%).[11]

Table 15–5. Prevalence of Voiding Symptoms in Patients with Prostatism Compared with Men without Protatism

SYMPTOMS	PROSTATISM (%)	FIFTH DECADE	NO PROSTATISM (%) SIXTH TO SEVENTH DECADES
Hesitancy	29–78	17	30
Intermittency	29	20	30
Weak stream	46–85	30	57
Terminal dribbling	68	56	51
Diuria	38–85	40	68
Nocturia	40–85	12	33
Urgency	32–68	40	48
Urge incontinence	16–30	9	16

From Sommer P, Nielsen KK, Bauer T, et al: Voiding patterns in men evaluated by a questionnaire survey. *Br J Urol* 1990; 65:155–160, Table II.

Urinary Incontinence

Bladder outlet obstruction may result in either overflow or urgency incontinence. Overflow incontinence characteristically occurs in the large-capacity decompensated bladder and may occur as a result of either functional or structural obstruction or from poor detrusor contractility. Leakage occurs when intravesical pressure exceeds urethral resistance. Overflow may mimic stress incontinence; however, diagnosis is clinched by abdominal palpation of a distended bladder and the presence of an elevated postvoid residual. Enuresis may be an early urinary sign of the presence of overflow incontinence.

Urgency incontinence is frequently associated with outlet obstruction and is generally due to detrusor instability. When an unstable contraction occurs, the bladder neck opens automatically and continence must be maintained by the volitional contraction of the distal/external sphincter (Fig. 15–14). If for any reason external sphincteric contraction is delayed or is deficient, incontinence will occur.

Particularly in the elderly population, cognitive or functional impairment, or other physical and environmental impediments to reaching the bathroom may result in an inability to act in a timely fashion when the unstable contraction occurs; incontinence is then inevitable. Anticholinergic medication may improve instability; however, if it is used in the setting of outlet obstruction, voiding efficiency will worsen, with the possibility of urinary retention. Following the relief of obstruction, these medications may be very useful in managing persistent irritative symptoms while awaiting their spontaneous improvement.

Urologic Pain

Dysuria, or pain in voiding, may occur in association with outlet obstruction. More commonly, it indicates the presence of infection or inflammation, the incidence of which may be increased in the face of outlet obstruction as a result of increased residual urine and urinary statis, which allows for

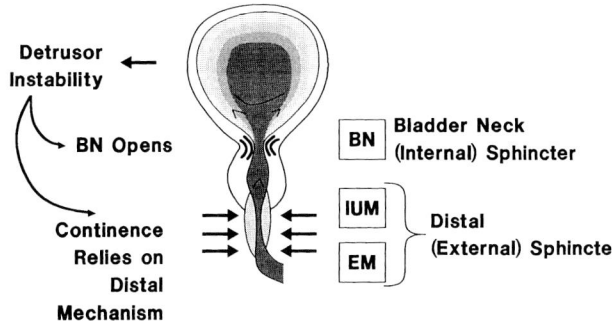

Figure 15–14. Continence is maintained by the external sphincter mechanism when the bladder neck is open in conjunction with an unstable detrusor contraction. BN, bladder neck; EM, extrinsic mechanism of the external sphincter; IUM, intrinsic mechanism of the external sphincter.

bacterial incubation. Some patients with obstruction complain of suprapubic pain relieved by voiding, presumably because of distention of the hypertrophied, somewhat inelastic bladder. Perineal discomfort can also herald prostatic disease and often accompanies prostatitis. Flank pain is uncommon in outlet obstruction but can be due to obstructive hydroureteronephrosis or upper tract infection.

Hematuria

Hematuria can occur as a result of the superficial varices that often are seen on an enlarged prostatic adenoma. The hematuria will be gross, total, and painless and will occur in the setting of obstructive symptoms. It may also result from infection, malignancy, stones, and so on; thus its occurrence must never be minimized and must be appropriately investigated.

Urinary Retention

Urinary retention is the sudden occurrence of a total inability to void, and it may result from bladder outlet obstruction or from loss of detrusor contractility. In the latter event neurogenic, myogenic, pharmacologic, or psychogenic causes may be responsible. In men with prostate outlet obstruction neither prostatic size nor the duration of symptoms is a good predictor of who will develop acute urinary retention (AUR).[12,13] It often develops in patients with minimal or recent-onset symptoms and is rare in patients with well-established symptoms. The precipitating insult may be alcohol ingestion, infection, medications such as antihistamines, or overdistention. Out of 212 patients with prostate outlet obstructive symptoms followed by Craigen et al, 89 (42%) presented in AUR, with 66% of these complaining of obstructive voiding symptoms of less than 3 months' duration.[14] Of the remaining 123 patients followed for 7 years only 10% subsequently developed AUR. Ball et al followed 107 patients with relatively stable obstructive voiding symptoms and only two patients developed AUR.[15] Acute urinary retention is usually an indication for surgical intervention. Breum et al found that 90% of patients presenting with acute urinary retention required surgery by 1 year,[16] whereas Craigen et al found that only 58% required surgery within 3 years.[14] Initial management should be catheter drainage followed by at least one voiding trial, because acute retention is reversible in some patients.

Symptom Scores

Because voiding symptoms alone do not accurately predict the presence or severity of outlet obstruction, systems have been developed that quantify the severity of individual symptoms and combine the results into a single score. These methods were devised to evaluate patients prior to surgery, to analyze outcome data following therapy, and to compare results from various treatment options. Two early symptom-scoring systems include the Boyarsky scoring system[17] and the Madsen–Iversen system.[18]

The Boyarsky system was developed at the instigation of the Food and Drug Administration (FDA) in 1976 to provide guidelines for investigating BPH. It evaluated the severity of nine voiding symptoms, scoring them from 0 to 3 for a total possible score of 27 points. The Madsen–Iversen scoring system, developed in 1983, rated force of stream, straining to void, hesitancy, intermittency, bladder emptying, stress incontinence or postvoid dribbling, urgency, frequency, and nocturia. These symptoms were each scored from 0 to 4. Patients scoring less than 10 were mildly symptomatic, those scoring 10 to 20 were moderately symptomatic, and those above 20 were severely symptomatic. The symptom score also combined objective evidence of outlet obstruction. Because symptons in these two systems were not weighted by objective data and had significant overlap with etiologies other than outlet obstruction, and because there was subjective variability regarding patients' perceptions of symptom severity, their application was severely limited.

Both Jensen et al[19] and Sommer et al[20] used calculated obstructive, irritative, and total scores (modified Madsen–Iversen score) to evaluate patients with and without prostatism. Jensen noted that all categories of symptoms scores were significantly higher in patients with prostatism than in age-matched men without prostatism. Sommer, using the same system, found approximately 20% of men in the fifth through seventh decades of life without subjective prostatism had total scores greater than 9, which was equal in severity to those in men undergoing prostatectomy!

In 1990 the American Urologic Association (AUA) established a Measurement Committee to develop a prostate symptom severity score. Barry et al developed a self-administered, seven-question symptom index (Table 15–6).[21,22] Each question on the AUA Sympton Index was rated from 0 to 5, producing a possible maximal score of 35. Symptoms were ranked by score as being mild (0 to 7), moderate (8 to 19), or severe (20 to 35). This system has been shown to be internally consistent and to correlate strongly with patients' global ratings of their urinary difficulties.[21–23] Unfortunately, the initial tests to determine the validity of the AUA scoring system was flawed by the selection of subjects. Men were selected by urologists as most likely to have prostatism as a result of a BPH comparison with younger, relatively asymptomatic patients. Chancellor et al compared urodynamic findings and AUA Symptom Index scores in 57 consecutive men and found no difference between obstructed symptomatic and unobstructed symptomatic (detrusor dysfunction) patients.[24] This was also reported by Allen and Kreder.[25] Additionally, Chancellor and Rivas reported 35 urodynamically unobstructed women with symptomatic

Table 15-6. About Your Urinary Activities

CIRCLE YOUR SCORE FOR EACH BELOW.

	NONE	1 TIME	2 TIMES	3 TIMES	4 TIMES	5 OR MORE TIMES
❶ Over the last month or so, how many times did you most typically get up to urinate from the time you went to bed at night until the time you got up in the morning?	0	1	2	3	4	5

	NOT AT ALL	LESS THAN 1 TIME IN 5	LESS THAN HALF THE TIME	ABOUT HALF THE TIME	MORE THAN HALF THE TIME	ALMOST ALWAYS
❷ Over the past month or so, how often have you had a sensation of not emptying your bladder completely after you finished urinating?	0	1	2	3	4	5
❸ Over the past month or so, how often have you had to urinate again less than two hours after you finished urinating?	0	1	2	3	4	5
❹ Over the past month or so, how often have you found that you stopped and started again several times when you urinated?	0	1	2	3	4	5
❺ Over the past month or so, how often have you found it difficult to postpone urination?	0	1	2	3	4	5
❻ Over the past month or so, how often have you had a weak urinary stream?	0	1	2	3	4	5
❼ Over the past month or so, how often have you had to push or strain to begin urination?	0	1	2	3	4	5

Total Symptom Score = Sum of Questions 1 to 7 = ☐

From the American Urological Association (AUA) Symptom Index for BPH.

voiding complaints to also have high index scores (mean of 17.5, range: 4 to 33)![26]

Despite the AUA System Index's inability to diagnose bladder outlet obstruction when used alone and the lack of correlation between urodynamic signs of obstruction, this system still has three important uses. It is a good initial patient evaluation to determine need for further investigation, it can be used to monitor surgical overuse, and it can effectively grade treatment outcome. One study of 27 men with symptomatic BPH who had an AUA Symptom Index score before and after prostatectomy showed mean scores to decrease from 17.6 to 7.1—a seemingly highly significant result.[27]

PHYSICAL EXAMINATION

Men with voiding problems due to BPH are often elderly and may have systemic conditions such as cardiovascular and pulmonary disease, and evidence of this must be sought during general physical examination. Abdominal palpation may identify the presence of a flank or abdominal mass, bladder distention, or hernia. The specific urologic examination includes the external genitalia in the male and a vaginal examination in the female. In men examination of the course of the urethra may reveal evidence of underlying urethral stricture disease in the form of induration and scarring or fistulas to the perineum. The vaginal examination in women must include a digital pelvic and a speculum examination, looking particularly for evidence of vaginal prolapse, which may result in voiding dysfunction because of distortion of the outlet. Vaginal mucosal atrophy suggests hormonal deficiency that may affect urethral function.

The digital rectal examination addresses both the presence of other rectal pathology, the innervation of the anal sphincter, and specifically evaluates the prostate gland. The prostate's size, shape, surface characteristics, and consistency are important. Prostatic size is estimated, recognizing the notorious inaccuracy of this measure and the fact that neither the size nor the architecture of the prostate gland can rule out either obstruction or carcinoma.[28] In the patient with prostate outlet obstruction, however, a particularly large gland may indicate the need for open surgical treatment.

The neurologic examination is important in both the male and female patient with voiding symptoms, emphasis being placed on the examination of the S2,3,4 dermatomes.

Residual Urine

The estimation of residual urine volume is important in the urologic evaluation of the patient with recurrent infection, incontinence, or suspected outlet obstruction. The volume can be determined by either catheterization or bladder ultrasonography (a reliable and a less invasive method). In patients with outlet obstruction its presence implies bladder decompensation. Poor detrusor contractility or other etiology, such as neurogenic bladder dysfunction, can also cause increased residual urine volumes. Bruskewitz and associates found that the residual volume did not correlate with symptoms, endoscopic findings, or urodynamic measurements in patients with obstruction.[5] They also noted a wide variation in residual urine in the same patients with BPH when measured repetitively. Although a residual urine volume of 50 mL or greater is probably abnormal, single determination can be inaccurate. Low residual urine volume may also be found in patients with significant outlet obstruction (Figure 15–15).[29]

LABORATORY STUDIES

Urinalysis and urine culture are indicated in patients with voiding symptoms. Although hematuria, either gross or microscopic, may occur in patients with outlet obstruction due to either BPH or urethral stricture disease, it may also be evidence of urologic malignancy, stones, and other benign lesions. Inefficient bladder emptying caused by outflow obstruction may result in urinary tract infection, which may lower the sensory threshold, leading to pain, irritative symptoms, and aggravating detrusor hyperactivity. A urine cytology should be obtained in older patients with irritative symptoms and in any patient with hematuria.

A complete blood count might detect anemia or infection. Serum chemistries are also important, especially to assess renal function. Although an elevated creatinine may occur for many reasons and is seen more frequently in the elderly, it also can indicate significant outlet obstruction. If the elevated serum creatinine improves following catheter drainage of the bladder, prostatectomy may be indicated. Significant azotemia is uncommon in obstructive BPH or urethral stricture disease, but upper tract dilation and damage can result from progressive bladder decompensation, a rising postvoid residual, and infection.

The level of serum prostate specific antigen (PSA) should be checked in patients being evaluated for voiding symptoms, those with an abnormal or suspicious digital rectal examination, those with a positive family history, and routinely in patients between the ages of 50 and 70 years with an expected 10-year survival. Its more discriminating use in those patients more than 70 years of age is debated. Both BPH and prostate cancer can elevate the PSA. Using a PSA threshold of 4.0 ng/mL (Hybritech assay), the sensitivity for detecting adenocarcinoma of the prostate is approximately 70%, and the specificity is only about 50%.[30] The use of PSA density, determined by dividing the serum PSA value by the estimated prostatic volume is measured by transrectal ultrasound (TRUS), may be able to differentiate small volume prostate cancer from BPH. Benson and associates evaluated 533 patients. Assuming prostate cancer prevalence at 18.4%, a PSA density value of 0.15 corresponds to a 12% probability of finding cancer.[31] Another factor may be the increase in serum PSA over time, which is referred to as PSA velocity. The rate of increase is usually higher in prostate cancer than in BPH. A PSA velocity of more than 0.75 ng/mL per year can differentiate cancer from BPH with a specificity of greater than 90%; however, the sensitivity remains low.[32] High grade tumors may not make as much PSA and can invalidate the preceding equations. Suspicion of prostate cancer for any reason should prompt further investigation.

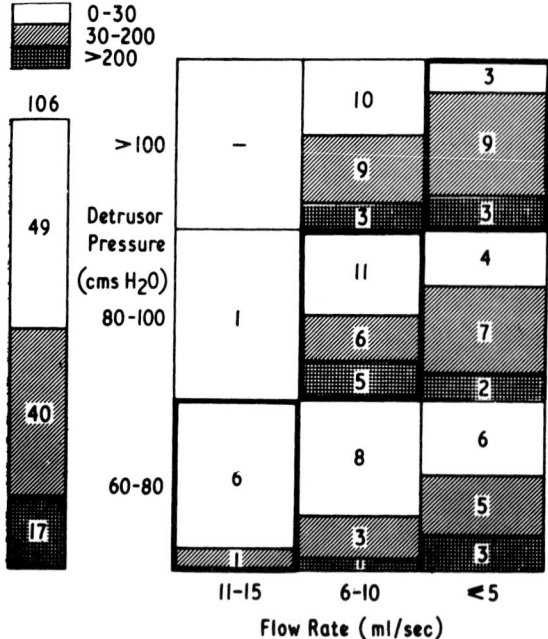

Figure 15–15. Residual urine volume related to the severity of prostatic obstruction. One hundred six patients with prostatic obstruction are grouped according to urodynamic micturition study results and the volume of their residual urine. It is evident that the degree of outlet obstruction as assessed by their voiding pressure and urine flow rate does not correlate with the volume of residual urine. (From Turner-Warwick R, Whiteside CG, Arnold EP, et al: A urodynamic view of prostatic obstruction and the results of prostatectomy. *Br J Urol* 1973;45:631.)

ENDOSCOPY

Cystourethroscopy can provide important information about urethral, prostatic, and bladder morphology but cannot always accurately diagnose infravesical obstruction. No studies have shown a significant correlation between bladder trabeculation and urodynamic evidence or severity of outflow obstruction.[33-35] However, despite its limitations and inability to characterize a dynamic system, certain clinically pertinent information may be obtained. No data have objectively correlated visual appearance of the prostatic urethra with outflow obstruction in patients with BPH.[27] It can identify structural obstructions such as that due to urethral stricture or bladder neck contracture, and it can give some useful information in men with BPH. The length of the prostatic urethra is normally less than 3 cm, and significant increase in this length may affect the surgical approach to prostatectomy. Endoscopy of the bladder is essential if hematuria is present and also should record trabeculation, diverticula, bladder neck morphology, position of the ureteral orifices, prostatic median lobe presence, stricture disease, malignancy, and bladder stones.

RADIOGRAPHIC IMAGING

Historically, excretory urography (intravenous pyelogram [IVP]), retrograde urethrography, and voiding cystourethrography were included in the evaluation of outlet obstruction. Currently, their use is limited to those cases where specific indications exist. Ultrasonography—a noninvasive method of imaging the prostate, bladder, and kidneys—has achieved wider application. Table 15–7 lists urographic alterations seen in outlet obstruction.

Plain Abdominal Radiograph

The plain abdominal radiograph provides surprisingly little information in patients complaining of obstructive voiding symptoms and is rarely indicated. It may be obtained to rule out spina bifida occulta or spinal abnormalities in patients with neurogenic bladder dysfunction, and may be performed in those with strong indications for the presence of calculi in either the lower or upper urinary tract.

Intravenous Pyelogram (IVP)

Excretory urography is no longer routinely indicated in the evaluation of outlet obstruction, for fewer than 5% of patients with prostatism will demonstrate hydronephrosis on IVP.[36,37] It is only a crude measure of renal function, a factor better studied by other specific tests. When excretory urography is performed in patients with outlet obstruction, the features generally sought are upper tract dilatation, prostatic encroachment on the bladder base, calculi, bladder wall thickening and trabeculation, elevated postvoid residual, and bladder diverticula.

Table 15–7. Urographic Alterations Attributable to BPH

Kidney
  Parenchymal atrophy secondary to long-term pyelocaliectasis
  Prominence of fetal lobations with atrophy
  Extravasation of contrast medium

Pelvis and calyces
  Mild, moderate, or severe pyelocaliectasis (hydronephrosis). (Recovery varies with time and degree of obstruction.)
  Degree of hydronephrosis (and resultant parenchymal atrophy) is greater with an intrarenal pelvis; that is, large extrarenal pelvis may diminish degree of caliectasis.

Ureters
  Tortuous, redundant, dilated (atonic) ureters
  Diminished or ineffectual peristalsis
  Elevation (cranial) of distal ureters (fishhook, J hook, or hockey stick deformity)
  Asymmetry of findings if there is subtrigonal compression by large adenoma

Bladder
  Increased size secondary to urinary retention
  Elevation of bladder base; smooth; irregular; may be asymmetric
  Thickened bladder wall (2 to 3 mm is normal)
  Trabeculated mucosal pattern (minimal or coarse)
  Cellule or diverticulum formation (mild or diffuse)
    Diverticula may be multiple and exceed size of bladder
    Hypotonic; poor emptying; varied postvoiding residual

Prostate
  Seen indirectly as result of bladder floor deformity
  Bladder indentation (varies)
  Intravesical component (median lobe enlargement)
  Distortion of bladder neck and elongation of posterior urethra
  Trigonal or intraureteric ridge enlargement or effacement

From McClennan BL: Diagnostic imaging evaluation of benign prostatic hyperplasia. *Urol Clin North Am* 1990;17(3):523.

Retrograde Urethrography

This is a most important study in the patient with suspected urethral stricture disease in whom it will localize and characterize the stricture and assist in formulation of a treatment plan. The study should visualize the entire urethra, and if this is not possible an antegrade voiding study may be necessary either by the voiding film following excretory urography or through a suprapubic cystotomy. This is especially important in posterior urethral distraction defects following pelvic fracture urethral injury in whom bladder neck competence and the length of the distraction are important considerations. Other urologic conditions producing voiding symptoms or outlet obstruction that may be evaluated by retrograde urethrography include urethral diverticulum, fistula, abscess, and trauma. Retrograde urethrography is not performed routinely in the evaluation of patients with outlet obstruction.

Voiding Cystourethrography

Historically, voiding cystourethography has been performed to diagnose reflux, but it finds particular value in the visualization of the bladder outlet in patients with bladder outlet obstruction. Ideally, it is performed under fluoroscopy, "spot" films being exposed to document representative events. Its value is enhanced by the simultaneous monitoring of urodynamic events, a study called videourodynamics, which is discussed later. Alone, a voiding cystourethrogram is not indicated in the routine evaluation of patients with suspected outlet obstruction.[27]

Ultrasonography

Ultrasonography is noninvasive, fast, and safe, and has several applications in the evaluation of bladder outlet obstruction. Small, hand-held units can rapidly measure residual urine volume. More sophisticated apparatus is used to image the upper tracts to look for hydronephrosis, calculi, or renal masses, and the study is especially valuable when renal function is impaired and the use of intravenous contrast material is contraindicated.

Transrectal ultrasonography is most valuable for the examination of the prostate, providing the best cross-sectional anatomic depiction of the gland.[38] In uncomplicated BPH the gland is usually spherical or ellipsoid and a formula can be used to calculate its size. The formula to determine the volume of an ellipse or a prolated ellipse (Vol = $L \times W \times D \times \pi/6$) can be used to calculate prostatic volume, and because prostate specific gravity ranges from 1.0 to 1.5, prostatic weight in grams can be estimated by multiplying volume by specific gravity.[39] This calculation can be used to determine PSA density.

In patients with a clinical suspicion of prostate carcinoma transrectal ultrasound-guided biopsy is now mandatory. Prostate carcinoma usually arises in the peripheral zone of the prostate but may occasionally arise in the transition zone.[40] When the tumor is small the image is most often hypoechoic, but as its volume increases its appearance can be variable.[41,42] Occasionally, hypoechoic or hyperechoic areas can be seen in BPH, probably representing either microcalculi or corpora amylacea.[43]

Although ultrasonography can identify BPH, help diagnose prostate carcinoma, and document residual urine and hydronephrosis, it does not predict or give direct objective evidence of bladder outlet obstruction, and so the decision to treat should rarely be based on its findings alone. Routine use of renal or transrectal ultrasonography, unless directed by clinical suspicion of cancer or renal disease, is not indicated in the evaluation of the patient with bladder outlet obstruction.

URODYNAMIC EVALUATION

Although symptoms, symptom scores, physical examination, and laboratory studies provide needed clinical data, they cannot alone accurately diagnose bladder outlet obstruction or identify whether a patient's complaints and manifestations arise from obstruction or another lower urinary tract condition. Similarly, radiographic imaging and endoscopy are limited by the fact that they generally provide a static evaluation of a dynamic problem. Urodynamic study is the optimal method used to diagnose bladder and outlet obstruction, and the studies performed may range from simple uroflowmetry to videourodynamic study (Table 15–8). These studies are discussed in Chapter 3, but their role in the identification and characterization of bladder outlet obstruction will be presented here.

Cystometry

Filling cystometry is the graphic representation of bladder pressure as a function of increasing volume. Because this test characterizes only the filling phase, it does not have a specific role in the diagnosis of bladder outlet obstruction. Detrusor instability is defined as an involuntary phasic detrusor contraction of any pressure associated with symptoms of urge and/or leakage occurring while the patient is attempting to inhibit micturition.[44] Clinically, the unstable bladder presents with a symptom complex of frequency, nocturia, urgency, and urge incontinence, known collectively as the "urge syndrome," which is frequently seen in patients with bladder outlet obstruction. Provocative filling cystometry demonstrates detrusor instability in 55 to 80% of patients with prostate outlet obstruction, and the incidence decreases to 22 to 50% (slightly less than half) following transurethral prostatectomy (TURP).[45,46] Only one series has shown men with a greater degree of obstruction by urodynamic criteria to have a greater incidence of instability.[47]

Studies of human and animal detrusor muscle preparations with obstruction and instability have generated several

Table 15–8. Urodynamic Armamentarium

Uroflowmetry
Cystometry
Pressure–flow studies
Videourodynamics
Ambulatory urodynamics
Urethral pressure studies
Sphincter EMG

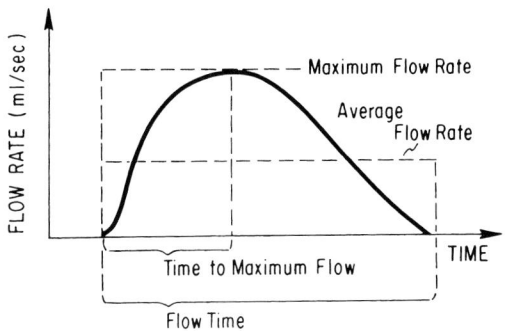

Figure 15-16. Idealized uroflow curve identifying frequently measured variables.

tomy.[50] Moreover, preoperative cytometry has not been shown to have any preoperative prognostic value for the outcome of prostatectomy and is of no clinical value in diagnosing bladder outflow obstruction.[49-52]

Uroflowmetry

Uroflowmetry is a commonly used, noninvasive, and inexpensive test that measures urinary flow, defined as the voided volume per unit time (mL/sec). For improved interpretability more than one flow rate should be obtained because several factors, including voided volume, emotional stress, and degree of abdominal straining, may cause varying results. The parameters generated include total voiding time, time to peak flow, mean flow rate, and peak flow rate (Fig. 15-16). Peak flow rate (Q_{max}) correlates best with the presence of outlet obstruction, with the other parameters providing lesser value in the assessment.[49] Peak flow varies with the volume voided, and it is generally accepted that voided volumes of less than 150 mL generate inaccurate flow patterns and parameters.[53-55] For this reason several nomograms have been constructed to allow for the comparison of flow rates regardless of voided volume.[49] Siroky et al constructed a nomogram from 300 flow rates in 80 normal men, and 98% of patients with documented outlet obstruction had nomogram corrected flow rate values beyond 2 standard deviations from the mean (Fig. 15-17).[55] Abrams and Griffiths have also constructed a flow rate nomogram and have in the past arbitrarily set the limit for a normal flow rate at ≥15 mL/sec on a minimum voided volume of 150 mL and an obstructed flow rate at ≤10 mL/sec; measurements between these two limits were considered equivocal.[56] The morphology of the uroflow curve may also reveal valuable information, the con-

hypotheses as to the cause and relationship.[48] The explanation enjoying the most support is that of postjunctional supersensitivity probably resulting from partial parasympathetic denervation. Other possible contributing factors include altered adrenoceptor function, afferent nerve dysfunction, an imbalance of peptide neurotransmitters, and a primary or acquired myogenic defect.[48]

Most studies show that both preoperative and postoperative detrusor instability correlate with irritative symptom scores and are associated with continued symptoms following surgery.[49] Persistence of instability following relief of obstruction may be a result of a failure of the detrusor to recover, regardless of cause, or may be due to the instability resulting from an etiology other than obstruction, such as age-related decreased cortical inhibition. No reliable cystometric predictor has been found that determines whether detrusor instability will resolve following surgery. Some patients with chronic retention and high-pressure bladder contractions may have a good prognosis after prostatec-

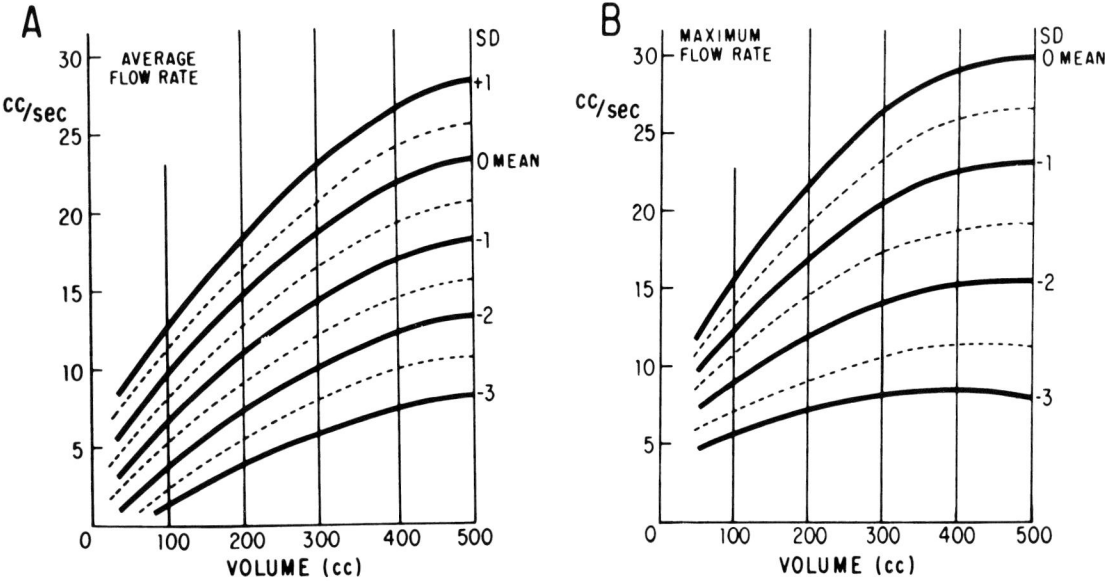

Figure 15-17. Flow rate nomogram relating average flow rate and maximum flow rates to volume voided. (From the flow rate nomogram: I. development. Siroky MB, Olsson CA, Krane RJ: *J Urol* 1979;122:665.

tour in the presence of abdominal straining being quite typical.

A normal-appearing flow curve and peak flow rate do not exclude the presence of bladder outlet obstruction, 17 to 25% of patients referred with symptoms of prostatism having high-flow obstruction.[57,58] This may be due to detrusor compensation in the face of significant obstruction, and in this setting, the incidence of persistent postoperative detrusor instability may be high and adversely affect outcome.[59]

A major problem with uroflowmetry is its inability to distinguish between a poor flow resulting from infravesical obstruction and that due to impaired detrusor contractility. Several studies have addressed the ability of uroflowmetry or corrected uroflowmetry to predict the presence of outlet obstruction. Schafer reported that only 75% of patients with obstruction according to the Siroky nomogram had outflow obstruction based on Passive Urethral Resistance Relation (PURR, computer-assisted pressure/flow relation).[60] Chancellor et al, using the Abrams–Griffiths method, demonstrated that uroflowmetry could not distinguish between outflow obstruction and impaired detrusor contractility.[61] Nielsen et al, summarizing data collected by Jensen and Schou, demonstrated that uroflowmetry alone is insufficient in diagnosing infravesical obstruction.[49] Despite these misgivings, it continues to be extensively used because it is noninvasive, easy, and useful as a screening tool in the evaluation of patients with suspected outlet obstruction.

Pressure–Flow Studies

Recognizing the previously mentioned limitations in the identification of bladder outlet obstruction, pressure–flow studies offer the next best hope for its accurate diagnosis. These studies ideally require the simultaneous recording of detrusor pressure and urine flow rate during volitional voiding (see Chapter 3 for a detailed description). Detrusor pressure (Pdet) cannot be measured directly but is obtained by subtracting abdominal pressure (Pabd) from total bladder pressure (Pves), this subtraction being done electronically by the urodynamic equipment. Abdominal pressure is also not directly measureable but is approximated by recording rectal pressure.

A number of variables may be recorded during pressure flow study, including the opening pressure, pressure at peak flow, maximum micturition pressure, and so on (Fig. 15–18). Unfortunately, there is no consensus regarding a critical value for pressure and flow that is diagnostic for obstruction. Although it is certainly true to say that there would be little argument that obstruction existed in a patient in whom Pdet was 100 cm H_2O at Qmax of 10 mL/sec, there would be less agreement in a patient with a pressure of 50 cm H_2O and flow rate of 10 mL/sec. Recognizing this dilemma, Blaivas suggested that obstruction is suggested by a pressure–flow study in which low flow occurs despite a detrusor contraction of adequate force, duration, and speed regardless of the actual numerical values. Fortu-

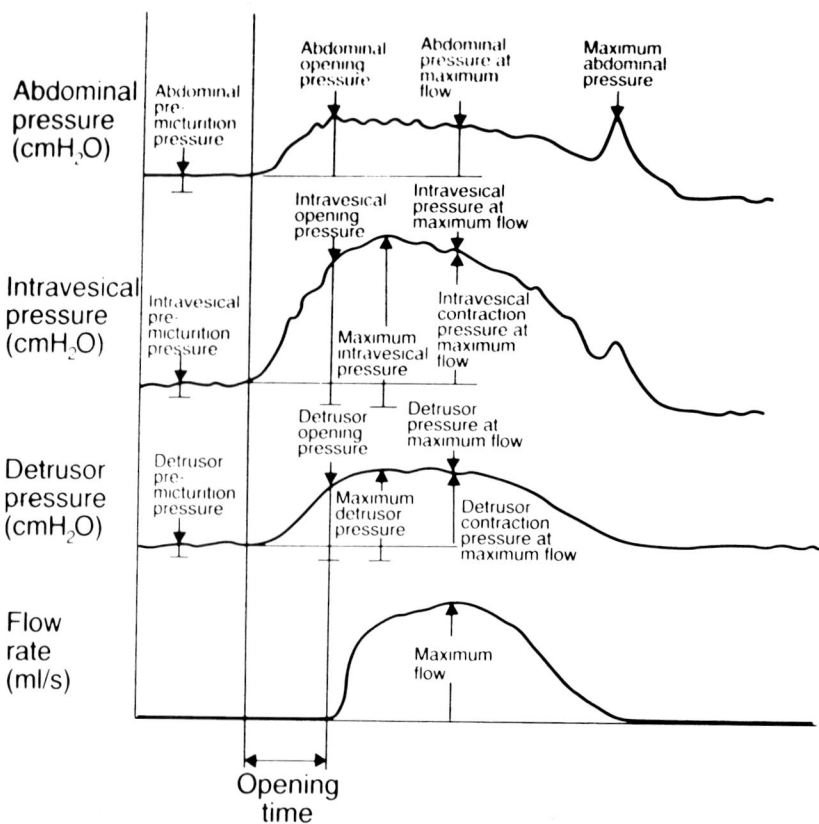

Figure 15–18. Frequently measured variables during pressure–flow micturition studies.

nately, in the majority of cases studied the urodynamic data are diagnostic.

Other methods devised to assist in the diagnosis of bladder outlet obstruction using pressure–flow data include the calculation of a urethral resistance factor.[62] Such equations assumed laminar flow through a rigid tube, and despite their accuracy in straightforward cases of high-pressure–low-flow and low-pressure–high-flow examples, the urethral resistance factors could not reliably distinguish between cases in the borderline area.[56] Hence their use has been abandoned by the International Continence Society's Standardization Committee.[62]

Computer-Assisted Analysis of Pressure–Flow Data

In the early 1970s Griffiths developed the Urethral Resistance Relation.[63–65] This was based on the principle that the urethra is a distensible, elastic tube and that a flow-controlling zone of maximal resistance exists. This concept graphically describes the relationship between detrusor pressure and urinary flow in order to define the lowest point of resistance for micturition. This point, the flow-controlling zone, is presumed to be situated at the pelvic floor under physiologic conditions.[66] When bladder outlet obstruction exists, the site of obstruction becomes the flow-controlling zone.[65,67] Abrams and Griffiths developed the pressure–flow rate nomogram plotting detrusor pressure (Pdet) versus maximal flow (Qmax)[56] (Fig. 15–19).[56] The three areas on the graph are an obstructed, unobstructed, and equivocal area. If the result of the patient being evaluated fell into the equivocal area a plot was drawn with values recorded throughout the entire micturition (Fig. 15–20). The mean slope and maximal detrusor pressure were then analyzed. If the average slope was less than 2 cm H_2O/mL^{-1} sec^{-1} and the detrusor pressure was less than 40 cm H_2O when flow ended, the patient was not obstructed, whereas if the average slope was greater than 2 cm H_2O/mL^{-1} sec^{-1}, and the detrusor

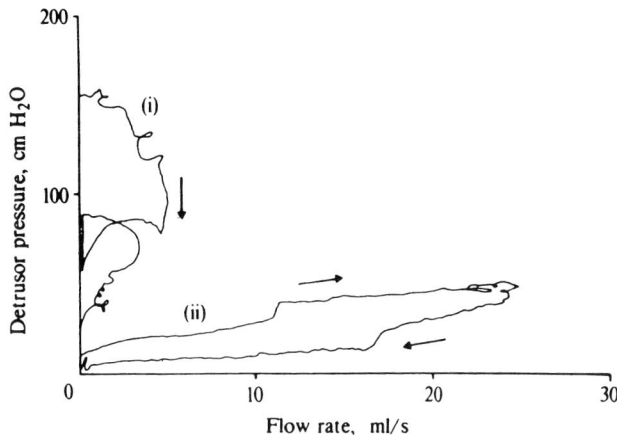

Figure 15–20. Detrusor pressure–flow plots, obtained during micturition of two males. Obviously obstructed (i) and nonobstructed (ii) plots are shown. In these cases it is easy to see from the shape of the plots that the patients are obstructed (low flow rate, high detrusor pressure) and not obstructed (high flow rate, low detrusor pressure), respectively. (From Abrams PH, Griffiths DJ: The assessment of prostatic obstruction from urodynamic measurements and from residual urine. *Br J Urol* 1979;51:129–134.)

pressure was greater than 40 cm H_2O when flow ended, the patient was classified as obstructed.

Jensen and associates, using this Abrams and Griffiths definition of outlet obstruction (using computer analysis of simultaneous pressure/flow plots), performed a prospective, preoperatively blind study on a group of patients selected for TURP based on standard clinical criteria.[68] Several important results were noted. Although there were statistically significant differences between the obstructed and unobstructed groups preoperatively, there were no differences postoperatively. Further urodynamic analysis showed that prostatectomy did not significantly change voiding in the unobstructed group, whereas all the obstructed patients became unobstructed.[49] When subjective outcome after TURP was related to preoperative assessment, the obstructed men had a success rate of 93%, whereas the success rate in the unobstructed group was 78%. The success rate for TURP in unobstructed men not only indicates a high placebo effect, but also suggests that TURP may benefit the patient by an unknown mechanism, possibly affecting sensory input in view of the fact that urodynamic parameters were unaffected. Despite this phenomenon, pressure–flow study and particularly its further elaboration and interpretation using computerized analysis are important from both a diagnostic and prognostic standpoint, and certainly in analyzing outcome from prostatectomy.[49]

Several other authors have used theoretical modeling and computer analysis of pressure–flow data to describe more accurately the physical phenomenon of bladder outlet obstruction. Schafer defined urethral resistance by a formula that includes the cross-sectional area of the urethra (A) and the minimal opening pressure (Pmuo) ($Q \sim A \cdot \sqrt{Pdet - Pmuo}$). Fluid will flow through a tube from a

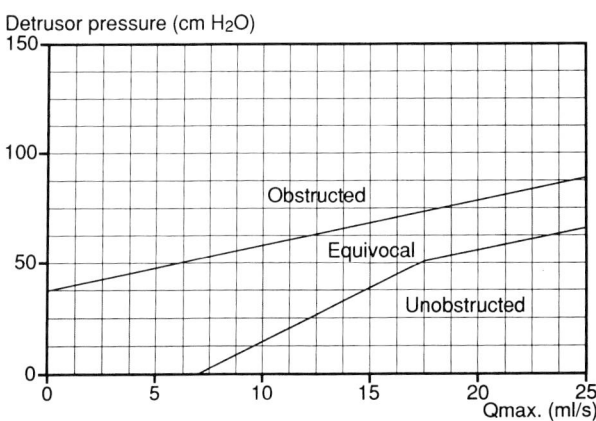

Figure 15–19. Abrams and Griffiths nomogram. (From Abrams PH, Griffiths DJ: The assessment of prostatic obstruction from urodynamic measurements and from residual urine. *Br J Urol* 1979; 51:129–134.)

higher to lower pressure; the velocity will be proportional to the difference. This equation demonstrates that flow (Q) depends on several factors: The cross-sectional area (A) and the detrusor pressure (Pdet) less the pressure required to open the system at the elastic flow-controlling zone (Pmuo, the urethral opening pressure).[66,69] Minimal opening pressure is the pressure at which flow commences and is the measure of the degree of compressive obstruction. The constrictive component of BPH is somewhat ignored. This is again based on the urethra as a distensible tube with a flow-controlling zone (the relaxed bladder neck under pathologic conditions).

The balance of mechanical energy during micturition involves the combination of the contractile ability of the detrusor and the characterization of urethral resistance at the outlet that can be described in a pressure–flow graph (Fig. 15–21). Specific types of obstruction involve changes in the lumen size and opening pressure and are represented by constrictive (i.e., stricture) or compressive (i.e., BPH) patterns of obstruction (Fig. 15–22).[66] When pressure and flow are plotted against each other for each moment of time and analyzed by a computer, assuming the urethra remains passive throughout micturition, the resulting curve is the passive urethral resistance relation (PURR), which defines bladder outlet obstruction by the Pmuo. To simplify the results of the analysis of PURR further, a straight line, the "linear PURR," can be constructed. A nomogram was developed with zones representing increasing degrees of obstruction that can be easily applied to clinical urodynamic evaluations (Fig. 15–23).

Rollema and Mastrigt, also using a urethral resistance model defined by an elastic tube with a flow-controlling zone, developed a computer program—CLIM[3,70,71] (Fig. 15–24). The program uses the detrusor contractility parameter W and considers detrusor pressure, flow rate, and bladder volume throughout micturition. Obstruction parameters URA and U/L have been introduced and characterize the pressure–flow plot as one value that quantifies the degree of obstruction. The parameter URA is defined as the intersection of the quadratic urethral resistance relation with the pressure axis of the pressure–flow plot, whereas the parameter U/L is the maximum extrapolated rate of increase in isometric pressure. Rollema and Mastrigt, using CLIM, prospectively performed preoperatively blind pressure–flow studies on patients selected for TURP by conventional clinical criteria. These patients were assigned as being either obstructed or unobstructed according to Abrams and Griffiths's methods and then by urethral parameters URA and U/L.[70] The two systems gave the same diagnoses consistently, although URA was a more quantitative measure.[49]

At present no computerized model seems to have demonstrated superiority over Abrams and Griffiths's definition.[49] However, this may change as these factors become more precise, simplified, and easier to use. The argument that computer calculation is too complicated and cumbersome is becoming invalid as the use of computer software increases daily.

Videourodynamics

Videourodynamic study marries electronic urodynamic study with simultaneous intermittent fluoroscopic screening of the bladder and outlet at strategic points in the study. This requires a major investment in equipment, for the study is performed on a fluoroscopy table. Its major value is in the identification of the location of the obstruction. This is particularly important in complex cases, such as those with suspected functional bladder neck obstruction. In the male with prostatic obstruction, the prostatic urethra appears elongated and the urinary stream may appear bifurcated within the prostatic fossa. In the man with equivocal pressure–flow data this feature may clinch the diagnosis. In the patient with neurogenic sphincter dysfunction, the bladder neck or distal sphincter may demonstrate poor relaxation.

Sphincter Electromyography (EMG)

Electromyography of the pelvic floor and sphincters is performed to examine sphincter activity during bladder filling and voiding (see Chapter 3). However, in neurologically normal patients with obstructive symptoms it provides little additional information. It finds valuable use in the assessment of the patient with neurogenic bladder dysfunction in whom it may identify dyssynergic contraction or inappro-

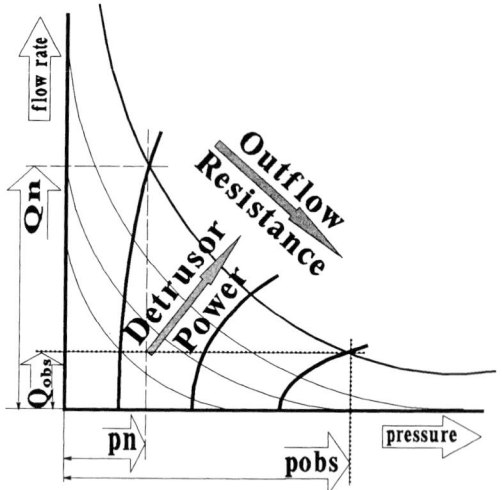

Figure 15–21. Energy balance of micturition. Regardless of the complexity of the pathophysiology of voiding, it is a mechanical balance between the detrusor as energy source and the bladder outlet as energy converter that determines voiding dynamics. This can be precisely described in a pressure–flow graph where any outflow condition, as well as detrusor strength, in its most simple form, can be represented by hyperbolic and parabolic lines, respectively, and directions of functional changes can be clearly identified. On the basis of this simple mechanical model, urodynamic data analysis quantifies the contribution of the outlet and the detrusor separately and thus the resultant micturition balance. (From Schafer W: Principles and clinical application of advanced urodynamic analysis of voiding function. *Urol Clin North Am* 1990;17(3):553–566.)

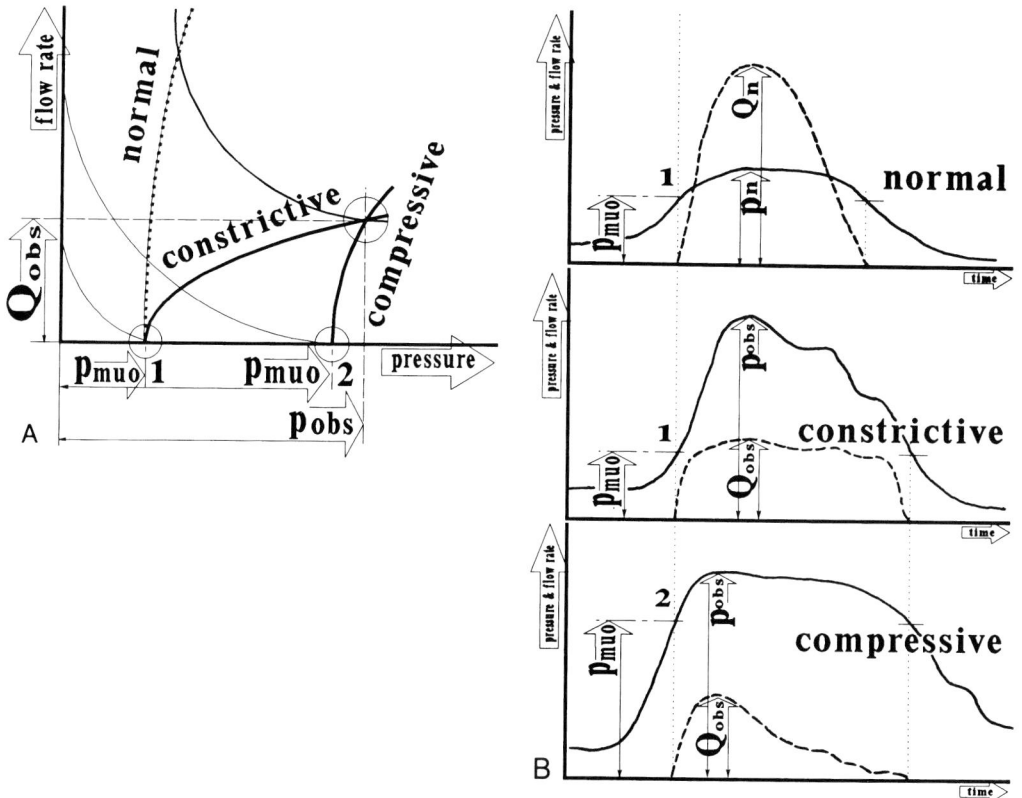

Figure 15–22. Specific types of obstruction. Features that establish outflow condition, the opening pressure (Pmuo), and the effective size can be altered separately, leading to distinct forms of obstruction. If the effective size is reduced, such as in a rigid stricture, the outflow curve becomes flatter (**A**). This results in the typical voiding pattern of a constrictive obstruction with the plateaulike flow rate curve (**B**). If only the urethral opening pressure is elevated, the curve is shifted to the higher pressure (**A**). This compressive obstruction creates the pattern commonly found in BPH. Because Pmuo determines the detrusor contraction strength necessary to initiate and maintain voiding, it is easy to see why in a compressive obstruction, even with the same flow and pressure as in a constrictive obstruction, retention and large residual urine volumes are likely to occur. (From Schafer W: Principles and clinical application of advanced urodynamic analysis of voiding function. *Urol Clin North Am* 1990;17(3):553–566.)

priate nonrelaxation of the distal sphincter mechanism during the voiding contraction.

Micturitional Urethral Pressure Profile

Simple perfusion urethral pressure profilometry has no value in the assessment of bladder outlet obstruction.[72] Yalla and associates, however, have pioneered in the use of the micturitional urethral pressure profile, which examines the bladder and urethral pressures simultaneously during voiding,[73] and good correlation has been found between this study and pressure–flow data in men with bladder outlet obstruction.[73,74]

SPECIFIC ETIOLOGIES

Benign Prostatic Hyperplasia

Benign prostatic hyperplasia (BPH) is one of the most common conditions afflicting the elderly male. Traditionally, its diagnosis and treatment relied heavily on symptoms and clinical findings that often correlated poorly with the severity of bladder outlet obstruction, and indeed in many outlet obstruction did not exist. The constellation of voiding symptoms referred to as prostatism includes both irritative and obstructive symptoms. However, conditions other than obstruction can cause these same symptoms. These include impaired detrusor contractility, detrusor instability, and sensory urgency. Even in those patients who do have obstruction it is probable that only about 25% present solely with symptoms of impaired voiding, the majority having symptoms related to the resultant detrusor instability.[75]

Prospective studies have demonstrated that the symptoms of prostatism fluctuate considerably with time.[12,14,15] Craigen and associates, following 60 patients with moderate presenting symptoms of prostatism, found 48% to have only minimal voiding symptoms at final follow-up 4 to 7 years later.[12] Ball and coworkers reported a similar series of 107 patients with prostatism in whom surgery was not initially performed.[15] After 5 years only 10 had required surgery. Of

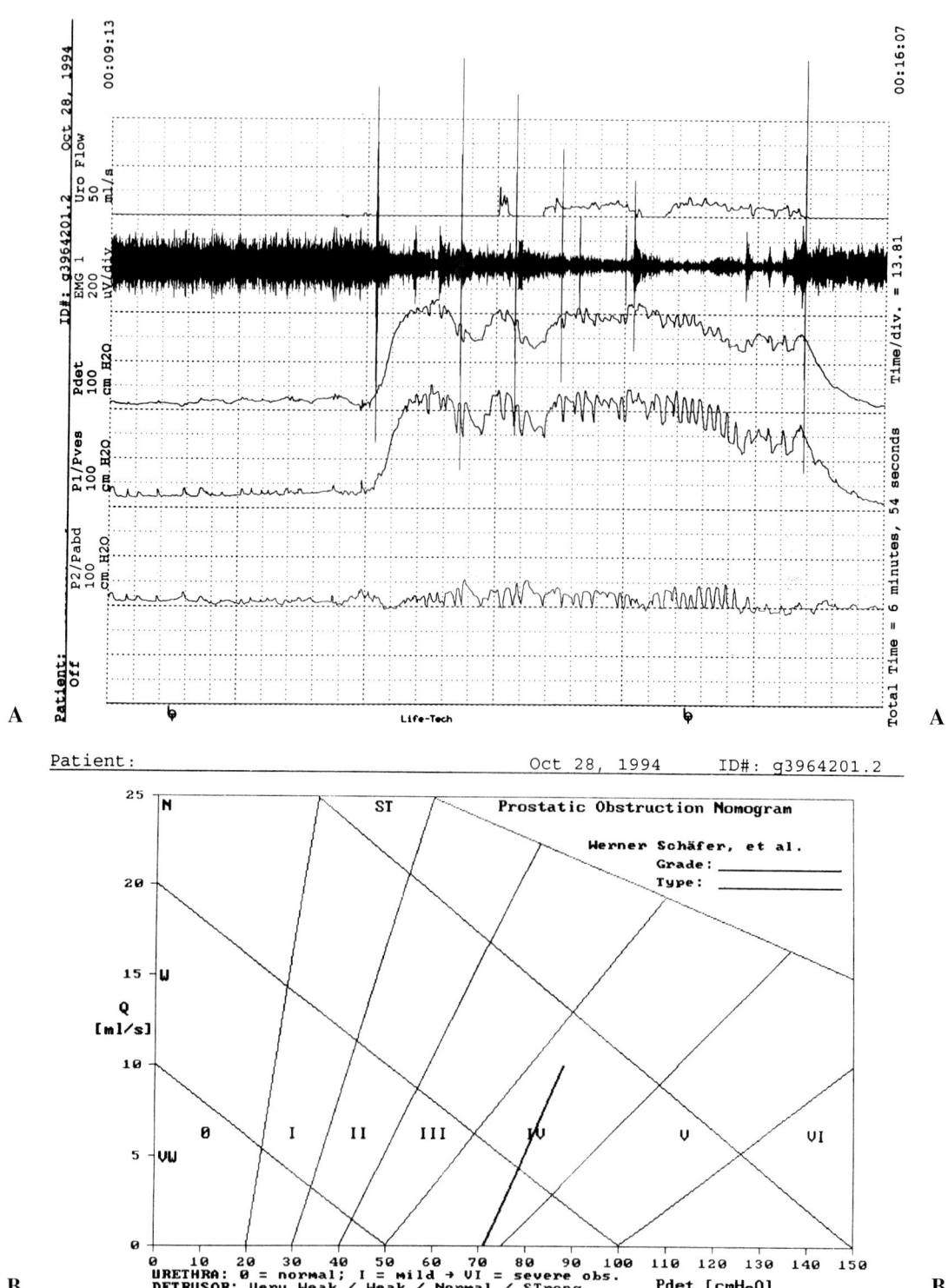

Figure 15–23. (A) Pressure–flow study of an elderly male with symptoms of prostatism. Study demonstrates an unstable detrusor contraction preceding high pressure–low flow voiding representative of bladder outlet obstruction. (B) Schaeffer nomogram of the patient in (A) demonstrating obstructive voiding.

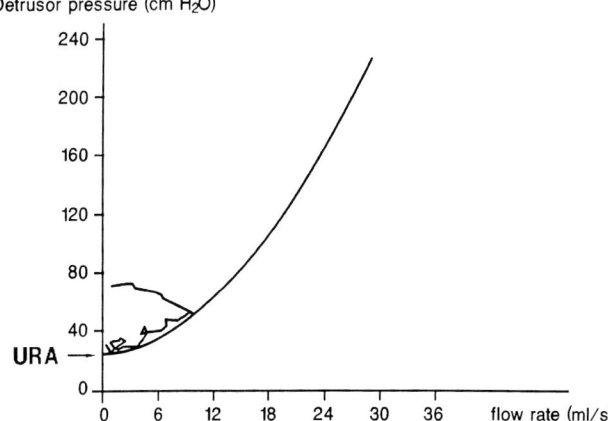

Figure 15–24. Detrusor pressure–flow plot of male patient with "prostatism," analyzed by the computer program Dx/CLIM. The value of the urethral resistance parameter URA is indicated on the y-axis. In this case the patient is obstructed (high value of URA). (From Rollema HJ, Mastrigt RV: Improved indication and follow-up in transurethral resection of the prostate using the computer program CLIM: a prospective study. *J Urol* 1992;148:111–116.)

the remaining 97 patients, symptoms had increased in 16, remained the same in 50, and improved in 31. Hence it is clear that moderate symptoms of prostatism can not only stabilize but substantially improve over time.

Treatment carries a high cost not just in the United States, where more than 300,000 transurethral prostatectomies (TURP) are performed annually,[76] but to the 15 to 30% of patients who do not benefit symptomatically from surgical intervention.[77,78] The indications for treatment to relieve infravesical obstruction are not straightforward except in patients with complications such as upper tract obstruction/dilatation or detrusor decompensation. Other relatively unequivocal indications include retention, recurrent infection, bleeding, and stones. Most patients who undergo treatment, however, have uncomplicated prostatism. Because uncomplicated prostatism may be due to several other factors in the elderly male and unobstructive BPH is so prevalent in this age group, accurate diagnosis appears to be critical, and urodynamic study is currently the best way to achieve this. Transurethral resection of the prostate for symptoms is not benign. Some 15 to 30% of patients do not have a favorable outcome.[79–81] Complications after TURP include incontinence (0.4 to 3.3%),[82] urethral stricture (16.4 to 22%),[83] bladder neck contracture (>15%),[84] and impotence (3.5 to 10.2%).[82] As stated earlier, prostatism can result from other causes, and symptoms can improve over time[14,15] or in response to placebo effect (reported from 40 to 60% in some studies).[79–81] An accurate diagnosis is important to a successful outcome both medically and economically.

Recently, recommendations have been put forth by the AHCPR as to the initial evaluation of all patients presenting with prostatism.[27] They recommend history, AUA Symptom Index, physical examination, urinalysis, and a creatinine serum in all patients. Optional tests include PSA, uroflowmetry, postvoid residual urine measurement, pressure–flow studies, and endoscopy (optional later if invasive treatment is planned). Tests not recommended in routine cases are IVP, ultrasonography, filling cystometry (CMG), and routine endoscopy.

Outlet Obstruction in Women

Bladder outlet obstruction in women is uncommon, but when it does occur it most often follows anti-incontinence or other pelvic surgery. Functional obstruction caused by sphincter dyssynergia is rare in the neurologically normal woman and is best diagnosed by videourodynamic study. More often voiding dysfunction is due to poor detrusor contractility. The incidence of obstruction following cystourethropexy has been reported to be between 2.5 and 24%,[85–87] and Raz believes that it is a frequently overlooked event.[86]

The diagnosis is best made by careful analysis of the chronological events. These are usually those of a woman with stress incontinence and no voiding problems who undergoes cystourethropexy and subsequently develops bladder instability symptoms and inefficient voiding. Physical examination and endoscopy generally confirm an acute retropubic urethral axis. A urodynamic evaluation can be helpful in establishing the etiology of the voiding dysfunction (outflow obstruction versus detrusor failure), but the diagnosis and particularly the decision to correct the problem surgically are based primarily on the clinical factors.[87,88]

Management will initially be expectant, using anticholinergic medications and clean intermittent catheterization if needed. If symptoms persist urethrolysis is often curative and may be performed using a variety of approaches. In a reported series of surgical revisions of obstructive cystourethropexies, resolution of symptoms of instability ranged from 50 to 90%.[86,88] In some women with vaginal prolapse, a large cystocele may also cause obstructed voiding and detrusor instability symptoms.[89]

Bladder Neck Obstruction

Bladder outlet obstruction due to bladder neck dysfunction in neurologically normal men has been well established.[90–97] Its incidence is unknown because of poor recognition and misdiagnosis. The etiology also remains unclear but has been attributed to bladder neck hypertrophy, fibrosis, or detrusor–bladder neck dyssynergia.[95] However, once anatomic etiologies have been ruled out by endoscopy and urethrography, functional obstruction is most likely due to an imbalance of adrenergic innervation,[98,99] a hypothesis supported by the response to alpha adrenolytic treatment.[96,100] Bladder neck dysfunction is not regarded as neuropathic; detrusor–bladder neck dyssynergia in neurologically impaired men actually is quite rare.[101]

Diagnosis is best made using videourodynamic study showing a failure of the bladder neck to open despite an adequate detrusor contraction (Fig. 15–25). Ideally, the pres-

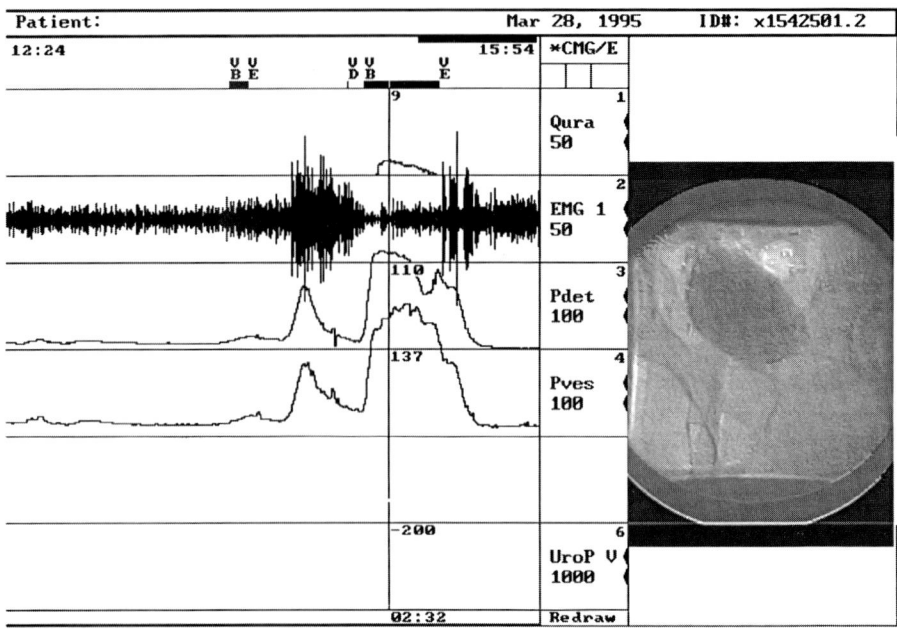

Figure 15–25. A videourodynamics study in a man with bladder outlet obstruction. The pressure–flow study shows classic features. The simultaneous video demonstrates poor bladder neck opening and identifies the site of obstruction.

sure–flow study should be unequivocally obstructive, although this is not always the case.

Definitive treatment of functional bladder neck obstruction is by endoscopic bladder neck incision.[90,92-94,96,98] A unilateral incision at the 5 or 7 o'clock position is used to preserve antegrade ejaculation; this procedure requires minimal convalescence, and is highly effective.[98] Chapple and Turner-Warwick report no recurrence of bladder neck obstruction or development of bladder neck contracture in their series of more than 200 cases and the incidence of decrease in ejaculate.[98] Nonsurgical management uses alpha adrenergic blockade and has been shown to be efficacious in some series.[96,99,100]

Neurogenic Obstruction

Neurogenic functional bladder outlet obstruction can occur at two levels, the bladder neck (proximal or internal sphincter) and the external (distal) sphincter.[101]

BLADDER NECK DYSSYNERGIA

Inappropriate contraction or failure of relaxation of the smooth muscle at the bladder neck has been described by Krane and Olsson in 6 of 52 patients with neuropathic vesical dysfunction.[102] The condition occurred in patients with hyperreflexic bladders, and they called it "sympathetic dyssynergia" and suggested it was due to inappropriate adrenergic stimulation. Diagnosis was based on pressure–flow studies demonstrating outlet obstruction together with simultaneous voiding cystourethrography identifying the location of the obstruction to be at the closed bladder neck. Therapy was either alpha-adrenergic blockage or endoscopic incision. In our experience this entity is uncommon in the neurogenic population.

DETRUSOR–SPHINCTER DYSSYNERGIA OF THE EXTERNAL SPHINCTER

Neuropathic obstruction at the external sphincter can manifest either as poor relaxation or as active contraction at the time of detrusor contraction.[103] The most recognizable form of functional neurogenic infravesical obstruction occurring at the striated sphincter level is in patients with suprasacral spinal cord lesions below the pons, in whom there is a loss of coordination between the detrusor and the external sphincter, called detrusor–sphincter dyssynergia (DSD). In addition to spinal cord injury, other neurologic diseases, including multiple sclerosis, which frequently affects the spinal cord, can produce DSD.[104] Clinically, these patients empty the bladder inefficiently, there are changes in bladder morphology, and eventually upper tract dilation and damage occurs. Treatment options involve two alternate philosophies.

One alternative is to accept the detrusor hyperreflexia and to promote bladder emptying by aiming therapy at the external sphincter. Pharmacologic agents have been used to relax the sphincter but have met with limited success. Other alternatives include the use of endoscopically implanted stents and external sphincterotomy. In any of these events the resulting involuntary voiding/incontinence is managed using condom catheters in the male, which introduce a problem of their own because of skin breakdown. This option is not appropriate in women, for obvious reasons. The second alternative is to accept the sphincter dyssynergia for the continence it provides and to inhibit the involuntary bladder contractions or use other methods to improve the bladder as a storage reservoir, and then perform clean, intermittent catheterization to empty the bladder. Methods used include anticholinergic pharmacotherapy, augmentation enterocystoplasty, detrusor myomectomy, and denervation procedures. There is no single optimal technique, and individualization of care is essential.

Mechanical Obstruction

PROSTATE CANCER

Locally advanced prostate cancer can cause outlet obstruction. Diagnosis is based on digital rectal examination, PSA determination, ultrasound-guided biopsy, and endoscopy. Treatment may utilize hormonal ablation, endoscopic resection, radiation therapy, or surgical excision.

URETHRAL STRICTURE DISEASE

The result of urethral injury, regardless of etiology, is the formation of scar that may reduce the caliber of the urethral lumen and result in stricture. Historically, the major cause was gonococcal infection, but in the developed world, with access to antibiotics and education, trauma is now the leading cause. Urethral strictures generally present with the symptoms of obstructed voiding. Because the process of urethral cicatrization may be very slow, the slowing of the stream may be insidious, and delayed recognition is not uncommon. In some cases the process is very rapid and readily recognized, such as in the postmeatal stricture that occurs following transurethral resection of the prostate. Other presentations of urethral stricture include urinary tract infections, urethral bleeding, epididymitis, and in some communities, periurethral phlegmon, or urethrocutaneous fistula. In older men there is occasionally some difficulty in deciding whether the symptoms are due to the stricture or prostate enlargement. In such cases it is judicious to reassess the patient after urethral dilatation to determine which of the two pathologies is the cause of the voiding difficulty.

Diagnosis depends on accurate visualization of the full extent of the stricture by radiologic studies and/or endoscopy. Excretory urography or renal ultrasonography is ideally performed at the time of diagnosis of significant and long-standing urethral strictures. Bladder and upper tract changes are uncommon but may be important in the overall care of the patient, and sometimes the excreted contrast can be voided as a "poor man's" cystourethrogram to delineate the urethra proximal to the stricture. Retrograde urethrography, however, is the mainstay of the radiographic investigation of stricture disease. The urethrogram should not only delineate the stricture but also show the urethra proximal and distal to it (Fig. 15–26). The length, caliber, location, multiplicity, and proximity of the stricture to the sphincter should all be identified. Combined retrograde ure-

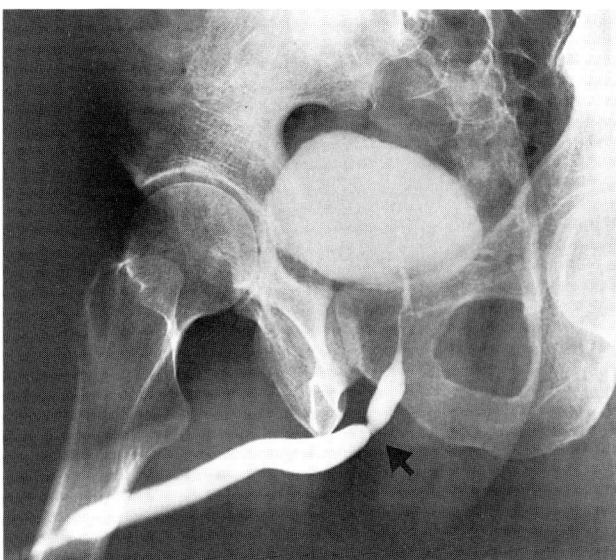

Figure 15–26. Retrograde urethrogram showing short bulbar urethral stricture.

throgram-voiding cystourethrogram is indispensable in the evaluation of the obliterative urethral defect that allows pelvic trauma (Fig. 15–27). The sonographic urethrogram has been reported to be equally efficacious and in some ways superior as a diagnostic modality when compared with the standard retrograde urethrogram. The stated advantages include the identification of the extent and thickness of periurethral fibrosis and spongiofibrosis, the accurate measurement of urethral luminal size, and the noninvasive nature of the study.[105–107] Magnetic resonance imaging has also been described for the evaluation of pelvic fracture urethral distraction defects prior to surgery.[106] Although urethrography is the mainstay of investigation and identifies the important characteristics necessary for treatment selection, endoscopy is still valuable. "Gray" urethra, where spongiofibrosis extends beyond the limits of the definitive stricture, may not be apparent radiographically but is often evident urethroscopically and will inform the surgeon of the needed limits of his repair.

The management of urethral stricture disease involves a thorough discussion of options, including dilation, optical urethrotomy, and surgical repair. The modern approach has steadily moved away from repeated instrumentations toward an earlier open surgical intervention.

Treatment of Lower Urinary Tract Obstruction

A full and complete discussion of the treatment options, indications, advantages and disadvantages, and expected outcomes is beyond the scope of this chapter. The management of mechanical obstruction of the lower urinary tract is generally one of surgical intervention to remove the impediment. Neurogenic or functional outlet obstruction is often

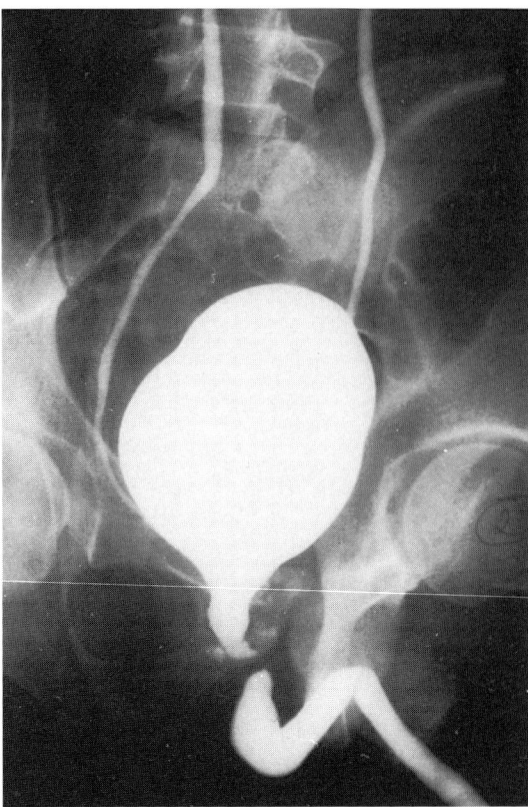

Figure 15–27. A combined retrograde urethrogram and voiding cystourethrogram in a patient with a pelvic fracture urethral distraction defect. This film demonstrates the length of the defect and the healthy appearance of the anterior urethra. Competence of the bladder neck, essential for continence after repair, is demonstrated by x-ray exposure prior to the "voiding" film.

initially treated pharmacologically, together with clean, intermittent catheterization. Surgical options are usually reserved for patients who fail conservative therapy, especially those with damaged or imperiled upper tracts.

In the management of outlet obstruction due to benign prostatic hypertrophy the diagnosis must first be proved objectively. Because prostate size, symptoms, residual urine, IVP, and endoscopic assessment of prostatic and bladder characteristics have been shown to be unrelated to the severity of infravesical obstruction, only pressure–flow studies can reliably delineate obstructed from unobstructed voiding. Treatment of symptomatic BPH includes watchful waiting, pharmacologic agents such as finasteride and alpha-adrenergic blockers, and a variety of surgical procedures, where TURP remains the gold standard.

REFERENCES

1. Larsson G, Abrams P, Victor A: The frequency/volume chart in detrusor instability. *Neurourol Urodyn* 1991;10:533–543.
2. Abrams PH, Farrar DJ, Turner-Warwick R, et al: The results of prostatectomy: a symptomatic and urodynamic analysis of 142 patients. *J Urol* 1979;121:640.
3. Rollema JH, Mastrigt R: Objective analysis of prostatism: clinical application of the computer program CLIM. *Neurourol Urodyn* 1991;10:71–76.
4. Coolsaet B, Blok C: Detrusor properties related to prostatism. *Neurourol Urodyn* 1986;5:435.
5. Bruskewitz RC, Iversen P, Madsen PO: Value of postvoid residual urine determination in evaluation of protatism. *Urology* 1982;20:602.
6. Christensen MM, Bruskewitz RC: Clinical manifestations of benign prostatic hyperplasia and indications for therapeutic intervention. *Urol Clin North Am* 1990;17(3):509–516.
7. Martin KW: Prostatectomy: a discourse on the indications for and the choice of operations. *Ann Coll Surg Engl* 1973; 52:304.
8. Abrams PH, Feneley RCL: The significance of the symptoms associated with bladder outflow obstruction. *Urol Int* 1978; 33:171.
9. Walsh PC: Benign prostatic hyperplasia. In Walsh PC, Gittes RF, Perlmutter AD, et al, eds. *Campbell's Urology.* 4th ed, vol 2. Philadelphia: WB Saunders, 1979;949–964.
10. Stephenson TP, Farrar DJ: Urodynamic study of 15 patients with postmicturition dribble. *Urology* 1977;9(4):404–406.
11. Hald T: Urodynamics in benign prostatic hyperplasia: a survey. *Prostate* 1989;2:69.
12. Birkoff JD, Wiederhorn AR, Hamilton ML, Zinsser HH: Natural history of benign prostatic hypertrophy and acute urinary retention. *Urology* 1976;7:48–52.
13. Powell PH, Smith PJB, Feneley RCL: The identification of patients at risk from acute urinary retention. *Br J Urol* 1980; 52:520.
14. Craigen AA, Hickling JB, Saunders CRG, Carpenter RG: Natural history of prostatic obstruction. *J R Coll Gen Pract* 1969;18:226–232.
15. Ball AJ, Feneley RCL, Abrams PH: The natural history of prostatism. *Br J Urol* 1981;53:613–616.
16. Breum L. Klarskov P, Munck LK, et al: Significance of acute urinary retention due to infravesical obstruction. *Scand J Urol Nephrol* 1982;16:21.
17. Boyarsky S, Jones G, Paulson DF, et al: A new look at bladder neck obstruction by the Food and Drug Administration: guidelines for investigation of benign prostatic hypertrophy. *Trans Am Assoc Genitourin Surg* 1977;68:29–32.
18. Madsen PO, Iversen P: A point system for selecting operative candidates. In: Hinman F, ed. *Benign Prostatic Hypertrophy.* New York: Springer-Verlag, 1983;763–765.
19. Jensen KME, Jorgensen JB, Morgensen P, Bille-Brahe NE: Some clinical aspects of uroflowmetry in elderly males. *Scand J Urol Nephrol* 1986;20:93–99.
20. Sommer P, Nielsen KK, Bauer T, Kristensen ES, Hermann GG, et al: Voiding patterns in men evaluated by a questionnaire survey. *Br J Urol* 1990;65:155–160.
21. Barry MJ, Fowler FJ, O'Leary MP, et al: The Measurement Committee of the American Urological Association: the American Urological Association symptom index for benign prostatic hyperplasia. *J Urol* 1992;148:1549–1557.
22. Barry MJ, Fowler JF, O'Leary MP, Bruskewitz RC, et al: The Measurement Committee of the American Urological Association: correlation of the American Urological Association symptom index with self-administered versions of the Madsen-Iversen, Boyarsky and Maine medical assessment program symptom indexes. *J Urol* 1992;148:1558–1563.
23. O'Leary MP, Barry MJ, Fowler FJ: Hard measures of subjective outcomes: validating symptom indexes in urology. *J Urol* 1992;148:1546–1548.
24. Chancellor MB, Rivas DA, Keeley FX, et al: Similarity of

the American Urologic Association symptom index among men with benign prostate hyperplasia (BPH), urethral obstuction not due to BPH and detrusor hyperreflexia without outlet obstruction. *Br J Urol* 1994;74:200–203.

25. Allen VJ, Kreder KJ: Bladder outlet obstruction in males in the setting of voluntary versus involuntary detrusor contractions. *J Urol* 1995;153:452A.

26. Chancellor MB, Rivas DA: American Urologic Association symptom index for women with voiding symptoms: lack of index specificity for benign prostatic hyperplasia. *J Urol* 1993;150:1706–1709.

27. McConnell JD, Barry MJ, Bruskewitz RC, et al: *Benign Prostatic Hyperplasia: Diagnosis and Treatment*. Clinical Practice Guideline, No. 8. AHCPR Publication No. 94-0582, Rockville: Agency for Health Care Policy and Research, Public Health Service, US Department of Health and Human Services, February 1994;29–34.

28. Galatius H, Hansen RI: Rectal estimation of prostatic size. *Ugeskr Laeger* 1983;145:824–825.

29. Turner-Warwick RT, Whiteside CG, Worth PHL, et al; A urodynamic view of bladder neck obstruction. *Br J Urol* 1973;45:44–59.

30. Catalona WJ, et al: Measurement of prostate-specific antigen in serum as a screening test for prostate cancer. *N Engl J Med* 1991;324:1156.

31. Benson MC, Whang IS, Olsson CA, et al: Use of prostate specific antigen density to enhance predictive value of intermediate levels of serum prostate specific antigen. *J Urol* 1992;147:817.

32. Carter HB, Pearson JC, Metter EJ, et al: Longitudinal evaluation of prostate specific antigen levels in men with and without prostate disease. *JAMA* 1993;150:106.

33. Nielsen KK, Kristensen ES, Pedersen OS, et al: Prostatectomy symptomatological, uroflowmetric and cystometric changes after operation and correlation between symptoms, cystometry, cystourethroscopy and flow measurements. *Ugeskr Laeger* 1986;148:70–74.

34. Andersen JT, Nordling J: Prostatism: II. The correlation between cystourethroscopic, cystometric and urodynamic findings. *Scand J Urol Nephrol* 1980;14:23–27.

35. Abrams PH, Roylance J, Feneley RCL: Excretion urography in the investigation of prostatism. *Br J Urol* 1976;48:681–684.

36. Andersen JT, Jacobsen O, Strandgaard L: The diagnostic value of intravenous pyelography in infravesical obstruction in males. *Scand J Urol Nephrol* 1977;11:225–230.

37. Butler MR, Donnelly B, Komaranchat A: Intravenous urography in evaluation of acute retention. *Br J Urol* 1978;12:464–466.

38. Rifkin MD: Ultrasound of the prostate: applications and indications. *J Suisse Med* 1991;121(9):282–291.

39. Rifkin MD: The prostate and seminal vesicles. In: *Diagnostic Imaging of the Lower Genitourinary Tract*. New York: Raven Press, 1985;121.

40. McNeal JE: Normal anatomy of the prostate and changes in benign prostatic hypertrophy and carcinoma. *Semin Ultrasound CT MR* 1988;9(5):329.

41. Resnick MI: Transrectal ultrasonography of the prostate. In Rous JN, ed. *Urology Annual 1988*. East Norwalk, CT: Appleton-Century Crofts, 1988.

42. Rifkin MD, Friedland GW, Shortliffe L: Prostatic evaluation by transrectal endosonography: detection of carcinoma. *Radiology* 1986;158:85.

43. Waterhouse RL, Resnick MI: The use of transrectal ultrasonography in the evaluation of patients with prostatic carcinoma. *J Urol* 1989;141:233.

44. Abrams PH, Blaivas JG, Stanton SL, Anderson JT: Standardization of terminology of lower urinary tract function. *Neurourol Urodyn* 1988;7:403–428.

45. Abrams P: Detrusor instability and bladder outlet obstruction. *Neurourol Urodyn* 1985;4:317–328.

46. Moore KH, Sutherst JR: Response to treatment of detrusor instability in relation to psychoneurotic status. *Br J Urol* 1990;66:486–490.

47. Cucchi A: Detrusor instability and bladder outflow obstruction: evidence for a correlation between the severity of obstruction and the presence of instability. *Br J Urol* 1988;61:420.

48. Chapple CR, Smith D: The pathophysiological changes in the bladder obstructed by benign prostatic hyperplasia. *Br J Urol* 1994;73:117–123.

49. Neilsen KK, Nording J, Hald T: Critical review of the diagnosis of prostatic obstruction. *Neurourol Urodyn* 1994;13:201–217.

50. Dorflinger T, Frimodt-Moller PC, Bruskewitz RC, et al: The significance of uninhibited detrusor contractions in prostatism. *J Urol* 1985;133:819–821.

51. Jensen KM-E, Jorgensen JB, Morgensen P: Urodynamics in prostatism: III. Prognostic value of medium-fill water cystometry. *Scand J Urol Nephrol* 1988;114 (suppl):78–83.

52. Balslev-Jorgensen J, Jensen KM-E, Morgensen P: Significance of predominantly irritative symptomatology before a prostatic operation. *J Urol* 1990;143:739–741.

53. Siroky MB, Olsson CA, Krane RJ: The flow rate nomogram: I. development. *J Urol* 1979;122:665.

54. Drach GW, Layton TN, Binard WJ: Male peak urinary flow rate: relationships to volume voided and age. *J Urol* 1979;122:210.

55. Siroky MB, Olsson CA, Krane RJ: The flow rate nomogram: II. Clinical correlation. *J Urol* 1980;123:208.

56. Abrams PH, Griffiths DJ: The assessment of prostatic obstruction from urodynamic measurements and from residual urine. *Br J Urol* 1979;51:129–134.

57. Gerstenberg TC, Andersen JK, Klarskov P, et al: High flow infravesical obstruction in men: symptomatology, urodynamics and the results of surgery. *J Urol* 1982;127:943–945.

58. Iversen P, Bruskewitz RC, Jensen KM-E, Madsen PO: Transurethral prostatic resection in the treatment of prostatism with high urinary flow. *J Urol* 1983;129:995–997.

59. Jensen KM-E, Jorgensen JB, Morgensen P: Urodynamics in prostatism: I. prognostic value of uroflowmetry. *Scand J Urol Nephrol* 1988;114 (suppl):63–71.

60. Schafer W, Noppeney R, Rubben H, Lutzeyer W: The value of free flow rate and pressure/flow studies in the routine investigation of BPH patients. *Neurourol Urodyn* 1988;7:219–221.

61. Chancellor MB, Blaivis JG, Kaplan SA, Axelrod S: Bladder outlet obstruction versus impaired detrusor contractility: the role of uroflow. *J Urol* 1991;145:810–812.

62. Bates P, Bradley WE, Glen E, et al: The standardization of terminology of lower urinary tract function. *J Urol* 1979;121:551–554.

63. Griffiths DJ: Hydrodynamics of male micturition: I. Therapy of steady state flow through elastic walled tubes. *Med Biol Eng* 1971;7:201–215.

64. Griffiths DJ: Hydrodynamics of male micturition: II. Measurements of stream parameters and urethral elasticity. *Med Biol Eng* 1971;9:589–596.

65. Griffiths DJ: The mechanics of the urethra and of micturition. *Br J Urol* 1973;45:496–507.

66. Schafer W: Principles and clinical application of advanced urodynamic analysis of voiding function. *Urol Clin North Am* 1990;17(3): 553–566.

67. Blaivis JG: Urodynamic techniques and dysfunction. In:

Yalla S, McGuire E, Elbadawi A, et al, eds. *Principles and Practice of Urodynamics and Neurourology.* New York: Macmillan, 1988;155–198.
68. Jensen KM-E, Jorgensen JB, Morgensen P: Urodynamics in prostatism: II. Prognostic value of pressure-flow study combined with stop-flow test. *Scand J Urol Nephrol* 1988;176 (suppl 114):72–77.
69. Schafer W: Urethral resistance? Urodynamic concepts of physiological and pathological bladder outlet function during voiding. *Neurourol Urodyn* 1985;4:161–201.
70. Rollema HJ, Mastrigt RV: Improved indication and follow-up in transurethral resection of the prostate using the computer program CLIM: a prospective study. *J Urol* 1992; 148:111–116.
71. Mastrigt RV, Rollema HJ: Urethral resistance and urinary bladder contractility before and after transurethral resection of the prostate as determined by the computer program CLIM *Neurourol Urodyn* 1988;7:226–228.
72. Abrams PH: Perfusion urethral profilometry. *Urol Clin North Am* 1979;6:103.
73. Yalla SV, Sharma GVRK, Barsamian EM: Micturitional static urethral pressure profile: a method of recording urethral pressure profile during voiding and the implications. *J Urol* 1980;124:649–656.
74. Desmond AD, Ramayya GR: Comparison of pressure/flow studies with micturitional urethral pressure profiles in the diagnosis of urinary outflow obstruction. *Br J Urol* 1988; 61:224–229.
75. Webster GD, Carson CC: Bladder outlet obstruction. In: Resnick MI, Older RA, eds. *Diagnosis of Genitourinary Disease.* New York: Thieme-Stratton, 1982;227–248.
76. Holtgrewe HL, Mebust WK, Dowd JB, et al: Transurethral prostatectomy: practice aspects of the dominant operation in American urology. *J Urol* 1989;141:348–353.
77. Frimodt-Moller PC, Jensen KME, Iversen P, Madsen PO, Bruskewitz RC: Analysis of presenting symptoms in prostatism. *J Urol* 1984;132:272.
78. Blaivas JG: Urodynamics: the second generation. *J Urol* 1983;129:783.
79. Bensen H, Epstein MD: The placebo effect. *JAMA* 1976; 232:12.
80. Caine M, Perlberg S, Gordon R: The treatment of benign prostatic hypertrophy with flutamide (SCH 13521)—a placebo-controlled study. *J Urol* 1975;114:564.
81. Abrams PH: A double-blind trial of the effects of cancidin on patients with benign prostatic hypertrophy. *Br J Urol* 1977;49:67.
82. Mebust WK, Holtgrewe HL, Cockett ATK, Peters PC: Transurethral prostatectomy: immediate and postoperative complications. A cooperative study of 13 participating institutions evaluating 3885 patients. *J Urol* 1988;141:243–247.
83. Nielsen KK, Nordling J: Urethral stricture following transurethral prostatectomy. *Urology* 1990;35:18–24.
84. Caine M: Late results and complications of prostatectomy. In: Hinman F Jr, ed. *Benign Prostatic Hypertrophy.* New York: Springer-Verlag, 1983;971–978.
85. Juma S, Sdrales L: Etiology of urinary retention after bladder neck suspension. *J Urol* 1993;149(752):401A.
86. Nitti VW, Raz S: Obstruction following anti-incontinence procedures: diagnosis and treatment with transvaginal urethrolysis. *J Urol* 1994;152:93–98.
87. Cardoza LD, Stanton SL, Williams JE: Detrusor instability following surgery for genuine stress incontinence. *Br J Urol* 1979;51:204.

88. Webster GD, Kreder KJ: Voiding dysfunction following cystourethropexy: its evaluation and management. *J Urol* 1990; 144:670–673.
89. McGuire EM: The urodynamic examination of the incontinent patient. In: Krane RJ, Siroky MB, eds. *Clinical Neurourology,* Boston: Little Brown, 1991;289–297.
90. Turner-Warwick R, Whiteside CG, Worth PHL, Milroy EJG, Bates CP: A urodynamic view of the clinical problems associated with bladder neck dysfunction and its treatment by endoscopic incision and transtrigonal posterior prostatectomy. *Br J Urol* 1973;45:44–59.
91. Bates CP, Arnold EP, Griffiths DJ: The nature of the abnormality in bladder neck obstruction. *Br J Urol* 1975;47:651–656.
92. Webster GD, Lockhart JL, Older RA: The evaluation of bladder neck dysfunction. *J Urol* 1980;123:196–198.
93. Kaplan SA, Te AE, Jacobs BZ: Urodynamic evidence of vesical neck obstruction in men with misdiagnosed chronic nonbacterial prostatitis and the therapeutic role of endoscopic incision of the bladder neck. *J Urol* 1994;152:2063–2065.
94. Christensen MG, Nordling J, Andersen JT, Hald T: Functional bladder neck obstruction: results of endoscopic bladder neck incision in 131 consecutive patients. *Br J Urol* 1985; 57:60–62.
95. Norlen LJ, Blaivis J: Unsuspected proximal urethral obstruction in young and middle-aged men. *J Urol* 1986;135:972–976.
96. Mishra VK, Kumar A, Kapoor R, Srivastava A, Bhandari M: Functional bladder neck obstruction in males: a progressive disorder. *Eur Urol* 1992;22:123–129.
97. Gilja I, Kovacic M, Radej M, Parazajder J: Functional obstruction of bladder neck in men. *Neurourol Urodyn* 1989; 8:433–438.
98. Chapple C, Turner-Warwick R: Bladder outflow obstruction in the male. In: Mundy AR, Stephenson TP, Wein AJ, eds. *Urodynamics: Principles, Practice and Application.* 2nd ed. London: Churchill Livingstone, 1994;223–256.
99. Awad SA, Downie J, Lywood DW, Young RA, Jarzylo SV: Sympathetic activity in the proximal urethra in patients with urinary obstruction. *J Urol* 1976;115:545–549.
100. Hedlund H, Andersson KE: Effects of prazosin in men with symptoms of bladder neck obstruction and a non-hyperplastic prostate. *Scand J Urol Nephrol* 1989;23:251–254.
101. Turner-Warwick R: Observations on the function and dysfunction of the sphincter and detrusor mechanisms. *Urol Clin North Am* 1979;6:13–30.
102. Krane RJ, Olsson CA: Phenoxybenzamine in neurogenic bladder dysfunction: II. Clinical considerations. *J Urol* 1973; 110:653.
103. Kaplan SA, Chancellor MB, Blaivis JG: Bladder and sphincter behavior in patients with spinal cord lesions. *J Urol* 1991; 146 (1):113–117.
104. Blaivas JG: The neurophysiology of micturition: a clinical study of 550 patients. *J Urol* 1982;127:958.
105. Gluck CD, Bundy AL, Fine C, et al: Sonographic urethrogram: comparison to roentgenographic techniques in 22 patients. *J Urol* 1988;140:1404–1408.
106. McAninch JW, Laing FC, Jeffrey RB: Sonourethrography in the evaluation of urethral strictures: a preliminary report. *J Urol* 1988;139:294–297.
107. Merkle W, Wayner W: Sonography of the distal male urethra—a new diagnostic procedure for urethral strictures: results of a retrospective study. *J Urol* 1988;140:1409–1411.

16 Cystic Disease of the Kidney

Kenneth A. Kropp, Steven Arrowsmith

If only because of their ubiquity, renal cysts present a special challenge in urologic diagnosis. Renal cysts are extraordinarily common; autopsy studies have shown that at least half of the population over the age of 50 has renal cysts.[1] In the past, the presence of cysts of the kidney generally went undetected, because they rarely cause symptoms and are nearly never of themselves of serious consequence to the patient. In 12,500 admissions to the Brady Urologic Institute prior to 1926, not one case of renal cyst was identified.[2] Radiographic studies occasionally demonstrated these lesions; however, the comparatively low resolution of the available modalities revealed only the tip of an iceberg of pathology. As the use of CT scanning and ultrasonography became widespread, a Pandora's box was opened for the urologist. As these studies are done to evaluate other clinical problems, cystic lesions of the kidney were noted in a large percentage of patients.

The association between cysts of the kidney and malignancy has long been recognized. As large numbers of patients with renal cysts were studied both in autopsy series and in groups of patients who underwent surgical exploration for renal cyst, between 2.1 and 3.5% were found to have coexistent cyst and tumor.[3-6] In 1980 Lang[7] stated that 5.5% of asymptomatic space-occupying lesions of the kidney were ultimately determined to be malignant. Because the main differential in diagnosis for a simple renal cyst is malignancy, the delineation of the nature of the mass is imperative.

The urologist therefore is often placed in the uncomfortable position of attempting to design and justify an expensive and potentially morbid workup to evaluate a lesion of which the patient was totally unaware, a lesion found when looking for something else, with the goal being not so much to prove what the lesion is as to prove what it is not.

A wide variety of diagnostic tests has been employed and myriad decision-making schema have been set forth in an effort to minimize the risk of missing malignant lesions, minimize the risk to the patient from the studies themselves, and keep costs under control.

In the 1970s much of the attention devoted to the topic of renal cysts in the literature concerned the question of whether newer diagnostic modalities (CT and ultrasound) could reliably diagnose the simple renal cyst. This anxiety has largely been put to rest because many good studies have been published that demonstrated that when rigidly applied criteria are employed, both CT and ultrasound have a diagnostic accuracy approaching 100%.[8-10] Subsequent work has helped to define an ever-increasing range of cystic lesions that can be safely labeled as benign disease.

In this chapter we will attempt to clarify the issues surrounding the diagnostic approach to cystic lesions of the kidney. The special cases of autosomal dominant and autosomal recessive polycystic kidney disease will not be considered separately.

THE SIMPLE CYST

A "classic" simple cyst might be described as follows: The site of origin is usually the renal cortex, where it may distort the renal outline if it reaches sufficient diameter to displace the renal capsule. Cysts are lined by a single layer of epithelial cells and are surrounded by a paper-thin lamellated fibrous capsule. They are filled with straw-colored transudative fluid. Cysts are usually small, are often single, generally do not have any internal structure, and do not communicate with the renal collecting system. Simple cysts do not cause symptoms, do not affect renal function,[11] and do not cause any other particular morbidity.

Unfortunately, abundant exceptions exist to all the preceding statements. Cysts may arise deep in the cortex or in the renal medulla, where they may be more difficult to detect. The cyst lining may be thrown up into papillary projections, and the capsule of the cyst may vary greatly in thickness. The appearance of cyst fluid can vary, from clear to pastelike. Multiple simple renal cysts can coexist in the same kidney. Cysts can be septated or even multiloculated. Hypertension, urinary obstruction, hematuria, and pain have all been associated with the presence of simple renal cysts. As a pathologic entity, the simple renal cyst is rare in childhood but very common in adults, suggesting that this is an acquired rather than a congenital condition.

In its classic form, the simple cyst presents very low risk for malignancy. Well-defined criteria have been developed for each radiographic modality that allow the physician to assign renal masses to this low-risk group. What are the modality-specific criteria for the diagnosis of simple renal cyst?

Intravenous Pyelography

Although many renal masses are initially discovered in the course of an intravenous urogram, the intravenous pyelogram (IVP) is not adequate as the sole diagnostic modality to establish the diagnosis of renal cyst.[12,13] Because the study depends largely upon the radiographic appearance of contrast excreted into the renal collecting system, this study is best suited to detect lesions located within the collecting system itself, rather than parenchymal lesions such as the renal cyst. The IVP is also incapable of distinguishing solid and fluid-filled lesions. Therefore the IVP usually serves as a portal of entry into the diagnostic cascade built around the evaluation of renal masses, rather than a mainstay of the diagnosis of simple cysts.

Radionuclide Studies

Functioning renal cortical tissue can be delineated using radionuclide imaging techniques; therefore the technique has been employed in evaluation of renal masses suspected of being a simple cyst.[14,15] Obviously, it would be expected that the amount of radiopharmaceutical detectable in the region of a renal cyst would be reduced, resulting in a photon-deficient area on renal scan. However, the resolution of this technique is not adequate to distinguish simple cyst from potentially lethal lesions such as cystic tumor. The renal scan, although initially an important part of early diagnostic protocols in the diagnosis of renal cyst, has been supplanted by newer superior imaging modalities.

Nephrotomography

Before the CT scan became widely available, the nephrotomogram played a pivotal role in the evaluation of renal masses suspected of being cysts. Through the 1960s and 1970s, a number of large series corroborated the accuracy of this modality in the diagnosis of renal cysts.[16–19] With the use of the infusion technique and the application of rigid diagnostic criteria,[20] diagnostic accuracy was 96 to 100%. The diagnostic criteria required for the diagnosis of renal cyst are given in Table 16–1. Given the limitations of the study, including the requirement that the lesion be peripherally placed and the potential for contrast-associated morbidity, the nephrotomogram, although currently overarched by newer methods, is still a good method for diagnosing renal cysts.

Renal Arteriography

Another mainstay in the evaluation of renal masses through the 1960s and 1970s was the renal arteriogram. Again, there was abundant evidence in the literature to support the safety and accuracy of this technique.[21–26] The utility of the study was based on the property that renal cysts are hypovascular and most renal tumors are hypervascular. Unfortunately, a significant percentage of renal tumors, especially those of papillary histology, are hypovascular. Therefore when there are angiographic errors in diagnosis, it is possible to mislabel a hypovascular renal tumor as a renal cyst. Overall, the accuracy of renal angiography when used alone in the evaluation of renal cysts is on the order of 85%,[23,27] which no longer compares favorably with currently available diagnostic technology. Therefore arteriography should no longer be considered a first-line study to evaluate a suspected cyst. (Arteriographic criteria for a simple cyst are given in Table 16–2.)

Cyst Puncture

There is a very large body of experience in the literature concerning the use of cyst puncture–aspiration in the evaluation of renal masses.[28–32] Cyst puncture has the advantage of the potential for providing radiographic, biochemical, and cytologic information about the mass. By employing this multipronged attack, the risk of missing malignant lesions is greatly reduced. Criteria for the diagnosis of simple renal cyst are listed in Table 16–3. Histochemical and cytologic examinations of the cyst fluid are necessary because of the considerable overlap in the gross character of fluid from benign and malignant lesions. Clear fluid can be aspirated from cystic tumors,[33] and simple cysts may have dark or even oily aspirates.[34] The caveat that the size of the cyst on cystography must equal the size of the mass being evaluated alludes to the fact that renal tumors can have a cystic center. In this setting, a smooth-walled cavity might be demonstrated, but the size of the cyst would be less than the total size of the renal mass.

Table 16–1. Nephrotomographic Criteria for Simple Cyst (Bosniak)

1. The lesion must be peripherally placed so that at least 25% extends outside the cortex of the kidney.
2. The wall of the lesion must be thin.
3. The lesion must be lucent, compared to the surrounding tissues, and not more dense than on the scout tomogram (with no contrast medium).
4. The lesion must be well visualized in 360 degrees and should have a sharp demarcation from the adjacent renal parenchyma on at least some of the "cuts."

Table 16–2. Arteriographic Criteria for Simple Cyst

1. Lesion should be avascular (no "puddling" of contrast or abnormal tumor vessels).
2. There should be no opacification of lesion during nephrogram phase.
3. Lesion should have a smooth margin and sharp demarcation from surrounding parenchyma.
4. Sharp rim should be outlined by a few thin blood vessels abutting the central defect.

Table 16–3. Cyst Puncture Criteria for Simple Cyst

1. Fluid character:
   a. Grossly clear
   b. Only trace fat
   c. Only trace protein
   d. Normal or low LDH
   e. Low urea content
2. Cytology: no abnormal cells
3. Radiographic:
   a. Smooth-walled cyst cavity
   b. No filling defects
   c. Size of contrast-filled cyst equal to the size of the mass on prior films

When all criteria for simple cyst are met, including histochemical, cytologic, and radiographic criteria, this study is highly accurate. To our knowledge, there has never been a report of a false-negative (i.e., a tumor erroneously labeled as a cyst) when all these criteria suggested a benign cyst.

The procedure is safe, with a reported incidence of major complications of 0.75%.[35] Initial fears concerning the possibility of seeding the needle tract with malignant cells have not been borne out.[36]

Because of the high degree of accuracy and relative safety of this procedure, cyst puncture and aspiration should live on as a valuable adjunct in the evaluation of renal masses.

Surgery

All the diagnostic modalities discussed thus far were developed in the hope of forever eliminating the need for surgical exploration to rule out renal malignancy. In 1967 Kropp et al[37] were the first to raise concern about the routine use of surgical exploration in the evaluation of renal cysts, citing an operative mortality rate of 1.6% and a rate of morbidity of 30%. In a comparison between cyst puncture and renal exploration, Zelch[38] reported an operative mortality rate of 11% in flank exploration for renal cyst. Although subsequent reports have presented a more acceptable rate of morbidity and mortality for surgical approach to the diagnosis of renal cyst,[39] the invasiveness of this approach remains a legitimate concern.

One would think that open surgery would represent the gold standard in diagnosis of renal masses, yet even renal exploration has had reports of false-negative results.[40] Unfortunately, the only infallible diagnostic maneuver that can be performed is to remove the entire kidney for the pathologist to examine.

Since renal cysts do not require operative intervention on therapeutic grounds, exploration for cyst must be thought of as a diagnostic maneuver. In view of the accuracy of newer diagnostic methods to be discussed next, surgical exploration should be thought of as a step to be taken when other methods with less potential for morbidity have failed to rule out malignancy in a suspected cyst. However, if the urologist is faced with a lesion whose diagnostic character remains equivocal after the application of other studies, surgery should be performed without hesitation.

Ultrasound

In the late 1960s with the development of primitive A-mode ultrasound equipment, the value of ultrasonography in the evaluation of renal masses began to be appreciated.[41,42] A-mode equipment gave only rough representations of sound patterns on an oscilloscope screen, yet even in early reports, diagnostic accuracy in renal cyst was more than 90%. In the early 1970s B-mode scanning improved resolution and as experience in ultrasonography grew, accuracy continued to climb.[43–46] Today ultrasound examination is one of the cornerstones in the diagnostic approach to renal cysts.

Ultrasonographic criteria for the diagnosis of simple cyst are given in Table 16–4. Performance and interpretation of the renal ultrasound are subject to a greater degree of dependency upon operator technique than are other studies. However, differences in operator confidence and technique tend to be reflected in a greater percentage of masses being labeled as indeterminate.[47] In contrast to angiography, which might underdiagnose malignant lesions, lack of operator confidence in the performance of ultrasonography, then, would place lesions in a category where they would be studied more closely by other means.

Because of its high degree of accuracy in distinguishing cyst from tumor, and the lack of potential morbidity to the patient, ultrasonography is an excellent first-line study in the evaluation of cystic renal masses.

CT CRITERIA FOR SIMPLE CYST

The other giant in the armamentarium in the diagnosis of renal cyst is CT. This method combines the advantages of provision of excellent anatomic detail with the added benefit of the ability to objectively quantify the density of fluid contained in a cystic lesion. The criteria for the CT diagnosis of simple cyst are shown in Table 16–5.[48] While not as dependent upon operator technique, certain technical factors may limit the accuracy of CT diagnosis, including detector miscalibration, partial volume effect, slow scan time, and streak effect.[49] However, if diagnostic criteria are religiously upheld, the accuracy rate of CT in the diagnosis of simple cyst has been reported to be nearly 100%.[47] In spite of these and other optimistic reports on the accuracy of CT in recent mass

Table 16–4. Ultrasound Criteria for Simple Cyst

1. Increased through-transmission of sound
2. No internal echoes
3. Sharply demarcated, smooth walls with far-wall enhancement
4. Comparison with adjacent echoic structure such as the gall bladder

Table 16–5. Computed Tomography (CT) Criteria for Simple Cyst

1. Sharp margination and demarcation from surrounding renal parenchyma
2. Smooth thin wall
3. Water density content (0–20 HU) that is homogeneous throughout
4. No enhancement following administration of contrast

diagnosis, we annually see 1 or 2 mistakenly diagnosed "renal cysts" at our local urology conferences.

Magnetic Resonance Imaging

Magnetic resonance imaging (MRI) is an exciting technology with a wide range of clinical applications. MRI has been employed to image renal masses[49] with encouraging results. Basic MRI criteria for the diagnosis of simple renal cyst are given in Table 16–6.[50] As a clinical tool, MRI continues to be in a state of refinement and evolution. Shortcomings include problems with motion artifact and the inability to detect calcification within soft tissue.[49] With the advent of new high-field-strength imaging sequences, newer MRI contrast materials, and other innovations in technique, MRI holds great promise as another highly sensitive diagnostic tool to be used in this clinical setting.[51] However, because of its expense and the relatively smaller fund of clinical experience compared to CT and ultrasound, MRI remains a second-line study to be employed as an adjunct in difficult diagnostic settings.

Other Techniques

A number of less familiar techniques have been proposed as being of value in the diagnosis of renal cyst. Prophetic of the explosion of laparoscopy in the 1990s was the report, published in 1976, of examination of the cyst cavity using a cystoscope.[52] In this study Roberts reported his experience in 27 patients of direct examination of the cyst cavity after percutaneous insertion of a trocar into the cyst. This was felt to be a useful adjunct to cyst puncture and cystography. As experience with laparoscopic technique grows, this idea may see a rebirth.

An idea less likely to be revived is retroperitoneal pneumography. This method saw its heyday in the 1940s and 1950s. A gas (air, CO_2, or even helium) was insufflated either directly into the flank or by a presacral route. This maneuver greatly improved the resolution of the structures of the retroperitoneum on plain radiographs. Although useful in determining the presence or absence of a renal mass, the technique could not distinguish cyst from tumor. After a number of deaths from air embolism, retroperitoneal pneumography itself died.

If a given lesion falls within the strict diagnostic guidelines for the diagnosis of simple cyst, whether by nephrotomography, complete cyst puncture–aspiration study, ultrasound, CT, or MRI, the workup can end at that point. Fortunately, any of these diagnostic methods will reliably detect whether a mass is clearly a cyst or clearly solid. But what about lesions that do not fall clearly into either category?

THE INDETERMINATE LESION

By definition, any finding not consistent with the modality-specific diagnostic criteria for either simple cyst or malignancy falls into the "indeterminate" category. Common radiologic findings that place a given renal mass into this category include the presence of calcification, increased density or echogenicity of the center of the lesion, thickening or nodularity of the cyst wall, septations within the cyst, or multilocularity. In the past, any of these findings would have mandated surgical exploration if strict diagnostic guidelines were followed. However, with increased experience in newer diagnostic tools, some lesions within this indeterminate group can still be classified as benign with reasonable accuracy. Bosniak[53] suggested a four-tiered classification system for cystic lesions of the kidney. Category I lesions meet rigidly applied diagnostic criteria for simple cyst. Category II lesions are "benign cystic lesions that are minimally complicated and for which experience is being accumulated that will allow surgery to be avoided if possible." Further down the road to despair are category III lesions, which exhibit some malignant characteristic that mandates surgical exploration. Finally, category IV lesions are cystic masses that are clearly malignant. Fortunately, the "gray-zone" lesions of categories II and III are not common. For example, of masses evaluated by CT scan, less than 10% fall into this indeterminate class.[54]

The recent literature has provided several reviews on the subject of the diagnostically problematic renal cyst[49,55] Each of these reviews addresses the following findings that place a lesion in category II or III.

Calcification

Amis et al[56] have stated that about 20% of cystic lesions with calcification ultimately prove to be malignant but that less than 5% of renal cysts are calcified. If calcification is noted, the best study to further evaluate the mass is CT.[54]

Table 16–6. MRI Criteria for Simple Cyst

1. Well-marginated oval or round lesion
2. Imperceptible cyst wall
3. No contrast enhancement
4. Homogeneous low-signal-intensity (dark) mass on T1 images; increased intensity on T2-weighted images

Ultrasound becomes much less useful in this setting because sound waves tend to reverberate from calcifications of the posterior cyst wall, making interpretation of the nature of the internal structure of the mass difficult or impossible. Hartman et al[49] have stated that any of the following findings would exclude a cystic mass with calcification from being considered benign and would give the mass a category III rating: thick, irregular calcification; soft-tissue mass extending beyond the area of calcification; increased density of the center of the mass (i.e., not water density); thickening of the cyst wall in noncalcified areas; and contrast enhancement of any portion of the mass. On the other hand, if there is only a small amount of calcification within the wall or septum of a cyst, there is no soft-tissue mass, there is no contrast enhancement, and the central portion of the lesion is of water density, then in their view, the lesion may still be safely labeled as benign (category II).

Internal Structure

Septations within the cyst cavity are often seen. Although they may be seen on either CT or ultrasound, a septated cystic lesion is probably best evaluated with ultrasound.[54] When is the presence of septation an ominous sign that mandates further more aggressive evaluation? Bosniak[53] answers that cysts may still be considered in category II if the septations are not too numerous and not too thick, and then hurries to admit that these parameters are not easy to define objectively. Hartman[49] specifies that septae greater than 1 mm in thickness or those with solid elements at septal attachment require surgical intervention. As previously stated, the presence of fine calcification of the septum is still consistent with a benign lesion.

Increased Density

Although one of the diagnostic criteria for the CT diagnosis of renal cyst is density equal to that of water, increased density does not necessarily exclude a diagnosis of benign cyst. These lesions may be associated with old hemorrhage or inflammation, but they are especially common in autosomal dominant polycystic kidney disease. Bosniak[53] has offered the following criteria by which high-density cysts may still be considered as benign lesions: (1) the lesion must be perfectly smooth, round, shaply marginated, and homogeneous; (2) the lesion must not enhance upon the intravenous administration of contrast material and its configuration must remain unchanged; (3) the lesion must be 3 cm or less in size. Larger lesions may still be considered benign if upon ultrasound examination they meet all criteria for the diagnosis of simple cyst.

Cyst Wall Abnormalities: Thickening or Nodularity

While there may be modifying circumstances which allow the clinician to avoid surgical exploration in the face of other worrisome findings, the presence of any nodularity or thickening of the cyst wall by with CT or ultrasound is disqualifying for the assignment of a diagnosis of benign cyst.

CONCLUSIONS

The urologist today has a large armamentarium of diagnostic tests at his disposal for the evaluation of renal mass lesions. Which asymptomatic renal mass to pursue with diagnostic tests is a judgment call best made by the urologist. Although well over 90% of renal masses can be correctly diagnosed without surgery, which renal mass to explore is again a decision best made by the clinician most knowledgeable about renal masses, the urologist.

REFERENCES

1. Kissane JM: Congenital malformations. In: Heptinstall RH, ed. *Pathology of the Kidney*, 3rd ed. Boston: Little, Brown, 1983; 83–140.
2. Young HH, Davis DM: *Young's Practice of Urology*. Philadelphia: WB Saunders, 1926.
3. Lang EK: Coexistence of cyst and tumor in the same kidney. *Radiology* 1971;101:7.
4. Emmet JL, Levine SR, Woolner LB: Co-existence of renal cyst and tumor: incidence in 1,007 cases. *Br J Urol* 1963;35:403.
5. Brannan W, Miller W, Crisler M: Coexistence of renal neoplasms. *South Med J* 1962;55:749.
6. Ambrose SS, Lewis LL, O'Brien DP, Walton KN, Ross JR: Unsuspected renal tumors associated with renal cysts. *J Urol* 1977;117:704.
7. Lang EK: Roentgenologic approach to the diagnosis and management of cystic lesions of the kidney: is cyst exploration mandatory? *Urol Clin North Am* 1980;7(3):677.
8. Limgard DA, Lawson TL: Accuracy of ultrasound in predicting the nature of renal masses. *J Urol*, 1979;122:724.
9. McClennan BL, Stanley RJ, Melson GL, Levitt RG, Sagel SS: CT of the renal cyst: is aspiration necessary? *AJR* 1979; 133:671.
10. Clayman, RV, Williams RD, Fraley EE: The pursuit of the renal mass. *N Engl J Med* 1979;300:72.
11. Roth JK, Roberts JA: Benign renal cysts and renal function. *J Urol* 1980;123:625.
12. Pollack HM, Goldberg BB, Bogash M: Changing concepts in the diagnosis and management of renal cysts. *J Urol* 1974; 111:326.
13. Lang EK: Roentgenographic assessment of asymptomatic renal lesions. *Radiology* 1973;109:257.
14. Pollack HM, Edell S, Morales JO: Radionuclide imaging of renal pseudotumors. *Radiology* 1974;111:639.
15. Stewart BH, Haynie TP, Noeal M, Carr EA: Role of scintillation scanning in diagnosis of renal tumors. *J Urol* 1962; 87:782.
16. Peterson CC, Jackson JH, Moore JG: A re-evaluation of nephrotomography stressing the limitations of the procedure. *J Urol* 1968;98:721.
17. Chynn KY, Evans JA: Nephrotomography in the differentiation of renal cyst from neoplasm: a review of 500 cases. *J Urol* 1960;83:21.
18. Lillard RL, Keyting WS, Daywitt AL: Four phase nephroto-

mography in the diagnosis of renal cysts and tumors. *AJR* 1967;99:593.
19. Witten DM, Greene LF, Emmet JL: An evaluation of nephrotomography in urologic diagnosis. *AJR* 1963;90:115.
20. Bosniak MA: Nephrotomography: a relatively unappreciated but extremely valuable diagnostic tool. *Radiology* 1974; 113:313.
21. Melicow MM, Becker JA: Radiographic simulation of certain solid tumors of the renal corpus to renal cyst. *J Urol* 1967; 97:592.
22. McLaughlin III, AP, Talner LB, Leopold GR, McCullough DL: Avascular renal cell carcinoma: varied pathologic and angiographic features. *J Urol* 1974;111:587.
23. Watson RC, Fleming RJ, Evans JA: Arteriography in the diagnosis of renal carcinoma. *Radiology* 1968;91:888.
24. Young JM, Morrow JW: Problems in interpretation of angiograms in renal mass lesions. *J Urol* 1972;107:925.
25. Meaney TF: Errors in angiographic diagnosis of renal masses. *Radiology* 1969;93:361.
26. Leitner WA, Anderson EE, Weber CH, Grimes JH, Johnsrude IS: Limitations of arteriography in renal mass evaluation. *Arch Intern Med* 1972;130:868.
27. Lang EK: The accuracy of roentgenographic techniques in the diagnosis of renal mass lesions. *Radiology* 1971;98:119.
28. Harris RD, Goergen TG, Talner LB: The bloody renal cyst aspirate: a diagnostic dilemma. *J Urol* 1972;114:832.
29. Jean WD, Penry JB, Roylance J: Renal puncture. *Clin Radiol* 1972;32:298.
30. Wheeler BC: Use of the aspirating needle in the diagnosis of solitary renal cyst. *N Engl J Med* 1942;226:55.
31. Thornbury JR: Needle aspiration of avascular renal lesions. *Radiology* 1972;105:299.
32. Navari RM, Ploth DW, Tatum RK: Renal adenocarcinoma associated with simple cysts. *JAMA* 1981;246:1808.
33. Lang EK: Coexistence of cyst and tumor in the same kidney. *Diag Radiol* 1971;101:7.
34. Wettlaufer JN, Modarelli RO: Triple contrast percutaneous nephrocystography and analysis of cyst aspirate. *Urology* 1978; 7(3):373.
35. Lang EK: Renal cyst puncture and aspiration: a survey of complications. *AJR* 1977;128:723.
36. von Schreeb T, Arner O, Skovsted G, Wikstad N: Renal adenocarcinoma: is there risk of spreading tumour cells in diagnostic puncture? *Scand J Urol Nephrol* 1967;1:270.
37. Kropp KA, Grayhack JT, and Wendel RM: Morbidity and mortality of renal exploration for cyst. *Surg Gynecol Obstet* 1967;125:803.
38. Zelch J, Lalli AF, Stewart BH, Daughtry JD: Complications of renal cyst exploration versus renal mass aspiration. *Urology* 1976;7:244.
39. Stanisic TH, Babcock JR, Grayhack JR: Morbidity and mortality of renal exploration for cyst. *Surg Gynecol Obstet* 1977; 145:733.
40. Rehm RA, Taylor WN, Taylor JN: Renal cyst associated with carcinoma. *J Urol* 1961;86:307.
41. Goldberg BB, Ostrum BJ, Isard HJ: Nephrosonography: ultrasound differentiation of renal masses. *Radiology* 1968; 90:1113.
42. Goldberg BB, Pollack HM: Differentiation of renal masses using A-mode ultrasound. *J Urol* 1971;105:765.
43. Leopold GR, Talner LB, Asher WM, Gosink BB, Gittes RF: Renal ultrasonography: an updated approach to the diagnosis of renal cyst. *Radiology* 1973;109:671.
44. King DL: Renal ultrasonography: an aid in the clinical evaluation of renal masses. *Radiology* 1972;105:633.
45. Asher WM, Leopold GR: A streamlined approach to renal mass lesions with renal echogram. *J Urol* 1972;108:205.
46. Barnett E, Morley P: Ultrasound in the investigation of space-occupying lesion of the urinary tract. *Br J Urol* 1971;44:733.
47. Pollack HM, Banner MP, Arger PH, et al: The accuracy of gray-scale renal ultrasonography in differentiating cystic neoplasms from benign cysts. *Radiology* 1982;143:741.
48. McClennan BL, Stanley RJ, Melson GL, Levitt RG, Sagel SS: CT of the renal cyst: is cyst aspiration necessary. *AJR* 1979; 133:671.
49. Hricak H, Williams RD, Moon KL, et al: Nuclear magnetic resonance imaging of the kidney: renal masses. *Radiology* 1983;147:765.
50. Hartman DS, Aronson S, Frazer H: Current imaging of indeterminate renal masses. *Radiol Clin North Am* 1991;29:475.
51. Semelka RC, Shoenut JC, Kroeker MA, et al: Renal lesion: controlled comparison between CT and 1.5T MR imaging with non-enhanced and gadolinium-enhanced fat-suppressed spin-echo and breath-hold FLASH techniques. *Radiology* 1992; 182:425.
52. Roberts JA: Renal cystoscopy. *Urology* 1974;7:537.
53. Bosniak MA: The current radiologic approach to renal cysts. *Radiology* 1986;158:1.
54. Balfe DM, McClennan BL, Stanley RJ, et al: Evaluation of renal masses considered indeterminate on computed tomography. *Radiology* 1982;142:421.
55. Dalla-Palma L, and Pozzi-Mucelli R: Problematic renal masses in ultrasonography and computed tomography. *Clin Imag* 1990;14:83.
56. Amis ES, Cronan JJ, Yoder IC, et al: Renal cysts: curios and caveats. *Urol Radiol* 1982;4:199.

17 The Complex Cystic Mass

Robert A. Older, Marguerite C. Lippert

Typical renal cysts and obvious solid renal masses do not present a diagnostic problem. The complex cystic mass, however, often creates a diagnostic dilemma. To deal with cystic lesions it is necessary to establish clear diagnostic criteria and to perform optimal imaging studies to evaluate these criteria. This will optimize our ability to identify lesions that are clearly benign or malignant and reduce the number placed in an indeterminate category.

Despite using multiple imaging techniques, the etiology of these complex cystic masses cannot always be determined. Management in these instances will be surgical, unless clinically contraindicated. The type of surgery may be affected by the likelihood that a lesion is malignant or benign. Imaging therefore has two goals: (1) to accurately place as many lesions as possible into groups that are "determinate" and for which therapy is clear and (2) to determine, if possible, whether a lesion placed in an indeterminate category has a high or low probability of malignancy. This second goal is not always easily achieved. To reach these goals studies must be performed and interpreted carefully. This will reduce incorrect diagnoses resulting from improper performance or interpretation. Attention to detail is necessary to diagnose these complex lesions accurately.

A classification of cystic mass lesions helps to define criteria for differentiating benign from malignant lesions. The best current classification is that developed by Bosniak.[1,2] This classification considers both ultrasound (US) and computed tomographic (CT) criteria, and the principles can be expanded to magnetic resonance imaging (MRI).

- Class 1: Uncomplicated simple cysts: no further workup needed.
- Class 2: Minimally complicated benign cysts: cysts with thin (1 mm or less) septations; cysts with thin, fine calcifications; high-density cysts and infected cysts. Most need no follow-up, but those lesions toward the more suspicious end of the group do deserve follow-up (subgroup IIF).[3]
- Class 3: More complicated and suspicious lesions such as those with thick, irregular calcifications; multiple thick septa; thick walls; nonenhancing nodularity; or multiloculated mass. These lesions can be benign or malignant, and many require surgical intervention.[3]
- Class 4: Clearly malignant lesions with cystic components such as lesions with solid portions, enhancing or large areas of nodularity, or enhancing or nonuniform thick wall.

CLASSES 1 AND 2

Ultrasound is often the first imaging study to characterize a lesion. Class 1 lesions are anechoic, with smooth walls and good through transmission (Fig. 17–1). A class 2 cystic lesion may have thin septations demonstrated with ultrasound (Fig. 17–2).

To avoid diagnostic errors due to technique, equipment must be properly adjusted. Gain settings that are too high can make a cystic lesion appear solid, whereas low settings can mask true internal echos. If experience with an ultrasound unit is limited, comparison with known cystic structures such as the bladder or gallbladder will help adjust gain settings. It is important to understand the limitations of ultrasound in general and specifically for the equipment being used. Body habitus can significantly affect visualization of renal lesions, particularly on the left side, where it is more difficult to obtain a good acoustic window. Small lesions are more difficult to define and should not be considered simple cysts unless they are well seen and well characterized. A lesion not clearly visualized with US should be evaluated with CT.

In adults the kidneys can be evaluated with either a 3.5-Mhz or a 5-Mhz transducer, depending on body size. The 5-Mhz transducer will provide better detail but in a larger patient may not have sufficient tissue penetration. Often the combination of both transducers is helpful.

On computed tomography class 1 or 2 cystic lesions must have (1) low density (i.e., 0 to 20 HU), (2) sharp margins, (3) smooth walls, and (4) no evidence of enhancement following administration of iodinated contrast (Fig. 17–3). Thin septa (pencil line) are acceptable for class 2 but not thick or nodular septa (Fig. 17–4). Thin, curvilinear calcification also places a lesion in class 2, and this finding is best demonstrated with CT (Fig. 17–5). Calcification will produce acoustic shadowing and limit visualization of the mass with ultrasound.

A special example of a class 2 lesion is the "high-density cyst," which has a density range of 40 to 100 HU[4] and is often of higher density than the surrounding unenhanced renal parenchyma (Fig. 17–6). The high density can be due to

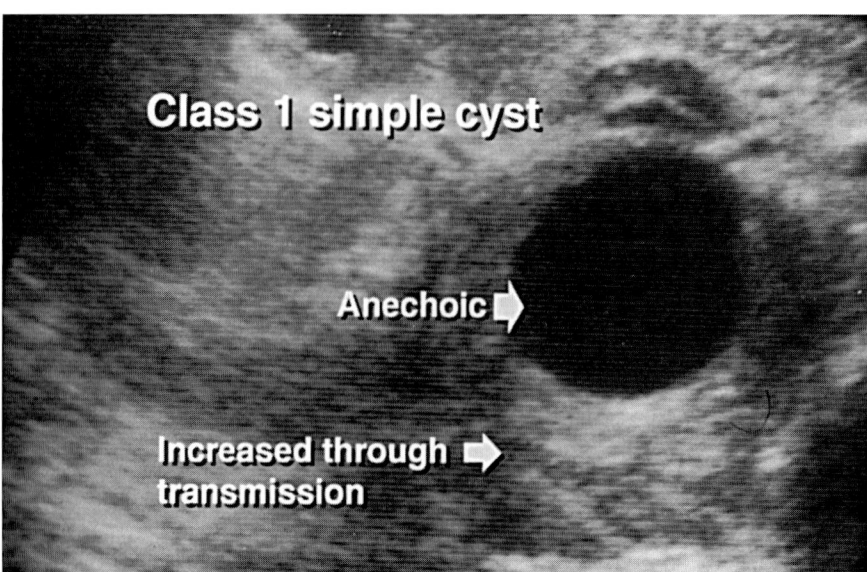

Figure 17–1. Ultrasound of a simple class 1 renal cyst. The lesion is anechoic with smooth walls and good through transmission.

proteinaceous material, hemorrhage, colloid formation, or elevated iron content.[4] High-density cysts are common in autosomal dominant polycystic disease[4] and in acquired renal cystic disease.[5] This type of lesion is often first noted on CT, but an unenhanced or enhanced CT alone is not sufficient for diagnosis because of the high baseline density of these lesions. Both pre- and postcontrast studies with thin sections are necessary to exclude enhancement. CT criteria for a benign lesion include a smooth, homogeneous, and sharply marginated lesion less than 3 cm in size. There must be no enhancement and at least one-fourth of the lesion must extend outside the kidney to allow evaluation of the wall.

US findings of an anechoic lesion typical for a simple cyst can also be considered as confirmation that the high-density lesion is benign. Unfortunately, many high-density cysts have internal echoes and decreased through transmission, probably because of hemorrhagic contents.[4,6,7] Bosniak found that many hyperdense cysts appear solid on US because of products resulting from hemorrhage, with only 50% showing the appearance of a simple cyst. In instances where the two imaging modalities did not agree, he considered CT more reliable than US, with the single most important criterion being the presence or absence of enhancement following contrast administration.[6,8]

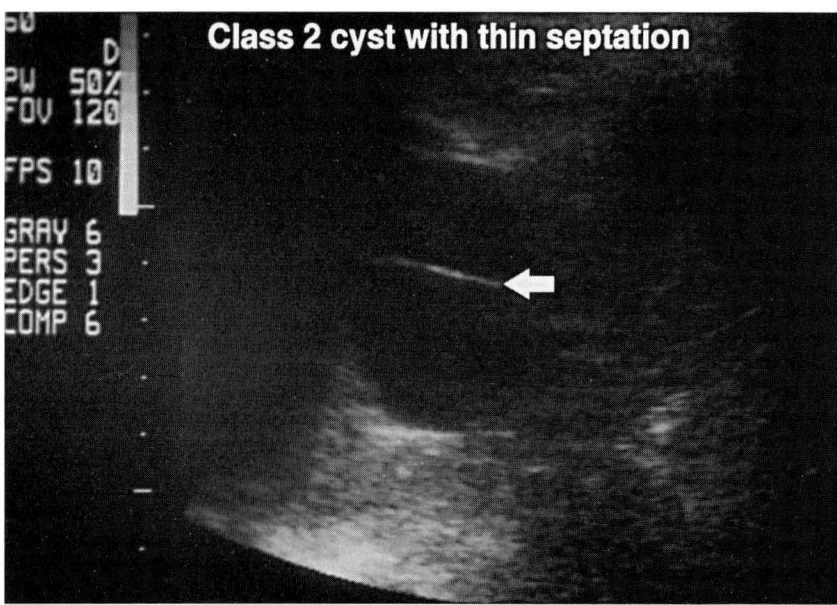

Figure 17–2. Class 2 cyst containing a thin septation.

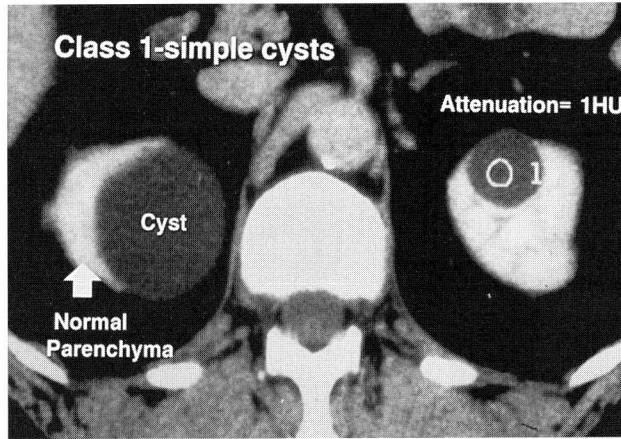

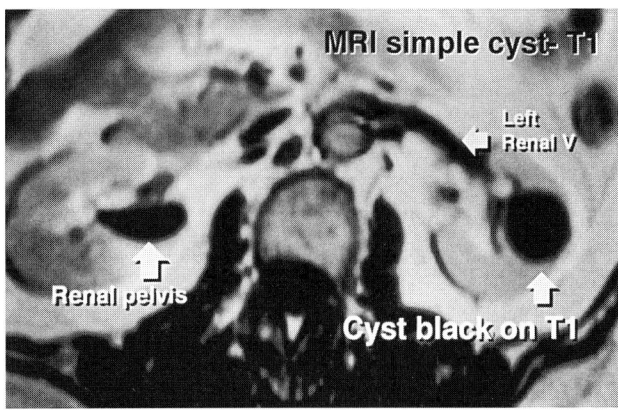

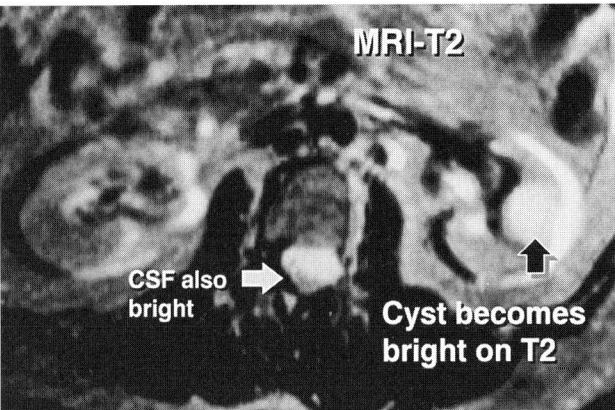

Figure 17–3. (A) Simple cysts on enhanced CT with low attenuation (1 HU), sharp margins, and no enhancement. (B) MRI of a simple cyst in a different patient. Sharply defined lesion with homogeneous low intensity on T1 similar to CSF. (C) T2-weighted MRI shows the cyst as high intensity.

The presence of a ''solid''-appearing lesion with US, however, should not be disregarded, especially if CT is suboptimal technically or not conclusive. Foster[9] found ultrasound correctly identified small (<3 cm) cysts and carcinomas when thin-section bolus CT showed equivocal enhancement. If CT is equivocal for enhancement and ultrasound shows a solid lesion, malignancy cannot be excluded and surgery should be considered. If, however, the lesion

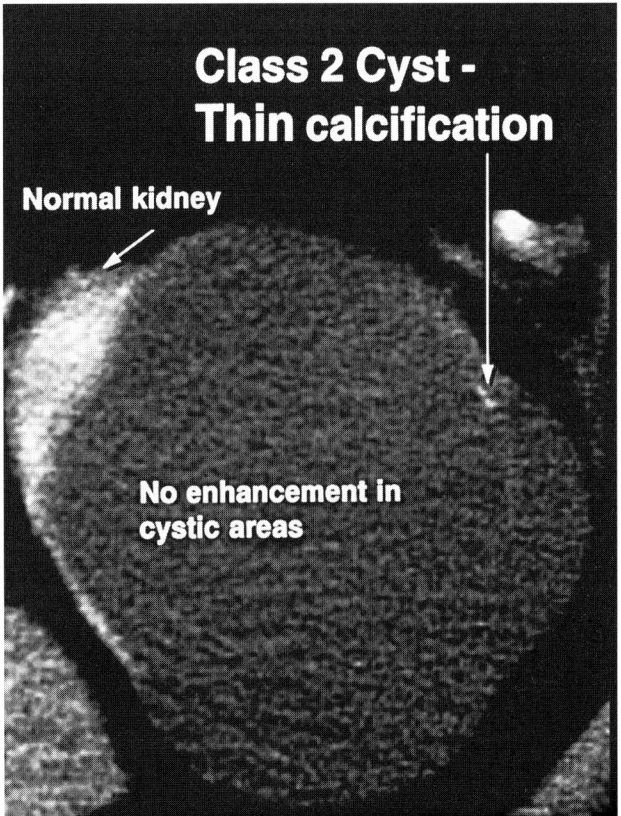

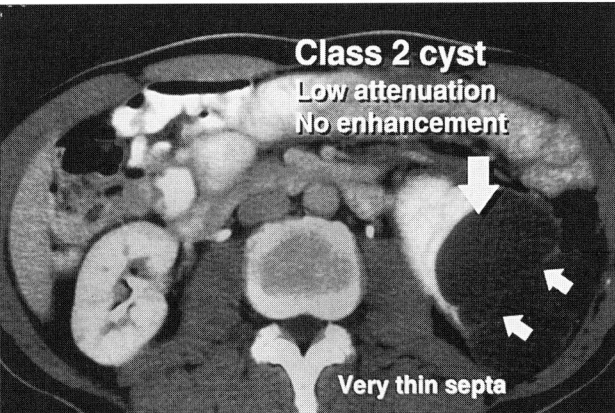

Figure 17–4. Class 2 cyst on computed tomography. Fine septations are visible, but the lesion is of homogeneous low density, has thin walls, and has no enhancement.

Figure 17–5. Class 2 cyst with thin calcification on CT.

appears solid with ultrasound but is a typical high-density lesion without enhancement on CT, follow-up is reasonable (class 2F). Levine found that most hemorrhagic cysts larger than 2 cm resolved on follow-up imaging.[5] Another option for evaluating a discrepancy between CT and US findings is cyst puncture.[2]

Experience with the hyperdense cystic lesion is limited in the literature, and the incidence of carcinoma with this appearance is unknown. Malignant lesions meeting the criteria for a benign hyperdense cyst have been described,[4] and these lesions should be treated cautiously.

CLASS 3

Class 3 lesions are complicated by thick (Fig. 17–7), nodular, or multiple septa; thick or irregular calcification; and thick or mildly nodular walls. The difficulty with class 3 lesions is that they can be benign or malignant and the imaging features cannot always differentiate one from the other. In a small series of class 3 lesions approximately 50% were malignant and 50% benign.[2] Enhancement is not considered a component of a class 3 lesion, and it is the goal of CT or MRI to demonstrate whether or not enhancement is present. Enhancement will place a lesion into class 4.

Prior to the use of CT, calcification of a mass lesion, especially nonperipheral, was found to have a strong relationship to renal cell carcinoma, and for many years any type of renal mass calcification was considered suspicious for malignancy.[10] With the increased sensitivity of computed tomography benign calcifications are more often detected.

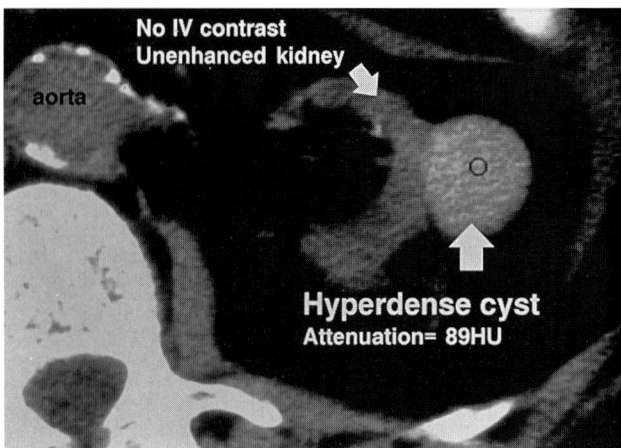

Figure 17–6. High-density cyst on CT: cyst measures 89 HU; cyst density greater than unenhanced renal parenchyma.

Thin, curvilinear calcification is present in benign cystic lesions, and it is now thought that only thick or irregular calcifications are suggestive of carcinoma. Even these thick calcifications are not always malignant (Fig. 17–8), but they often require surgical intervention to exclude carcinoma (Fig. 17–9). In this group of patients, clinical factors and history will play a major role in therapeutic decisions as well as imaging findings. Calcification associated with abnormal soft tissue (Fig. 17–10) increases the possibility of malignancy.

Nodularity within a cystic mass may represent tumor or a benign process (Fig. 17–11A). Enhancement of the nodule

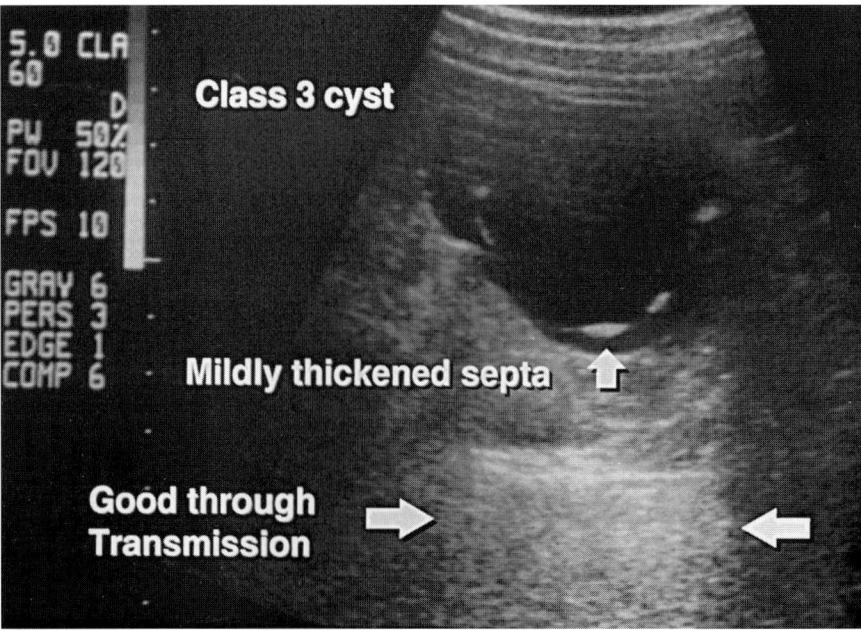

Figure 17–7. Class 3 cyst. Ultrasound shows slightly thickened septa.

The Complex Cystic Mass 353

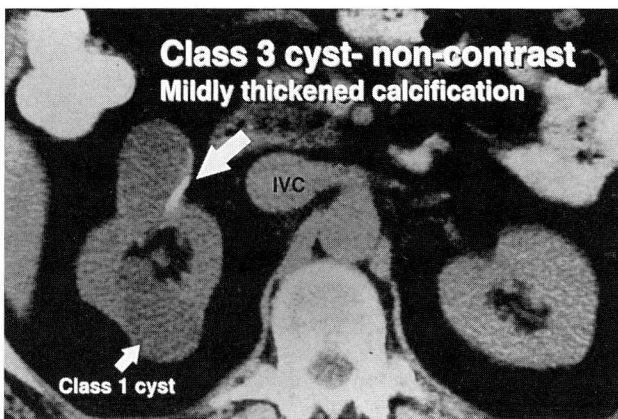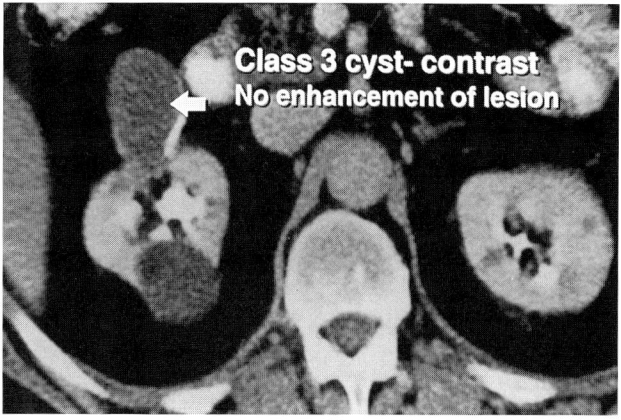

Figure 17–8. (A) Class 3 cyst with slightly thickened calcification on CT. All other features suggested a benign cyst. (B) No enhancement was present and the mass showed no change with follow-up.

in Figure 11A would indicate a class 4 surgical lesion. MRI (Fig. 17–11B) was performed because a prior contrast reaction precluded enhanced CT. This study showed hemorrhagic fluid but no enhancement following GDPA administration. Follow-up 2 months later showed the nodule had reduced in size, indicating a benign process (Fig. 17–11C). In this patient MRI was used to clarify a difficult case and may have significant potential in this regard.[11–13] MRI is most useful in patients with renal failure, contrast allergy, or other contraindications to enhanced CT.[14]

Multilocular lesions are class 3 by definition but often show characteristics of a class 4 lesion, as will be discussed later. A multilocular mass may represent a benign multilocular cystic nephroma, and in the right clinical population

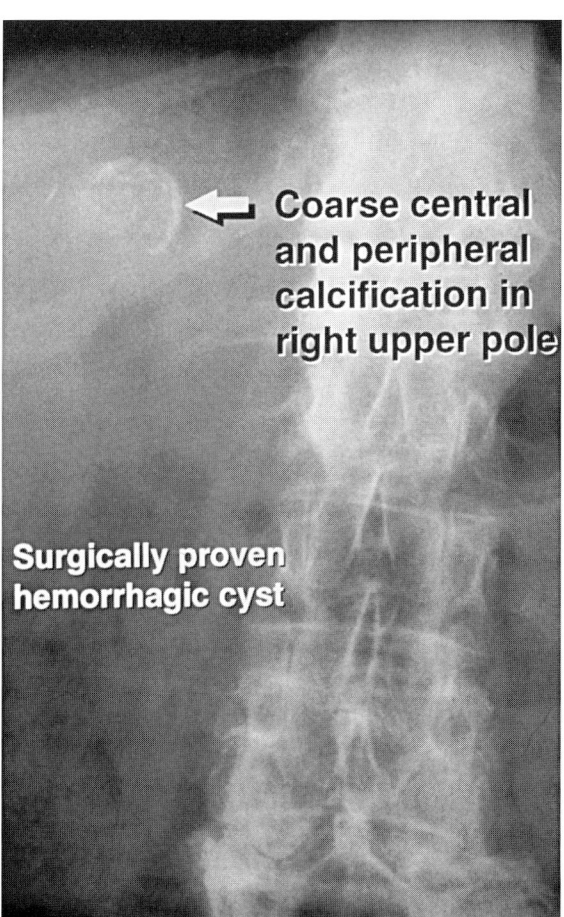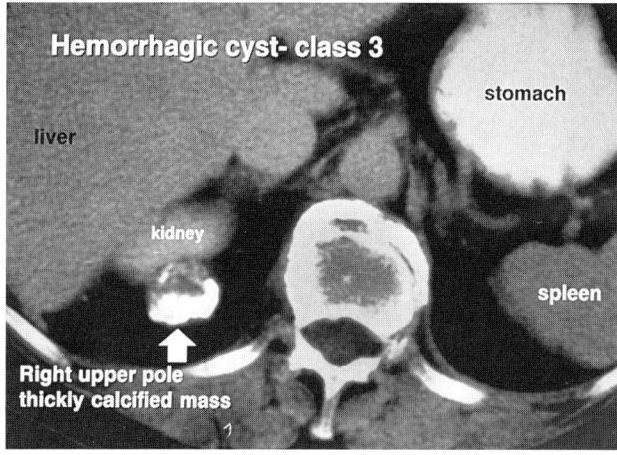

Figure 17–9. (A) Dense circular-appearing calcification initially noted on abdominal film. (B) CT confirmed an associated soft-tissue mass that led to partial nephrectomy. This proved to be a hemorrhagic cyst.

354 Diagnosis of Genitourinary Disease

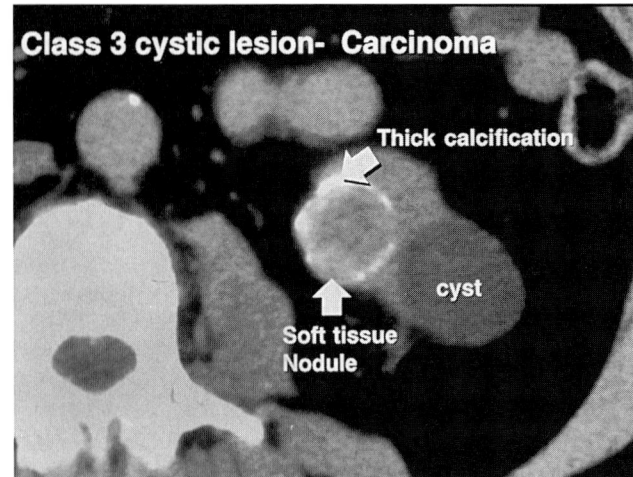

Figure 17–10. Thick calcification associated with nodular soft tissue. Surgery revealed carcinoma.

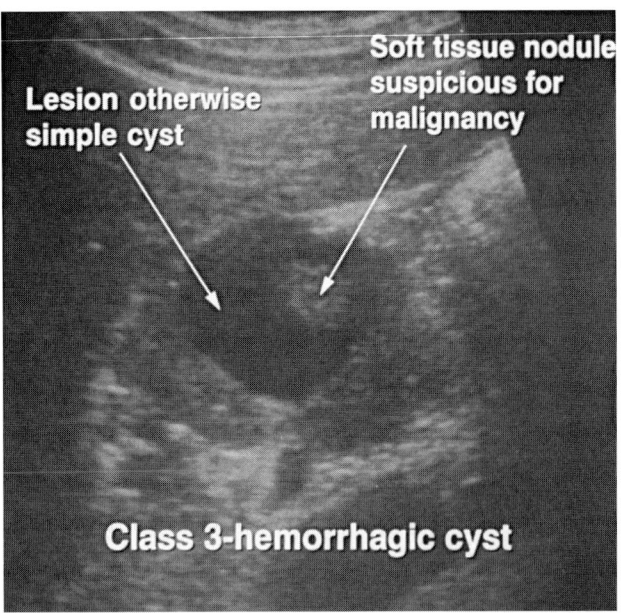

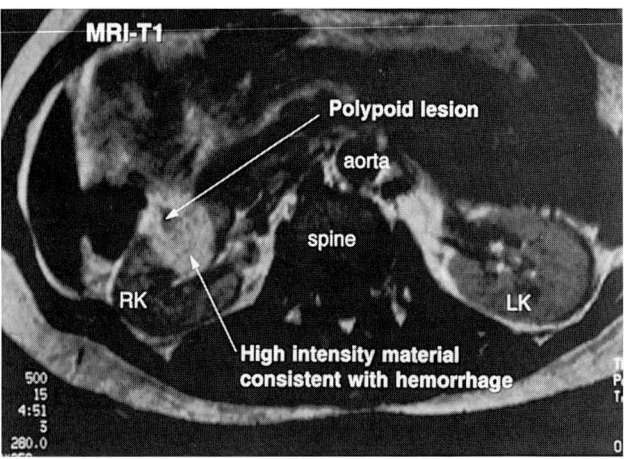

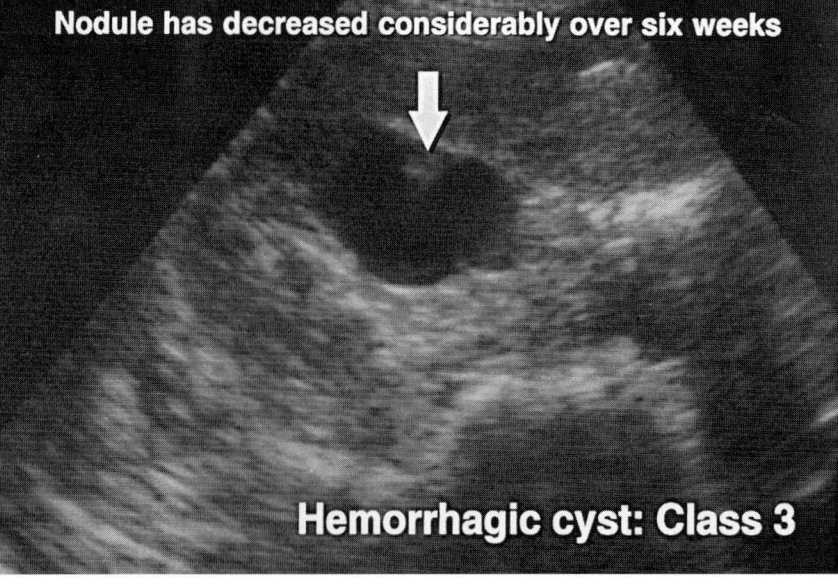

Figure 17–11. (A) Well-circumscribed nodularity noted in an otherwise cystic-appearing lesion with ultrasound. (B) MRI performed because of prior severe allergic reaction to iodinated contrast demonstrated hemorrhagic fluid but no enhancement of nodule. (C) Follow-up ultrasound showed marked reduction in the nodule, indicating a benign process.

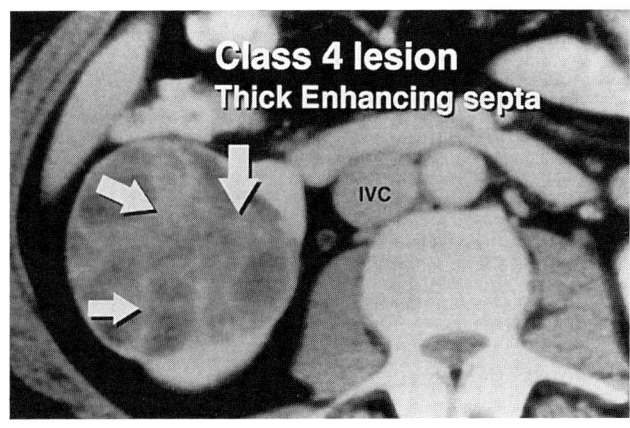

Figure 17–12. Enhanced CT scan of multilocular renal cell carcinoma shows multiple thickened and enhancing septations.

(i.e., males up to 4 years old and middle-aged females 50 to 60 years old) this diagnosis should be considered. Dalla-Palma noted thick septa with prominent enhancement (>30 HU) in multilocular renal cell carcinoma but only faint enhancement in thin septa in multilocular cystic nephroma. Vegetations were seen in carcinoma, but not in multilocular cystic nephroma.[15] When areas of thick septal enhancement are present (Figs. 17–12, 17–13), the mass becomes a class 4 lesion.

CLASS 4

Enhancement places a lesion in class 4, but the degree of enhancement can vary. Figure 17–14 shows a thick-walled cystic lesion with several areas of peripheral enhancement indicating carcinoma. Enhancement is much less apparent in Figure 17–15, in which the lesion is almost totally cystic. Only a small area of peripheral enhancement indicates the true nature of this renal cell carcinoma. To diagnose this type of lesion correctly, thin-section CT scans (4 to 5 mm) both before and after contrast are necessary. With less than optimal CT technique the focal enhancement could have been missed and the mass considered a benign cyst. Pariety and colleagues found at least one area of enhancement in all 15 of the cystic carcinomas in their series but concur that the enhancement may be visible only on a single scan, with the remainder of the lesion appearing as a simple cyst.[16]

DIAGNOSTIC PITFALLS

The following lists some diagnostic pitfalls of US and CT:

1. Ultrasound
   a. Improper gain settings.
   b. Limited visualization of a lesion.
2. Computed tomograpy
   a. Failure to obtain true pre- and postcontrast studies
      (1) Contrast mistaken for calcification (Fig. 17–16)
      (2) Calcification missed (Fig. 17–17)
      (3) Enhancement missed
   b. CT sections too thick
      (1) Enhancement missed
   c. Poor contrast bolus
   d. Failure to obtain measurements
      (1) Visual observation alone can be misleading
   e. Incorrect area of measurement
      (1) It is crucial that the most suspicious area be measured for possible enhancement. Measurement of the central portion of a lesion alone is not sufficient and can lead to an incorrect diagnosis (Fig. 17–18).
   f. Nonspecificity of enhancement
      (1) Enhancement is the main criterion for determining malignancy in a cystic mass, but unfortunately it is not specific. Lesions with enhancement will not

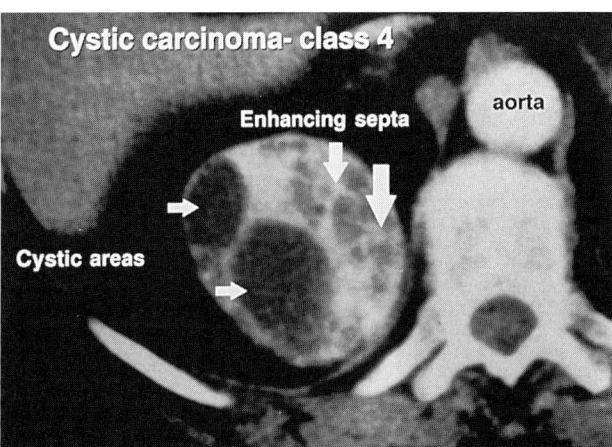

Figure 17–13. US (**A**) and CT (**B**) of a multilocular lesion shows several well-defined cystic spaces, but more peripherally thickened enhancing septa indicate renal cell carcinoma.

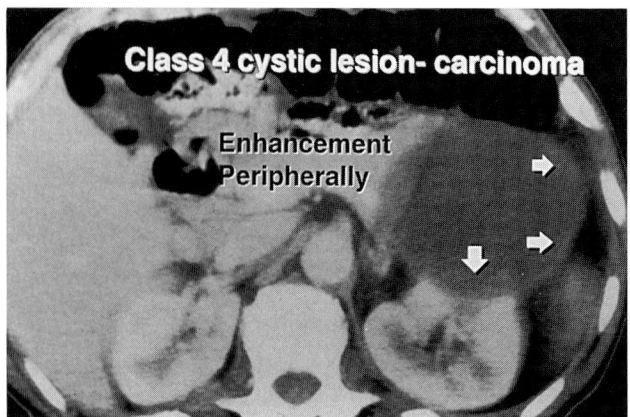

Figure 17–14. Thick-walled cystic lesion with multiple areas of peripheral enhancement.

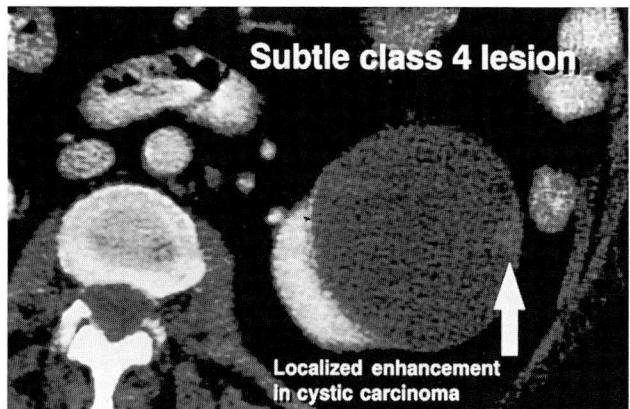

Figure 17–15. Predominantly cystic renal mass. Small area of peripheral enhancement (arrows) indicating the true etiology, renal cell carcinoma.

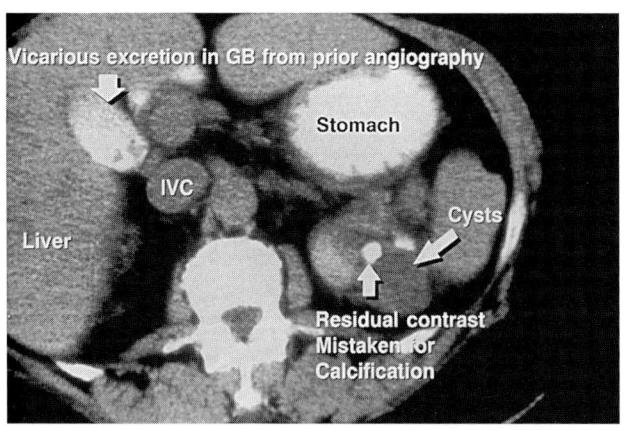
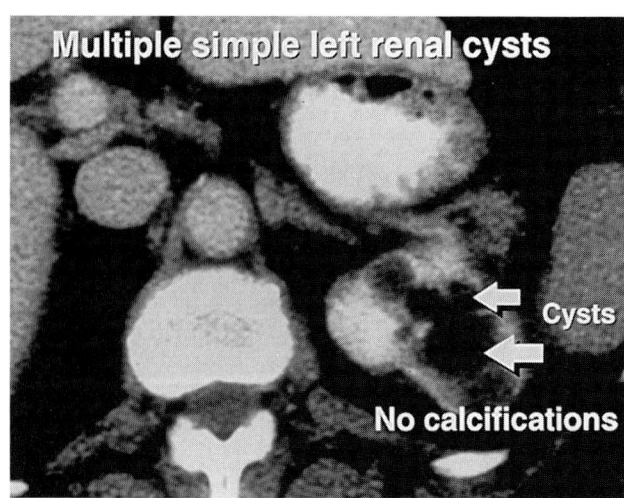

Figure 17–16. **(A)** "Unenhanced" CT 1 day following peripheral angiography—residual contrast mistaken for thick calcification. Note vicarious excretion in gallbladder. **(B)** Follow-up enhanced scan shows no abnormal calcification.

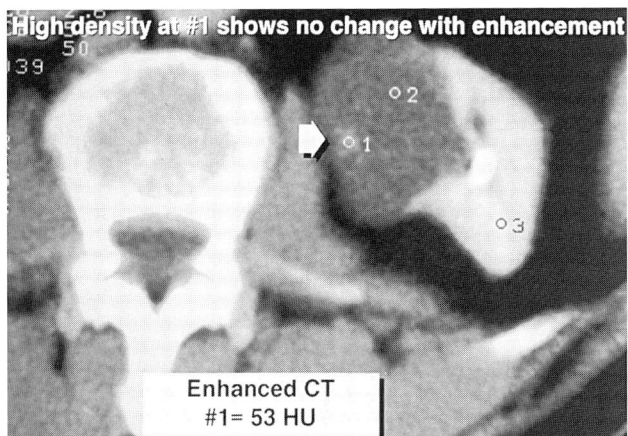 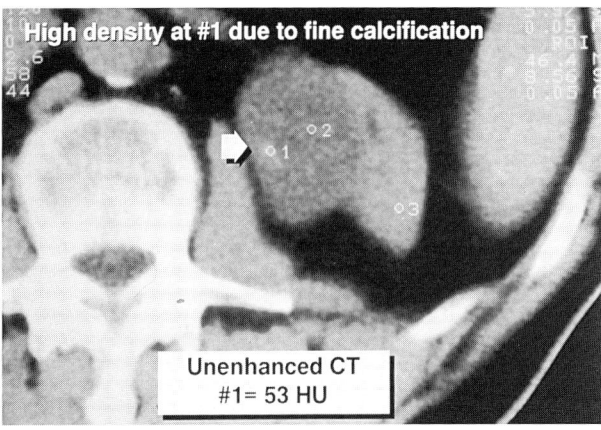

Figure 17–17. Complex class 3 cyst (**A**). Tiny area of increased attenuation (53 HU) could be mistaken for enhancement without precontrast study (**B**) showing that the high attenuation is due to fine calcification.

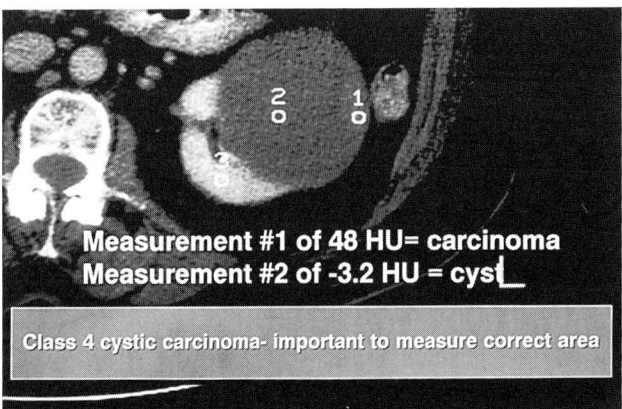

Figure 17–18. Cystic renal cell carcinoma left kidney. Central measurements give a false impression of a benign cystic mass. Measurements need to be made in the more suspicious area peripherally. (Same patient as is shown in Fig. 17–15.)

all prove to be malignant. Inflammatory masses and certain complex cysts can demonstrate enhancement (Fig. 17–19). An abnormal vascular lesion can also lead to apparent enhancement, suggesting malignancy (Fig. 17–20).

OTHER PROCEDURES

The basic imaging studies used in evaluating cystic masses are ultrasound and CT. MRI may be of benefit, especially in an institution where there is considerable experience with this imaging modality. In patients in whom iodinated contrast cannot be used, gadolinium–DTPA-enhanced MRI can be used to evaluate the presence or absence of enhancement.

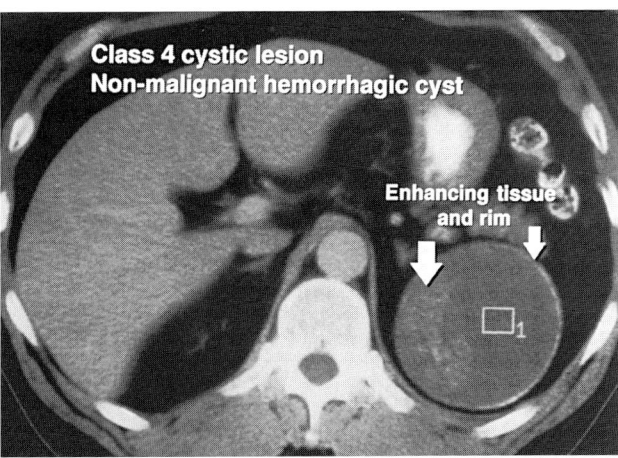

Figure 17–19. Thick-walled cystic lesion with enhancing material in the periphery of the lesion. This proved not to be renal cell carcinoma but rather a complicated hemorrhagic cyst.

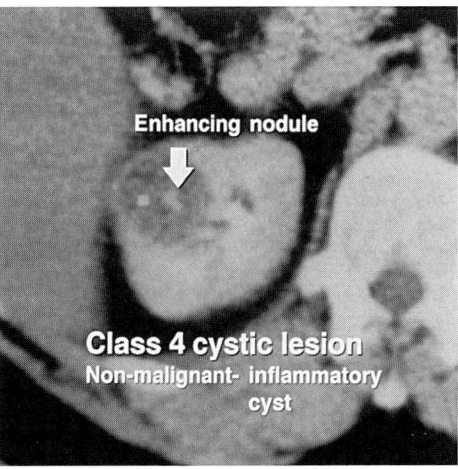

Figure 17–20. Benign cystic lesion with small area of central enhancement. This was considered suspicious for malignancy but proved to be an inflammatory cyst with a large anomalous central vessel producing the area of central enhancement.

Figure 17–21. (**A**) CT of subcapsular hematoma caused by renal cell carcinoma. (**B**) Selective renal angiogram. Neovascularity confirmed malignancy in a suspicious area on CT.

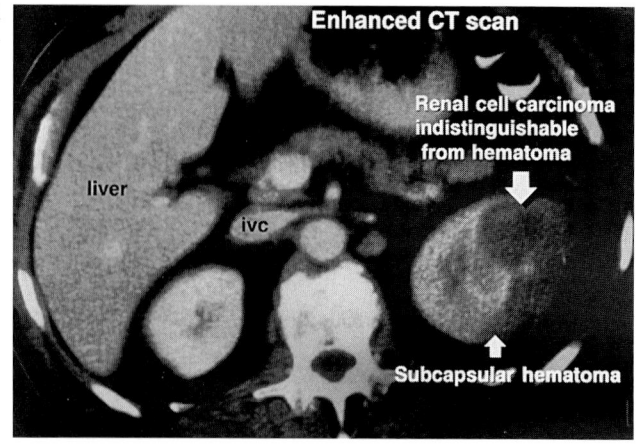

Figure 17–22. (**A**) CT of adult dominant polycystic kidney disease. Solid-appearing mass was not present on the previous scan. (**B**) Subtraction arteriography clearly demonstrates tumor neovascularity in the mass, indicating renal cell carcinoma.

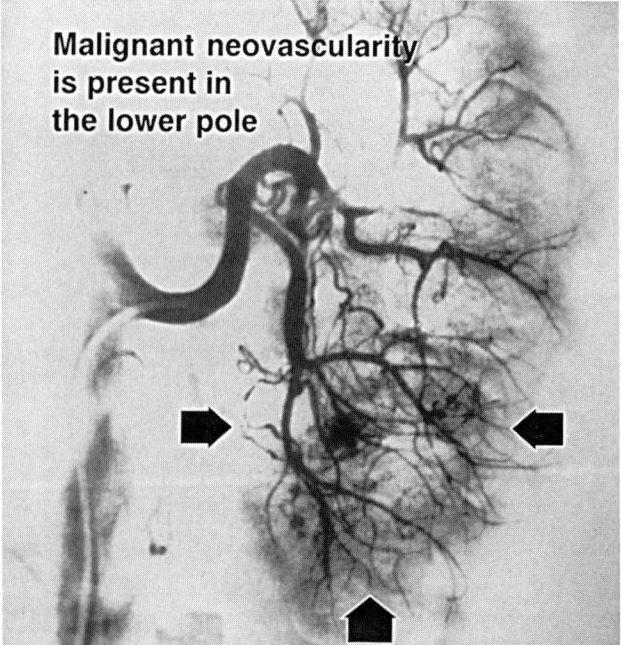

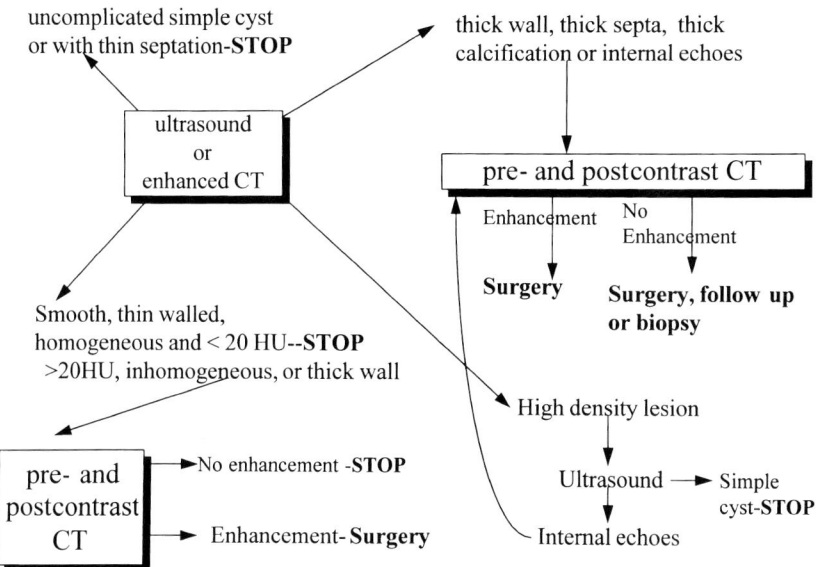

Figure 17–23. Schematic for renal mass evaluation.

GD-DTPA can safely be used in patients allergic to iodinated contrast or in renal failure.[3,14]

Spiral CT, the newest and fastest type of CT scanner, may help in small lesions. Its speed allows the images to be obtained in a single breath-hold and eliminates artifacts related to respiratory motion. This can reduce volume averaging with the potential for more accurate density measurements. Spiral CT, however, may actually be too fast, obtaining the images before optimal medullary enhancement. Either a loading dose of contrast or delayed scans may be needed to visualize the renal parenchymal completely.[17]

Angiography is infrequently used for diagnosis of a renal lesion. It should not be completely forgotten, however, and in some instances it can provide significant information. The demonstration of even a small area of tumor vascularity can confirm the diagnosis of renal cell carcinoma. We have, on occasion, found this useful, such as in a patient with tumor-related subcapsular hemorrhage (Fig. 17–21). The hematoma made the carcinoma less apparent on ultrasound and CT, but angiographically demonstrated neovascularity identified the malignancy. A hemorrhagic cyst in adult dominant polycystic kidney disease can appear solid with both CT and ultrasound and mimic a renal cell carcinoma. Enhancement with either CT or MRI will identify a carcinoma in most cases, but in questionable cases selective renal angiography can be of help (Fig. 17–22). Biopsy is not usually performed in complex cystic masses.[18] Clear fluid, even with negative cytology, does not conclusively exclude carcinoma.[3,18] However, in a case in which the surgeon wishes to avoid an open surgical procedure for clinical reasons, a negative biopsy may be reassuring, and a positive biopsy would clearly indicate the need for surgery.[19]

As with all renal lesions, evidence of spread outside the renal capsule or to lymphatic or venous structures should be evaluated because such spread may clarify an otherwise indeterminate lesion.

The schematic in Figure 17–23 summarizes our basic approach to the cystic mass.

REFERENCES

1. Bosniak MA: The current radiological approach to renal cysts. *Radiology* 1986;158:1–10.
2. Aronson S, Frazier HA, Baluch JD, et al: Cystic renal masses: usefulness of the Bosniak classification. *Urol Radiol* 1991; 13:83–90.
3. Bosniak MA: Problems in the radiologic diagnosis of renal parenchymal tumors. *Urol Clin North Am* 1993;20:217–230.
4. Hartman DS, Ellsworth W III, Laskin WB, Brody JM, et al: Cystic renal cell carcinoma: CT findings simulating a benign hyperdense cyst. *AJR* 1992;159:1235–1237.
5. Levine E, Slusher SL, Grantham JJ, Wetzel LH: Natural history of acquired renal cystic disease in dialysis patients: a prospective longitudinal CT study. *AJR* 1991;156:501–506.
6. Bosniak MA: Difficulties in classifying cystic lesions of the kidney. *Urol Radiol* 1991;13:91–93.
7. Sussman S, Cochran ST, Pagini JJ, McArdle C, et al: Hyperdense renal masses: a CT manifestation of hemorrhagic renal cysts. *Radiology* 1984;150:207–211.
8. Bosniak MA: Questions and answers. *AJR* 1994;163:216.
9. Foster WL Jr, Roberts L Jr, Halvorsen RA, Dunnick NR: Sonography of small renal masses with indeterminacy density characteristics on computed tomography. *Urol Radiol* 1988; 10:59–67.
10. Daniels WW, Hartman GW, Witten DM, et al: Calcified renal masses: a review of ten years experience at the Mayo Clinic. *Radiology* 1972;103:503–508.
11. Rominger MB, Kenney PJ, Morgan DE, et al: Gadolinium-enhanced MR imaging of renal masses. *Radiographics* 1992; 12:1097–1116.

12. Semelka RC, Hricak H, Stevens SK, et al: Combined gadolinium-enhanced and fat-saturation MR imaging of renal masses. *Radiology* 1991;178:803–809.
13. Brown ED, Semelka RC: Magnetic resonance imaging of the urinary tract. In: Resnick M, Older R, eds. *Diagnosis of Genitourinary Disease*. New York: Thieme, 1997.
14. Rofsky NM, Weinreb JC, Bosniak MA, et al: Renal lesion characterization with Gadolinium-enhanced MR imaging: efficacy and safety in patients with renal insufficiency. *Radiology* 1991;180:85–89.
15. Dalla-Palma L, Pozzi-Mucelli F, di Donna A, et al: Cystic renal tumors: US and CT findings. *Urol Radiol* 1990;12:67–73.
16. Parienty RA, Pradel J, Parienty I: Cystic renal cancers: CT characteristics. *Radiology* 1985;157:741–744.
17. Herts BR, Einstein DM, Paushter DM: Spiral CT of the abdomen: artifacts and potential pitfalls. *AJR* 1993;161:1185–1190.
18. Amis EA Jr, Cronan JJ, Pfister RC: Needle puncture of cystic renal masses: a survey of the Society of Uroradiology. *AJR* 1987;148:197–299.
19. Nicefero JR, Coughlin BF: Diagnosis of renal cell carcinoma: value of fine-needle aspiration cytology in patients with metastases or contraindications to nephrectomy. *AJR* 1993;161:1303–1305.

18 Benign and Malignant Tumors of the Upper Urinary Tract

Marguerite C. Lippert, Robert A. Older

Renal parenchymal masses include simple cysts, malignant tumors, benign tumors, and complex cysts. Renal cell carcinoma represents 85 to 90% of renal neoplasms, whereas urothelial cancers make up 7 to 8%. With the advent of CT scanning, ultrasonography, and MRI, diagnosis and staging of renal masses have changed dramatically in the last 15 years.

IMAGING TECHNIQUES

Imaging studies in the evaluation of renal parenchymal tumors are divided into three categories: (1) studies used primarily for the detection of renal masses, (2) studies used primarily to characterize the renal mass, and (3) studies used for staging. These groups overlap, but in general, methods of detection include

1. Excretory urography with tomography
2. Ultrasound
3. Computed tomography (CT)

Although CT is also the primary method of characterization of lesions, it has been playing a large role in detection of masses because of its sensitivity.[1]

Studies used for characterization of a renal mass are

1. Computed tomography
2. Ultrasound
3. Magnetic resonance imaging (MRI)
4. Percutaneous biopsy
5. Arteriography

Staging is accomplished with

1. Computed tomography
2. MRI
3. Angiography and venography
4. Bone scans
5. Chest radiographs

An approach to the evaluation of renal masses is presented in Figure 18–1.

Isotope Renal Scans

Nuclear scanning is a helpful adjunct when faced with an excretory urogram that is not clearly normal or abnormal. The goal is to differentiate a renal pseudotumor, such as prominent lobulation or hypertrophied columns of Bertin, from a true renal mass. Isotope renal scanning makes this distinction by separating functioning from nonfunctioning renal tissue. Scanning is performed with technetium-dimercaptosuccinate (DMSA). After an early vascular phase, the DMSA concentrates only within functioning renal parenchyma. Normal renal tissue will show radioactivity, whereas a mass (tumor or cyst) appears as a "cold" spot (Fig. 18–2).[2] Studies have shown a high accuracy for this distinction,[3] and technical improvement, including SPECT, should improve this further.

RENAL CELL CARCINOMA

Renal cell carcinoma accounts for 85% of renal neoplasms. It occurs most commonly in individuals between the ages of 40 and 60 and is twice as common in males as females. It is unilateral 97% of the time but can be bilateral and multiple in less common genetic syndromes such as Von Hippel–Lindau disease.

Presentation

Clinical presentation of renal cell carcinoma has changed dramatically over the last 15 years with the increased usage of CT scanning, ultrasonography, and MRI of the abdomen to evaluate patients with unrelated and related complaints. Therefore two-thirds of localized renal cell carcinoma is detected incidentally by such imaging studies in patients with no symptoms from their tumor.

The classic triad of pain, flank mass, and hematuria is rare but suggestive of advanced disease. Thirty to 50% of patients present with hematuria and about 40% present with flank pain. The pain can be colicky, from passage of blood clots; constant and dull, from invasion of surrounding areas; or sharp, from tumor hemorrhage.

362 Diagnosis of Genitourinary Disease

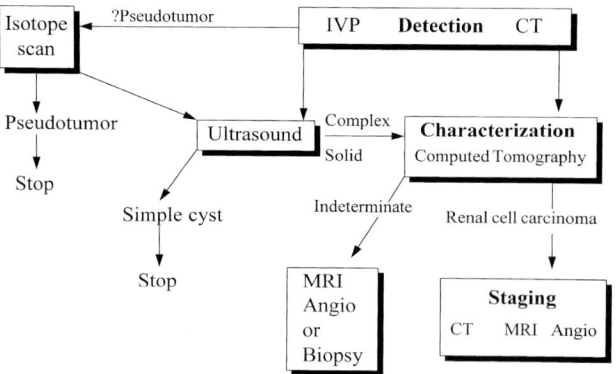

Figure 18–1. Schematic representation of renal mass evaluation.

About 10 to 40% of patients can present with paraneoplastic syndromes.[4] Weight loss, cachexia, and fatigue can be the presenting symptoms but do not necessarily represent metastatic disease, just as the other paraneoplastic syndromes do not. Secretion of renin or reninlike substances may account for the 22% of patients who are hypertensive at presentation. Elevated levels of erythropoietin by tumor cells may account for the 3% of patients who present with polycythemia. Secretion of a parathyroid hormone–related protein accounts for some of the 10% of patients presenting with hypercalcemia. Others may have bone metastases. A suspected hepatotoxic product from tumor cells may account for the 10 to 14% of all renal cell carcinoma patients who present with Stauffer's syndrome,[5] in which patients have abnormal liver function tests and fever but no liver metastases. A pyrogenic factor may account for the 20% of patients who present with pyrexia. Other, rarer paraneoplastic syndromes include alterations of serum glucose by production of glucagon or insulin. If the paraneoplastic syndrome disappears after a nephrectomy, metastases are less likely.

Thirty percent of patients may have distant metastases at the time of presentation. Symptoms from bone or brain metastases may be the presenting symptoms.

Examination

Although rare, a palpable flank mass may be present. A varicocele, especially left-sided and of sudden onset, should be sought in a male patient and may mean occlusion of the renal vein or inferior vena cava by tumor thrombus. Cachexia and hypertension may be present, as described earlier in the paraneoplastic syndromes. Rarely, high-output cardiac failure results from a large arteriovenous fistula within the tumor.

Laboratory Studies

There are no laboratory findings specific to renal cell carcinoma, but patients can present with anemia from chronic disease, polycythemia, hypercalcemia, and hyperglycemia, and in Stauffer's syndrome they can present with an elevated alkaline phosphatase, elevated $alpha_2$-globulin, and a prolonged prothrombin time. Erythrocyte sedimentation rate may be elevated in half of presenting patients. Urine cytology is rarely helpful except perhaps in rare, poorly differentiated tumors diffusely infiltrating the renal parenchyma.

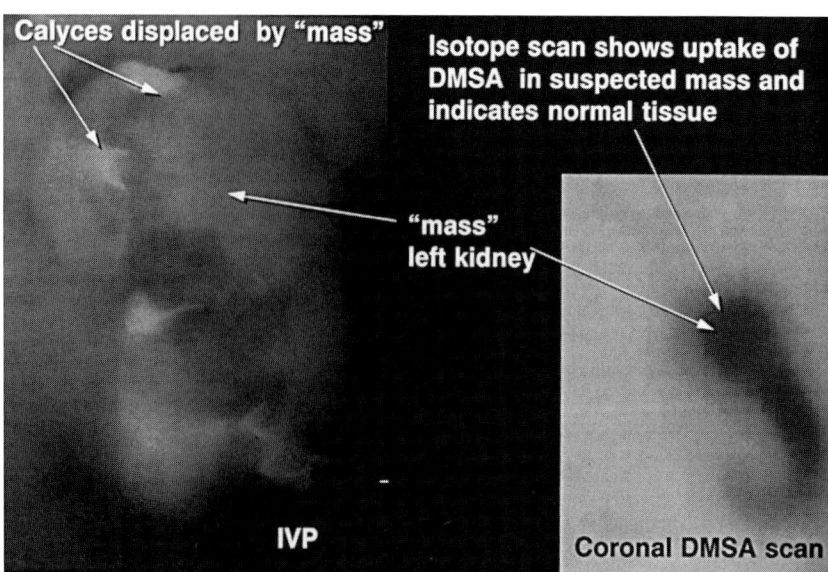

Figure 18–2. Use of the isotope scan (DMSA) to verify a pseudotumor as the etiology of a mass suspected on urography.

Imaging: Diagnosis and Staging

EXCRETORY UROGRAPHY

The preliminary radiograph routinely obtained during excretory urography may provide significant information by showing areas of calcification in a mass. The pattern of calcification is helpful in diagnosis. Calcium in a punctate or mottled pattern within a renal mass suggests malignancy. Thin, peripheral calcification is more commonly found with a benign lesion. Any calcified renal lesion, regardless of the characteristics of the calcification, must be further evaluated, and the best study for this is CT. Because of its greater sensitivity for detecting calcium, CT has altered our approach to the calcified lesion. Thin peripheral calcification in an otherwise cystic unenhanced mass is no longer regarded as suspicious for carcinoma, whereas thick, punctate, or central calcification is suspicious, especially if associated with solid tissue.

On nephrogram films taken immediately after injection of contrast medium the entire renal outline can be visualized in most patients, and this is essential to detection of small parenchymal lesions.[6] The routine addition of linear tomography to excretory urography affords improved visualization of the renal parenchyma and thereby greatly enhances the diagnostic capacity of this study. Urography without tomography should not be used when evaluating hematuria or a possible renal mass. Urography is often used as the first study to evaluate hematuria. Even the tomography, however, the sensitivity of urography for detecting renal masses is significantly less than CT, especially for small lesions.[1,7] If urography is negative, CT should follow unless the source of bleeding is found elsewhere, such as in the bladder.

Renal cell carcinoma can present in multiple ways on the urogram. There may be

1. Splaying, elongation, or distortion of the collecting system
2. Lucent mass in parenchyma
3. Hyperdense vascular mass
4. Obliteration of a segment of the renal outline
5. Failure of opacification of a portion of the collecting system
6. Enlargement of the total renal mass
7. Visualization of collateral vessels
8. Change in the renal axis.

Figure 18–3 represents a composite of some of the many urographic presentations of renal cell carcinoma.

ULTRASOUND

Both excretory urography and ultrasound are used as primary studies for evaluation of hematuria or suspected renal mass. If detected with urography a lesion will be evaluated with ultrasound unless clearly a solid or vascular lesion. Demonstration of a simple cyst with ultrasound will terminate the evaluation. Most renal cell carcinomas have internal echogenicity similar to the kidney parenchyma (isoechoic) (Fig. 18–4) or less often, approximately 10%, lower than the renal parenchyma (hypoechoic).[8] In addition to a solid appearance on gray-scale ultrasound, Doppler and color Doppler ultrasound can be used to characterize a lesion further. A Doppler shift frequency of 2.5 kHz or greater has been suggested as an indicator of malignancy because high-frequency Doppler shift is encountered in malignant renal masses but infrequently in benign lesions.[9] We have not routinely evaluated our solid masses with Doppler ultrasound.

If a solid lesion is detected with ultrasound, evaluation of the renal vein and inferior vena cava (IVC) will be performed to look for venous extension. In essentially all cases, however, we will proceed to CT, MRI, or angiography for diagnostic confirmation and staging. Ultrasound can provide visualization of portions of the venous structures but does not provide a complete assessment of the venous structures, lymph nodes, or adjacent viscera.

Recently, the concept of renal cell carcinoma as a hypoechoic or isoechoic lesion has been challenged. A significant number of renal cell carcinomas present as hyperechoic masses (Fig. 8–5),[10,11] an appearance traditionally thought to represent an angiomyolipoma. This has reduced the confidence level of the ultrasound examination for angiomyolipoma and necessitates further studies in these cases.

Ultrasound can be used as a screening study for hematuria, but neither ultrasound nor urography has the sensitivity of CT. Although there is some evidence that US may be more sensitive than urography for a renal mass,[1] US does not provide adequate visualization of the collecting system and therefore does not routinely detect lesions such as transitional cell carcinoma or papillary necrosis.

COMPUTED TOMOGRAPHY

The primary diagnostic study for renal cell carcinoma is CT, with an overall diagnostic accuracy of close to 95% for a dynamic contrast-enhanced study.[12] Although generally used as a second line study, a CT urogram can be used as a first-line study in patients with hematuria.[13] This combines urography with a limited CT and, if technically and financially feasible, is an excellent concept because the combination of routine radiographs and CT could provide optimal evaluation of both the renal parenchyma and collecting structures.

In most situations, however, CT will be used for diagnosis and staging or a previously detected lesion. On an unenhanced CT scan renal cell carcinoma may have an attenuation similar to (isodense), less than (hypodense), or greater than (hyperdense) the normal renal parenchyma.[14,15] The

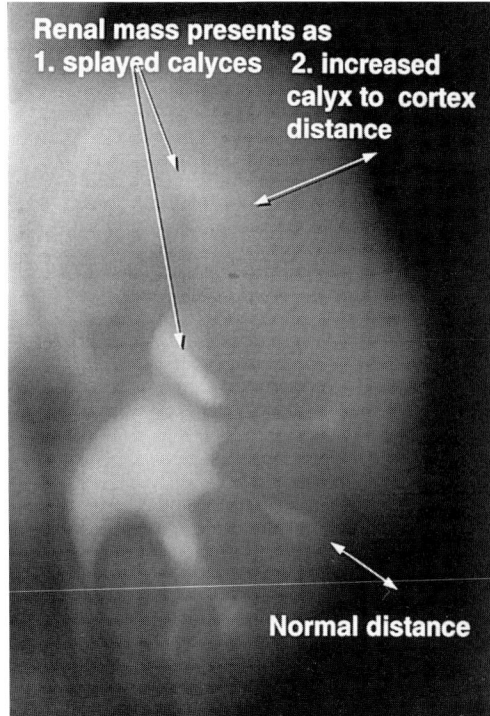
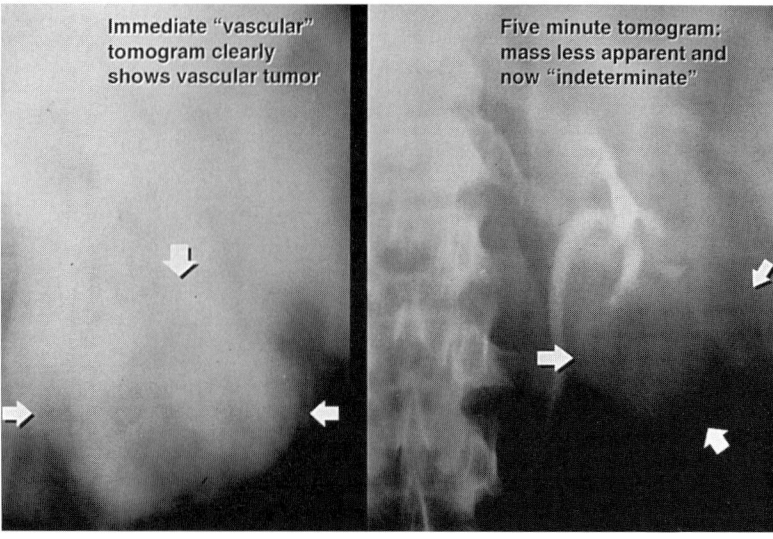
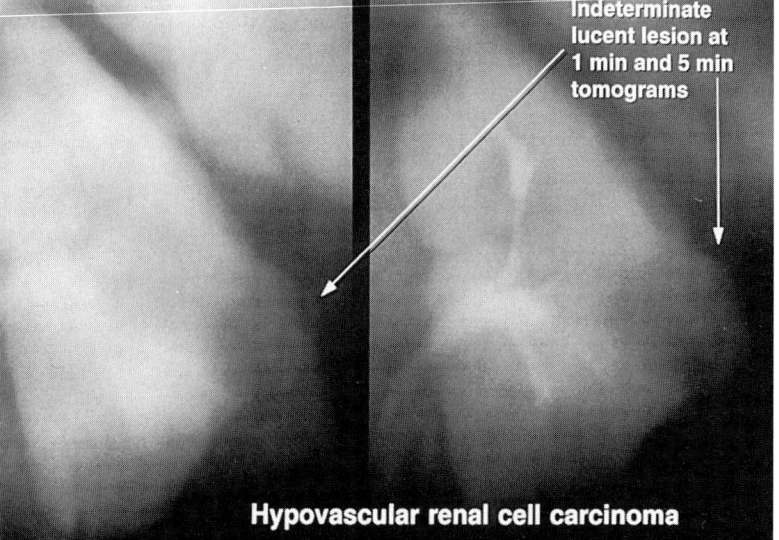
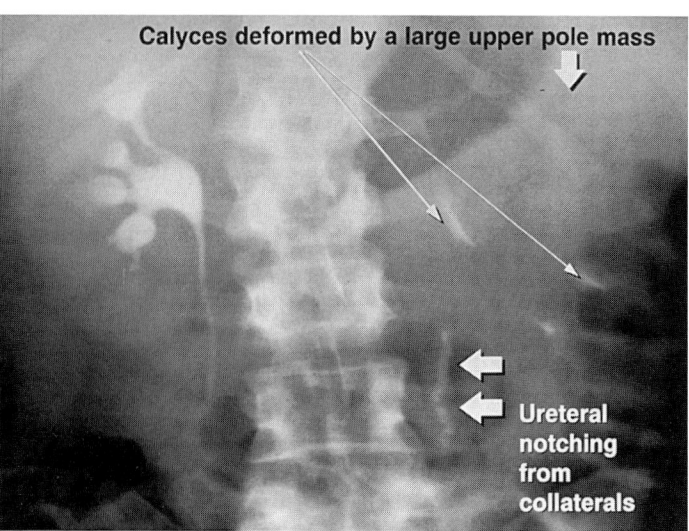

Figure 18–3. Urographic presentations of renal cell carcinoma. (**A**) Calyceal splaying and increase in the distance from the calyces to the apparent outer margin of the kidney. (**B**) Vascular blush on early tomograms with calyceal splaying on late tomograms. (**C**) Hypovascular mass with cortical bulge. (**D**), (**E**) Gross architectural distortion with evidence of collateral flow.

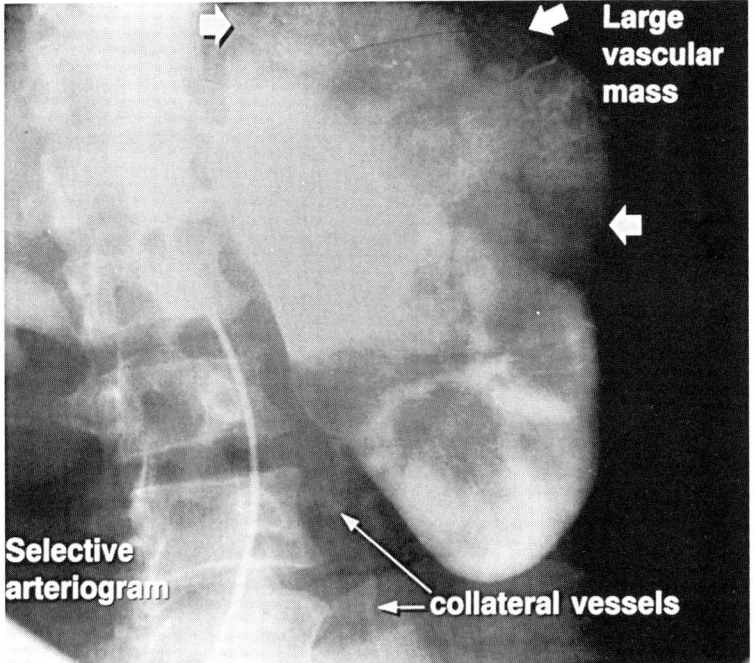
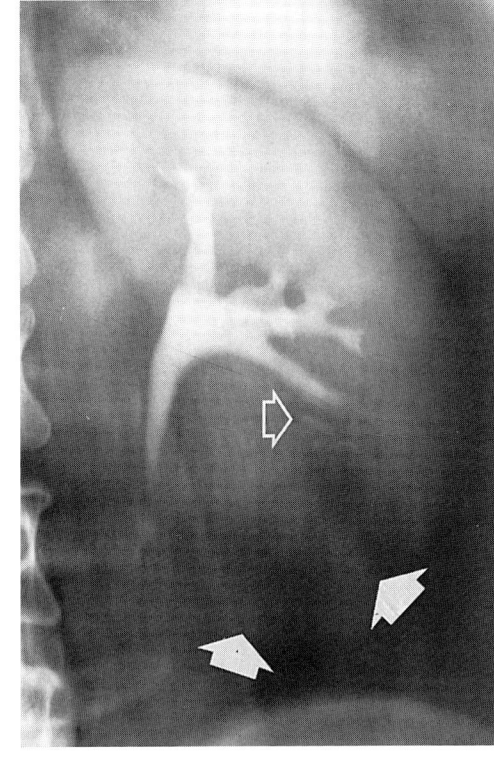

Figure 18–3 Continued (F) Mild calyceal compression (open white arrow) and increased parenchymal thickness left lower pole (white arrow). (G) Renal enlargement with nonvisualization of the collecting structures related to renal vein involvement.

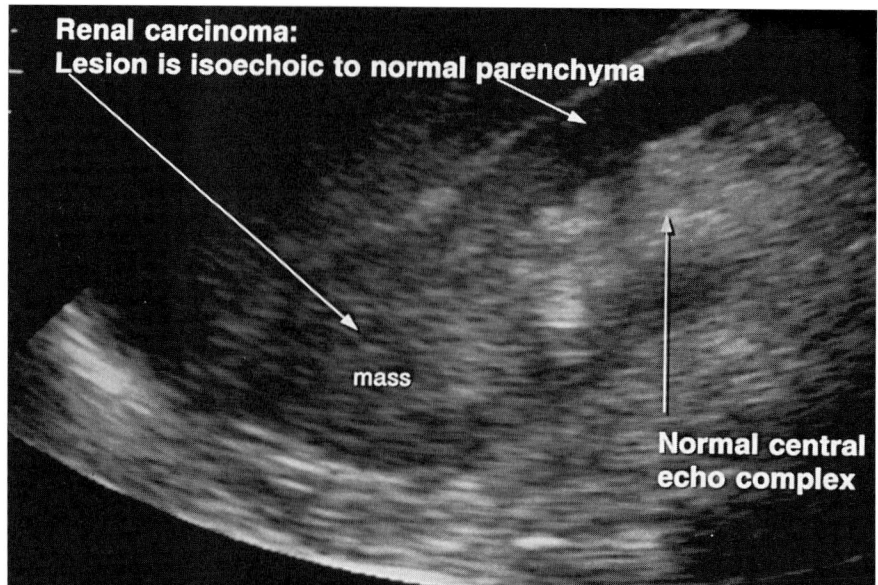

Figure 18–4. Ultrasound of isoechoic renal cell carcinoma.

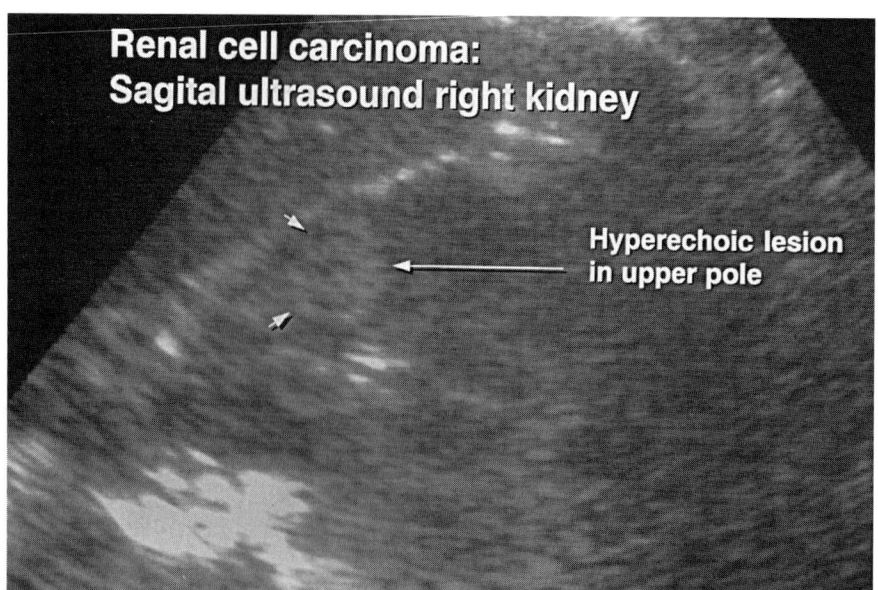

Figure 18–5. Ultrasound of hyperechoic renal cell carcinoma.

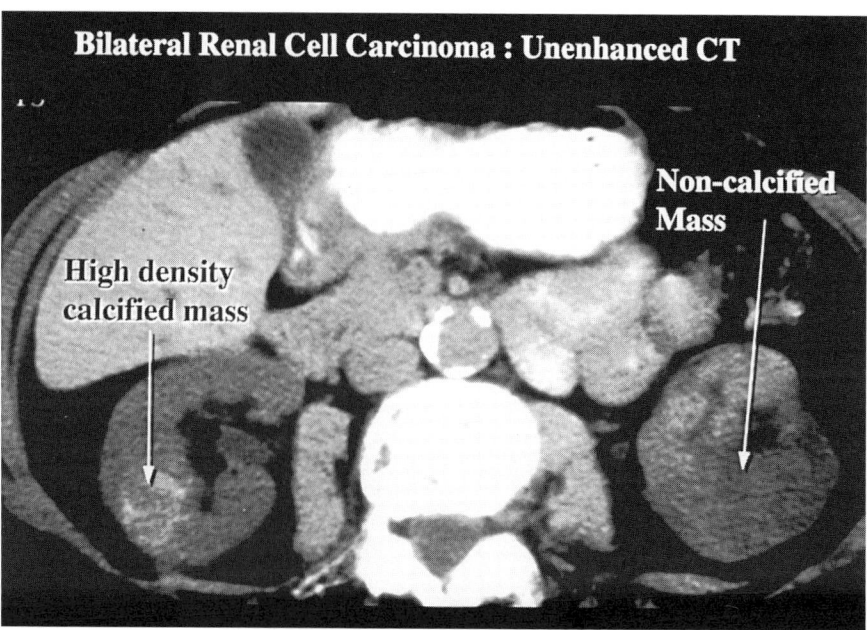

Figure 18–6. High-density renal cell carcinoma secondary to fine calcification.

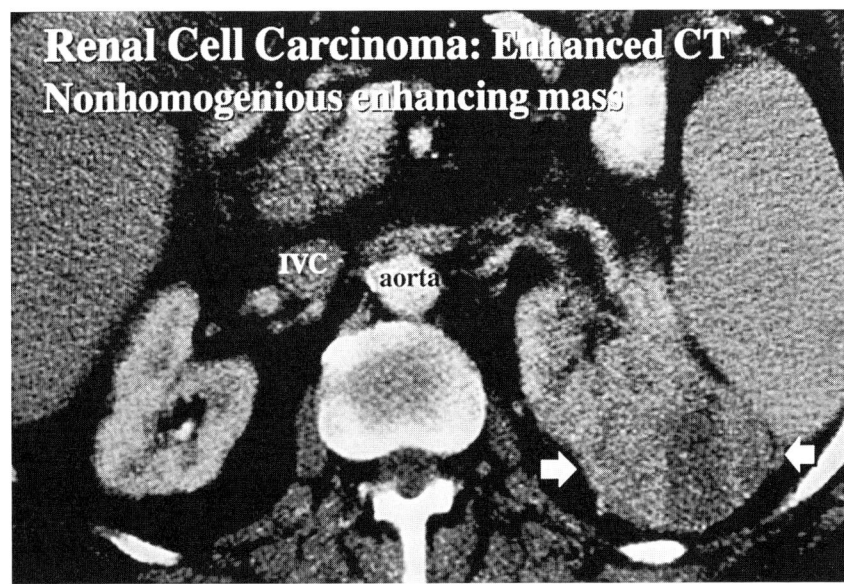

Figure 18–7. Dynamic enhanced CT of renal cell carcinoma. Heterogeneous enhancement with areas of density equal to and less than adjacent normal parenchyma.

presence of necrosis, calcification, or hemorrhage will affect the appearance of the lesion.[14] Calcification or hemorrhage may produce hyperdense areas within a lesion[16] (Fig. 18–6), whereas necrotic tissue is usually hypodense. Calcification can be found in 31% of renal cell carcinomas.[14]

Renal cell carcinoma will usually be apparent by its distortion of the renal outline or internal architecture, but a small or infiltrating lesion may not alter the shape of the kidney[14] and may go undetected with an unenhanced scan. The accuracy of CT diminishes if contrast is not used,[12] and enhancement therefore is always used unless clinically contraindicated by allergy or renal failure. If contrast cannot be used, MRI becomes the preferred study for both diagnosis and staging.[12]

The appearance of renal cell carcinoma following contrast enhancement will vary, depending on the vascularity of the tumor, its degree of necrosis, and technical factors such as the amount and speed of contrast injection and timing of the image acquisition. Following the initial dynamic arterial phase, renal cell carcinoma usually shows heterogeneous enhancement that is less than the adjacent normal renal parenchyma (Figs. 18–7, 18–8).[14] The degree of enhancement is most often sufficient to be visually detectable, but hypovascular lesions may enhance very little and be detectable only by a change in measured CT attenuation coefficients (Fig. 18–9).

Highly vascular lesions, on the other hand, may have enhancement equal to or greater than the normal parenchyma if images are obtained in a dynamic fashion during the rapid

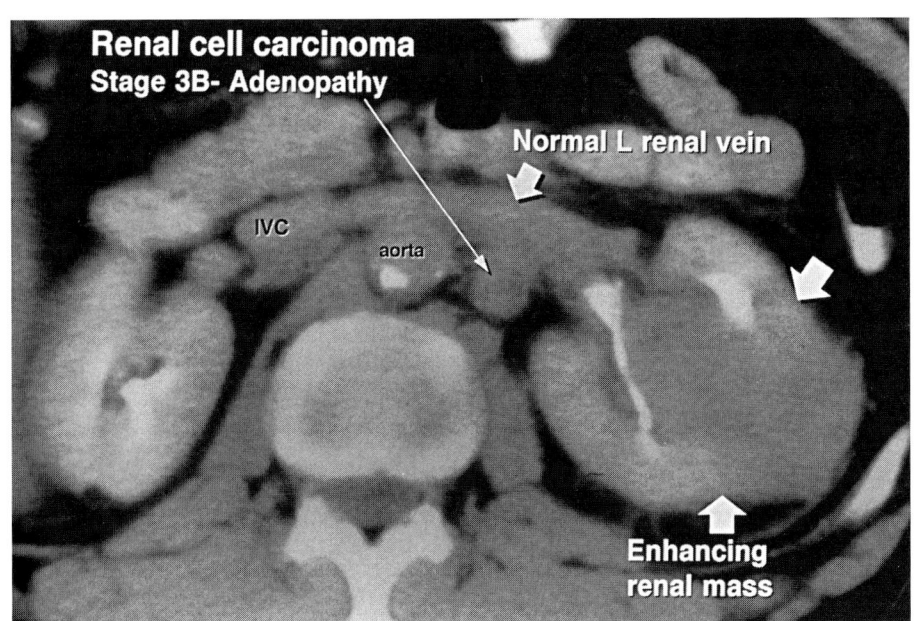

Figure 18–8. Nondynamic enhanced CT of renal cell carcinoma left kidney. The mass is of lower density than adjacent normal parenchyma and also deforms the central collecting structures. Adenopathy is present.

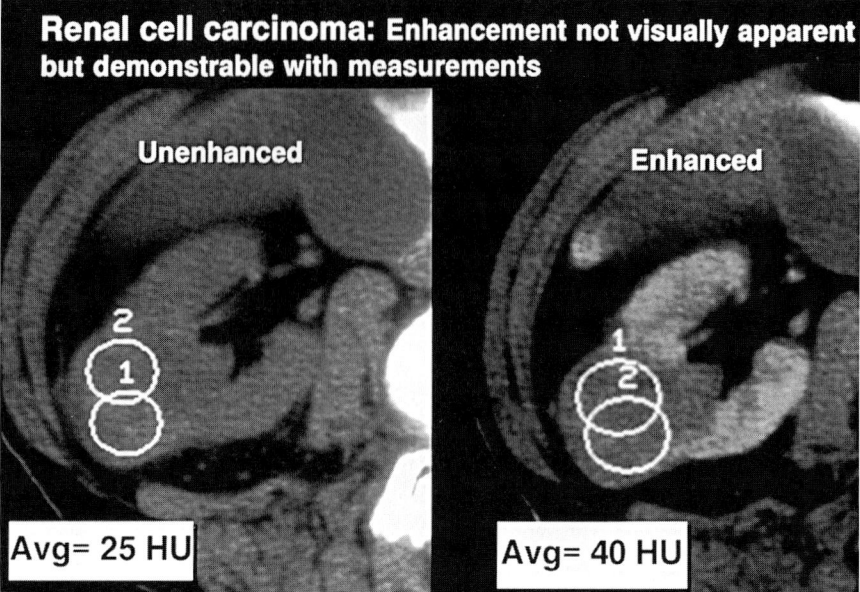

Figure 18–9. CT of renal cell carcinoma. Enhancement not visually apparent and the change between unenhanced and enhanced attenuation values only detected using region of interest measurements.

mechanical injection of contrast (Fig. 18–10). Many current scanners obtain renal images during the cortical nephrogram phase before maximal tubular concentration of the contrast by the kidney and with attenuation coefficients primarily dependent on the degree of vascularity. A very vascular renal cell carcinoma may equal or even exceed the density of the adjacent normal renal parenchyma. This is most likely to occur with rapid spiral scanners, which scan the entire abdomen in a single breath-hold. Spiral scanning is unlikely to miss a vascular tumor, but small or central hypovascular lesions could be missed if delayed images to visualize the entire renal parenchyma are not obtained.[17] Infiltrating lesions may show a diffuse alteration of architecture without a well-defined mass (Fig. 18–11).

STAGING

In the past, clinical staging was based on the Robson system,[18] but currently the tumor, node metastasis (TNM) system[19] allows better international comparison of treatment results (Table 18–1). Both classifications are still used in clinical practice.

Overall staging accuracy for CT has been as high as 91%. Most staging errors occur when differentiating stage I from stage II lesions. Errors are related to difficulties in separating inflammatory changes from tumor infiltration or small vessels from lymphatic involvement with tumor.[15] Perinephric stranding is not specific and is often not due to spread of tumor.[19] A discrete soft-tissue mass in the perinephric space, however, is a reliable indicator of at least stage II disease (Fig. 18–12). Perinephric abnormalities are more likely with increasing size of the tumor, being uncommon with lesions of less than 3 cm.[14] Minimal or microscopic extension into the perinephric fat cannot be detected, and this further reduces the ability of CT to differentiate stage I from stage II lesions.[15,20]

Other stages are more easily differentiated with much higher accuracy,[20] and CT is currently the best study for separating stage I and II lesions from higher stages,[12] which clinically is most important. CT, if performed in a dynamic fashion, is reliable for detection of thrombus in the IVC and often the renal vein (stage IIIA) (Fig. 18–13).[12,21] A filling defect in the vein is the most conclusive evidence of thrombus, most of which are tumor thrombi (Fig. 18–14). Enhancement within the vein or thrombus is due to tumor vessels and indicates a tumor thrombus rather than a bland thrombus (Fig. 18–15).[19] Enhancement of the IVC wall suggests adherence or invasion of tumor.[12] Renal vein enlargement is suggestive of tumor involvement (Fig. 18–16) but is not a reliable criterion.[21] This finding alone has both a high false-positive and a high false-negative rate. A vascular tumor can increase the size of the vein simply through increased flow, producing a false-positive study, and tumor thrombus can be present in the renal vein without enlargement.[19] Although very accurate in detecting thrombus in the IVC, CT is clearly less accurate than MRI or cavography in determining the cephalic extent of the thrombus. Because this is important for surgical planning, MRI or cavography of patients with IVC thrombus on CT is warranted.[22]

Stage IIIB lesions involve local lymph nodes, and when enlarged these are readily demonstrated with CT (Fig. 18–17), as are cases involving both the nodes and veins (Stage IIIC). Limited lymph node involvement will not always be detected by CT scanning, whereas seemingly involved lymph nodes can occasionally be normal at surgery. Using a size criterion of 1 cm or greater, false-positive rates have

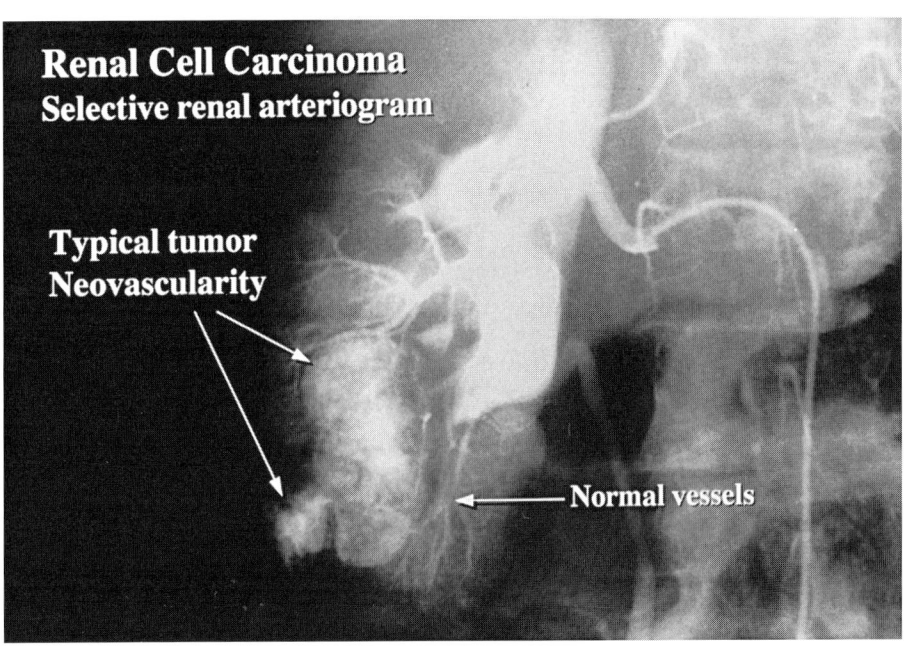

Figure 18–10. (A) CT of bilateral renal cell carcinoma (same patient as Fig. 18–6). Right lesion is highly vascular and isodense to normal parenchyma, whereas left lesion is hypodense. (B) Selective right renal angiogram of the right-sided tumor shows typical neovascularity.

ranged from 3 to 43% and appear to be higher with greater tumor necrosis.[19] Extension through the perirenal fat and Gerota's fascia (stage IV) is detectable (see Fig. 18–12), but care must be taken not to overcall minimal changes.

Abdominal CT imaging will also demonstrate involvement of adjacent structures such as adrenal, liver, spleen, or colon. Distant metastasis can appear anywhere, but common sites, listed in order are lung, bone, brain, liver, and subcutaneous tissue. Bone scanning is appropriate to rule out bone metastases in patients with bone pain, hypercalcemia, or an elevated alkaline phosphatase. Lung metastases can be evaluated with a routine chest radiograph. However, because chest CT is more sensitive for mediastinal adenopathy and lung metastases 3 to 5 mm in size, chest CT scanning is appropriate for patients with renal vein or IVC involvement, suspected regional lymph node involvement, or large tumors.

MAGNETIC RESONANCE IMAGING

Magnetic resonance imaging (MRI) is used primarily for staging renal cell carcinoma. It provides noninvasive imaging of the vasculature and is an alternative to venography for determining involvement and extension of tumor in the renal vein and IVC. MRI has shown an accuracy of up to 96% for venous and lymph node involvement and may be superior to CT for overall staging (see Fig. 18–16C).[12,23,24]

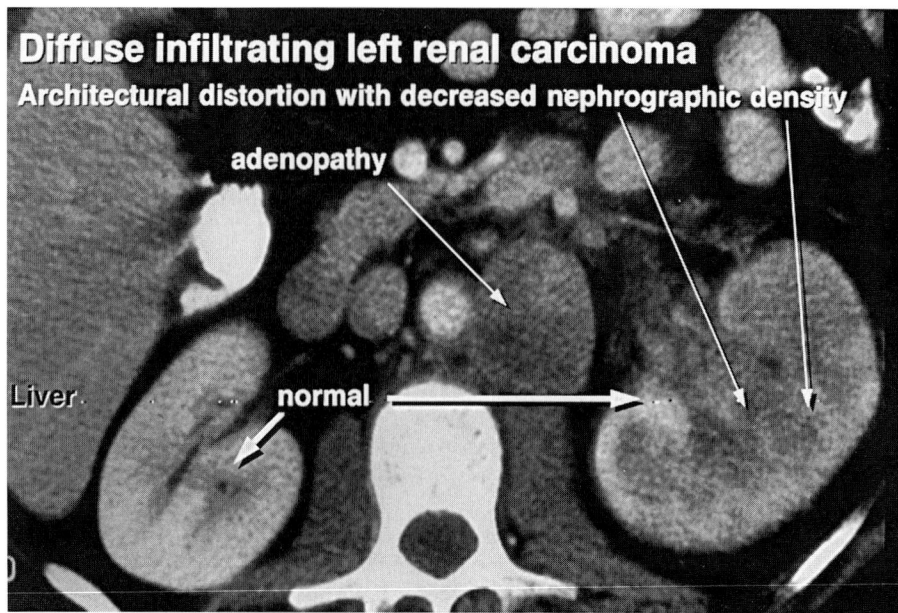

Figure 18–11. Dynamic enhanced CT of diffuse infiltrating renal cell carcinoma. Decreased nephrogram with no well-defined mass. Prominent adenopathy also present.

Table 18–1. Clinical Staging of Tumors

ROBSON STAGE	DESCRIPTION	TNM STAGE
I	Tumor contained within renal capsule	
	Small tumor (<2.4 cm)	T1
	Large tumor (>2.5 cm)	T2
II	Tumor spread to perinephric fat	T3a
IIIA	Venous tumor thrombus	
	Renal vein tumor thrombus only	T3b
	Infradiaphragmatic caval thrombus	T3c
	Supradiaphragmatic caval thrombus	T4b
IIIB	Regional lymph node metastasis	N1-N3
IIIC	Venous tumor thrombus and regional lymph node metastasis	
IVA	Direct invasion of adjacent organs outside Gerota's fascia	T4a
IVB	Distant metastasis	M1a–M1d, N4

Modified with permission from Zagoria.[19]

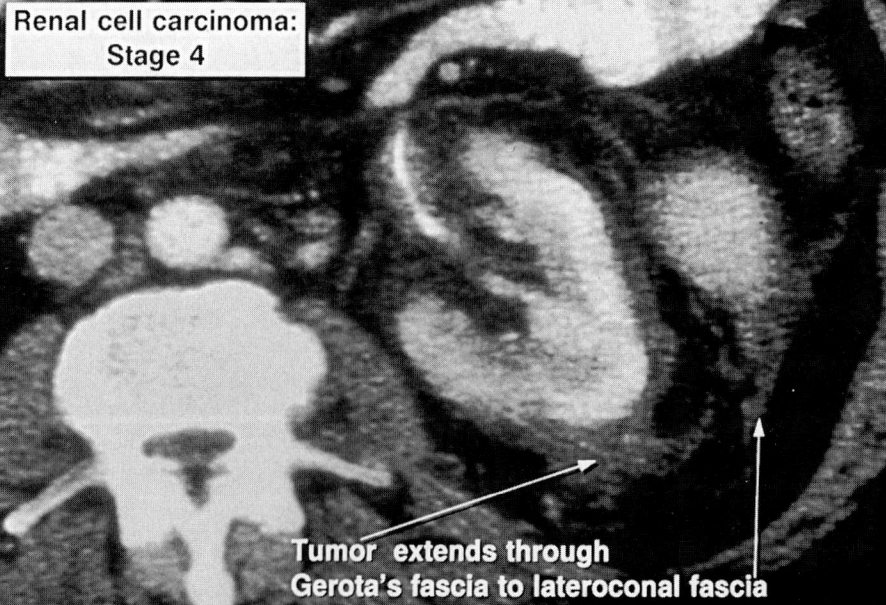

Figure 18–12. CT of stage IV left-sided renal cell carcinoma. The bulk of the tumor mass is better seen in Fig. 18–7.

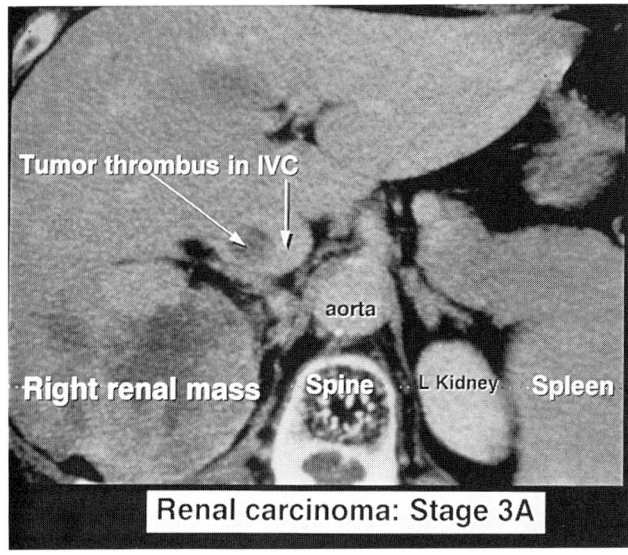

Figure 18–13. CT of renal cell carcinoma with IVC involvement.

As with CT, MRI depends primarily on nodal size for identification of abnormal nodes and has an accuracy similar to that of CT. MRI, however, is better for distinguishing nodes from adjacent vessels.[19] Although CT is able to detect most tumor thrombi, the superior margin of the thrombus is not clearly shown with CT but is seen in essentially all MRI cases (Fig. 18–18).[23,25] The ability of MRI to provide direct sagittal and coronal images is an advantage in evaluating venous extent.[19] MRI also demonstrates increased signal intensity in tumor thrombus on postcontrast (gadolinium) scans, whereas CT only occasionally shows this feature.[23] Myneni, using gradient recall acquisition in the steady state (GRASS), was able to differentiate tumor from blood thrombus accurately in all eight cases in which it was used.[25] Tumor invasion of the wall of the vena cava can also be detected with MRI.[25] In experienced hands MRI can be as accurate as cavography, and in many institutions it has replaced cavography.[24,22]

MRI is an evolving technology using multiple differing sequences. The ability to detect and localize tumor thrombus may depend on the sequences chosen. Standard spin-echo sequences may be degraded by a number of artifacts, and the use of other sequences such as gradient-recalled echo (GRE) or gradient-recalled acquisition in the steady state

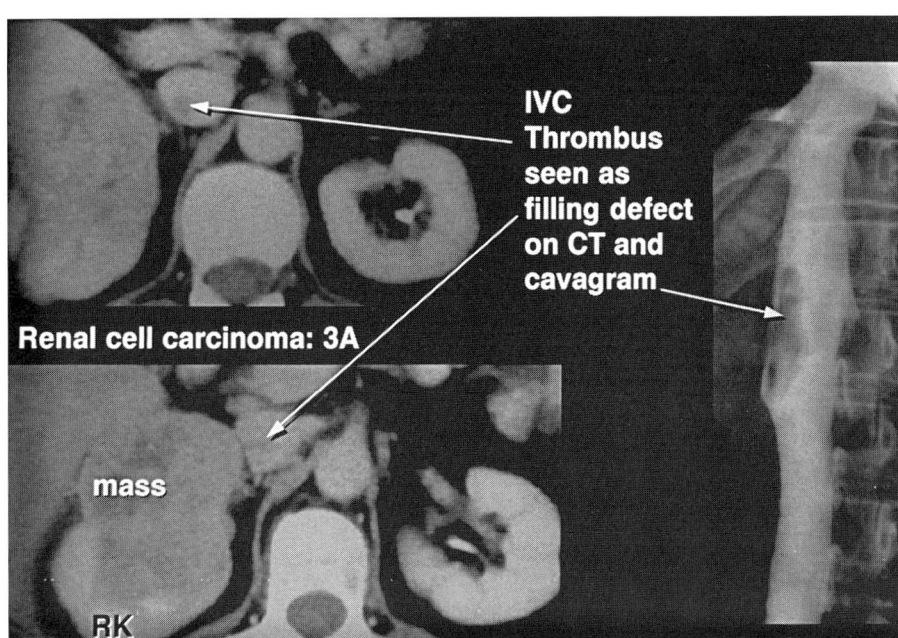

Figure 18–14. CT and venogram demonstrating tumor extension to the IVC.

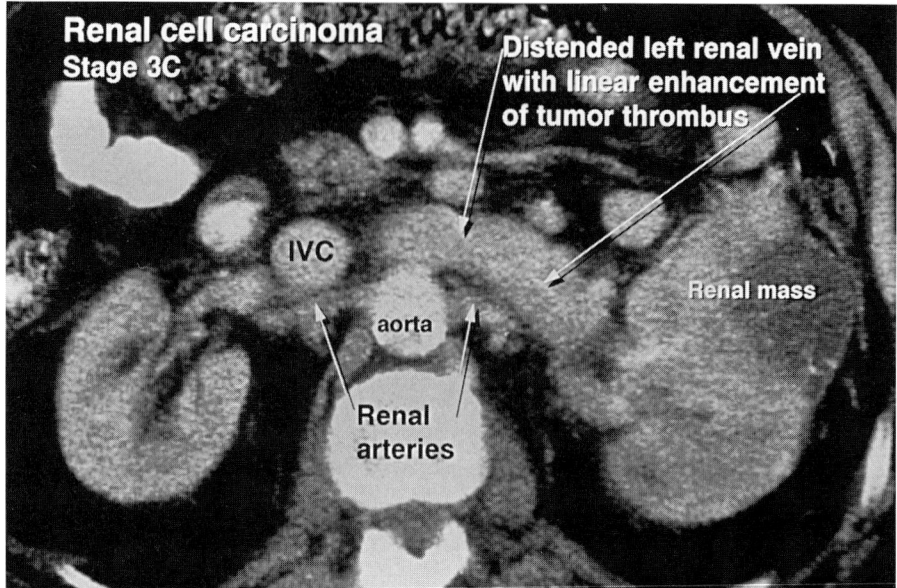

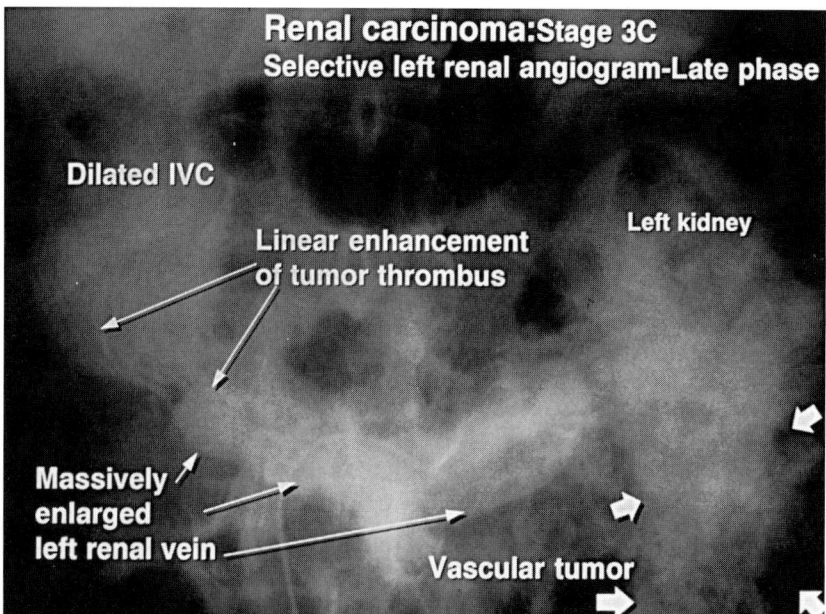

Figure 18–15. Tumor involvement of the left renal vein. (**A**) CT shows an enlarged vein with areas of abnormal enhancement. (**B**) Late-phase arteriogram confirms the massively enlarged left renal vein with linear enhancement of the tumor thrombus. This can be seen extending into the vena cava.

(GRASS) may provide improved detection and localization of tumor thrombus. For thrombus suspected of being in the right atrium, cine or cardiac gated MRI images may be necessary to overcome motion artifact, but even this may not detect all atrial tumors.[25,26] Cavography therefore is still indicated if there is any doubt about extension into the right atrium.[27]

MRI currently has limited use in the diagnosis of renal cell carcinoma. This is related to cost, availability, experience, and the limited detection of small intraparenchymal lesions.[12] Semelka in a recent series found MRI to be as accurate as CT for detecting renal masses and attributes his better results compared to earlier studies to improvements in MR technique and the use of enhancement with gadolinium. He agrees, however, that cost considerations may limit the routine use of MR in the evaluation of renal carcinoma.[23] In most cases CT will provide the necessary information with less expense.

In instances where contrast-enchanced CT cannot be used because of allergy or renal failure, MRI provides an accurate and safe alternative.[23] Enchanced MRI with gadolinium can be used in patients with renal failure and has no cross reactivity with iodinated contrast.[28,29] The use of gadolinium enhancement during MRI increases the detection and improves characterization of mass lesions as compared to unenhanced images.[30] MRI may also prove useful in providing anatomic vascular information prior to surgery. Oka, using noncontrast MR angiography, was able to demonstrate the great vessels and main renal vessels in 17 patients with renal call carcinoma.[31]

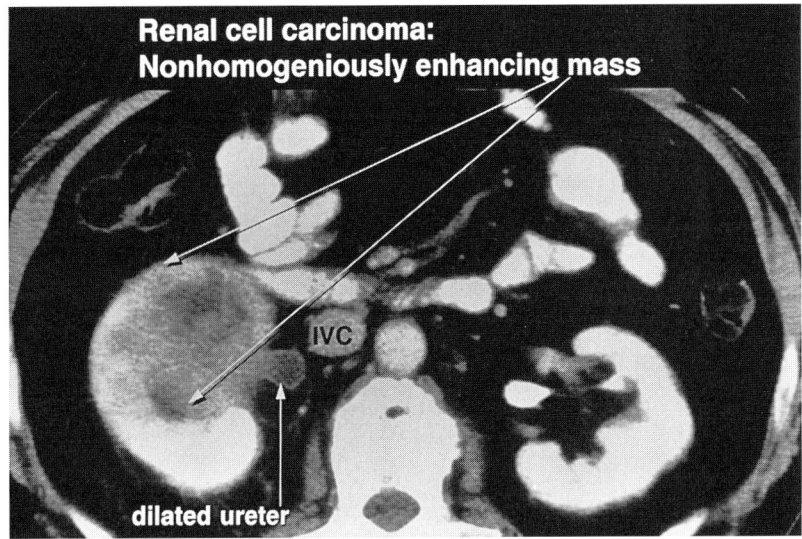

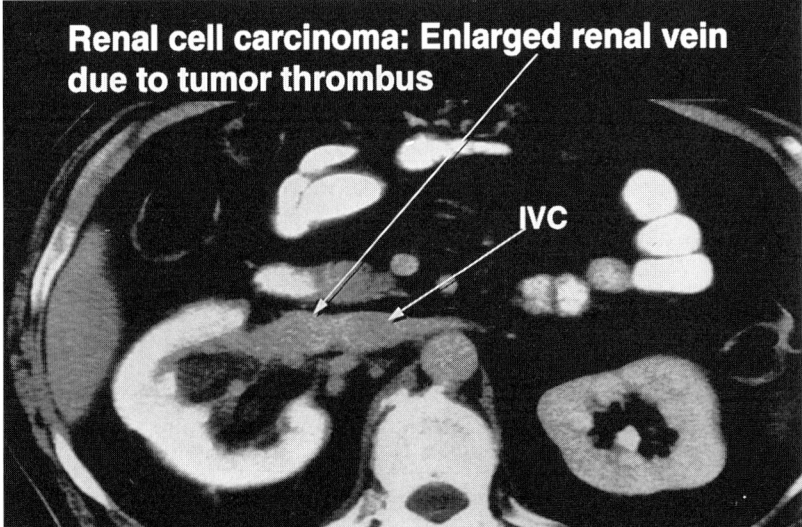

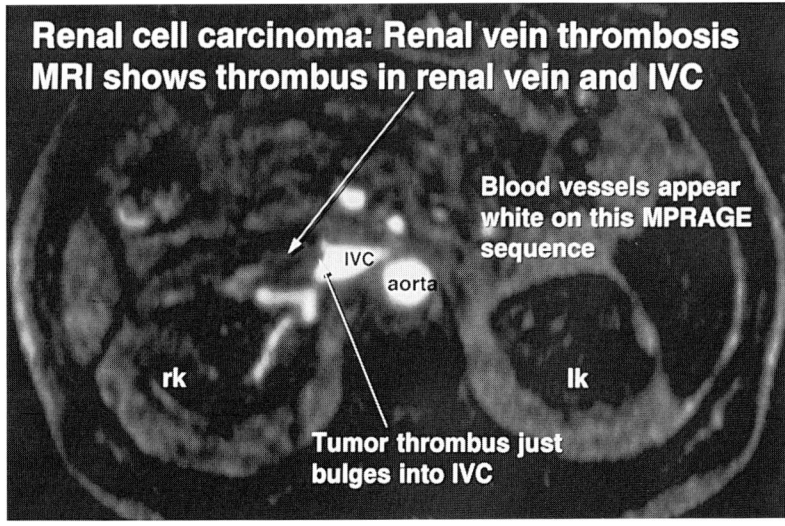

Figure 18-16. Renal cell carcinoma. (**A**) CT demonstrates a mass and (**B**) an enlarged right renal vein but a specific thrombus is not identified. (**C**) MRI shows thrombus filling the renal vein and just barely extending into the inferior vena cava.

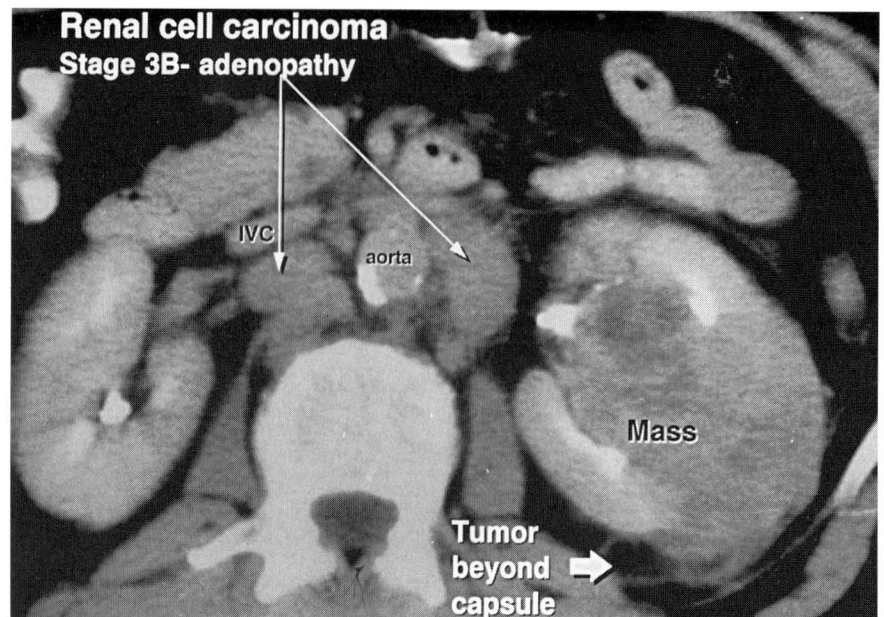

Figure 18–17 Renal cell carcinoma with bilateral para-aortic adenopathy as well as extension into the perinephric fat.

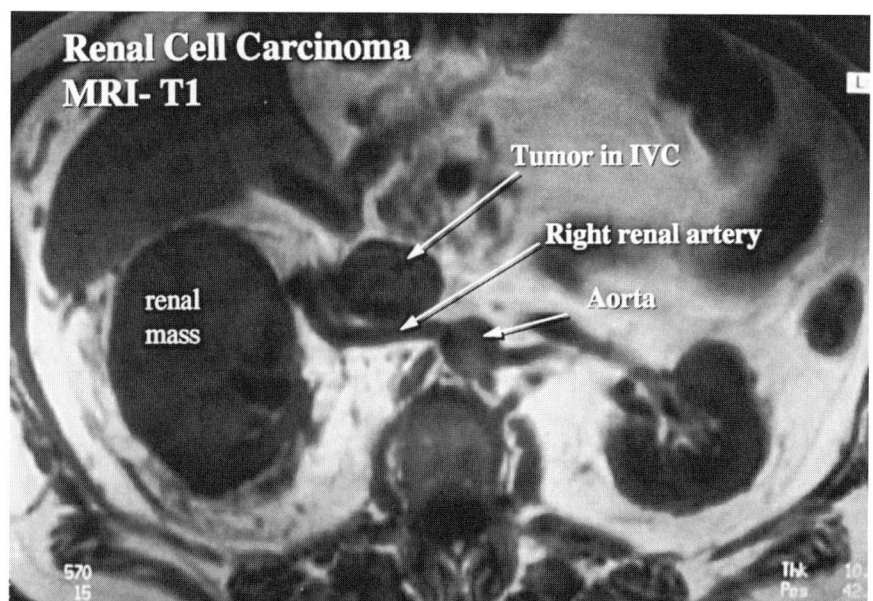

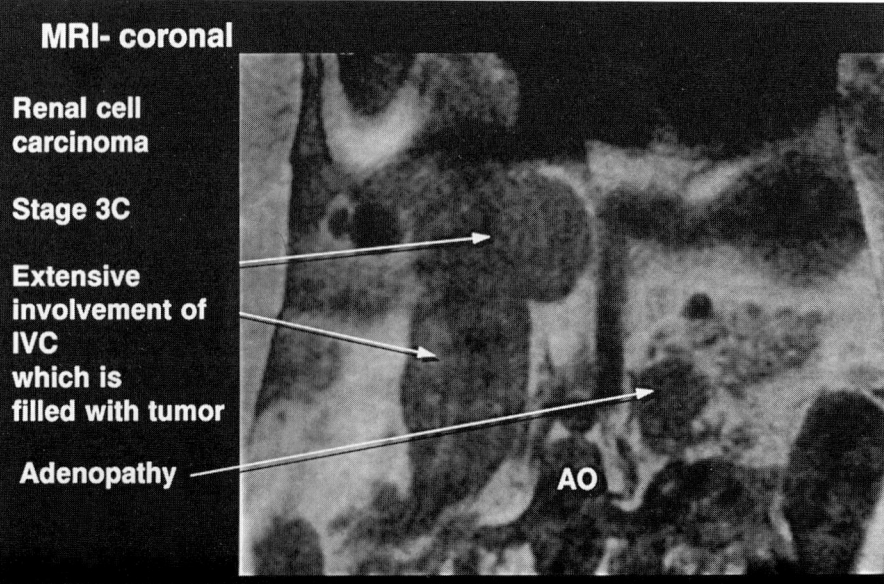

Figure 18–18. (**A**) Renal cell carcinoma MRI. T1-weighted axial image shows a large right renal mass and tumor thrombus in the inferior vena cava. (**B**) Renal cell carcinoma (different patient). MRI shows extensive involvement with tumor in an enlarged inferior vena cava.

Benign and Malignant Tumors of the Upper Urinary Tract

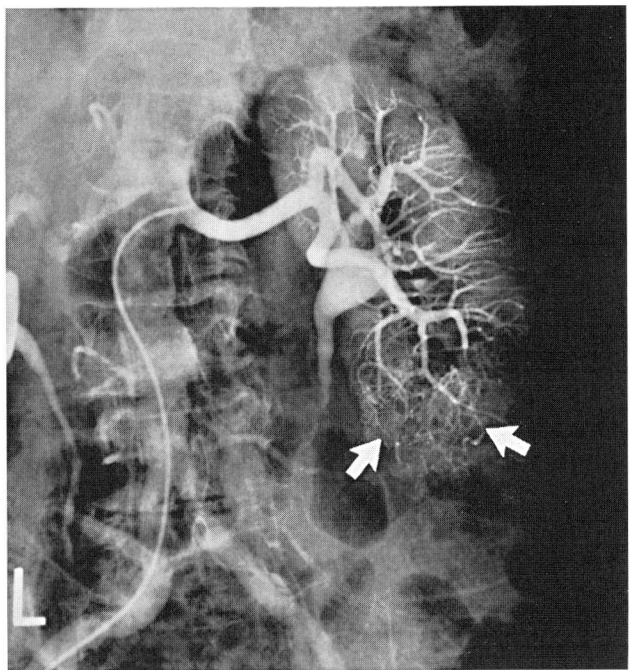 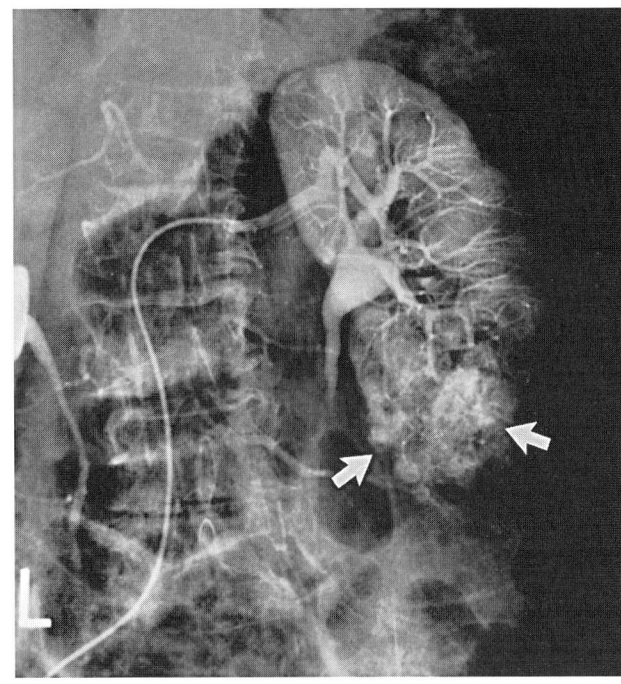

Figure 18–19. Selective left renal arteriogram of a patient with renal cell carcinoma. Typical tumor neovascularity (arrows) is seen both on the early (**A**) and late (**B**) phases of the study.

ANGIOGRAPHY

Angiography, once the primary study for the diagnosis of renal cell carcinoma, is seldom used for diagnostic purposes. More often arteriography is used to provide a vascular roadmap and venography is used to evaluate venous extent of tumor into the renal veins or IVC. Even venous extent is becoming less the province of angiography and more that of MRI. Although invasive, venography in experienced hands provides consistent and accurate assessment of venous tumor extent. It is particularly useful in cases with equivocal MRI findings or in patients in whom MRI cannot be performed for technical reasons.[19]

Most renal cell carcinomas are highly vascular tumors that are easily demonstrated with arteriography. Neovascularity with irregular vessels, pooling of contrast, and A-V shunting are often present (Fig. 18–19). Diagnostic problems arise, however, in cases of hypovascular or avascular tumors where angiography may be normal in the presence of even a moderate-sized lesion. Angiography, however, can still be of diagnostic value, especially in cases where other modalities are difficult to use. The demonstration of tumor vascularity, even if minimal, can resolve a diagnostic dilemma (Fig. 18–20).

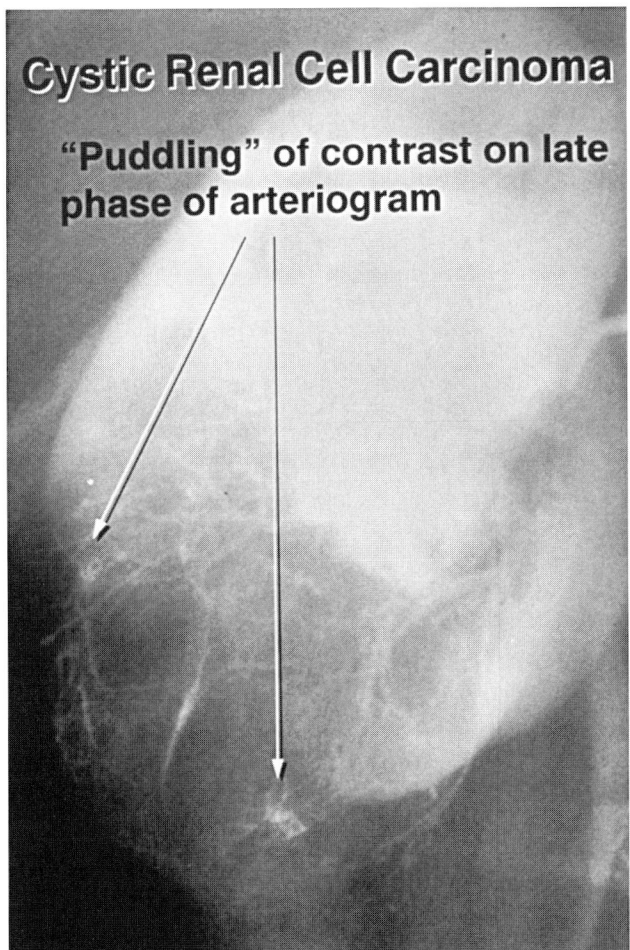

Figure 18–20. Hypovascular renal cell carcinoma with minimal neovascularity.

PERCUTANEOUS NEEDLE ASPIRATION OR BIOPSY

There is little need for biopsy because the vast majority of solid renal lesions represent renal cell carcinoma. This procedure is reserved for instances where therapeutic approach might be altered. Atypical lesions suggesting lymphoma or possible metastatic disease in a patient with a known primary lesion are instances where biopsy can be of benefit. Infiltrating lesions, such as transitional cell carcinoma, may also benefit from biopsy because the surgical approach will be altered. Biopsy is occasionally used for complex cystic masses, although the results for this are often inconclusive and do not eliminate the need for surgery.[32,33]

UROTHELIAL CANCERS OF THE KIDNEY AND URETER

Urothelial cancers of the renal collecting system and pelvis account for 5 to 10% of renal tumors but for only 5% of all urothelial cancers. Ureteral cancers are far less common and account for only 1% of the tumors of the upper urinary tracts. Urothelial renal cancers are three times more common in men than in women, and urothelial ureteral cancers occur twice as frequently in men. Peak incidence of urothelial upper tract tumors is in the sixth and seventh decades. Patients with urothelial upper tract tumors have a 30 to 75% incidence of prior or later bladder cancer, so that bladder evaluation is paramount.

Symptoms and Signs

Microscopic or gross hematuria occurs in 60 to 75% of patients at presentation. Patients (30%) can present with flank pain, which can be acute, from passages of clots, or dull. Fifteen percent of patients are asymptomatic but diagnosed by an imaging study done coincidentally. Advanced stage accounts for 7 to 10% of presenting patients who may have a palpable flank mass, anorexia, or weight loss.

Diagnostic Evaluation

UROGRAPHY–PYELOGRAPHY

Excretory urography has long been the initial study for suspected transitional cell carcinoma and continues in this role despite the development of multiple alternate imaging techniques. Often it is not specifically transitional cell carcinoma that is suspected, but hematuria of unknown cause that leads to the urogram being obtained. Transitional cell carcinoma (TCC) can have multiple presentations with urography. Deformity of the pelvocalyceal system or an irregular filling defect is the most common appearance (Fig. 18–21). Hydronephrosis caused by obstruction, decreased function of the affected kidney,[34] and calyceal amputation are other presentations.[35] The "goblet" sign (Fig. 18–22C) resulting from ureteral dilatation below a urothelial malignancy has an appearance different from ureteral calculi, which would narrow the ureter by virtue of associated edema.[35]

The ability of urography to detect lesions will depend not only on the size and location of the abnormality, but also on the quality of the urogram. Sufficient contrast media (75 to 100mL) is needed to produce complete filling and distention of the pelvocalyceal system. Trendelenburg position and external compression also improve filling of the collecting structures and lesion detection. Tomography or oblique views may be necessary when overlying bowel content obsures the kidneys. Despite all efforts, a urogram may not be optimal, and if there is suspicion of a significant filling defect, retrograde pyelography can be used. After obtaining the upper tract cytology at cystoscopy, retrograde ureteropyelograms are done with bulb tip catheters in an attempt to fill the entire ureter and renal pelvis. The catheter tips are placed just within the ureteral orifices so that even distal ureteral tumors can be seen as filling defects. Care should be taken not to introduce air bubbles, and fluoroscopy is helpful to know when the collecting system is full but extravasation has not occurred. This will provide better filling of the pelvocalyceal system, detect lesions not apparent on urography, and provide a means of obtaining cytologies (Figs. 18–22, 18–23A). Paivansolo found a detection rate of 61% (11/17) for urography and 89% (8/9) for retrograde pyelography.[34] Retrograde pyelography is of particular value when tumor involvement has resulted in a nonfunctioning kidney.[35]

ULTRASOUND

Ultrasound has limited use in the evaluation of transitional cell carcinoma; its detection rate is well below those of other imaging modalities.[34] Although large lesions are apparent with ultrasound (Fig. 18–24 A,B),[36] small lesions in nondilated calyces can easily be overlooked. Probably the greatest value of ultrasound in the evaluation of a filling defect is to demonstrate if it is a stone rather than a tumor. Rarely, a high-grade transitional cell carcinoma may be sufficiently echogenic to mimic a stone.[35,37]

COMPUTED TOMOGRAPHY

Computed tomography, although not used as extensively for transitional cell carcinoma as renal cell carcinoma, can provide considerable information helpful in diagnosis and staging of lesions. On an unenhanced scan transitional cell carcinoma will have a density (30 to 48 HU) greater than fat or urine and similar to the renal parenchyma.[38] Almost all urothelial tumors are less dense than stones, allowing differentiation on an unenhanced scan. In general, the density of transitional cell carcinoma is less than that of a blood clot (50 to 65 HU),[35] but this differentiation cannot be consistently relied upon.[34]

Following the intravenous administration of iodinated contrast media, transitional cell carcinoma will enhance (10 to 40 HU), but generally less than renal cell carcinoma.[38] Most lesions will present as a mass or as thickening of the renal pelvis or ureter (see Figs. 18–23, 18–24).[39] Nyman detected 24 of 28 pelvic tumors as compared to 17/28 at urography and 12/14 with retrograde pyelography. Nineteen

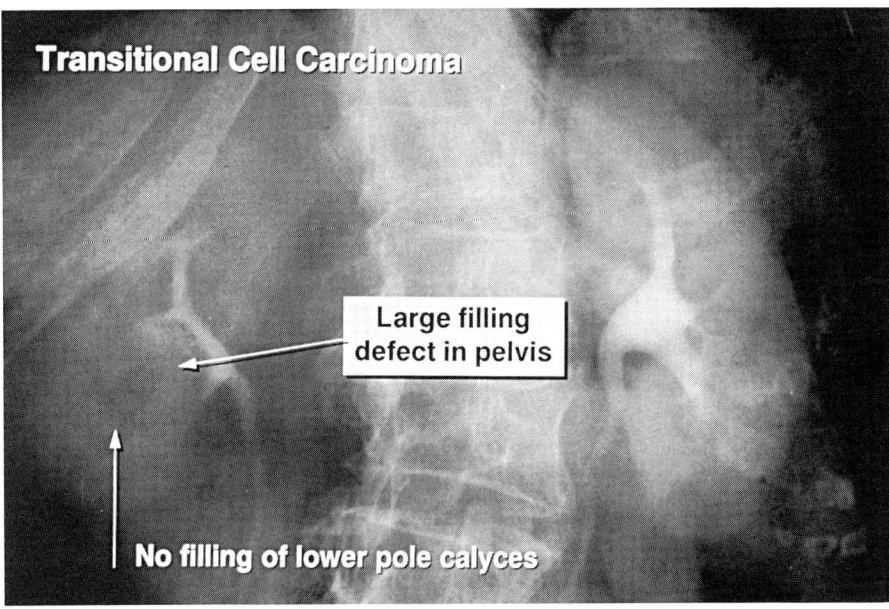

Figure 18–21. Excretory urogram of transitional cell carcinoma of the infundibulum (**A**) and renal pelvis (**B**).

lesions presented as slightly enhancing discrete masses in the renal pelvis. Five lesions distorted the renal pelvis without a well-defined mass.[38] Baron, in a study of 24 lesions, found a sessile mass in 12, ureteral wall thickening in 5, and infiltration of the renal parenchyma in 7.[40] Pelvocalyceal irregularity, infundibular stenosis, hydronephrosis, nonvisualization,[35] and a focal segmental delayed nephrogram caused by obstruction are other presentations.[41]

In contrast to the more common papillary transitional cell carcinoma, which presents as relatively discrete filling defects, nonpapillary transitional cell carcinoma tends to be invasive into the adjacent renal parenchyma or surrounding fat (Fig. 18–25). Invasive transitional cell carcinoma may grow along the normal intrarenal structures with minimal, if any, mass effect.[42] An infiltrating lesion with extension of the tumor into the renal parenchyma is more difficult to separate from renal cell carcinoma, but a central location and lack of distortion of the renal shape favor transitional cell carcinoma.[35] Poorly defined margins, obliteration of the central sinus fat, and an entrapped or obliterated collecting system are also features favoring the diagnosis of transitional cell carcinoma (see Fig. 18–24C).[42]

Although uncommon, large, infiltrating-type transitional cell carcinomas may produce an appearance difficult to distinguish from renal cell carcinoma, lymphoma, or metastatic disease. The lesions can be central or peripheral with no mass effect on the renal sinus or renal contour. Adenopathy, involvement of the veins, and calcification can occur. In this type of lesion needle biopsy may be necessary to differentiate transitional cell carcinoma from other malignancies.[36]

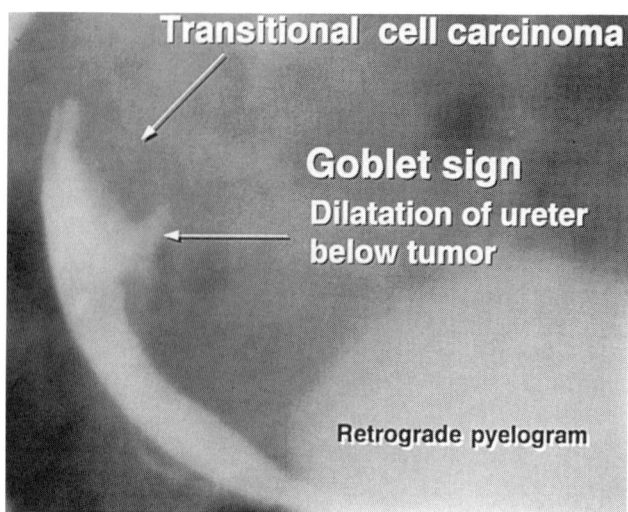

Figure 18–22. Transitional cell carcinoma of the ureters in three different patients.

CYSTOSCOPY

Cystoscopy is paramount to eliminate any associated bladder tumors as well as to note bloody urine effluxing from either ureteral orifice in a patient with gross hematuria.

CYTOLOGY

Voided cytology is simple, but may miss upper tract tumors. If an abnormality on IVP suggests which upper tract has an abnormality, ureteral catheterization to obtain upper tract urine for cytology at the time of cystoscopy is appropriate. Saline barbotage improves the chance of diagnosing an upper tract tumor because more cells are procured.

ANTEGRADE PYELOGRAPHY

Percutaneous antegrade pyelography is an option that is controversial because of the theoretical concern of tracking tumor cells along the percutaneous site. However, tumor cells have not been found to be a problem in percutaneous nephroscopy tracts to treat urothelial upper tract tumors.

BRUSH BIOPSY

Retrograde brushing of a radiographic upper tract filling defect through a ureteral catheter under fluoroscopic guidance more reliably obtains cells for cytologic analysis than simply collecting urine for upper tract cytologic analysis. Urine for cytology can be obtained from the ureteral catheter after the brushing instead of a barbotage.

URETEROSCOPY

Ureteroscopy is an accurate diagnostic method to visualize as well as biopsy ureteral urothelial tumors. Flexible ureteroscopes are similarly helpful for renal urothelial tumors, although nephroscopy has also been used to visualize and biopsy. Because of the concern of perforation of the collec-

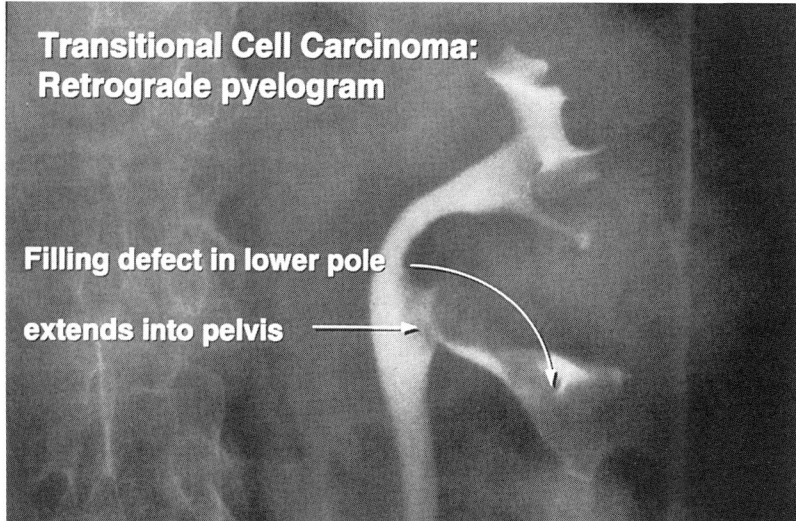

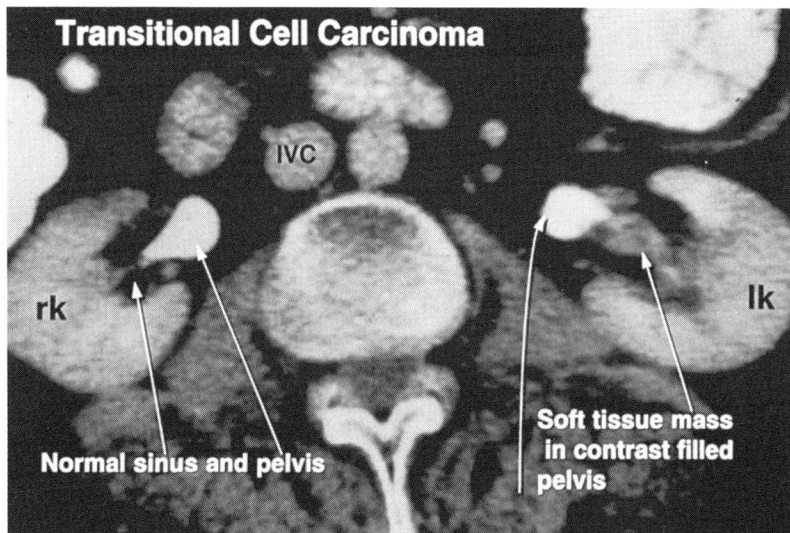

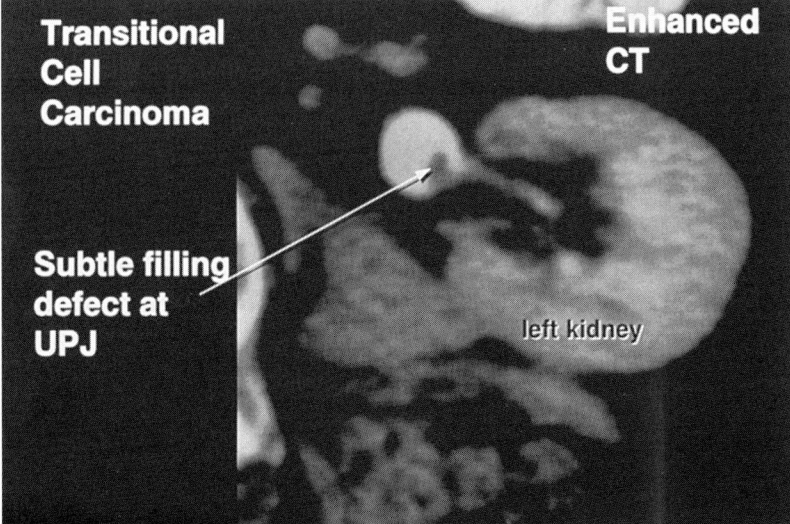

Figure 18–23. (A) Retrogram pyelogram demonstrating a lower-pole lesion poorly seen on urography. Enhanced CT shows this lesion as a soft-tissue density in the renal pelvis (B) and producing a filling defect in the lower pelvis (C).

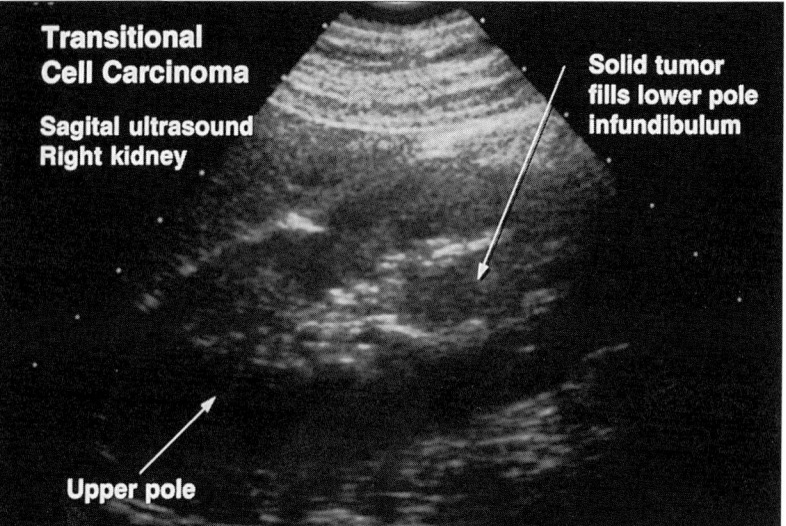
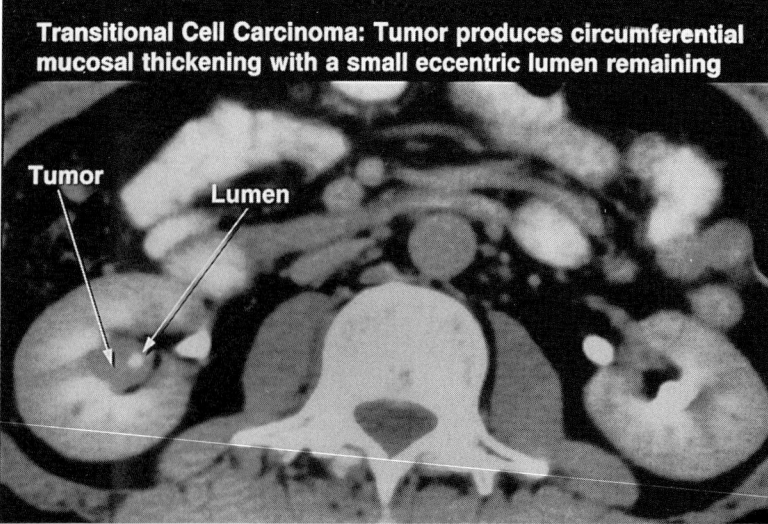

Figure 18–24. (A) Transitional cell carcinoma producing a defect in the right lower calyces with urography. Ultrasound (B) shows solid tissue separating the normally compact central echoes in the right lower pole. Narrowing of the contrast-filled lumen is clearly seen on CT (C).

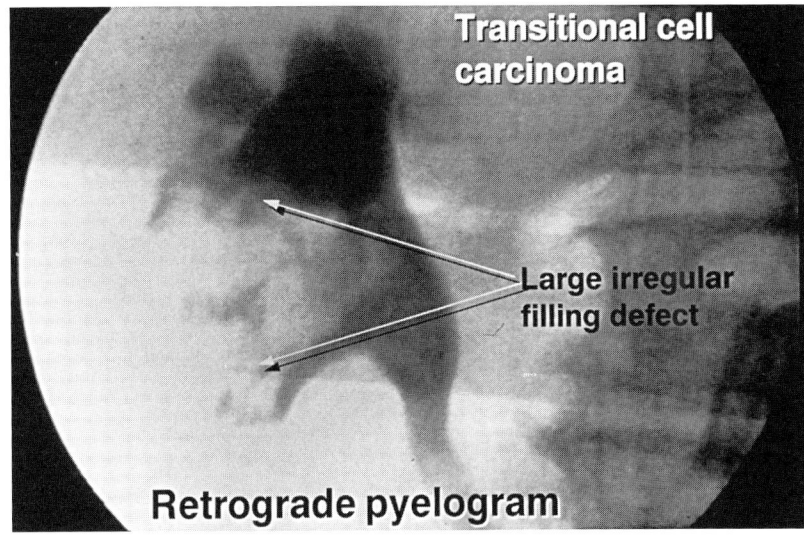

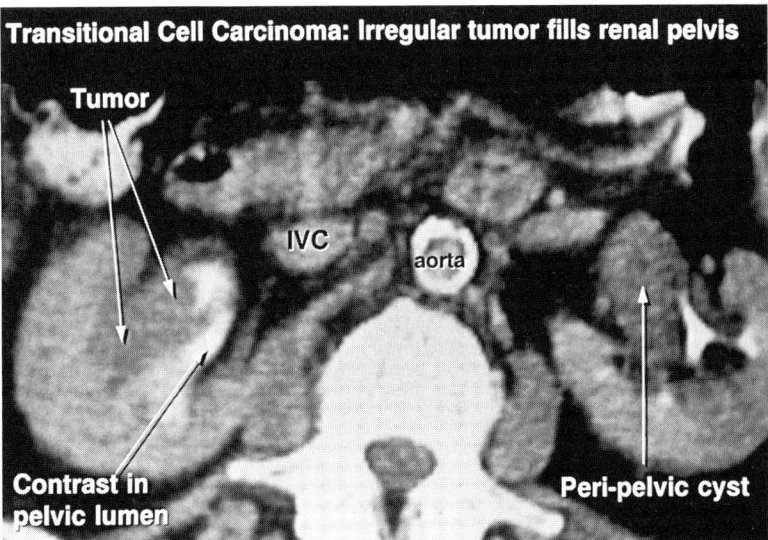

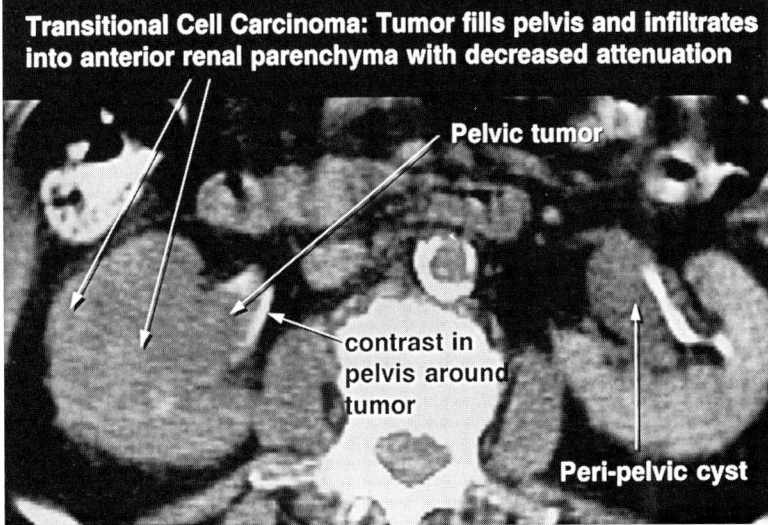

Figure 18–25. Large, irregular filling defect seen on a retrograde spot film (**A**) is shown by CT (**B**, **C**) not only to involve the renal pelvis but also to extend into the renal parenchyma.

tion system during ureteroscopy and the possible spillage of tumor cells, ureteroscopy is reserved for those patients with a positive upper tract cytology but no radiographic lesion or other diagnostic dilemmas. An obvious filling defect on a retrograde pyelogram plus a positive cytology from that ureter would be adequate evidence for treatment. Ureteroscopy would then not be necessary for further management decisions unless some type of renal or ureteral sparing surgery was desirable such that other tumors would need to be excluded or biopsy was necessary to determine grade.

STAGING

Staging is based on the depth of tumor invasion. Pathologic staging is most accurate, but clinical staging preoperatively should include an abdominal CT to assess local extent of tumor as well as lymphadenopathy. If the tumor is large or other than low grade, chest radiography or CT and bone scan are necessary to rule out metastatic lesions to lung and bone.

CT is accurate in detection of transitional cell carcinoma but of limited use for staging. Periureteral streaking is a nonspecific finding more often representing nonmalignant change rather than tumor extension. Staging is most accurate when it demonstrates actual tumor extension through the wall of the pelvis or ureter.[39] CT is able to detect infiltration of the renal parenchyma either by distortion of the normal architecture or by the presence of a solid mass lesion.[38] Baron was able to detect renal parenchymal invasion with CT but was less successful in detecting adenopathy resulting from normal-sized nodes containing malignancy. CT cannot separate tumors limited to the mucosa from those with muscle invasion.[40] As with renal cell carcinoma CT is accurate in detecting abnormal lymph nodes if they are enlarged.[38]

MRI has not been used extensively for transitional cell carcinoma, but in a small series it demonstrated greater sensitivity for detection of transitional cell carcinoma than CT. Staging was similar for the two modalities.[43]

BENIGN RENAL TUMORS

Adenoma

Renal adenomas are common findings at autopsy, radiographic imaging, and nephrectomy for other causes. Controversy stems from Bell's publication of 62 renal adenomas less than 3 cm in diameter of which only three had metastasized.[44] Subsequent publications[45] show no histologic distinguishing features between renal adenomas and renal cell carcinomas. They also occur twice as commonly in men as in women.

Patients are asymptomatic and there are no features distinguishing them from renal cell carcinoma except their size (<3 cm), absence of calcifications, and necrotic centers. Therefore these tumors are usually treated as malignant tumors.

Oncocytoma

Renal oncocytoma is a benign tumor with characteristic pathologic findings, no clinical findings, and suggestive but not reliable radiographic findings. Oncocytomas make up 3 to 5% of renal tumors,[46] are twice as common in men as in women, and are most common in the ages between 40 and 60. Because patients are asymptomatic at presentation, these tumors are typically found by coincidental radiographic imaging.

Classic gross pathologic findings include a central stellate scar and encapsulation. No areas of necrosis are seen. Microscopic findings reveal large eosinophilic cells with granular cytoplasm, but they are to be distinguished from granular renal cell carcinoma. They are typically unilateral but can rarely be bilateral or synchronous. They can be large and are more commonly found at other body sites, such as the adrenal, parathyroid, thyroid, and salivary glands.

IMAGING

Certain imaging features have been described for an oncocytoma. When studied with enhanced CT these lesions are generally homogeneous and may have a central stellate hypodensity (33%) (Fig. 18–26A).[47] With ultrasound they are often homogeneous except for the area of the central scar, an inconsistent sonographic finding (6 to 25%) (Fig. 18–26B).[47,48] This ultrasound appearance, however, is not specific. Renal cell carcinoma, although usually heterogeneous, can have a very uniform appearance indistinguishable from oncocytoma. Although only approximately 6% of renal cell carcinomas have a homogeneous ultrasound appearance, the incidence of renal cell carcinoma is so much greater than oncocytoma that such a homogeneous mass is as likely to be carcinoma as oncocytomas if it is less than 5.5 cm.[49] An area of central necrosis can mimic the central scar of oncocytoma.

In a recent retrospective analysis of oncocytoma and renal carcinoma, CT features were unreliable in differentiating oncocytoma from carcinoma. The criteria of homogeneity and central low density were poor predictors of oncocytoma for both small and large tumors.[50]

An angiographic pattern, the "spoke-wheel," has been attributed to oncocytoma (Fig. 18–26C), and although this pattern may increase the possibility that a mass is an oncocytoma, it is not a specific finding, also being present in renal cell carcinoma (Fig. 18–27).[51,52] The imaging features of oncocytoma are suggestive but not diagnostic of oncocytoma. They should raise suspicion of this entity and in the proper clinical setting they may alter the surgical approach to a lesion.

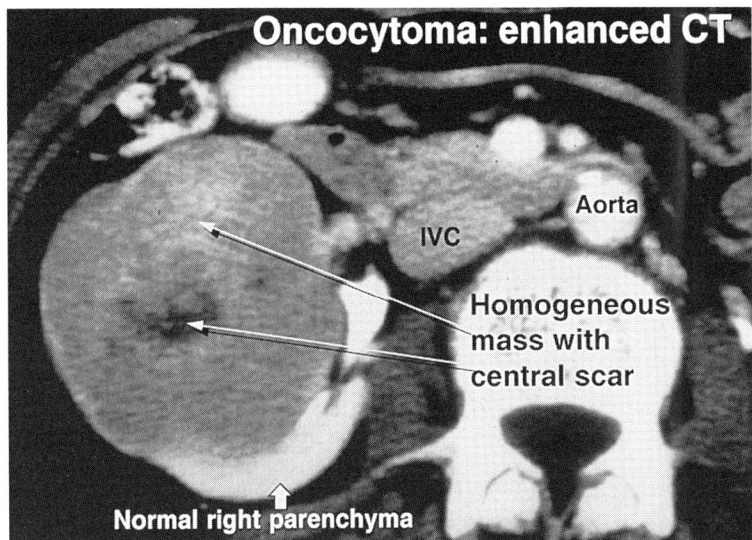

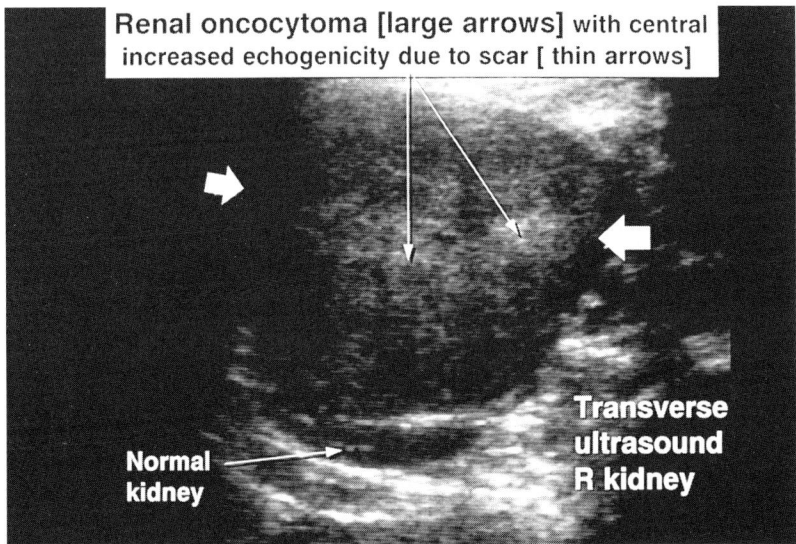

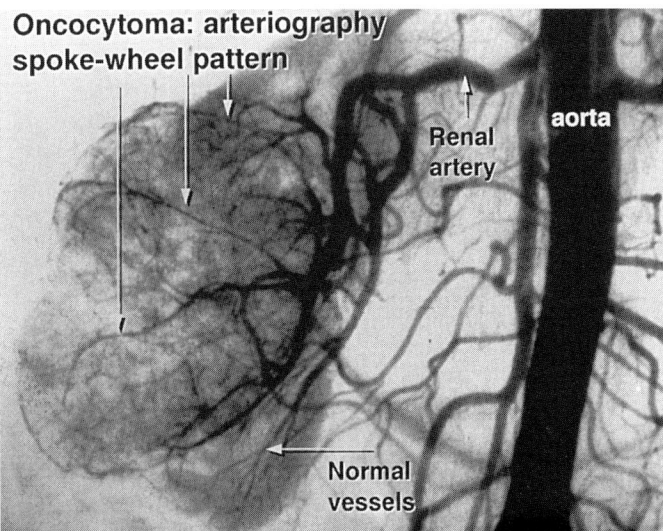

Figure 18–26. Oncocytoma demonstrated by CT (**A**) ultrasound (**B**) and arteriography (**C**).

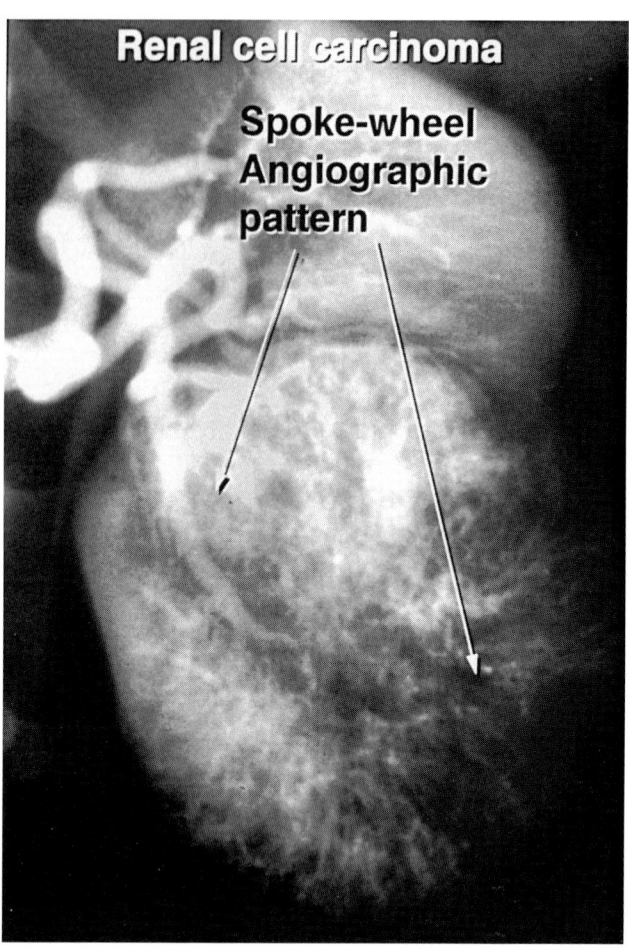

Figure 18–27. Selective left renal arteriogram of a renal cell carcinoma with a "spoke–wheel" angiographic pattern.

Because of unreliable radiographic findings, unreliable flow–cytometry findings,[53] and the possible but rare presence of renal cell carcinoma in the same kidney, oncocytomas are typically treated with excision.

Renal Angiomyolipomas (Hamartomas)

Renal angiomyolipomas are benign renal tumors with characteristic pathologic findings, characteristic radiologic findings, and a variable presentation. They can occur sporadically or as part of tuberous sclerosis, an autosomal dominant syndrome. If sporadic, they occur four times more commonly in women than in men and are usually single.

Half of patients with renal angiomyolipomas have some or all stigmata of tuberous sclerosis, which includes adenomatous sebaceum of the face, brain gliosis, mental retardation, seizures, and angiomyolipomas of the retina, brain, heart, lung, bone, pancreas, or liver. Eighty percent of these patients have renal angiomyolipomas, which are mostly bilateral. In these patients the tumors are often found as part of the routine imaging done for patients diagnosed with tuberous sclerosis.

In sporadic cases, patients can present with massive hemorrhage, flank pain, and hypotension. Alternatively, incidental detection can occur when patients are imaged for other complaints or appropriate detection made when patients are imaged for vague abdominal symptoms from large tumors.

Characteristic histologic findings include components of mature fat cells, abnormal blood vessels, and smooth vessels, although proportions can vary significantly, so that 80% of patients may have minimal fat component.

IMAGING

The demonstration of fat within a renal tumor by any type of imaging has for years been considered a sign of a benign angiomyolipoma.[54] There are case reports of fat engulfed by a renal cell carcinoma mimicking an angiomyolipoma,[55] proven cases of fat within a renal cell carcinoma,[56,57,58] liposarcomas of the kidney,[59,60] and fat within an oncocytoma due to engulfment of surrounding fat.[61] These are, however, rare occurrences and should not alter the basic concept that demonstrable fat within a renal mass indicates a benign angiomyolipoma.[62] Occasional reported cases of fat actually within a renal cell carcinoma had other suspicious imaging features such as extension to the vena cava[56] or malignant-appearing calcifications.[57,58] To focus on the rare occurrences mentioned earlier would necessitate surgery for many benign lesions and would almost certainly do more harm than good. The main question therefore is not the significance of a fat-containing lesion, but what can be accepted as imaging proof that fat is present.

A hyperechoic lesion seen on ultrasound is most often an angiomyolipoma with the increased echogenicity produced by either fat or vascular structures in the mass (Fig. 18–28). CT has not always confirmed the presence of fat, even in proven angiomyolipomas.[63–65] In view of this and the previously reported low incidence of hyperechoic renal cell carcinomas,[8] it is tempting to consider a hyperechoic lesion an angiomyolipoma even if fat is not conclusively demonstrated with CT. Our own (unpublished) experience over the past few years has suggested that the hyperechoic form of renal cell carcinoma was more common than heretofore believed (Fig. 18–29), and recent published studies have confirmed this. A Japanese study showed a 60% incidence of small (<3 cm) hyperechoic renal cell carcinomas.[10] Similar high incidences of hyperechoic renal cell carcinomas have been confirmed with subsequent studies in the United States.[11] A hyperechoic lesion therefore cannot be considered a benign angiomyolipoma without further proof of the presence of fat. This is most often done with CT, a study highly sensitive for detection of the low-density fat (Figs. 18–30, 18–31). The study must be done carefully, however, within 4- to 5-mm sections to detect small amounts of fat. Scans at 10 mm will not consistently detect small amounts of fat, and scans as thin as 2 mm can improve detection of fat in small suspicious areas. It is also important that precontrast scans be obtained because the enhancement that occurs in an angiomyolipoma can mask the presence of fat.[66,67] The value chosen to verify that fat is present varies among authors, but a reasonable number to use is −30 HU.[67]

Some authors have used pixel mapping to detect fat,[66,67] a method which is time consuming, but may obviate surgery if fat is detected (Fig. 18–32). This involves printing out the actual CT measurements of each pixel in a specific region of interest. This reduces averaging of tissues and shows negative numbers that might otherwise be obscured. Because a single pixel with a negative attenuation value may be artifactual at least three adjacent negative pixels are required before concluding fat is present.[66,67] Recent studies with thin sections have detected fat in the vast majority of lesions.[68] Failure to detect fat within a lesion with current CT technology is therefore considered suspicious for malignancy. Surgery is probably warranted, realizing that some of these lesions may still prove to be angiomyolipomas.[64]

As an alternate to CT, MRI can be used for detection of fat (Fig. 18–31B and Fig. 18–33). MRI is probably as sensitive as CT, but there is less experience with MRI. In one series MRI detected fat in five of six cases and was more sensitive than 8- to 10-mm-thick CT images, but it was not compared against thin-section CT.[69] A lesion first detected with CT or MRI showing unequivocal fat can be considered benign. A hyperechoic lesion detected with CT can only be considered a benign angiomyolipoma after confirmation of intratumoral fat with CT or MRI.

Because these tumors can be multicentric, they are managed conservatively. If they spontaneously hemorrhage or are large and symptomatic, angioinfarction is appropriate treatment.[70]

Other Benign Renal Tumors

Fibromas have been described in a medullary location as occurring in more than 35% of autopsy studies[71] and are frequently bilateral. They are rarely diagnosed during a patient's lifetime because they would have to grow to quite a large size to be clinically obvious.

Lipomas are rare but are more likely to occur in middle-aged women. They can be quite large and present with pain and/or hematuria.

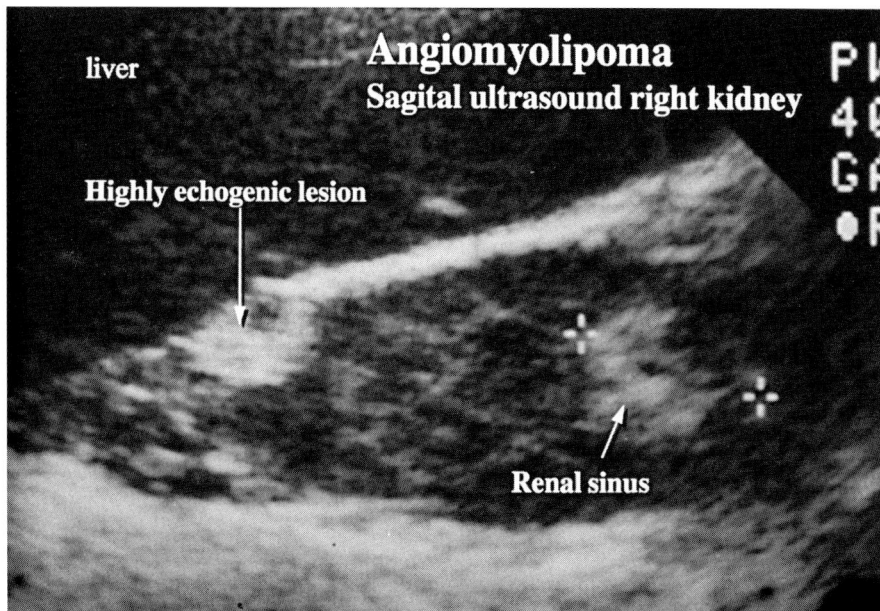

Figure 18–28. Ultrasound study of a typical small hyperechoic angiomyolipoma.

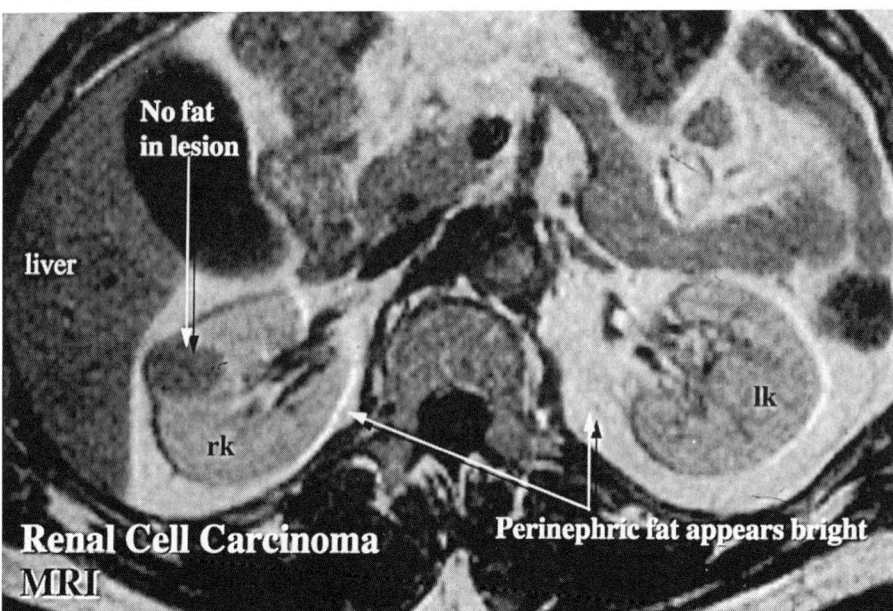

Figure 18–29. (A) Ultrasound examination of small hyperechoic renal cell carcinoma. (B) MRI of this hyperechoic lesion failed to demonstrate fat within the tumor.

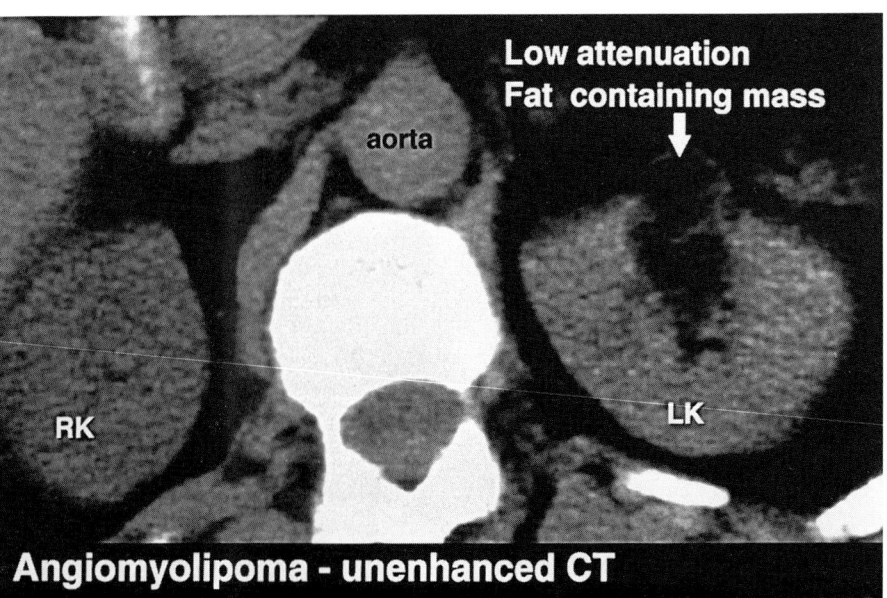

Figure 18–30. Typical fat-containing angiomyolipoma with unenhanced CT.

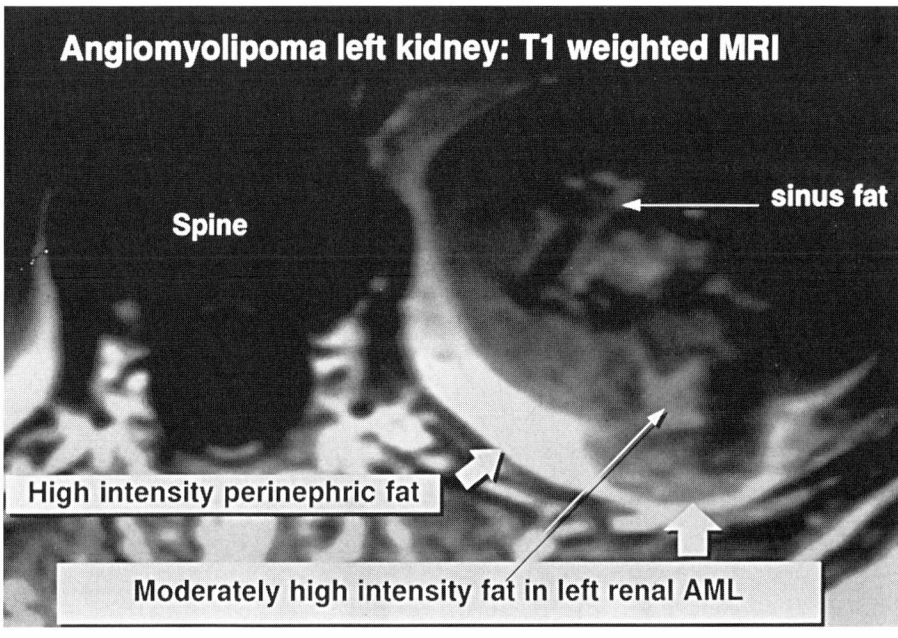

Figure 18–31. CT enhanced (**A**) shows a fat-containing lesion extending into the renal hilus. Pathologically proven angiomyolipoma. T1-weighted MRI of this same lesion (**B**) shows the fat as a bright signal.

Leiomyomas are asymptomatic, diagnosed at autopsy, and less than 1 cm in size. Juxtaglomerular cell tumors are benign, are extremely rare, but can present with severe hypertension and hypokalemia. These tumors are typically 2 to 3 cm in size. Histologically, the tumors resemble hemangiopericytomas and secrete renin.

SECONDARY MALIGNANT RENAL TUMORS

Hematogenous dissemination of other solid malignancies to the kidneys occurs late in these cancers and therefore was previously diagnosed at autopsy. However, because patients are imaged after treatment failures, metastases to the kidneys can be detected but are rarely symptomatic. Lung, breast, and pancreatic cancers are the most common solid tumors to spread hematogenously to the kidneys.

IMAGING

Honda compared the CT findings of patients with pathologically proven metastatic renal lesions with those of renal cell carcinoma. They used 14 criteria and statistically analyzed the value of each of these in separating metastatic lesions from renal cell carcinoma. They found number, size, shape, and laterality to be the most useful criteria. Of renal cell carcinomas, 96% were solitary, but only 47% of metastases were solitary. Metastases were smaller (less than 3 cm),

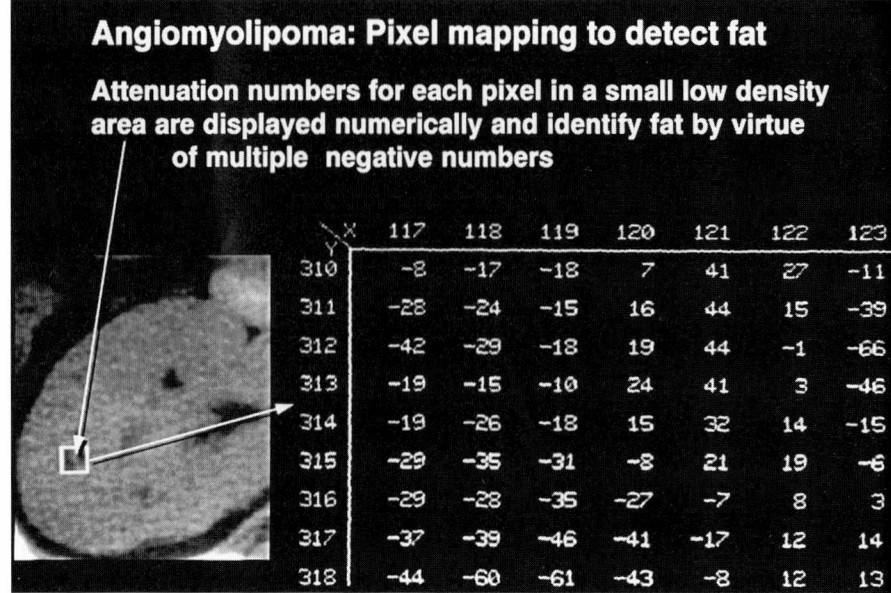

Figure 18-32. Pixel mapping used to identify a small amount of fat in a pathologically proven angiomyolipoma.

and 25% had a wedge shape, which is not found in renal cell carcinoma (Fig.18-34). Perirenal involvement occurred in metastatic disease, but was far more common with renal cell carcinoma.[72] Most metastatic lesions will present as multiple, bilateral enhancing lesions that may be well defined or infiltrative. Multiplicity favors metastatic disease, but there is no specific CT appearance for an individual metastatic lesion to separate it from renal cell carcinoma.[73] A metastatic lesion can be solitary, large, and indistinguishable from renal cell carcinoma.[74] In patients with known malignancy elsewhere, a new single renal lesion is four times more likely to be a metastatic lesion than renal cell carcinoma. In a patient with widespread disease, biopsy to prove metastatic versus renal cell carcinoma is probably not indicated. However, it can be helpful in a patient with a known primary but no other evidence of metastatic disease.[73]

Lymphoma, leukemia, and multiple myeloma are the most common hematologic malignancies to spread hematogenously to the kidneys. Before effective chemotherapy, asymptomatic renal involvement was common and usually represented disease elsewhere.

Lymphomatous involvement of the kidneys is almost always associated with generalized disease, making diagnosis less difficult.[75] Abdominal adenopathy, however, is not always present, and its absence does not exclude renal lymphoma. This is particularly true in patients with long-standing disease who have been previously treated. Cohan and colleagues found retroperitoneal adenopathy in only 41% of

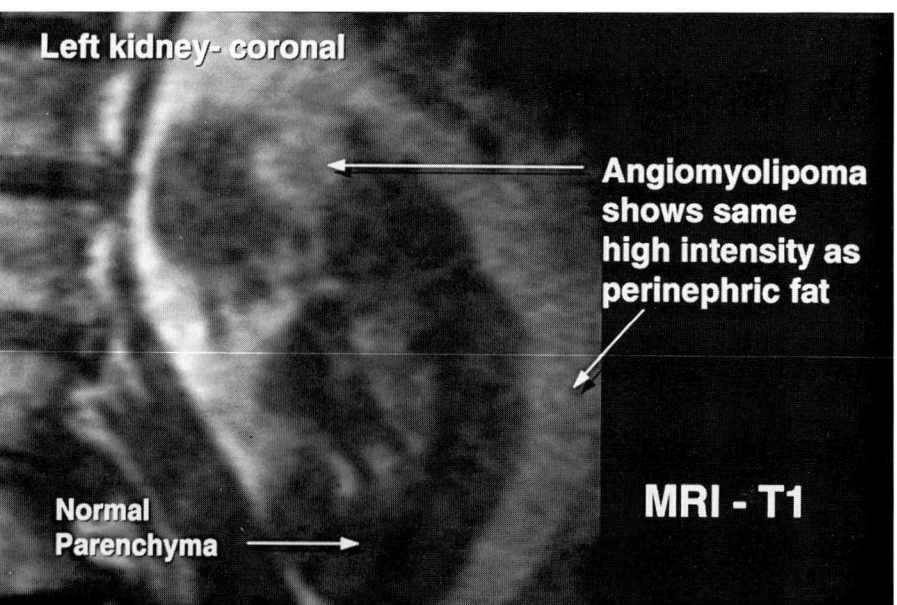

Figure 18-33. Coronal MRI demonstrating an incidentally detected angiomyolipoma.

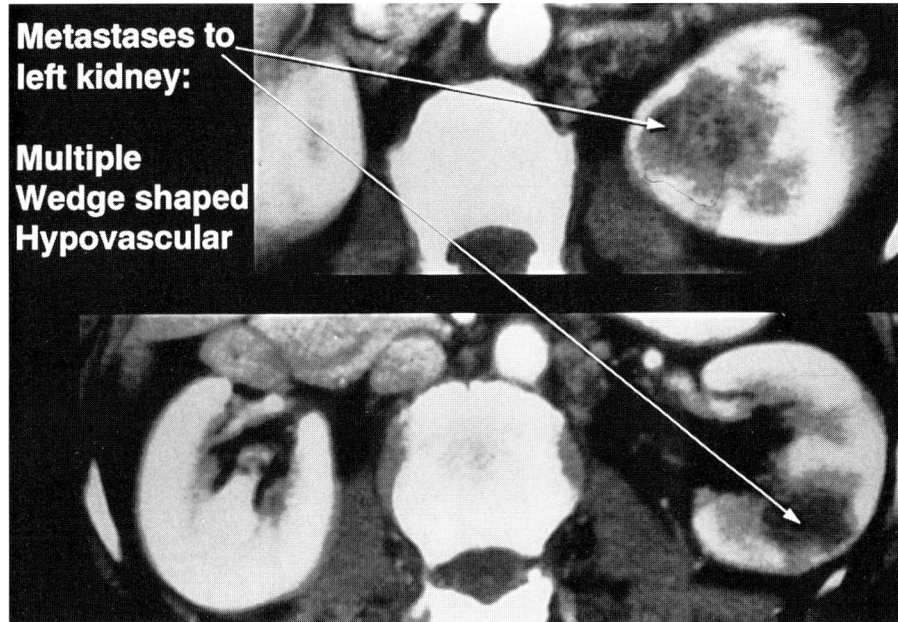

Figure 18–34. Breast carcinoma metastatic to the left kidney.

their patients in whom renal lymphoma presented as bilateral renal masses.[76] Reznek and colleagues also noted an absence of retroperitoneal adenopathy in 43% of their cases, including initial presentations as well as follow-up patients.[77] Although the most common renal presentation is multiple bilateral masses (Fig. 18–35), the kidneys can be involved by direct invasion of adjacent retroperitoneal masses (Fig. 18–36), diffuse infiltration, or a single mass.[75–77]

In instances of multiple bilateral masses the renal outline may be abnormal or there may be nephromegaly with a normal contour. An enhanced study is necessary to demonstrate the lesions, which enhance less than the normal renal parenchyma.[78] Perinephric disease is usually associated with renal involvement but can occur without obvious involvement of the kidney.[76–77] In instances where the diagnosis is not clear and the possibility of renal cell carcinoma exists, needle biopsy is useful to separate these entities that require different therapy.

NONNEOPLASTIC DIFFERENTIAL DIAGNOSIS

In the evaluation of "mass" lesions of the kidney it is important to recognize two abnormalities that are nonneoplastic but that can be confused with renal cell carcinoma. These

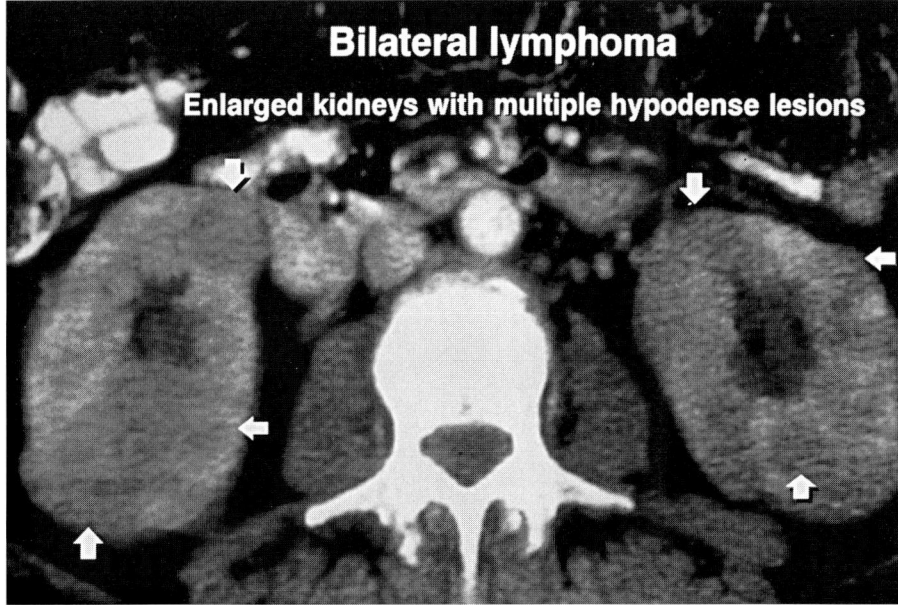

Figure 18–35. CT of renal lymphoma with multiple lesions bilaterally.

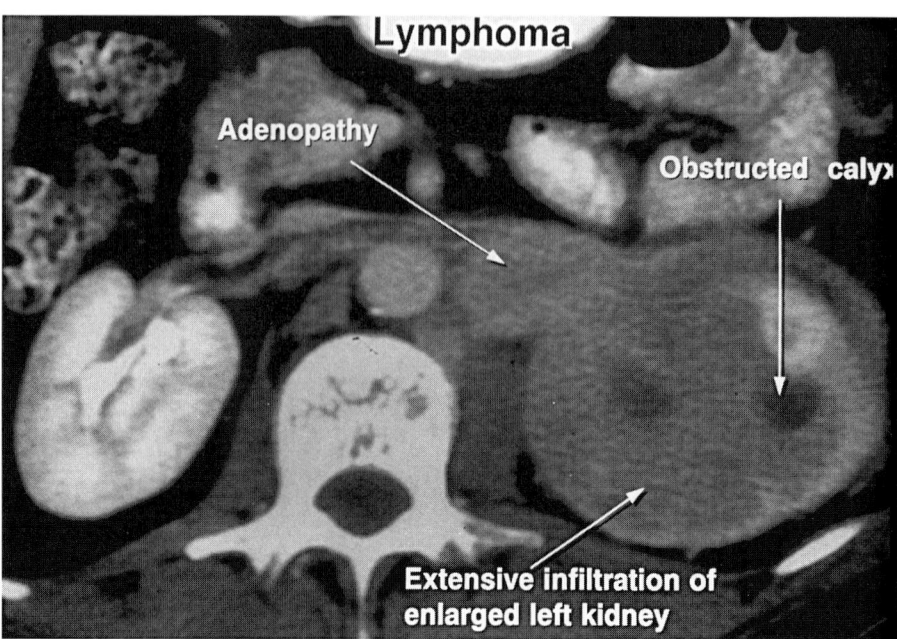

Figure 18–36. CT of lymphoma involving para-aortic nodes and extending into the left kidney.

are renal infarct and focal areas of acute pyelonephritis. Renal infarction produces an area of diminished to absent enhancement on CT. There is often rim enhancement because of intact capsular vessels. It does not, however, produce a true mass effect. The adjacent structures are not displaced or distorted, and the collecting structures exist unchanged in the midst of the "mass." The lesion is sharply demarcated from the remaining parenchyma, with minimal, if any, alteration in the renal contour (Fig. 18–37). A follow-up scan in 6 to 8 weeks will often show development of focal scarring.

Focal pyelonephritis can produce a mass on both ultrasound and CT. The lesion will be relatively isodense on unenhanced scans and will show diminished enhancement as compared to normal parenchyma. The clinical picture is often the key to diagnosis, but in addition the CT appearance of the remainder of the kidney is a clue to the diagnosis. Other changes of pyelonephritis are often present. A coarsely striated nephrogram, possibly with other areas of focal diminished enhancement, suggests pyelonephritis (Fig. 18–38). If there is doubt, a follow-up scan after antibiotic therapy will show resolution of the lesions.

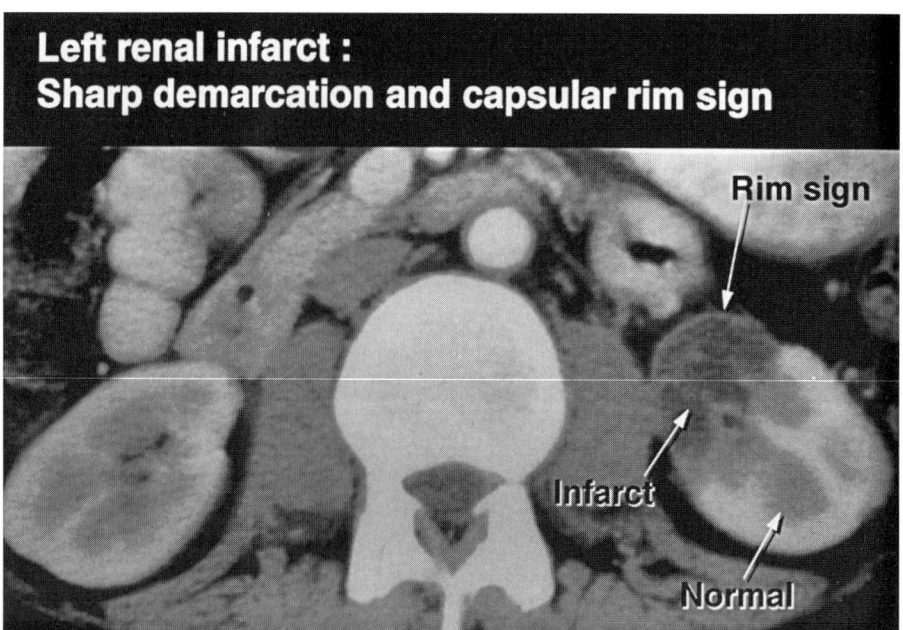

Figure 18–37. Enhanced CT of left renal infarct.

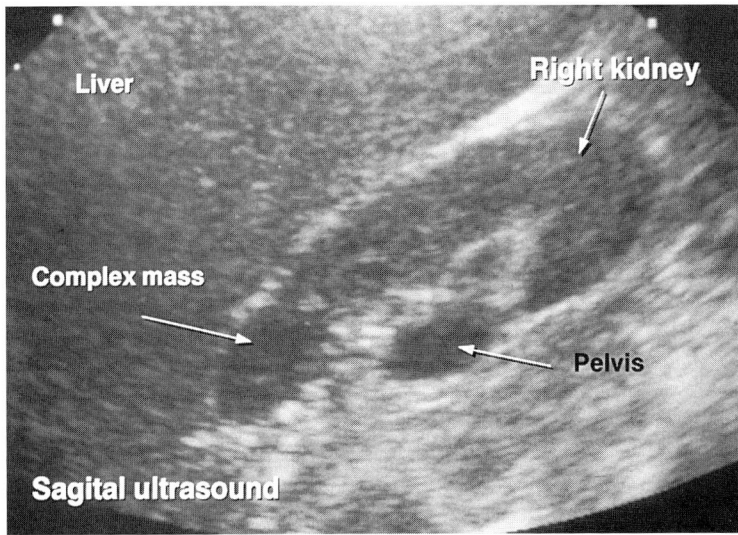

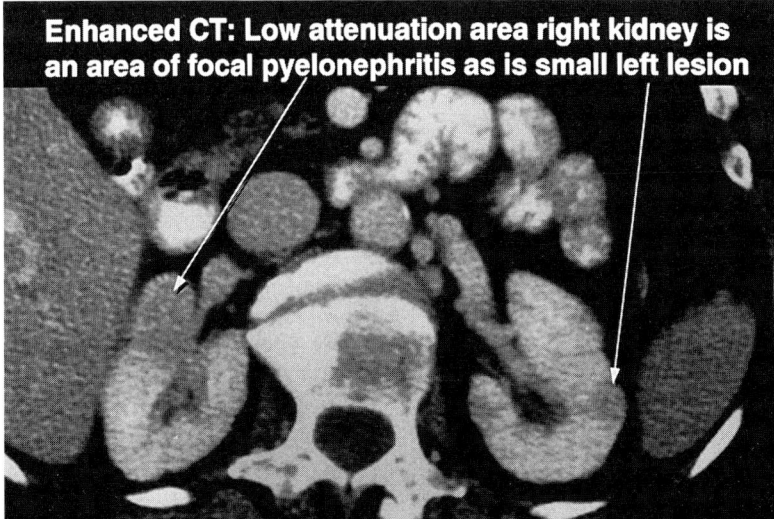

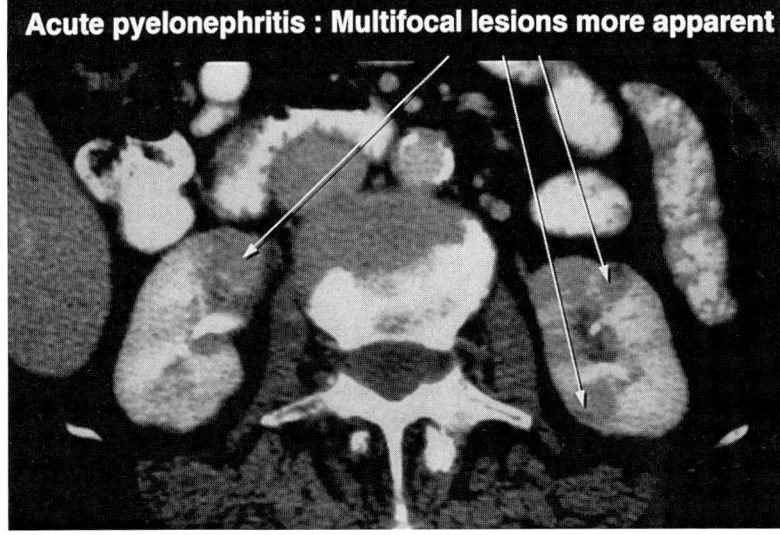

Figure 18–38. Pyelonephritis. Ultrasound (**A**) showed a complex-appearing mass in the upper pole with an otherwise normal right kidney. Enhanced CT (**B**, **C**) showed this focal lesion to be one of many hypodense areas representing pyelonephritis. Follow-up CT showed resolution of these abnormalities.

REFERENCES

1. Warshauer DM, McCarthy SM, Street L, et al: Detection of renal masses: sensitivities and specificities of excretory urography/linear tomography, US, and CT. *Radiology* 1988; 169:363–365.
2. Pollack HM, Edel LS, Morales JO: Radionuclide imaging in renal pseudotumors. *Radiology* 1974;111:639.
3. Older RA, et al: Accuracy of radionuclide imaging in distinguishing renal masses from normal variants. *Radiology* 1980; 136:443–448.
4. Sufrin G, Chasan S, Golio A, Murphy GP: Paraneoplastic and serologic syndromes or renal adenocarcinoma. *Semin Urol* 1989;7:158.
5. Stauffer MH: Nephrogenic hepatosplenomegaly (abstract). *Gastroenterology* 1961;40:694.
6. Older RA, Mclelland R, Cleeve DM, Moore AV, Webster GD: Importance of routine vascular nephrotomography in excretory urography. *Urology* 1980;15:312–317.
7. Demos TC, Schoffer M, Love L, Waters WB, Moncada R: Normal excretory urography in patients with primary kidney neoplasms. *Urol Radiol* 1985;7:75–79.
8. Charboneau JW, Hattery RR, Ernst EC III, James EM, Williamson B Jr, Hartman GW: Spectrum of sonographic findings in 125 renal masses other than benign simple cyst. *AJR* 1983; 140:87–94.
9. Kier R, Taylor KJW, Feylock AL, Ramos I. Renal masses: characterization with doppler US. *Radiology* 1990;176:703–707.
10. Yamashita Y, Takahashi M, Watanabe O, et al: Small renal cell carcinoma: pathologic and radiologic correlation. *Radiology* 1992;184:493–498.
11. Forman HP, Middleton WD, Melson GL, McClennan BL: Hyperechoic renal cell carcinomas: increase in detection at US. *Radiology* 1993;188:431–434.
12. McClennan BL, Deyoe LA: The imaging evaluation of renal cell carcinoma: diagnosis and staging. *Radiol Clin North Am* 1994;32:55–69.
13. Rosenfield, personal communication.
14. Zagoria RJ, Wolfman NT, Karstead N, Hinn GC, Dyer RB, Chen YM: CT features of renal cell carcinoma with emphasis on relation to tumor size. *Invest Radiol* 1990;25:261–266.
15. Fein AB, Lee JKT, Balfe DM, Heiken JP, et al: Diagnosis and staging of renal cell carcinoma: a comparison of MR imaging and CT. *AJR* 1987;148:749–753.
16. Schweden FJ, Schild HH, Riedmiller H: Renal tumors in adults. In: Schild HH, Schweden FJ, Lane EK, eds. *Computed Tomography in Urology*, New York: Thieme, 1992;135–176.
17. Herts BR, Einstein DM, Paushter DM: Spiral CT of the abdomen: artifacts and potential pitfalls. *AJR* 1993;161:1185–1990.
18. Robson CJ, Churchill BM, Anderson W: The results of radical nephrectomy for renal cell carcinoma. *Trans Am Assoc Genitourin Surg* 1968;60:122.
19. Zagoria RJ, Bechtold RE, Dyer RB: Staging of renal adenocarcinoma: role of various imaging procedures. *AJR* 1995; 164:363–370.
20. Johnson CD, Dunnick NR, Cohan RH, Illescas FF: Renal adenocarcinoma: CT staging of 100 tumors. *AJR* 1987;148:59–63.
21. Zeman RK, Cronan JJ, Rosenfield AT, Lynch JH, Jaffee MH, Clark LR: Renal cell carcinoma: dynamic thin-section CT assessment of vascular invasion and tumor vascularity. *Radiology* 1988;167:393–396.
22. Goldfarb DA, Novick AC, Lorig R, Bretan PN, et al: Magnetic resonance imaging for assessment of vena caval tumor thrombi: a comparative study with venacavography and computerized tomography scanning. *J Urol* 1990;144;1100–1104.
23. Semelka RC, Shoenut JP, Magro CM, Kroeker MA, MacMahon R, Greenberg HM. Renal cancer staging: comparison of contrast-enhanced CT and gadolinium-enhanced fat-suppressed spin-echo and gradient-echo MR imaging. *J Magn Reson Imaging* 1993;3:597–602.
24. Kabala JE, Gillatt DA, Persad RA, Penry JB, Gingell JC, Chadwick D: Magnetic resonance imaging in the staging of renal cell carcinoma. *Br J Radiol* 1991;64:683–689.
25. Myneni L, Hricak H, Carroll PR: Magnetic resonance imaging of renal cell carcinoma with extension into the vena cava: staging accuracy and recent advances. *Br J Urol* 1991;68:571–578.
26. Roubidoux MA, Dunnick NR, Sostman HD, Leder RA: Renal carcinoma: detection of venous extension with gradient-echo MR imaging. *Radiology* 1992;182:269–272.
27. Straton CS, Libertino JA, Larsen CA: Is magnetic resonance imaging alone accurate enough in staging renal cell carcinoma? *Urology* 1992;40:351–353.
28. Rofsky NM, Weinreb JC, Bosniak MA, et al: Renal lesion characterization with gadolinium-enhanced MR imaging: efficacy and safety in patients with renal insufficiency. *Radiology* 1991;180:85–89.
29. Terens WT, Gluck R, Golimbu M, Rofsky NM: Use of gadolinium-DTPA-enhanced MRI to characterize renal mass in patient with renal insufficiency. *Urology* 1992;40:152–154.
30. Eilenberg SS, Brown JJ, Lee JKT, Heiken JP, Mirowitz SA: Evaluation of renal masses with contrast enhanced rapid acquisition spin echo MR imaging. *Magn Reson Imaging* 1993; 11:7–6.
31. Oka T, Morimoto K, Shimoi M, Tsujimura A, et al: MR angiography of renal cell carcinoma. *Urol Int* 1993;50:198–202.
32. Amis EA Jr, Cronan JJ, Pfister RC: Needle puncture of cystic renal masses: a survey of the Society of Uroradiology. *AJR* 1987;148:197–299.
33. Nicefero JR, Coughlin BF: Diagnosis of renal cell carcinoma. Value of fine-needle aspiration cytology in patients with metastases or contraindications to nephrectomy. *AJR* 1993; 161:1303–1305.
34. Paivansalo M, Merikanto J, Myllyla V, Hellstrom P, Kallionen M, Jalovaara P: Radiological and cytological detection of renal pelvic transitional-cell carcinoma. *Rofo Fortschr Geb Rontgenstr Neuen Bildgeb Verfahr* 1990;153:266–270.
35. Leder RA, Dunnick RD: Transitional cell carcinoma of the pelvicalices and ureter. *AJR* 1990;155:713–722.
36. Bree RL, Schultz SR, Hayes R: Large infiltrating renal transitional cell carcinomas: CT and ultrasound features. *J Comput Assist Tomogr* 1990;14:381–385.
37. Janetschek G, Putz A, Feichtinger H: Renal transitional cell carcinoma mimicking stone echoes. *J Ultrasound Med* 1988; 7:83–86.
38. Nyman U, Oldbring J, Aspelin P. CT of carcinoma of the renal pelvis. *Acta Radiol* 1992;33:31–38.
39. Badalament RA, Bennett WF, Bova JG, Kenworthy PR, et al: Computed tomography of primary transitional cell carcinoma of upper urinary tracts. *Urology* 1992;40:71–75.
40. Baron RL, McClennan BL, Lee JKT, Lawson TL: Computed tomography of transitional-cell carcinoma of the renal pelvis and ureter. *Radiology* 1982;144:125–130.
41. Eamann S, Stanley RJ, Lloyd K: Focal obstruction nephrogram: an unusual CT appearance of a transitional cell carcinoma. *J Comput Assist Tomogr* 1984;8:1019–1022.
42. Fukuya T, Honda H, Nakata H, Egashira K, et al: Computed tomographic findings of invasive transitional cell carcinoma in the kidney. *Radiat Med* 1994;12:6–10.
43. Huang CL, Liu GC, Sheu RS, Huang CH: Magnetic resonance imaging and computed tomography of transitional cell carci-

noma of renal pelvis and ureter. *Kaohsiung J Med Sci* 1994; 10:194–202.
44. Bell ET: *Renal Disease*, 2nd ed. Philadelphia: Lea and Febiger, 1950:435.
45. Bennington JL, Beckwith JB: Tumors of the kidney, renal pelvis and ureter. In: *Atlas of Tumor Pathology*. Washington, DC: Armed Forces Institute of Pathology, 1975, Facs. 12.
46. Lieber MM, Tsukamoto T: Renal oncocytoma. In: deKernion JB, Pavone-Macalusa M, eds. *Tumor of the Kidney*. Baltimore: Williams & Wilkins, 1986;257.
47. Quinn MJ, Hartman DS, Friedman AC, et al: Renal oncocytoma: new observations. *Radiology* 1984;153:49–53.
48. Tikkakoski T, Paivansalo M, Alanen A, et al: Radiologic findings in renal oncocytoma. *Acta Radiol* 1991;32 (Fasc. 5):363–367.
49. Goiney RC, Goldenberg L, Cooperberg PL, et al: Renal oncocytomas: sonographic analysis of 14 cases. *AJR* 1984;143:1001–1004.
50. Davidson AJ, Hayes WS, Hartman DS, et al: Renal oncocytoma and carcinoma: failure of differentiation with CT: *Radiology* 1993;86:693–696.
51. Older RA, Cleeve D, Fetter B, Jackson D: "Spoke-wheel" angiographic pattern in renal masses: nonspecificity. *Radiology* 1978;128–836.
52. Ambos MA, Bosniak MA, Quentin VJ, Madayag MA, Lefleur RS: Angiographic patterns in renal oncocytoma. *Radiology* 1978;129:615–622.
53. Rainwater LM, Farrow GM, Lieber NM: Flow cytometry of renal cell oncocytoma: common occurrence of deoxyribonucleic acid polyploidy and aneuploidy. *J. Urol* 1986;135:1167.
54. Bosniak MA: Angiomyolipoma (hamartoma) of the kidney: a preoperative diagnosis is possible in virtually every case. *Urol Radiol* 1981;3:135–142.
55. Prando A: Intratumoral fat in a renal cell carcinoma. *AJR* 1991;156:871 (letter).
56. Radin DR, Chandrasoma P: CT demonstration of fat density in renal cell carcinoma. *Acta Radiol* 1992;33:365–367.
57. Helenon O, Chretien Y, Paraf F, Melki P, Denys A, Moreau JF: Renal cell carcinoma containing fat: demonstration with CT. *Radiology* 1993;188:429–430.
58. Strotzer M, Lehner KB, Becker K: Detection of fat in a renal cell carcinoma mimicking angiomyolipoma. *Radiology* 1993;188:427–428.
59. Cano JY, D'Altorio RA: Renal liposarcoma: case report. *J Urol* 1976;115:747–749.
60. Mayes DC, Fechner RE, Gillenwater JY: Renal liposarcoma. *Am J Surg Pathol* 1990;14:268–273.
61. Curry NS, Schabel SI, Garvin AJ, Fish G: Intratumoral fat in a renal oncocytoma mimicking angiomyolipoma. *AJR* 1990;154:307–308.
62. Davidson AJ, Davis CJ: Fat in renal adenocarcinoma: never say never. *Radiology* 1993;188:316.
63. Paivansalo M, Lahde S, Hyvarinen S, et al: Renal angiomyolipoma ultrasonographic, CT, angiographic and histologic correlation. *Acta Radiol* 1991;32(Fasc 3):239–243.
64. Okamura K, Hasegawa S, Kuriki O, Saito M, Sahashi M, Miyake K: Small hyperechoic renal tumors displaying no fat content on CT. *Urol Int* 1992;49:175–178.
65. Hartman DS, Goldman SM, Friedman AC, Davis CJ, et al: Angiomyolipoma: ultrasonic–pathologic correlation. *Radiology* 1981;139:451–458.
66. Takahashi K, Masanori H, Okubo RS, Hyodo H, et al: CT pixel mapping in the diagnosis of small angiomyolipomas of the kidneys. *J Comp Assist Tomogr* 1993;17:98–101.
67. Kurosaki Y, Tanaka Y, Kuramoto K, Itai Y: Improved CT fat detection in small kidney angiomyolipomas using thin sections and single voxel measurements. *J Comp Assist Tomogr* 1993;17:745–748.
68. Yamashita Y, Ueno S, Makita O, et al: Hyperechoic renal tumors: anaechoic rim and intratumoral cysts in US differentiation of renal cell carcinoma from angiomyolipoma. *Radiology* 1993;188:179–183.
69. Uhlenbrock D, Fisher C, Beyer K: Angiomyolipoma of the kidney, comparison between magnetic resonance imaging, computed tomography, and ultrasonography for diagnosis. *Acta Radiol* 1988;29(Fasc 5):523–526.
70. Oesterling JE, Fishman EK, Goldman SM, Marshall FF: The management of renal angiomyolipoma. *J Urol* 1986;135:1121.
71. Bensib SM; Pathologic features of renal parenchymal tumors. In: Culp DA, Loening SA, eds. *Genitourinary Oncology*. Philadelphia: Lea & Febiger, 1985;185.
72. Honda H, Coffman CE, Berbaum KS, Barloon TJ, Masuda K: CT analysis of metastatic neoplasms of the kidney. *Acta Radiol* 1992;33:39–44.
73. Volpe JP, Choyke PL: The radiologic evaluation of renal metastases. *Crit Rev Diagn Imaging* 1990;30:219–246.
74. Choyke PL, White ME, Zeman RK, Jaffe MH, Clark LR: Renal metastases: clinicopathologic and radiologic correlation. *Radiology* 1987;162:359–363.
75. Bosniak MA: Problems in the radiologic diagnosis for renal parenchymal tumors. *Urol Clin North Am* 1993;20:217–230.
76. Cohan RH, Dunnick NR, Leder RA, Baker ME: Computed tomography of renal lymphoma. *J Comput Assist Tomogr* 1990;14:933–938.
77. Reznek RH, Mootoosamy I, Webb JAW, Richards MA: CT in renal and perirenal lymphoma: a further look. *Clin Radiol* 1990;42:233–238.
78. Heiken JP, Gold RP, Schnur MJ, King DI, Bashist B, Glazer HS: Computed tomography of renal lymphoma with ultrasound correlation. *J Comput Assist Tomogr* 1983;7:245–250.

19 Benign and Malignant Tumors of the Lower Urinary Tract

Gabriel P. Haas, David J. Grignon, James E. Montie

BENIGN AND MALIGNANT TUMORS OF THE BLADDER

The urinary bladder is a complex extraperitoneal structure that functions both to store and to expel urine voluntarily. It is lined by transitional epithelium normally no more than seven cells thick. Deep to the mucosa are thick layers of smooth muscle, the detrusor and the trigone, depending on the anatomic location, which can be subdivided histologically into inner longitudinal, middle circular, and outer longitudinal layers. These layers are covered by an outer serosal adventitia consisting of connective tissue and, on the superior portion of the bladder, by the peritoneum. The vast majority of tumors arising from the bladder originate from the mucosal layer and are, potentially malignant. Tumors involving the muscular layers are either primary sarcomas or, much more frequently, invasive epithelial tumors. A variety of symptoms may indicate the presence of a bladder tumor, and radiologic tests may confirm the presence of an abnormality. Cytology may be useful in detection of the pathologic condition, and it may identify the nature of the lesion. However, most of the pathologic findings must be confirmed by direct visualization during cystoscopy, and the ultimate identification depends on tissue diagnosis. Further radiologic studies will then lead to clinical staging for appropriate treatment.

Before an in-depth review of the modalities used to diagnose bladder lesions, a brief review of the variety of pathologic conditions encountered in the bladder is indicated.

Benign Tumors of the Bladder

TRANSITIONAL CELL PAPILLOMA

The diagnosis of a completely resected mucosal lesion as a papilloma is very controversial among pathologists. The controversy originates with the histologic criteria that differentiate this lesion from low-grade bladder cancer. Currently, most authorities readily accept the occurrence of such lesions, which account for 2 to 3% of papillary transitional cell tumors.[1,2] These lesions are small, usually unifocal, and characterized by delicate fibrovascular stalks covered by cytologically and architecturally normal transitional cell epithelium.[2] These tumors occur in a younger age group than transitional cell carcinomas overall. Recurrences are common (up to 70%), and ultimate development of a change in the character of the lesion and subsequent development of invasive disease has been seen in up to 7% of patients.[1] When seen during cystoscopy, the mass appears as a delicate papillary structure that virtually floats in the bladder on a fine stalk.

INVERTED PAPILLOMA

Inverted papillomas are estimated to account for less than 1% of urothelial tumors of the urinary bladder and can occur at any age; most patients, however, are middle-aged, with a median age of 55 years.[3] Inverted papillomas are more common in males and most often present with hematuria and/or irritative symptoms, but occasionally they produce obstructive symptoms.[3] Some authors have suggested that these represent genuine neoplasms[4]; others have related their origin to proliferative urothelial lesions such as cystitis glandularis and cystitis cystica.[5] Ultrastructural studies have shown features similar to normal transitional epithelium and the epithelium of low-grade papillary tumors.[6]

At cystoscopy the majority of lesions in the urinary bladder are localized to the trigone. They are characteristically pedunculated or sessile with a smooth surface. Most are small (<3 cm), but lesions of up to 8 cm have been reported.[7] Most reported cases have been single, but occasional multifocal lesions have been described.

Urine cytology is not particularly helpful in establishing the benign nature of the lesion because the findings have been reported in many cases to indicate the presence of "suspicious" or "atypical" features.[3]

Inverted papillomas are usually removed by transurethral resection and the diagnosis is established following histologic review. The natural history of inverted papilloma is benign with only rare examples of recurrence documented.[3] Nevertheless, reports of an association of transitional cell cancer and inverted papilloma have been reported[8]; thus periodic follow-up of resected lesions is indicated.

VILLOUS ADENOMA

A few well-documented examples exist of tumors arising in the urinary bladder that have been histologically identical to villous adenoma of the colon.[9] Similar lesions have more frequently been described in the urachus. The tumors appear cystoscopically as exophytic papillary masses. Histologically, the lesions have an exophytic, papillary architecture, with the fronds covered by columnar mucus-secreting epithelium with goblet cells. No recurrences have developed in any of the reported cases.

The differential diagnosis in such cases includes florid cystitis glandularis (polypoid cystitis glandularis) and well-differentiated adenocarcinoma.

MESENCHYMAL NEOPLASMS

Benign mesenchymal neoplasms are uncommon in the urinary bladder with the vast majority represented by leiomyomas (estimated to be 35%[10]), hemangiomas, and neurofibromas. Benign mesenchymal tumors account for only 0.9% of primary bladder lesions. Rare examples of a variety of other benign mesenchymal tumors can be found in the literature, including granular cell tumors, lymphangioma, benign fibrous histiocytoma, and ganglioneuroma.

NEPHROGENIC ADENOMA

Nephrogenic adenoma is an infrequent, glandular-appearing lesion whose histologic appearance is similar to primitive renal collecting tubules.[11] Most authorities consider it to be metaplastic rather than neoplastic. It is more common in males and is thought to arise from metaplasia secondary to chronic inflammation or infection. Although it may have an infiltrative character and may recur following resection, the lesion does not metastasize and is considered benign.

Malignant Tumors of the Bladder

More than 95% of all bladder malignancies are epithelial in origin. The three basic types of carcinoma are transitional cell carcinoma (TCC), squamous cell carcinoma, and adenocarcinoma. At times, mixed-histology tumors may be present, and occasionally it may be problematic to identify the original histologic derivation. Carcinoid tumors, small cell carcinoma, malignant lymphoma, plasmacytoma, germ cell tumor, carcinosarcoma, and melanoma are very rare primary lesions of the bladder. The remainder of the tumors may have mesodermal origins or are metastatic lesions.

ETIOLOGY AND PATHOGENESIS

A broad knowledge of the etiologic agents contributing to the development of bladder cancer is helpful in anticipating the correct diagnosis. The exact mechanism of carcinogenesis remains uncertain in most cases, although new data regarding the role of cytogenetics, oncogenes, and suppressor genes are opening up new understanding of possible mechanims.

It has been estimated that one-third of all bladder cancer cases are related to tobacco smoke exposure.[12] Cigarette smokers have been shown to have a two- to fourfold increase in bladder cancer risk when compared to nonsmokers.[13] Although nitrosamines and 2-naphthylamine, known bladder carcinogens, are present in cigarette smoke, the exact pathogenesis of the increased risk in tobacco smokers remains unknown. Histologic studies on the bladders of smokers and nonsmokers have shown increased numbers of atypical cells and increased thickness of the basal layer in smokers.[14]

Occupational exposure is thought to account for another third of bladder cancer cases in North America. Workers in the dye industry who are exposed to benzidine (4,4-diaminobiphenyl) and 2-naphthylamine (aromatic amines) have 10 to 50 times higher death rates from bladder cancer than the unexposed population. Others linked to bladder cancer are auto workers, railway workers, metal machine workers, drill press operators, electrical and electronics workers, plumbers, painters, truck drivers, leather workers, rubber workers, and others.[15,16]

The data linking analgesic use to bladder cancer are not as strong as those for renal pelvis tumors, but a weak association does exist between phenacetin use and bladder cancer. The risk becomes significant only when high total doses in the 2000-g range are reached.[17]

Numerous reports have appeared in the literature regarding the role of cyclophosphamide in bladder cancer. A cumulative risk of 10.7% at 12 years has been reported, with a latency period of 65 to 141 months.[18] The development of bladder cancer is believed to be due to the accumulation of acrolein, a degradation product of cyclophosphamide. Although the majority of reported tumors have been transitional cell carcinomas, examples of squamous cell carcinoma, adenocarcinoma, and leiomyosarcoma have been described.

The development of bladder carcinomas has been reported in patients with prior exposure to radiation therapy. The risk of transitional cell carcinoma has been reported to be increased two- to fourfold in women previously treated with radiation therapy for cervical carcinoma.[19] The time interval between radiation exposure and development of bladder cancer may be as long as 20.5 years.[19] Most patients present with high-grade, advanced disease without a prior history of superficial disease. In addition to transitional cell carcinoma, examples of adenocarcinoma and primary bladder sarcoma have been described in patients with prior histories of radiation exposure.[19]

Some studies have suggested an increased risk of bladder cancer in coffee and tea drinkers,[20] but the relationship is weak.

Human papilloma virus infection, which has been implicated as an important factor in tumors of the anogenital region and upper respiratory tract, has been considered in bladder cancer, with conflicting results. Using in situ DNA hybridization and polymerase chain reaction, Kerley and coworkers[21] found HPV DNA in only one of 27 bladder cancers studied. In contrast, Anwar and colleagues[22] found evidence of HPV DNA in 81% of carcinomas studied (39 of 48). Until more consistent evidence becomes available, the significance of HPV in bladder carcinogenesis remains uncertain.

Patients with recurrent infections, infected diverticula, pyocystis in a diverted bladder, and long-standing indwelling catheters are at an increased risk for the development of bladder cancer. It is also more common to see the less frequently found tumor types in this population, such as adenocarcinomas and squamous cell cancer.

The incidence of squamous cell cancer of the bladder is rare in Western countries; however, it is the most frequently encountered histology in regions of the world where *Schistosoma haematobium* is endemic.

Molecular cytogenetic studies utilizing a variety of techniques have provided considerable insight into potential tumor suppressor gene involvement in bladder cancer. Commonly reported numerical abnormalities have included loss of chromosome 9 and trisomy of chromosome 7.[23] Loss of the Y chromosome has been another frequent finding and can be correlated with a worse outcome.[23] A deletion on the long arm of chromosome 9 (9q-) has been reported in up to 50% of all transitional cell carcinomas independent of stage and grade.[23,24] These results indicate that a tumor suppressor gene may be located at this site, which is critical in the development of transitional cell carcinoma. It has been suggested that this is an early event, and it may be the first cytogenetic event in this process.[23] Other frequently reported structural alterations have involved chromosomes 1 and 5.[23] Fluorescence in situ hybridization studies have demonstrated abnormalities of chromosomes 1, 7, 9, 11, 15, and 17.[23] These have proven particularly valuable in evaluating low-grade papillary tumors.

Loss-of-heterozygosity studies have revealed loss of material on chromosomes 1p, 1q, 3p, 5q, 6q, 9q, 11p, 13q, 17p, and 18q.[23,24] Involvement of 13q and 17p implicates the retinoblastoma and p53 suppressor genes in bladder cancer.

Despite reports of a few familial clusters of cases there is little evidence to suggest that significant numbers of bladder cancers are related to heredity.[25] The possibility that some or all such occurrences reflect some common environmental exposure is difficult to exclude.

Pathology of Malignant Lesions

TRANSITIONAL CELL CANCER

Most patients with bladder cancer are between 50 and 80 years of age and are male by a ratio of 3 or 4 to 1. Eighty percent of the lesions are superficial at initial presentation. The clinical and pathologic staging of bladder cancer is critical in the process of therapeutic decision making. Traditionally, bladder cancers have been divided clinically into "superficial" and "invasive" disease. The superficial group includes all tumors that have not invaded into the muscularis propria of the bladder (stages Ta, TIS, and T1). However, tumors invading the lamina propria (T1) demonstrate a biological potential different from, and less favorable than, tumors not penetrating the basement membrane. Invasive tumors include those that have extended to involve the muscularis propria or deeper (T2, T3, and T4).

The fundamental goal of local staging is to determine whether muscularis propria invasion has or has not occurred. This is the single most important piece of information for therapeutic decision making. The most useful test in this determination is a transurethral resection of the tumor (TURBT) with histologic assessment for the presence or absence of muscle invasion. The bimanual examination performed at the time of cystoscopy is also helpful in that palpable tumors are almost always muscle invasive. Various imaging modalities (computed tomography, magnetic resonance imaging, and ultrasound) may be of value as adjuncts, but for the most part they are not particularly sensitive in detecting early muscle invasion.

For patients with muscle-invasive disease, the extent of the disease then becomes important in therapeutic decision making. Local extension beyond the confines of the urinary bladder may result in unresectability, and so imaging studies aimed at documenting local extension into perivesical soft tissues or adjacent organs are frequently performed.

Also of importance is the use of biopsies and transurethral resections of the prostate gland to document the degree of involvement, if any, of this organ.[26] Several studies have documented the relatively high rate of involvement of the prostate gland by transitional cell carcinoma in selected subgroups of patients. In patients with muscle-invasive bladder cancer, the frequency of involvement of the prostate gland approaches 50%.[27] This is particularly true in patients who have multifocal carcinoma in situ associated with the invasive tumor.

More recently, authors have suggested that the degree of prostate involvement should be considered in assigning a stage to such patients: (1) tumors confined to the prostatic urothelial lining, (2) tumors extending into ducts and acini but confined by the basement membrane, and (3) tumors with stromal invasion. This may have significant therapeutic and prognostic implications. The presence of stromal invasion indicates a need for aggressive therapy; therefore the presence or absence of this feature needs to be documented pathologically in all such specimens. Patients with stromal invasion in the prostate gland have a much higher likelihood of developing metastatic disease than patients whose prostatic involvement is in situ only. The presence of extensive prostatic urethral involvement also indicates a group of patients at high risk for urethral recurrence, and some authors recommend urethrectomy at the time of cystoprostatectomy for these patients.[28]

Finally, the evaluation of regional or distant metastases is important in guiding therapy. Of greatest interest is the assessment of regional lymph node status. Various imaging modalities are available for this (computed tomography, magnetic resonance imaging, ultrasound, and lymphangiography), but ultimately, pelvic lymphadenectomy remains the most accurate. Computed tomography is the most widely used imaging tool for this purpose, and in patients with gross ("incurable") nodal involvement fine-needle aspiration has a role to play in confirming the presence of tumor. In most cases, however, the node dissection is performed at the time of cystectomy. Evidence in the literature suggests that at least some patients with limited nodal disease may be cured by the lymph node dissection.[29]

Carcinoma in situ (CIS) may be associated with existing papillary or sessile tumors or can occur independent of other transitional cell tumors. The typical presentation is with dysuria, pain (perineal, penile, suprapubic), frequency, hematuria, or sterile pyuria; occasionally, they may be asymptomatic. In some cases the clinical presentation can mimic that of interstitial cystitis. This is extremely significant; in the Mayo Clinic experience, 23% of men initially considered to have interstitial cystitis were found to have CIS (in contrast to 1.3% of women).[30] In most cases the disease is multifocal. Cystoscopically, the bladder mucosa is characteristically red and velvety, although it may appear essentially normal.

In random bladder biopsies from patients with synchronous bladder tumors or taken during follow-up of bladder cancer patients, the recognition of a denuded pattern is extremely important. It is insufficient for the pathologist simply to sign out such a biopsy as "negative" without first obtaining levels on the biopsy and second indicating in the report that the surface epithelium is completely absent. Recuts may well demonstrate involvement of Brunns nests or foci of preserved surface epithelium in such cases. Correlation with urine cytology results can be extremely helpful, with positive cytology in most cases having this growth pattern.

Studies of blood group antigen expression in CIS have shown loss of normal A, B, and H antigens in CIS.[31] In one report CEA immunostaining was frequently found in CIS, in contrast to normal urothelium, where it was absent.[31] DNA ploidy studies by both image analysis and flow cytometry have demonstrated a high frequency of aneuploidy.[32]

Numerous studies have confirmed the high risk of progression for CIS with development of invasive disease in as many as 83% of cases.[31,33] Observations in the cystectomy specimens of patients with carcinoma in situ only have revealed foci of microinvasion in 34% of bladders and muscle-invasive disease in up to 9%.[34] Five-year survival for patients with CIS treated by radical surgery has ranged from 85 to 100%.[33,34]

Papillary tumors are characterized by an exophytic growth pattern. The tumors can be single or multiple and range from small, fingerlike projections to larger, complex lesions resulting in a nearly solid appearance. In most series approximately two-thirds are single and one-third are multiple at the time of presentation. The documentation of single versus multiple tumors is significant as patients with multiple tumors have a higher risk of recurrence and progression. Tumors arise most often on the lateral and posterior walls and least often on the dome.[35]

Nonpapillary transitional cell carcinomas show a range of gross appearances from polypoid to sessile to ulcerated and infiltrative. In some cases the polypoid or sessile growth patterns can be associated with a stalk. A discrete polypoid pattern is characteristic of the sarcomatoid variant. On sectioning, the tumors tend to be solid, gray-white and infiltrative.

Tumors in the urinary bladder having both a malignant epithelial and a malignant spindle cell component have been called carcinosarcoma or sarcomatoid carcinoma. These tumors affect males more frequently than females (by a ratio of 2 or 3 to 1) and tend to occur in an older age group (seventh and eighth decades), with only rare examples described in patients under the age of 50 years. The most frequent presentation is hematuria, although irritative and obstructive symptoms can occur.

Sarcomatoid transitional cancers are usually exophytic and often have a polypoid and/or pedunculated growth pattern. Occasionally, a sessile pattern is evident. Most are large, with cases of up to 12 cm reported. Histologically, the tumors are characterized by a mixture of carcinoma with a malignant spindle cell component. In most cases the spindle cell element has been found to express cytokeratin[36] at least focally. Other epithelial markers such as epithelial membrane antigen may also be expressed, although less consistently.[37] Coexpression of vimentin in the spindle cell component has been found by most.[36,37] Occasionally, the spindle cells have expressed muscle-specific actin, but studied cases have been negative for desmin.[37]

Prognostic Markers

DNA Content (Ploidy). Extensive work has been done to evaluate the value and significance of DNA content analysis in transitional cell carcinomas. In general, studies of tumor tissue have consistently demonstrated a strong correlation between the presence of DNA aneuploidy and high-grade and advanced stage.[38] One exception to the latter is transitional cell carcinoma in situ, which has been found to be DNA aneuploid in up to 100% of cases. The correlation with grade has been particularly striking in papillary transitional cell carcinoma. Blomjous et al[39] detected DNA aneuploidy in no instances of grade 1, 61% of grade 2, and 100% of grade 3 tumors. They also found the frequency of aneuploidy to increase from 14% in stage Ta lesions to 83% in muscle-invasive (stages T2 to T4) tumors.

DNA ploidy has repeatedly been shown to be a significant prognostic indicator for transitional cell carcinomas in general.[38,39] For noninvasive (Ta) and invasive tumors not involving the muscularis propria (T1) treated conservatively, DNA content is a powerful indicator of the potential for recurrence and progression.[39] Because 73 to 97% of muscle-invasive tumors are DNA aneuploid, DNA content is of less value as a prognostic marker for this group of patients.[40]

More recently, studies have suggested that the presence of a DNA aneuploid population predicts for a better response to radiation therapy[40] or to combined radiation therapy and chemotherapy in the setting of bladder preservation.

Cellular Proliferation. Assessment of cellular proliferation in transitional cell carcinoma has been performed with many different methodologies, including mitoses counting, flow cytometry (S-phase fraction), proliferating cell nuclear antigen (PCNA), Ki-67, and bromodeoxyuridine. For the most part these studies have shown a positive correlation between increased proliferation and higher grade and stage. In studies with outcome data, a positive correlation with prognosis has also been demonstrated.[38]

Morphometry. A large body of literature exists in relation to nuclear morphometric studies of transitional cell carcinoma. Many investigators have used measurements of nuclear size, nuclear area, and others to improve on the subjective grading of these tumors.[41] Others have assessed the prognostic significance of these indices.[42]

Basement Membrane Status. Several studies have evaluated the importance of basement membrane in bladder cancer.[43] These have utilized immunohistochemistry and antibodies directed against type IV collagen and laminin. Interestingly, these have shown that in some cases of invasive transitional cell carcinoma, an intact basement membrane surrounds the invasive tumor nests, whereas in others this is completely absent. The pattern of basement membrane staining has been shown to correlate with survival. The 5-year survival for patients with tumors having intact basement membranes is 61% compared to 32% for those with patchy or absent staining.[43]

Blood Group Antigens. Normal transitional epithelium expresses A, B, and precursor H antigens, as well as the related M, N, T, and Lewis antigens. Loss of blood group antigen staining correlates with histologic grade and may indicate an increased risk for progression. This technique has not gained widespread acceptance in clinical practice.

Other Antigens. Both class I and class II HLA antigens have been shown to be expressed by some invasive transitional cell carcinomas.[44] An inverse correlation between class I HLA antigen expression and stage and survival has been reported recently. Patients with HLA class I antigen–positive tumors had a 5-year survival of 74% compared with 36% for patients with negative tumors.

Growth Factors. Expression of the epidermal growth factor receptor has been shown to correlate with the histologic grade and stage of transitional cell carcinomas of the urinary bladder.[45] In lower-stage tumors, positivity for epidermal growth factor receptor (EGFR) has been correlated with recurrence and progression, and in higher-stage tumors, with decreased survival.

Oncogenes. Increased ras oncogene expression has been demonstrated in dysplastic and malignant urothelium.[46] To date, however, no role as a prognostic marker has been delineated.

The HER-2\neu oncogene (c-erB-2) has also been shown to be expressed in a significant proportion of transitional cell carcinomas.[47] This oncogene encodes for a membrane protein that is a receptor related to the epidermal growth factor receptor. Most studies have demonstrated a correlation between c-erB-2 expression and histologic grade and stage and in some stories a correlation with prognosis. In contrast, a recent study found an inverse relationship between c-erB-2 expression and survival.[48] Cases with increased c-erB-2 expression have been found to have increased mRNA expression, although not all cases with increased mRNA expression show increased protein expression.[47]

Suppressor Genes. There is presently tremendous interest in two of the known suppressor genes and their potential role as prognostic indicators in bladder cancer. Mutations of the p53 suppressor gene have been well documented in transitional cell carcinoma.[49] These mutations have been shown to be associated with allelic deletion on chromosome 17p, the site of the p53 suppressor gene.[50] Several groups have demonstrated a positive correlation between p53 abnormalities and tumor stage. Recent studies have also indicated a higher risk for progression of stage pT1 tumors, which harbor p53 mutations.[49]

Loss of the retinoblastoma suppressor gene product has also been demonstrated in bladder cancers.[51] Loss of this suppressor gene is almost exclusively seen in high-grade tumors. Recent reports have shown a significant correlation between loss of retinoblastoma suppressor gene protein expression and decreased survival in patients with transitional cell carcinoma.[52]

Follow-up. Follow-up in these patients is somewhat dependent on the characteristics of the tumor, but most patients are followed with repeat cystoscopies (with urine and bladder wash cytologies and biopsy as indicated) every 3 months for 2 years, decreasing to every 6 months for the next 2 years and yearly thereafter. Up to 5% of patients develop upper tract tumors[53]; therefore upper tract studies are generally recommended on a yearly basis.

SQUAMOUS CELL CARCINOMA

Clinical Features. The proportion of bladder tumors represented by squamous cell carcinoma shows significant geographic variation. In areas of the world where schistosomiasis is endemic, squamous cell carcinoma accounts for up to 73% of all bladder cancers.[54] In contrast, in series from England and the United States, this tumor makes up 3% to

6% of bladder malignancies. Most patients present with hematuria and/or irritative symptoms. Rare cases with associated hypercalcemia have been described. A high proportion of patients have advanced disease at the time of diagnosis.

Etiology and Pathogenesis. Many patients with squamous cell carcinoma have a long-standing history of irritation related to infection, stones, long-term indwelling catheter, or urinary retention. The presence of long-standing keratinizing squamous metaplasia (leukoplakia) has long been recognized as a risk factor for the development of squamous cell carcinoma. A significant number of tumors arising in bladder diverticula are also squamous in type. A small number of tumors arising in bladder exstrophy are squamous cell carcinomas. Tumors of the urachus can also be squamous in type. Squamous cell cancer is the most common bladder cancer in geographic areas where schistosomiasis is endemic.

Schistosome infection is a major worldwide medical problem. Of the three major *Schistosoma* species pathogenetic to humans—*S. mansoni*, *S. japonicum*, and *S. haematobium*—only *haematobium* is associated with bladder cancer. In Egypt, where carcinoma of the urinary bladder is the major oncologic problem, schistosome eggs were identified in the bladder wall in 902 of 1095 squamous cell cancer cases (82%).[54]

Most tumors are bulky, polypoid, solid, necrotic masses, sometimes filling the lumen of the bladder; others are predominantly flat and irregularly bordered. The presence of necrotic material on the surface seems to be relatively constant.

Microscopic Pathology. The tumors range from well differentiated with well-defined islands of squamous cells showing keratin production, prominent intercellular bridges, and minimal nuclear pleomorphism to poorly differentiated tumors with marked nuclear pleomorphism and only focal evidence of squamous differentiation. Squamous metaplasia is identifiable in the adjacent epithelium in 17 to 60% of cases.

Rare examples of tumors showing features of verrucous carcinoma have been described. It should be noted that in a background of schistosomiasis, verrucous carcinoma is not nearly so uncommon, accounting for 3% of bladder cancers in one series.[54] These are characterized by an exophytic, papillary, or "warty" gross appearance; acanthosis and papillomatosis of the epithelium; minimal nuclear or architectural atypia; and rounded, pushing, deep margins. In other locations this histology has been associated with a relatively nonaggressive behavior. Follow-up in the three cases reported in the urinary bladder has shown no recurrence or progression after 3, 24, and 36 months.

Verrucous carcinoma at other sites has been linked to human papillomavirus infection. One of the reported cases in the urinary bladder developed in a background of long-standing anogenital condyloma acuminata, suggesting a possible link with the bladder tumor. Condyloma acuminata are not uncommon in the urinary bladder and have been shown to contain HPV.[55] The role of HPV infection in the development of bladder carcinomas in general remains uncertain, with conflicting studies reported.[21,22]

Survival. Overall the prognosis for patients with these tumors has been poor, with 5-year survival rates ranging from 7.4 to 50%.

The biological behavior of these tumors is different from that of transitional cell carcinoma. In most patients deaths are related to local recurrence rather than to metastatic disease. When metastases do occur, they show a striking predilection for bone involvement.

ADENOCARCINOMA

Primary adenocarcinoma accounts for less than 1% of malignant bladder tumors. Primary adenocarcinoma of the urinary bladder has been divided into two major categories: those arising in the urachus and those developing in the urinary bladder proper.

Urachal Adenocarcinoma

Diagnostic Criteria. The separation of urachal from nonurachal adenocarcinoma remains a clinicopathologic diagnosis. Various criteria for the establishment of a urachal origin have been proposed over the years, including location in the bladder dome, primary involvement of muscle or deeper structures, presence of a suprapelvic mass, tumor growth in the bladder wall extending into the space of Retzius, sharp demarcation between tumor and normal surface epithelium, an intact or ulcerated epithelium, absence of cystitis cystica or glandularis elsewhere in the bladder, and documentation of the presence of urachal remnants.

Clinical Features. Adenocarcinoma of the urachus may be seen over a wide age range, with the youngest case reported in a 15-year-old female.[56] The majority are seen in the fifth and sixth decades of life, with a mean age of 50.6 years. This is approximately 10 years younger than those of nonurachal origin. The male-to-female ratio is 1.8 to 1, a lower ratio than the 2.6 to 1 for nonurachal adenocarcinomas.[57] The most frequent presentation is hematuria (71%), with lesser numbers complaining of pain (42%), irritative symptoms (40%), mucusuria (25%), and umbilical discharge (2%).

Etiology/Pathogenesis. A variety of pathogenetic mechanisms have been suggested as accounting for the propensity of tumors of the urachus to be adenocarcinomas. Most authors generally accept intestinal metaplasia of the urachal epithelium as the origin.

Gross Pathology. Most urachal adenocarcinomas form discrete masses in the dome of the bladder. The tumors appear to have an epicenter in the wall of the bladder, rather than being mucosally based, as is typical for nonurachal tumors. The bladder mucosa may be intact or ulcerated. The cut surface may be solid or, more frequently, may have a glistening, mucoid appearance because of abundant mucus production. In some cases the tumor extends along the urachal tract, and there may be associated tumor within the abdominal wall.

Microscopic Pathology. Urachal adenocarcinomas can show a variety of histologic appearances. Most commonly, the tumors are of a mucinous (colloid) type, with nests and single cells floating in extravasated mucin. Individual cells may have a signet ring morphology or may be more columnar with cytoplasmic mucin. The next most frequent pattern is enteric, with features typical of colorectal adenocarcinomas. These tumors may contain Panethlike cells and argyrophil (neuroendocrine) cells. In one study the reported 5-year survivals were 61 and 31% for urachal and nonurachal tumors, respectively ($p = 0.07$). The 10-year survival for the urachal cases was 46%.[57]

Nonurachal Adenocarcinoma

Clinical Features. Nonurachal adenocarcinomas account for 61 to 80% of primary bladder adenocarcinomas.[57] These tumors can occur over a wide age range, with a mean of 59.4 years. They are more common in males than in females (2.6:1). Hematuria is the most common presentation (88%), followed by irritative symptoms (48%) and, rarely, mucusuria (2%). The tumors are often advanced, with metastatic disease in up to 40% of patients at the time of presentation.[57]

Etiology/Pathogenesis. It has generally been accepted that primary nonurachal adenocarcinomas in most cases arise from metaplasia of the transitional epithelium. Supportive evidence comes from cases shown to arise in patients with long-standing diffuse intestinalization of the bladder mucosa associated with a nonfunctioning bladder, chronic irritation, obstruction, or cystocele. In patients with adenocarcinoma the presence of cystitis glandularis has been reported in 14 to 67% of cases. This is also considered to be the mechanism in patients with exstrophy. Most malignancies arising in association with exstrophy have been adenocarcinomas, although occasional examples of squamous cell carcinoma and transitional cell carcinoma have been described. The risk for development of adenocarcinoma in patients with exstrophy ranges from 4.1 to 7.1%. There is also an increased risk of adenocarcinoma in patients with pelvic lipomatosis, and this too has been attributed to the association with cystitis glandularis. Adenocarcinomas can also arise in association with infection by *Schistosoma haematobium*. Finally, there have been rare examples of adenocarcinoma and adenosarcoma arising in association with endometriosis involving the bladder.

Gross Pathology. Gross features of primary nonurachal adenocarcinomas range from exophytic and papillary to solid and sessile to ulcerating and infiltrative. The signet ring variant frequently shows diffuse thickening of the bladder wall, producing a linitis plastica–like appearance. In this group the mucosa has often shown no involvement by the neoplasm.

Differential Diagnosis. The differential diagnosis of adenocarcinoma is extensive. First, the possibility of a benign condition that is mimicking adenocarcinoma needs to be excluded. In unusual cases extravasation of mucus can be seen, and in these cases careful evaluation for malignant cells is necessary. Patients with long-standing intestinal metaplasia are at risk for the development of adenocarcinoma, and such cases should be carefully evaluated for early evidence of neoplastic transformation. Rare examples of villous adenomas arising in the urinary bladder proper are reported. These show the cytologic and architectural atypia of adenomatous epithelium but lack the stromal invasion of adenocarcinoma. Nephrogenic adenoma also must be considered in the differential diagnosis. These lesions have a mixed papillary and tubular architecture, often associated with the presence of "hobnail" cells. Involvement of the urinary bladder in patients with endometriosis is not rare. The histology is similar to that of endometriosis, with variable amounts of endometrial glands and stroma with hemosiderin-laden macrophages. The diagnosis should not be difficult.

Prognosis. The prognosis for these tumors has generally been considered to be dismal. The overall 5- and 10-year survival rates for the 48 cases of nonurachal adenocarcinoma reported by Grignon et al[57] were 31% and 28%, respectively. These data indicated that most patients dying of this tumor do so in the first 5 years, with late recurrences and death being uncommon. The 5-year survival for patients with stage B disease was 76%, indicating the potential curability of earlier-stage disease.

Small Cell Carcinoma

Clinical Features. Small cell carcinomas, histologically identical to those occurring in the lung, are being reported with increasing frequency.[58] The tumor is estimated to account for about 0.5% of bladder malignancies. It develops much more frequently in men than in women and is a tumor of older patients. Hematuria is by far the most frequent presentation (90% of cases), with symptoms of bladder irritability or obstruction occurring infrequently. Patients frequently present with locally advanced or metastatic disease. Paraneoplastic syndromes—including ectopic ACTH production, hypercalcemia, and hypophosphatemia—have been observed infrequently. At least four cases have been documented to arise in bladder diverticula, and one case has been documented in a patient with prior augmentation cystoplasty.

Pathogenesis. Several theories concerning the histogenesis of these tumors have been presented. The most often cited and currently favored is that these tumors arise from multipotential undifferentiated or stem cells present in the urothelium. The frequent association of this lesion with other histologic variants such as transitional cell carcinoma or adenocarcinoma has been cited as evidence in favor of this theory. A second possibility is that the tumor arises from neuroendocrine cells that can be found in normal or metaplastic urothelium. Finally, the possibility of origin from an as yet undefined population of submucosal neuroendocrine cells has been raised.

Gross Pathology. No specific features separate small cell carcinoma from other carcinomas of the urinary bladder. These tumors have ranged in size from 2-cm polypoid lesions to solid masses of up to 10 cm. They can develop at any location, including the dome and within diverticula. Ulceration of the overlying mucosa has been described in some cases.

Microscopic Pathology. The tumors fulfill the light-microscopic criteria for a diagnosis of small cell carcinoma of the lung. They can show either an oat cell or an intermediate cell pattern, and frequently both are present at the same time. The oat cell type is characterized by a relatively uniform population of cells with scant cytoplasm and hyperchromatic nuclei with dispersed chromatin and absent or inconspicuous nucleoli. The intermediate cell type has more abundant cytoplasm, with larger nuclei having a lesser degree of hyperchromasia but similar chromatin and nucleolar features. In some cases this pattern is associated with a more spindled architectural appearance. Both types show extensive necrosis, prominent nuclear molding, and frequent mitoses.

Between 23 and 67% of cases have been reported to be mixed with other histologic patterns.[59] A transitional cell carcinoma component has been reported most often, but glandular or squamous differentiation has often been observed. One case of small cell carcinoma arose in association with a urachal adenocarcinoma. In at least 11 cases the adjacent urothelium has shown severe dysplasia or transitional cell carcinoma in situ.[59]

In most cases evidence of neuroendocrine differentiation can be found with neuron-specific enolase immunoreactivity. Although most cases are cytokeratin positive, some are nonreactive.

Differential Diagnosis. The major differential diagnoses are small cell carcinoma from another site involving the bladder and malignant lymphoma. Small cell carcinomas histologically identical to those of the bladder may arise in the prostate gland. In about 50% of cases these have an associated adenocarcinoma component; positive staining of this element for prostate specific antigen (PSA) or prostatic acid phosphatase (PAP) would confirm a prostatic origin. The small cell component usually is negative for PSA and PAP in prostatic tumors, and so in pure cases clinical correlation may be essential to resolving this differential. Metastases from other sites also need to be considered. Interestingly, symptomatic bladder metastases from bronchogenic small cell carcinoma is rare, but clinical correlation is necessary to exclude this possibility. The identification of a transitional cell component, including transitional cell carcinoma in situ, would strongly support a primary bladder origin.[59]

The aggressive nature of this tumor has been noted repeatedly in the literature. Overall survival has been poor in reported cases, although recent reports indicate that these tumors may be particularly sensitive to chemotherapy.[59]

Malignant Melanoma. Primary malignant melanoma is a rare tumor of the urinary bladder; 11 cases have been reported to date.[60] These tumors occur more frequently in females (8:3) in the sixth to seventh decades (range 46 to 81 years, median 57 years) and most often present with gross hematuria (64%) followed by metastases (27%). Pathologically, the gross appearance is most often described as dark brown to black, polypoid or fungating, and solid to infiltrating. Some cases had a flat or "macular" appearance. They have been reported in all parts of the bladder, with size ranging from 5 mm to 8 cm. Histologically, all have conformed to the usual appearance of melanoma, with large malignant cells arranged in nests and showing varying amounts of pigment. All cases studied to date by immunohistochemistry have shown positivity for S100 protein and HMB45.[60] The major problem diagnostically with such cases is proving that the lesion is not a metastasis. Metastatic melanoma involves the bladder much more commonly than primary tumors. In a comprehensive review of malignant melanoma of the genitourinary tract, Stein and Kendall[61] noted that between 14 and 22% of patients dying with metastatic melanoma have bladder involvement. The following criteria have been proposed for primary lesions: (1) the clinical history should be negative for a previous skin lesion; (2) careful examination of the entire skin surface, including use of a Woods light to exclude a depigmented area that may represent a regressed melanoma, must be done; (3) comprehensive clinical studies should exclude an ophthalmic or other visceral primary site; (4) the pattern of metastases or recurrence should be consistent with a primary bladder lesion, rather than with disseminated metastatic disease; and (5) atypical melanocytes should be present in the mucosa adjacent to the tumor nodule.[61]

Pheochromocytoma. Nearly 200 cases of bladder pheochromocytomas have been described.[62] Paraganglionic tissue within the wall of the bladder has been described.[63] Paragangliomas occur from childhood to old age and are found equally in males and females. Rare examples in association with neurofibromatosis, intestinal carcinoid, and long-term dialysis have been reported.

Patients characteristically present with symptoms referable to catecholamine excess (tachycardia, hypertension, headaches, fainting, and dizziness). Hematuria is relatively

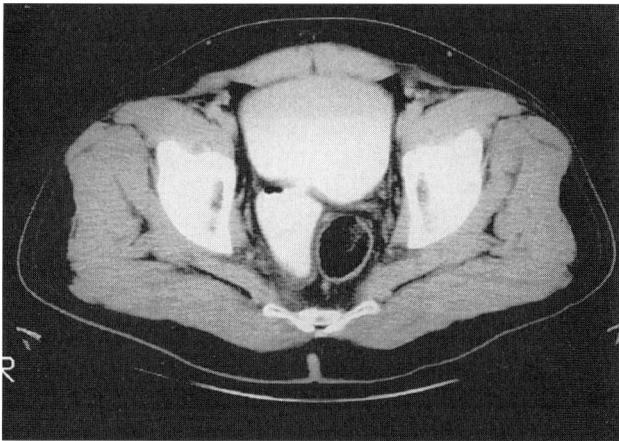

Figure 19–4. Irregularity of posterolateral aspect of large right-sided bladder diverticulum. This proved to be a poorly differentiated transitional cell carcinoma with invasion into perivesical soft tissue.

Mesenchymal tumors appear quite solid, well demarcated and smooth, except in rare instances of ulceration (Fig. 19–6). Stippled calcification in the area of the dome of the bladder on x-ray or CT scan may suggest a urachal carcinoma.[74]

CT scan is also used for evaluating the pelvic lymph nodes. The sensitivity and specificity of the study are 65 and 90%, respectively.[75,76] When enlarged nodes are present a CT-guided needle biopsy may provide histologic confirmation of the clinical diagnosis. In this respect, CT has completely replaced lymphangiography in the detection of metastatic lesion.

MRI. Magnetic resonance imaging may be useful for staging tumors larger than 1 or 2 cm. The intraluminal component of the lesion is depicted as higher intensity than urine on T1-weighted images; however, the invasive component,

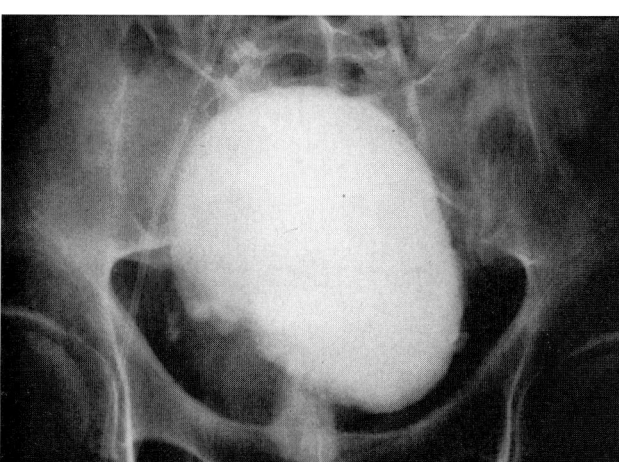

Figure 19–5. Distortion of (R) posterior aspect of bladder secondary to deeply invasive transitional cell carcinoma bladder with associated mass palpable on examination under anesthesia, clinical stage T3b.

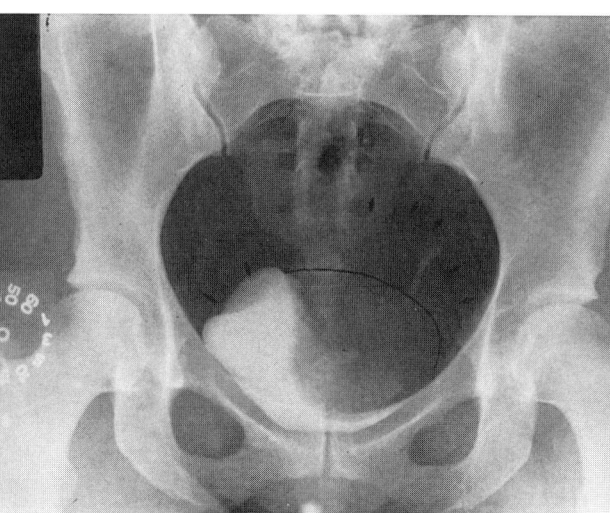

Figure 19–6. Bladder indented by mass in wall of bladder that proved to be leiomyoma. Radiographic appearance indicative only of mural or extramural mass.

if present, is demonstrated as a high-intensity region disrupting the low signal originating from the bladder wall on a T2-weighted image. As noted earlier with CT scan, inflammatory lesions may mimic tumor invasion.[77]

MRI is considered as good or slightly more accurate in the staging of bladder malignancies than CT scan.[77–80] It is more accurate in detecting involvement of the seminal vesicles or the prostate. On the other hand, loops of bowel may be mistaken for adenopathy. Overall, MRI is considered nearly equivalent to CT scan for detecting adenopathy and should be reserved for difficult cases.

MRI is also valuable in the diagnosis of pheochromocytoma. The lesion has a moderate intensity on T1-weighted images and is hyperintense on T2-weighted images. The presence of the lesion may be confirmed with radioiodine-labeled metaiodobenzylguanidine (MIBG) nuclear imaging.

Nuclear Scan. With the advent of the CT scan, liver–spleen scans to evaluate for hepatic metastases are of historical interest only. The use of bone scan to rule out bony metastatic lesions is somewhat controversial. Although bladder cancer does have a propensity for bone metastases and the test may be useful for following future therapy, it is rarely abnormal in the face of normal liver function tests, particularly alkaline phosphatase. Nevertheless, there is at least anecdotal evidence that some patients may develop advanced bony disease despite normal blood test results.

In conclusion, the recommended diagnostic studies for a patient suspected of having a bladder tumor include a thorough history and physical examination, urine cytology, upper tract evaluation with intravenous pyelography or ultrasound/retrograde pyelography, and cystoscopy with possible biopsy of suspicious areas. The metastatic workup for patients with newly diagnosed invasive bladder cancer is a

Tumors of the Lower Urinary Tract 405

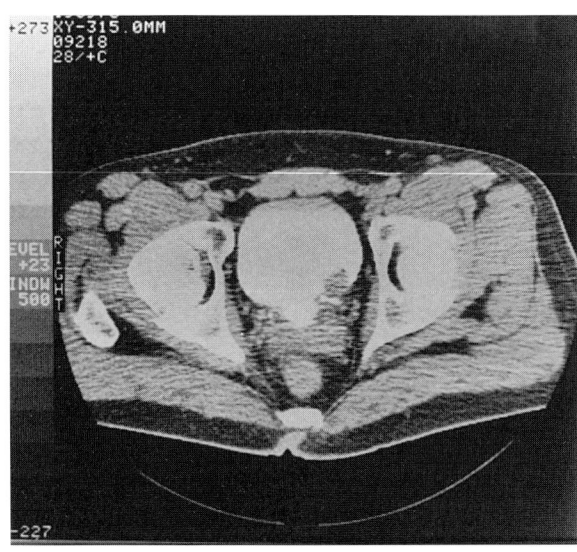

Figure 19–1. (A) IVP demonstrating slight dilation of lower (L) ureter; bowel gas overlying bladder obscures vision of bladder. (B) CT scan of same case shows filling defect in bladder secondary to well-differentiated noninvasive transitional cell carcinoma. This case illustrates (1) partial obstruction (L) ureteral orifice without invasion; (2) limitations of IVP in identification of filling defect in bladder; and (3) unreliability of CT scan to predict pathologic stage. Patient was managed with transurethral resection only.

material. Tumors projecting into the lumen of the bladder may be identified as denser than urine but less dense than the urographic contrast (see Fig. 19–1B). Thickening of the bladder wall is a sign of an infiltrative lesion. However, this evaluation may be misleading after recent resection or extensive biopsy; it is most valuable prior to significant instrumentation (Figs. 19–3, 19–4). CT is not reliable to differentiate superficial muscle invasion from either noninvasive neoplasms or deeply invasive ones, but significant extravesical involvement can be suspected if thickening of the bladder wall, loss of delineation of the outer contour, or infiltration of the perivesical fat plane is seen (Fig. 19–5).

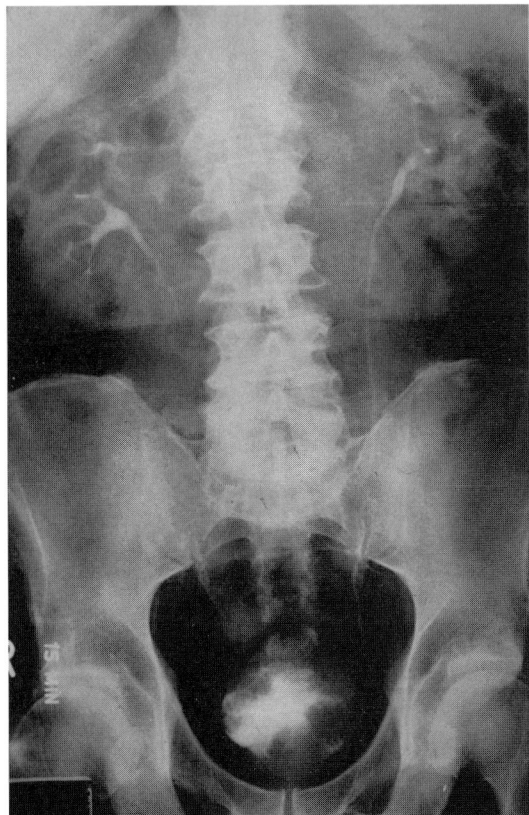

Figure 19–2. Multiple irregular filling defects in bladder secondary to several papillary TCC, all noninvasive.

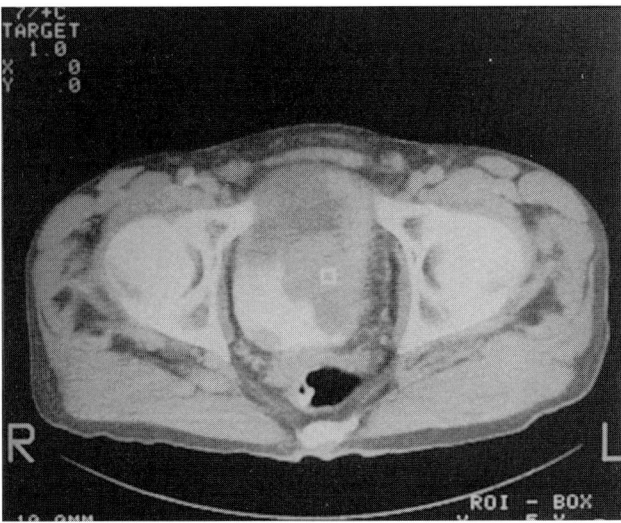

Figure 19–3. Large filling defect on left side of bladder secondary to T1 transitional cell carcinoma bladder. Irregularity of bladder wall and confirmatory evidence of intramural invasion.

the detection of the bladder primary. A thorough history and physical examination, including a bimanual pelvic examination under anesthesia, are integral parts of the patient's evaluation.

Cytology. The cytologic examination of urine (voided, catheterized, and washed) has become an indispensable tool in the management of bladder cancer patients. The major contributions of urine cytology relate to the follow-up and monitoring of therapy response in bladder cancer patients. Although urine cytology has proven to be of value as a diagnostic tool in screening high-risk patient populations,[65–67] its use has not been advocated in more widespread applications.

Cells from well-differentiated tumors are less likely to shed and appear in voided urine specimens. Urine cytology is more sensitive in patients with high-grade tumors; however, the false-negative rate may still be as high as 20%. False-positive findings caused by inflammation or prior therapy occur in 1 to 12% of cases. To avoid cellular degeneration in urine that remained in the bladder for prolonged periods of time, the first voided specimen of the day should not be used. Likewise, osmotic changes resulting from contrast media may cause minor difficulties in interpretation.

Saline bladder washing is more accurate even for low-grade lesions because the cells are mechanically displaced and are better preserved.

An abnormal urine cytology should be followed up by cystoscopy. If no specific lesions can be identified, random bladder biopsies, including the prostatic urethra, should be performed. If, despite a positive cytology report, all biopsy material is negative, the upper urinary tracts should be evaluated by imaging with contrast and selective ureteral cytology. Furthermore, if there is a discrepancy between high-grade malignancy defined by cytology and the visual and/or histologic confirmation of only low-grade tumor(s), random biopsies are indicated because additional areas of carcinoma in situ should be suspected.

Cytology is also a useful way to follow an individual after radical cystectomy whose urethra was not removed. Urethral washing every 3 to 6 months should be analyzed for cytologic abnormalities in the initial postoperative period.

Flow Cytometry. Detection of abnormal DNA content by flow cytometry is an additional tool in the armamentarium of bladder cancer detection. The best results are obtained on bladder barbotage specimens.

Cystoscopy. Cystoscopic evaluation is the primary diagnostic tool in patients suspected of having a bladder tumor. This permits direct visualization of the bladder mucosa and biopsy of suspicious lesions as well as random biopsies of normal mucosa in selected patients. Bladder wash specimens obtained at the time of cystoscopic evaluation also provide useful cytologic material.

The role of random biopsies has evolved over the past several years. Recognition of the importance of identifying associated urothelial dysplasia and carcinoma in situ in patients with "superficial" disease led to recommendations that all patients have random mucosal biopsies. More recently, the low yield in patients with low-grade tumors has led several authors to suggest that random biopsies be restricted to those patients with grade 2 or 3 tumors, or to patients with stage T1 disease.[68]

Cystogram and Excretory Urography. All patients being evaluated for possible bladder tumor require some assessment of the upper tracts. This is important to screen for the presence of upper tract disease as the cause of the presenting symptom (hematuria) and to exclude coexistent upper tract disease in patients with demonstrated urinary bladder cancer. For the diagnosis of the bladder tumor, however, the excretory urograph is not sufficiently sensitive to be a reliable indicator of bladder pathology; however, it is an important tool for ruling out the presence of an upper tract abnormality (Fig. 19–1). The larger the tumor, the more likely it is to show up on the study (Fig. 19–2). Voiding cystograms may demonstrate a bladder-filling defect in larger tumors and aid in localization of involvement.

In patients in whom an intravenous contrast study is contraindicated, renal ultrasonography and retrograde pyeloureterography may accomplish the same goals. The risk to patients who may have allergic reactions can be diminished by the use of new hypoallergenic contrast materials and pretreatment with steroids and benadryl.

Transurethral Ultrasound for Diagnosis and Staging. Transabdominal bladder sonography is commonly available and can detect 80 to 95% of bladder tumors larger than 5 mm but only 33% of smaller lesions.[69–73] Bladder diverticula that may be inaccessible to cystoscopy may be visualized by ultrasound. Appropriate bladder distention is essential for a good-quality study. Bladder tumors appear denser than urine but are slightly hypoechoic when compared with the normal bladder wall. Invasive tumors should be suspected when the hypoechoic mass appears to disrupt the echogenic bladder wall.[73] The differential diagnosis for false-positive findings includes bladder wall trabeculation, inflammatory lesions, blood clots, and less frequently, stones or prostate lesions. Mesenchymal tumors generally appear as more solid masses than mucosal malignancies.

Ultrasound may also suggest the presence of hydronephrosis. The evaluation should include both the distal ureters and the kidneys.

Transurethral ultrasound is most useful for evaluating tumors confined to the bladder wall and is less so for extravesical extension.[69]

CT. Computerized tomography is generally reserved for the staging of known invasive lesions rather than for primary diagnosis. The bladder needs to be distended by contrast

common, and the combination of paroxysmal hypertension with painless hematuria at the time of micturition is practically pathognomonic. Diagnosis is usually confirmed by measurements of catecholamines and their metabolites in urine and serum. 131I-MIBG scintigraphy may confirm the suspected lesion in the urinary bladder.

Grossly, the tumors are located intramurally. There is an apparent predilection for the trigone and anterior wall or dome.[62] The overlying mucosa may be intact or ulcerated and are usually well circumscribed, lobulated, and pink to yellow-brown. Size ranges from 0.2 to 15 cm, with two-thirds being less than 4 cm.

Histologically, the tumor is composed of cells arranged in discrete nests separated by a prominent sinusoidal vascular network. Individual cells have abundant pale eosinophilic to clear cytoplasm with central nuclei. Nuclei tend to have finely distributed chromatin but may show considerable variation in size, with nuclear atypia present to some degree in most cases. Mitoses are generally infrequent, and necrosis is not prominent.

The most useful immunohistochemical studies of bladder paraganglioma are the consistent lack of immunoreactivity for cytokeratin and the positive reaction to neuroendocrine markers.

Malignant Mesenchymal Tumors. Primary sarcomas of the urinary bladder are uncommon tumors that show a distinctive age distribution in terms of the types of tumors seen. Rhabdomyosarcoma is the most frequent tumor of the bladder in childhood; leiomyosarcoma is the most frequent in adults.

Rhabdomyosarcoma accounts for between 4 and 8% of all malignant tumors in children below the age of 15 years.[64] Only rare examples have been described in adult patients. Not all malignant neoplasms of the bladder in children are rhabdomyosarcomas, however. Examples of other sarcoma types and a variety of epithelial tumors have also been described. Rhabdomyosarcoma occurs more frequently in males (3:2), with most developing before 5 years of age. They most often present because of hematuria or bladder neck obstruction. Cystoscopically, the characteristic finding is of a polypoid mass filling the lumen. Grossly, these tumors are characteristically polypoid masses and may be single or multiple, producing the ''sarcoma botryoides'' appearance. The trigone is the preferred location.

Histologically, most are embryonal in type, with a diffuse infiltration of small, blue, round cells with scant cytoplasm. In the sarcoma botryoides type, the cells are more scattered in a loose myxoid stroma with a compact collection of rhabdomyoblasts beneath the surface epithelium. Although rare rhabdoid or strap cells containing cross striations may be found, most cases require immunohistochemistry or electron-microscopic examination to confirm the diagnosis.

Leiomyosarcoma is the most common malignant mesenchymal tumor of the bladder in adults, with 64 well-documented cases published in the English literature. There has been a wide age range (7 to 81 years), with a mean age of 52 years. Nine of the cases occurred in patients under the age of 21 years. Several cases have been reported following cyclophosphamide therapy. The most common presentation has been hematuria followed by obstructive symptoms.

Grossly, the tumors are most often lobulated or polypoid and may be ulcerated. A ''mushroom shape'' at cystoscopy has been said to be typical. Most tumors are in the 2- to 5-cm range, but masses up to 13 cm have been described.

Histologically, most have the typical appearance of leiomyosarcoma, with interweaving fascicles of spindle-shaped cells having long, blunt-ended nuclei and eosinophilic cytoplasm. Nuclear pleomorphism is variable, as is the mitotic rate. Necrosis may be present. In a few cases a myxoid histology has predominated; an epithelioid histology also has been described.

Other rare mesenchymal tumors that have been reported include malignant fibrous histiocytoma, primary osteosarcoma, fibrosarcoma, angiosarcoma, hemangiopericytoma, liposarcoma, rhabdoid tumor, and lymphoreticular tumors such as malignant lymphoma, plasmacytoma, or leukemia.

Metastatic Tumors. Most secondary tumors involving the bladder result from direct invasion from malignancies in adjacent structures; the rest are metastases from distant organs. Malignant melanoma (38%) and tumors of the stomach (23%), breast (11%), kidney (10%), and lung (8%) are the most common sources of metastases.

Symptoms related to the urinary bladder usually develop late in the course of known progressive disease; however, cases have been reported where the bladder finding was the first evidence of a metastatic tumor. In one case of breast cancer the urinary bladder was the only site of metastasis. In rare examples of malignant melanoma to the bladder, sufficient melanoma pigment was released to darken the urine.

Metastasis should be suspected in any case of a bladder tumor where the histology is nonurothelial. In cases of pure adenocarcinoma or squamous cell carcinoma, clinical correlation is necessary to exclude the possibility of secondary involvement. In squamous carcinoma the finding of keratinizing squamous dysplasia in the adjacent epithelium would support a bladder primary. Most cases of secondary involvement by prostatic adenocarcinoma can be readily recognized by the distinctive histology of the tumor and the impression confirmed with immunohistochemistry. Involvement by malignant melanoma is almost always secondary, although rare examples of primary melanoma at this site do occur.

DIAGNOSIS OF BLADDER TUMORS

By far the most common presenting symptom of bladder cancer is painless hematuria, present in 70 to 90% of patients. Irritative symptoms, including frequency, urgency, and dysuria, may be seen in up to 20% of cases. Less frequently, patients complain of flank pain secondary to ureteral obstruction, lower-extremity edema caused by lymphatic obstruction, or symptoms related to pelvic mass. Rarely, patients may present with metastatic disease prior to

BENIGN AND MALIGNANT TUMORS OF THE URETHRA

Urethral Cancer in the Male

Unlike most other genitourinary malignancies, urethral cancer is more common among females than among males. The most common presenting symptoms in men are signs of bladder outlet obstruction, and the condition may present as stricture disease. Urethral discharge, bleeding, and a palpable mass are other frequent findings. The etiology of urethral carcinoma is uncertain; however, a large number of cases are associated with long-standing, chronic irritation, such as recurrent stricture disease, fistulas, and abscesses. Human papilloma virus infection has also been considered as a possible etiologic agent for the development of urethral cancer.

Most male urethral cancers arise in the bulbomembranous urethra; the next most common site is the penile urethra. These lesions generally have squamous cell histology. Approximately 7% of urethral tumors arise in the prostatic urethra, have a transitional cell histology, and are associated with transitional cell cancer of the bladder. Bleeding is the most common presentation of prostatic urethral cancer. Six percent of the lesions are adenocarcinomas located in the prostatic and bulbomembranous segments and are thought to originate from periurethral glands.

Evaluation should include a thorough physical examination of the penis, perineum, and inguinal lymph nodes. Retrograde urethrogram may demonstrate an elongated, irregular urethral stricture typical of the appearance of carcinoma. Cystoscopy and biopsy are essential for diagnosis. Urinary cytology may be helpful, particularly with transitional cell cancer of the prostatic urethra. If this diagnosis is made, complete evaluation of the bladder, including random biopsies, should be performed. Staging studies should also include computerized tomography of the inguinal and pelvic nodal areas, chest x-ray, and bone scan in advanced cases. Unlike penile cancer, enlarged inguinal nodes associated with diagnosed urethral cancer usually signify metastatic disease rather than infection; thus they should be biopsied. We have had good success with aspiration cytology of enlarged lymph nodes.

Miscellaneous Benign Lesions

Condyloma acuminata is a sexually transmitted disease resulting from papilloma virus infection. When present in the urethra, the lesion may mimic a urethral tumor, although its fleshy, wartlike appearance should alert the urologist to the diagnosis. The condition is most likely to involve the urethral meatus, followed by the distal urethra. More proximal lesions and bladder involvement are rare. The diagnosis is made by evaluating the biopsy specimen following urethroscopy, with the pathologist looking for typical koilocytotic changes. These may also be present on urine cytology. It should be kept in mind that the male urethra may be a common reservoir for human papilloma virus, even in the absence of visible lesions.

Polyps of the urethra are benign mucosal lesions that cannot be distinguished from low-grade malignancy on visual evaluation; however, they lack the histologic criteria for cancer. They may present with a symptomatology similar to that of urethral cancer, or they may be incidental findings obtained during the workup of other urinary tract disorders.

Urethral diverticula are neither tumors nor evidence of malignancy; however, they may present as a palpable mass in both the male and the female. Thus they should be considered in the differential diagnosis. The lesions consist of epithelium-lined pouches that communicate with the urethral lumen by a narrow neck. They may be congenital in young patients; however, in the adult, they are thought to be the consequence of chronic inflammation, infection, and obstruction of the periurethral glands. Some may be large and harbor infection, stones, and even urethral cancer. Urethral pain and symptoms of irritation, such as frequency, urgency, dysuria, and incontinence, may be presenting signs. A palpable mass or obstructive symptoms characterizes the larger diverticula. The presence of chronic infection after the rest of the urinary tract has been ruled out as a source should also raise the possibility of the diagnosis. Physical examination should include thorough palpation of the urethra. Cystoscopy is often negative when the diverticulum is collapsed; however, simultaneous palpation of the mass may demonstrate the opening. A urethrogram with a double balloon catheter that occludes both the bladder neck and external meatus, thereby raising the intraurethral pressure, may be very useful. Other methods that may be helpful include the voiding urethrograph and urethral ultrasound (transvaginal in the female).

Urethral Cancer in the Female

The female urethra is lined by transitional epithelium in its proximal one-third and by squamous epithelium in the distal two-thirds. Consequently, tumors arising in the proximal third tend to be transitional cell cancers; in the distal part they are usually squamous cell cancers. Most of the transitional cell cancers are associated with similar malignancy in the bladder; however, occasionally primary lesions may arise. Adenocarcinomas may also arise from the proximal portion, another very rare event.

The pathogenesis of urethral cancer in the female varies according to the histology of the lesion. Transitional cell cancers are thought to result from a cause similar to that of bladder cancer. Squamous cell cancers most likely result from chronic irritation. There is an increased association of the condition with urethral diverticula, and urinary stasis is thought to be responsible for the increase in frequency.

Hematuria or the appearance of blood on the tissue paper used to clean the perineum following voiding may be the first sign of an abnormality. Symptoms of urgency often accompany proximal urethral tumors, and advanced cases may present with obstructive findings. Many of the symptoms are nonspecific and relate to chronic inflammation.

Physical examination may reveal the presence of a palpable mass. A bimanual examination is mandatory and careful attention should be directed at the inguinal nodes. Cystoscopy and biopsy of the lesion should lead to the definitive diagnosis. Staging workup is similar to that performed in males.

Urethral Caruncle

Urethral caruncle is a benign lesion present exclusively in the distal female urethra. The tumors have a round, reddish, fleshy appearance and generally originate from the posterior surface of the urethral meatus. They are usually less than 0.5 cm in size but may have an irregular surface, inflamed or even ulcerated. They are most common in postmenopausal women and may be incidental to atrophy of the surrounding vaginal mucosa. An association has also been made with chronic irritation and infection; however, these conditions may also be related to a lack of sufficient estrogen in postmenopausal patients. Although some patients may present with spotting, discomfort, or obstructive symptoms, most cases are completely asymptomatic and are diagnosed on routine pelvic examination.

Evaluation of urethral caruncles should include thorough visual inspection, bimanual examination, and cystoscopy. Suspicious lesions should be biopsied. The major concern is to rule out the presence of urethral carcinoma. The differential diagnosis also includes several other benign conditions, such as condylomas, hemangiomas, or urethral prolapse.

REFERENCES

1. Deming CL: The biological behavior of transitional cell papilloma of the bladder. *J Urol* 1950;63:815–820.
2. Koss LG: *Tumors of the Urinary Bladder.* Washington, DC: Armed Forces Institute of Pathology, 1974; 1–115.
3. Caro DJ, Tessler A: Inverted papilloma of the bladder: a distinct urologic lesion. *Cancer* 1978;42:708–713.
4. Cameron KM, Lupton CH: Inverted papilloma of the lower urinary tract. *Br J Urol* 1976;48:567–577.
5. Kunze E, Schauer A, Schmitt M: Histology and histogenesis of two different types of inverted urothelial papillomas. *Cancer* 1983;51:348–358.
6. Alroy J, Miller AW III, John S, James KK, Gould VE: Inverted papilloma of the urinary bladder. *Cancer* 1980;46:64–70.
7. Tannenbaum M: Inverted papilloma: urothelial tumor of benign biological potential. *Urology* 1976;7:76–79.
8. Renfer LG, Kelley L, Belville WD: Inverted papilloma of the urinary tract: histogenesis, recurrence and associated malignancy. *J Urol* 1988;140:832–834.
9. Channer JL, Williams JL, Henry L: Villous adenoma of the bladder. *J Clin Pathol* 1993;46:450–452.
10. Jacobs MA, Bavendam TG, Leach GE: Bladder leiomyoma. *Urology* 1989;34:56–57.
11. Ford TF, Watson GM, Cameron KM: Adenomatous metaplasia (nephrogenic adenoma) of urothelium: an analysis of 70 cases. *Br J Urol* 1985;57:427–433.
12. Howe GR, Burch JD, Miller AB, et al: Tobacco use, occupation, coffee, various nutrients, and bladder cancer. *J Natl Cancer Inst* 1980;64:701.
13. Clavel J, Cordier S, Boccon-Gibod L, et al: Tobacco and bladder cancer in males: increased risk for inhalers and smokers of black tobacco. *Int J Cancer* 1989;44:605.
14. Auerbach O, Garfinkel L: Histologic changes in the urinary bladder in relation to cigarette smoking and use of artificial sweeteners. *Cancer* 1989;64:983–987.
15. Silverman DT, Levin LI, Hoover RN, et al: Occupational risks of bladder cancer in the United States. I. White men. *J Natl Cancer Inst* 1989;81:1472.
16. Silverman DT, Levin LI, Hoover RN, et al: Occupational risks of bladder cancer in the United States. II. Nonwhite men. *J Natl Cancer Inst* 1989;81:1480.
17. Fokkens W: Phenacetin abuse related to bladder cancer. *Environ Res* 1979;20:192–198.
18. Pedersen-Bjergaard J, Ersbøll J, Hansen VL, et al: Carcinoma of the urinary bladder after treatment with cyclophosphamide for non-Hodgkin's lymphoma. *N Engl J Med* 1988;318:1028–1032.
19. Sella A, Dexeus FH, Chong C, Ro JY, Logothetis CJ: Radiation therapy-associated invasive bladder tumors. *Urology* 1989;33:185–188.
20. Ciccone G, Vineis P: Coffee drinking and bladder cancer. *Cancer Lett* 1988;41:45.
21. Kerley SW, Persons DL, Fishback JL: Human papillomavirus and carcinoma of the urinary bladder. *Modern Pathol* 1991;4:316–319.
22. Anwar K, Naiki H, Nakakuki K, Inuzuka M: High frequency of human papillomavirus infection in carcinoma of the urinary bladder. *Cancer* 1992;70:1967–1973.
23. Sandberg AA, Berger CS: Review of chromosome studies in urological tumors. II. Cytogenetics and molecular genetics of bladder cancer. *J Urol* 1994;151:545–560.
24. Knowles MA, Elder PA, Williamson M, Cairns JP, Shaw ME, Law MG: Allelotype of human bladder cancer. *Cancer Res* 1994;54:531–538.
25. McCullough DL, Lamm DL, McLaughlin AP III: Familial transitional cell carcinoma of the bladder. *J Urol* 1975;113:629.
26. Rikken CHM, van Helsdingen PJRO, Kazzaz BA: Are biopsies from the prostatic urethra useful in patients with superficial bladder carcinoma? *Br J Urol* 1987;59:145–147.
27. Wood DP Jr, Montie JE, Pontes JE, Medendorp VS, Levin HS: Transitional cell carcinoma of the prostate in cystoprostatectomy specimens removed for bladder cancer. *J Urol* 1989;141:346–349.
28. Richie JP, Skinner DG: Carcinoma in situ of the urethra associated with bladder carcinoma: the role of urethrectomy. *J Urol* 1978;119:80–81.
29. Skinner DG: Management of invasive bladder cancer: a meticulous pelvic node dissection can make a difference. *J Urol* 1982;128:34–36.
30. Young RH, Wick MR: Transitional cell carcinoma of the urinary bladder with pseudosarcomatous stroma. *Am J Clin Pathol* 1989;90:96–99.

31. Sanchez-Fernandez de Sevilla C, Quadreny M, Salom G, Bacete P, Bosch L: Morphometric and immunohistochemical characterization of bladder carcinoma in situ and its preneoplastic lesions. *Eur Urol* 1992;21:5–9.
32. Norming U, Tribukait B, Gustafson H, Nyman CR, Wang N, Wijkström H: Deoxyribonucleic acid profile and tumor progression in primary carcinoma in situ of the bladder: a study of 63 patients with grade 3 lesions. *J Urol* 1992;147:11–15.
33. Malkowicz SB, Nichols P, Lieskovsky G, Boyd SD, Huffman J, Skinner DG: The role of cystectomy in the management of high grade superficial bladder cancer (PA, P1, PIS and P2). *J Urol* 1990;144:641.
34. Amling CL, Thrasher JB, Dodge RK, Frazier HA, Robertson JE, Paulson DF: Radical cystectomy for stages TA, TIS and T1 transitional cell carcinoma of the bladder. *J Urol* 1994;151:31–36.
35. Stephenson WT, Holmes FF, Noble MJ, Gerald KB: Analysis of bladder carcinoma by subsite. *Cancer* 1990;66:1630–1635.
36. Young RH, Wick MR, Mills SE: Sarcomatoid carcinoma of the urinary bladder: a clinicopathological analysis of 12 cases and review of the literature. *Am J Clin Pathol* 1988;90:653–661.
37. Bannach B, Grignon DJ, Shum DT: Sarcomatoid transitional cell carcinoma vs pseudosarcomatous stromal reaction in bladder carcinoma. *J Urol Pathol* 1993;1:105–119.
38. Lipponen PK, Collan Y, Eskelinen MJ, Pesonen E, Sotarauta M, Nordling S: Comparison of morphometry and DNA flow cytometry with standard prognostic factors in bladder cancer. *Br J Urol* 1990;65:589–597.
39. Blomjous CEM, Schipper NW, Baak JPA, Van Galen EM, De Voogt HJ, Meyer CJLM: Retrospective study of prognostic importance of DNA flow cytometry of urinary bladder carcinoma. *J Clin Pathol* 1988;41:21–25.
40. Jacobsen A, Pettersen EO, Åmellem O, Berner A, Ous S, Fossa SD: The prognostic significance of deoxyribonucleic acid flow cytometry in muscle invasive bladder carcinoma treated with preoperative irradiation and cystectomy. *J Urol* 1992;147:34–37.
41. DeSanctis PN, Tannenbaum M, Tannenbaum S, Olsson C: Morphologic quantitation of nuclear size in various grades of transitional cell carcinoma of urinary bladder. *Urology* 1982;20:196–199.
42. Blomjous CEM, Vos W, Schipper NW, Uyterlinde AM, Baak JPA, De Voogt HJ, Meijer CJLM: The prognostic significance of selective nuclear morphometry in urinary bladder carcinoma. *Hum Pathol* 1990;21:409–413.
43. Schapers RFM, Pauwels RPE, Havenith MG, Smeets AWGB, van den Brandt PA, Bosman FT: Prognostic significance of type IV collagen and laminin immunoreactivity in urothelial carcinomas of the bladder. *Cancer* 1990;66:2583–2588.
44. Stefanini GF, Bercovich E, Mazzeo V, et al: Class I and class II HLA antigen expression by transitional cell carcinoma of the bladder: correlation with T-cell infiltration and BCG treatment. *J Urol* 1989;141:1449–1453.
45. Neal DE, Smith K, Fennelly JA, Bennett MK, Hall PR, Harris AL: Epidermal growth factor receptor in human bladder cancer: a comparison of immunohistochemistry and ligand binding. *J Urol* 1989;141:517–521.
46. Meyers FJ, Gumerlock PH, Kokoris SP, Devere RW, McCormick F: Human bladder and colon carcinomas contain activated ras p21. *Cancer* 1989;63:2177–2181.
47. Wood DP Jr, Wartinger DD, Reuter V, Cordon-Cardo C, Fair WR, Chaganti RSK: DNA, RNA and immunohistochemical characterization of the HER-2/neu oncogene in transitional cell carcinoma of the bladder. *J Urol* 1991;146:1398–1401.
48. Nguyen PL, Swanson PE, Jaszcz W, et al: Expression of epidermal growth factor receptor in invasive transitional cell carcinoma of the urinary bladder: a multivariate survival analysis. *Am J Clin Pathol* 1994;101:166–176.
49. Sarkis AS, Dalbagni G, Cordon-Cardo C, et al: Nuclear overexpression of p53 protein in transitional cell bladder carcinoma: a marker for disease progression. *J Natl Cancer Inst* 1993;85:53–59.
50. Olumi AF, Tsai YC, Nichols PW, et al: Allelic loss of chromosome 17p distinguishes high grade from low grade transitional cell carcinoma of the bladder. *Cancer Res* 1990;50:7081–7083.
51. Ishikawa J, Xu H-J, Hu S-X, et al: Inactivation of the retinoblastoma gene in human bladder and renal cell carcinomas. *Cancer Res* 1991;51:5736–5743.
52. Logothetis CJ, Xu H-J, Ro JY, et al: Altered expression of retinoblastoma protein and known prognostic variables in locally advanced bladder cancer. *J Natl Cancer Inst* 1992;84:1256–1261.
53. Koontz WW, Prout GR, Jr, Smith W, et al: The use of intravesical thiotepa in the management of non-invasive carcinoma of the bladder. *J Urol* 1981;125:307.
54. El-Bolkainy MN, Mokhtar NM, Ghoneim MA, Hussein MH: The impact of schistosomiasis on the pathology of bladder carcinoma. *Cancer* 1981;48:2643–2648.
55. Del Mistro A, Koss LG, Braunstein J, Bennett BD, Saccomano G, Simons KM: Condylomata acuminata of the urinary bladder. *Am J Surg Pathol* 1988;12:205–215.
56. Cornil C, Reynolds CT, Kickham CJE: Carcinoma of the urachus. *J Urol* 1967;98:93–95.
57. Grignon DJ, Ro JY, Ayala AG, Johnson DE, Ordóñez NG: Primary adenocarcinoma of the urinary bladder: a clinicopathologic analysis of 72 cases. *Cancer* 1991;67:2165–2172.
58. Oesterling JE, Brendler CB, Burgers JK, Marshall FF, Epstein JI: Advanced small cell carcinoma of the bladder: successful treatment with combined radical cystoprostatectomy and adjuvant methotrexate, vinblastine, doxorubicin and cisplatin chemotherapy. *Cancer* 1990;65:1928–1936.
59. Grignon DJ, Ro JY, Ayala AG, et al: Small cell carcinoma of the urinary bladder: a clinicopathologic analysis of 22 cases. *Cancer* 1992;69:527–536.
60. Van Ahlen H, Nicolas V, Lenz W, Boldt I, Bockisch A, Vahlensieck W: Primary melanoma of urinary bladder. *Urology* 1992;40:550–554.
61. Stein DS, Kendall AR: Malignant melanoma of the genitourinary tract. *J Urol* 1984;132:859–868.
62. Thrasher JB, Rajan RR, Perez LM, Humphrey PA, Anderson EE: Pheochromocytoma of urinary bladder: contemporary methods of diagnosis and treatment options. *Urology* 1993;41:435–439.
63. Rode J, Bentley A, Parkinson C: Paraganglion cells of urinary bladder and prostate: potential diagnostic problem. *J Clin Pathol* 1990;43:13–16.
64. Kaplan WE, Firlit CF, Berger RM: Genitourinary rhabdomyosarcoma. *J Urol* 1983;130:116–119.
65. Crabbe JG, Cresdee WD, Scott TS, Williams MH: The cytologic diagnosis of bladder tumor amongst dyestuff workers. *Br J Indust Med* 1956;13:270.
66. Melamed MR, Koss LG, Ricci A, Whitmore WF: Cytohistologic observations on developing carcinoma of the urinary bladder in man. *Cancer* 1960;13:67.
67. Gamarra MC, Zein T: Cytologic spectrum of bladder cancer. *Urology* 1984;23:23–26.
68. Paulson J, Metwalli N, Wu B, Nochomovitz L: Transitional cell carcinoma of bladder with features of inverted papilloma. *Lab Invest* 1988;58:71A. Abstract.

69. Choyke PL, Thickman D, Kressel HY, et al: Controversies in the radiologic diagnosis of pelvic malignancies. *Radiol Clin North Am* 1985;23:531–549.
70. Abu-Yousef MM, Narayana AS, Franken EA, Jr, Brown RC: Urinary bladder tumors studied by cystosonography. I. Detection. *Radiology* 1984;153:223–226.
71. Denkhaus H, Crone-Muzebrock W, Huland H: Noninvasive ultrasound in detecting and staging bladder carcinoma. *Urol Radiol* 1985;7:121–131.
72. Itzchak Y, Singer D, Fischelovitch Y: Ultrasonographic assessment of bladder tumors: I. Tumor detection. *J Urol* 1981;126:31–33.
73. Cronan JJ, Simeone JF, Pfister RC, et al: Cystosonography in the detection of bladder tumors: a prospective and retrospective study. *J Ultrasound Med* 1982;1:237–241.
74. Kwok-Liu JP, Zikman JM, Cockshott WP: Carcinoma of the urachus: the role of computed tomography. *Radiology* 1980;137:731–734.
75. Lang EK: Neoplasms of the bladder, prostate and urethra. *Semin Roentgenol* 1983;18:288–298.
76. Weinerman PM, Arger PH, Coleman BG, et al: Pelvic adenopathy from bladder and prostate carcinoma: detection by rapid-sequence computed tomography. *AJR* 1983;140:95–99.
77. Fisher MR, Hricak H, Tanagho EA: Urinary bladder MR imaging: II. Neoplasm. *Radiology* 1985;157:471–477.
78. Dooms GC, Hricak H: Magnetic resonance imaging of the pelvis: prostate and urinary bladder. *Urol Radiol* 1986;8:156–165.
79. Lee JKT, Rholl KS: MRI of the bladder and prostate. *AJR* 1986;147:732–736.
80. Amendola MA, Glazer GM, Grossman HB, et al: Staging of bladder carcinoma: MRI-CT-surgical correlation. *AJR* 1986;146:2279–1183.

20 Renal Tumors in Children

Sandip P. Vasavada, Juan G. Corrales, Jack S. Elder

In children renal tumors are nearly always malignant. Exceptions include angiomyolipoma, which, in children, occurs most commonly in children with tuberous sclerosis, and congenital mesoblastic nephroma, which is a tumor of neonates and young infants. This chapter will review the various malignant and nonmalignant tumors that cause a solid renal mass in children.

WILMS' TUMOR

Incidence

Wilms' tumor represents the most common renal malignancy in the pediatric population. In the United States, approximately 450 to 500 children develop Wilms' tumor each year. Overall, Wilms' tumor accounts for 80% of all genitourinary cancers in children less than 15 years of age. More than 90% of all Wilms' tumor cases are seen prior to age 7, with a peak incidence between ages 3 and 4 years. Males and females are equally affected.

Pathogenesis

Wilms' tumor is presumed to be secondary to an abnormal proliferation of metanephric blastema, and these tumors are thought to have both hereditary and nonhereditary origins. Knudson and Strong proposed a two-hit mutational model to separate Wilms' tumor into these two tumor types. It is believed that children with the ''hereditary'' form have a genetic susceptibility and a constitutional lesion that is either inherited or from a somatic mutation. These kidneys are thought to undergo oncogenesis in the germ cell stage, and only one subsequent event is required for tumorigenesis. In contrast, for the development of a sporadic tumor two separate and independent somatic events are necessary. This model has further been confirmed by the observation in several tumors that inactivation of both alleles of a tumor suppressor gene is required for oncogenesis.[1] Overall, most Wilms' tumor cases appear to be sporadic.

The finding of several associated anomalies with Wilms' tumor linked this disease with a specific genetic locus that appears to be inactivated or mutated to result in a Wilms' tumor. Karyotypic analysis of several children with WAGR syndrome (Wilms' tumor, aniridia, genitourinary malformations, and mental retardation) demonstrated deletions on the short arm of chromosome 11. Subsequent studies have confirmed the Wilms' tumor suppressor gene (WT 1) location at 11p13.[2] The WT 1 protein encodes a transcription factor 45 to 49 kd in size whose function appears to be consistent with that of a tumor suppressor gene.[3] Recent studies indicate that WT 1 is critical to renal development in both mouse and human systems.[4] WT 1 has been detected in high levels in the developing renal blastemic cells, renal vesicles, and glomerular epithelium.[5] Furthermore, severe genitourinary and mesothelial abnormalities result in animals with deletions in one allele of the WT 1 tumor suppressor gene.[6] Further studies have shown a second Wilms' tumor locus at 11p15, known as WT 2, and this has been linked to cases of Beckwith–Wiedemann syndrome.[7]

Although Wilms' tumor has been studied extensively with respect to putative oncogenes, only the tumor suppressor gene p53 has yielded any relation with WT 1 or Wilms' tumor. Bardeesy et al showed that p53 expression correlated with anaplastic tumor histology and the patients had a poorer disease specific survival rate as compared to p53 negative patients.[8] Maheswaren has demonstrated a physical and functional interaction between WT 1 and p53 indicating that the two may act synergistically or regulate each other's expression through a variety of growth factors.[9]

Presentation

The majority of patients with Wilms' tumor present with a palpable abdominal or flank mass. Physical examination classically reveals a smooth, firm, nontender mass, as compared with the irregular mass of neuroblastoma. Microscopic hematuria is present in 30 to 50% of children, with a smaller percentage having gross hematuria. Approximately 50% are hypertensive. The differential diagnosis is the same as that for any childhood abdominal mass and is summarized in Table 20–1.

Associated Anomalies

As many as 15% of children with Wilms' tumor have an associated anomaly. If one of these conditions or anomalies is recognized early in childhood, serial screening with ultrasound is recommended to detect the presence of Wilms' tumor before it becomes symptomatic.[10]

Table 20–1. Differential Diagnosis of Childhood Abdominal Mass

RENAL CAUSES	NONRENAL CAUSES
Wilms' tumor	Mesenteric/choledochal cyst
Multicystic dysplastic kidney	Intestinal duplication cyst
Hydronephrosis	Splenomegaly
Polycystic kidney	Neuroblastoma
Congenital mesoblastic nephroma	Rhabdomyosarcoma
	Lymphoma
	Hepatoblastoma

Hemihypertrophy. Hemihypertrophy is a partial or complete asymmetry of the body. This condition affects one in 14,000 in the general population and is found in 3% of children with a Wilms' tumor. The hypertrophied side is not necessarily the same as the one afflicted with the Wilms' tumor.

Denys–Drash Syndrome. The Denys–Drash syndrome syndrome consists of Wilms' tumor in association with intersex disorders and mesangial sclerosis. Well over 90% of patients have incidence of point mutations in the WT 1 gene. Interestingly, the phenotypic effects of this point mutation are far more deleterious than those resulting from complete deletion of WT 1, as in patients with the WAGR syndrome.[11]

Beckwith–Wiedemann Syndrome. The Beckwith–Wiedemann syndrome consists of an enlargement of several organs in the body, including kidney, liver, pancreas, and adrenal cortex. Many of these patients have hemihypertrophy as well as microcephaly, mental retardation, and macroglossia. Approximately 10% develop associated malignancies of the adrenal cortex, liver, and kidney.[12]

Genitourinary Anomalies. A wide variety of genitourinary anomalies occur in children with Wilms' tumor, including hypospadias, cryptorchidism, pseudohermaphroditism, and renal duplication, ectopia, and fusion (e.g., horseshoe kidney) anomalies.

Aniridia. The incidence of aniridia in the general population is 1 in 50,000, whereas 1 to 2% of children with Wilms' tumor have aniridia. Wilms' tumor appears to be associated with sporadic rather than familial aniridia and has a significant correlation with Wilms' tumor in children with the 11p deletion. In 1984 Narahara described the WAGR syndrome, consisting of Wilms' tumor, aniridia, genitourinary anomalies, and mental retardation.[13]

Imaging Studies

Ultrasound. Renal ultrasound often is the initial study in the evaluation of a child with an abdominal mass arising from a Wilms' tumor. Sonography typically demonstrates a solid intrarenal mass (Fig. 20–1). At times calcification or cystic areas may appear within the mass. Additionally, ultrasound permits evaluation of the renal vein and/or the vena cava to identify tumor thrombus and therefore allow appropriate therapeutic management.

Intravenous Pyelogram. In the past the intravenous pyelogram (IVP) often was used to evaluate children with a Wilms' tumor, but currently other forms of upper tract imaging are used more often. Characteristically, the tumor

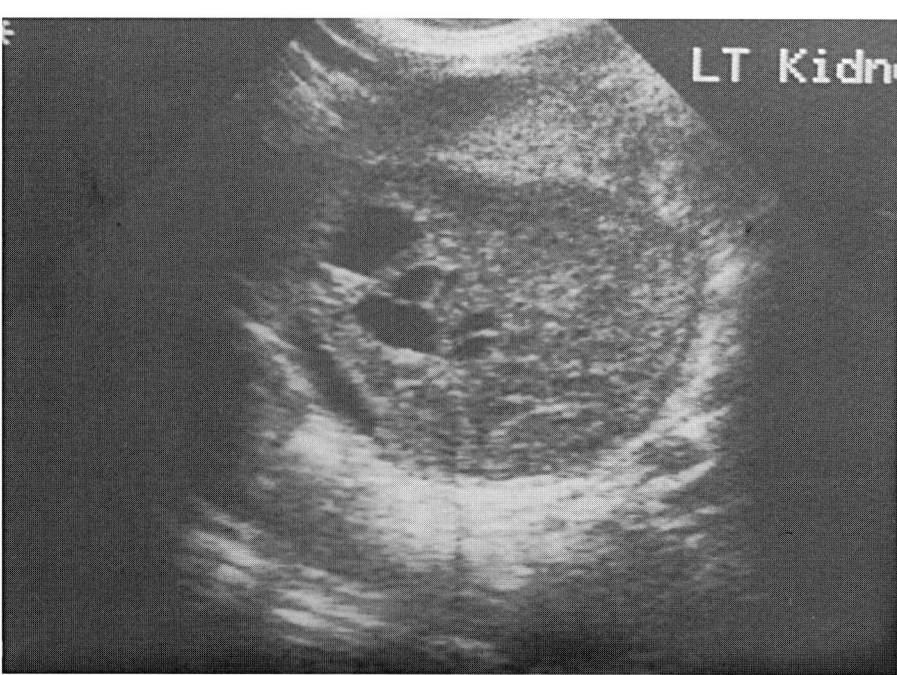

Figure 20–1. Ultrasound of Wilms' tumor showing solid mass with areas of necrosis.

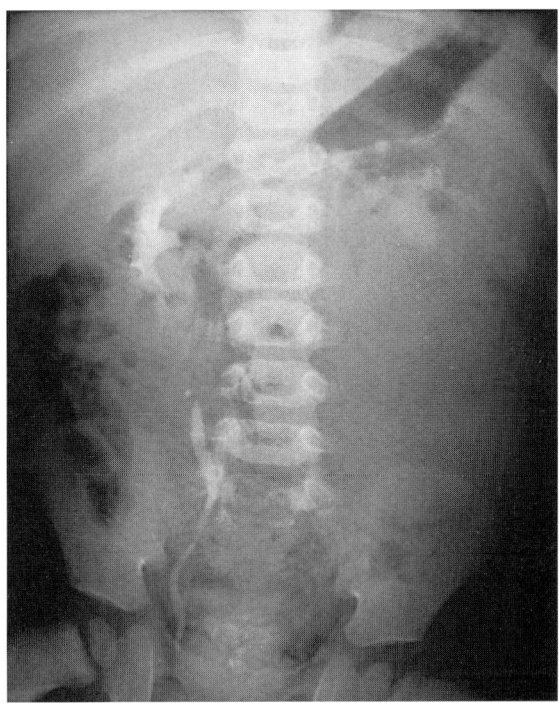

Figure 20–2. IVP showing large left abdominal mass with nonfunction of the left kidney. Patient had left Wilms' tumor.

causes distortion of the calyces with presence of a mass effect in the kidney. Rarely, a peripheral "eggshell" calcification from old hemorrhage is visualized. Nonvisualization of the affected kidney may be a sign of complete renal pelvic or ureteral obstruction, renal vein obstruction by tumor, or complete replacement of the kidney by tumor (Fig. 20–2). The IVP also allows assessment of contralateral renal function as well as evaluation of the possibility of bilateral Wilms' tumors.

Computed Tomography Scan. Despite the widespread use of computed tomography scan (CT), its role in the imaging of Wilms' tumor is limited (Fig. 20–3, A & B). Although it often presents precise anatomic delineation of structures in the kidney and retroperitoneum, its predictive value with respect to overall surgical staging has not yet been determined.[14] Furthermore, limitations of the CT scan include difficulty in assessing liver invasion and tumor thrombus extension. CT scan may have a role in differentiating neuroblastoma from Wilms' tumor.

Magnetic Resonance Imaging. Magnetic resonance imaging (MRI) has shown a great deal of promise as the newest imaging modality for the evaluation of Wilms' tumor, particularly because it demonstrates the extent of tumor thrombus in the vena cava.[15]

Arteriography. Arteriography is used only if the mass is not clearly intrarenal, the mass is so small that it cannot be assessed by other imaging studies, the mass is in a solitary kidney, or there are bilateral Wilms' tumors and partial nephrectomy is planned (Fig. 20–3C). Inferior venacavography is not used except in unusual cases because ultrasound and MRI demonstrate the extent of vena caval involvement.

Laboratory Tests

The standard laboratory evaluation in children with a suspected Wilms' tumor includes the complete blood count, renal and liver function panels, and a urinalysis. When neuroblastoma is suspected in the diagnosis, urinary or serum catecholamines should be measured also. To aid further in this important distinction, one may obtain catecholamine metabolite levels (urinary homovanillic acid [HMA] or vanillamandelic acid [VMA]) or serum ferritin or neuron-specific enolase (NSE).

Currently, efforts are under way to identify tumor markers that could either detect or monitor the activity of a previously diagnosed Wilms' tumor. For example, elevated hyaluronic acid levels have been found in 74% of prenephrectomy urine specimens.[16] Similarly, elevated serum prorenin levels may be found in patients with Wilms' tumor.[17]

Pathology

The histopathology of Wilms' tumor has a central role with tumor stage in determining the prognosis in these patients. Classically, Wilms' tumor is encapsulated within a segment of the kidney, and the mass distorts the calyceal anatomy and often contains elements of necrosis. Approximately 20% of tumors are myxomatous, with soft areas often intertwined with hyaline cartilaginous tissue.

Microscopically, Wilms' tumor has three elements—including undifferentiated blastema, primitive glomeruli and tubules, and embryonic mesenchyme—that form a swirl of nephrogenic cells upon a spindle cell stromal framework. In addition, the tumor may contain striated muscle, smooth muscle, collagenous fibrous tissue, cartilage, bone, and fat cells.[18] The diagnosis depends on the identification of primitive glomeruli and abortive tubules in the mesenchymal spindle cell framework.

Recently, there has been interest in measuring nuclear roundness in cells from these tumors to predict outcome. In one study of children with favorable histology, the authors were able to identify favorable characteristics in children with stage III and IV tumors, but not children with stage I or II tumors.[19]

The National Wilms' Tumor Study Group (NWTS) has helped further classify each pathologic subtype and identify favorable and unfavorable histologies based on survival statistics. The favorable subtypes represent the majority of Wilms' tumor cases encountered, and favorable histology refers to the classic triphasic appearance of Wilms' tumor. Unfavorable subtypes represent less than 10% of all Wilms' tumors; however, they account for more than 39% of the deaths caused by Wilms' tumor.[20]

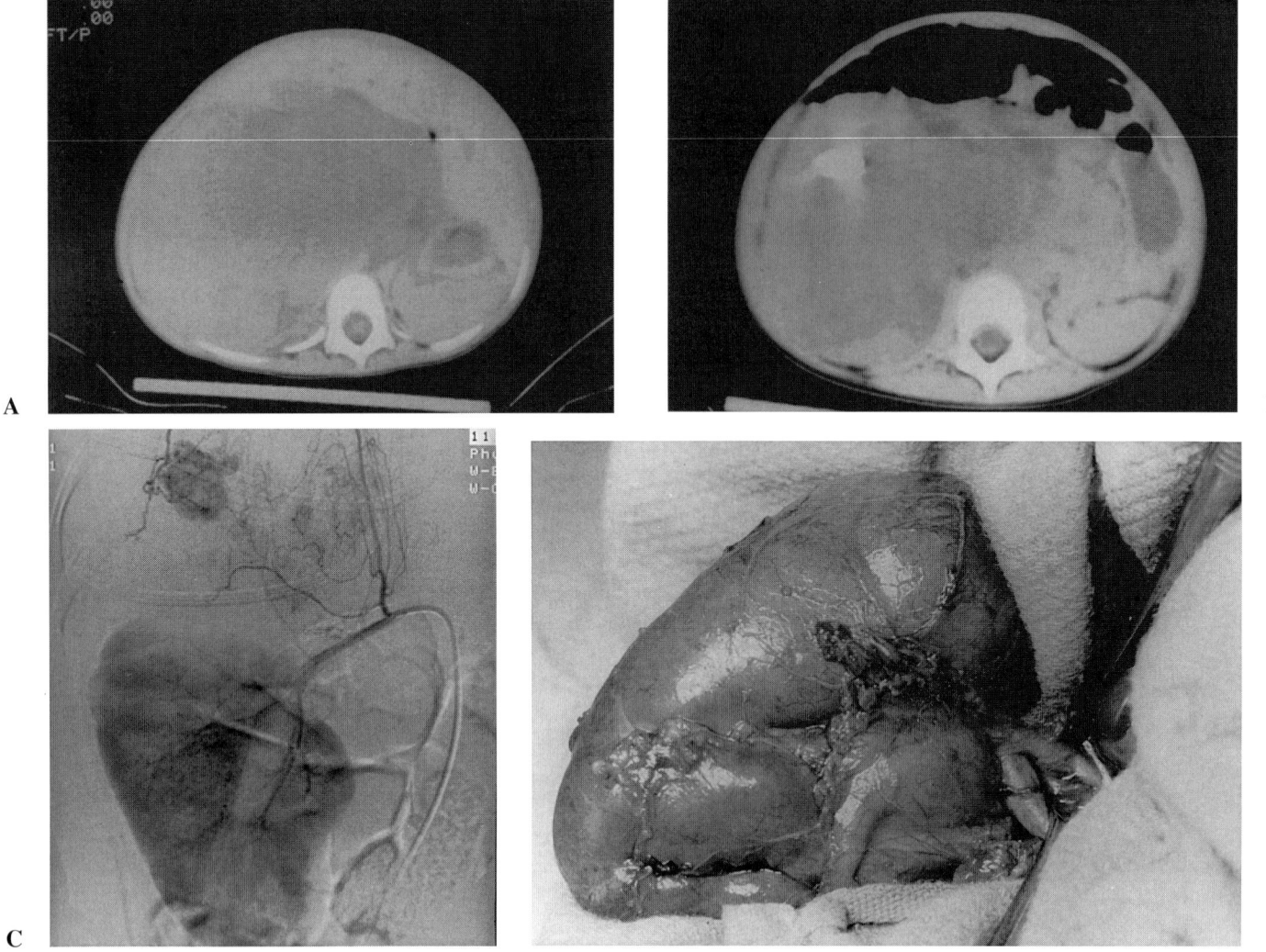

Figure 20–3. Patient with Wilms' tumor in solitary right kidney. (**A, B**) CT scan shows large right-sided renal tumor. (**C**) Arteriogram shows large upper pole mass. (**D**) Isolated kidney with upper pole mass (arrow).

Unfavorable Subtypes

Anaplastic tumors are generally found in older children. They exhibit extreme hyperchromatism and abnormal mitotic figures. If the anaplastic component is present in less than 10% of the specimen, it is considered to be focal, whereas if it is present in more than 10%, it is termed *diffuse*. There is some evidence that focal anaplasia has a much better prognosis than diffuse lesions.[21] Although relapse-free survival has been 27 to 55% in the past, a recent single institution report shows that adding cyclophosphamide to the usual three-drug regimen may increase survival even more.[20]

Sarcomatous tumors account for approximately 3% of all Wilms' tumors. Histologically, these tumors tend to have minimally prominent nucleoli and scant cytoplasm; architecturally, they demonstrate a spindle cell pattern. The tumor occurs more commonly in males and is termed the bone-metastasizing renal tumor of childhood (clear cell sarcoma of the kidney, CCSK).

Rhabdoid tumors make up less than 2% of all Wilms' tumor cases and are currently classified out of the Wilms' tumor category. The tumor is composed of large cells that are suggestive of rhabdomyoblasts, and no muscle cells are present. These tumors do have a tendency for central nervous system metastases. The survival rate is less than 20%.[22]

Favorable Subtypes

Several renal tumors have been categorized as favorable subtypes yet actually are not classic Wilms' tumors.

Congenital mesoblastic nephroma (CMN) occurs in neonates and young infants and usually has a benign course when properly excised. This tumor is discussed later in this chapter.

Multiocular cysts appear cystic, contain no normal renal tissue, and have interlocular septae that contain either fibrous tissue or embryonic tissue separating adjacent loculi. They usually have a bimodal age distribution, with one peak in the pediatric age group and the other in the middle adulthood. These kidneys are not neoplastic, but they may contain a Wilms' tumor. Because it is difficult to distinguish these tumors from cystic Wilms' tumor, excision generally is performed.[23]

Rhabdomyosarcomas represent a rare but favorable variant of Wilms' tumors.

Nephrogenic Rests

Knudson and Strong proposed a "two-hit" process whereby lesions that harbor a Wilms' tumor precursor are induced after a second insult as part of oncogenesis. Consistent with this theory is the concept of nephrogenic rests. These rests represent embryologic precursors that persist postnatally and can be induced to form a Wilms' tumor. The nephrogenic rests are further subcategorized into intralobar (ILNR) and perilobar (PLNR) rests based on chronology of development and location within the kidney. During renal development, the medullary portions form earlier than the lobar periphery. It follows that tumors arising in the periphery tend to be in younger patients than those in the central or medullary portions of the kidney. To confirm this, Beckwith and others have extensively studied these rests and their relation to Wilms' tumors and determined that the majority of these rests undergo involution with time and become inconsequential.[24] An important variant, however, undergoes some change and becomes hyperplastic or neoplastic. Beckwith has reported a 41% incidence of Wilms' tumors in association with nephrogenic rests.[24] Furthermore, in the bilateral Wilms' tumors, nearly 100% contained nephrogenic rests, particularly the peripheral type. Subsequent studies have shown an association between ILNR and metachronous tumor formation, ILNR and WAGR syndrome, and ILNR and Denys–Drash syndrome.[14]

Staging

A number of staging systems have been proposed for Wilms' tumors; however, the clinicopathologic system developed by NWTS is now widely accepted as the best (Table 20–2).

Surgical Management

In a child with suspected Wilms' tumor the preferred surgical approach is a transperitoneal incision that will allow optimal exposure of the entire abdomen and simultaneous exposure of the contralateral kidney. This approach generally is accomplished through a transverse abdominal incision 2 to 3 cm above the umbilicus. The initial step is to determine the extent of the tumor by palpating the intraabdominal contents as well as paraortic and hilar lymph nodes and vena cava.[25] Exploration of the contralateral kid-

Table 20–2. National Wilms' Tumor Staging System

Stage I:	Tumor limited to kidney and completely excised. The surface of the renal capsule is intact. Tumor was not ruptured before or during removal. There is no residual tumor apparent beyond the margins of resection.
Stage II:	Tumor extends beyond the kidney but is completely removed. There is regional extension of the tumor (i.e., penetration through the outer surface of the renal capsule into perirenal soft tissue). Vessels outside the kidney substance are infiltrated or contain tumor thrombus. The tumor may have undergone biopsy or there has been local spillage of tumor confined to the flank. There is no residual tumor apparent at or beyond the margins of excision.
Stage III:	Residual nonhematogenous tumor confined to abdomen. Any one or more of the following occur: a. Lymph nodes on biopsy are found to be involved in the hilus, the periaortic chains, or beyond. b. There has been diffuse peritoneal contamination by tumor, such as by spillage or tumor beyond the flank before or during surgery, or by tumor growth that has penetrated through the peritoneal surface. c. Implants are found on the peritoneal surfaces. d. The tumor extends beyond the surgical margins either microscopically or grossly. e. The tumor is not completely resectable because of local infiltration into vital structures.
Stage IV:	Hematogenous metastases. Deposits beyond stage III (e.g., lung, liver, bone, and brain).
Stage V:	Bilateral renal involvement at diagnosis. An attempt should be made to stage each side according to the preceding criteria on the basis of extent of disease before biopsy.

ney is necessary to be absolutely certain that it is normal, because if the child has bilateral involvement, then chemotherapy is administered prior to surgical excision. Contralateral renal exploration includes opening Gerota's fascia and exposing both the anterior and posterior surfaces of the kidney. Next, radical nephrectomy is performed if the tumor appears resectable along with a sampling of regional lymph nodes to stage the disease further. A formal lymph node dissection is not required, as this does not alter overall patient survival. The renal vein and inferior vena cava should be palpated prior to vessel ligation to exclude intravascular tumor extension.

Every effort should be made to avoid tumor spillage, because this complication may increase the potential for relapse in the abdomen.[26] Minor tumor spillage makes the tumor at least stage II and major spillage makes the tumor at least stage III (see Table 20–2), which may require more intensive postoperative therapy. It is advisable to place metal surgical clips at the edge of the tumor bed to assist the radiation therapist in forming the proper treatment zones, should radiotherapy be necessary.

Although Wilms' tumors may be enormous, the complication rate following radical nephrectomy is relatively low. Ritchey et al reviewed 1910 patients enrolled in NWTS-3 and found that 132 (7%) developed small bowel obstruction (usually because of adhesions or intussusception), 17 (0.9%) had significant intraoperative hypotension, 5 (0.3%) had cardiac arrest, and 9 (0.5%) died from operative complications.[27]

If a tumor appears unresectable, the tumor should be biopsied and chemotherapy with or without radiotherapy should be instituted, followed by tumor excision. Ritchey et al report 5% of patients were found to have an unresectable tumor.[28] All patients received actinomycin D and vincristine; doxorubicin with or without cyclophosphamide also was administered to one-third of the patients. Approximately one-third received radiation therapy. Long-term survival correlated with the response to the initial trial of chemotherapy. All who demonstrated a complete response were alive at 4 years, whereas 79% with a partial response and 63% with no response were alive at 4 years.[28]

Chemotherapy

Most chemotherapy regimens are instituted soon after bowel function resumes postoperatively. Patients with stage I favorable histology are treated for 24 weeks, whereas others are treated for 65 weeks. Most current regimens are based on the findings of the previous NWTS conclusions and are the basis for the NWTS IV drug regimen. This includes a combination of actinomycin D, vincristine, and doxorubicin. Actinomycin D and vincristine are given to stage I and II patients with the addition of the third agent, doxorubicin, for the stage III and IV patients or any patient with unfavorable histology (anaplasia).

It is important to monitor blood counts because acute hematologic toxicity may occur as a result of the chemotherapy agents. Doxorubicin is well known to cause cardiac toxicity and has resulted in death in several cases; therefore careful monitoring is essential when this drug is administered.

Radiation Therapy

Radiation therapy is reserved for patients with stage III or IV tumors or for those with stage II to IV tumors and unfavorable histology. No children with stage I or II tumors and favorable histology receive radiation therapy. Similarly, anaplastic stage I tumors do not receive irradiation. Stage III tumors with favorable histology receive approximately 1000 cGy to the tumor bed, and if there is abdominal dissemination, to the entire abdomen. Anaplastic stage II to IV tumors receive higher doses of radiation to the same areas as the more favorable tumors.

National Wilms' Tumor Studies

Because relatively few children have Wilms' tumor, it is difficult for most single institutions to acquire enough patients to study new forms of therapy. The National Wilms' Tumor Study (NWTS) was initiated in 1969 and has allowed collaborative evaluation of treatment regimens by children's hospitals throughout the United States. It has provided important information concerning factors that affect prognosis and outcome in Wilms' tumor patients. The basis for therapy is that nephrectomy is performed in most cases and postoperative chemotherapy with or without radiation therapy is administered. Exceptions to this principle include children with bilateral Wilms' tumor or unresectable Wilms' tumor, in whom biopsy is performed, followed by chemotherapy with or without radiation therapy and subsequent tumor removal.

Three NWTS studies have been performed to date, and the fourth is almost complete.

NWTS I ran from 1969 to 1974 and several important observations were made. NWTS I showed that for stage I tumors actinomycin D for 15 months was effective chemotherapy and that there was no survival advantage for routine radiotherapy. Furthermore, the combination of actinomycin D and vincristine was more beneficial than either one alone. It was also shown that a limited tumor spill did not affect survival and that patients with local tumor spillage or patients who underwent tumor biopsy were best served by local flank irradiation rather than by whole abdomen irradiation.[14]

NWTS II ran from 1974 to 1979. This study showed that administration of vincristine and actinomycin D for 6 months following removal of stage I tumors was as effective as 15 months of postoperative chemotherapy. It also confirmed the adverse effect of local nodal disease on patient prognosis.

NWTS III was conducted from 1979 to 1985 and showed that in patients with stage II tumors, radiotherapy was unnecessary. In stage III tumors radiotherapy with 1000 cGy was as effective as that with 2000 cGy. All patients with positive lymph nodes were upstaged to stage III, as there was an 82% survival for those with negative nodes versus a 54% survival for those with positive nodes. In patients with stage II and III tumors, no additional benefit was achieved from adding doxorubicin to the treatment regimen (Table 20–3).[29]

Table 20–3. Survival in Wilms' Tumor (NWTS-3)

STAGE	HISTOLOGY	4-YR POSTNEPHRECTOMY SURVIVAL (%)
I	Favorable	97
II	Favorable	92
III	Favorable	84
IV	Favorable	83
I–III	Unfavorable	68
IV	Unfavorable	55

Based on D'Angio GJ, Breslow N, Beckwith JB, et al: The treatment of Wilms' tumor: results of the Third National Wilms' Tumor Study. *Cancer* 1989; 64: 349.

Table 4–4. Treatment Scheme for NWTS-4

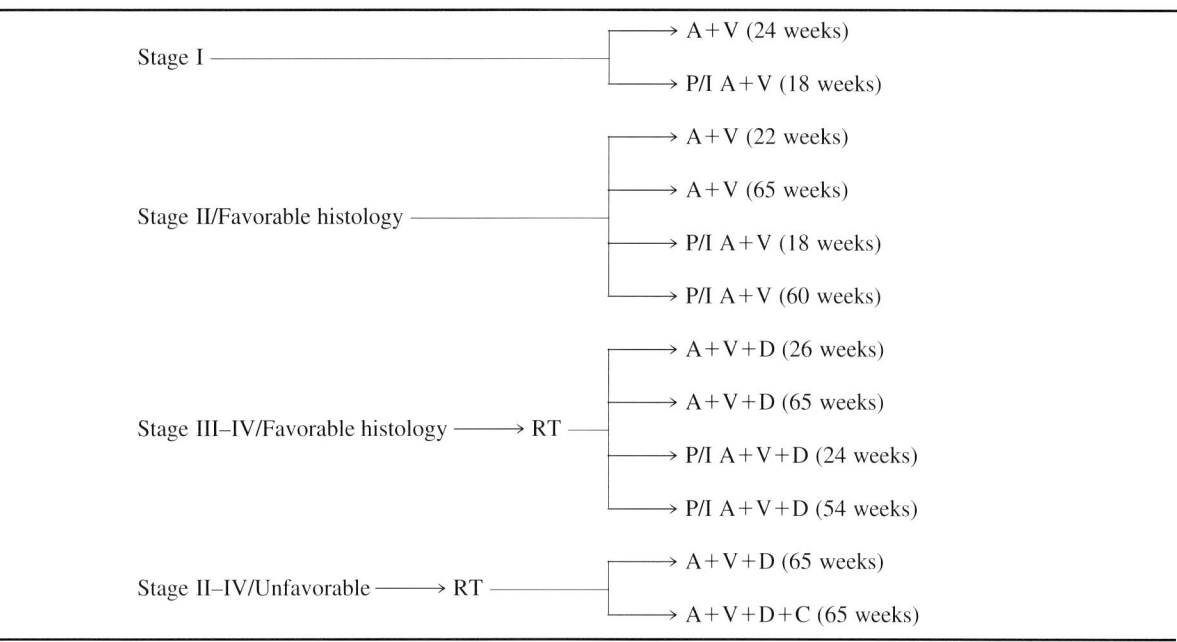

Postoperative treatment protocol for NWTS-4. A = actinomycin D; V = vincristine sulfate; D = doxorubicin; C = cyclophosphamide; P/I = pulsed, intensive therapy; RT = radiation therapy.

NWTS IV aims to improve the overall outcome of patients with unfavorable histology while limiting therapy for those with less aggressive tumors. Accordingly, stage I favorable histology and stage I anaplastic tumors (unfavorable histology) receive no radiation therapy or cyclophosphamide. Stage II favorable-histology tumors are treated without radiation therapy or doxorubicin. Pulse dose chemotherapy is being studied for its possible efficacy in these patients. Stage III tumors of favorable histology receive 1000 cGy of flank irradiation, and doxorubicin is added to the chemotherapy regimen. For stage IV tumors a continued aggressive multidrug chemotherapeutic approach is utilized. Additionally, pulmonary irradiation is administered for the lung metastases (Table 20–4).

Small Stage I Wilms' Tumor

In children less than 2 years old with a stage I Wilms' tumor, favorable histology, less than 550 g, the prognosis is significantly better than that in children with a larger tumor.[30] There is preliminary evidence that these children may not even need postoperative chemotherapy.[31]

Bilateral Wilms' tumor

Approximately 5% of children with a Wilms' tumor have bilateral disease (Fig. 20–4). The patient characteristics and tumor behavior in children with bilateral Wilms' tumor are different from those with a unilateral Wilms' tumor. For example, children with bilateral disease tend to present at a younger age, have a higher incidence of associated anomalies, and are more likely to have a family history of genitourinary cancer.[14] Beckwith and associates reported that all bilateral Wilms' tumor cases exhibited nephrogenic rests and that they were predominantly PLNR in synchronous cases and ILNR in metachronous cases.[24] The prognosis of patients with synchronous tumors is better than that of those with metachronous tumors and is greater than 76% for 3 years.[32] The improved survival is in part due to aggressive chemotherapy regimens.

In children with bilateral Wilms' tumor the initial procedure is to perform a laparotomy and to biopsy the tumors in both kidneys, to stage the lymph nodes, and, if there is favorable histology, to administer chemotherapy. Following chemotherapy, a partial nephrectomy or excisional biopsy is done if all tumors can be safely removed. If this does not appear to be the case, additional chemotherapy with or without radiotherapy is instituted. In this setting, a third-look operation is carried out within 6 months of therapy to biopsy or definitively treat any residual disease. The advantage of this approach is that it spares renal units and lessens the overall tumor burden prior to surgical treatment. If there is unfavorable histology in the initial specimen in a child with bilateral disease, sparing of renal function is of secondary importance and initial tumor removal followed by three-drug chemotherapy and second-look laparotomy is recommended. Survival for children with synchronous bilateral Wilms' tumor is approximately 80%.

Patients with bilateral Wilms' tumors need close follow-up, even long term, as late recurrences have been documented as late as 4.6 years posttherapy.[32]

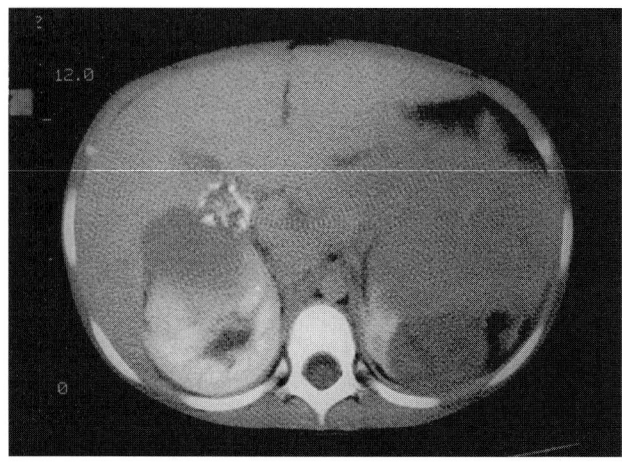

Figure 20–4. Bilateral Wilms' tumor. (**A, B**) CT scan shows large bilateral renal masses. Patient underwent bilateral biopsy and chemotherapy. (**C**) Following chemotherapy, CT scan shows single right renal mass (calcified) and two masses on left side (arrows). Patient underwent bilateral partial nephrectomy.

International Society of Pediatric Oncology Trials: Preoperative Chemotherapy

In the International Society of Pediatric Oncology (SIOP) trials, children with Wilms' tumor are treated with chemotherapy before and after nephrectomy, rather than undergoing nephrectomy followed by chemotherapy, as is done in the NWTS. The goal is to downstage the tumor with chemotherapy, possibly allowing renal-sparing surgery. In the most recent study all children underwent identical preoperative chemotherapy with actinomycin D and vincristine. The 2-year relapse-free survival was 92% in stage I tumors, 75% for stage II (negative lymph nodes), 49% in stage II (positive lymph nodes), and 77% for stage III.[33] Other groups also have reported similar results with chemotherapy with or without radiation therapy given before and after nephrectomy.[34,35] The limitations of this approach are the initial biopsy, which is intended to make the diagnosis of Wilms' tumor and to determine whether the patient has favorable or unfavorable histology, and staging, which is clinical rather than pathologic. In the SIOP trial, half of the children with stage II tumors were randomized to receive radiation therapy, and none developed an abdominal recurrence, whereas a significant number of abdominal recurrences occurred in those with stage II tumors who did not receive postoperative radiation.[33] This finding suggests that children may not receive adequate postoperative therapy if the tumor is significantly downstaged.

Complications of Chemotherapy and Radiation Therapy

Therapy of Wilms' tumors involves a great deal of potential morbidity, and those at particular risk include infants. In a review of the NWTS in 1989, toxicity and infection accounted for 15% of all deaths, although most were part of salvage regimens.[29] Nonetheless, many of these complications can be avoided if the patients are closely monitored.

Hematologic Toxicity. Acute hematologic toxicity is seen in Wilms' tumor patients, mostly as a result of the bone marrow suppression from the alkylating agents. For this reason it is essential to monitor the blood counts regularly.

Gastrointestinal Toxicity. Gastrointestinal toxicity occurs rather frequently and may result from either chemotherapy or radiation therapy, especially in younger children. Radiation enteritis causes a late onset of vomiting and diarrhea with abdominal distention.

Hepatic Toxicity. Hepatotoxicity results most commonly from radiation therapy of right-sided tumors. The liver dysfunction may result in liver enlargement, thrombocytopenia, or ascites.

Orthopedic Complications. In the past most orthopedic complications occurred in children less than 2 years old and in those treated with orthovoltage radiation therapy. In one study, 10- to 40-degree scoliosis occurred in 58%; 30- to 60-degree kyphosis, in 3%; lower rib hypoplasia, in 55%; and limb length inequality, in 10%. There was an overall incidence of bone growth abnormalities in 84%.[36] Current forms of megavoltage radiation appear to be less likely to cause these late orthopedic deformities.

Pulmonary Complications. Pulmonary complications result from the combination of chemotherapy, lung irradiation, and infection. Generally, the symptoms are limited to a fever or mild cough. The frequency of these complications is decreasing with closer monitoring of therapy.

Renal Complications. Renal complications may occur from radiation therapy to the remaining kidney, with microhematuria, azotemia, and edema. Fortunately, most of these complications are not long term, and follow-up studies have shown minimal residual effect on kidney function.

Reproductive Complications. Increases in perinatal mortality and in low birth weight were seen in the offspring of female survivors of Wilms' tumor who received abdominal radiation.[37] The male patients had no untoward effects. Therefore it appears that female survivors of Wilms' tumor are at increased risk for reproductive problems and that their offspring are at increased risk for clinically significant birth defects. The effect of radiation on the ovary and testis is well known, and Scott has shown evidence of ovarian failure in postpubertal females with poor secondary sexual characteristics and elevated FSH and LH levels.[38] The testis may manifest oligospermia.

Secondary Neoplasms. In patients treated for Wilms' tumor, the probability of developing a secondary neoplasm is 8 to 17% over a 5- to 25-year period.[39,40] Evans et al showed a higher incidence of secondary benign and malignant neoplasms in patients who received radiation therapy.[41] The most common benign tumor is an osseous/chondromatous tumor, and a wide variety of malignant tumors can occur, including various sarcomas, hepatomas, and leukemias.

Neonatal Wilms' Tumor

In neonates Wilms' tumor is extremely rare. Rather, the tumor is much more likely to be a congenital mesoblastic nephroma (see later). However, 15 neonatal Wilms' tumors have been identified, three of which were noted on antenatal ultrasound examination.[42] All the patients underwent primary excision of the tumor; 80% were stage I, 20% were stage II, and all had favorable histology. Ten patients received postoperative chemotherapy, and one was given radiation therapy; all are alive 8 months to 13 years postoperatively. Of the five not receiving postoperative chemotherapy, one developed a relapse and died at 16 months despite receiving chemotherapy.

Adult Wilms' Tumor

Adult Wilms' tumors usually affect young adults. In one series, the median age was 33 years and the patients typically presented with pain, abdominal or flank mass, or hematuria.[43] Although these patients often admitted to experiencing these symptoms for several years prior to seeking consultation, remarkably, less than 15% presented with metastatic disease. An aggressive multimodality treatment approach has resulted in good survival rates in these patients. Most current recommendations agree that initial therapy is radical nephrectomy for diagnosis followed by radiation therapy postoperatively, including the lung fields if pulmonary metastases are present. Subsequently, chemotherapy consisting of actinomycin D and vincristine is administered. This regimen has yielded disease-free survival rates of 40 to 50% after 18 months of therapy, with half of these patients being disease-free more than 5 years. Ultimately, however, prognosis partly depends on the stage at time of presentation. Patients with stage III and IV disease have fared far worse than those with more localized disease.

CONGENITAL MESOBLASTIC NEPHROMA

Epidemiology

Congenital mesoblastic nephroma (CMN) was described by Bolande et al as a neonatal renal tumor that is distinguishable from Wilms' tumor in its morphology and relatively benign behavior.[44] This tumor develops in approximately one in 500,000 infants[45] and accounts for less than 3% of pediatric renal neoplasms.[46] CMN usually is diagnosed at birth or within the first 3 months of life, whereas Wilms' tumor has a peak incidence between 2 and 3 years of age. CMN accounts for the vast majority of neonatal renal tumors.

Etiopathogenesis

Controversy exists about the origin of CMN. During early embryogenesis the totipotential renal blastema is mainly stromagenic. Snyder et al related tumor development to the two-hit theory for pathogenesis of Wilms' tumor and suggested that if neoplasia is induced during the early stromagenic phase, a conventional CMN might result.[47] If persistent stromal elements last into the newborn period, a second step in tumor induction could result in a CMN cellular variant (sarcoma). Another theory is that the tumor originates from uninduced nephrogenic mesenchyme.[48]

Another observation is that trisomy 11 is common in many CMN tumors,[49] particularly those with the "cellular" and "mixed" histologic subtypes of CMN. It has been proposed that insulin-like growth factor II (IGFII) gene, which has been mapped to the short arm of chromosome 11 and is expressed in mesenchymal cells during kidney development, may play a key role in the acquisition of the growth properties of neoplasia.[49]

Pathology

Three histologic types of CMN have been described: the classic pattern of CMN, the "cellular" or atypical variant, and a third type, which shows mixed features. A rare cystic variety also has been described.[50]

Classically, an involved kidney is greatly enlarged and distorted by the tumor. The mass has a slightly bulging cut surface that has a whorled, coarsely trabeculated appearance, similar to a uterine leiomyoma. Typical size ranges from 0.6 to 9.0 cm. Cellular CMNs are softer than the classic type and show areas of hemorrhage, necrosis, and cystic degeneration.

Classic CMN is composed of uniform spindle-shaped cells arranged in interlacing bundles. The cells have pale eosinophilic cytoplasm and ovoid, enlongated vesicular nuclei with inconspicuous nucleoli. Foci of extramedullary hematopoiesis are frequently observed. Areas resembling hemangiopericytoma may be present also. Mitotic activity ranges from 0 to 1 mitotic figures per 10 high-power fields (HPFs).

The cellular variant contains diffuse sheets of closely packed cells with scanty cytoplasm. Thin-walled vascular spaces are scattered throughout these neoplasms. Mitotic activity ranges from 8–10 to 25–30 mitotic figures per 10 HPFs in the most active areas. Necrosis and hemorrhage are commonly present.

Tumors with combined histologic classic and cellular features show variable cellularity ranging from fibroleiomyomatous paucicellular to highly cellular areas with increased mitotic activity. In other cases the two components are clearly demarcated or the cellular component may exhibit an unusual degree of anaplasia.[51]

Immunohistochemical studies have shown that classic and cellular CMN often contain actin, desmin, and acidic fibroblastic growth factor, a potent stimulator of mesenchymal cell proliferation.[51] In addition, immunoreactive renin staining often is present in surgical specimens, particularly in the areas of renal cortex entrapped within the tumor, presumably accounting for the common finding of preoperative hypertension in these patients.[52] In flow cytometric studies, classic CMN and cellular CMN are diploid, whereas the cellular component of the combined tumor exhibits aneuploid DNA stemlines.[51]

Clinical Features and Diagnosis

CMN usually presents as an asymptomatic abdominal mass in the newborn period or early infancy, although recent reports show that CMN may be detected using prenatal ultrasound.[46] CMN may be associated with polyhydramnios.[46,53] The tumors are more common on the left side.

Renin-mediated hypertension is common in infants with CMN. Recent immunochemical studies in removed kidneys indicate that renin production by CMN cells is minimal and is highest in areas of renal cortex entrapped by the tumor.[52,54]

The behavior of this tumor is not well understood. In the majority of the cases CMN is a relatively benign lesion, but local invasion, recurrence, and metastases to the lung and brain can occur.[55,56] The cellular variant is thought by some to be more likely to exhibit aggressive characteristics.[55] Furthermore, most of the infants with aggressive lesions are more than 3 months old.[57] Consequently, infants more than 3 months of age with a CMN cellular variant or atypical histologic features should be considered for adjunctive therapy following radical nephrectomy.[56]

CMN and Wilms' Tumor

There are several differences between CMN and Wilms' tumor:

1. CMN usually is diagnosed at birth or within the first 3 months of life, whereas Wilms' tumor has a peak incidence between 2 and 3 years.
2. Wilms' tumor is a primitive embryonal neoplasm that is thought to develop from residual metanephric blastema and histologically mimics different stages of renal development, whereas CMN typically consists of spindle cells that resemble primitive mesenchymal tissue of less definite derivation with few or no neoplastic epithelial cells.
3. Clinically, CMN usually is cured by surgery alone, whereas Wilms' tumors have a propensity to recur or metastasize if not treated with systemic chemotherapy.
4. Both CMN and Wilms' tumors arise from primitive renal cells. Molecular analysis of these tumors, however, demonstrates significant differences. Wilms' tumor frequently is associated with loss of heterozygosity at chromosome bands 11p13 and/or 11p15, but CMN is not. IGF-II, N-myc oncogene, and WT 1 (the putative Wilms' tumor supressor gene located at chromosome 11p13) are highly expressed in Wilms' tumors and fetal kidneys. IGF-II is detected readily in CMN, but N-myc and WT 1 are not detected in CMN.[45] The difference between CMN and Wilms' tumor may be the time point at which mutagenesis occurs.[47]
5. Bilateral renal involvement is much more common in children with Wilms' tumor than in those with CMN, in which it is extremely rare.

Diagnosis

In selected cases, prenatal diagnosis can be made by ultrasound, which shows a solid renal mass.[46] In the newborn and infant the abdominal mass is the key to diagnosis, and the tumor usually is confirmed by ultrasound. Abdominal and chest computed tomography (or MRI) are done to stage this neoplasm preoperatively. MRI of the head also should be done if central nervous system metastases are suspected (Fig. 20–5).

Treatment and Follow-up

Both the classic and cellular variants of CMN usually are curable by radical nephrectomy. Unlike Wilms' tumor, there is not a tendency for bilateral renal involvement. Adjuvant therapy is not required for most patients with this neoplasm. Recurrent or metastatic tumors may occur, usually to the lungs or brain, and close observation of these patients is quite important. Follow-up examination should include abdominal, chest, and brain examination.

Routine cytogenetic examination could identify specific chromosomal markers of those neoplasms with more aggressive behavior, in which case chemotherapy should be considered.

RENAL ANGIOMYOLIPOMA (HAMARTOMA)

Renal angiomyolipoma is a benign mesenchymal nodule consisting of blood vessels with thickened walls, smooth muscle, and adipose tissue. Renal angiomyolipoma occurs in two forms: isolated or as a part of tuberous sclerosis (TSC) complex. Between 20 and 40% of angiomyolipomas occur

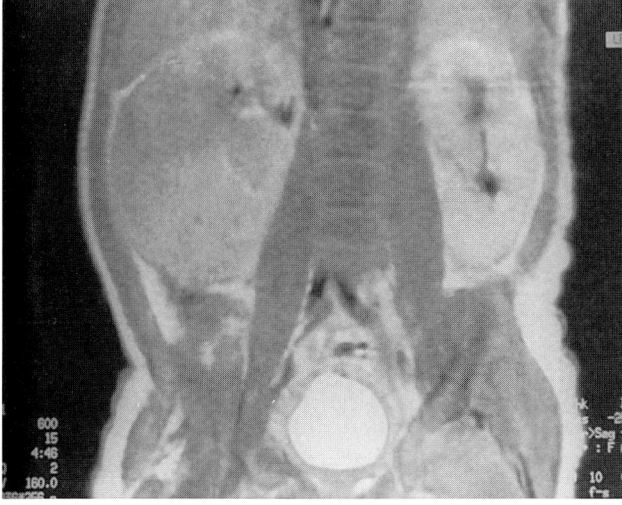

Figure 20–5. MRI of congenital mesoblastic nephroma, right kidney.

in individuals with tuberous sclerosis, and 40 to 80% of tuberous sclerosis patients develop an angiomyolipoma.[58] In children, however, angiomyolipoma occurs almost exclusively in those with tuberous sclerosis. Angiomyolipoma is predominant in women, with a female-to-male ratio of 3 or 4 to 1, in those with and in those without tuberous sclerosis.[58] The prevalence of tuberous sclerosis is approximately 1 in 10,000.[59] Although as many as 50% of these patients may develop an angiomyolipoma, distinguishing this tumor from renal cell carcinoma and other renal tumors is important.[60]

Etiology

Histologically, the two forms of renal angiomyolipoma are indistinguishable, raising the hypothesis that solitary angiomyolipoma may be atypical variants of the tuberous sclerosis complex.

Tuberous sclerosis is an autosomal dominant condition with genetic locus heterogeneity. Half of patients are mentally retarded, and most have seizures and one of the characteristic dermatologic lesions, including adenoma sebaceum (facial angiofibromas), hypopigmented macules (ash leaf patches), shagreen patches, and ungual fibromas. Involvement can occur in areas other than the kidney, including cortical tubers, subependymal nodules, retinal astrocytomas, and cardiac rhabdomyomas. Two major gene loci have been identified, including chromosome 9q34 (TSC1) and 16p13.3 (TSC2). These may act as growth suppressor genes analogous to the two-hit model of the traditional tumor suppressor gene in the Knudson hypothesis.[61]

Clinical Manifestations

Renal angiomyolipomas with tuberous sclerosis are rare in children less than 5 years old. In the pediatric population, they are more common between 6 and 10 years, and most common in patients older than 10 years.[62] In children there are often multiple tumors of various sizes that occur in both kidneys, as compared to the isolated, unilateral, solitary, symptomatic, moderate-sized tumor, which is usually predominant in middle-aged women.[58]

The pattern of presentation has changed because more asymptomatic lesions are being discovered incidentally by renal ultrasound and CT. Symptoms and signs may occur with increasing size of the tumor(s) and resultant compression of surrounding tissue; they include abdominal or flank pain, hematuria, hemmorrhage, or anemia.

Approximately 80% of patients with diagnosis of renal angiomyolipoma have some or all of the other stigmata of tuberous sclerosis. The renal lesions commonly associated with TSC are angiomyolipoma and renal cyst. Renal cysts are more common in children with TSC and are often small and scattered. If there is severe involvement, with numerous and large cysts, hypertension or end-stage renal disease may occur.[63]

Natural History

The natural history of renal angiomyolipoma in children is not well understood. However, tumor size seems to be a good parameter, because those that are more than 4 cm in diameter are more likely to be symptomatic and require treatment, whereas smaller lesions generally can be followed, with surgical intervention rarely necessary.[64] Most angiomyolipomas in patients with tuberous sclerosis are multiple and bilateral. Progressive tumor growth can cause destruction of the renal parenchyma to the point that with multiple or bilateral tumors it can lead to renal failure.[62]

Pathology

Angiomyolipomas are very vascular tumors, consisting of smooth muscle, adipose tissue, and blood vessels with thickened walls. The tumors are grossly circumscribed but not encapsulated. They range in size from small punctate tubers to a huge mass exceeding 20 cm in diameter, with the mean diameter being approximately 9 cm. The amount of fat in the tumor varies. Very fat lesions are yellow, whereas more muscular tumors are pink and fleshy. Growth toward the hilum can lead to renal pelvic and calyceal compression and occasionally invasion of the renal veins.

Microscopic examination shows fat necrosis and collections of xanthoma cells. The fat and smooth muscle cells of the tumors interdigitate with normal renal parenchyma at the margins of the tumor, which is not encapsulated. The blood vessels either lack elastic tissue or contain abnormally distributed elastic tissue, possibly explaining their propensity to rupture. The smooth muscle cells often contain atypical, large, hyperchromatic nuclei. The presence of mitotic activity may cause concern and even result in a mistaken diagnosis of malignancy. Progressive metastatic disease from angiomyolipomas has not been demonstrated.[63]

Diagnosis

Angiomyolipoma is diagnosed most often by sonography or CT. Sonography is the usual screening method. It typically shows the tumor as echodense, because of the fatty tissue, and well circumscribed. Similarly, CT may provide the correct diagnosis if an adequate amount of fatty tissue is present.[65] However, some angiomyolipomas contain only a tiny amount of fat, which can be easily overlooked by ultrasound or CT.[66] A renal biopsy is rarely necessary. The use of thin cuts on nonenhanced CT scans improves the chances of detecting and measuring these small areas of fat. If the muscular portion of the tumor predominates, these techniques do not guarantee a specific diagnosis, because with sonography a low sonodense pattern may appear, and with

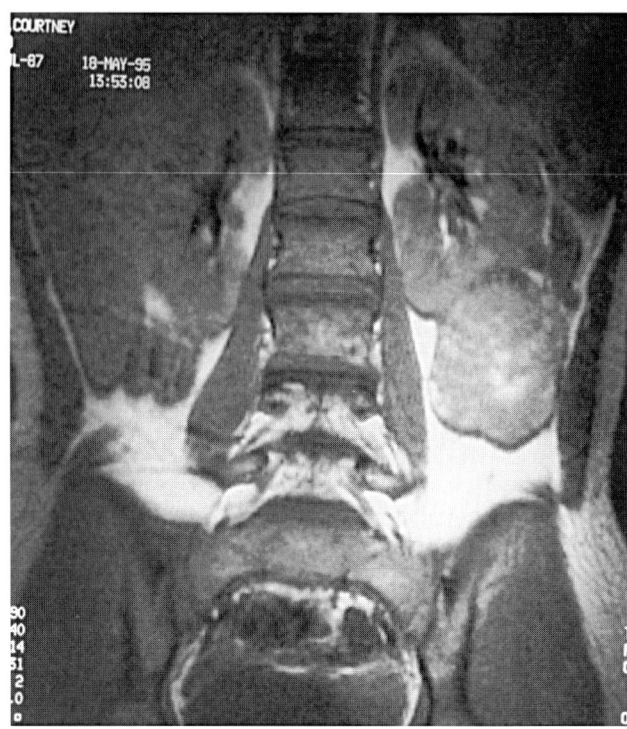

Figure 20–6. MRI of patient with tuberous scleorosis and 6-cm angiomyolipoma on lower pole of left kidney. Patient underwent partial nephrectomy.

CT angiomyolipomas may display a density comparable to carcinoma.

The characteristic pattern on MRI depends on the amount of fatty tissue in the tumor, which corresponds to a high signal intensity in T1-weighted images and a lower intensity in T2-weighted images (Fig. 20–6).[65] When angiomyolipoma is composed of little fat and contains large amounts of smooth muscle, the signal intensity in MRI alters and may have the appearance of a carcinoma. Gadolinium-enhanced MRI may provide even better resolution.[67]

In summary, in children, the initial ultrasound diagnosis of renal angiomyolipoma should be confirmed by CT scan or MRI. It is also necessary to search for other internal stigmata of TSC.

Treatment

The risks of untreated angiomyolipoma include development of abdominal or flank pain, palpable mass, hemorrhage, hematuria, anemia, and hypertension.[64] However, these complications occur primarily in individuals with tumors more than 4 cm in diameter. Nonoperative treatment is recommended in most children with renal angiomylipoma. If the tumor is smaller than 4 cm, follow-up by ultrasound every 6 to 12 months is mandatory, because at least 27% may grow.[64] However, if the lesion(s) is larger than 4 cm, selective angiographic embolization or partial nephrectomy may be necessary, particularly if serial imaging studies demonstrate that the tumor is growing.[60,64]

In patients with tuberous sclerosis, angiomyolipomas are usually multiple and bilateral or associated with renal cysts. They present at a younger age, are more likely to be symptomatic, tend to be larger, and are more likely to grow. Consequently, it is important to preserve as much functional renal tissue as possible if hemorrhage occurs. Because renal cell carcinoma is uncommon in the pediatric population, total nephrectomy with an incorrect preoperative diagnosis of malignant tumor is unlikely.

RENAL CELL CARCINOMA

Older children with solid renal tumors may have a renal cell carcinoma. Radiographically, renal cell carcinoma cannot be distinguished from Wilms' tumor. Although the natural history of renal cell carcinoma appears to be similar in children and adults, it may have a more favorable prognosis below the age of 10 years.[68]

REFERENCES

1. Comings DE: A general theory of carcinogenesis. *Proc Natl Acad Sci USA* 1973; 70:3324.
2. Bonetta L, Kuehn SE, Huang A, et al: Wilms' tumor locus on 11p13 defined by multiple CpG island associated transcripts. *Science* 1990; 250:994.
3. Coppes MJ, Haber DA, Grundy PE: Genetic events in the development of Wilms' tumor. *N Engl J Med* 1994; 331:586.
4. Rackley RR, Flenniken AM, Kuriyan NP, et al: Expression of the Wilms' tumor suppressor gene WT 1 during mouse embryogenesis. *Cell Growth Differ* 1993; 4:1023.
5. Pritchard-Jones K, Fleming S, Davidson D, et al: The candidate Wilms' tumor gene is involved in genitourinary development. *Nature* 1990; 346:194.
6. Kreidberg JA, Sariola H, Loring JM, et al: WT 1 is required for early kidney development. 1993; *Cell* 74:679.
7. Ping AJ, Reeve AE, Law DJ, et al: Genetic linkage of Beckwith-Wiedemann syndrome to 11p15. *Am J Hum Genet* 1989; 44:720.
8. Bardeesy N, Falkoff D, Petruzzi MK, et al: Anaplastic Wilms' tumor, a subtype displaying poor prognosis, harbours p53 mutations. *Nat Genet* 1994; 7:91.
9. Maheswaran S, Park S, Bernard A, et al: Physical and functional interaction between WT 1 and p53 proteins. *Genetics* 1993; 90:5100.
10. Green DM, Breslow NE, Beckwith JB, et al: Screening of children with hemihypertrophy, aniridia, and Beckwith-Wiedemann syndrome in patients with Wilms' tumor: a report from the National Wilms' Tumor Study. *Med Pediatr Oncol* 1993; 21:188.
11. Coppes MJ, Huff V, Pelletier J: Denys–Drash syndrome: relating a clinical disorder to genetic alterations in the tumor suppressor gene WT 1. *J Pediatr* 1993; 123:673.
12. Sotelo-Avila C, Gonzalez-Cruzzi F, deMello D, et al: Complete and incomplete forms of Beckwith-Wiedemann syndrome: their oncogenic potential. *J Pediatr* 1980; 96:47.
13. Narahara K, Kikkawa K, Kimira S, et al: Regional mapping of catalase and Wilms' tumor: aniridia, genitourinary abnormalities, and mental retardation triad loci to the chromosome segment 11p1305 p1306. *Hum Genet* 1984; 66:181.
14. Snyder HM, III, D'Angio GJ, Evans AE, et al: Pediatric oncology. In: Walsh PC, Retik AB, Stamey TA, Vaughan ED, eds. *Campbell's Urology*, 6th ed. Philadelphia: WB Saunders, 1992; 1967.
15. Weese DL, Applebaum H, Taber P: Mapping intravascular extension of Wilms' tumor with magnetic resonance imaging. *J Pediatr Surg* 1991; 26:64.
16. Lin RY, Argenta PA, Sullivan KM, et al: Urinary hyaluronic acid is a Wilms' tumor marker. *J Pediatr Surg* 1995; 30:304.
17. Leckie BJ, Birnie G, Carachi R: Renin in Wilms' tumor: prorenin as an indicator. *J Clin Endocrinol Metab* 1994; 79:1742.
18. Robbins SL, Cotran RS, Kumar V: *Pathologic Basis of Disease*, 3rd ed. Philadelphia: WB Saunders, 1984; 1957.
19. Partin AW, Yoo JK, Crooks D, et al: Prediction of disease-free survival after therapy in Wilms' tumor using nuclear morphometric techniques. *J Pediatr Surg* 1994; 29:457.
20. Corey SJ, Anderson JW, Vawter GF, et al: Improved survival for children with anaplastic Wilms' tumors. *Cancer* 1991; 68:970.
21. Green DM, Beckwith JB, Breslow NE, et al: Treatment of children with stages II to IV anaplastic Wilms' tumor: a report from the National Wilms' Tumor Study Group. *J Clin Oncol* 1994; 12:2126.
22. Weeks DA, Beckwith JB, Luckey DW: Relapse associated variables in stage I favorable histology Wilms' tumor: a report of the National Wilms' tumor study. *Cancer* 1987; 60:1204.
23. Castillo OA, Boyle ET, Jr, Kramer SA: Multilocular cysts of kidney: a study of 29 patients and review of literature. *Urology* 1991; 37:156.
24. Beckwith JB, Norkool P, Breslow N, et al: Clinical observations in children with clear cell sarcoma of the kidney. *Proc Am Assoc Cancer Res* 1986; 27:200, Abstract.
25. Othersen HB, de Lorimier A, Hrabovsky E, et al: Surgical evaluation of lymph node metastases in Wilms' tumor. *J Pediatr Surg* 1990; 25:330.
26. Breslow N, Churchill G, Beckwith JB, et al: Prognosis for Wilms' tumor patients with non-metastatic disease at diagnosis: results of the Second National Wilms' tumor study. *J Clin Oncol* 1985; 3:521.
27. Ritchey ML, Kelalis PP, Breslow N, et al: Surgical complications after nephrectomy for Wilms' tumor. *Surg Gynecol Obstet* 1992; 175:507.
28. Ritchey ML, Pringle KC, Breslow NE, et al: Management and outcome of inoperable Wilms' tumor: a report of National Wilms' Tumor Study-3. *Ann Surg* 1994; 220:683.
29. D'Angio GJ, Breslow N, Beckwith JB, et al: The treatment of Wilms' tumor: results of the Third National Wilms' Tumor Study. *Cancer* 1989; 64:349.
30. Green DM, Breslow NE, Beckwith JB, et al: Treatment outcome in patients less than 2 years of age with small, stage I, favorable-histology Wilms' tumors: a report from the National Wilms' Tumor Study. *J Clin Oncol* 1993; 11:91.
31. Larsen E, Perez-Atayde A, Green DM, et al: Surgery only for the treatment of patients with stage I (Cassady) Wilms' tumor. *Cancer* 1990; 66:264.
32. Montgomery BT, Kelalis PP, Blute ML, et al: Extended follow-up of bilateral Wilms' tumor: results of the National Wilms' Tumor Study. *J Urol* 1991; 146:514.
33. Tournade MF, Com-Nougue C, Voute PA, et al: Results of the Sixth International Society of Pediatric Oncology Wilms' Tumor Trial and Study: a risk-adapted therapeutic approach in Wilms' tumor. *J Clin Oncol* 1993; 11:1014.

34. Dykes EH, Marwaha RK, Dicks-Mireaux C, et al: Risks and benefits of percutaneous biopsy and primary chemotherapy in advanced Wilms' tumour. *J Pediatr Surg* 1991; 26:610.
35. Greenberg M, Burnweit C, Filler R, et al: Preoperative chemotherapy for children with Wilms' tumor. *J Pediatr Surg* 1991; 26:949.
36. Rate WR, Butler MS, Robertson WW, et al: Late orthopedic effects in children with Wilms' tumor treated with abdominal radiation. *Med Pediatr Oncol* 1991; 19:265.
37. Li FP, Gimbrere K, Gelber RD, et al: Outcome of pregnancy in survivors of Wilms' tumor. *JAMA* 1987; 257:216.
38. Scott JS: Pubertal development in children treated for nephroblastoma. *J Pediatr Surg* 1981; 16:122.
39. Li FP, Cassady JR, Jaffe N: Risk of second tumors in survivors of childhood cancers. *Cancer* 1975; 35:1230.
40. Hartley AL, Birch JM, Blair V, et al: Second primary neoplasms in a population-based series of patients diagnosed with renal tumours in childhood. *Med Pediatr Oncol* 1994; 22:318.
41. Evans AE, Norkook P, Evans MS, et al: Late effects of treatment for Wilms' tumor: a report from the National Wilms' Tumor Study Group. *Cancer* 1991; 67:331.
42. Ritchey ML, Azizkhan RG, Beckwith JB, et al: Neonatal Wilms' tumor. *J Pediatr Surg* 1995; 30:856.
43. Kilton L, Matthews MJ, Cohen MH: Adult Wilms' tumor: a report of prolonged survival and review of the literature. *J Urol* 1980; 124:1.
44. Bolande RP, Brough AJ, Izant RJ: Congenital mesoblastic nephroma of infancy: a report of eight cases and the relationship to Wilms' tumor. *Pediatrics* 1967; 40:272.
45. Tomlinson GL, Argyle JC, Velasco G, et al: Molecular characterization of congenital mesoblastic nephroma and its distinction from Wilms' tumor. *Cancer* 1992; 70:2358.
46. Matsumura M, Nishi T, Sasaki Y, et al: Prenatal diagnosis and treatment strategy for congenital mesoblastic nephroma. *J Pediatr Surg* 1993; 28:1607.
47. Snyder HM, III, Lack EE, Chetty-Baktavizian A, et al: Congenital mesoblastic nephroma: relationship to other renal tumors of infancy. *J Urol* 1981; 126:513.
48. Nadasdy T, Roth J, Johnson DL, et al: Congenital mesoblastic nephroma: an immunohistochemical and lectin study. *Hum Pathol* 1993; 24:413.
49. Mascarello JT, Cajulis TR, Krous HF, et al: Presence or absence of trisomy 11 is correlated with histologic subtype of congenital mesoblastic nephroma. *Cancer Genet Cytogenet* 1994; 77:50.
50. Vujavic GM: Congenital cystic mesoblastic nephroma: a rare cystic renal tumour of childhood. *Scand J Urol Nephrol* 1992; 26:315.
51. Pettinato G, Manivel JC, Wick MR, et al: Classical and cellular (atypical) congenital mesoblastic nephroma: a clinicopathologic, ultrastructural, immunohistochemical, and flow cytometric study. *Hum Pathol* 1989; 20:682.
52. Malone PS, Duffy PG, Ransley PG, et al: Congenital mesoblastic nephroma, renin production, and hypertension. *J Pediatr Surg* 1989; 24:599.
53. Ohmichi M, Tasaka K, Sugita N, et al: Hydramnios associated with congenital mesoblastic nephroma: case report. *Obstet Gynecol* 1989; 74:469.
54. Tsuchida Y, Shimizu K, Hata J, et al: Renin production in congenital mesoblastic nephroma in comparison with that in Wilms' tumor. *Pediatr Pathol* 1993; 13:155.
55. Joshi VV, Kasznica J, Walters TR: Atypical mesoblastic nephroma: pathological characterization of a potentially aggressive variant of conventional congenital mesoblastic nephroma. *Arch Pathol Lab Med* 1986; 110:100.
56. Heidelberger KP, Ritchey ML, Dauser RC, et al: Congenital mesoblastic nephroma metastatic to the brain. *Cancer* 1993; 72:2499.
57. Gormley TS, Skoog SJ, Jones RV, et al: Cellular congenital mesoblastic nephroma: what are the options? *J Urol* 1989; 142:479.
58. Kennelly MJ, Grossman HB, Cho KJ: Outcome analysis of 42 cases of renal angiomyolipoma. *J Urol* 1994; 152:1988.
59. Wiederholt WD, Gomez MR, Kurland LT: Incidence and prevalence of tuberous sclerosis in Rochester, Minnesota, 1950 through 1982. *Neurology* 1985; 35:600.
60. Van Baal JG, Smits NJ, Keeman JN, et al: The evolution of renal angiomyolipomas in patients with tuberous sclerosis. *J Urol* 1994; 152:35.
61. Green AJ, Johnson PH, Yates JRW: The tuberous sclerosis gene on chromosome 9q34 acts as a growth suppressor. *Hum Mol. Genet* 1994; 3:1833.
62. Tallarigo C, Baldassarre G, Bianchi G, et al: Diagnostic and therapeutic problems in multicentric and renal angiomyolipoma. *J Urol* 1992; 148:1880.
63. Bernstein J, Robbins TO: Renal involvement in tuberous sclerosis. *Ann NY Acad Sci* 1991; 615:36.
64. Steiner MS, Goldman SM, Fishman EK, et al: The natural history of renal angiomyolipoma. *J Urol* 1993; 150:1782.
65. Uhlenbrock D, Fischer C, Beyer HK. Angiomyolipoma of the kidney: comparison between magnetic resonance imaging, computed tomography, and ultrasonography for diagnosis. *Acta Radiol* 1988; 29:523.
66. Trigaux JP, Pauls C, Van Beers B: Atypical renal hamartomas: ultrasonography, computed tomography, and angiographic findings. *J Clin Ultrasound* 1993; 21:41.
67. Hooper LD, Mergo PJ, Ros PR: Multiple hepatorenal angiomyolipomas: diagnosis with fat suppression, gadolinium-enhanced MRI. *Abdom Imag* 1994; 19:549.
68. Broecker B: Renal cell carcinoma in children. *Urology* 1991; 38:54.

21 Section 1: Upper Urinary Tract Trauma

Hunter Wessells, Jack W. McAninch

The kidney is the most commonly injured genitourinary organ; 8 to 10% of abdominal trauma is associated with renal trauma.[1] Ureteral injury caused by external violence is rare, with most ureteral injuries being iatrogenic. The diagnosis and treatment of upper urinary tract trauma depend on the mechanism of injury, the age of the patient, and the clinical presentation. In this chapter we will review the diagnosis and management of external violence injuries to the adrenal gland, kidney, ureteropelvic junction, and ureter. Appropriate intervention is required to prevent bleeding, obstruction, loss of function, extravasation of urine, and potentially life-threatening sepsis.[2]

ADRENAL TRAUMA

Because of its small size and protected location in the retroperitoneum, the adrenal gland is rarely injured. The majority of reports of adrenal injury in the literature consist of autopsy and radiologic detection of adrenal hemorrhage as a result of blunt trauma.[3,4] A recent report of 14 cases of adrenal trauma included ten caused by penetrating injuries.[5] Adrenal injuries in all cases were detected during either operative or radiographic staging of associated injuries. All patients in this study had extensive associated injuries, a high incidence of shock, and a significant transfusion requirement. There were two deaths. Twelve of the patients required surgery: five underwent adrenalectomy, and the other seven had debridement and hemostatic repair of the adrenal lacerations. There were no documented cases of adrenal insufficiency, and the postoperative course was dictated by the associated injuries.

RENAL TRAUMA

Renal injuries can be divided into two categories based on mechanism of injury: blunt and penetrating. Although the same classification of renal injuries is used in both types of trauma, the clinical and radiographic evaluation differs, as does the need for surgical intervention. Once the decision to operate has been made, the surgical approach and reconstructive techniques are identical.

Blunt Renal Trauma: Initial Evaluation

Blunt trauma accounts for 80 to 90% of renal injuries; motor vehicle accidents, falls, sports injuries, external violence, and assaults are the usual causes. Blunt trauma accounts for a greater proportion of renal injuries in the rural setting compared to urban hospitals.[6] However, only a small percentage will require surgery.[2] Injury can occur as a result of direct blows or deceleration; if the mechanism involves a high-speed motor vehicle or a fall from a significant height, the damage can be extensive. Excessive stretch on the renal artery can cause intimal injury and thrombosis.[2] Associated intra-abdominal injuries are common in such cases, as are shock, loss of conciousness, and multiple bony fractures. An algorithm for the evaluation and management of blunt renal trauma is depicted in Figure 21–1.

HISTORY

In blunt renal trauma the history is important to determine the mechanism of injury and the magnitude of forces involved. Any injury caused by a rapid deceleration can cause major vascular and parenchymal damage, even in the absence of symptoms or physical findings. Pain in the abdomen or flanks should make one suspect renal trauma. Gross hematuria is an indicator of renal injury, although it can be absent and does not correlate with the extent of injury.[7]

PHYSICAL EXAMINATION

The kidney is protected superiorly by the bony thorax.[8] Therefore lower rib fractures, vertebral fractures, transverse process fractures, and flank contusions indicate the possibility of blunt renal injury. An abdominal mass, upper abdominal tenderness, or distention may be due to injury to the kidney or other intra-abdominal organs.

URINALYSIS

Urinalysis should be obtained as soon as possible because hematuria indicates renal injury. A catheterized urine specimen should be obtained if the patient is severely injured. More than five red blood cells per high-power field or a positive urine dipstick implies injury to the kidney, although not the severity.

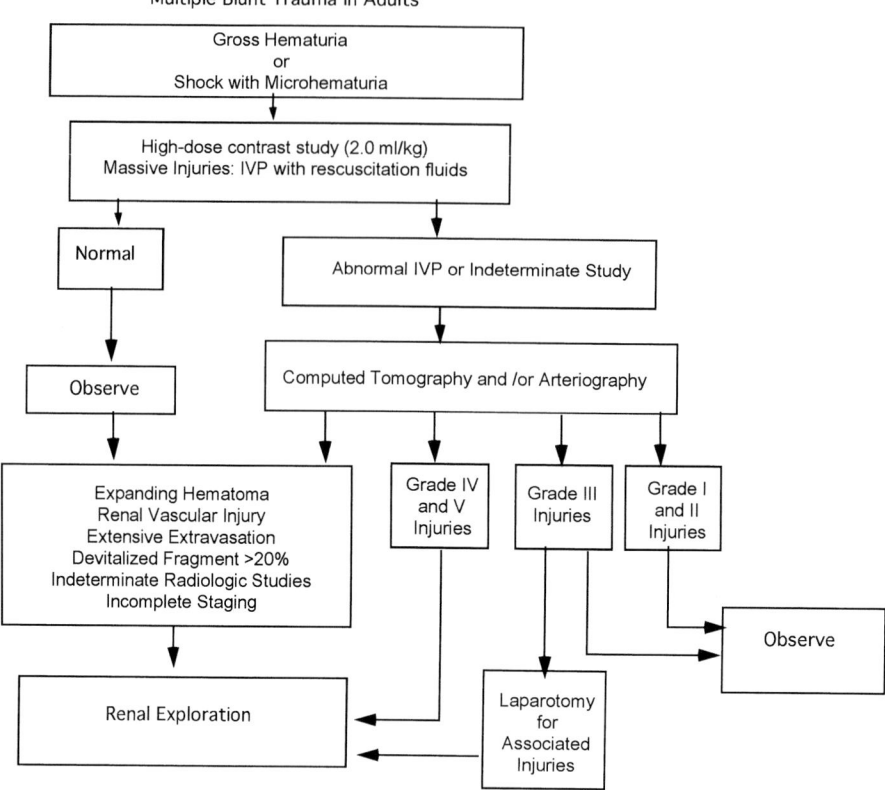

Figure 21-1. Algorithm for the evaluation and management of blunt renal trauma.

Because arterial thrombosis can occur without microhematuria in 28% of cases[9] and not all patients with hematuria have significant renal injury, guidelines for imaging have been developed. In a prospective study of 1007 patients with blunt trauma only those with gross hematuria or microscopic hematuria in the presence of shock (systolic blood pressure < 90 mm Hg) had significant renal injuries. The authors concluded that patients with blunt trauma, microscopic hematuria, and no shock who do not have associated major intra-abdominal injuries can be managed safely without further imaging studies.[10] Major deceleration injuries, signs of an acute abdomen, and suspected liver or spleen injury require imaging by the trauma surgeon that includes the kidneys. Additionally, all pediatric blunt renal trauma requires imaging to stage the extent of renal injury completely.

Penetrating Renal Trauma: Initial Evaluation

Penetrating renal injuries constitute between 10 and 20% of all renal injuries; most are due to gunshot wounds or stab wounds. Virtually all gunshot wounds to the kidney have associated organ injury.[11] In one series stab wounds had associated nonrenal injuries in 77% of cases, although the location of the entrance may affect the incidence of intra-abdominal injuries.[11,12] Most penetrating renal trauma requires operation.[13] At San Francisco General Hospital a nonoperative approach is used in 25 to 50% of cases, all of which are well staged with minor injuries.[2,10,14] An algorithm for the evaluation and management of penetrating renal trauma is outlined in Figure 21-2.

HISTORY

Information regarding the caliber of the weapon and therefore its muzzle velocity helps determine the extent of tissue damage. As muzzle velocity increases, the local tissue damage increases, along with the need for debridement. Most common handguns cause only localized tissue injury. Bullets of the expanding variety cause markedly increased soft-tissue injury.[15]

Information concerning the instrument used in a stab wound should be elicited, specifically the length of the knife, degree of contamination, and whether it was removed intact.

PHYSICAL EXAMINATION

Penetrating wounds to the flank or upper abdomen suggest renal trauma. Entrance and exit wounds should be noted. In the case of stab wounds, some authors have noted a lower incidence of associated injuries when the entrance site is dorsal to the posterior axillary line.[12]

URINALYSIS

Most patients with stab wounds and gunshot wounds to the kidney have hematuria, although its absence does not rule out a significant injury.[16,17] Therefore, regardless of the

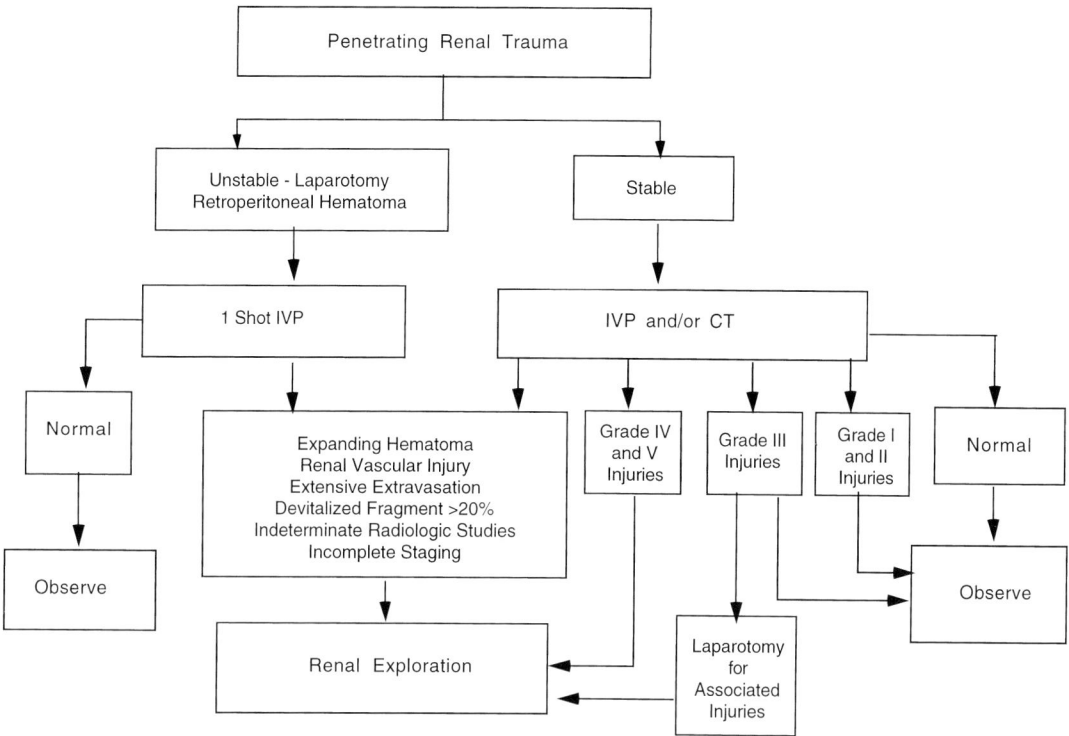

Figure 21-2. Algorithm for the evaluation and management of penetrating renal trauma.

findings on urinalysis, all patients with suspected penetrating renal trauma require complete radiographic or surgical staging.

Classification of Renal Injuries

Renal injuries, whether due to blunt or penetrating trauma, are classified according to severity. The five grades of renal injury as defined by the Organ Injury Scaling Committee of the American Association for the Surgery of Trauma are described in Table 21-1 and Figure 21-3.[18] They can also be divided into minor and major injuries. Minor injuries account for the majority of blunt renal trauma and consist of contusions, small hematomas, and superficial lacerations (grades I and II). These do not involve the deep parenchyma or collecting system and rarely require intervention. Major injuries include deep parenchymal lacerations and collecting system involvement, implying extravasation and more severe bleeding. Vascular injuries and shattered kidneys are also major injuries. This classification system is based on a complete definition of the extent of injury using symptoms, signs, imaging studies, surgery if necessary, and autopsy results to stage the renal injury.

Table 21-1. Classification of Renal Injuries

GRADE	DESCRIPTION OF INJURY
1	Contusion: hematuria with normal radiological studies
	Hematoma: subcapsular and nonexpanding
2	Hematoma: perirenal, confined to retroperitoneum
	Laceration < 1 cm depth without extravasation
3	Laceration > 1 cm depth without collecting system injury or extravasation
4	Laceration: through renal cortex, medulla, collecting system
	Vascular: renal artery or vein injury; contained hemorrhage
5	Laceration: shattered destroyed kidney
	Vascular: renal arterial and venous avulsion

Drawn from Moore EE, et al.[18]

Radiographic Staging of Blunt and Penetrating Renal Trauma

Complete staging of a renal injury is necessary before it can be determined whether surgical intervention is indicated rather than observation. All penetrating renal trauma and all pediatric renal trauma require radiographic imaging. Blunt trauma in the adult requires radiographic staging if gross hematuria or microhematuria with shock is present. When the mechanism of injury is deceleration, imaging of the urinary tract is also mandatory. Only adults with blunt trauma, with microhematuria, and without shock can be managed without imaging of the urinary tract.[10]

The first radiologic study in the stable patient is the high-dose intravenous pyelogram (IVP). Two mg/kg of contrast is recommended. A normal IVP does not need further evaluation. This study should include tomograms to define the

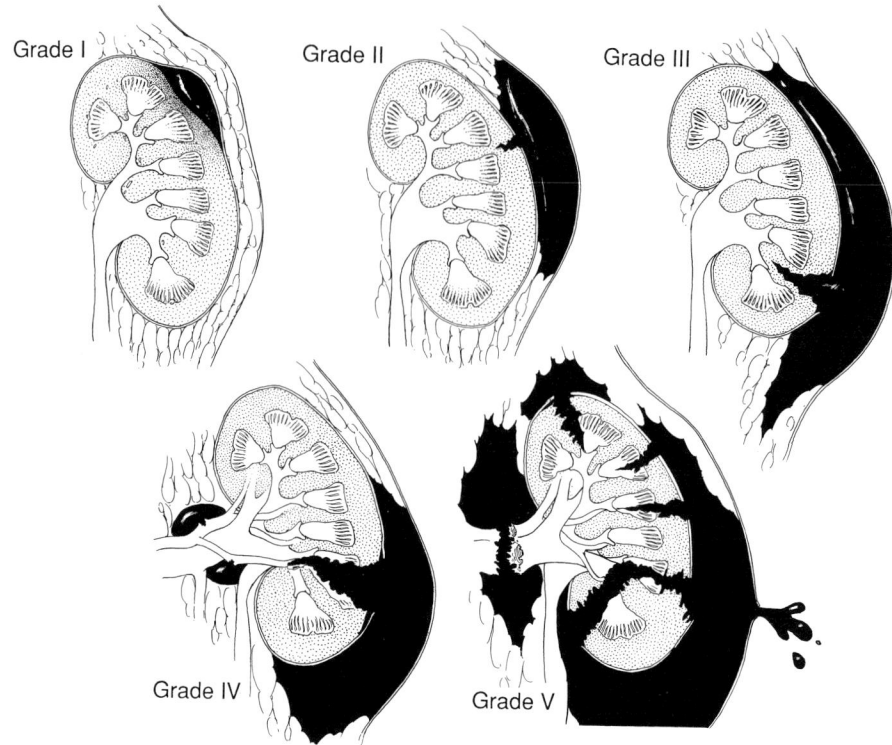

Figure 21-3. Classification of renal injuries. (Based on Moore EE, Shackford SR, Pachter HL, McAninch JW, et al: Organ injury scaling: spleen, liver, kidney. *J Trauma* 1989; 29:1664–1666.

parenchymal integrity as well as visualization of the collecting system, renal pelvis, and ureters. Evidence of major injury is an indication for renal exploration. An indeterminate IVP should be further evaluated with computed tomography (CT). Contrast-enhanced CT will adequately stage renal injuries, including renal arterial injury.[19] CT can show the depth of lacerations, extravasation, devitalized fragments, retroperitoneal hematoma, and any associated intra-abdominal injuries (Fig. 21-4).[20] In the patient undergoing CT evaluation of intra-abdominal trauma, intravenous contrast administration provides the necessary imaging of the kidneys. The IVP is not required in these instances.

The unstable patient requires a different approach to renal imaging. An infusion IVP can be obtained in the resuscitation area. One film 10 minutes after contrast injection should adequately demonstrate the renal outline and the collecting system. If the patient requires immediate laparotomy and the trauma surgeon encounters a retroperitoneal hematoma, an on-table IVP is recommended prior to exploration of the involved kidney. The 10-minute film will assure the presence of a functioning contralateral kidney. Major injuries and indeterminate studies need to be further evaluated, and exploration is the final step in staging the injury. Although the final surgical staging may reveal an injury that could have been managed conservatively, we have successfully repaired these kidneys. No nephrectomies have occurred under these circumstances.

Arteriography has been supplanted to a large extent by computed tomography. If CT cannot clearly exclude a renal arterial injury, arteriography is indicated. In centers where CT is not available arteriography will image renal lacerations and arterial injury adequately.[2] Another use for arteriography is to allow selective angioembolization of segmental renal arterial injuries in patients with severe blunt trauma, stab wounds, or delayed bleeding.[21-23]

Indications for Operation

Indications for renal exploration are controversial but can be divided into absolute and relative indications (Fig. 21-5). Absolute indications include vascular injury, expanding retroperitoneal hematoma, pulsatile hematoma, and extensive urinary extravasation.[24] Extravasation itself may not require intervention, but it implies a significant parenchymal injury. Relative indications include nonviable renal parenchyma in excess of 20% of the kidney and incomplete staging resulting from emergency laparotomy. Penetrating injuries to the kidney require exploration in all cases unless complete radiographic staging confirms the presence of a minor injury without any associated organ injuries.

Indications for Nonoperative Management

Adults with blunt trauma, microscopic hematuria, no deceleration injury, and no shock can be discharged without radiographic studies. Patients with well-staged minor injuries can also go home unless they have gross hematuria. Patients with gross hematuria should remain at bedrest in the hospital until the bleeding resolves; if the urine remains clear with activity, they can be discharged. If gross hematuria persists

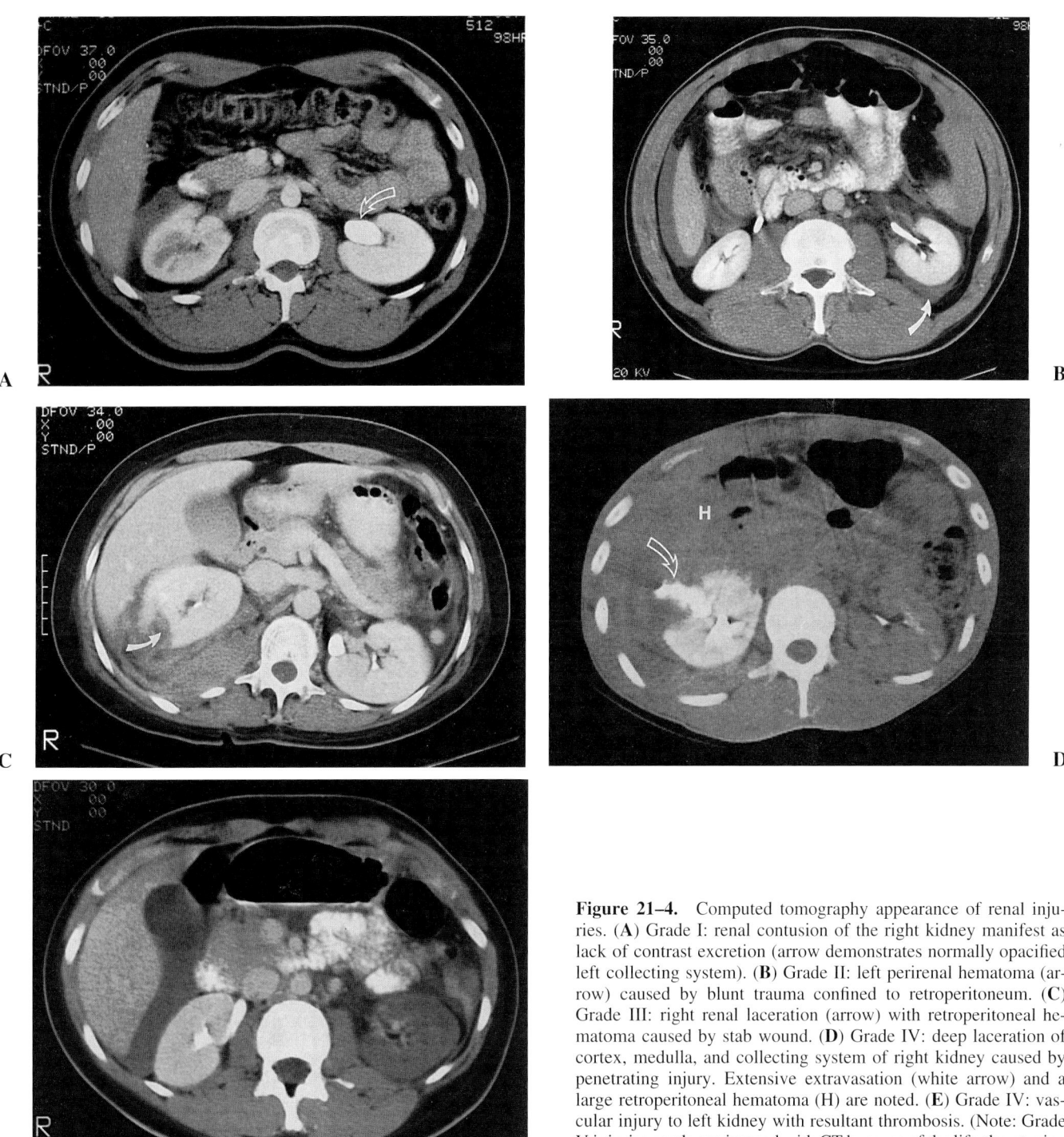

Figure 21–4. Computed tomography appearance of renal injuries. (**A**) Grade I: renal contusion of the right kidney manifest as lack of contrast excretion (arrow demonstrates normally opacified left collecting system). (**B**) Grade II: left perirenal hematoma (arrow) caused by blunt trauma confined to retroperitoneum. (**C**) Grade III: right renal laceration (arrow) with retroperitoneal hematoma caused by stab wound. (**D**) Grade IV: deep laceration of cortex, medulla, and collecting system of right kidney caused by penetrating injury. Extensive extravasation (white arrow) and a large retroperitoneal hematoma (H) are noted. (**E**) Grade IV: vascular injury to left kidney with resultant thrombosis. (Note: Grade V injuries rarely are imaged with CT because of the life-threatening nature of injuries and need for immediate intervention.)

or returns with ambulation, repeat imaging with CT or arteriography is recommended.[2]

The management of more significant blunt renal injuries is controversial. With improved staging and a defined set of indications for exploration only 2.1% of patients require surgery for blunt trauma at our trauma center.[14] It is clear that many severely injured kidneys can be managed nonoperatively.[25,26] However, the risks of delayed bleeding, persistent extravasation, and sepsis must be considered when a major renal injury is not repaired immediately. Husmann and associates reported a much higher complication rate in patients with concomitant blunt renal and intraperitoneal injuries when expectant rather than surgical management was chosen.[27] Because almost all patients with intra-abdominal injuries undergo laparotomy by the trauma surgeon, it affords the opportunity to explore and repair the injured kidney.

```
INDICATIONS FOR OPERATION FOR RENAL TRAUMA

ABSOLUTE INDICATIONS

Expanding Retroperitoneal Hematoma
Pulsatile Hematoma
Vascular Injury
Extensive Extravasation

RELATIVE INDICATIONS

Devitalized Fragment >20% of the Kidney
Laparotomy for Associated Injuries
Incomplete Staging of Renal Injury
```

Figure 21–5. Indications for renal exploration after trauma.

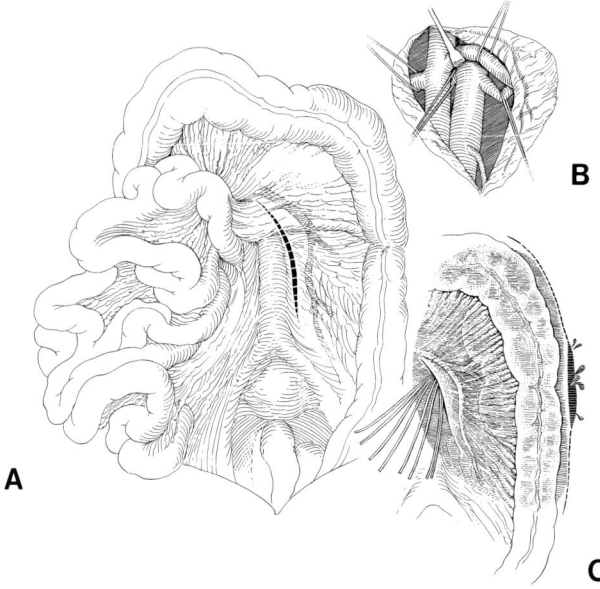

Figure 21–6. Operative approach to the renal vasculature. (**A**) Bowel retracted cephalad to expose posterior parietal peritoneum, which is incised medial to the inferior mesenteric vein. (**B**) Vessels exposed and loops in place. (**C**) White line of Toldt incised lateral to the colon and hematoma entered. (From McAninch JW, Carroll PR: Renal trauma: kidney preservation through improved vascular control—a refined approach. *J Trauma* 1982; 22:285–290. With permission.)

When we explored blunt renal injuries the nephrectomy rate was 12.9%.[14]

A minority of penetrating injuries of the kidney can be managed nonoperatively if complete radiographic staging is possible; contusions and minor lacerations can be observed. Incomplete definition of the extent of injury mandates surgical exploration. Laparotomy is often necessary for the treatment of other injuries, in which case the kidney should be explored and reconstructed. Presently at our institution we explore 45% of stab wounds and 75% of gunshot wounds.[14]

Operative Repair of Renal Injuries

APPROACH

The midline transperitoneal approach to the traumatized kidney has been largely responsible for the reduction in nephrectomy rates.[28] It allows early renal vascular isolation and detection of associated injuries. The incision is made from xyphoid to pubis. After exploration of the abdomen the ligament of Treitz is exposed and the posterior peritoneum overlying the aorta is incised medial to the inferior mesenteric vein (Fig. 21–6). Even in the face of large hematomas dissection over the midabdominal aorta is safe. After exposure of the renal artery and vein, vessel loops are passed to allow immediate access to the renal vasculature.

Once vascular control is gained the colon is resected medially by incising the line of Toldt. Complete exposure of the kidney can be achieved by bluntly dissecting through the hematoma. Examination of the entire kidney, vessels, collecting system, and ureter is mandatory. If massive bleeding occurs the artery should be occluded with a vascular clamp or Rummel tourniquet.

RECONSTRUCTIVE TECHNIQUES

The principles involved in the repair of renal injuries include debridement of nonviable tissue, hemostasis, closure of the collecting system, and coverage of the defect. The amount of tissue debrided depends on the location of the injury as well as the mechanism of injury. Stab wounds generally cause less tissue destruction than gunshot wounds. Debridement is performed sharply with a scalpel to remove any nonviable tissue. The renal capsule should be preserved to aid in subsequent closure of the renal defect. Polar injuries are best debrided by partial nephrectomy (Fig. 21–7). Central defects are best debrided and closed by renorrhaphy (Fig. 21–8). In blunt trauma large devitalized segments may require debridement.

Hemostasis is obtained by figure-of-eight suture ligature of the bleeding vessels with fine, absorbable monofilament on a tapered needle. Manual compression of the kidney during this portion of the procedure will usually control hemorrhage, but occlusion of the renal artery is simple if the vessels have been previously isolated. Closing the defect will often overcome venous pressure and stop venous bleeding. Cautery or hemostatic agents may also be useful in stopping minor bleeding points.

The collecting system should be closed with a running 4–0 chromic suture. A watertight closure of the collecting system does not need internal stenting. If the closure is suspect or if the renal pelvis or ureter is repaired, a double J stent or nephrostomy tube is advisable. Retroperitoneal drains are used routinely.

Defects in the renal parenchyma may be closed primarily in many cases. Interrupted simple or mattress 3–0 chromic

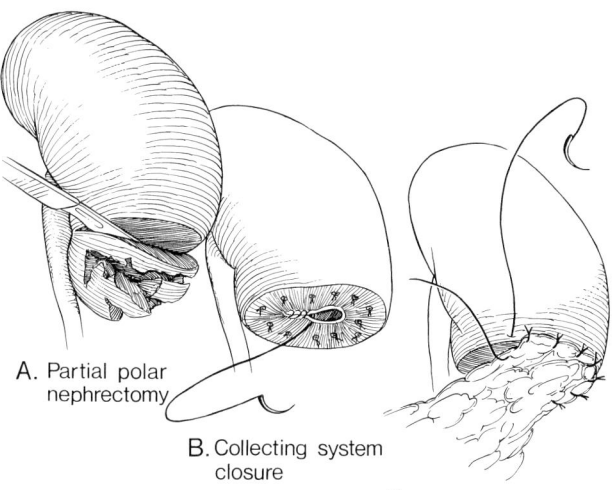

Figure 21–7. Reconstruction of renal polar injury with partial nephrectomy. (**A**) Debridement of nonviable tissue. (**B**) Ligation of vessels and closure of collecting system. (**C**) Coverage of defect with omental pedicle flap.

sutures through the capsule can close small defects. If a capsule is not available, the defect can be covered with an omental pedicle flap, a perinephric fat flap, a dexon patch or wrap, or a free peritoneal graft.

The thrombosed or lacerated main renal artery can be reconstructed by excision and primary repair, saphenous vein graft interposition, prosthetic graft, or rarely autotransplantation. Segmental arterial lacerations can be repaired primarily using an interrupted vascular technique; when deep parenchymal lacerations also occur, partial nephrectomy is indicated. Venous injuries may be more difficult to detect even with CT. Injury to the main renal vein can be repaired with fine vascular sutures once total vascular control has been achieved. Complete disruption of the vein associated with massive bleeding usually mandates nephrectomy. Segmental renal vein injuries can be ligated because of the existence of intrarenal venous collaterals.

POSTOPERATIVE CARE

Patients are managed just as they would be after any major intra-abdominal procedure. Nasogastric tube decompression is continued until the return of peristalsis. Urethral catheter drainage is maintained until the patient is stable and can void. If drains are left in the retroperitoneum, removal within 48 hours is usually possible unless leakage is evident. Persistent urinary extravasation after 5 to 7 days may occur because of poor collecting system closure or ureteral obstruction from clots.[2] Intravenous urography is helpful in these situations. Continued closed drainage of the area and relief of ureteral obstruction will allow closure of the leak.

Hematuria usually resolves within 24 to 48 hours after renal repair, at which point the patient may be allowed to ambulate. Serial hematocrit determination is useful in unstable patients. Patients can be discharged once they can tolerate a regular diet and can ambulate freely.

Follow-up is essential to document the resolution of hematuria and monitor blood pressure. An IVP or nucleotide

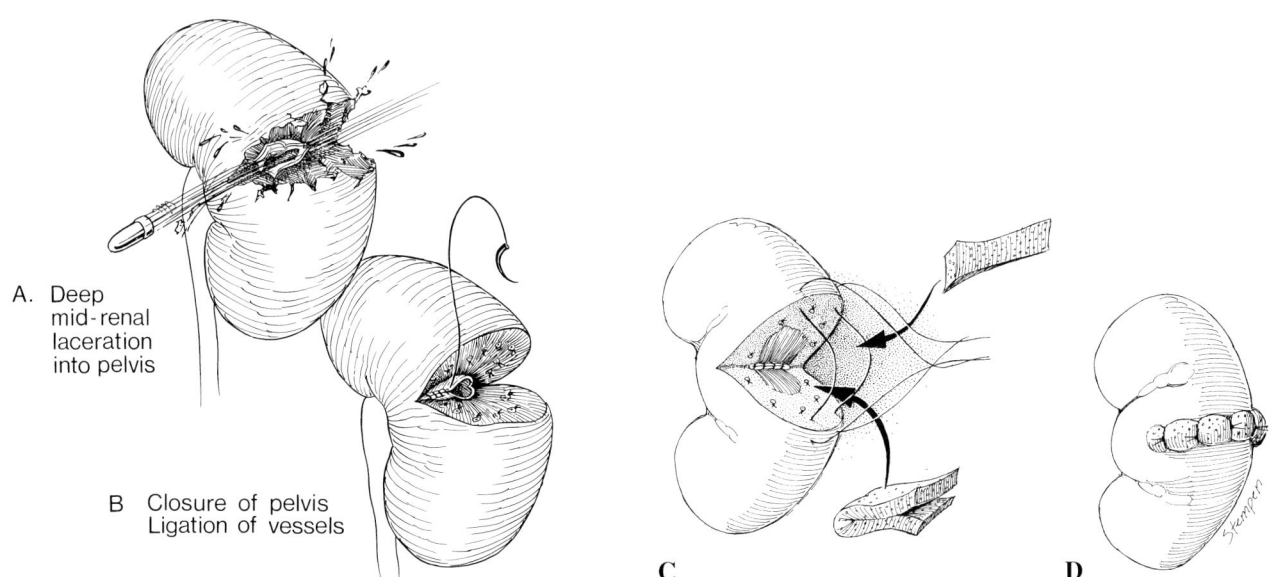

Figure 21–8. Reconstruction of midpole renal injury with renorrhaphy: (**A**) Typical deep laceration involving collecting system. (**B**) Debridement, hemostasis, and collecting system closure. (**C**) Placement of gelatin sponge bolsters and capsular sutures. (**D**) Final reapproximation.

renal scan at 3 months postinjury will assess function and possible obstruction of the reconstructed kidney.

COMPLICATIONS

Complications may develop as a result of surgical intervention as well as the decision not to operate. The reported complication rate varies widely, ranging from 3 to 20%;[28] complications are rare in our experience. The most common early complications are delayed bleeding, urinoma, fistula, abscess, and hypertension. These usually occur within 4 weeks of injury. Delayed bleeding is most likely within the first 2 weeks, and if heavy may require transfusion or exploration. Urinoma may form as a result of untreated extravasation or as a postoperative complication. Urinary fistulas may occur in association with undrained collections or as a result of necrosis of tissue devitalized by the blast effect of gunshot wounds. Abscesses of the retroperitoneum are associated with high fever and sepsis; CT can provide accurate diagnosis and allow percutaneous drainage in selected cases. Prompt surgical drainage is necessary in those not amenable to interventional techniques. Hypertension in the early postoperative period is usually transient and does not require treatment.

Late complications include delayed hypertension, arteriovenous fistula, hydronephrosis, chronic pyelonephritis, and calculus formation.[1] Hypertension after renal injury has been reported in 0.7 to 33% of patients. The causes include renovascular hypertension due to an ischemic segment; arteriovenous fistula; and scarring resulting in a Page kidney.[29] If medical management fails, surgical correction is necessary. Obstruction due to scarring in the region of the renal pelvis and ureter can lead to stone formation and chronic infection.

URETERAL INJURIES

Renal pelvis and ureteral injuries due to external violence make up less than 1% of all urologic trauma. Almost all of these are the result of penetrating wounds, although blunt trauma is associated with ureteropelvic junction disruption, especially in children. The diagnosis can be difficult because of the lack of physical signs of injury, and delayed presentation is not uncommon. One-third to one-half of ureteral injuries are not recognized immediately.[30,31] Therefore a high index of suspicion is always necessary to avoid the late complications of urinoma, sepsis, and nephrectomy.

Mechanism of Injury

Gunshot wounds account for 95% of traumatic ureteral injuries.[32] High-velocity bullets can cause major damage to the ureter as a result of the blast effect. These injuries may not become apparent until several days have passed and necrosis occurs.[2] Stab wounds are another frequent cause of ureteral injury. Blunt injuries of the ureter occur in two populations: pediatric trauma and severe deceleration injuries. The pediatric ureter can be injured by hyperextension of the more flexible spine with avulsion of the ureter at the ureteropelvic junction (UPJ).[32] In adults blunt ureteral injuries are associated with deceleration injury, falls from great heights, and multisystem trauma.[30,31] Iatrogenic injuries secondary to pelvic surgery and ureteroscopy comprise the other major cause of ureteral trauma but will not be discussed here.

Diagnosis

The history and physical examination provide little information regarding ureteral injuries. Signs and symptoms related to associated injuries predominate. Patients usually have gross or microscopic hematuria, but in 10 to 30% it will be absent. Therefore a high index of suspicion is necessary to immediately recognize injuries to the ureter.[33,34]

Contrast-enhanced imaging of the ureter is indicated in all cases of penetrating injury in proximity to the ureter.[35] However, radiographic studies may miss ureteral injuries. Intravenous urography is variably succesful in recognizing ureteral injuries: extravasation of contrast in the retroperitoneum is the most typical appearance (Fig. 21–9A). Hypotension or renal injury may cause delayed excretion of contrast. Presti et al found only three of 18 urograms to be diagnostic of ureteral trauma, whereas Guerriero reports easy recognition of the injury in 90% of cases.[33,36] Computed tomography has rarely been used in the diagnosis of acute ureteral trauma. Extravasation of contrast medial to the renal pelvis suggests ureteropelvic junction injury. CT is very useful to identify urine collections from injuries as well as the site of contrast extravasation (Fig. 21–9B). It must be stressed that without a high index of suspicion ureteral injuries will be missed.

Many patients with ureteral trauma will require immediate laparotomy for associated organ injury, and only a limited IVP will be possible. A nondiagnostic IVP is one of the few good indications for retrograde pyelography if the patient is stable or laparotomy is not planned. Direct intraoperative assessment of ureteral integrity is often required; inspection of the ureter for peristalsis and contusion is mandatory if in proximity to an injury. Adjunct methods such as injection of indigo carmine intravenously or directly into the collecting system may help identify injury.

Indications for Exploration

All injuries to the ureter that are immediately recognized should be repaired surgically. Delayed injuries may be surgically repaired if they are discovered within 10 to 14 days and are not associated with obstruction, infection, abscess,

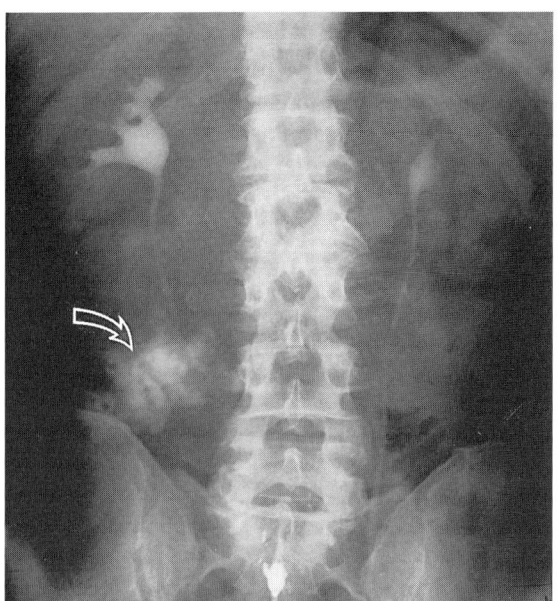 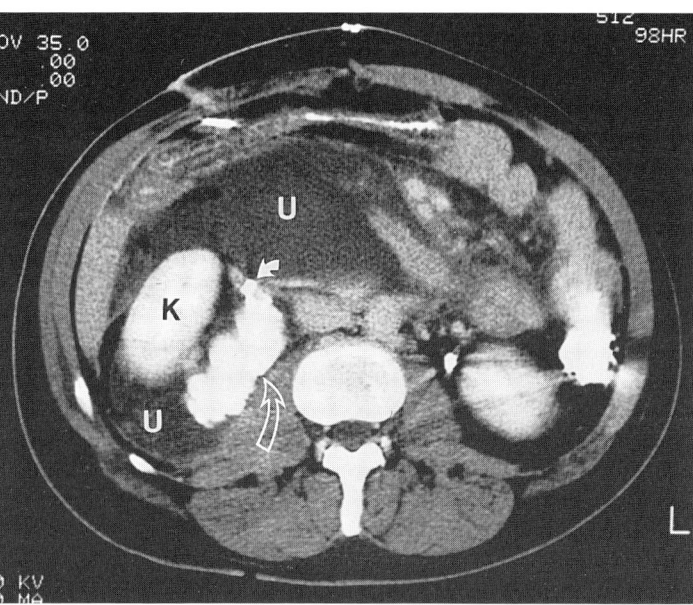

Figure 21-9. (A) Intravenous pyelogram demonstrating ureteral injury after stab wound to the back. Note extensive extravasation of contrast in the region of the midureter on the right (white arrow). (B) Computed tomography demonstrating extravasation of contrast from right upper ureteral injury not recognized at time of laparotomy. Note extravasation (open arrow) from the ureter (white arrow) medial to the kidney (K), as well as large urinoma (U).

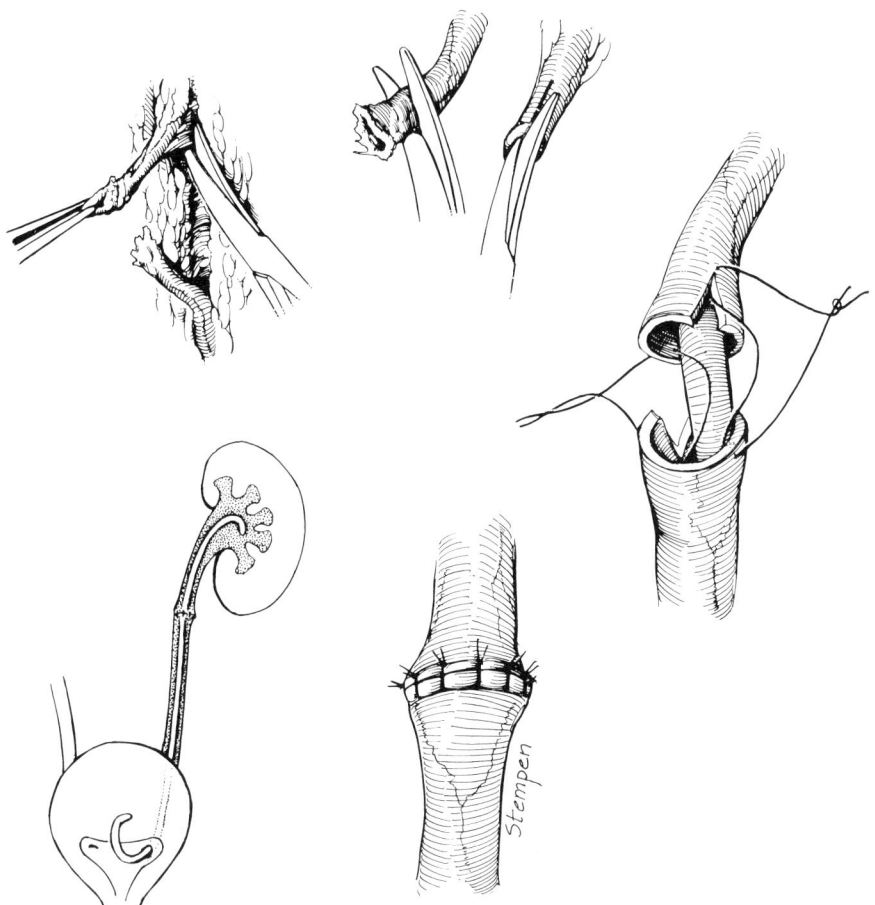

Figure 21-10. Ureteroureterostomy: debridement, spatulation, and precise mucosal apposition performed over an internal ureteral stent. (From Presti JC, Carroll PR: Intraoperative management of the injured ureter. In: Schrock TR ed., *Perspectives in Colon and Rectal Surgery*. St. Louis: Quality Medical Publishers, 1988. With permission.)

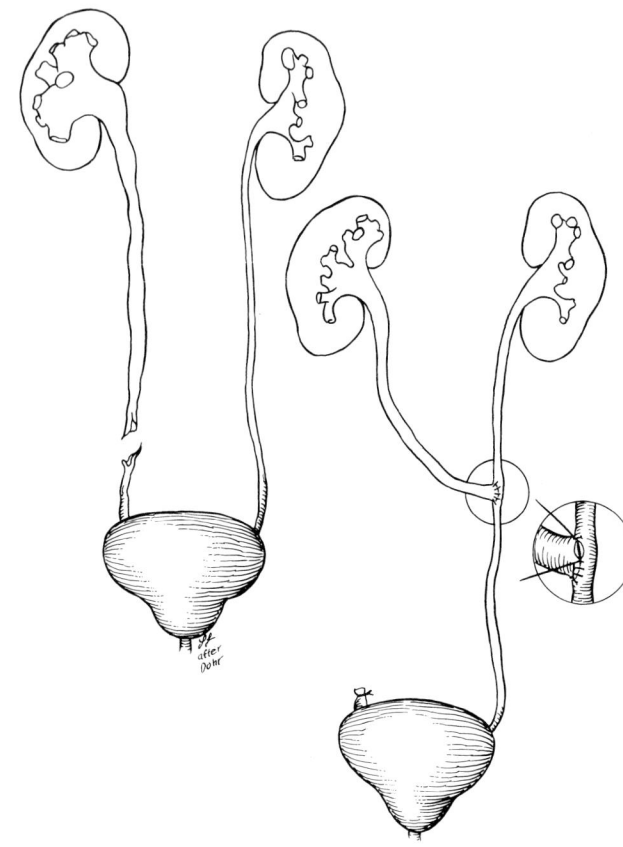

Figure 21–11. Transureteroureterostomy: debridement of ureter, ligation of distal stump, and running closure of transureteroureterostomy. (From McAninch JW: Injuries to the urinary system. In: Blaidsell WF, Trunkey DD, eds. *Trauma Management: Abdominal Trauma, 1.* New York: Thieme Stratton, 1982; 199. With permission.)

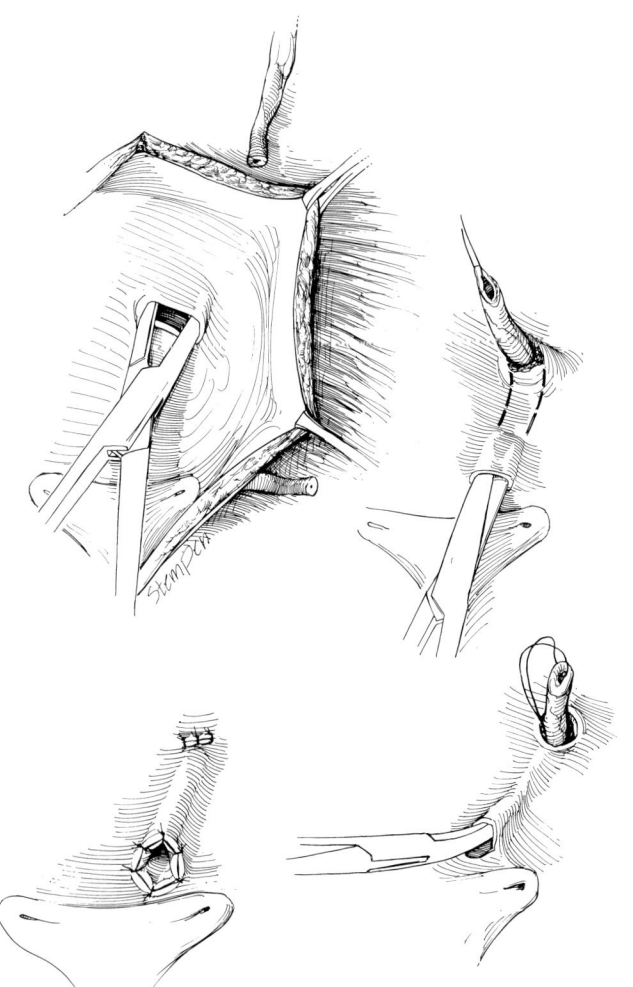

Figure 21–12. Ureteral reimplantation. Creation of neohiatus, development of submucosal tunnel, positioning of ureter through tunnel, and final appearance. (From Presti JC, Carroll PR: Intraoperative management of the injured ureter. In: Schrock TR, ed. *Perspectives in Colon and Rectal Surgery.* St. Louis: Quality Medical Publishers, 1988. With permission.)

or urinoma. In those instances percutaneous nephrostomy and ureteral stenting may allow healing, whereas an open approach may result in nephrectomy. If extravasation or stricture persists, delayed reconstruction in 3 to 6 months is indicated.

Operative Repair of Ureteral Injuries

The reconstruction of ureteral injuries is possible in a high percentage of cases if recognized early and repaired according to general reconstructive principles. These include debridement of devitalized tissue, a spatulated tension-free anastamosis, watertight closure, mucosal approximation, ureteral stenting, coverage of the repair with vascularized tissue, and appropriate drainage. The exact techniques vary according to the mechanism of injury, location of the injury, and whether the transection is partial or complete. Partial transections due to stab wounds can be closed primarily with interrupted 5–0 chromic or vicryl.

Ureteropelvic junction disruption is treated by debridement and primary reanastomosis of the renal pelvis and ureter, as for a pyeloplasty. A ureteral stent and nephrostomy tube are recommended, and a drain should be left in the perinephric space.

Injuries to the abdominal ureter can usually be repaired primarily as depicted in Figure 21–10. Debridement of necrotic tissue, spatulation of both ends, and ureteroureterostomy over a double J stent are feasible in most instances. Interrupted fine absorbable suture should be used. In cases of concomitant bowel or pancreatic injury the omentum should be mobilized and placed between the ureteral repair and other structures. A Penrose-type drain should be placed in the retroperitoneum in all cases. Large defects caused by high-velocity missiles may require transureteroureterostomy (Fig. 21–11). This can be performed at the time of initial injury or may be delayed if the patient's condition precludes immediate reconstruction. The injured ureter is passed behind the mesocolon to the contralateral side, where a 1-cm ureterotomy is made on the medial aspect of the intact opposite ureter. Interrupted or running techniques using 5–0 absorbable suture are acceptable. Both ureters should be stented and a retroperitoneal drain left adjacent to the anastomosis.

Lower ureteral injuries in the pelvis are best repaired by ureteral reimplantation. This avoids dependence on the variable blood supply of the distal ureter. The ureter should be brought into the bladder and spatulated prior to anastomosis to the bladder mucosa with 4–0 absorbable suture (Fig. 21–12). Creation of a submucosal tunnel is desirable to prevent reflux. To achieve a tension-free anastomosis with longer defects, a psoas hitch (Fig. 21–13) may be necessary. If the bladder is not injured a Boari flap can bridge even longer defects (Fig. 21–14). If there is significant bladder damage caused by a gunshot wound, a transureteroureterostomy is preferable. A ureteral stent should always be used; the bladder is closed in two layers and a drain is placed in the space of Retzius. In females a Foley catheter is sufficient for bladder drainage, but in males a suprapubic catheter is recommended as well.

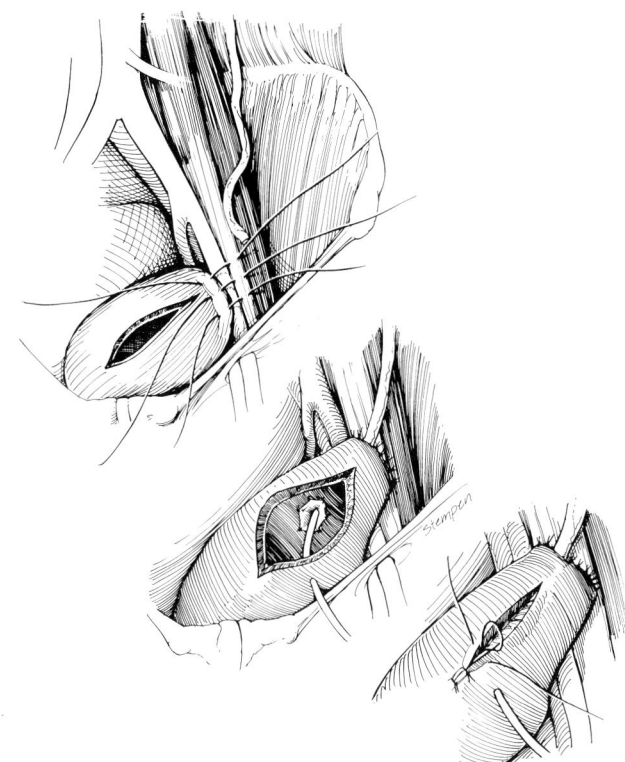

Figure 21–13. Ureteral reimplantation with vesicopsoas hitch. Mobilized bladder anchored to central tendon of psoas muscle; reimplantation of ureter medially; closure of cystotomy. (From Presti JC, Carroll PR: Intraoperative management of the injured ureter. In: Schrock TR, ed. *Perspectives in Colon and Rectal Surgery.* St. Louis: Quality Medical Publishers, 1988. With permission.)

Postoperative Care

Bladder drainage should be maintained for at least 7 days. Cystography should be performed prior to the removal of the bladder catheter. If voiding is normal without increase in drain output, the perivesical drain can be removed. If pediatric feeding tubes are used, a contrast study can be performed at 7 to 10 days, prior to removal of the stent. Double J stents should be removed at 3 or 4 weeks. Follow-up intravenous urography 1 month after stent removal is necessary to rule out obstruction. Obstruction can be asymptomatic, and therefore repeat imaging at 1 year is advisable.

Complications

Complications may occur because of delay in diagnosis or as a result of inadequate healing of surgical repairs. Delayed

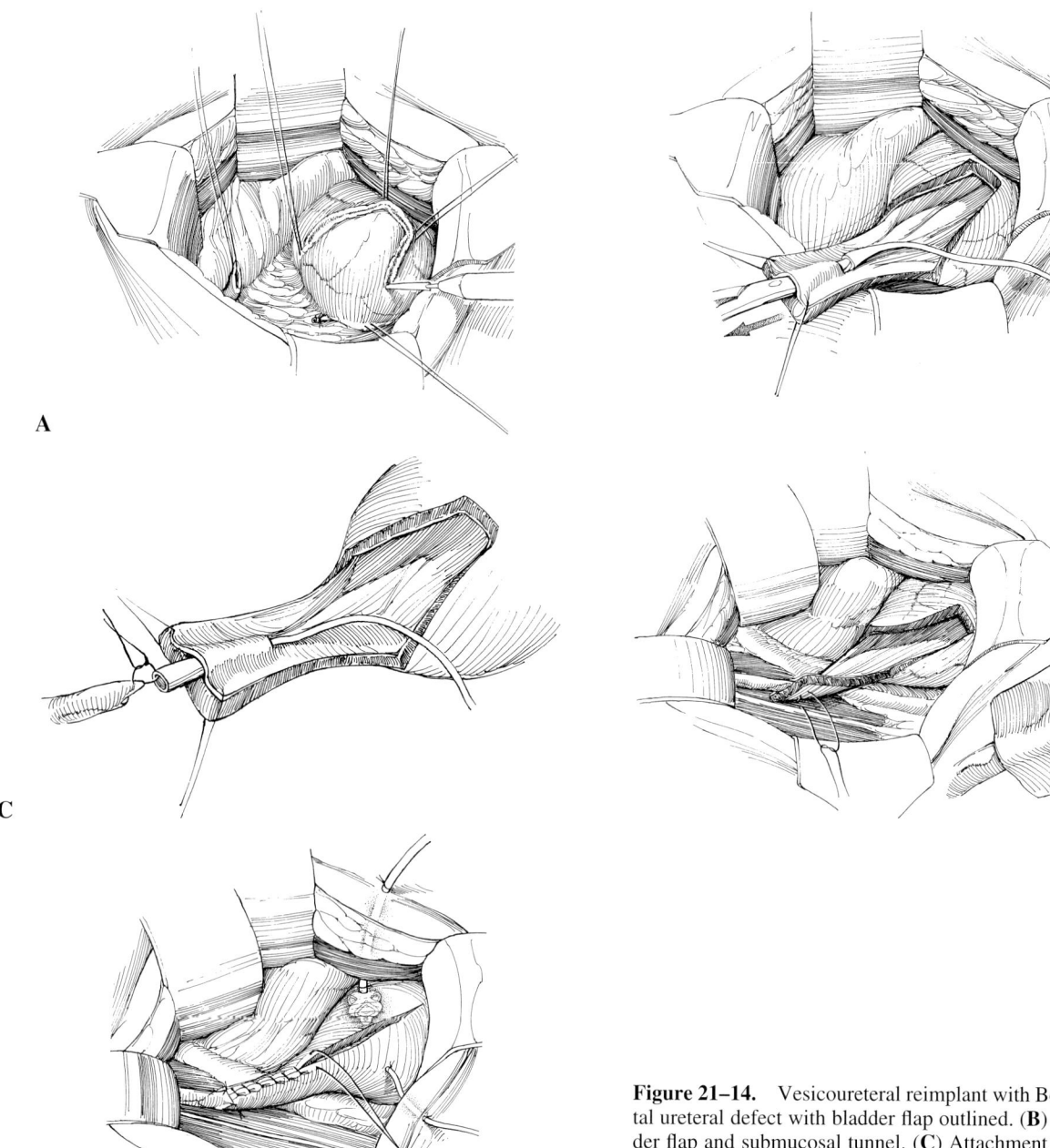

Figure 21–14. Vesicoureteral reimplant with Boari flap. (**A**) Distal ureteral defect with bladder flap outlined. (**B**) Creation of bladder flap and submucosal tunnel. (**C**) Attachment of ureter to catheter to allow positioning through tunnel. (**D**) Fixation of flap to psoas minor and spatulated anastomosis. (**E**) Bladder flap closure as tube. (From Hinman F Jr: *Atlas of Urologic Surgery*. Philadelphia: WB Saunders, 1989. With permission.)

recognition of UPJ disruption was associated with a significantly higher rate of complication and nephrectomy in a literature review by Boone et al.[31] The sequelae of missed ureteral injury include abscess, urinoma, fistula, and obstruction. These entities may present with a nonspecific picture of ileus, fever, and flank pain.

After operative reconstruction hydronephrosis may develop as a result of stricture, retroperitoneal fibrosis, or urinoma. A slow leak from a repair may result in urinoma formation; if this becomes infected, sepsis will result. Fistula formation implies obstruction and usually responds to ureteral stenting. Urinary tract infections must be treated promptly in these patients to prevent ascending involvement of the kidney and retroperitoneum.

REFERENCES

1. McAninch JW : Renal injuries. In: Gillenwater JY, Grayhack JT, Howards SS, Duckett JW, eds. *Adult and Pediatric Urology*. St Louis: Mosby Year Book, 1991.

2. McAninch JW: In Maddox KL, Moore EE, Feliciano DV, eds. Genitourinary trauma, Stamford, CT: Appleton & Lange, 1988; 537–552.
3. Sevitt S: Post-traumatic adrenal apoplexy. *J Clin Pathol* 1955; 8: 194.
4. Murphy BJ, Casillas J, Yrizarry JM: Traumatic adrenal hemorrhage: radiologic findings. *Radiology* 1988; 169: 703.
5. Gomez RG, McAninch JW, Carroll PR: Adrenal gland trauma: diagnosis and management. *J Trauma* 1993; 35: 870–874.
6. Krieger JN, Algood CB, Mason JT, et al: Urological trauma in Pacific Northwest: etiology, distribution, management and outcome. *J Urol* 1984; 132: 70–73.
7. Bright TC, White K, Peters PC: Significance of hematuria after trauma. *J Urol* 1978; 120: 455–456.
8. Moore KL: *Clinically Oriented Anatomy*. Baltimore: Williams & Wilkins, 1980.
9. Stables DP, Fouche RF, Van Niekerk JP, et al: Traumatic renal artery occlusion. *J Urol* 1976; 115: 229.
10. Mee SL, McAninch JW, Robinson AL, et al: Radiographic assessment of renal trauma: a 10 year prospective study of patient selection. *J Urol* 1989; 141: 1095–1098.
11. Sagalowsky AI, McConnell JD, Peters PC: Renal trauma requiring surgery: an analysis of 185 cases. *J Trauma* 1983; 23: 128–131.
12. Bernath AS, Schutte H, Fernandes RRD, et al: Stab wounds of the kidney: conservative management in flank penetration. *J Urol* 1983; 129: 468–470.
13. Carroll PR, McAninch JW: Operative indications in penetrating renal trauma. *J Trauma* 1985; 25: 587–593.
14. McAninch JW, Carroll PR, Klosterman PW, et al: Renal reconstruction after injury. *J Urol* 1991; 145: 932–937.
15. Fackler ML: Wound ballistics. In: Trunkey DD, Lewis FR, eds. *Current Therapy of Trauma*. St Louis: Mosby Year Book, 1991.
16. Eastham JA, Wilson TG, Ahlering TE: Urological evaluation and management of renal proximity stab wounds. *J Urol* 1993; 150: 1771–1773.
17. McAninch JW, Carroll PR, Armenakas NA, et al: Renal gunshot wounds: methods of salvage and reconstruction. *J Trauma* 1993; 35: 279–283.
18. Moore EE, Shackford SR, Pachter HL, et al: Organ injury scaling: spleen, liver, kidney. *J Trauma* 1989; 29: 1664–1666.
19. Steinberg DL, Jeffrey RF, Federle MP, et al: Computed tomography appearance of renal pedicle injury. *J Urol* 1984; 132: 1163.
20. Bretan PN, McAninch JW, Federle MP, et al: Computed tomographic staging of renal trauma: 85 consecutive cases. *J Urol* 1986; 136: 561.
21. Kantor A, Sclafani JA, Scalea T, et al: The role of interventional radiology in the management of genitourinary trauma. *Urol Clin North Am* 1989; 16: 255–266.
22. DeBock L, Verhagen PF: Selective embolization in the treatment of severe blunt renal trauma. *Neth J Surg* 1989; 41: 31–34.
23. Eastham JA, Wilson TG, Larsen DW, et al: Angiographic embolization of renal stab wounds. *J Urol* 1992; 148: 268.
24. McAninch JW, Carroll PR: Renal trauma: kidney preservation through improved vascular control—a refined approach. *J Trauma* 1982; 22: 285–289.
25. Husmann DA, Morris JS: Attempted nonoperative management of blunt renal trauma extending through the corticomedullary junction: the short-term and long-term sequelae. *J Urol* 1990; 143: 682–684.
26. Cass AS, Luxenberg M, Gleich P, et al: Long-term results of conservative and surgical management of blunt renal lacerations. *Br J Urol* 1987; 59: 17.
27. Husmann DA, Gilling PJ, Perry MO, et al: Major renal lacerations with a devitalized fragment following blunt abdominal trauma: a comparison between nonoperative (expectant) versus surgical management. *J Urol* 1993; 150: 1774–1777.
28. Scott RF, Selzman HM: Complications of nephrectomy: review of 450 patients and a description of a modification of the transperitoneal approach. *J Urol* 1966; 95: 307–312.
29. Peterson NE: Complications of renal trauma. *Urol Clin North Am* 1989; 16: 221–236.
30. Campbell EW Jr, Filderman PS, Jacobs SC: Ureteral injury due to blunt and penetrating trauma. *Urology* 1992; 40: 216–220.
31. Boone TB, Gilling PJ, Husmann DA: Ureteropelvic junction disruption following blunt abdominal trauma. *J Urol* 1993; 150: 33–36.
32. Corriere JN: Ureteral injuries. In: Gillenwater JY, Grayhack JT, Howards SS, Duckett JW, eds. *Adult and Pediatric Urology*. St. Louis: Mosby Year Book, 1991; 491–498.
33. Presti JC, Carroll PR, McAninch JW: Ureteral and renal pelvic injuries from external trauma: diagnosis and management. *J Trauma* 1989; 29: 370–374.
34. Carlton CE Jr, Scott RJ, Guthrie AG: The initial management of ureteral injuries: a report of 78 cases. *J Urol* 1971; 105: 335–340.
35. Carroll PR, Dixon CM, McAninch JW: The management of renal and ureteral trauma. In: Blaidsell FW, Trunkey DD, eds. *Abdominal Trauma*. New York: Thieme Medical Publishers, 1993; 250–276.
36. Guerriero WG: Ureteral injury. *Urol Clin North Am* 1989; 16: 237–248.

21 Section 2: Lower Urinary Tract Trauma

J. Patrick Spirnak

CLINICAL SIGNIFICANCE

Traumatic bladder injury occurs either as a direct result of external violence or as an iatrogenic complication during the course of any pelvic operative procedure. When recognized promptly and properly repaired, bladder injury seldom leads to significant postoperative morbidity; however, when undiagnosed or improperly managed, bladder injury may lead to pelvic abscess with sepsis, urinary ascites, or formation of fistulas. These complications usually require additional surgical intervention.

Urethral injury can also occur either as a direct result of external violence or as a result of surgical manipulation. Although urethral disruption in itself is seldom life-threatening, complications such as the formation of strictures can lead to chronic patient morbidity.

ANATOMY

The bony pelvis represents a formidable protective structure for the bladder, prostate, and portions of the male urethra that are contained within. Because the pelvis is a ring, it is not possible to have a single isolated fracture without fracture, dislocation, or diastasis at a second location.[1]

The urinary bladder is an extraperitoneal musculomembranous sac that functions primarily as a urine storage reservoir. In children it is predominantly an abdominal organ lying just beneath the anterior abdominal wall. The bladder assumes its normal adult position as a pelvic organ beneath the symphysis pubis at about the sixth year of life. In men the bladder neck is contiguous with the prostate and is firmly fixed to the posterior surface of the symphysis pubis by the dense puboprostatic ligaments. In females the pubovesical ligaments attach the bladder directly to the pubic symphysis. Inferiorly, the pelvic floor provides the primary support of the bladder. Posteriorly, the base of the bladder is supported by the rectum and is fixed in position by the rectovesical ligaments. In females, similar support is provided by the vagina and uterus. Anteriorly, the medial and paired lateral umbilical ligaments provide support. With the exception of the fixed bladder neck, the remainder of the bladder is free to move and expand in response to bladder filling, and it assumes a globular shape when distended. The superior surface or dome is the least supported as well as the weakest part of the bladder.[2] It is the only surface covered by peritoneum.

The male urethra is divided into anterior and posterior portions. The posterior urethra consists of the prostatic and membranous segments. The prostatic urethra averages 3.0 cm in length and traverses the prostate gland between the bladder neck and verumontanum. The membranous urethra traverses and is firmly fixed to the urogenital diaphragm. It is about 2.0 to 2.5 cm in length. Injury to the posterior urethra in association with pelvic fracture involves the prostatomembranous urethra and is usually associated with pubic rami or symphysis fractures.

Anatomic descriptions of the urogenital diaphragm (triangular ligament, external urinary sphincter) and its relations to the prostate and prostatic urethra vary.[3-5] One concept views the urogenital diaphragm as a thick layer of skeletal muscle sandwiched between two separate fascial layers that span the pubic arch.[6] The apex of the prostate rests on the superior fascial layers, with the prostate being connected to the urogenital diaphragm only by the membranous urethra. When the posterior urethra is traumatically disrupted, it is believed to occur at the level of the natural cleavage plane between the prostate and the superior fascial layers of the urogenital diaphragm.[5] However, anatomic and radiographic studies by Colapinto and McCallum have refuted this classic concept.[4] In cadaveric studies, those workers demonstrated the prostate and urogenital diaphragm to be a single unit with striated muscle extending from the urogenital diaphragm into the prostatic substance. They did not identify a superior layer of fascia distinctly separating the two structures. Contrary to earlier beliefs, the weakest point was actually at the inferior surface of the urogenital diaphragm or at the bulbomembranous urethral junction and not at the prostatomembranous urethral junction. Using cadavers, Colapinto and McCallum experimentally demonstrated the prostate, membranous urethra, and urogenital diaphragm to remain as an anatomic unit during forceful avulsion of the urethra. Radiographic evidence substantiates this theory.[4,7] Patients with complete urethral disruption may demonstrate extravasation into the perineum, a finding one would not expect if the urogenital diaphragm were intact.

Colles's perineal fascia is a continuation of Scarpa's abdominal fascia and of the scrotal dartos fascia.[8] It attaches posteriorly to the urogenital diaphragm, inferior rami of the pubis, and ischium. Laterally, it attaches to the fascia lata of

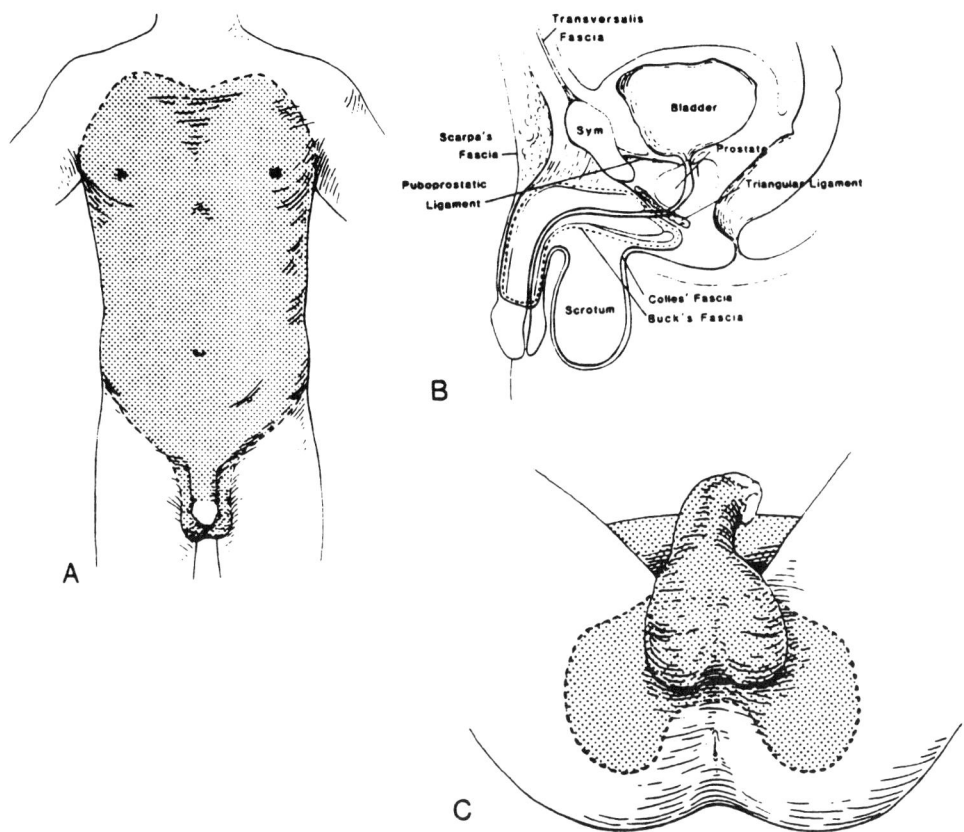

Figure 21–15. (A) The normal male pelvis showing the relationship of the pelvic structures to the associated perineal fascia. (B, C) Potential path of urinary extravasation following the attachments of Colles' fascia. Note the classic appearance of the perineal butterfly hematoma diagnostic of urethral disruption.

the thigh and superiorly to the coracoclavicular fascia. It is of significance only in defining the potential path or urinary extravasation, should the urogenital diaphragm or Buck's penile fascia be disrupted. Urine and blood may extend posteriorly into the perineum and scrotum, yielding the classic butterfly hematoma, or anteriorly to the level of the clavicle. (Fig. 21–15).[9]

ETIOLOGY AND MECHANISM OF UROLOGIC INJURY

Motor vehicle accidents, particularly those involving pedestrians or motorcyclists, are responsibile for the vast majority of pelvic fractures. Less common causes are falls from heights, sporting accidents, and industrial crush injuries.

The incidence of urethral injuries associated with pelvic fracture in men ranges from 1.4 to 11%.[10] Urethral injuries are rare in females, presumably because the urethra is not attached to the pubis.[11] Pokorny and associates have described four mechanisms responsible for urethral injury in pelvic trauma.[12] Three involve shearing forces generated at the time of pelvic disruption. The fourth involves direct laceration by a displaced bony spicule, which is believed to be a rare occurrence.

Bladder rupture occurs in approximately 5 to 10% of patients with pelvic fracture.[7] The injury may be extraperitoneal (50 to 85%), intraperitoneal (15 to 45%), or, rarely, both (none to 12%).[7] Classically, an intraperitoneal rupture consists of a large horizontal tear through the dome of the bladder. The injury is believed to occur with the bladder full as a result of a blow delivered to the lower abdomen. The intravesical pressure becomes acutely elevated, and the bladder perforates at its weakest point. Oliver and Taguchi experimentally demonstrated the bladder dome to be the least supported by adjacent structures and the area of the bladder wall where the muscle fibers are most widely separated, thus making the dome the weakest and most frequent site of intraperitoneal perforation.[2]

Extraperitoneal bladder rupture in association with pelvic fracture usually involves the anterolateral aspect near the bladder neck. Until recently, extraperitoneal perforation was believed to result exclusively from direct penetration of the bladder wall by a bony spicule or by disruption of the ligamentous attachments between the bladder and pelvis.[13,14] However, Carroll and McAninch noted only 35% of the bladder injuries in their series to be on the same side as the pelvic fracture.[15] Cass and Luxenberg reported similar findings[16] and proposed a second mechanism of injury. With the bladder empty, severe lower abdominal trauma may cause bursting or extraperitoneal perforation similar to that which occurs with the bladder full. Thus the pelvic fracture associated with extraperitoneal perforation may be coincidental rather than causative, as initially thought.

Combined urethral and bladder injuries complicated about 1% of pelvic fractures.

DIAGNOSIS

Signs and Symptoms

All patients with pelvic fracture should be suspected of having a urologic injury. Gross hematuria or blood at the urethral meatus are the most common findings in severe urologic injury. As the male urethra tears, the bulbocavernosus muscle contracts, and blood is forced out the urethral meatus. An inability to urinate may be seen in patients with a bladder perforation or a urethral injury; however, more common causes in the trauma victim include an empty bladder or simply an inability to void on command because of pain or shock from the fractured pelvis. Perineal or genital swelling resulting from extravasation of blood or urine may be present. The classic perineal butterfly hematoma is diagnostic of urethral disruption but may not be present in patients examined shortly after the injury. Rectal examination is imperative and may reveal an "absent" prostate, a pelvic hematoma, or more important, an associated rectal laceration. Abdominal tenderness suggests intraperitoneal extravasation of urine or concomitant intra-abdominal visceral injury and warrants further diagnostic evaluation.

WHO NEEDS TO BE EVALUATED?

It has been suggested that all patients with pelvic fracture[17] or pelvic fracture associated with microscopic hematuria undergo radiographic evaluation of the lower urinary tract to rule out urethral or bladder injury.[12,18] Antoci and Schiff in 1982 reviewed 234 patients with pelvic fracture and found 120 patients with microscopic hematuria.[19] All underwent urologic evaluation, which failed to yield a single instance of bladder or urethral perforation. Their review of the literature also failed to reveal a single case of a patient with a pelvic fracture and concomitant microscopic hematuria who had a significant lower urinary tract injury. Fallon has reported similar findings.[20] It would appear that the finding of microscopic hematuria in the absence of other urologic signs and symptoms is a poor predictor of the presence of a significant urologic injury in pelvic fracture patients. Urologic evaluation consisting of a retrograde urethrogram and cystogram is recommended in all male patients with pelvic fractures associated with gross hematuria or blood at the meatus, perineal swelling, nonpalpable prostate, or inability to urinate.

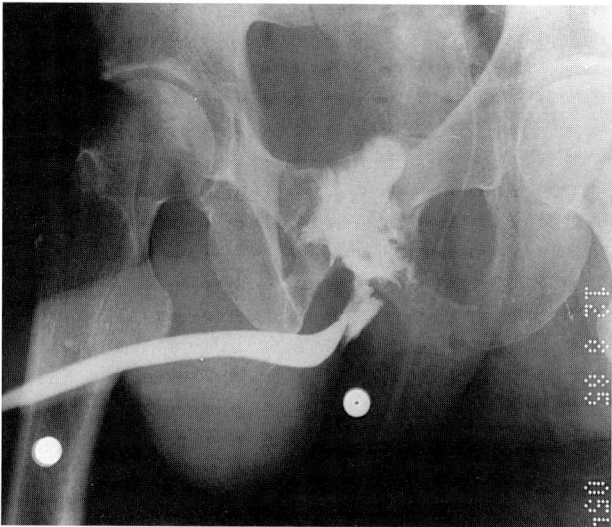

Figure 21–17. Retrograde urethrogram demonstrating complete urethral disruption. Note the absence of bladder filling.

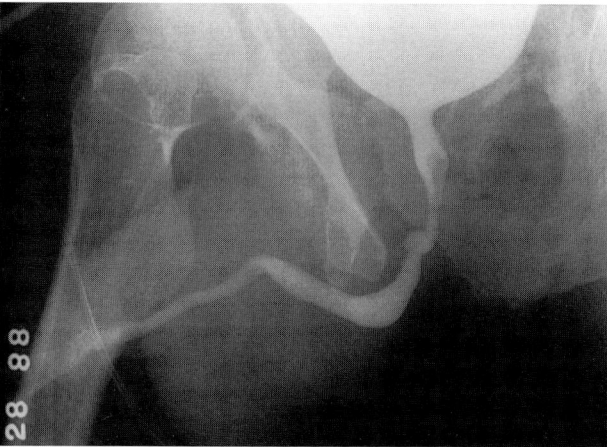

Figure 21–16. Retrograde urethrogram demonstrating free flow of contrast into the bladder without extravasation.

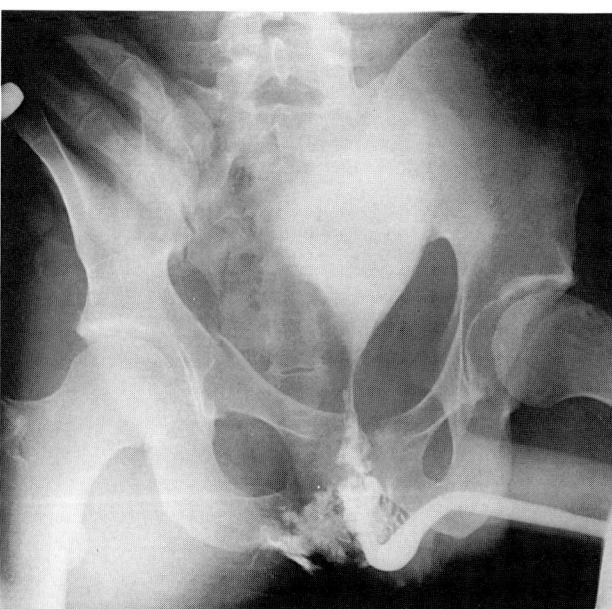

Figure 21–18. Retrograde urethrogram demonstrating a partial urethral disruption. Note extravasation of contrast and partial filling of the bladder.

Radiographic Evaluation of the Male Urethra

To avoid converting a partial urethral tear into a complete disruption, trauma victims with suspected lower urinary tract injuries should not undergo urethral catheterization until the integrity of the urethra has been radiographically demonstrated. Ideally, a retrograde urethrogram is performed with the patient in the oblique position with the penis stretched perpendicular to the femur. By positioning the patient obliquely, foreshortening of the bulbous urethra is avoided, and the entire urethra may be adequately examined. However, it is not always possible to position all trauma victims obliquely. In such cases, a urethrogram adequate to rule out urethral disruption may be obtained with the patient flat by placing the penis on stretch perpendicular to the lower extremity. Water-soluble contrast medium (30 to 40 mL) is instilled into the urethra through a 14F Foley catheter placed into the distal urethra and inflated with 2 to 3 mL of sterile water. A film is obtained while the last 10 mL is being instilled. If the urethra is normal (i.e., no sign of extravasation), the catheter is advanced into the bladder and a cystogram is performed (Fig. 21–16).

Extravasation of contrast medium without filling of the bladder is diagnostic of a complete urethral disruption (Fig. 21–17). Partial urethral disruption is diagnosed in the presence of extravasation with partial filling of the bladder (Fig. 21–18).

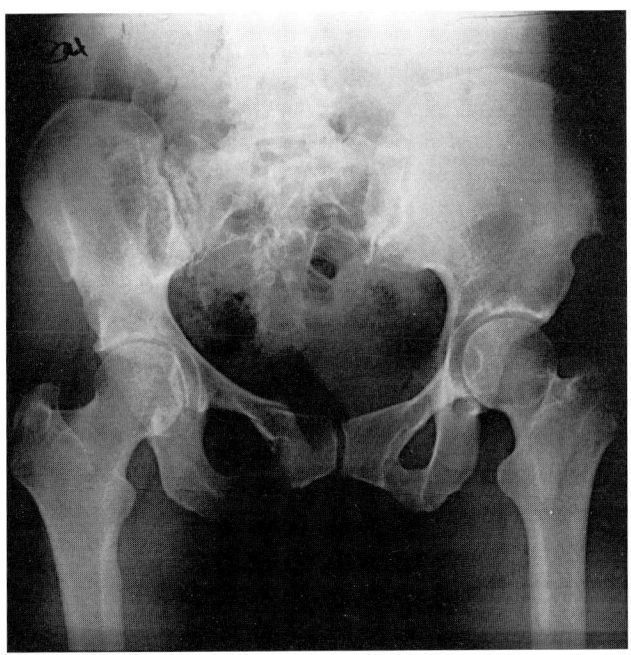
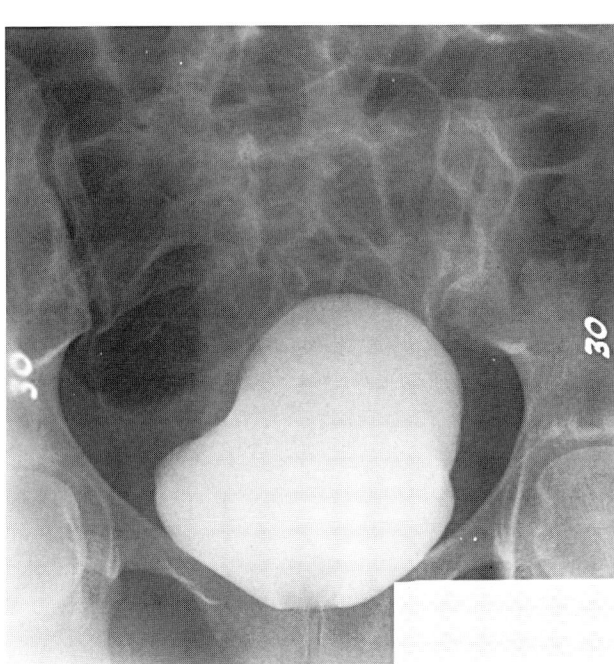
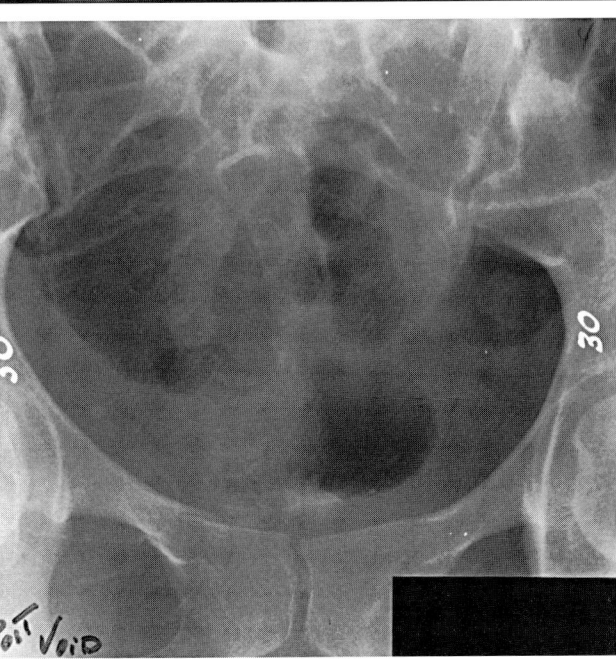

Figure 21–19. A normal cystogram. (**A**) Plain film demonstrating pelvic fracture. (**B**) Anteroposterior film showing a filled bladder. (**C**) Drainage film showing absence of extravasated contrast.

Bladder Evaluation

In male patients, after urethral trauma has been ruled out, the catheter is advanced into the bladder and a cystogram is performed. In females the urethra is examined and a 16F Foley catheter is placed.

Cystography when properly performed has an accuracy rate approaching 100%.[21] To avoid false-negative results, the bladder must be distended. The importance of bladder distention was demonstrated by Weyrauch and Peterfy when they demonstrated false-negative results in dogs with bladder lacerations 2 cm in length after inadequate bladder filling.[22] After a plain film of the abdomen and pelvis is obtained (Fig. 21–19A), the bladder is filled under gravity with dilute contrast (300 to 400 mL). A bulb syringe is attached to the Foley and contrast is administered until the bladder is full or until a detrusor contraction occurs. Bladder filling under fluoroscopy is helpful but is usually not practical in the trauma setting. With the bladder full an anteroposterior film is obtained (Fig. 21–19B). The bladder is then emptied and a drainage film is obtained (Fig. 21–19C). Small amounts of extravasation not seen behind a contrast-filled bladder are readily identified on the drainage film.

Cystographic findings diagnostic of an extraperitoneal bladder perforation include a teardrop-shaped bladder secondary to compression by a pelvic hematoma associated with the extravasation of contrast medium confined to the pelvis. Radiographically, the extravasation may range from flamelike wisps or linear streaks to large stellate or sunburst patterns, which may be more obvious on the postdrainage film (Fig. 21–20). Radiographically, intraperitoneal bladder perforation may produce diffuse extravasation of contrast medium throughout the peritoneal cavity with no discernible pattern. Extravasated contrast may accumulate in the dependent portion of the pelvis, obscuring the superior aspect of the bladder and producing an hourglass configuration. Contrast may also accumulate in the paracolic gutters or beneath the diaphragm (Fig. 21–21).

Treatment

Intraperitoneal perforation of the bladder requires prompt surgical exploration and bladder repair. The treatment of extraperitoneal perforation is currently controversial. Tears associated with minimal urinary extravasation are managed by urethral catheter drainage. Indications for bladder exploration and closure include poor drainage caused by clots, persistent extravasation, or fever. If the patient is undergoing surgical exploration for other causes, the bladder is explored and repaired. A cystogram is repeated prior to catheter removal.

Partial urethral disruption is treated by either suprapubic urinary diversion or urethral catheter drainage. To avoid converting a partial tear into a complete tear, no one other

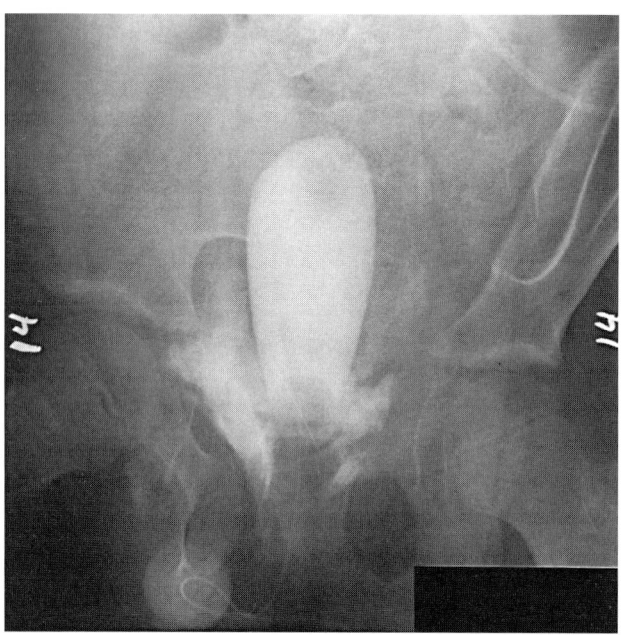
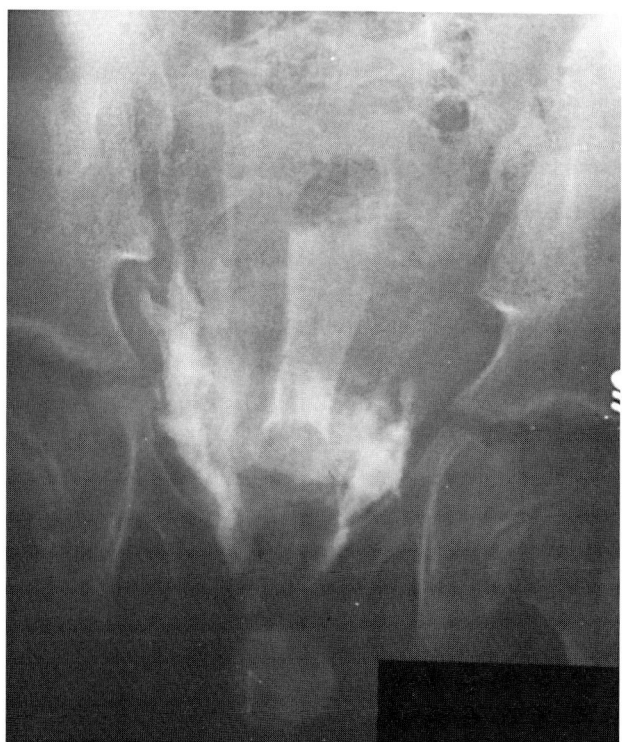

Figure 21–20. Cystographic appearance of extraperitoneal bladder perforation. (**A**) Note the teardrop deformity caused by extrinsic compression by the pelvic hematoma and the flamelike wisps of extravasation confined to the pelvis. (**B**) Drainage film demonstrates persistence of extravasation.

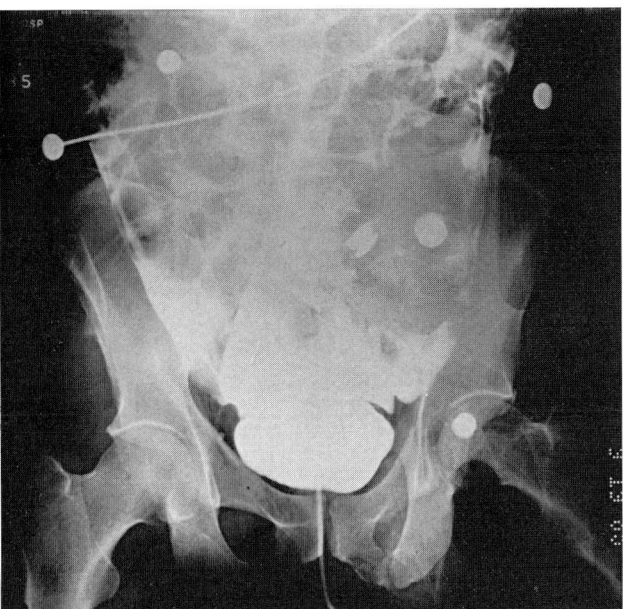

Figure 21-21. Cystographic appearance of intraperitoneal bladder perforation. Note extravasated contrast throughout the peritoneal cavity.

than a urologist should attempt urethral catheterization. The management of complete urethral disruption is controversial. We favor immediate catheter realignment. Others divert the urine through a suprapubic catheter and perform elective urethroplasty 3 to 6 months after the injury.

REFERENCES

1. Ward RE, Clark DG: Management of pelvic fractures. *Radiol Clin North Am* 1981; 19:167.
2. Oliver JA, Taguchi Y: Rupture of the full bladder. *Br J Urol* 1964; 36:524.
3. Chilton CP, Turner-Warwick R: The relationship of the male distal urethral sphincter mechanism to the pelvic floor musculature. *Ann R Coll Surg Engl* 1985; 67:54.
4. Colapinto V, McCallum RW: Injury to the male posterior urethra in fracture pelvis: a new classification. *J Urol* 1977; 118:575.
5. Peters PC, Bright TC III: Management of trauma to the urinary tract. *Adv Surg* 1976; 10:197.
6. Colapinto V: Trauma to the pelvis: urethral injury. *Clin Orthop* 1980; 151:46.
7. Wolk DJ, Sandler CM, Corriere JN Jr: Extraperitoneal bladder rupture without pelvic fracture. *J Urol* 1985; 134:1199.
8. Wesson MB: Fasciae of the urogenital triangle. *JAMA* 1923; 81:2024.
9. Bright TC III, Peters PC: Injuries to the bladder and urethra. In: Harrison JH, Gittes RF, Perlmutter AD, et al, eds.: *Campbell's Urology*, 4th ed. Philadelphia: WB Saunders, 1978; 906.
10. Sandler CM, Harris JH Jr, Corriere JN Jr, et al: Posterior urethral injuries after pelvic fractures. *AJR* 1981; 137:1233.
11. Kaiser TF, Farrow FC: Injury of the bladder and prostatomembranous urethra associated with fracture of the bony pelvis. *Surg Gynecol Obstet* 1965; 120:99.
12. Pokorny M, Pontes JE, Pierce JM: Urologic injuries associated with pelvic trauma. *J Urol* 1979; 121:455.
13. Brosman SA, Fay R: Diagnosis and management of bladder trauma. *J Trauma* 1973; 13:929.
14. Morehouse DD, MacKinnon KJ: Urologic injuries associated with pelvic fractures. *J Trauma* 1969; 9:479.
15. Carroll PR, McAninch JW: Major bladder trauma: mechanisms of injury and a unified method of diagnosis and repair. *J Urol* 1984; 132:254.
16. Cass AS, Luxenberg M: Features of 164 bladder ruptures. *J Urol* 1987; 138:743.
17. Moy HN: Lower urinary tract injuries. *Br J Urol* 1970; 42:739.
18. Clark SS, Prudencio RF: Lower urinary tract injuries associated with pelvic fractures: diagnosis and management. *Surg Clin North Am* 1972; 52: 183.
19. Antoci JP, Schiff M Jr: Bladder and urethral injuries in patients with pelvic fractures. *J Urol* 1982; 128:25.
20. Fallon B, Wendt JC, Hawtrey CE: Urological injury and assessment in patients with fractured pelvis. *J Urol* 1984; 132:712.
21. Carroll PR, McAninch JW: Major bladder trauma: the accuracy of cystography. *J Urol* 1983; 130:887.
22. Weyrauch HM Jr, Peterfy RA: Tests for leakage in the early diagnosis of the ruptured bladder. *J Urol* 1940; 44:264.

22 Diseases and Imaging of the Prostate

David S. Sandock, Martin I. Resnick

The prostate is susceptible to a wide variety of clinical diseases. These range from inflammatory and infectious to benign and malignant growth. The clinical assessment of these disease processes is often difficult and indirect. Though digital rectal examination remains the most direct method of evaluating the prostate, there are currently a wide variety of radiologic and hematologic tests to evaluate the prostate. Transrectal ultrasonography, computed tomography (CT), and magnetic resonance imaging (MRI) may all be of value, but each test has limitations of which the clinician must be aware. In addition, the explosion in the use of prostate specific antigen (PSA) has resulted in an increased referral of patients with prostatic disorders. Recently, two pharmacologic agents have been approved by the Food and Drug Administration (FDA) for the medical management of benign prostatic hyperplasia (BPH), as well as numerous new surgical options to transurethral resection of the prostate (TURP). Finally, the best treatment of carcinoma of the prostate is under considerable debate. This chapter will review the diagnosis of prostatic disorders with an emphasis on imaging studies. It will also review the current treatment strategies and controversies concerning the common prostatic disorders.

ANATOMY OF THE PROSTATE

The prostate is a small, pyramid-shaped gland that surrounds the urethra and is located between the bladder and urogenital diaphragm (Fig. 22–1). The prostate itself is surrounded by a tough fibrous capsule. The base of the prostate abuts the bladder neck and the apex lies distally at the external urethral sphincter. Posteriorly, the prostate is separated from the rectum by the anterior and posterior layers of Denonvillier's fascia. Anteriorly, the prostate is fixed to the bony pelvis by the puboprostatic ligaments. The deep dorsal vein of the penis continues along the anterior surface of the prostate as the venous plexus of Santorini. The nerves to corpus cavernosa of the penis travel along the posterolateral surfaces of the prostate. The verumontanum lies along the posterior prostatic urethra and contains the openings of the ejaculatory ducts. The seminal vesicles lie posterior to the bladder and join the vas deferentia to form the ejaculatory duct.

The prostate is composed of several regions comprising different areas of glandular and nonglandular tissue (Fig. 22–2).[1] The glandular region is divided into three zones (peripheral, transition, and central) and the periurethral glands. The nonglandular region is located in the anteromedial portion of the gland and is composed of fibromuscular stroma. The periurethral glands make up about 1% of prostatic glandular tissue and are located in the smooth muscle of the urethra in the preprostatic sphincter. Benign hyperplasia in the periurethral glands leads to an enlarged middle lobe.[2,3]

The peripheral zone lies posteriorly and laterally in the prostate. The glandular architecture consists of small, round acini amid loosely woven, randomly oriented stroma. Approximately 70% of the prostate gland lies in the peripheral zone. This zone does not undergo benign hyperplasia but is the site of origin of 70% of all prostate carcinoma.

The transition zone is located on both sides of the distal two-thirds of the proximal urethral segment.[4] This is the main site of origin of benign prostatic hyperplasia (BPH). In young men this zone represents approximately 5% of prostatic volume, whereas in older men with BPH the transition zone may comprise 90% of the prostate gland. Approximately 20% of prostate cancer originates in this zone.

The central zone surrounds the ejaculatory ducts as they travel through the prostate tissue to the verumontanum. This zone comprises most of the prostatic tissue at the base of the prostate and narrows as it approaches the opening of the ejaculatory ducts into the verumontanum. The central zone compromises approximately 25% of the prostate and is the site of origin of about 10% of carcinomas.

The main arterial supply to the prostate is from the inferior vesical artery, although it also receives some flow from the obturator and inferior gluteal arteries. The venous drainage of the prostate is via veins paired to the previously named arteries as well as to the anterior prostatic plexus, which drains into the hypogastric veins. Lymphatic drainage from the prostate is to the obturator, external iliac, and internal iliac lymph node groups. Further lymph node drainage travels to the common iliac and preaortic nodes.

PHYSICAL EXAMINATION OF THE PROSTATE

Palpation of the prostate may be performed in the lateral decubitus position, or more commonly, with the patient

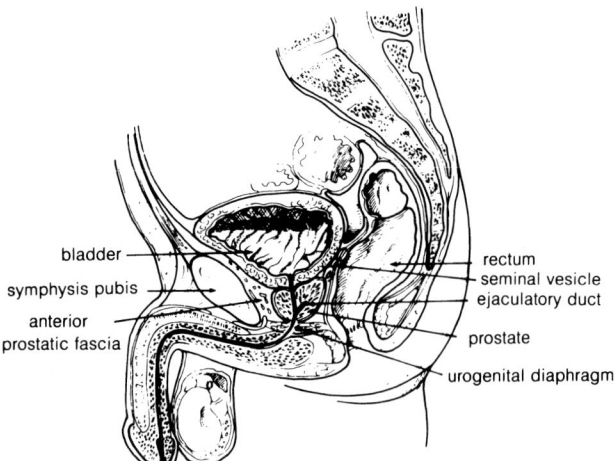

Figure 22–1. Prostate and anatomic relations. Midsagittal section of the male pelvis demonstrating the relationships of the prostate to adjacent structures.

standing and bending over the examination table. The anus should be visually examined for disorders. As the gloved, well-lubricated finger is inserted, rectal tone should be assessed. The apex of the prostate gland is palpated first, followed by both sides of the gland all the way to the base. The consistency of normal prostate tissue is similar to that of the contracted thenar muscles. Increased firmness, nodules, asymmetry, tenderness, bogginess, and loss of normal architecture (loss of median sulcus or sharp lateral borders) are all considered abnormal.

IMAGING OF THE NORMAL PROSTATE

Transrectal Ultrasound of the Prostate

Ultrasound technology was first applied to the prostate in 1951 by Wild and Reid.[5] The images were very poor using the time amplitude echogram technology available at that time and little prostate ultrasonography was performed until the introduction of transrectal B-mode ultrasonography by Wantabe 17 years later.[6] In 1969 Boyce et al developed a hand-held transrectal ultrasound (TRUS) probe, replacing the older chair-mounted models.[7] King et al reported the first large series of transrectal ultrasonography findings.[8] The introduction of gray-scale imaging by Boyce and Resnick led to the introduction of more clinically useful images.[9] The addition of high-frequency transducers, real-time imaging,

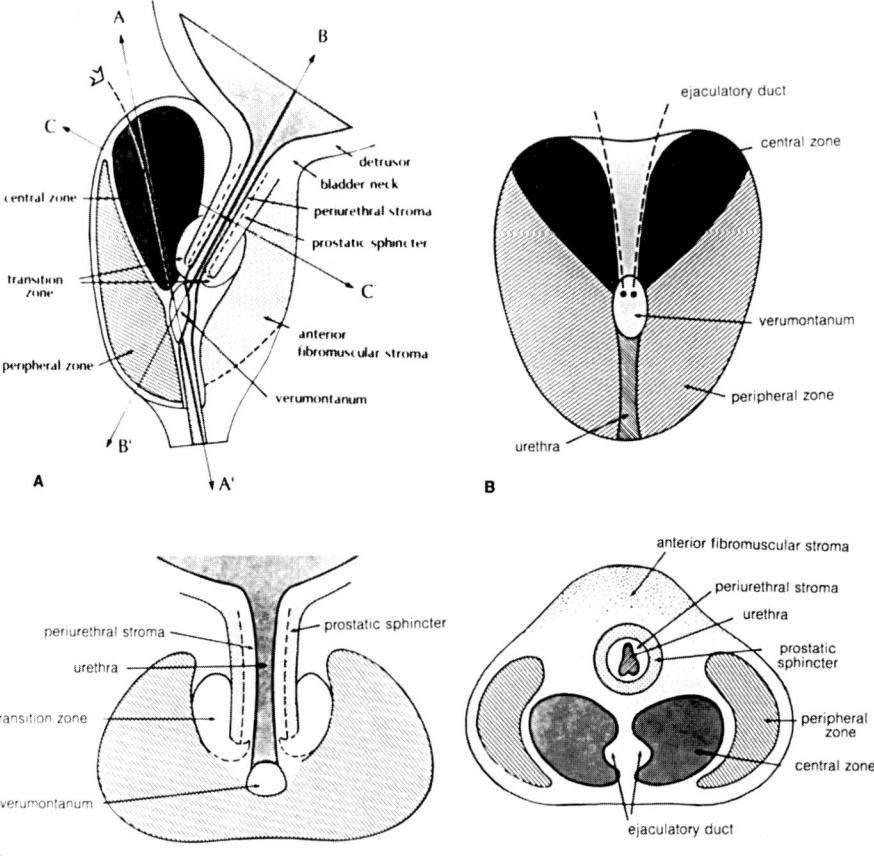

Figure 22–2. Diagrammatic representations of prostatic internal architecture. **(A)** Midsagittal plane. Note that the open arrow points to course of ejaculatory ducts. **(B)** Coronal section along A–A'. **(C)** Oblique section along B–B'. **(D)** Transverse section along C–C'. (Redrawn from McNeal JE: Normal and pathologic anatomy of the prostate. *Urology* 1981;17 (suppl):11.

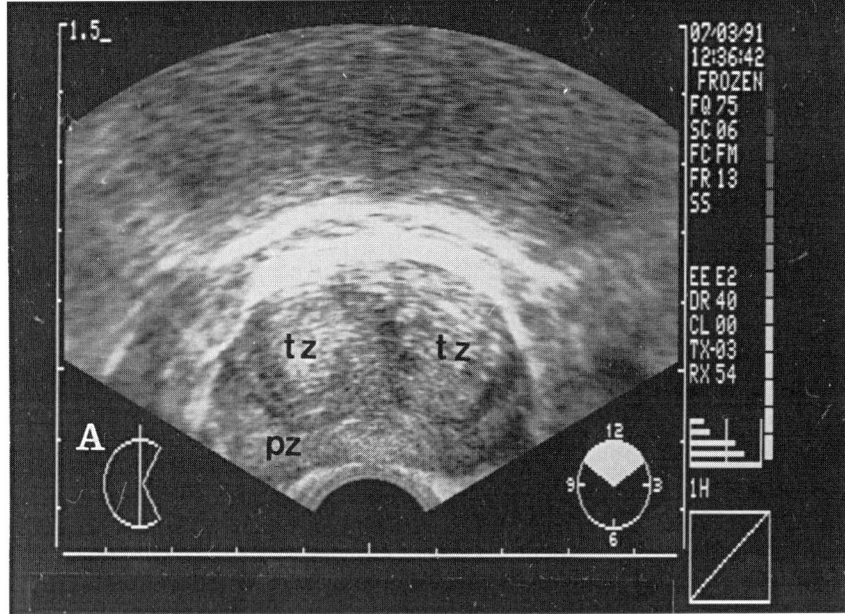

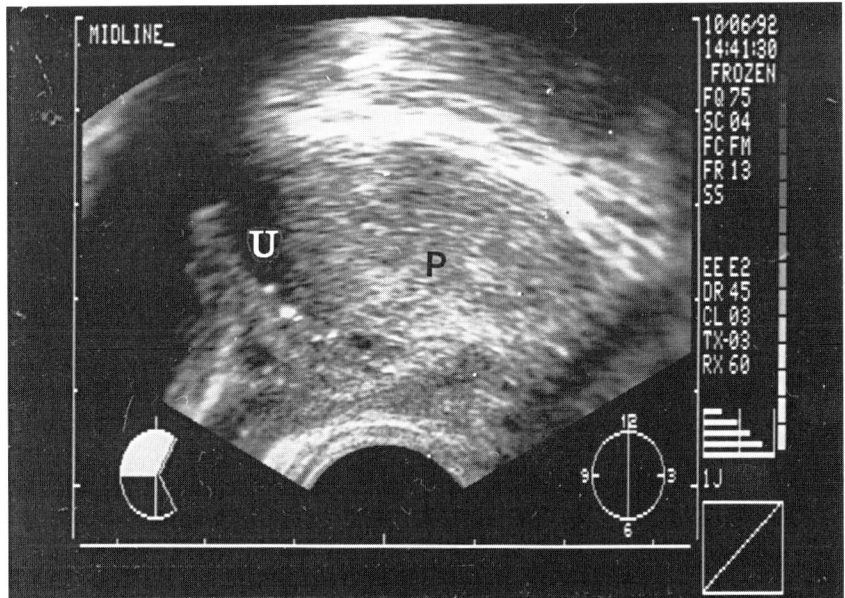

Figure 22–3. Normal prostate. Transrectal ultrasound revealing the zonal anatomy of the prostate. **(A)** Transverse (t.z. = transition zone, p.z. = peripheral zone). **(B)** Midline sagittal (P = prostate, U = urethra).

and sophisticated computers has enabled the development of today's portable ultrasound machines.

The sonographic appearance of the normal prostate follows its zonal anatomy (Fig. 22–3). The prostate appears ellipsoid in shape and is surrounded by a distinct continuous capsule. The peripheral zone is considered isoechoic, and other zones and lesions are compared in echogenicity to the peripheral zone. The normal prostate tissue appears homogeneous with TRUS. The seminal vesicles are visualized posterior to the bladder and have a slightly hypoechoic sonographic appearance. On transverse images the transverse diameter is normally greater than the anteroposterior dimension.

Computed Tomography of the Prostate

Computed tomography (CT) is used to generate a two-dimensional image in the transverse plane of a section of the body. The technology involved is based on the fact that an x-ray beam is differentially attenuated, depending on the density of tissue that it passes through. By passing numerous x-ray beams through the body utilizing a circular array of scanners, a computer is able to produce a two-dimensional representation of that "slice" of the body. The densities of tissues in the body are represented visually in the CT images in shades of gray and numerically in Hounsfield units (HU). Water is assigned a Hounsfield number of zero and appears as neutral gray. Air appears black and is assigned negative

1000 HU; at the opposite end of the scale, petrus bone is positive 1000 HU.

Computed tomography is able to demonstrate size, contour, and density, but internal architecture appears homogeneous and the capsule is not seen separately from the parenchyma.[10] CT is also unable to differentiate prostatic tissue reliably from the levator ani muscles or the rectum.[11] Because their Hounsfield units overlap, CT cannot distinguish between benign and malignant disease.

Magnetic Resonance Imaging of the Prostate

Magnetic resonance imaging (MRI) is an imaging technique that produces tomographic images in all three planes without the use of ionizing radiation. MRI takes advantage of the spin properties of the hydrogen nucleus, which is abundant in human tissue. When these nuclei are subjected to an external magnetic field, they exhibit a spinning and wobbling motion termed *precession*. When a radiofrequency is applied, the net magnetization of the objects in study may be tipped 90 to 180 degrees. A receiver coil picks up voltage changes caused by changes in the magnetic field and a computer generates an image. MRI scanning is useful because different body tissues have different magnetic properties.

Magnetic relaxation is the return to an equilibrium state after the application of an excitation pulse. The T2 relaxation time refers to the decay of the transverse component of the magnetization; the T1 relaxation refers to the regrowth of the longitudinal component of the magnetization after excitation. Different body tissues display different intensities in T1 and T2 imaging based on their respective relaxation times. Endorectal surface coils have improved the image quality for MRI of the prostate.[12]

MRI, unlike CT, is able to delineate some of the intraprostatic architecture. T1-weighted images reveal the prostate as a homogeneous structure of medium signal intensity. T2 images, however, reveal the zonal anatomy of the prostate. On T2-weighted images, the peripheral zone appears hyperintense. The seminal vesicles also appear hyperintense, and the prostatic capsule appears lower in intensity than the gland itself and is well demarcated in the normal prostate.[13] T1-weighted images are most useful for delineation of the periprostatic veins, neurovascular bundles, and lymph nodes.[14]

INFLAMMATORY DISEASE OF THE PROSTATE

Acute Bacterial Prostatitis

DEFINITION AND ETIOLOGY

Acute bacterial prostatitis is a bacterial infection of the prostate usually caused by aerobic gram-negative bacteria. Ascent of infected urine through the urethra and reflux into the prostatic ducts is the most common route of infection, but direct hematogenous and lymphatogenous spread may also occur. Acute prostatitis is usually associated with acute cystitis, and urinary retention is not uncommon.

CLINICAL FINDINGS

Acute bacterial prostatitis is usually an acute febrile illness accompanied by chills, malaise, low back or perineal pain, irritative voiding symptoms (frequency, urgency, dysuria), occasional obstructive voiding symptoms (straining, hesitancy, retention), and myalgia.

Physical examination reveals a warm, tender, enlarged, and partly indurated prostate. Urine culture is performed instead of expressed prostatic secretion culture, because prostatic massage may lead to bacteremia and sepsis.

TRUS is usually not performed in acute prostatitis secondary to the risk of causing bacteremia. When performed, the findings are quite nonspecific. When secondary to surgical manipulation, the findings are usually periurethral, as opposed to nonsurgical etiologies, in which the findings are more peripherally located.[15] The typical finding is an enlarged gland with multiple hypoechoic areas caused by inflammation and edema. Color Doppler imaging in acute prostatitis demonstrates increased blood flow.[16,17] Acute prostatitis does not appear differently from the normal prostate on MRI.

TREATMENT

Patients with acute bacterial prostatitis should be treated with antibiotics as soon as possible. Almost all antibiotics easily diffuse into the prostate in the inflamed state, and trimetheprim-sulfamethoxazole is a good empiric choice. Patients should be treated with oral antibiotics for 10 to 14 days to decrease the chances of developing chronic bacterial prostatitis or prostatic abscess. If a patient appears bacteremic, he should be hospitalized and parenteral antibiotics should be administered. Patients should not be instrumented through the urethra in the acute condition. Patients in urinary retention should therefore be managed with placement of a suprapubic catheter.

Chronic Bacterial Prostatitis

DEFINITION AND ETIOLOGY

Chronic bacterial prostatitis is a nonacute infection of the prostate generally caused by the same organisms that lead to acute bacterial prostatitis. Although chronic bacterial prostatitis may result as a complication of acute bacterial prostatitis, there may be no prior history of the acute form of the disease.

CLINICAL FINDINGS

The symptoms in chronic bacterial prostatitis are extremely variable, ranging form irritative voiding symptoms to chronic perineal or low back pain. Some patients are asymptomatic and are only found after finding unsuspected bacteriuria. On examination the prostate may feel boggy, indurated, or normal.

DIAGNOSIS

Typically, the diagnosis is made by positive culture of expressed prostatic secretions in the face of a negative urine culture. If TRUS is performed in a patient with chronic prostatitis, nonspecific findings of focal or diffuse, hyper- or hypoechoic regions may be seen (Fig. 22–4).[18] Calcifications are readily seen by TRUS and are a sign of chronic prostatitis. On MRI, however, chronic prostatitis appears as areas of low intensity indistinguishable from carcinoma of the prostate.[19]

TREATMENT

Trimethoprim-sulfamethoxazole (TMP-SMX) has traditionally been the first-line antibiotic for chronic nonbacterial prostatitis because of its ability to cross the noninflamed lipid barrier of the prostatic epithelial cells. TMP-SMX has been shown to cure 30 to 40% of patients when treated for 12 weeks.[20] Fluoroquinolones (e.g., ciprofloxacin, norfloxacin) have also been shown to be effective at treating refractory chronic bacterial prostatitis.[21] Patients who cannot be cured, may be treated with chronic prophylactic antibiotics (e.g., TMP-SMX, nitrofurantoin).

Chronic Nonbacterial Prostatitis

Chronic nonbacterial prostatitis is the most common of all the prostatitis syndromes. Patients with this condition present a clinical picture similar to that of patients with chronic bacterial prostatitis. However, no organisms can be cultured, and the patients generally have no history of urinary tract infection. Organisms of such genera as *Mycoplasma, Chlamydia, Trichomonas,* and *Ureaplasma*, and viruses have been sought as etiologic agents, but the search has been to no avail. Extensive work has attempted to prove *C. trachomatis* or *U. urealyticum* to be the cause of chronic nonbacterial prostatitis, but no conclusive proof has been found. At present, the origin of this problem is unknown. Clinical evaluation is similar to that of chronic bacterial prostatitis, but only inflammatory cells are seen with expressed prostatic secretion, and all cultures are negative.

Although a trial of doxycycline may be administered, treatment is usually supportive and may not be successful. Patients may benefit symptomatically from frequent sitz baths and anti-inflammatory medications. Alpha-1 antagonists, as used in patients with BPH, may help relieve symptoms as well.

Prostadynia

Prostadynia patients have symptoms of chronic prostatitis, but prostate examination and expressed secretions are completely normal. No inflammatory cells are present, and again cultures remain negative. There is some evidence that when these patients are studied urodynamically, they show some degree of functional obstruction of the bladder neck or internal sphincter.[22] Because this area of the urinary tract is predominantly innervated with alpha-1 receptors, alpha-1 antagonists may be tried. Others believe that some patients with this syndrome have a tension myalgia of the pelvic floor and prescribe muscle relaxants. Finally, in some patients, emotional or psychiatric problems predominate, and referral to a psychiatrist is recommended.

Prostatic Abscess

Prostatic abscess is a relatively uncommon infection of the prostate. It may be a complication of chronic prostatitis or occur independently. Prostatic abscess is more common in men with diabetes, chronic renal failure, and conditions of immunosuppression and in those undergoing urethral instrumentation or chronic catheterization.[23] The prostate is usually enlarged, but tenderness and fluctuation are unreliable signs and are seen in less than one-third of cases. Consequently, imaging plays a large part in diagnosis of prostatic abscess.

On TRUS, prostatic abscesses are seen as irregularly shaped, hypoechoic masses, with or without internal echoes (Fig. 22–5). With CT, prostatic abscesses appear as a single or multilocular area of low attenuation, and on MRI, prostatic abscess may appear as intermediate or high signal intensity. MRI is not typically used to diagnose inflammatory diseases of the prostate.

Although treatment includes antibiotics, most cases require drainage. Transurethral incision or resection is currently the best method of draining a prostatic abscess. An-

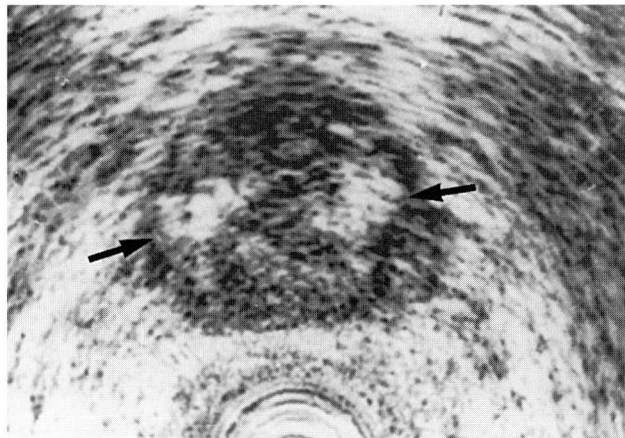

Figure 22–4. Chronic prostatitis. Transrectal ultrasound of the prostate demonstrating an enlarged gland with ill-defined margins. Hyperechoic areas represent prostatic calculi (arrows).

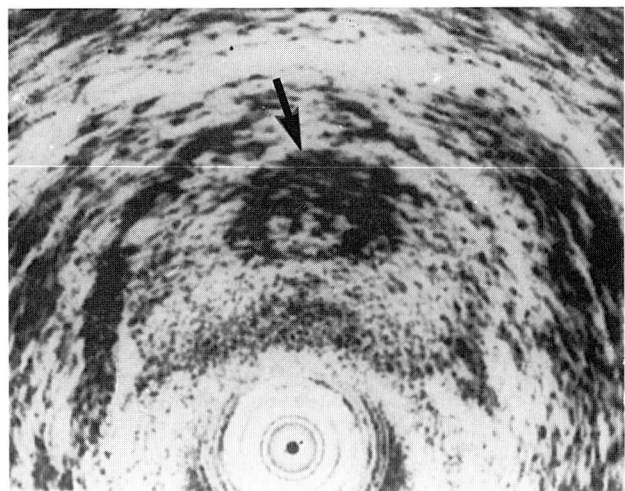

Figure 22–5. Prostatic abscess. Transrectal ultrasound of the prostate demonstrating a hypoechoic region near the center of the gland (arrow). Internal echoes are seen and the borders are indistinct.

tibiotics are directed at gram-negative bacteria, unless culture results point to a different etiologic agent.

BENIGN PROSTATIC HYPERPLASIA

Definition and Etiology

Benign prostatic hyperplasia (BPH), or benign enlargement of the prostate, occurs in most men as they age. The one exception occurs in males castrated prior to puberty. The prostate changes very little in size from birth until puberty, but after puberty, the prostate grows approximately 1.6 g per year until the third decade, after which it grows about 0.4 g per year.[24] As early as 30 years of age, nodules begin to form in the periurethral tissue and transition zone of the prostate. The nodules in the transition zone continue to enlarge throughout life and make up the bulk of BPH tissue. Although the etiology of BPH is most likely multifactorial, evidence supports androgens (testosterone) and estrogens as a strong influence.

Clinical Findings and Diagnosis

Patients with BPH experience symptoms caused by the effects that enlargement and increased tone of the prostate

Table 22–1. AUA Symptom Questionnaire

AUA SYMPTOM SCORE (Circle 1 number on each line)							
7 Questions to be answered:	not at all	less than 1 time in 5	less than half the time	about half the time	more than half the time	almost always	
1. Over the past month, how often have you had a sensation of not emptying your bladder completely after you finished urinating?	0	1	2	3	4	5	
2. Over the past month, how often have you had to urinate again less than two hours after you finished urinating?	0	1	2	3	4	5	
3. Over the past month, how often have you found you stopped and started again several times when you urinated?	0	1	2	3	4	5	
4. Over the past month, how often have you found it difficult to postpone urination?	0	1	2	3	4	5	
5. Over the past month, how often have you had a weak urinary stream?	0	1	2	3	4	5	
6. Over the past month, how often have you had to push or strain to begin urination?	0	1	2	3	4	5	
	none	1 time	2 times	3 times	4 times	5 or more times	
7. Over the past month, how many times did you most typically get up to urinate from the time you went to bed at night until the time you got up in the morning?	0	1	2	3	4	5	
						Total Score: _____	

have on the lower urinary tract. The mechanical obstruction of the enlarged gland is referred to as the static component of obstruction, and the increased tone of the prostatic smooth muscle is called the dynamic component of obstruction. Symptoms may be classified as obstructive (hesitancy, decreased force, intermittency, terminal dribbling, incomplete evacuation, and retention) or irritative (frequency, nocturia, urgency, and dysuria). Several systems have developed objective criteria in an attempt to quantify these symptoms and monitor a patient's response to therapy. The American Urological Association (AUA) symptom score is shown in Table 22–1. On physical examination, the prostate should be noted for size, contour, and consistency. The prostate in BPH is generally enlarged and feels rubbery. It should be noted that a large prostate may be nonobstructing and a smaller gland may result in significant obstruction. Any evidence of carcinoma should be investigated appropriately.

Beyond the history and physical examination, a urinalysis and serum creatinine are the only other required tests for evaluating patients with BPH. Optional tests to be performed at the urologist's discretion include prostate specific antigen (PSA), uroflow and postvoid residual, upper urinary tract imaging, and cystoscopy. The latter group of tests need not be performed routinely, but only with suspicion of a specific problem. An algorithm of the diagnosis and management of BPH is shown in Figure 22–6.[25] Cystoscopy is generally performed at the time of surgery, if at all. Cystoscopy is not required or able to diagnose obstruction, but it may be performed in the office if there is a question of stricture or bladder neck contracture or if an operative approach must be planned.

Imaging

With transrectal ultrasonography, the prostate with BPH appears more rounded than ellipsoid in shape (Fig. 22–7). The capsule remains clearly demarcated but may appear thickened secondary to compression of the peripheral zone from the enlarging adenoma. The prostate tissue in BPH may appear sonographically as enlargement of the relatively hypoechoic central zone or as heterogeneous, well-delineated BPH nodules. Focal nodules may compress or distort the capsule but should not disrupt the capsule.[26] Volume may be easily calculated with TRUS, which is useful for diagnosis and follow-up of medical therapy. CT usually depicts BPH as an enlarged homogeneous gland with smooth margins.

Although not a primary imaging modality for BPH, there are typical findings on MRI (Fig. 22–8). As the transition zone grows with BPH, the peripheral zone (hyperintense on T2 images) is compressed, and in extreme cases only a thin rim of peripheral zone remains. Nodules of varying signal intensity are seen in the central gland. Stromal BPH has an intermediate signal intensity, whereas a high signal intensity is seen with glandular BPH. Carcinoma in the central gland is indistinguishable from BPH.

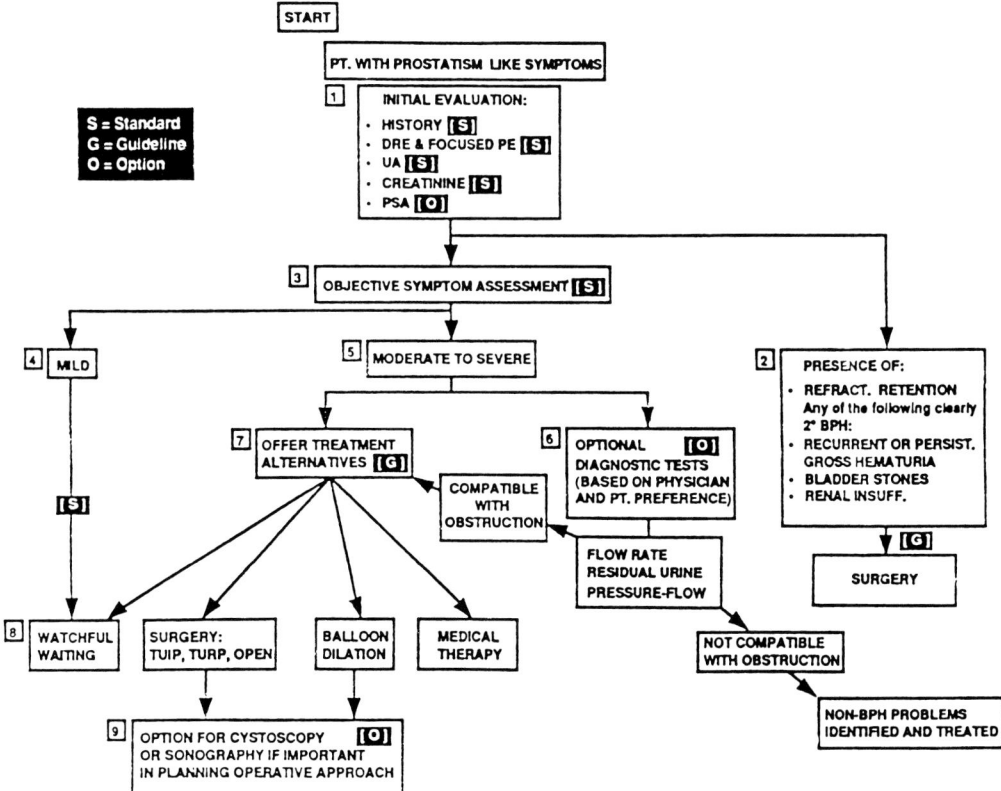

Figure 22–6. BPH management algorithm. (Reproduced with permission from BPH: patient care policies/guidelines. Mebust WK: *AUA Updates* 1993;12(29).

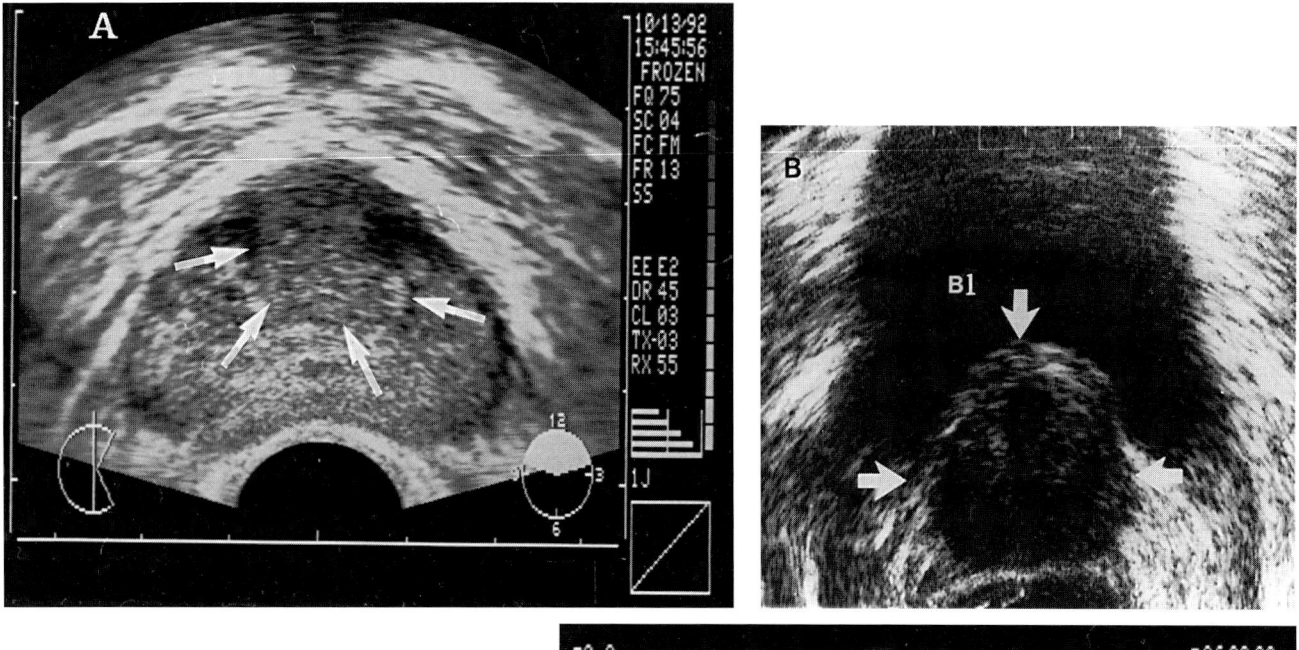
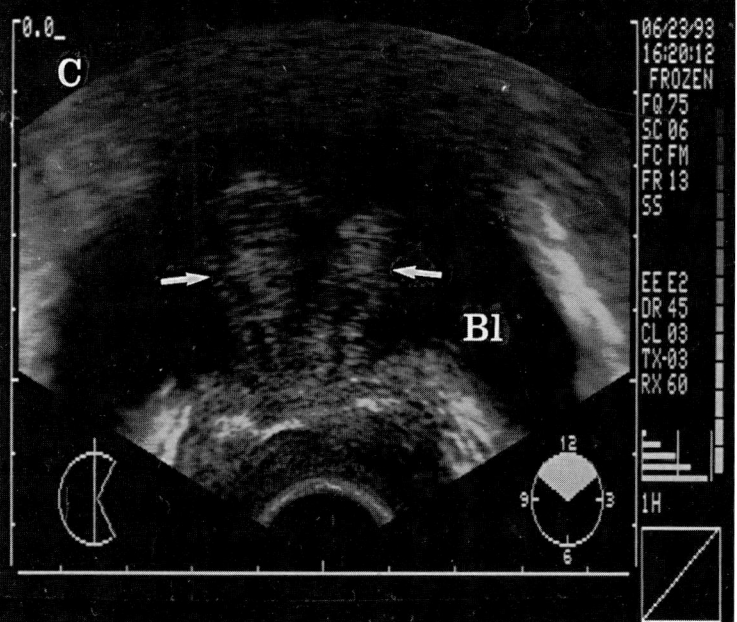

Figure 22–7. BPH. Transrectal ultrasound reveals various aspects of BPH. (A) Early BPH. The central zone is enlarged (arrows). (B) An enlarged ellipsoid-shaped prostate is seen with total glandular BPH (arrows). (C) Middle lobe enlargement (arrows) with extension into the bladder (Bl) is seen.

Treatment

With an extremely prevalent disease like BPH, decisions need to be made about who needs treatment. Absolute indications for treatment include acute urinary retention, bladder stones, recurrent urinary tract infection, recurrent hematuria, hydronephrosis, and azotemia. A more common indication for treatment is symptoms that are sufficiently bothersome that the patient wishes to be treated. With the advent of nonsurgical options for treatment, patients may be more willing to undergo treatment at an earlier stage. The treatment of BPH has changed dramatically in the past few years with the introduction of pharmacologic management and a multitude of new surgical options.

In men with mild symptoms only, observation alone is an option, as many men can tolerate their symptom once reassured that they are not due to cancer. Currently, two classes of medications are being used for the treatment of BPH: alpha-1 antagonists (terazosin, doxazosin) and 5-alpha reductase inhibitors (finasteride). The rationale for using alpha-1 antagonists is due to the high incidence of alpha-1 receptors in the prostate and bladder neck. Blocking these receptors decreases the tone of the prostate, or in other words, decreases the dynamic component of prostatic obstruction. This therapy is not curative, but it does help the patient symptomatically and objectively with increased flow rates and relief of symptoms. A recent study compared 237 men with clinical BPH randomly placed on terazosin (Hy-

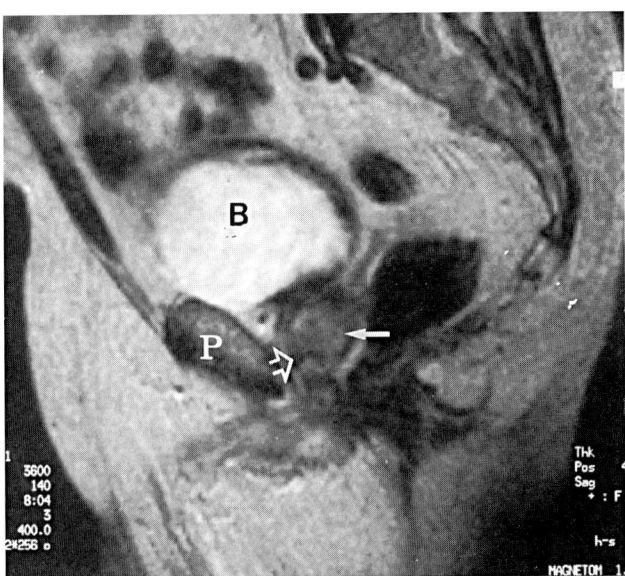

Figure 22–8. BPH. MRI reveals enlargement of the central zone of the prostate (solid arrow) with compression of the surrounding peripheral zone (open arrow). (P = pubis, B = bladder.) (Courtesy of RA Older.)

trin) or placebo.[27] Patients were randomized to receive 2, 5, or 10 mg terazosin or placebo. All treatment groups had significantly decreased symptom scores, and patients receiving 10 mg terazosin had a significant increase in peak flow compared to the placebo group. Terazosin has recently received FDA approval for the treatment of BPH.

5-Alpha reductase inhibitors reduce the androgenic stimulation of the prostate gland by inhibiting the conversion of testosterone to dihydrotestosterone (DHT). One randomized study comprised of 895 men placed patients on finasteride or placebo. At 1 year the treated patients (5 mg finasteride daily) had a 2.5 decrease in their total symptom score ($p < .05$), compared to a 1.0 decrease in the placebo group. The peak flow rate increased by 1.6 mL/sec in the treatment group ($p < .01$) compared to no change in the placebo group. Finasteride effects on symptoms appear to work by decreasing prostatic size, thereby decreasing the static component of obstruction. The prostate generally decreases in size by approximately 20 to 25% by 6 to 12 months. It should be noted that PSA is approximately halved with the use of finasteride. An upper limit of 2.0 should therefore be used for PSA analysis, and PSA velocity may be particularly useful in this situation. Continuous use of finasteride results in a persistent decrease in symptoms. Finasteride (Proscar) was the first medication to be approved by the FDA for the treatment of BPH. With the availability of both alpha-1 antagonists and finasteride primary care physicians are now taking a larger role in the management of patients with BPH.

In patients with more severe symptoms, or the previously mentioned absolute indications for treatment, pharmacologic management of the prostate is inadequate and intervention is necessary. Transurethral resection of the prostate (TURP) and open simple prostatectomy have long been the gold standards for treatment of small to medium and large obstructing prostates. TURP is a highly effective treatment, but it is not without its morbidity. About 2% of patients have some incontinence, impotence may be expected in approximately 5%, and operative mortality is approximately 0.2%.[28] Transurethral incision of the prostate (TUIP) was really the first surgical alternative to TURP, first introduced into the United States in 1973.[29] TUIP is quicker and easier to perform than TURP, offers a shorter hospital stay, and may be ideal for prostates of less than 20 g.[30]

More recently, lasers have been added to the urologist's armamentarium for ablation of prostatic tissue. Transurethral ultrasound-guided, laser-induced prostatectomy (TULIP) and visual laser ablation of the prostate (VLAP) are the two main systems at present. TULIP is performed with a right-angle-firing laser device that is housed inside a balloon placed intraurethrally and whose location is confirmed by digital palpation and ultrasonic localization. The laser fiber is connected to a standard ND-YAG laser. The prostatic tissue is not vaporized or ablated, but shrinks secondary to coagulation necrosis. Consequently, the effects are not immediate. Recently, a large multicenter study was published on results of TULIP.[31] Of 150 patients treated, there were no intraoperative complications, no cases of TUR syndrome, and no necessity for blood transfusion; average hospital stay was 1.7 days. Six-month follow-up was available on 63 patients. Mean peak flow rates increased from 6.7 mL/sec to 11.9 mL/sec, and mean symptom scores decreased from 18.8 to 6.1. Although the results are promising, long-term randomized studies comparing different treatment modalities are still needed.

VLAP is performed through a standard cystoscope under direct vision. As with TULIP, the procedure utilizes a right-angle fiber and a ND-YAG laser source. Norris et al recently reported their experience with VLAP in 108 patients.[32] With follow-up of 6 months, mean AUA symptom scores decreased by 12.6 (97 patients) and mean peak flow rates increased by 4.9 mL/sec (75 patients). No patient required blood transfusion or had an intraoperative complication. All but three patients were discharged home (with a catheter for 5 to 7 days) the day of the procedure. As with TULIP, this procedure seems promising, but long-term controlled studies are needed. Studies are under way utilizing contact lasers that vaporize tissue, but as with other new procedures long-term follow-up studies are lacking.

Prostatic intraurethral stents represent an entirely different method of managing the obstructing prostate. Instead of removing the prostatic tissue, the intraurethral stent holds the prostatic urethra open and becomes epithelialized. Although most studies have had good success in elderly, debilitated, poor surgical candidates, only one study has placed stents in BPH patients routinely. This study reports the use of the Urolume endoprosthesis in 95 healthy BPH patients.[33] At 12-month follow-up mean symptom scores decreased from 15 to 6.3 and mean peak flow increased from 8.6 to 15.6

mL/sec. Mean postvoid residual decreased significantly as well. These stents will probably find a niche in the treatment of BPH patients. The stents also have promise in the treatment of refractory urethral strictures and in spinal cord patients with external sphincter detrusor dyssynergia.[33]

Several other modalities for treating patients with symptomatic BPH are also available. Balloon dilation of the prostate has been tested and does not appear to have significant long-term benefit. Other therapies currently being investigated include hyperthermia (heating the prostate to 45°C), high-intensity focused ultrasound, microwave, and low-frequency microwave therapies. All are in the early stages of testing.

CARCINOMA OF THE PROSTATE

Adenocarcinoma of the prostate is the most common male malignancy and the second leading cause of death in men. Approximately 134,000 new cases are diagnosed annually, and autopsy studies reveal an even higher incidence. Frankes demonstrated an autopsy incidence of 30% in men more than 50 years of age, and the incidence in older men is even higher.[34] Scardino et al calculated that a 50-year-old man had a 42% lifetime risk of developing histologic evidence of prostate cancer, a 9.5% chance of developing clinical prostate cancer, and a 2.9% lifetime chance of dying of the disease.[35] This can be aptly explained by the extremely slow doubling time of prostatic carcinoma. At present, there is no way to predict which tumors will behave more aggressively. Although no specific etiologic agent is known for prostate cancer, both genetic and environmental agents appear to play a role, and testosterone is thought to act as a tumor promoter.[36]

Screening

Although localized cancer of the prostate is potentially curable, once the cancer has spread, treatment options are limited to slowing the progress of the disease. Screening for prostate cancer prior to the development of metastases is an attractive notion. An ideal screening test must be highly sensitive if it is to identify as many patients as possible. It should also have high sensitivity, specificity, and positive and negative predictive values to be most useful. A screening test should be economically feasible as well. The population to be screened also has to fulfill certain requirements. There must be a high enough incidence in asymptomatic patients for screening to be worthwhile. The aggressiveness of the disease must be accounted for, and there should be good treatment for patients who have the disease.

Screening for prostate cancer should be directed at patients at highest risk and at those who will benefit most from diagnosis and subsequent treatment. With prostate cancer, screening should be directed at patients from 40 or 50 years old (depending on family history) to those 70 to 75 years of age.[37]

Prostate cancer varies greatly in its aggressiveness. Most cancers with a volume of less than 1 cm^3 do not metastasize,[38] and those less than 4 cm^3 in volume are localized in 94% of cases.[39–41] Stamey et al have proposed that tumors with volume less than 0.5 cm^3 will not achieve clinical significance due to the slow doubling time of prostate cancer.[42] Stamey has also stated that only one of 380 men with the prostate cancer will die of the disease.[43] Based on these data, screening for prostate cancer should be directed at finding more aggressive tumors between 0.5 and 4 cm^3 total volume. Unfortunately, there is no method to differentiate the indolent tumors from the aggressive ones.[44]

PSA SCREENING

The American Cancer Society recommends that men over the age of 50 have an annual PSA and digital rectal examination (DRE). But PSA is not a perfect screening tool. Recently, Oesterling performed a statistical review of the literature and found that PSA was a poor predictor of prostate cancer when used alone.[45] A value of greater than 4.0 ng/mL had a 49% positive predictive value (PPV), and for a value of 10.0 or greater the PPV increased to only 75%. Based on this review, Oesterling concluded that PSA had neither the sensitivity nor the specificity to stand alone as a screening study.

The use of PSA combined with digital rectal examination (DRE) and TRUS clearly increases the accuracy of diagnosis of carcinoma of the prostate. Cooner et al studied 1807 patients with PSA, DRE, and TRUS and found that a PSA of more than 10.0 ng/mL had a PPV of 80%, whereas patients with a PSA of less than 4.0 ng/mL and a normal DRE rarely had prostate cancer.[46] Rommel et al performed PSA, DRE, and TRUS with biopsy on 2020 patients referred for a suspicion of prostate cancer.[47] They found that patients with an abnormal DRE and a PSA between 4.0 and 10.0 and those with a PSA of more than 10 ng/mL had positive predictive values of 32 and 68%, respectively. They also found that if patients with PSA levels of less than 4 ng/mL and a normal DRE had not been biopsied, only 1% of the prostate cancers in their study would have been missed. Catalona et al studied 1653 men over 50 years of age with a screening PSA.[48] Men with an elevated PSA underwent DRE and TRUS followed by TRUS-directed biopsy if either was abnormal. Eighty-five men were biopsied with a PSA between 4 and 9.9 ng/mL. Nineteen (24%) of these men had positive biopsies. All 19 were clinically localized, but only 10 of the 17 (59%) who underwent radical prostatectomy were pathologically confined. Brawer et al studied 1249 men over 50 years of age with screening PSA.[49] Of these men, 187 (15.9%) had an elevated PSA and 105 (56.2%) underwent DRE and TRUS-guided biopsy. A total 32 carcinomas (32.5%) were found and more than one-third had a normal rectal examination. Brawer et al concluded that PSA is a useful adjunct to DRE in the initial evaluation of patients with suspected prostate cancer but caution that the long-term effect on morbidity and mortality of earlier detection of prostate cancer is unknown.

PSA density (PSAD) and PSA velocity are two values that may increase the sensitivity and specificity of PSA in the diagnosis of prostate cancer. PSAD is calculated by dividing the patient's PSA by the volume of the prostate. (An assumption of 1 cm^3 volume equaling 1 g of prostate tissue is used.) Benson et al studied 61 patients and found a mean PSAD of 0.581 in prostate cancer patients and 0.044 in patients with BPH.[50] Of the 34 patients with a PSAD above 0.1, 33 had cancer, whereas only one of 20 patients with BPH had a PSAD above 0.1. In another study of PSAD, 2020 patients were evaluated with PSA, PSAD, DRE, and TRUS with biopsy.[47] These authors stated that in men under 80 with a PSA below 20 ng/mL, a PSAD above 0.14 was the strongest predictor of prostate cancer. Brawer et al, however, were not able to predict which patients would have a positive biopsy using 218 patients utilizing PSAD.[51] They found that PSAD was no better than serum PSA in predicting the presence or absence of prostatic carcinoma.

PSA velocity refers to the change in PSA over time. Carter et al demonstrated that PSA increased at a faster rate in men with prostate cancer than in those with BPH and had a specificity of 90%.[52] Brawer et al studied PSA velocity in 701 patients in the second year of a PSA screening study.[53] They found that an annual PSA increase of 20% may identify men at risk for prostate cancer even if the actual PSA value is less than 4.0 ng/mL and that patients identified may be detected at an earlier stage and are more likely to have organ-confined disease.

TRUS SCREENING

Thompson stated that a screening test for prostate cancer should have a specificity of 95% or greater.[54] Early studies showed that TRUS has a sensitivity of 60 to 85% and a specificity of 41 to 79%.[55] Two recent studies with pathologic correlation demonstrate very poor sensitivity and specificity of TRUS alone for diagnosing prostate cancer. Coffield et al performed TRUS on 148 autopsy specimens with no clinical diagnosis of prostate cancer and found a sensitivity of 32% and a specificity of 63%.[56] They stated that diagnosis would have been increased if PSA had been used. Another study correlated preoperative TRUS with pathologic findings after cystoprostatectomy in 51 patients with no suspicion of prostate cancer.[57] TRUS may detect smaller, nonpalpable tumors. One study demonstrated that tumors found by TRUS averaged 1.8 cm^3 in volume as opposed to 6 cm^3 in those found by DRE.[58] In a study of 1807 men Cooner et al found that a combination of abnormal DRE and PSA of more than 4 had a positive predictive value of 60%.[46]

The addition of an abnormal TRUS only increased the value to 62%. These data show that TRUS alone is not an adequate test for screening for carcinoma of the prostate.

SCREENING IN SUMMARY

Traditionally, DRE alone was used in checking or screening men for prostate cancer. When PSA is added approximately twice as many cancers may be found. The effect of finding these additional cancers on long-term morbidity and mortality remains to be seen. Large, controlled screening studies are currently under way by the National Cancer Institute. Men with an abnormal prostate on DRE with a life expectancy of more than 10 years should undergo directed and systematic biopsies. Most authors agree that men with a PSA of more than 10.0 ng/mL should also undergo biopsy regardless of DRE. However, the management of men with a normal DRE and a PSA between 4.0 and 10.0 ng/mL is more controversial. Although some would biopsy these patients, others, such as Stamey, follow them with DRE and PSA over time.[59] Until large-scale, prospective, randomized trials are completed, the value of screening for prostate cancer remains unknown.

Grading

Currently, the Gleason's grading system is the one most commonly used in the United States.[60] This system grades adenocarcinoma of the prostate from 1 to 5 based solely on architectural criteria. A grade of 1 signifies a well-differentiated tumor, whereas 5 represents poorly differentiated tumors. The Gleason's sum represents the grade of the largest area of tumor plus the grade of the second largest area of tumor. The range therefore is from 2 to 10.

Staging of Carcinoma of the Prostate

Although for several decades the Jewett system and its modifications have been most commonly utilized, currently the trend is toward the use of the tumor, nodes, metastases (TNM) system. The TNM system of classification of prostate cancer staging is seen in Table 22–2.

PHYSICAL EXAMINATION

Physical examination of the prostate (DRE) has been shown in numerous studies to be inaccurate at staging carcinoma of the prostate. The main problem is in differentiating between extracapsular disease (T3) and carcinoma confined to the prostate (T2). In addition, DRE is usually unable to determine seminal vesicle invasion (T3c) and obviously is unable to detect lymph node metastases (N1-N3) because of their location deep in the pelvis.

Table 22–2

Primary Tumor (T) Stage
  TX: Primary tumor cannot be assessed
  T0: No evidence of primary tumor
  T1: Clinically inapparent tumor (not palpable)
    T1a: Incidental, less than 5% of tissue resected
    T1b: Incidental, more than 5% of tissue resected
    T1c: Tumor identified by needle biopsy (i.e., with increased PSA)
  T2: Tumor palpable, confined within prostate
    T2a: Tumor involves half of a lobe or less
    T2b: Tumor involves more than half a lobe, but not both lobes
    T2c: Tumor involves both lobes
  T3: Tumor extends through prostatic capsule
    T3a: Unilateral capsular extension
    T3b: Bilateral capsular extension
    T3c: Tumor invades seminal vesicle(s)
  T4: Tumor fixed or invades adjacent structures
    T4a: Tumor invades bladder neck, external sphincter, or rectum
    T4b: Tumor invades levator ani or is fixed to pelvic wall

Regional Lymph Nodes (N) Stage
  NX: Nodes cannot be assessed
  N0: No regional lymph node metastases
  N1: Tumor in single node, 2 cm or less
  N2: Tumor in single node, between 2 cm and 5 cm in size or multiple lymph node involvement, all less than 5 cm
  N3: Tumor involvement in a node greater than 5 cm

Distant Metastases (M) Stage
  MX: Presence of metastases cannot be assessed
  M0: No evidence of distant metastases
  M1: Distant metastases present
    M1a: Nonregional lymph nodes
    M1b: Bone(s)
    M1c: Other sites

PSA AND STAGING

Although not exact, PSA is a useful aid in staging of carcinoma of the prostate. In general, PSA increases with increasing stage; however, the overlap between stages is great.[45,61,62] Patients with PSA of more than 70.0 ng/mL are likely to have extracapsular disease.[45] Another series of 301 patients undergoing radical prostatectomy revealed that the difference in PSA of less than 10.0 ng/mL versus more than 50.0 ng/mL predicted a 0 versus a 45% incidence of lymph node metastases, and a 5 versus 73% incidence of seminal vesicle invasion.[63] PSA is also somewhat predictive of bone metastases. Oesterling et al retrospectively reviewed 561 patients with recently diagnosed prostate cancer; only three (0.005%) patients with a PSA of less than 10.0 ng/mL had a positive bone scan.[33] In addition, of the 467 patients with a PSA of less than 8.0 ng/mL, none had a positive bone scan. Oesterling et al concluded that patients with prostate cancer, a PSA of less than 10 ng/mL, and no skeletal symptoms do not require a bone scan.

PROSTATIC ACID PHOSPHATASE AND STAGING

Prostatic acid phosphatase (PAP) was the main marker assessing for patients for prostate cancer from the early 1940s until the recent emergence of PSA. PAP is a member of the acid phosphatase family (enzymes that hydrolyze phosphate esters to produce inorganic phosphates) and is produced in the epithelial cells of the prostate. PAP may be elevated as a result of prostate cancer, BPH, acute prostatitis, and prostatic infarct. Currently available assays have some cross-reactivity with other acid phosphatases and may lead to false-positive results.

In prostate cancer patients, PAP is increased in direct proportion to stage of the cancer; however, the ranges are broad, and exact staging is impossible. In addition, poorly differentiated tumor cells secrete less PAP than do well-differentiated cancer cells. This leads to a false-negative rate of 15 to 40% in patients with metastatic disease.[45] Patients with localized prostate cancer (T1 and T2) may also have mildly elevated enzymatic PAP and should not be denied the benefit of curative therapy. Some authors consider an elevated PAP as evidence of metastatic disease not yet clinically apparent and have termed this stage D0. Lymph node dissection may be of diagnostic help in this situation.

TRANSRECTAL ULTRASOUND

The sonographic appearance of carcinoma of the prostate on TRUS is highly variable. Early studies utilizing B-mode and gray-scale technology indicated that carcinoma had a hyperechoic appearance.[8,9] As technology improved it was recognized that most sonographically visible tumors are hypoechoic lesions, but some may appear hyperechoic, isoechoic, or heterogeneous[64,65] (Fig. 22–9). The majority of carcinomas of the prostate visualized have irregular margins and are located in the peripheral zone. In studies with pathologic correlation prostate cancer appeared hypoechoic in 65 to 84% of cases and isoechoic in 16 to 35%.[66–68] Shinohara et al, in a study with 292 men with biopsy proven carcinoma of the prostate, demonstrated that the percent of men with hypoechoic lesions increased with increasing suspicion of cancer on DRE.[67] Only 33% of men with normal DRE had hypoechoic lesions, whereas 79 and 90% of men with firm and nodular prostates on DRE had hypoechoic lesions. There is some evidence that early carcinomas are of low echogenicity and become more echogenic as they grow and locally invade normal tissue.[64] Another report stated that smaller tumors tended to be isoechoic, whereas larger tumors took on a hypoechoic appearance.[69] Hypoechoic lesions may also be caused by benign etiologies such as cysts, infarcts, inflammatory conditions, and blood vessels, which can lead to confusion in diagnosis.[55]

Careful imaging of the prostatic capsule and seminal vesicles may provide signs of cancer of the prostate. Locally invasive carcinoma will often disrupt or deform the normally

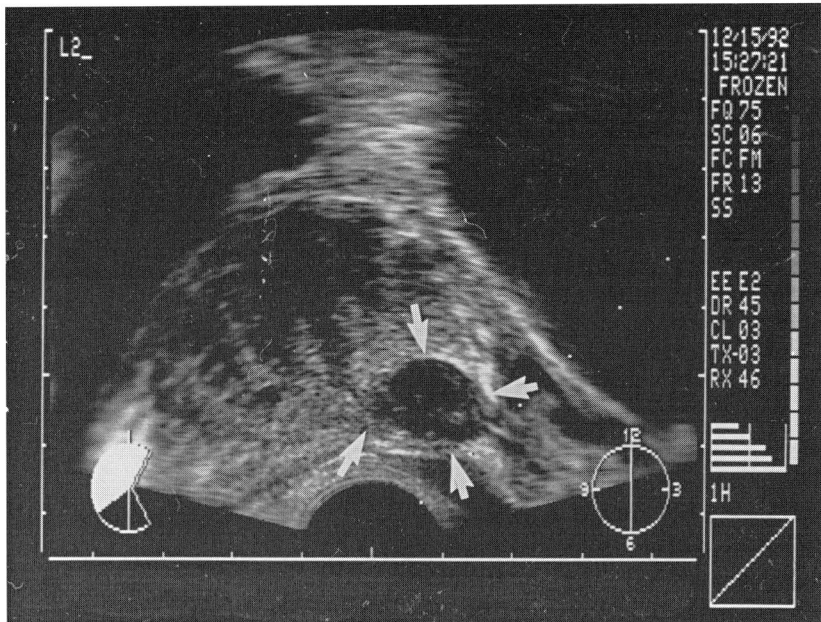

Figure 22–9. Prostate cancer. Transrectal ultrasound reveals a hypoechoic region (arrows) in the peripheral zone. Biopsy revealed adenocarcinoma of the prostate.

continuous hyperechoic prostatic margin (Fig. 22–10). In addition, hypoechoic strands adjacent to the prostate may signify extension of the carcinoma into the periprostatic fat. Asymmetry or enlargement of one of the seminal vesicles may signify gross invasion of the carcinoma. Microinvasive disease of the seminal vesicle is not visible sonographically.[70]

TRANSRECTAL ULTRASOUND STAGING

Transrectal ultrasound can be of use in staging carcinoma of the prostate. Although it is not perfect, TRUS has been shown to be more accurate than the approximately 50% accurate DRE in determining extracapsular extension.[71] TRUS has been shown to predict extracapsular extension with a sensitivity of from 69 to 89% and a specificity of from 91 to 100%.[70,72,73] Rifkin et al found that TRUS correctly staged 66% of patients with advanced disease and 46% of those with localized disease.[74] Seminal vesicle invasion is predicted with sensitivities of from 29 to 92% and specificities of from 80 to 100%.[70,75,76]

Volume of tumor has been shown to be an indicator of extracapsular tumor extension, seminal vesicle invasion, and nodal metastases. In a series of radical prostatectomy spec-

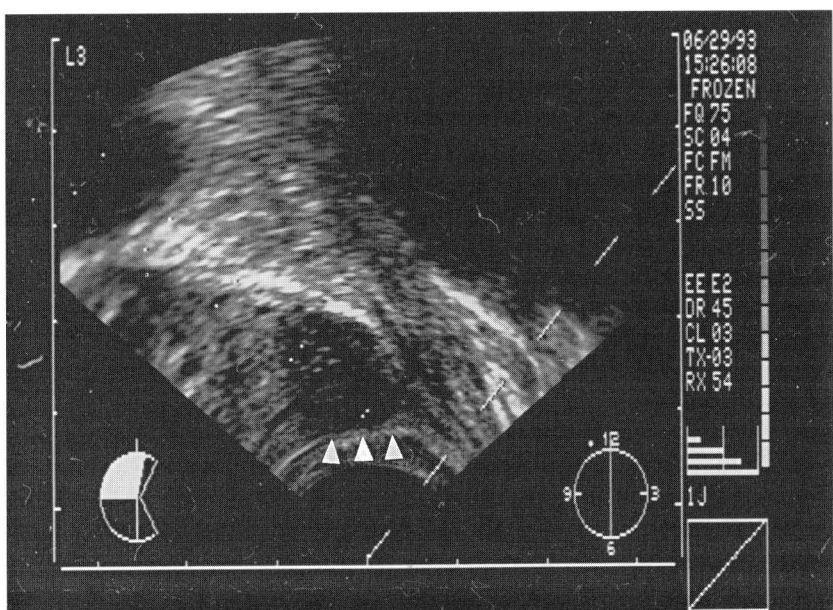

Figure 22–10. Prostate cancer. Transrectal ultrasound reveals a bulging prostatic capsule (arrows) adjacent to a hypoechoic lesion that proved to be prostate cancer on biopsy.

imens, capsular penetration was found in only 7% of those less than 4 cm³ in volume and in 86% of tumors of more than 12 cm³.[40] Similar results were found with seminal vesicle invasion in 82% of tumors with a volume of more than 12 cm³ and in only 6% of those with a volume of less than 4 cm³. Lymph node metastases were present in 46% of cases with tumor volume above 12 cm³ and in only 1% of cases with tumor volumes below 4 cm³.[40] Unfortunately, although TRUS can accurately predict prostate gland volume,[41] TRUS cancer volume measurements do not correlate well pathologically.[77]

TRUS AND BIOPSY FOR STAGING AND DIAGNOSIS

Although sonographic signs of prostate cancer are relatively nonspecific, TRUS is a useful aid in performing biopsy of the prostate. Ultrasound-guided biopsy of the prostate has been performed by both perineal and transrectal routes[78,79]; however, the transrectal route is currently most popular. Patients are given oral antibiotics the night before and 2 to 3 days following biopsy. A cleansing enema is administered the morning of the biopsy, which aids in visualization and reduces bacterial seeding. A needle fits through a channel in the ultrasound probe, and needle placement is guided visually with real-time ultrasound. In most instances a spring-loaded device is used to assist the biopsy (Fig. 22–11).

Although biopsy of only hypoechoic lesions would miss approximately 20% of prostate cancers,[68] biopsying hypoechoic lesions combined with systematic sextant biopsies has been shown to be quite accurate.[80] In comparing biopsy with DRE and TRUS, Lippermann et al concluded that performing random sextant biopsies was the critical issue, not the method of biopsy.[81] Although findings at TRUS may direct one's biopsy location, the decision to biopsy a patient with suspected prostate cancer (abnormal PSA or DRE) should be made prior to inserting the ultrasound probe, and systematic sextant biopsies should be performed in all cases. TRUS provides an accurate method for needle direction in both directed and random sextant biopsies in patients with palpable lesions or those with normal DRE and an elevated PSA.[17]

CT APPEARANCE AND STAGING

CT has very limited usefulness in the staging of patients with carcinoma of the prostate. CT can provide evidence of extraprostatic extension and lymphadenopathy, but accuracy is poor. Signs of extraprostatic cancer on CT include unilateral levator ani enlargement, rectal wall thickening, and apparent invasion of the bladder base and seminal vesicles. CT accuracy in diagnosing extracapsular extension ranges from 48 to 67%.[82–84] Sensitivity in these studies ranged from 48 to 68%. Most of the inaccuracy was due to understaging.

CT has been used to evaluate for the presence of pelvic lymph node metastases. In this setting CT is used to find lymph nodes larger than 1 cm. Caution must be exercised, though, because lymph nodes may be enlarged secondary to inflammatory conditions. Studies vary dramatically, with sensitivity of finding positive lymph nodes reported from none to 93% and overall accuracy from 77 to 93%.[83,85] CT is useful in the placement of transperineal iodine 125 prostate implants[86] and in the evaluation of distant metastases from carcinoma of the prostate. CT has also been used to

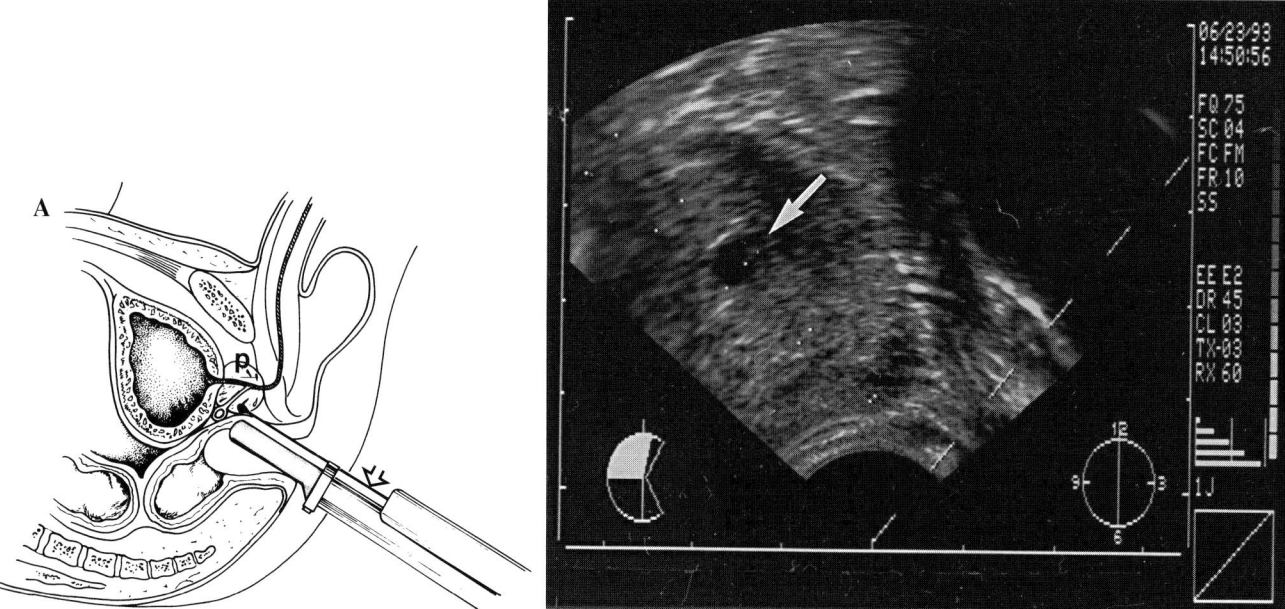

Figure 22–11. Prostate cancer. (**A**) Diagram representing the transrectal ultrasound probe with biopsy needle directed into the prostate. (**B**) A path is delineated (dotted line) for guiding biopsy needle through the peripheral hypoechoic lesion (arrow).

assist in prostate biopsy in patients following abdominoperineal resection who have an elevated PSA and suspected prostate cancer.[87]

MRI APPEARANCE AND STAGING

Because of better image quality (see earlier), most current MRI studies of the prostate use the endorectal coil technique instead of whole-body scanners. The characteristic appearance of prostate cancer on MRI is best seen on T2-weighted images (Fig. 22–12). The carcinoma appears as areas of decreased signal intensity amid the high-signal-intensity peripheral zone. This finding is nonspecific and may be seen with chronic prostatitis and BPH with prostatic infarcts. Carcinoma of the prostate in other zones is not distinguishable from the surrounding prostate. Because of its low specificity, low sensitivity in the central regions of the prostate, and high cost, MRI would be a poor screening test for prostate cancer.

MRI is more useful in the detection of extracapsular extension of a known carcinoma than in its original diagnosis. Gross tumor extension into the periprostatic fat is seen best on T1-weighted images (Fig. 22–13), whereas seminal vesicle invasion is best seen on T2-weighted images (Fig. 22–14).[14] The accuracy of MRI at detecting extra-prostatic cancer varies with the site of spread. Tempany et al studied invasion of the neurovascular bundles and found a sensitivity of 68% and a specificity of only 59%.[88] One study was able to differentiate stage T2 (organ confined) from T3 (extracapsular) and N+ (lymph-node-positive) disease with an accuracy of 89%.[89] Another study revealed a sensitivity of 69% and a specificity of 95% for seminal vesicle invasion seen on MRI.[90] Rifkin et al, in a large, multicenter study of 231 patients utilizing MRI, TRUS, and surgical staging,

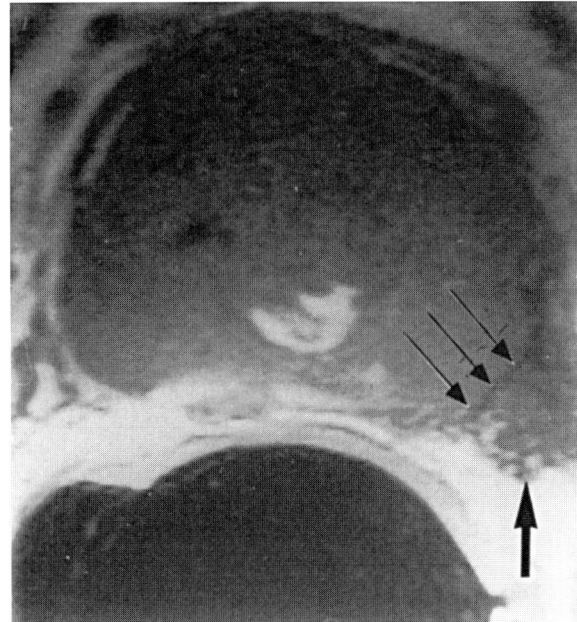

Figure 22–13. Prostate cancer. MRI (T1 weighted) demonstrates prostate cancer extending into the periprostatic fat (thick arrow). The prostatic capsule is seen clearly (narrow arrows).

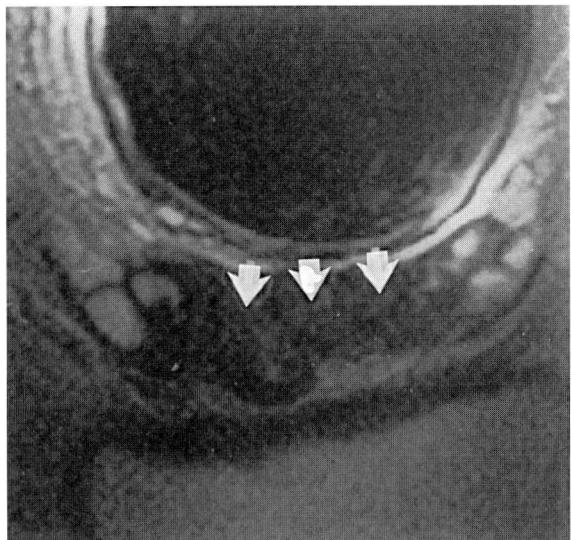

Figure 22–14. Prostate cancer. MRI (T2 weighted) demonstrates prostate cancer extending into the seminal vesicles (arrows).

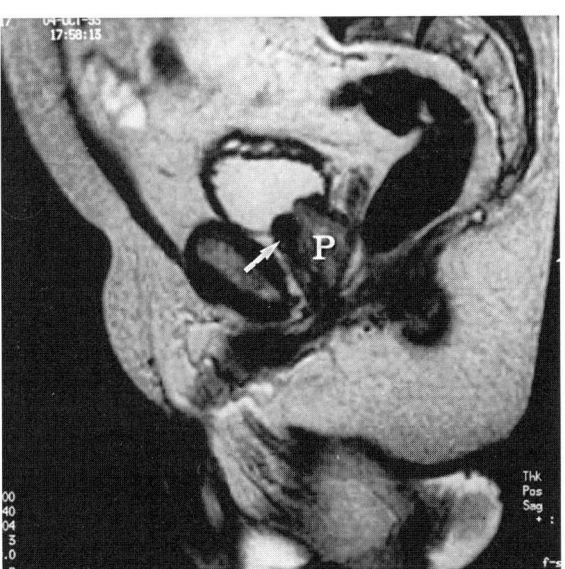

Figure 22–12. Prostate cancer. MRI (T2 weighted) demonstrates prostate cancer as a hypointense lesion (arrow). (P = prostate.) (Courtesy of RA Older.)

demonstrated that MRI was more accurate with advanced disease.[74] MRI correctly staged 77% of advanced prostate cancer cases and only 45% of localized cases. Rifkin et al concluded that both MRI and TRUS were inaccurate at staging carcinoma of the prostate secondary to the inability of either imaging modality to detect the presence of microscopic metastases. MRI has also been shown not to be of help in the detection of microscopic lymph node metastases.

LAPAROSCOPIC STAGING

Bilateral pelvis lymph node dissection is currently the standard method of assessing the early metastases of prostate cancer. This procedure has traditionally been performed through a lower abdominal incision, either in conjunction with radical prostatectomy or as a separate procedure. Recently, laparoscopic technique has been applied to urology and has led to the development of laparoscopic pelvis lymph node dissection.[91,92] Although this technique has a steep learning curve and takes longer than open lymph node dissection, the laparoscopic approach has the benefit of a shorter hospital stay, decreased blood loss, and decreased postoperative narcotics use; it has also been shown to be effective at achieving an adequate node sampling.[93,94] This is an ideal procedure for patients with suspected positive lymph node metastases and for those undergoing radical perineal prostatectomy or radiation therapy.

Treatment

At present, radical prostatectomy and bilateral pelvic lymph node dissection is the gold standard for treatment of localized carcinoma of the prostate. Other options include radiation therapy (external beam and radioactive seed implants), cryotherapy, and observation alone.

EXTERNAL BEAM IRRADIATION

External beam irradiation involves directing high-dose ionizing radiation at the prostate and surrounding area in the pelvis. Rapidly proliferating tissues like the prostate cancer are more sensitive to the radiation. This therapy seems to have the advantage of being able to treat local extracapsular disease, which would not be amenable to treatment by radical prostatectomy. Unfortunately, cure rates are not as high as one would like. Catalona found treatment failure in one-fourth to one-third of patients with T1 to T3 prostate cancer (50 to 65% metastatic).[95] Kabalin et al performed TRUS biopsies in 27 patients 5 years after external beam irradiation and found a 93% positive biopsy rate, including 20 of 22 with a normal DRE.[96] Overall survival was found to be approximately 60% for patients with T1 and T2 disease at 10 years follow-up.[97] Patients in this series were biopsied at 2 years of follow-up and found to be positive in 38, 59, and 74% of small T2, large T2, and T3 patients, respectively. This form of prostate cancer treatment has an alarmingly high positive biopsy rate after treatment, although some patients have demonstrated long-term disease-free survival. Kaplan et al studied 117 patients with serial PSA measurements after external beam irradiation for carcinoma of the prostate.[98] Only 44 (37.6%) of the 117 patients had biochemical progression, but 30 of those (68%) rapidly progressed to have clinical progression. They concluded that greatly elevated pretreatment PSA, large local tumors, advanced local disease, and high Gleason score were all predictors for progressive disease.

Radiation therapy is not without its morbidity. Up to 20% of patients will have some gastrointestinal side effects, ranging from diarrhea, rectal bleeding, and fecal incontinence to intestinal obstruction and fistula formation. Irritative voiding symptoms are seen in 10 to 15% of patients. Most of the complications are relatively minor and decrease with time. Impotence is seen in up to 14% of cases.

INTERSTITIAL SEED RADIATION (BRACHYTHERAPY)

Interstitial seed implantation has not proven to be an effective form of therapy for prostate cancer. This technique involves placing radioactive "seeds" directly inside the prostate. Whitmore and Hilaris published their results of ^{125}I interstitial seed implantation with 10-year follow-up.[99] During the follow-up period, 40% of patients with T2a and 70% with T2b experienced progression of their disease. In general, a 10-year survival rate of approximately 60% can be expected in patients with stages T1 to T3 and negative lymph nodes treated with brachytherapy.[100,101] In general, local control with brachytherapy has been worse than that achieved with either radical prostatectomy or external beam radiation.[102] Newer isotopes are being studied that are being implanted more accurately with ultrasound techniques. Whether this approach will be beneficial remains to be determined.

RADICAL PROSTATECTOMY

Radical prostatectomy involves the surgical removal of the entire prostate and seminal vesicles. This procedure is routinely combined with bilateral lymph node dissection. In recent years the retropubic approach has been most frequently used because it allows for easy dissection and removal of the pelvic lymph nodes. Recently, with the popularization of laparoscopy, the radical perineal prostatectomy has had a resurgence in popularity.

Approximately 72% of patients with stage T2 prostate cancer may expect 10-year disease-free survival.[103–105] These numbers compare favorably with interstitial and external beam irradiation; however, ideally, prospective, randomized studies comparing radical prostatectomy, external beam irradiation, and expectant therapy need to be performed to determine the best treatment modalities for the various stages of carcinoma of the prostate.

Radical prostatectomy is also accompanied by morbidity. Incontinence is not uncommon. One recent study of 418 patients undergoing radical retropubic prostatectomy demonstrated a 15% incidence of grade 2 stress incontinence and 3% total incontinence.[106] Impotence is very common and increases with age. Intraoperative blood loss of more than 500 mL is not uncommon, even with excellent surgical technique. However, the use of autologous blood donation has greatly decreased the risks of heterologous blood transfusion.[106] Radical prostatectomy performed in patients with extracapsular disease is associated with a higher rate of recurrence than if performed in patients with organ-confined disease.[107,108] Risk factors for extracapsular disease have been reported to include PSA, PSAD, number of positive biopsies (an indirect indicator of tumor volume), and tumor volume.[109–111]

EXPECTANT MANAGEMENT

Recently, several authors have argued for observation, or expectant therapy, as a treatment modality for localized cancer of the prostate. Although this has always been an option, in most cases observation has been reserved for the extremely elderly, debilitated, and generally poor surgical candidates. These recent reports claim that the morbidity of radical prostatectomy outweighs its benefits. With the widespread use of PSA more and more cases of prostate cancer are being identified each year, and generally at earlier stages. Consequently, the critical issue becomes, ''Will this early detection and presumably treatment lead to a decrease in the mortality from carcinoma of the prostate, or will it lead to overtreatment and its undesired morbidity?''

All the current reports on expectant management are non-randomized and are generally based on a high selected group of patients. Selection criteria from some of the series include low stage and grade, absence of clinical symptoms, and a defined period of nonprogression. The Orebro study was reported on by Johansson et al.[112,113] Although this study reports on tumors of all grades, selection bias led to the majority (66%) of the patients having grade 1 tumors. In addition, one-third of the 233 patients had T1a disease, 15% were stage T1b, and 52% were T2. Also the mean age of this study group was 72 years of age. At 12.5 years of follow-up, death from prostate cancer occurred in 10% of patients; in 66% death occurred from other causes. The low death rate from prostate cancer in this study represents the predominant low grade and stage of this selected aged patient population. Of the 223 patients, 77 patients had progression of their disease. Sixty-four percent of progressions was local versus 36% progression to metastatic disease.

Handley et al reported on 278 patients managed with expectant therapy in the United Kingdom.[114] Patients of all grades and stages were represented in this study with the only entrance criterion being lack of symptoms. Nearly all these patients (95%) were diagnosed by TURP. The interesting aspect of this study was that more patients died of prostate cancer (45%) than died of other causes (5%). This can be explained by the broader entrance criteria and the fact that 19.4% of patients had metastatic disease at diagnosis.

Schellhammer recently compiled 10-year outcomes from five expectant management series.[115] For patients who would be candidates for radical prostatectomy in the United States (less than 70 years old, localized disease), he found 10-year metastases-free survival rates of 80 to 85%, which compares favorably with results of radical prostatectomy.

Long-term, prospective, randomized studies are necessary to definitively answer the questions of which treatment is best for patients with localized carcinoma of the prostate. Two studies are currently being conducted in Scandinavian countries: irradiation versus observation in Denmark and northern Sweden, and radical prostatectomy versus observation in Sweden and Finland.

REFERENCES

1. McNeal J: The prostate gland: morphology and pathology. *Monogr Urol* 1983;4:1.
2. Smith E, Resnick M: Imaging of the prostate. In: Lepor H, Lawson R, eds. *Prostatic Diseases*. Philadelphia: WB Saunders, 1993.
3. Muldoon L, Resnick M: Normal anatomy of the prostate. In: Resnick M, ed. *Prostatic Ultrasonography*. Philadelphia: BC Decker, 1990.
4. Cooner W: Anatomy of the prostate as seen by ultrasound. *AUA Updates* 1990;9(42).
5. Wild J, Reid J: Application of echo-ranging techniques to the structure of biopsy tissues. *Science*, 1951;115:226.
6. Wantabe H, Katoh H: Diagnostic application of the ultrasonography for the prostate. *J Urol* 1968;59:279.
7. Boyce W: History of prostatic ultrasonography. In: Resnick M, ed: *Prostatic Ultrasonography*. Philadelphia: BC Decker, 1990; 1–16.
8. King W, Wilkiemeyer R, Boyce W, McKinney W: Current status of prostatic ultrasonography. *JAMA*, 1973;226:444.
9. Resnick M, Willard J, Boyce W: Recent progress in ultrasonography of the bladder and prostate. *J Urol* 1977;117:444.
10. Arger P: Computed tomography of the lower urinary tract. *Urol Clin North Am* 1985;12:677.
11. Declecq G, Dennis L, Broos J, Appel R: Evaluation of lower urinary tract by transrectal ultrasonography. *Comput Tomogr* 1981;5:153.
12. Schnall M, Lenkinski R, Pollack H, Imai Y, Kressel H: Prostate: MR imaging with an endorectal surface coil. *Radiology* 1989;172:570.
13. Newhouse J: Clinical use of urinary tract magnetic resonance imaging. *Radiol Clin North Am* 1991;29:455.
14. Ramchandani P, Schnall M: Magnetic resonance imaging of the prostate. *Semin Roentgenol* 1993;28:74.
15. Rifkin M, Dahnert W, Kurtz A: State of the art: endorectal sonography of the prostate gland. *AJR* 1990;154:691.
16. Wantabe H: Transrectal sonography: a personal review and recent advances. *Scand J Urol Nephrol* 1991;137:75.
17. Rifkin M, Alexander A, Helinek T, Merton D: Color Doppler as an adjunct to prostate ultrasound. *Scand J Urol Nephrol* 1991;137(suppl):85.
18. Rifkin M: Prostate Ultrasound. *Semin Ultrasound CT MR* 1988;9:352.
19. Schiebler M, Tomaszewski J, Bezzi M: Prostatic carcinoma and benign prostatic hyperplasia: correlation of high resolution MR and histopathologic findings. *Radiology* 1989;172:131.
20. Meares E: Prostatitis: review of pharmacokinetics and therapy. *Rev Infect Dis* 1982;4:475.
21. Lim D, Schaeffer A: Prostatitis syndromes. *AUA Updates*, 1993;12(1).
22. Barbalias G: Prostadynia or painful male urethral syndrome? *Urology* 1990;36:146.
23. Weinberger M, Cytron S, Servadio C: Prostatic abscess in the antibiotic era. *Rev Infect Dis* 1988;10:239.

24. Berry S: The development of human benign prostatic hyperplasia with age. *J Urol* 1984;132:474.
25. Mebust W: BPH: patient care policies/guidelines. *AUA Updates* 1993;12(29).
26. Morse R, Resnick M: Imaging of the prostate. In: Paulson D, ed. *Prostatic Disorders*. Philadelphia: Lea & Febiger, 1989; 28.
27. Lepor H, Auerbach S, Puras-Baez A, et al: A randomized, placebo-controlled multicenter study of the efficacy and safety of terazosin in the treatment of benign prostatic hyperplasia. *J Urol* 1992;148:1467.
28. Mebust W: A review of TURP complications and the AUA National Cooperative Study. *AUA Updates* 1989;8(24).
29. Orandi A: Transurethral incision of the prostate. *J Urol* 1973; 110:229.
30. Bruskewitz R, Christensen M: Critical evaluation of transurethral resection and incision of the prostate. *Prostate* 1990; 3(suppl):27.
31. McCullough D, Roth R, Babayan R, et al: Transurethral ultrasound-guided laser induced prostatectomy: National Cooperative Study results. *J Urol* 1993;150:1607.
32. Norris J, Norris R, Lee R, Rubenstein M: Visual laser ablation of the prostate: clinical experience in 108 patients. *J Urol* 1993;150:1612.
33. Oesterling J: Stenting of the male lower urinary tract: a novel idea with much promise. *J Urol* 1993;150:1648. Editorial.
34. Frankes L: Latent carcinoma of the prostate. *J Pathol Biol*. 1954;68:603.
35. Scardino P, Weaver R, Hudson M: Early detection of prostate cancer. *Hum Pathol* 1992;23:211.
36. Bova G, Carter B, Bussemarkers M, et al: Homozygous deletion and frequent allelic loss of chromosome 8p22 loci in human prostate cancer. *Cancer Res* 1993;53:3869.
37. Resnick M: Transrectal ultrasound versus digitally directed prostatic biopsy: a comparative study. *J Urol* 1988;139:754.
38. McNeal J, Bostwick D, Minduchuk R: Patterns of progression in prostate cancer. *Lancet* 1986;1:60.
39. McNeal J, Villers A, Redwine E, Frieha F, Stamey T: Histologic differentiation, cancer volume and pelvic lymph node metastases in adenocarcinoma of the prostate. *Cancer* 1990; 66:1225.
40. McNeal J, Villers A, Redwine E, Frieha F, Stamey T: Capsular penetration in prostate cancer. *Am J Surg Pathol* 1990; 14:240.
41. Terris M, Stamey T: Determination of prostate volume by transrectal ultrasound. *J Urol* 1991;145:984.
42. Stamey T, Frieha F, McNeal J, Redwine E, Whitmore A, Schmid H: Relationship of tumor volume to clinical significance for treatment of prostate cancer. *J Urol* 1992; 147:303A.
43. Stamey T: Cancer of the prostate. *Mongr Urol* 1983;4:68.
44. Scardino P: Early detection of prostate cancer. *Urol Clin North Am* 1989;16:635.
45. Oesterling J: PSA: a critical assessment of the most useful tumor marker for carcinoma of the prostate. *J Urol* 1991; 145:907.
46. Cooner W, Mosely B, Rutherford C: Prostate cancer detection with ultrasonography, digital rectal exam and prostate specific antigen. *J Urol* 1990;143:1146.
47. Rommel F, Agusta V, Bresslin J, et al: The use of prostate specific antigen density in the diagnosis of prostate cancer in a community based urology practice. *J Urol* 1994; 151:88.
48. Catalona W, Smith D, Ratliff T, et al: Measurement of prostate specific antigen in serum as a screening test for prostate cancer. *N Engl J Med* 1991;324:1156.
49. Brawer M, Chetner M, Beatie J, Buchner J, Vessella R, Lange P: Screening for prostate carcinoma with prostate specific antigen. *J Urol* 1992;147:841.
50. Benson M, Whang I, Pantuck A, et al: Prostate specific antigen density: a means of distinguishing benign prostatic hyperplasia and prostate cancer. *J Urol* 1992;147:815.
51. Brawer M, Aramburu E, Chen G, Preston S, Ellis W: The inability of prostate specific antigen index to enhance the predictive value of prostate specific antigen in the diagnosis of prostate cancer. *J Urol* 1993;150:369.
52. Carter H, Pearson J, Metter E, et al: Longitudinal evaluation of prostate specific antigen levels in men with and without prostate disease. *JAMA* 1992;267:2215.
53. Brawer M, Beatie J, Wener M, Vessella R, Preston S, Lange P: Screening for prostatic carcinoma with PSA: results of the second year. *J Urol* 1993;150:106.
54. Thompson I: Screening for carcinoma of the prostate. *AUA Update* 1990;9:225.
55. Waterhouse R, Resnick M: The use of transrectal prostatic ultrasonography in the evaluation of patients with prostatic carcinoma. *J Urol* 1989;141:233.
56. Coffield K, Speights V, Brawn P, Riggs M: Ultrasound detection of prostate cancer in postmortem specimens with histopathologic correlation. *J Urol* 1992;147:882.
57. Terris M, Frieha F, McNeal J, Stamey T: Efficacy of transrectal ultrasound for identification of clinically undetected prostate cancer. *J Urol* 1991;146:78.
58. Greene D, Scardino P: Transrectal ultrasonography for prostate cancer. *PPO Update* 1990;4:1.
59. Stamey T: Diagnosis of prostate cancer: a personal view. *J Urol* 1992;147:830.
60. Gleason D: Histologic grading and staging of prostatic carcinoma. In: Tannenbaum M, ed. *Urologic Pathology: The Prostate*. Philadelphia: Lea & Febiger, 1977;171–197.
61. Stamey T, Yang N, McNeal J, Freiha F, Redwine E: Prostate specific antigen as a serum marker for adenocarcinoma of the prostate. *N Engl J Med* 1987;317:909.
62. Partin A, Carter H, Chan D, et al: Prostate specific antigen in the staging of localized prostate cancer: influence of tumor deafferentation, tumor volume and benign hyperplasia. *J Urol* 1990;143:747.
63. Stamey T, McNeal J: Adenocarcinoma of the prostate. In: Walsh P, Retik A, Stamey T, Vaughn E, eds. *Campbell's Urology*. Philadelphia: WB Saunders, 1992;1159–1221.
64. Rifkin M, Friedland G, Shortliffe L: Prostatic evaluation by transrectal endosonography: detection of carcinoma. *Radiology* 1986;158:85.
65. Lee F, Gray J, McCleary R, et al: Prostatic evaluation by transrectal sonography. *Radiology* 1986;158:91.
66. Dahnert W, Hamper U, Eggleston J, Walsh P, Sanders R: Prostatic evaluation by transrectal sonography with histopathologic correlation: the echogenic appearance of early carcinoma. *Radiology* 1988;158:97.
67. Shinohara K, Wheeler T, Scardino P: The appearance of prostate cancer on transrectal ultrasonography: correlation of imaging and pathologic examinations. *J Urol* 1989;142:76.
68. Hammerer P, Huland H: Systematic sextant biopsies in 651 patients referred for prostate evaluation. *J Urol* 1994;151:99.
69. Goldstein S, Gammelgard J, Holm H: Transrectal ultrasonic volume determination of the prostate—a preoperative and postoperative study. *J Urol* 1982;127:1115.
70. Pontes J, Eisenkraft S, Wantabe H, Ohe H, Saitoh M, Murphy G: Preoperative evaluation of localized prostatic carcinoma by transrectal ultrasonography. *J Urol* 1985;134:289.
71. Fujino A, Scardino P: Transrectal ultrasonography of prostate cancer: its value in staging and monitoring response to radiotherapy and chemotherapy. *J Urol* 1985;133:806.

72. Hamper U, Sheth S: Prostate ultrasonography. *Semin Roentgenol* 1993;28:57.
73. Perrapato S, Carothers G, Maatman T, Soechtig C: Comparing clinical staging plus transrectal ultrasound with surgical-pathologic staging of prostate cancer. *Urology* 1989; 33:103.
74. Rifkin M, Zerhouni E, Gatsonis C, et al: Comparison of magnetic resonance imaging and ultrasonography in staging early prostate cancer: results of a multi-institutional cooperative trial. *N Engl J Med* 1990;323:621.
75. Sorek P, McHugh T: Letter to the editor. *J Urol* 1986; 136:479.
76. Salo J, Kivisaari L, Rannikko S, et al: Computed tomography and transrectal ultrasound in the assessment of local extension of prostate cancer before radical prostatectomy. *J Urol* 1987; 137:435.
77. Terris M, McNeal J, Stamey T: Estimation of prostate cancer volume by transrectal ultrasound imaging. *J Urol* 1992; 147:855.
78. Holm H, Gammelgard J: Ultrasonically guided precise needle placement in the prostate and seminal vesicles. *J Urol* 1981; 125:385.
79. Resnick M: Ultrasound guided and digitally guided biopsies of the prostate. *J Endourol* 1989;3:177.
80. Hodge K, McNeal J, Terris M, Stamey T: Random systematic versus directed ultrasound guided transrectal core biopsies of the prostate. *J Urol* 1989;142:71.
81. Lippermann H, Ghiatas A, Sarosdy M: Systematic transrectal ultrasound guided prostate biopsy after negative digitally guided prostate biopsy. *J Urol,* 1992;147:827.
82. Mukamel E, Hannah J, Barbaric Z, DeKernion J: The value of computerized tomography scan and magnetic resonance imaging in staging prostatic carcinoma: comparison with the clinical and histological staging. *J Urol* 1986;136:1231.
83. Platt J, Bree R, Schwab R: The accuracy of CT in the staging of carcinoma of the prostate. *AJR* 1987;149(2):315.
84. Hricak H, Dooms G, Jeffrey R, et al: Prostatic carcinoma: staging by clinical assessment, CT and MRI imaging. *Radiology* 1987;162:331.
85. Hricak H, Thoeni R: Neoplasms of the prostate gland. In: Pollack HM, ed. *Clinical Urography, 2.* Philadelphia: WB Saunders, 1990;1381–1403.
86. Wallner K, Chiv-Tsao S, Kitendra R, et al: An improved method for computerized tomography planned transperineal 125 iodine prostate implants. *J Urol* 1991;146:90.
87. Krauss D, Clark K, Nsouli I, Amin R, Kelly C, Mortek M: Prostate biopsy in patients after prostatectomy. *J Urol* 1993; 149:604.
88. Tempany C, Rahmouni A, Epstein J, Walsh P, Zerhouni E: Invasion of the neurovascular bundle by prostate cancer: evaluation by MR imaging. *Radiology* 1991;181:107.
89. Biodetti P, Lee J, Ling D, Catalona W: Clinical stage B prostate carcinoma: staging with MR imaging. *Radiology* 1987; 162:325.
90. Bezzi M, Kressel H, Allen K, et al: Prostatic carcinoma: staging with MR at 1.5 T. *Radiology* 1988;169:339.
91. Schuessler W, Vancaille T, Reich H, Griffith D: Transperitoneal endosurgical lymphaenectomy in patients with localized prostate cancer. *J Urol* 1991;145:988.
92. Winfield H, See W, Donovan J, Loening S, Williams R: A new cancer staging technique: laparoscopic pelvic lymph node dissection. *J Urol* 1991;145(pt 2):215A. Abstract 12.
93. Kerbl K, Clayman R, Petros J, Chandhoke P, Gill I: Staging pelvic lymphadenectomy for prostate cancer: a comparison of laparoscopic and open techniques. *J Urol* 1993;150:396.
94. See W, Cohen M, Winfield H: Inverted V peritoneotomy significantly improves nodal yield in laparoscopic pelvic lymphadenectomy. *J Urol* 1993;149:772.
95. Catalona W: *Prostate Cancer.* New York: Grune & Stratton, 1984.
96. Kabalin J, Hodge K, McNeal J, Frieha K, Stamey T: Identification of residual cancer in the prostate following radiation therapy: role of transrectal ultrasound guided biopsy and PSA. *J Urol* 1989;142:136.
97. Bagshaw M: Potential for radiotherapy alone in prostatic cancer. *Cancer* 1985;55:2079.
98. Kaplan I, Cox R, Bagshaw M: Prostate specific antigen after external beam radiotherapy for prostate cancer: follow-up. *J Urol* 1993;149:519.
99. Whitmore W, Hilaris B: Treatment of localized prostate cancer by interstitial 125-I. In: Karr J, Yamanaka H, eds. *Prostate Cancer: The Second Tokyo Symposium.* New York: Elsevier Science Publishing, 1989;344.
100. Gervasi L: Prognostic significance of lymph node metastases in prostate cancer. *J Urol* 1989;142:332.
101. Fuks Z: The effect of local control on metastatic dissemination of carcinoma of the prostate: long-term results in patients treated with 125 iodine implantation. *Int J Radiat Oncol Biol Phys* 1991;21:537.
102. Smalley S, Noble M: Prostate brachytherapy: clinical results, complications and salvage therapy (Part II). *AUA Updates* 1992;11(34).
103. Gibbons J, Correa RJ, Brannen GE, et al: Total prostatectomy for clinically localized prostate cancer: long term results. *J Urol* 1989;141:564.
104. Myers R, Flemming T: Course of clinically localized adenocarcinoma of the prostate treated by radical prostatectomy. *Prostate* 1983;4:461.
105. Elder J, Jewett H, Walsh P: Radical perineal prostatectomy for clinical stage B2 carcinoma of the prostate. *J Urol* 1982; 127:704.
106. Hautmann R, Sauter T, Wenderoth U: Radical retropubic prostatectomy: morbidity and urinary continence in 418 consecutive cases. *Urology* 1994;43(2 suppl.):47.
107. Paulson D, Moul J, Walther P: Radical prostatectomy for clinical stage T1-2, N0, M0 prostatic adenocarcinoma. *J Urol* 1990;144:1180.
108. Stein A, DeKernion J, Smith R, Dorey F, Patel H: Prostate specific antigen levels after radical prostatectomy in patients with organ confined and locally extensive disease. *J Urol* 1992;147:942.
109. Ackerman D, Barry J, Wicklund R, Olson N, Lowe B: Analysis of risk factors associated with prostate cancer extension to the surgical margin and pelvic lymph node metastases at radical prostatectomy. *J Urol* 1993;150:1845.
110. Stamey T, Villers A, Frieha F, McNeal J, Link P, Frieha F: Positive surgical margins at radical prostatectomy: importance of the apical dissection. *J Urol* 1990;143:1166.
111. Voges G, McNeal J, Redwine E, Freiha E, Stamey T: Morphologic analysis of surgical margins with positive findings in prostatectomy for adenocarcinoma of the prostate. *Cancer* 1992;69:520.
112. Johansson J, Adami H, Andersson S, Bergstrom R, Holmperg L, Krusemo U: High 10-year survival rate in patients with early, untreated prostate cancer. *JAMA* 1992;267:2191.
113. Johansson J: Watchful waiting for early stage prostate cancer. *Urology* 1994;43:138.
114. Handley R, Carr T, Powell P, Hall R: Deferred treatment of prostate cancer. *Br J Urol* 1988;62:249.
115. Schellhammer P: Natural history of prostate cancer: an analysis of contemporary expectant therapy series. Visiting professor lecture, at Case Western Reserve University. January 8, 1994.

23 Disorders of the Scrotum and Its Contents

David S. Sandock, Thomas E. Herbener, Martin I. Resnick

The scrotum, a relatively small part of the body, houses several important organs that are subject to a large number of disease processes. This chapter consolidates the currently available clinical information concerning the diagnosis and treatment of intrascrotal pathologies. Current imaging strategies are discussed in general and for each specific pathologic condition.

ANATOMY OF THE SCROTUM

The scrotal wall is composed of skin, fascia, and muscle in layers analogous to those of the anterior abdominal wall. The layers form an elastic sack with a midline septum and each compartment houses a testis, epididymis, and distal spermatic cord. The outermost layer is the scrotal skin. This skin is thin, highly pigmented, rugated in texture, and contiguous to that of the abdomen and perineum. Beneath the skin is the dartos layer, which consists of fibrous, elastic, and smooth muscle components and is quite vascular. The dartos fascia is continuous with Scarpa's fascia in the abdomen and Colles' fascia in the perineum. Beneath the dartos layer is the external spermatic fascia, which is a direct continuation of the external abdominal oblique fascia in the abdomen. The next layer is the cremasteric fascia, which is a continuation of the internal oblique fascia. This layer frequently contains striated muscle that is responsible for retraction of the testicles. Beneath the cremasteric fascia is the internal spermatic fascia, which is a continuation of the transversalis fascia. The next two layers are the parietal and visceral layers of the tunica vaginalis, which are continuations of the anterior and posterior peritoneum. The visceral tunica vaginalis is closely adherent to the tunica albuginea of the testicle. There is a potential space between the two layers of tunica vaginalis that may fill with fluid (hydrocele) or blood (hematocele).

The scrotal wall blood supply is from the perineal, femoral, and inferior epigastric arteries. Its venous drainage parallels the arterial supply. The lymphatic drainage of the scrotal wall is to the superficial and subinguinal nodes. This lymphatic drainage pattern is separate from that of the testicles, a fact that becomes important in the management of patients with testicular cancer.

The spermatic cord travels through the inguinal canal and enters the scrotum through the external inguinal ring. The spermatic cord contains the testicular artery, the testicular veins (the pampiniform plexus), testicular lymphatics, and the vas deferens, with its artery and veins. The cord is enveloped by external spermatic fascia.

The average testis dimensions are 4 × 3 × 2.5 cm. The testis is covered by a thick, fibrous capsule called the tunica albuginea. Along the posterolateral surface of the testis lies the epididymis. The two are connected by the rete testis and efferent ductules of the testis. The vas deferens is continuous with the tail of the epididymis, lies posteromedial to the epididymis, and travels through the spermatic cord. The internal spermatic or testicular artery supplies the testis and epididymis. The epididymis also receives blood from the vasal artery.

The lymphatic drainage of the right and left testicle have been studied extensively and are of great clinical significance in the staging and treatment of patients with testicular cancer.[1] Lymphatic drainage from the left testicle drains predictably to the left external iliac, left common iliac, preaortic, and finally periaortic lymph nodes. Lymphatic drainage from the right testicle drains to the right external iliac, right common iliac, paracaval, preaortic, precaval, and finally interaortocaval lymph nodes. Right to left crossover metastases are common, but left to right crossover has not been observed.[1]

PHYSICAL EXAMINATION OF THE SCROTUM AND ITS CONTENTS

The patient should be examined in an upright position with the examiner sitting. Visual inspection of the scrotum should be carried out by first looking for skin lesions and general asymmetry. The testes should be palpated bimanually. Then size, tenderness, consistency, and location in the scrotum should be noted. All scrotal masses should be transilluminated by placing a light posterior to the scrotum and dimming the room lights; this helps to distinguish fluid-filled lesions (i.e., hydrocele, spermatocele) from solid lesions (i.e., tumor).

The epididymis is palpated posterolateral to the testis and should be examined for tenderness and mass lesions. The spermatic cord is most easily palpated by grasping it between one's thumb and index finger high in the scrotum. The vas deferens originates from the inferior pole of the epididymis and is usually palpable in the cord. The cremasteric reflex should be tested by lightly scratching the medial aspect of the upper thigh. This stimulates the ilioinguinal nerve, which causes the cremasteric muscle to contract, thereby raising the testicle. This reflex is commonly absent with torsion of the spermatic cord. The inguinal region should be palpated for lymph nodes.

TECHNIQUES OF IMAGING AND RADIOGRAPHIC ANATOMY OF THE SCROTUM

Ultrasound and Color Doppler Imaging

For scrotal sonography the patient is placed in the supine position in a warm room (to prevent testicular contraction) with a towel holding the penis out of the way in a cephalad position. High-frequency probes (7 to 10 MHz) are used for scrotal imaging.[2,3] With higher-frequency probes, better image resolution is achieved, but the sound waves do not penetrate as deeply. This is well suited for the relatively superficial structures of the scrotum.

With ultrasound imaging, the scrotal wall appears as a 2 to 8 mm thick hyperechoic band (Fig. 23–1).[4] The testes appear as symmetrical ovoid structures with homogeneous, medium level echogenicity within and a hyperechoic rim representing the tunica albuginea.[2,5,6] The head of the epididymis is seen adjacent to the posterior superior aspect of the testis and is similar in echogenicity.[4,7] The body and tail are more difficult to image sonographically. Benign cysts of the epididymis are seen in 40% of cases.[4] A small amount of fluid is commonly seen in between the layers of the tunica vaginalis and appears anechoic. Small amounts of fluid are physiologic and permit the testis to move freely, whereas larger amounts are pathologic and represent a hydrocele.[8]

Color Doppler imaging is a relatively new modality that allows the simultaneous viewing of real-time gray-scale imaging and an evaluation of arterial and venous blood flow (Fig. 23–2). The Doppler effect, or Doppler shift, refers to the alteration in frequency that occurs when a wave (i.e., sound wave) is reflected off a moving target. The net frequency of the returning wave is evaluated and compared to the original signal; then different colors are superimposed on the gray-scale image, depending on whether the reflected waves are of higher or lower frequency (i.e., the red blood cells are moving away from or toward the transducer. The ability to evaluate perfusion simultaneously with real-time anatomic imaging is of great value in scrotal imaging.

Magnetic Resonance Imaging of the Scrotum

For magnetic resonance imaging (MRI) of the scrotum, a body surface coil is placed in direct contact with the scrotum (Fig. 23–3). The scrotal wall is seen clearly on T2-weighted images as being composed of several layers. The normal testes appear intermediate in signal intensity on T1-weighted images and high in signal intensity on T2-weighted images.[9,10] The tunica albuginea is seen as a dark rim of low signal intensity.[11] The epididymis is isodense to the testis on T1 imaging and hypodense to the testis on T2 imaging.[9,10] On T2-weighted images, the vas deferens is readily identified with low-intensity walls and a high-intensity lumen.[11]

Nuclear Scintigraphy of the Scrotum

In a normal nuclear study of the scrotum, symmetrical activity is seen in both sides of the scrotum representing flow to both testicles.[12] The scrotal wall, testis, and epididymis are not individually distinguishable. The iliac and femoral vessels are easily identifiable; however, the spermatic cord is seldom visualized.

CONGENITAL ABNORMALITIES OF THE SCROTUM

Scrotal Hypoplasia

Scrotal hypoplasia may be unilateral or bilateral. The overlying skin is typically nonrugated, and the absence of one or both testes is common. Treatment consists of only cosmetic measures such as local testosterone cream and in some patients placement of a testicular prosthesis.

Bifid Scrotum and Penoscrotal Transposition

Bifid scrotum is a condition where there appear to be two separate hemiscrotums. This is usually associated with severe (perineal or penoscrotal) hypospadias. Scrotoplasty is performed 6 months after hypospadias repair.[13] Penoscrotal

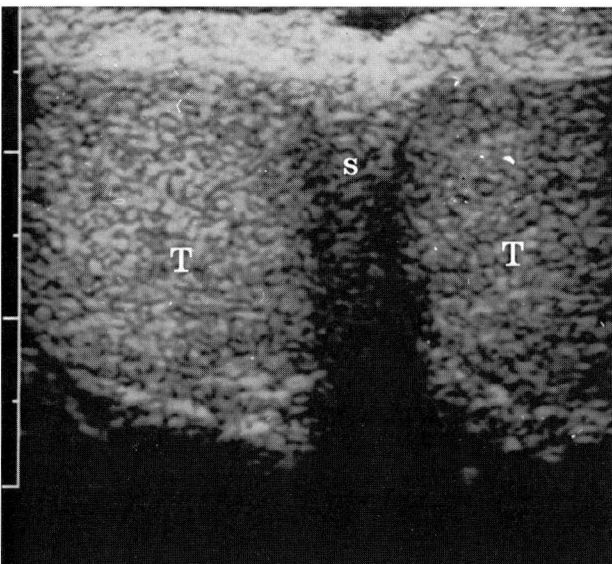

Figure 23–1. Normal testes (ultrasound). Normal testes (T) and intrascrotal septum (s) are seen. The testicular parenchyma has a homogeneous echogenicity.

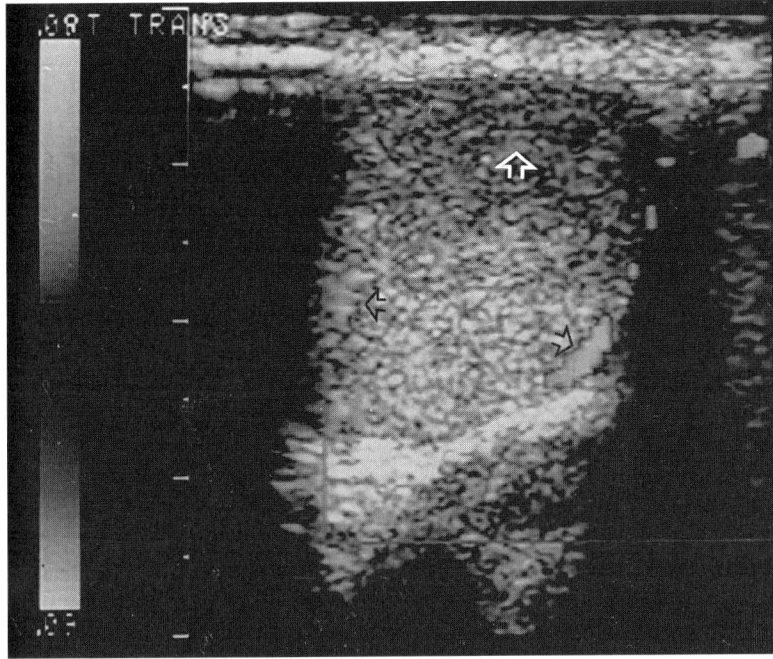

Figure 23–2. Normal testicular blood flow. Normal blood flow demonstrated (arrows) by color Doppler imaging (CDI). (Reproduced in black and white.)

transposition is either the most pronounced form of bifid scrotum or a separate entity. Although patients with penoscrotal transposition may be functionally normal, surgical correction should be performed for both psychological and cosmetic reasons.

Scrotal Ectopia

Scrotal ectopia is a rare congenital abnormality that refers to an anomalous position of the hemiscrotum. The ectopic scrotum may be anywhere from the groin to the perineum or from the inner thigh to the buttocks, but is most often suprainguinal.[14,15] The ipsilateral testis may be normal or dysplastic, and orchiopexy or orchiectomy may be performed as indicated. This condition may be associated with inguinal hernia, exstrophy, and cryptorchidism.[16] These patients should undergo a cryptorchidism workup as deemed necessary. Patients with the suprainguinal form have a high incidence of upper urinary tract abnormalities and should be screened with intravenous urography.

Scrotal Hemangiomas

Hemangiomas of the external genitalia account for approximately 1% of cutaneous hemangiomas and are much more common in females. Scrotal hemangiomas are rare, with fewer than 50 cases in the literature.[17] Cutaneous strawberry hemangiomas are the most common type; however, some intrascrotal hemangiomas may occur. The latter may require surgical excision because they tend not to involute, whereas the former rarely require treatment. Angiography, if performed, would demonstrate a proliferation of capillary and/or venous vessels, but generally need not be performed. Color Doppler ultrasound may aid in diagnosis of the intrascrotal hemangioma and is a completely noninvasive technique.

INFLAMMATORY PROCESSES

Epididymitis

DEFINITION AND ETIOLOGY

Acute epididymitis is an inflammation of the epididymis. The vast majority of cases are infectious in etiology, but acute epididymitis may also be secondary to trauma, reflux

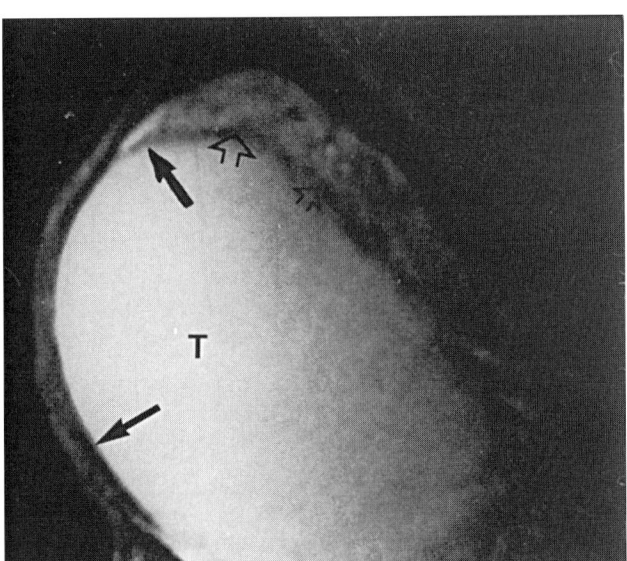

Figure 23–3. Normal testis (MRI, T2 weighted). The testis (T) is seen with high signal intensity. The epididymis is seen (open arrows) with mixed signal intensity, and the tunica albuginea (dark arrows) is seen with low signal intensity.

of sterile urine through the vas deferens, or use of the antiarrhythmic medication amiodorone.[18] Infectious cases are classified as sexually and nonsexually transmitted etiologies. In general, young boys, old men and postoperative patients from urologic procedures will have nonsexually transmitted epididymitis. The predominant etiologic organism is gramnegative coliform bacteria. Sexually active heterosexual men usually have either *Neisseria gonorrhoeae*, *Chlamydia trachomatis*, or both. These men are mainly less than 35 years old.[19] Sexually active homosexual men typically have gramnegative coliform bacteria. The underlying principle is that in any age or demographic group the most common etiology of epididymitis is the most common cause of bacteriuria or urethritis in that group.[20] In many cases an etiology may not be found.

CLINICAL FINDINGS

The primary symptoms of acute epididymitis include pain and swelling of the epididymis and scrotum. The patient may also experience symptoms of urethritis or prostatitis with dysuria and other irritative voiding symptoms. High fever is not uncommon. On physical examination, the epididymis is exquisitely tender, and a reactive hydrocele is commonly found. The ipsilateral testicle often becomes involved, leading to epididymo-orchitis.

DIAGNOSTIC TECHNIQUES

Diagnostic techniques should not only help confirm a diagnosis of epididymitis, but also help rule out torsion. Real-time gray-scale ultrasound findings are not specific. The epididymis is enlarged in size and is generally decreased in echogenicity because of inflammatory edema, but there may also be increased echogenicity.[21] There also may be thickening of the overlying scrotal skin. Color Doppler imaging is much more accurate in this setting. With color Doppler imaging of epididymitis, a marked increase in arterial blood flow is seen in most cases.[22,23] Ralls et al were able to differentiate epididymitis from other scrotal disorders with a sensitivity of 91% and a specificity of 100% using color Doppler imaging.[22] Wilbert et al found a sensitivity of 70% and a specificity of 88% in 10 patients with acute scrotal pain.[24] Hyperemia seen on color Doppler imaging seems to precede gray-scale findings. Hortsman et al found that 20% of the patients with clinical epididymitis demonstrated hyperemia using color Doppler, whereas gray-scale ultrasound was normal.[23] Color Doppler imaging may also demonstrate prominent venous flow in cases of acute epididymitis (Fig. 23–4), which is not seen in patients with a normal epididymis. Ultrasound also allows for the assessment of complications of epididymitis, such as abscess or pyelocele. Kim et al conducted radionuclide studies that also reveal increased blood flow in patients with acute epididymitis,[12] but this study is rarely performed with cases of suspected epididymitis.

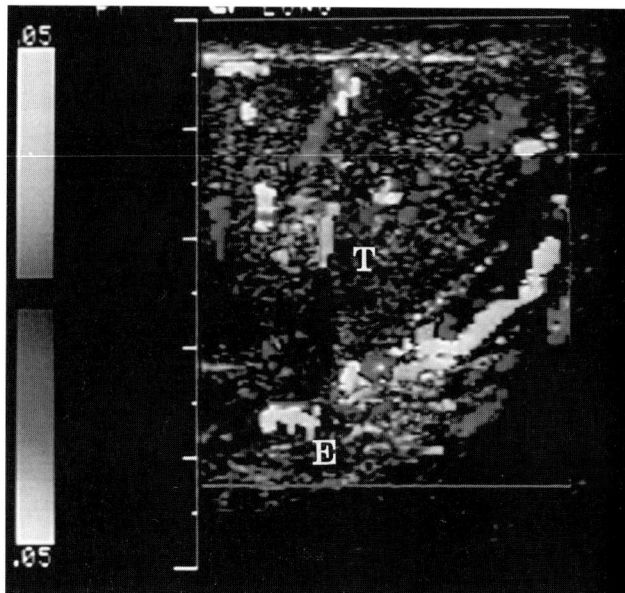

Figure 23–4. Epididymo-orchitis. The testis (T) and epididymis (E) are both grossly enlarged. Gray-scale ultrasound demonstrates decreased echogenicity, whereas the addition of color Doppler imaging (CDI) demonstrates reactive hyperemia.

THERAPY

Once the diagnosis has been made, treatment is directed at the causative organism, either based empirically or on culture. Patients with suspected sexually transmitted epididymo-orchitis should have a Gram stain and urethral smear culture. They should then receive 250 mg ceftriaxone intramuscularly and be started on a 10-day course of either oral tetracycline 500 mg q.i.d. or doxycycline 100 mg b.i.d. This combination drug therapy ensures coverage against both *N. gonorrhoeae* and *C. trachomatis*. If sexually transmitted disease is not suspected, a urine culture and sensitivity should be done and the patient should be started on a course of broad-spectrum antibiotics, such as trimethoprim/sulfamethoxazole or a quinolone. Nonsteroidal anti-inflammatory pain relievers may be of benefit. The patient should be instructed to rest as much as possible and keep his scrotum elevated on a towel when sitting or lying down.

Chronic Epididymitis

Chronic epididymitis represents an end-stage disease resultant from recurrent bouts of acute epididymitis. The epididymis becomes replaced with fibrous scar tissue and the patient typically has chronic mild pain or discomfort. On palpation the epididymis is indurated and may be tender. When examined with scrotal sonography, the epididymis appears either heterogeneous or hyperechoic.[25] Treatment is supportive unless symptoms are severe, in which case an epididymectomy may be performed.

Orchitis

DEFINITION AND ETIOLOGY

Orchitis, or inflammation of the testicle, is uncommon as an isolated process. Orchitis is much more likely to be secondary to epididymitis via direct extension and therefore to be part of epididymo-orchitis. When it does occur alone, the route of infection may be from hematogenous or lymphatic spread.

CLINICAL FINDINGS

The testicle is painful, tender, and enlarged, and a reactive hydrocele is often present. Fever, nausea, and vomiting are variably present.

DIAGNOSTIC TECHNIQUES

On scrotal sonography the testis appears enlarged and hypoechoic.[2] Occasionally, there are focal hypoechoic areas that may mimic tumor. If there is a strong clinical suspicion of orchitis, the patient may be treated appropriately and reimaged after his acute symptoms are gone. Reactive hydrocele is a common finding in acute orchitis. With color Doppler imaging (CDI), testicular hyperemia is seen, just as epididymal hyperemia is seen with acute epididymitis (Fig. 23–4).[23]

THERAPY

Treatment of acute orchitis is identical to that of acute epididymitis; each is a different expression of the same disease. (See the preceding discussion.)

MUMPS ORCHITIS

Mumps is the most common infectious etiology of acute orchitis and only occurs after puberty. The onset of mumps orchitis is rapid and occurs several days after mumps parotitis. The patient usually has a high fever, a swollen and erythematous scrotum, and lack of urinary symptoms. Acute mumps orchitis lasts approximately a week. Testicular atrophy may be noticed approximately a month after the acute phase. In about 30% of cases the testis is permanently damaged. If the damage occurs bilaterally, the patient may be rendered sterile. Treatment is supportive only. Fortunately, this disease is uncommon with today's immunization programs.

TORSION

Torsion of the Spermatic Cord

DEFINITION AND ETIOLOGY

Torsion of the spermatic cord is the twisting of the cord around its long axis. The incidence of torsion is one in 4000 in male patients less than 25 years old.[26,27] This is one of the true urologic emergencies, and if diagnosis is not made or therapy instituted quickly, the testicle will be lost. As the cord twists, there is at first venous blockage, followed by edema of the cord and scrotum and finally loss of arterial flow. It is generally agreed that a torsion of 720 degrees is necessary for a complete cessation of blood flow, both venous and arterial.[28,29] With complete torsion some damage to the seminiferous tubules can result within 1 or 2 hours; severe damage may occur by 4 hours; and often a nonviable testis results by 6 hours.[28–30] The cord may torse and detorse. Patients with onset of symptoms that last less than 24 hours do much better with respect to saving the testicle than patients with symptoms of more than 24 hours' duration.[31] Approximately two-thirds of torsions occur between the ages of 12 and 18 years, with the incidence slowly decreasing as age increases, although torsion may occur antenatally, neonatally, or at any time in adulthood. Certain patients are predisposed to torsion because of an abnormality of the insertion of the tunica vaginalis onto the spermatic cord. The tunica vaginalis completely invests the distal cord and testis in this case and allows the cord to rotate on its axis within the sac (intravaginal torsion). This abnormality is commonly referred to as the bell clapper deformity (Fig. 23–5) and is most often bilateral. In patients with a bell clapper deformity, there is probably also an initiating event, such as strenuous activity, trauma, or sexual activity, although in most cases there is no history of an initiating event. Forceful contraction of the cremasteric muscle may be the common mechanism of these precipitating events. Cryptorchid and malignant testes are also at an increased risk of torsion.[32] Antenatal (and neonatal) torsion has a different etiology. In this case the gubernaculum has not completely attached to the scrotum, the tunica vaginalis is loosely attached to the scrotum,[33] and the entire cord and vaginal sac twist (extravaginal torsion).

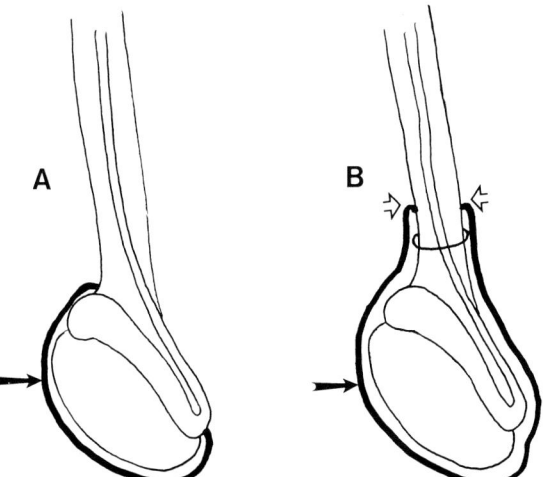

Figure 23–5. Bell clapper deformity. (**A**) Normal insertion of the tunica vaginalis (solid arrows). (**B**) The tunica vaginalis inserts high on the spermatic cord (open arrows), allowing intravaginal torsion of the cord.

CLINICAL FINDINGS

The patient usually has abrupt onset of unilateral testicular pain, followed by scrotal swelling and erythema. There may also be pain along the inguinal ligament and in the lower abdomen. Nausea and vomiting are commonly seen in patients with torsion. There are typically no urinary symptoms. Approximately 33 to 70% of patients admit to prior episodes of similar pain in the past that resolved spontaneously.[34] On physical examination there is a tender, swollen testicle that is usually high riding. The cremasteric reflex is usually absent, although this is not a reliable sign. There may be a leukocytosis, and urinalysis is normal. In cases of antenatal or neonatal torsion the patient is usually asymptomatic but may be irritable or not feel well.[35]

DIAGNOSTIC TECHNIQUES

During the physical examination an attempt may be made at manual detorsion. In most cases, as the cord torses, the anterior surface of the testis rotates toward the midline, and initial attempt at detorsion should be directed to turn the testicle in the opposite direction. If the patient immediately experiences relief of pain, a diagnosis is made. This is not a curative procedure, and a high percentage of patients will retorse. In this case orchiopexy should be performed electively within the next 24 hours.

Several imaging modalities may be of help in the diagnosis of torsion. It must be remembered that time is crucial, and if torsion is highly suspected or if imaging will cause a significant delay, the patient should be taken to the operating room for definitive treatment. The two imaging modalities commonly used are color Doppler imaging and nuclear scintigraphy.

Gray-scale ultrasound is not a reliable form of imaging, for the diagnosis of torsion of the spermatic cord as the acutely torsed testis may appear completely normal.[36,37] After a period of ischemia the testis may appear enlarged and hypoechoic; however, at this point the testis may be irreversibly damaged.[30,37] Ultrasound with color Doppler imaging is emerging as the best study for diagnosis of torsion of the spermatic cord. The classic findings of torsion of the spermatic cord with color Doppler imaging include the total absence of blood flow on the symptomatic side with normal blood flow on the contralateral side.[3] The latter finding serves as a control to ensure proper imaging technique. There is often increased blood flow in the peritesticular tissues, as this blood supply does not arrive in the scrotum via the spermatic cord.[23,38] Peritesticular hyperemia becomes more prominent with time and is analogous to the halo sign seen in late cases with nuclear scintigraphy. Color Doppler imaging is very accurate at diagnosing torsion of the spermatic cord, but it is not perfect. Sensitivity ranges from 82 to 89%, and specificity is 100% in most studies.[24,38–44] Pitfalls in diagnosis may occur with spontaneous detorsion where reactive hyperemia is seen or with incomplete torsion where decreased but not absent blood flow is seen. Color

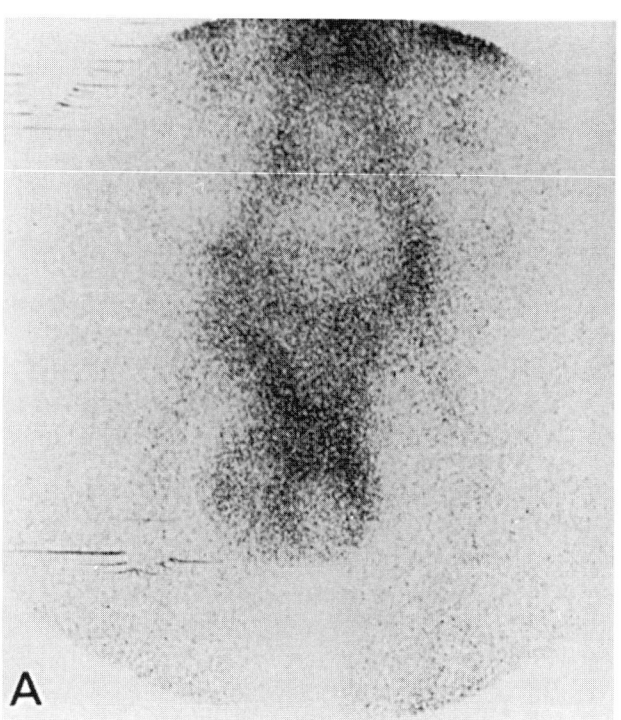

Figure 23–6. Nuclear scintigraphy torsed spermatic cord. A radionuclide scan reveals absence of perfusion to the left testis, suggesting torsion of the spermatic cord.

Doppler imaging is a noninvasive, quick, and very accurate imaging modality for evaluating torsion of the spermatic cord. The urologist must pay attention to the clinical impression based on physical examination and maintain a high degree of suspicion so as not to miss this very important diagnosis.

Nuclear scintigraphy was formerly the main imaging study of torsion of the spermatic cord. The findings vary according to the amount of time since the torsion and the degree of the torsion.[45] With acute torsion, there is decreased flow to the affected side (Fig. 23–6). In some cases, a nubbin sign is seen. This is an abrupt cutoff of activity at the level of the torsion. After approximately 7 hours, a halo sign is seen. This is seen with no activity centrally, representing the testis with no blood flow, and increased activity surrounding, representing the peritesticular hyperemia from the pudendal artery. After 24 hours this halo effect is even more pronounced.[12] Clinical studies have shown that color Doppler imaging is more accurate than nuclear scintigraphy for diagnosis of torsion of the spermatic cord,[38,41,42,44] as has a canine model study.[46] Because of the longer time it takes to perform nuclear scintigraphy and the increased accuracy of color Doppler imaging, the latter study is currently the study of choice for torsion of the spermatic cord if a study is to be performed at all.

THERAPY

Once a diagnosis of torsion is made or strongly suspected, the patient should be taken to the operating room for detorsion and orchiopexy as soon as possible. If the torsed testis is viable on detorsion, then orchiopexy is performed using nonabsorbable suture and "pexing" the testis in three locations. In all cases except neonatal torsion, the contralateral testis is also "pexed." In cases of neonatal or antenatal torsion, the contralateral testis rarely torses. In all cases if a nonviable testis is found, an orchiectomy is performed.

Torsion of the Testicular Appendages

The appendix testis and the appendix epididymis are vestigial remnants of the muellerian and mesonephric ducts. They are usually pedunculated and quite prone to torsion around their base. If left untreated, their natural history is to undergo ischemic necrosis and resorption. Their torsion causes pain but does not put the testis at risk. This is most common in boys under the age of 16 years, but many adult cases have been reported.[47] It is often difficult to differentiate this process from torsion of the spermatic cord.

The typical clinical picture is similar to that of torsion of the spermatic cord. If the patient presents early, a distinct 3- to 5-mm tender mass may be palpated at the superior pole of the testis or at the head of the epididymis. If the patient presents later, resultant edema of the scrotum makes it difficult to palpate this mass or to differentiate it from torsion of the spermatic cord. A blue dot sign on the overlying scrotum points toward torsion of one of the appendages.[48]

None of the preceding imaging modalities can reliably diagnose torsion of the appendages. Torsion of the appendices may lead to a reactive hyperemia that may mimic epididymo-orchitis on CDI. Therefore unless the diagnosis is convincingly made on clinical grounds, surgical exploration should be performed. The torsed appendage should be excised. Ipsilateral orchiopexy is probably not necessary[49] but may be performed. The contralateral hemiscrotum and testis should be left alone.

SCROTAL MASS LESIONS

Hydrocele

DEFINITION AND ETIOLOGY

A hydrocele is a collection of serous fluid between the two layers of the tunica vaginalis (Fig. 23–7). Hydroceles may be congenital or acquired. Congenital hydroceles are due to a prior or currently patent processus vaginalis and are the most common hydroceles in infants and children. In adults, hydroceles are secondary to infection, trauma, or malignancy, or they may be idiopathic.

CLINICAL FINDINGS

Patients with hydroceles present with a scrotal mass. Unless there is associated infection (i.e., epididymitis), there is usually no pain. If the mass is large, there may be a sensation of heaviness. On physical examination a cystic, nontender scrotal mass is found. This mass will transilluminate, differentiating it from other scrotal masses. The ipsilateral testicle is usually not palpable. In children with a communicating hydrocele, a history of a decrease in size on awakening and increase in size by night is common.

DIAGNOSTIC TECHNIQUES

Asymptomatic hydroceles do not have to be imaged unless there is a question of underlying testicular malignancy. If there is any question of underlying pathology, scrotal sonography should be performed. Gray-scale ultrasound is quite accurate at identifying testicular lesions that may not be palpable secondary to the hydrocele. The hydrocele itself is seen as an anechoic collection around the testicle (Fig. 23–8) but may have scattered echoes secondary to calculi, cholesterol crystals, or septations from inflammatory disease.[8] Other imaging modalities are not particularly useful for the evaluation of hydroceles.

THERAPY

Treatment of hydroceles is not necessary unless the patient is symptomatic. When performed, treatment consists of excising the tunica vaginalis. Aspiration is not an effective therapy and is only used for palliation in an unsuitable surgical candidate. Many hydroceles in children will resolve spontaneously. If persistent, they may be repaired through an inguinal approach. Associated inguinal hernia is common in children and may be repaired at the same time.

Varicocele

DEFINITION AND ETIOLOGY

A varicocele is a dilation of the testicular veins or pampiniform plexus in the spermatic cord (Fig. 23–7). Varicoceles are present in 10% of normal males and in approximately 30 to 40% of infertile males.[50–55] Left-sided varicoceles are much more common than right-sided ones (approximately 90% are left-sided) and are attributed to the drainage of the left testicular vein into the left renal vein as opposed to the inferior vena cava, as on the right. There is also a higher frequency of absent venous valves on the left side.[56] Varicoceles may be secondary to obstruction of the left renal vein, such as with renal cell carcinoma with a renal vein thrombus or retroperitoneal adenopathy. The sudden appearance of a varicocele should lead to an investigation of the retroperitoneum.

As stated earlier, varicoceles are associated with infertility. Approximately 56 to 90% of patients will have decreased sperm motility, and 25 to 67% will have oligospermia.[50,57] Semen parameters improve after varicocelectomy in approximately 65 to 70% of patients, but pregnancy rates are only 40 to 50%.[52,57–59] The main detrimental effect of the varicocele on spermatogenesis appears to be mediated by elevating the intrascrotal temperature.[55]

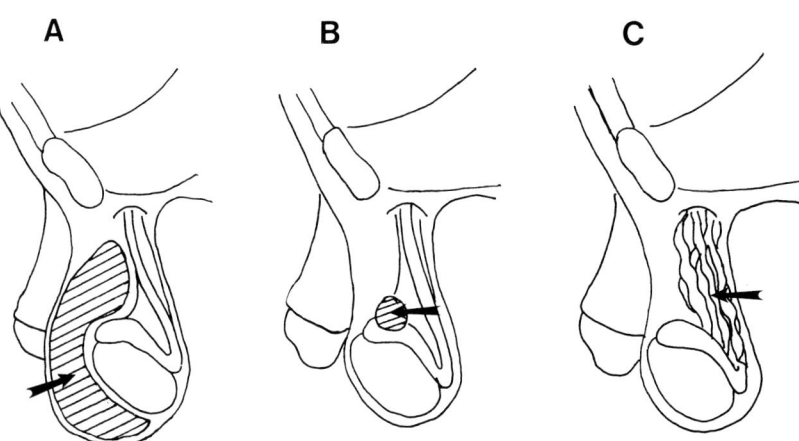

Figure 23–7. Intrascrotal swellings. **(A)** Hydrocele of the tunica vaginalis (arrow). **(B)** Spermatocele (arrow). **(C)** Varicocele (arrow).

CLINICAL FINDINGS

Most patients with varicoceles are asymptomatic. If symptomatic, the patient usually complains of a fullness or dull ache in the affected side or sides of the scrotum. On physical examination, the varicocele is palpated as enlarged soft scrotal mass with the consistency of a "bag of worms." Varicoceles are larger when the patient is standing and smaller when the patient lies down. Varicoceles are graded as follows:

> SUBCLINICAL: Visualized only with sophisticated imaging modalities (i.e., high-resolution sonography, color Doppler imaging); nonpalpable
> GRADE 1: Palpable only with Valsalva
> GRADE 2: Palpable without Valsalva
> GRADE 3: Visible without palpation

Ipsilateral testicular atrophy is present in varying degrees. Steeno et al found testicular atrophy in 34% of children with grade 2 varicocele and in 81% of children with grade 3 varicocele.[60]

DIAGNOSTIC TECHNIQUES

Although the incidence of clinically palpable varicocele is well known, the incidence of subclinical varicocele has yet to be established and is probably much higher. Palpable clinical varicoceles do not require imaging for diagnosis, but when imaging is desired, high-resolution gray-scale ultrasound is probably the best imaging modality (Fig. 23–9). The patient should be imaged in the supine and standing positions with and without Valsalva to reduce the number of false-negative scans. Typical gray-scale ultrasound findings include a prominence of veins in the pampiniform plexus, which increases in size during Valsalva. An increase of more than 1.0 mm during Valsalva relative to the relaxed upright position is considered a varicocele.[61] Other criteria

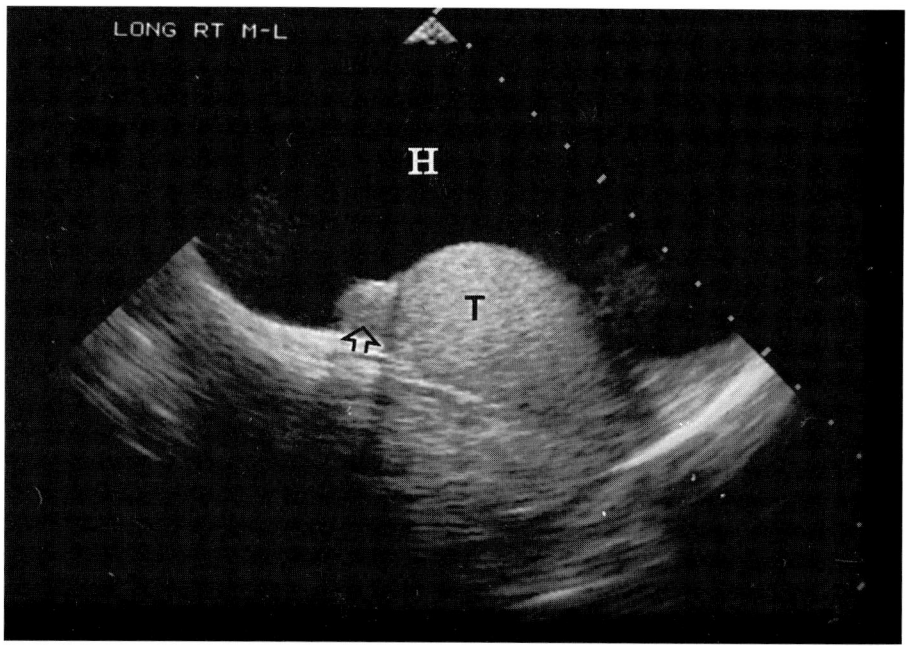

Figure 23–8. Hydrocele. A large simple hydrocele (H) is seen anterior to the testis (T) and epididymis (arrow).

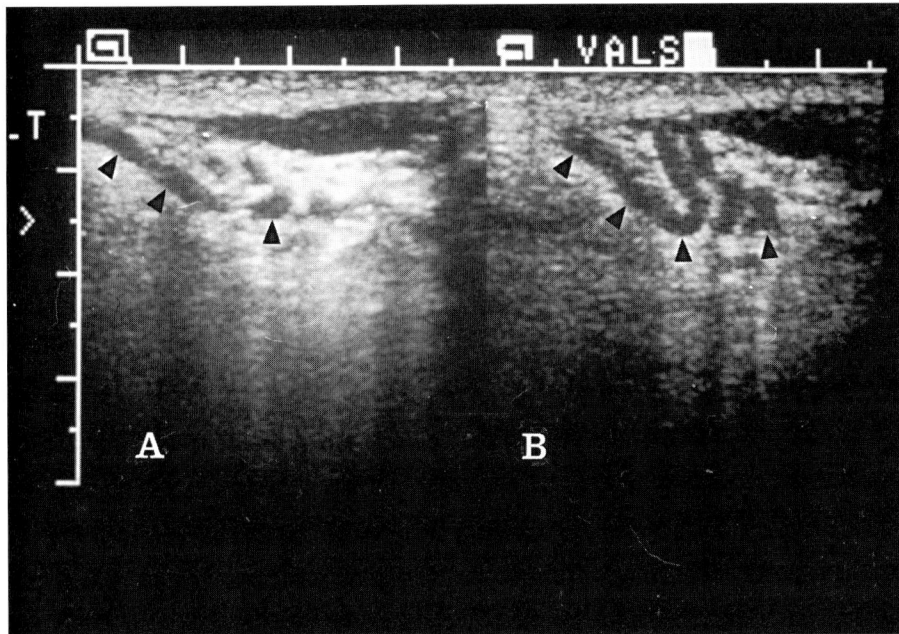

Figure 23–9. Varicocele. **(A)** Dilated veins (arrows) are seen. **(B)** The veins are enlarged with Valsalva.

diagnosing varicocele on ultrasound include veins larger than 2 mm without Valsalva and the presence of any veins caudal to the head of the epididymis.[8] Blood flow is seen dramatically with Valsalva in color Doppler imaging, and this appears to increase the diagnostic sensitivity.[62] Clinical and subclinical varicoceles may be imaged with nuclear scintigraphy.[63–66] Typcial findings include increased blood pool activity in the side with the varicocele. This technique offers no advantage over scrotal sonography.

THERAPY

Asymptomatic, long-standing varicoceles in fertile adults require no therapy. The exception is the sudden onset of a varicocele, as mentioned earlier, alerting the physician to the possibility of retroperitoneal tumor or adenopathy. Varicoceles in children and adolescents should be repaired in cases with evidence of testicular atrophy.

Once the decision to perform varicocelectomy is made, one must decide which approach to utilize. The goal in all approaches is to ligate and divide the dilated testicular veins and avoid injury to the testicular artery and lymphatic vessels. Currently, the inguinal approach is the most popular. This approach, which can be performed under local anesthesia, allows the spermatic cord to be brought into the field, facilitating identification and avoidance of the testicular artery and lymphatics. The operating microscope and Doppler stethoscope, which facilitate identification of the structures, may be utilized with this approach. Additionally, the testis may be delivered to identify posterior collaterals of the external spermatic and gubernacular veins. Utilization of these techniques leads to a decreased rate of hydrocele formation and varicocele recurrence.

Other approaches include high (retroperitoneal) ligation, transvenous radiographic embolization, and laparoscopic repair. High ligation is still a popular approach that offers the advantage of fewer vessels to ligate and the disadvantages of working in a small incision and more difficulty identifying the testicular artery and lymphatics. Radiographic embolization takes longer, has a higher recurrence rate, involves some potentially disastrous complications if the embolization coil migrates, and is, consequently, one of the least commonly employed approaches. The laparoscopic approach is becoming very popular as a quick, effective method of treating varicoceles. It does require general anesthesia and has a higher recurrence and hydrocele formation rate than the inguinal microscopic approach. There is also the risk of damage to the intra-abdominal organs and major vessels with laparoscopic trocar placement.

Spermatocele

Spermatoceles are small cystic masses palpated near the head of the epididymis. They are usually less than 1 cm in diameter, but they may be quite large. They contain sperm, usually nonviable, and arise from the tubules connecting the rete testis to the head of the epididymis. Because they are small and usually asymptomatic, most are found on physical examination. On examination, spermatoceles are rubbery to firm and transilluminate. If symptomatic, they may be excised. Ultrasound will reveal a small, cystic structure adjacent to but separate from the testicle (Fig. 23–10).

Hematocele

A hematocele is a collection of blood within the tunica vaginalis. It may follow trauma or may occur postoperatively,

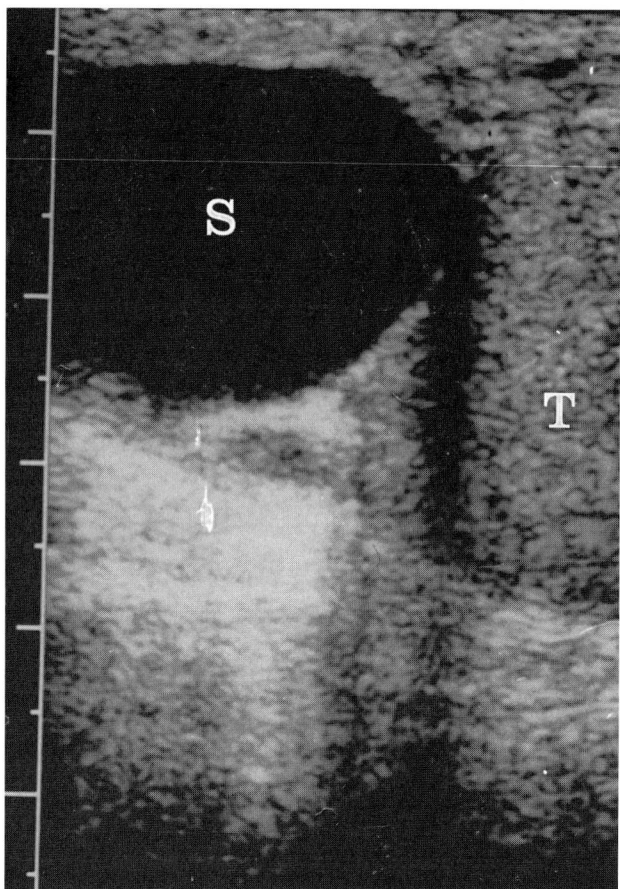

Figure 23–10. Spermatocele. A spermatocele is seen as a cystic structure (S) at the superior aspect of the testis (T).

after intrascrotal procedures. Hematoceles are strongly suspected based on history. On examination they do not transilluminate. Small, nonexpanding hematoceles may be treated conservatively with bedrest and scrotal elevation, but larger or expanding ones may require surgical drainage.

EXTRATESTICULAR LESIONS

Adenomatoid Tumors

Adenomatoid tumors make up 32% of all paratesticular tumors, making them the most common tumor of the paratesticular tissue.[67,68] Adenomatoid tumors in men usually arise from the epididymis (most commonly in the tail[69]) but may also arise from the testis, the tunica, or the spermatic cord.[70–73] These benign tumors generally occur in the third to forth decade of life. Most present as asymptomatic nodules, but up to 30% may present with pain.[74] There have been 10 cases reported on ultrasound findings with adenomatoid tumors in the scrotum.[75] The most common ultrasound finding is a hyperechoic, homogeneous mass, but hypoechoic and mixed echogenicity patterns have been seen as well. With the small number of cases and variable, nonspecific pattern displayed, it is impossible to make a definitive diagnosis with ultrasound. There is no literature on other imaging modalities and adenomatoid tumors. Because there have been no documented cases of metastases, treatment of these tumors is surgical excision.[76]

Cystadenoma of the Epididymis

Cystadenoma of the epididymis is a benign lesion arising from the efferent ductules in the epididymis. They are usually asymptomatic and are palpated most frequently in the head of the epididymis. They may be bilateral and have a higher incidence in patients with von Hippel–Lindau disease.[77] If symptomatic or found at scrotal exploration, they may be excised locally.

Rhabdomyosarcoma

Rhabdomyosarcoma of the paratesticular tissues may occur at any age but is most common in children and adolescents with two distinct incidence peaks at 4 and 16 years of age.[78] These tumors arise from undifferentiated mesenchymal cells and typically present as a large, painless scrotal swelling. Rhabdomyosarcoma spreads by lymphatic and hematogenous routes, and approximately one-third of patients have metastases at presentation.[79] The initial treatment is radical orchiectomy with adequate margins. Rhabdomyosarcoma is both radiation and chemotherapy sensitive, and chemotherapy has been shown to improve survival in patients with metastatic disease.[80]

Mesothelioma

Mesothelioma of the paratesticular tissues is an uncommon lesion with average age of presentation in the sixth decade. it usually presents as a painless scrotal mass, commonly associated with a hydrocele. Approximately 15% of patients have inguinal or abdominal metastases at the time of diagnosis.[81] Initial treatment is radical orchiectomy with adequate margins. The closeness of follow-up is dictated by the results of the original excision. Radiation and chemotherapy may be of help in patients with metastatic disease.

TUMORS OF THE TESTICLE

Incidence and Etiology

Testis tumors are the most common solid malignancy of males between the ages of 20 to 35 years,[82] accounting for 1 to 2% of neoplasms in males.[83] It is still relatively rare, with only two or three new cases per 100,000 males per year. The majority of tumors occur in three main age groups: during infancy, from adolescence to early adulthood, and over 50 years of age.[84]

There seem to be geographic, socioeconomic, and racial differences in the incidence of testis cancer. In Scandinavian countries, the incidence is more than 6 per 100,000 men, whereas in Japan the incidence is only 0.9 per 100,000 men.

Within a given race, higher socioeconomic classes have a higher rate of testicular cancer.[85,86] Nonwhites have lower rates than whites.[87] African-American males have an incidence of only 0.9 per 100,000, which may be due to a lower incidence of seminomas and teratomas.[88] Additionally, urban populations have a higher risk than rural populations.[89,90] Finally, the incidence of testis cancer seems to be increasing.[91]

Both congenital and acquired factors have been associated with tumors of the testis. Seven to 10% of patients with testis tumors have a history of cryptorchidism.[92] Early studies indicated a greater than 40-fold increase in incidence of testis tumor with cryptorchidism,[93] but more recent studies suggest an increase of between three and 14 times.[94–96] The risk is higher for intra-abdominal than for inguinal cryptorchid testes, and orchiopexy increases ease of detection, but it does not decrease the risk of testis cancer. Interestingly, 5 to 10% of patients with a cryptorchid testis who develop malignancy do so in the contralateral testis. Associations have been found between acquired causes, such as trauma and testicular atrophy, and testis cancer, but no causal relationships have been established.

Histologic Classification

SEMINOMATOUS GERM CELL NEOPLASMS

Seminoma is the most common histologic type of testis tumor in adults and represents 60 to 70% of germ cell tumors of the testis. The majority of patients present with low-stage disease, and all seminomas are extremely radiation sensitive. These facts help explain the greater than 90% overall cure rate with this histologic type.

There are three subtypes of seminoma: classic, anaplastic, and spermatocytic. Classic seminoma accounts for 85% of seminomas and is most common in the fourth decade of life. Syncytiotrophoblastic elements are seen in 10 to 15% of classic seminomas, which accounts for the incidence of increased beta-hCG in seminomas. Anaplastic seminoma is seen in 5 to 10% of seminoma cases and also is most common in the fourth decade of life. This subtype is the most locally and metastatically aggressive subtype of seminoma and accounts for 30% of seminoma deaths. Stage-for-stage anaplastic seminoma outcomes are the same as classic seminoma with treatment. Approximately 36% of anaplastic seminomas have an elevated beta-hCG. The third subtype is spermatocytic, which also accounts for 5 to 15% of seminomas. More than half of all men with this subtype are older than 50 years. Spermatocytic seminoma is the most favorable subtype, with metastases being rare.

NONSEMINOMATOUS GERM CELL TUMORS

Embryonal cell carcinoma represents approximately 20% of germ cell tumors of the testis. On presentation, these tumors tend to be small and irregularly shaped; they commonly invade the tunica vaginalis and spermatic cord. These are highly malignant tumors and tend to metastasize early.

Yolk sac carcinoma, also called infantile embryonal cell carcinoma, is the most common histologic type in infants and children. In adults it usually occurs in mixed histologies and is responsible for AFP (alpha fetoprotein) in these tumors.

Pure teratomas account for approximately 5% of germ cell tumors, but they are more commonly involved in mixed histologies. Teratocarcinoma, the combination of teratoma and embryonal cell carcinoma, makes up 25% of all testis tumors. Teratomas are seen in both adults and children and by definition contain at least two of the three germ cell derivatives. Teratomas are called mature or immature, based on the level of differentiation of their germ cell–derivative structures. When malignant transformation occurs, they are termed *malignant teratomas*.

Pure choriocarcinoma is rare, accounting for less than 1% of testicular neoplasms. Lesions in the testis are usually small and have central hemorrhage. Choriocarcinoma is an unusual testis tumor in that its primary mode of metastasis is hematologic. It tends to metastasize early despite the paradoxically small primary lesion.

NON–GERM CELL NEOPLASMS

Leydig cell tumors are rare, comprising less than 3% of testicular tumors. There are two age peaks of incidence, the first between 5 and 10 years and the second from 30 to 35 years. Prepubertal cases present with virilization, whereas about 30% of postpubertal tumors have virilizing effects. Approximately 15% are malignant, with all the malignancies occurring in adults. Initial treatment is radical orchiectomy, with benign forms needing no further therapy.

Sertoli cell tumors make up less than 1% of testicular neoplasms. These may occur at any age, with a third of cases in patients less than 10 years old and a third of patients between 20 and 45 years old. Patients usually present with a testicular mass, and 20 to 30% have associated gynecomastia. Malignancy is determined by the presence of metastases and occurs in 10 to 20% of patients. Malignancy may occur in children. The primary treatment in all cases is radical orchiectomy.

SECONDARY NEOPLASMS OF THE TESTIS

Lymphoma. Lymphoma is the most common testicular tumor in men over 50 years of age and accounts for 5% of all testicular tumors. It is the most common secondary tumor of the testis. Testicular lymphoma may be primary to the testis, an initial manifestation of extranodal disease, or a late manifestation of disseminated lymphoma.

Patients typically present with an enlarged, painless testicular mass. One-fourth of patients also have vague constitutional symptoms. About half have bilateral testicular lymphoma, although only 10% are synchronous.

Initial treatment is radical orchiectomy, which also provides tissue to establish the diagnosis. Staging and further treatment are usually carried out by the medical oncologist. Initial staging studies include a complete blood cell count and peripheral blood smear, abdominal and pelvic CT scan, chest x-ray, and bone scan.

Leukemia. The testis is the initial site of relapse in male children in remission from acute lymphocytic leukemia. Bilateral involvement is seen in about half of cases. Testis biopsy, not orchiectomy, is performed for diagnosis. Radiation to the testes is the appropriate initial treatment. These children also need further chemotherapy to prevent further relapse.

Metastases. Metastases to the testes are rare and are usually found at autopsy in patients with widely metastatic disease. Microscopically, the metastases invade the interstitium of the testis and typically spare the seminiferous tubules. The most common primary tumors that metastasize to the testis are melanoma and malignancies of the prostate, lung, gastrointestinal tract, and kidney.

BENIGN TESTICULAR TUMORS/LESIONS

Epidermoid cysts represent about 1% of all testicular neoplasms.[97] They are benign cysts composed of keratin-producing epithelium. Epidermoid cysts typically present as a painless scrotal mass or are found on routine examination, with only 15% presenting with pain. Unfortunately, most diagnoses are made by the pathologist, although some are recognized at radical orchiectomy and are excised locally. Preoperative diagnosis is difficult, and ultrasound images are variable and nonspecific. If the diagnosis is made prior to orchiectomy, local excision is adequate.[98,99]

Clinical Presentation of Primary Testicular Tumors

The most common presentation of a patient with a testis tumor is painless enlargement of the affected testis, which is noted by the patient or his sexual partner. Ten percent of patients will have acute pain secondary to bleeding or infarction of the tumor, and 30 to 40% will have a dull ache in the scrotum, lower abdomen, or perineum. Patients typically delay seeking treatment for 3 to 6 months after recognition of the problem.[100]

Approximately 10% of patients will present with symptoms secondary to metastatic disease. Back pain is the most common metastatic presentation and represents either retroperitoneal metastases impinging on nerve roots or skeletal metastases. Other metastatic presentations include gastrointestinal complaints secondary to retroduodenal metastases, central and peripheral nervous system manifestations, soft-tissue masses and lower-extremity swelling secondary to iliac or vena cava obstruction.

On physical examination, a firm, enlarged, painless testis is palpated. A reactive hydrocele is often present and occasionally may delay diagnosis of the testis tumor. Scrotal sonography is helpful in detection of testis tumors obscured by hydroceles. The abdomen should be palpated to search for evidence of retroperitoneal nodal metastases. The neck and inguinal region should be examined as well for enlarged lymph nodes. The chest should be examined because gynecomastia is present in 5% of patients with germ cell tumors and in a higher percentage of those with Leydig and Sertoli cell tumors.

Prior to radical orchiectomy, blood should be sent for beta-hCG and alpha fetoprotein (AFP). If these tumor markers are elevated prior to radical orchiectomy, they are very useful in evaluating treatment response and in follow-up evaluation for recurrences. AFP may be elevated with embryonal cell carcinoma, teratocarcinoma, and yolk sac tumor, but it is not elevated with pure seminoma or choriocarcinoma.[101] The half-life of AFP is 5 to 7 days. Beta-hCG is elevated in the serum of all patients with choriocarcinoma, in 50 to 60% of patients with embryonal or teratocarcinoma, and in 5 to 10% of patients with seminoma. The half-life of beta-hCG is 24 to 36 hours.

Imaging of Primary Testicular Tumors

Primary testicular tumors are best imaged and differentiated from other intrascrotal pathologies by scrotal sonography. The various histologic subtypes have characteristic findings on ultrasound (Fig. 23–11). Seminomas typically appear as homogeneous, hypoechoic, well-defined lesions within the testis.[2] The more aggressive embryonal cell carcinomas appear quite different. They are more heterogeneous in their echogenicity, representing area of necrosis and hemorrhage.[67] They also tend to have less-well-defined borders. Malignant teratomas frequently have echogenic foci representing calcifications, cartilage, and immature bone.[102] None of these ultrasound findings are pathognomatic of any type of testis tumor or even of malignancy itself.[9,73] Ultrasound also helps to identify small, nonpalpable tumors.[103]

MRI has also been used to image testicular tumors and may be of use if ultrasound is technically inadequate (Fig. 23–12).[9,104] Germ cell tumors of the testis appear hypointense to surrounding testicular tissue on T2-weighted images and isodense on T1-weighted images.[10] Seminomas may be differentiated from nonseminomatous germ cell tumors in some cases.[11] On T2-weighted MRI images, seminomas appear as homogeneous, low-signal masses, whereas nonseminomatous germ cell tumors appear heterogeneous and have a low-signal-intensity rim surrounding the mass.

Staging of Testicular Tumors

Clinical staging of patients with testicular cancer is important for both prognosis and treatment planning. Staging is

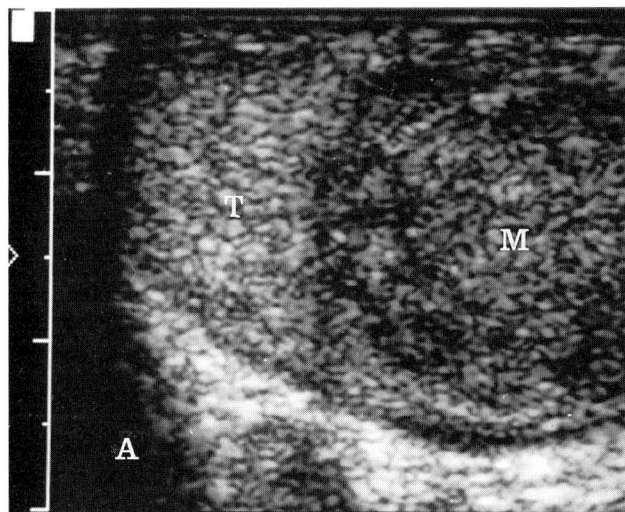
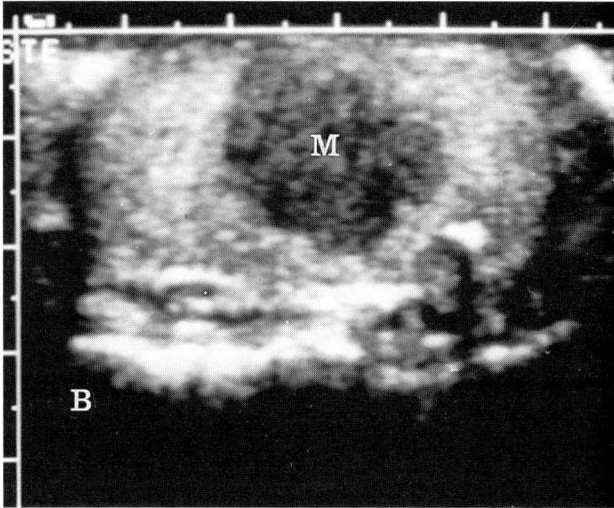

Figure 23–11. Testis tumors. **(A)** Embryonal cell carcinoma. This testicular mass (M) is large and compresses the surrounding normal testicular parenchyma (T). **(B)** Seminoma. A well-defined hypoechoic mass (M) is seen within the testis (T).

directed at the main sites of metastases. As described earlier, the initial metastases arrive at the retroperitoneum via the lymphatic system. The next most common site of metastases is the lung. Later, spread may occur to the liver, viscera, brain, and bone. When a tumor of the testis is suspected, initial staging studies consist of serum markers, scrotal sonography, CT of the abdomen and pelvis (this allows viewing of retroperitoneal adenopathy), chest x-ray, and possibly CT of the chest. Serum hCG and AFP are the only tests that must be performed prior to radical orchiectomy.

Many clinical staging systems have been developed over the years. Although the designations differ, the principle is the same in all. In the first stage the tumor is limited to the testis. In the second stage there are varying degrees of retroperitoneal lymph node disease. In the third stage metastatic disease occurs beyond the retroperitoneal lymph nodes. The American Joint Committee developed a TNM system to standardize both clinical and pathologic staging systems. The Skinner and Walter Reed staging systems are compared to the TNM system in Table 23–1.

Some departments advocate lymphangiography for staging of apparent clinical stage I (N0, M0) disease because up to 15% of these patients will have evidence of retroperitoneal metastases despite a negative clinical workup.[105] This study was performed prior to CT scanning, and many centers do not utilize lymphangiography.

As most patients with low-stage pure seminoma do not undergo retroperitoneal lymph node dissection (RPLND), treatment is based on clinical stage alone. Most clinical staging systems are modifications of the Boden and Gibb system.[106] The UCLA modification is shown in Table 23–2.[107]

Treatment

Initial treatment for tumors of the testis, regardless of histology, is radical inguinal orchiectomy with early control of the spermatic cord. This treatment allows for staging the tumor within the testis and for identifying the histology. The findings at orchiectomy have great significance in determining subsequent treatment needs. Patients should have orchiectomy as soon as possible, because length of time between diagnosis and treatment is directly related to pathologic stage.[108]

Figure 23–12. MRI testis tumor. A T2-weighted image reveals a low-signal-intensity mass (arrow) within the high-signal-intensity testis (T).

Table 23–1. TNM Staging of (NSGCT) Testicular Cancer

W.R.*	SKINNER	TNM
I	A	*T: Primary Tumor*
		TX: Cannot be assessed
		T0: No evidence of primary tumor
		Tis: Intratubular cancer (CIS)
		T1: Limited to testis
		T2: Invades beyond tunica albuginea or into epididymis
		T3: Invades spermatic cord
		T4: Invades scrotum
		N: Regional Lymph Nodes
		NX: Cannot be assessed
		N0: No regional lymph node metastases
IIA	B1	N1: Microscopic lymph node metastases
IIA	B1	N2a: Metastases in <=5 nodes, none >2 cm
IIB	B2	N2b: Metastases in >5 nodes, or any node >2 cm
IIC	B3	N3: Extranodal invasion
III	C	N4: Unresectable retroperitoneal metastases
		M: Distant Metastases
		MX: Cannot be assessed
		M0: No distant metastases
		M1: Distant metastases present

*W.R. = Walter Reed.

Seminoma

Seminoma is exquisitely radiosensitive. Patients with pure seminoma and low-stage disease (I and IIA) undergo radiation treatment to the ipsilateral inguinal and iliac regions as well as to the periaortic and pericaval regions up to the level of the diaphragm. These patients have a survival of greater than 90% at 5 years.[109,110] Patients with higher-stage disease are prone to significant rates of relapse if treated with radiation alone.[111]

Patients with higher-stage disease (IIB, III) and those with an elevated AFP (indicating nonseminomatous component) are treated with primary chemotherapy. Both seminomatous and nonseminomatous germ cell tumors are very effectively treated with platinum-based chemotherapy. Eighty-five to 90% of patients with high-stage seminoma achieve a complete response. Patients with residual retroperitoneal masses less than 3 cm in diameter may be observed with close follow-up because in 90% of cases this is fibrosis only. If the residual exceeds 3 cm, surgical excision should be performed.[112]

Nonseminomatous Germ Cell Tumor

Treatment of low-stage nonseminomatous germ cell tumor (NSGCT) is controversial. Traditional treatment in the United States for stage I (N0, M0) has been retroperitoneal lymph node dissection (RPLND). However, because 75% of these patients also have pathologic stage I, RPLND merely adds extra morbidity. When added to the fact that a high rate of cure is achieved with salvage chemotherapy, a case may be made for surveillance of these patients. Most recurrences occur in the first 2 years, and surveillance protocols are directed accordingly, with monthly serum markers, chest x-rays, and visits. Abdominal and pelvic CT scans are performed every 3 or 4 months.

If RPLND is chosen, a cure rate of approximately 95% may be attained in patients with pathologic N0 (stage I) disease. The decision must be made with the patient, balancing the exhaustive nature of a surveillance protocol with the possible morbidity of RPLND. Patients with pathologic stage IIA (N1, M0) NSGCT should receive two cycles of chemotherapy following RPLND. Patients with clinical stage IIA (N2a, M0) should also undergo RPLND followed by chemotherapy.

Patients with higher-stage disease should undergo primary platinum-based chemotherapy. Duration of chemotherapy is based on radiographic findings and normalization of serum markers. If AFP and hCG normalize but residual mass is demonstrated on CT scan, postchemotherapy RPLND should be performed. The pathology of this mass will be fibrosis in 40% of cases, teratoma in 20%, and residual tumor in 40%. Approximately 70% of patients with high-volume disease will be cured with the preceding protocol.

SCROTAL TRAUMA

Trauma to the scrotum may be delivered by either blunt or penetrating mechanisms. These two mechanisms of injury have different risks to the patient and are managed differently. All patients with penetrating injuries to the scrotum should be explored,[113] whether the mechanism of injury is gunshot wound, knife wound, or other. Aggressive debridement and appropriate repair should be performed based on findings. Blunt trauma, however, presents more of a challenge. Patients with a ruptured testis do much better with surgical repair than with conservative management, especially if performed less than 72 hours from the time of injury.[114,115]

Common mechanisms of blunt trauma to the scrotum include sports injuries, kicks to the groin, and injuries at work.

Table 23–2. UCLA Clinical Staging of Seminoma

I	Limited to the testis, epididymis, or spermatic cord
II	Metastases in the retroperitoneal nodes only
IIA	Retroperitoneal nodes <2 cm
IIB	Retroperitoneal nodes 2 to 10 cm
III	Supradiaphragmatic lymph node or visceral metastases

Adapted from Crawford D, Smith R, DeKernian J: Treatment of advanced seminoma with preradiation therapy. *J Urol* 1983;119:75.

Patients commonly present acutely with a swollen and tender scrotum. Physical examination can be quite difficult in this situation. It may be difficult to distinguish between injuries that require immediate operative therapy and those where the patient would do fine with conservative management. Conditions that require operative intervention include testicular rupture and the presence of a large hematocele.[116] Injuries such as scrotal wall hematomas and small, confined testicular hematomas may be observed.

Imaging of Blunt Scrotal Trauma

Scrotal sonography has proven to be a useful aid in the differentiation of scrotal injuries after blunt testicular trauma.[117-119] Hematoma of the scrotal wall is seen as thickening of the wall (Fig. 23-13). If this is the only injury, the patient may be managed conservatively. Rupture of the testis is seen as a disruption in the hyperechoic tunica albuginea. The ovoid shape of the testis may be lost, and if the rupture is severe, testicular parenchyma may be visualized extruding through the tunica albuginea. The sensitivity of detection of testicular rupture has been reported from 88 to 100%.[117,120,121] Hematocele may obscure rupture of the testes; however, significant hematoceles usually come to surgery as well.[120] Hematocele, if imaged immediately, appears similar to hydrocele, with hypoechoic pattern between the layers of the tunica vaginalis. As soon as the blood begins to clot, more echogenic foci are seen. Intratesticular hematomas appear as a hypoechoic region surrounded by normal testicular tissue. No evidence of testicular rupture should be evident. Color Doppler imaging (CDI) may also play a role in the evaluation of blunt trauma to the scrotum. Wilbert et al describe CDI findings in two patients with scrotal trauma.[24] One patient had increased perfusion; the second had decreased perfusion, although few details are presented. Future studies will decide the role of CDI in the setting. Although probably not clinically useful, intratesticular hematoma has been reported to have a high signal on T1 images and a mixed signal on T2 images.[11] Other imaging modalities are of little use in imaging the scrotum.

Treatment

Small intratesticular and scrotal wall hematomas may be managed conservatively with pain medication, scrotal elevation, and follow-up scrotal sonography. Any evidence of testicular rupture or significant hematocele requires surgical exploration. If the patient is taken to the operating room, the cord and testis should be thoroughly explored and any testicular rupture repaired. Necrotic tissue should be debrided aggressively. If the testis is deemed nonviable, orchiectomy should be performed. Both testes should be explored prior to the decision to proceed with orchiectomy. The operative management for penetrating scrotal injury is similar, with an extra emphasis on debridement and irrigation. Scrotal drains should be placed in cases with penetrating trauma.

UNDESCENDED TESTES

Definitions

Cryptorchidism is the failure of the testis to descend to its normal postnatal position in the scrotum. Several factors probably play a role in the maldescent of a testis. Absence or abnormalities of the gubernaculum may cause incomplete or abnormal descent. Lack of maternal gonadotropins may lead to incomplete descent, as testicular descent has been shown to be androgen mediated.[122] Intrinsic defects in the

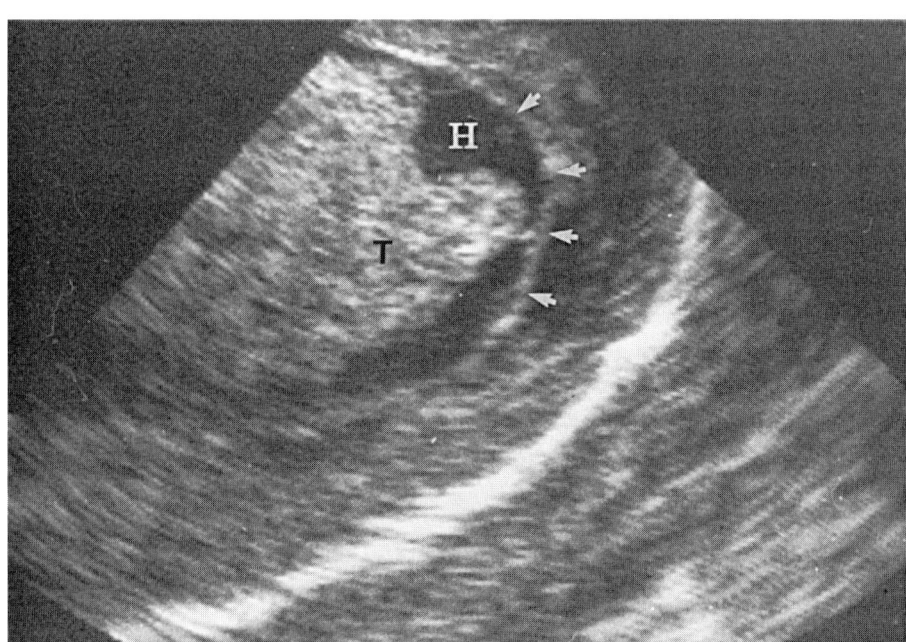

Figure 23-13. Hematoma of the testis. Hypoechoic hematoma (H) is seen adjacent to normal testicular parenchyma (T). The tunica albuginea is intact (arrows).

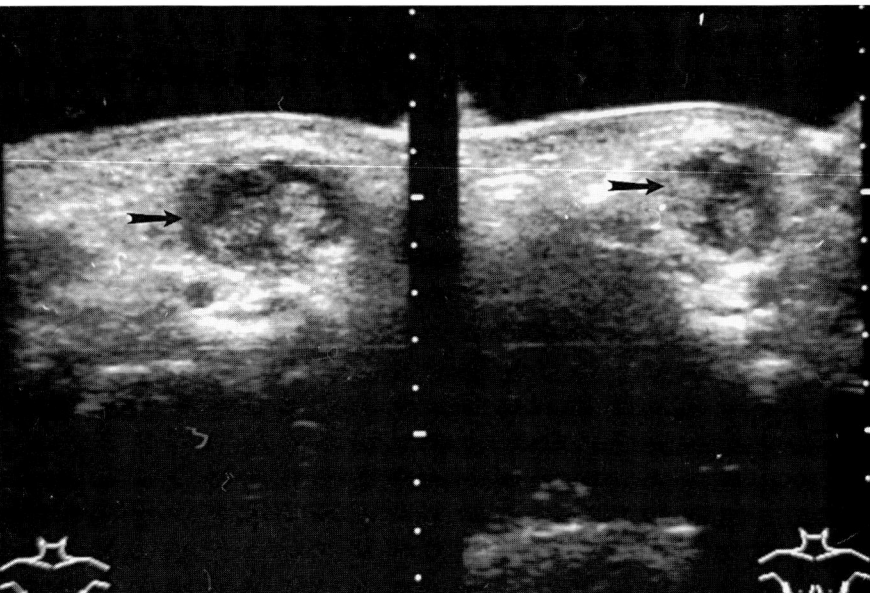

Figure 23–14. Torsed canalicular testis. The testis appears enlarged and hypoechoic on gray-scale ultrasound and is found in an ectopic position in the inguinal canal (arrow).

testis may make it androgen insensitive and lead to maldescent as well.

The cryptorchid testis may be intra-abdominal (proximal to the internal inguinal ring), canalicular (between the internal and external rings), or high scrotal in location (Fig. 23–14). If the testis is located outside the normal path of descent, it is termed *ectopic*. The ectopic testis may be suprapubic, penile, femoral, or perineal in location. The incidence of cryptorchidism is 30% in preterm male infants, 3.4% in full-term male infants, and 0.8% by 1 year of life.[35] One-third of boys have bilateral cryptorchidism, and 70% of unilateral cases are right sided. Patients with a suspected cryptorchid testis should be placed in a sitting cross-legged position and reexamined. Many retractile testes will spontaneously descend with this maneuver. These testes seldom require orchiopexy.

Cryptorchid testes are approximately 40 times more likely to develop a malignancy than normally descended testes.[93] Orchiopexy does not reduce this risk, but makes detection of malignancy much easier. A second reason to perform orchiopexy relates to fertility. The seminiferous tubules may undergo deleterious changes as early as the second year of life.[123,124]

Diagnosis

There are many techniques, ranging from physical examination to surgical laparotomy, to determine if an impalpable testis is absent or cryptorchid. Physical examination should be the first procedure performed to localize a cryptorchid testis. The examination should be performed in a warm room with the child as comfortable as possible. Careful palpation along the inguinal canal and high scrotum should be performed. Placing the child in a sitting position may help to identify a retractile testis.

Ultrasound may aid in diagnosis of a canalicular testis but is quite inaccurate in evaluating suspected abdominal testes. Ultrasound accuracy rates for diagnosis of intra-abdominal testes range from 13 to 85%.[125–127]

CT is also rather unsuccessful at diagnosing intra-abdominal testes. Accuracy rates of 33 to 50% have been reported.[125,128] CT also has the disadvantage of ionizing radiation and is difficult to perform in small children.

MRI has proven to be much more useful than CT (Fig. 23–15). Using both T1- and T2-weighted images increases diagnostic power, as the testis becomes hyperintense on T2 images. Sensitivities of up to 86% and specificities of 100% for intra-abdominal testis location have been achieved.[129] As with CT, small children generally require sedation in order to perform a study. Although MRI seems to be more useful than other imaging modalities, it may not be needed, given the wider use of laparoscopy.

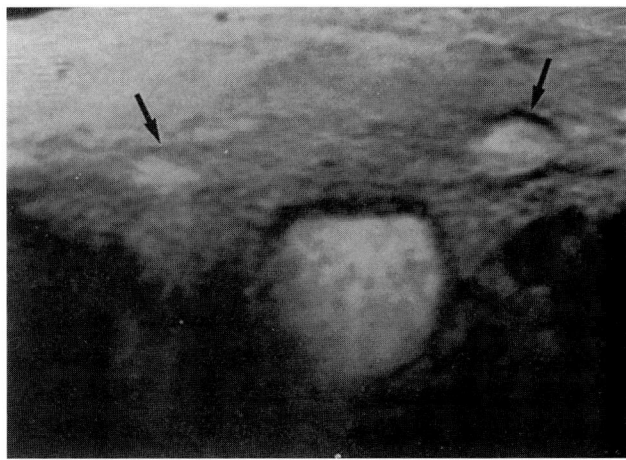

Figure 23–15. Undescended testes. T2-weighted MRI reveals high-intensity testes located in the inguinal canal (arrows).

Testicular venography and arteriography are invasive tests and are associated with significant morbidity.[130,131] They also have very significant false-positive and false-negative rates, leading to poor overall accuracy. Consequently, these tests are seldom performed.

Laparoscopy has evolved into an important modality for evaluation of the impalpable testicle. Of the impalpable testes, approximately 20 to 50% are absent.[132] Laparoscopy provides the best minimally invasive modality to ascertain the presence or absence of the cryptorchid testis. Laparoscopy may be scheduled during the same anesthetic as inguinal exploration and orchiopexy. The laparoscopic exploration for presence of an abdominal testis adds little time to the procedure and may even obviate the necessity for inguinal or open abdominal exploration.

Findings at laparoscopy may be divided into four categories. If a testis is found intra-abdominally, the question is answered and further treatment options are based on the level of the testis and the preference of the surgeon. In the second case, no testis, spermatic vessels, or vas deferens is found. In this situation a diagnosis of testicular agenesis is made and no further investigation is necessary. In the third case, no testis is seen, but the spermatic vessels and vas deferens are seen entering the internal inguinal ring. This finding necessitates an inguinal exploration. Orchiopexy or orchiectomy is performed based on the findings. In the final case, no testis is found, the vas deferens is seen entering the internal ring, and the spermatic vessels are atrophic. With the latter finding, some authors believe no inguinal exploration is necessary.[133,134] Rappe et al performed 10 inguinal explorations in this setting and found only one testis.[135] The one testis was atrophic and orchiectomy was performed.

Therapy

HORMONAL THERAPY

Hormonal therapy is the only form of medical management of cryptorchidism. The two available hormone treatments are hCG and Gn-RH (leutinizing hormone releasing factor). The hCG is given parenterally and works by stimulating Leydig cells to release testosterone and therefore promote descent of the testis. Success rates of 14 to 50% have been reported[136]; however, later studies show success rates of less than 10%.[132] hCG administration is painful, has some psychologic side effects, and may lead to genital enlargement. These side effects greatly limit its clinical usefulness. hCG may be administered to determine if the testis is retractile instead of truly cryptorchid.

Gn-RH is administered because of the belief that patients with cryptorchidism have a deficiency in Gn-RH secretion. This medication is administered via nasal inhaler and is much better tolerated. Success rates vary widely, from 6 to 70%.[122,137] This therapy is currently available in Europe, but not in the United States. Hormonal therapy may be tried, but few truly cryptorchid testes will descend. Patients with a truly cryptorchid testis should undergo orchiopexy at approximately 1 year of age.

THE PALPABLE UNDESCENDED TESTIS

For the palpable canalicular, or high scrotal, testis, an inguinal and testis orchiopexy may be performed through inguinal and scrotal incisions. If extra length is needed to place the testis low in the scrotum without tension, the spermatic vessels may be transected, or the Prentiss maneuver may be employed. The latter maneuver involves dissection along the floor of the inguinal canal and ligation of the inferior epigastric vessels.[138] The testis is then fixed in place in the scrotum.

THE IMPALPABLE TESTIS

Once an intra-abdominal testis is found via laparoscopy or open exploration, the surgeon must decide on either orchiectomy or one of a variety of orchiopexy techniques. Atrophic testes should be removed, as should any testis in a postpubertal male with a normal contralateral testis.[132] Options for treatment include two-staged orchiopexy, microvascular autotransplantation, Fowler–Stephens orchiopexy (the spermatic vessels are ligated several months prior to the planned orchiopexy, allowing for increased collaterals between the vasal and distal testicular arteries), one-stage Fowler–Stephens orchiopexy and laparoscopic-assisted first-stage Fowler–Stephens orchiopexy.[135]

REFERENCES

1. Donahue J, Zachary J, Maynard B: Distribution of nodal metastases in nonseminomatous testis cancer. *J Urol* 1982; 128:315.
2. Langer J: Ultrasound of the scrotum. *Semin Roentgenol* 1993; 28:5.
3. Mack L, Winter T: Scrotal Ultrasound. *ARRS Ultrasound Syllabus*. 1993:205.
4. Leung M, Godding G, Williams R: High resolution sonography of scrotal contents in asymptomatic subjects. *AJR* 1984;143:161.
5. Arger P, Mulhern C Jr, Coleman B: Prospective analysis of the value of scrotal ultrasound. *Radiology* 1981;141:763.
6. Carroll B, Gross D: High-frequency scrotal sonography. *AJR* 1983;140:511.
7. Rifkin M, Kurtz A, Goldberg B: Epididymis examined by ultrasound. *Radiology* 1984;151:187.
8. Doherty F: Ultrasound of the nonacute scrotum. *Semin Ultrasound CT MR* 1991;12:131.
9. Thurnher S, Hricak H, Carroll P, et al: Imaging the testis: comparison between MR imaging and US. *Radiology* 1988; 167:631.
10. Baker L, Hajek P, Burkhard T: MR imaging of the scrotum: normal anatomy. *Radiology* 1987;163:89.
11. Schnall M: Magnetic resonance imaging of the scrotum. *Semin Roentgenol* 1993;28:19.
12. Kim C, Zuckier L, Alavi A: The role of nuclear medicine in

the evaluation of the male genital tract. *Semin Roentgenol* 1993;28:31.
13. Elder J, Duckett J: Complications of hypospadias repair. In: Smith R, Ehrlich R, eds. *Complications of Urologic Surgery: Prevention and Management*. Philadelphia: WB Saunders, 1990;549.
14. Elder J, Jeffs R: Suprainguinal ectopic scrotum and associated anomalies. *Urology* 1982;127:336.
15. Lamm D, Kaplan G: Accessory and ectopic scrotum. *Urology* 1977;9:149.
16. Cunningham L, Keating M, Snyder H, Duckett J: Urologic manifestations of the popliteal pterygium syndrome. *J Urol* 1989;141:910.
17. Ray B, Clark S: Hemangioma of the scrotum. *Urology* 1976;8:502.
18. Gasparich J, Mason J, Greene H, et al: Amiodorone associated epididymitis: drug related epididymitis in the absence of infection. *J Urol* 1985;133:971.
19. Olier C, Sirot J: Role of chlamydiae in genital infections in men. *Semaine des Hopitaux* 1983;59:2719.
20. De Jong Z, Pontonnier F, Plante P, et al: The frequency of *Chlamydia trachomatis* in acute epididymitis. *Br J Urol* 1988;62:76.
21. Martin B, Conte J: Ultrasonography of the acute scrotum. *J Clin US* 1987;15:37.
22. Ralls P, Jensen M, Lee K, et al: Color Doppler sonography in acute epididymitis and orchitis. *J Clin US* 1990;18:383.
23. Hortsman W, Middleton W, Melson G: Scrotal inflammatory disease: color Doppler US findings. *Radiology* 1991;179:55.
24. Wilbert D, Schaerfe C, Stern W, et al: Evaluation of the acute scrotum by color coded Doppler ultrasonography. *J Urol* 1993;149:1475.
25. Blei L, Sihelnik S, Bloom D, et al: Ultrasonography analysis of chronic intratesticular pathology. *J Ultrasound Med* 1983;2:17.
26. Barada J, Weingarten J, Cromie W: Testicular salvage and age related in the presentation of testicular torsion. *J Urol* 1982;142:746.
27. Williamson R: Death in the scrotum: testicular torsion. *N Engl J Med* 1977;196:338.
28. Turner T, Howards S: Acute experimental testicular torsion: no effect on the contralateral testis. *J Androl* 1985;6:65.
29. Cosentino M, Rabinowitz R, Valvo J: The effect of prepubertal spermatic cord torsion on subsequent fertility in rats. *J Androl* 1984;5:833.
30. Bird K, Rosenfeld A, Taylor K: Ultrasonography in testicular torsion. *Radiology* 1983;147:527.
31. Leape, L: Torsion of the testis: invitation to error. *JAMA* 1967;200:669.
32. Pelander W, Luna G, Lilly J: Polyorchidism: case report and literature review. *J Urol* 1978;119:705.
33. Backhouse K: Embryology of testicular descent and maldescent. *Urol Clin North Am* 1982;9:315.
34. Cass A, Cass B, Verrarghaven K: Immediate exploration of the acute scrotum in young male subjects. *J Urol* 1980;124:829.
35. Scorer G, Farmington G: *Congenital Deformities of the Testis and Epididymis*. New York: Appleton-Century-Crofts, 1971.
36. Middleton W, Melson G: Testicular ischemia: color Doppler sonographic findings in five patients. *AJR* 1989;17:538.
37. Tumeh S, Benson C, Richie J: Acute diseases of the scrotum. *Semin Ultrasound CT MR* 1991;12:115.
38. Lerner R, Mevorach R, Hulbert W: Color Doppler US in the evaluation of acute scrotal disease. *Radiology* 1990;176:355.
39. Dewire D, Begun F, Lawson R, et al: Color Doppler ultrasonography in the evaluation of the acute scrotum. *J Urol* 1992;147:89.
40. Petros J, Andriole G, Kavoussi L, Middleton W: Color Doppler ultrasound (CDU) of normal and abnormal testes. *J Urol* (part 2) 1989;141:177A. Abstract 29.
41. Burks D, Markey B, Burkhard T, et al: Suspected testicular torsion and ischemia: evaluation with color Doppler sonography. *Radiology* 1990;175:815.
42. Zoeller G, Ringert R: Color-coded duplex sonography for the diagnosis of testicular torsion. *J Urol* 1991;146:1288.
43. Krieger J, Wang K, Mack L: Preliminary evaluation of color Doppler imaging for investigation of intrascrotal pathology. *J Urol* 1990;144:904.
44. Middleton W, Siegel B, Melson G, et al: Acute scrotal disorders: prospective comparison of color Doppler ultrasound and testicular scintography. *Radiology* 1990;177:177.
45. Holder L, Melloul M, Chen D: Current status of radionuclide scrotal imaging. *Semin Nucl Med* 1981;11:232.
46. Mevorach R, Lerner R: Use of color Doppler ultrasonography (CDU) in the diagnosis of scrotal pathology of uncertain etiologic basis. *J Ultrasound Med* 1993;12:200.
47. Altaffer L III, Steele S Jr: Torsion of the testicular appendages in men. *J Urol* 1980;124:56.
48. Dresner M: Torsed appendage. Diagnosis and management: blue dot sign. *Urology* 1973;1:63.
49. Holland J, Graham J, Ignatoff J: Conservative management of twisted testicular appendages. *J Urol* 1981;125:213.
50. Johnson DE, Pohl DR, Rivera-Correa H: Varicocele: an innocuous condition. *South Med J* 1970;63:34.
51. Macleod J: Further observations on the role of varicocele in human male infertility. *Fertil Steril* 1969;20:545.
52. Marks JL, McMahon R, Lipschultz LI: Predictive parameters of successful varicocele repair. *J Urol* 1986;136:609.
53. Aafjes J, Vijver J: Fertility of men with and without a varicocele. *Fertil Steril* 1985;43:901.
54. Pryor J, Howards S: Varicocele. *Urol Clin North Am* 1987;14:499.
55. Takihara H, Sakatoku J, Cockett A: The pathophysiology in varicocele in male infertility. *Fertil Steril* 1991;55:861.
56. Ahlberg N, Bartley O, Chidekel: Right and left gonadal veins: an anatomical and statistical study. *Acta Radiol* 1966;4:593.
57. Dubin L, Alemar R: Varicocelectomy as therapy in male infertility: a study of 504 cases. *J Urol* 1975;113:640.
58. Brown N: Miscellaneous tumors of the epithelial type. In: Pugh R, ed. *Pathology of the Testis*. Philadelphia: JB Lippincott, 1976:304.
59. Cockett A, Urry R, Dougherty K: The varicocele and semen characteristics. *J Urol* 1979;121:435.
60. Steeno O, Verstoppen G: Varicocele and the pathogenesis of the associated subfertility. *Andrologia* 1978;10:85.
61. Orda R, Sayfan J, Manor H, Witz E, Sofer Y: Diagnosis of varicocele and postoperative evaluation using inguinal ultrasonography. *Ann Surg* 1987;206:99.
62. Meacham R, Townsend R, Radmacher D, Drose J: The incidence of varicoceles in the general population when evaluated by physical examination, gray scale ultrasound, and color Doppler sonography. *J Urol* 1994;152:1535.
63. Harris J, Lipschultz L, Conoley P, et al: Radioisotope angiography in the diagnosis of varicocele. *Urology* 1980;16:69.
64. Wheatley J, Fajman W, Witten F: Clinical experience with radioisotope varicocele scan as a screening method for the detection of subclinical varicoceles. *J Urol* 1982;128:57.
65. Suga K, Ariyoshi I, Nakanishi T: Clinical study of varicocele by sequential scrotal scintography. *Andrologia* 1990;22:525.
66. Freund J, Handelsman D, Bautovich G: Detection of varicocele by radionuclide blood pool scanning. *Radiology* 1991;137:562.
67. Krone K, Carroll B: Scrotal ultrasound. *Radiol Clin North Am* 1983;21:595.

68. Phillips G, Abrams H, Kumari-Subaija S: Scrotal ultrasonography. In: Sanders R, Hill M, eds. *Ultrasound Annual 1983*. New York: Raven Press, 1983;207.
69. Longo V, McDonald J, Thompson G: Primary neoplasms of the epididymis. *JAMA* 1951;147:937.
70. Upton J, Das S: Benign intrascrotal neoplasms. *J Urol* 1986;135:504.
71. Kiely E, Flannagan A, Williams G: Intrascrotal adenomatoid tumors. *Br J Urol* 1987;60:225.
72. Rankin N: Adenomatoid tumors of the epididymis and tunica albuginea: two cases. *Br J Urol* 1986;28:187.
73. Tackett R, Lind D, Catalona W, Melson G: High resolution sonography in diagnosing testicular neoplasms: clinical significance of false positive scans. *J Urol* 1986;135:494.
74. Klerk D, Nime F: Adenomatoid tumors of the testicular and paratesticular tissue. *Urology* 1975;5:635.
75. Leonhardt W, Gooding G: Sonography of intrascrotal adenomatoid tumor. *Urology* 1992;39:90.
76. Richie J: Neoplasms of the testis. In: Walsh P, Retik A, Stamey T, Vaughn E, eds. *Campbell's Urology*, 6th ed. Philadelphia: WB Saunders, 1992;1254.
77. Price E: Papillary cystadenoma of the epididymis. *Arch Pathol* 1971;91:456.
78. Hamilton C, Pinkerton R, Horwich A: The management of paratesticular rhabdomyosarcoma. *Clin Radiol* 1989;40:314.
79. Steward L, Lioe T, Johnston S: Thirty-year review of intrascrotal rhabdomyosarcoma. *Br J Urol* 1991;68:418.
80. Grosfeld J, Weber T, Weetman R, Baener R: Rhabdomyosarcoma in childhood: analysis of survival in 98 cases. *J Pediatr Surg* 1983;18:141.
81. Kasdon E: Malignant mesothelioma of the tunica vaginalis propria testis: report of 2 cases. *Cancer* 1969;23:1144.
82. Patton J, Mallis N: Tumors of the testis. *J Urol* 1959;81:457.
83. Blandy J, Hope-Stone H, Dayan A: *Tumors of the Testicle*. New York: Grune & Stratton, 1970.
84. Droller M: Cancer of the testis: an overview. *Urol Clin North Am* 1980;7:731.
85. Graham S, Gibson R: Social epidemiology of cancer of the testis. *Cancer* 1972;29:1324.
86. Mack T, Henderson B: Cancer registries for special and general uses. In US–USSR Monograph, NIH Publ. No. 80-2044, 1980:57.
87. Teppo L: Testicular cancer in Finland. *Acta Pathol Microbiol Immunol Scand* 1973;(suppl):238.
88. Templeton A; Testicular neoplasms in Ugandan Africans. *Af J Med Med Sci* 1972;3:157.
89. Lipworth L, Daylan A: Rural preponderance of seminoma of the testis. *Cancer* 1969;23:1119.
90. Sharma K, Gaeta J, Bross I: Testicular tumors. *NY State J Med* 1972;72:2421.
91. Clemmesen J: Statistical studies in malignant neoplasms. *Acta Pathol Microbiol Scand* 1974;247(suppl):1.
92. Whitaker R: The management of the undescended testis. *Br J Hosp Med* 1970;4:25.
93. Gilbert J, Hamilton J: Studies in malignant testis tumors: incidence and nature of tumors in ectopic testes. *Surg Gynecol Obstet* 1940;71:731.
94. Farrer J, Walker A, Rajfer J: Management of the postpubertal cryptorchid testis. *J Urol* 1985;134:101.
95. Henderson B, Benton B, Jing J, et al: Risk factors for cancer of the testis in young men. *J Cancer* 1979;3:598.
96. Schottenfeld D, Warshauer M, Sherlock S, et al: The epidemiology of testicular cancer in young adults. *Am J Epidemiol* 1980;112:232.
97. Shah K, Maxted W, Chun B: Epidermoid cysts of the testis: a report of three cases and analysis of 141 cases from the world literature. *Cancer* 1981;47:577.
98. Ross J, Kay R, Elder J: Testis sparing surgery for pediatric epidermoid cysts of the testis. *J Urol* 1993;149:353.
99. Berger Y, Hajdu S, Herr H: Epidermoid cysts of the testis: role for conservative surgery. *J Urol* 1985;134:962.
100. Oliver R: Factors contributing to the delay in diagnosis of testicular tumors. *Br Med J* 1985;290:356.
101. Javadpour N: The role of biologic tumor markers in testicular cancer. *Cancer* 1980;45:1755.
102. Schwerk B, Schwerk W, Rodeck G: Testicular tumors: prospective analysis of real time ultrasound patterns and abdominal staging. *Radiology* 1987;164:369.
103. Fowler R, Chennells P, Ewing R: Scrotal ultrasonography: a clinical evaluation. *Br J Radiol* 1987;60:649.
104. Heiken J: Tumors of the testis and testicular adnexa. In: Pollack J, ed. *Clinical Urography*. Philadelphia: WB Saunders, 1989;1414.
105. Whitmore W Jr: The treatment of germinal tumors of the testis. In: *Proceedings of the 6th National Cancer Conference*. Philadelphia: JB Lippincott, 1970;219.
106. Boden G, Gibb R: Radiotherapy and testicular neoplasms. *Lancet* 1951;2:1195.
107. Crawford D, Smith R, DeKernian J: Treatment of advanced seminoma with preradiation therapy. *J Urol* 1983;119:75.
108. Bosl G, Vogelzang N, Goldman A, et al: Impact of delay in diagnosis on clinical stage of testicular cancer. *Lancet* 1981;2:970.
109. Dosoretz D, Shipley W, Blitzer P, et al: Megavoltage irradiation for pure testicular seminoma: results and pattern of failure. *Cancer* 1981;48:2184.
110. Peckham M, McElwain T: Radiotherapy of testicular tumors. *Proc R Soc Med* 1974;67:300.
111. Peckham M, Barret A, McElwain T, Hendry W, Raghaven D: Nonseminoma germ cell tumors (malignant teratoma) of the testis: results of treatment and analysis of prognostic factors. *Br J Urol* 1981;53:162.
112. Motzer R: Residual mass: an indication for further therapy in patients with advanced seminoma following systemic chemotherapy.
113. Gomez R, Castanheira A, McAninch J: Gunshot wounds to the male external genitalia. *J Urol* 1993;150:1147.
114. Gross M: Rupture of the testicle: the importance of early surgical treatment. *J Urol* 1969;101:196.
115. Cass A: Immediate radiological evaluation and early surgical management of genitourinary injuries from external trauma. *J Urol* 1979;122:772.
116. Cass A, Luxenberg M: Testicular injuries. *Urology* 1991;37:528.
117. Lewis C, Michell M: The use of real-time ultrasound in the management of scrotal trauma. *Br J Radiol* 1991;64:792.
118. Martinez-Pineiro L Jr, Cerezo E, Cozar J, et al: Value of testicular ultrasound in the evaluation of blunt scrotal trauma without haematocele. *Br J Urol* 1992;69:286.
119. Schaffer R: Ultrasonography of scrotal trauma. Review article. *Urol Radiol* 1985;7:245.
120. Kratzik C, Hainz A, Kuber W, et al: Has ultrasound influenced the therapy concept of blunt scrotal trauma? *J Urol* 1989;142:1243.
121. Fournier G, Laing F, Jeffrey R, McAninch W: High resolution scrotal ultrasonography: a highly sensitive but nonspecific technique. *J Urol* 1985;134:490.
122. Rajfer J: Hormonal therapy of cryptorchidism. A randomized double-blind study comparing hCG and gonadotropin releasing hormone. *N Engl J Med* 1986;314:466.
123. Zarzycki J, Szroeder J, Michalowski W: Ultrastructure of seminiferous tubule cells and interstitial cells in cryptorchid human testicles. *Acta Med Polon* 1977;18:385.

124. Hadziselimovic F: Cryptorchidism. *Adv Anat Embryol Cell Biol* 1977;53:3.
125. Hrebinko R, Bellinger M: The limited role of imaging techniques in managing children with undescended testes. *J Urol* 1993;150:458.
126. Madrazo B, Klugo R, Parks J, DiLoreto R: Ultrasonographic demonstration of undescended testes. *Radiology* 1979;133:181.
127. Komine S, Murayama M, Kinoshita N, et al: High resolution ultrasound examination in the diagnosis of the undescended testis in the inguinal region. *Acta Urol Jap* 1988;34:305.
128. Wolverson M, Jagannadharao B, Sundaram M, et al: CT in the localization of impalpable cryptorchid testes. *AJR* 1980;134:725.
129. Zobel B, Vicentini C, Masciocchi C: Magnetic resonance imaging in the localization of undescended abdominal testes. *Eur Urol* 1990;17:145.
130. Lowe H, Brock W: Laparoscopy for localization of the nonpalpable testis. *J Urol* 1983;131:728.
131. Green R Jr: Computerized axial tomography vs spermatic venography in the localization of the undescended testis. *Urology* 1985;26(5):513.
132. Elder J: Laparoscopy and the Fowler-Stephans orchiopexy in the management of the impalpable testis. *Urol Clin North Am* 1989;16:399.
133. Guiney E, Corbally M, Malone P: Laparoscopy and the management of the impalpable testis. *Br J Urol* 1989;63:313.
134. Castilho L: Laparoscopy for the nonpalpable testis: how to interpret the endoscopic findings. *J Urol* 1990;144:1215.
135. Rappe B, Zandberg A, De Vries J, et al: The value of laparoscopy in the management of the impalpable cryptorchid testis. *Eur Urol* 1992;21:164.
136. Job J, et al: Hormonal therapy of cryptorchidism with hCG. *Urol Clin North Am* 1982;9:405.
137. Hadziselimovic F: Long term effect of LH-RH analogue (Buserelin) on cryptorchid testes. *J Urol* 1987;138:1043.
138. Prentiss R, Weickgenant C, Moses J: Undescended testis. Surgical anatomy of the spermatic vessels, spermatic surgical triangles and lateral spermatic ligament. *J Urol* 1960;83:686.

24 New Tests for the Diagnosis of Erectile Dysfunction

Mark D. Stovsky, Allen D. Seftel, Thomas E. Herbener

GENERAL CONCEPTS

Insight into the basic physiology of male erectile function has grown significantly over the past several decades. With this knowledge has come a greater comprehension of the pathophysiologic mechanisms that contribute to erectile dysfunction. The proper evaluation and treatment of the patient must take into consideration not only the general distinction between organic and functional impotence but also the complex interrelationships that link these factors.

The efficient investigation of erectile dysfunction begins with a thorough understanding of its underlying causes. The normal physiologic mechanisms leading to tumescence require the coordinated action of the penile arterial and cavernosal tissue systems working in concert with spinal and cortical (supraspinal) neural pathways. Essentially, any process that affects penile arterial inflow, venous outflow, cavernosal or tunical tissue structure and performance, or penile neurologic function can produce erectile dysfunction. Psychogenic, pharmacologic, and endocrine abnormalities represent secondary, contributing elements that must also be studied to formulate an appropriate course of treatment. Treatment options are goal directed and often complex. With proper guidance, reassurance, and counseling, the majority of patients will realize a successful outcome.

This chapter focuses upon new diagnostic tests for impotence. We have purposefully avoided a discussion of the current therapeutic options available for the impotent male. Inasmuch as the current as well as the new diagnostic tests appear to center upon the neurovascular evaluation, we concentrate our discussion of diagnostic tests on vasculogenic and neurogenic impotence.

VASCULOGENIC IMPOTENCE

Arteriogenic Impotence

In general, the arterial system of the penis is supplied by paired internal pudendal vessels that are the terminal branches of the internal iliac arteries. The internal pudendal arteries give rise to the common penile arteries, which divide to form the dorsal, bulbourethral, and cavernosal arteries. The cavernosal arteries supply the erectile tissue and cavernosal sinusoids through the helicine arteries. Erection is heralded by a form of stimulation (e.g., sensory, pharmacologic, cortical) that results in penile arterial cavernosal and helicine smooth muscle relaxation and increased flow. The rate of inflow is dependent on several key factors, including the patency of the arterial tree, the degree of smooth muscle relaxation (arterial and cavernosal tissue), and the venous outflow resistance.[1-3] Anatomically, any abnormality that limits blood flow within the abdominal aorta or the penile arterial system (internal pudendal, penile, or helicine arteries) can lead to arteriogenic erectile dysfunction ("failure to fill").

The principal causes of penile arterial insufficiency have a bimodal demographic distribution. In the population ranging from ages 35 and above, the causes of arteriogenic impotence are associated with atherosclerosis and peripheral vascular disease, including hypertension, diabetes mellitus, tobacco smoking, and hypercholesterolemia/hyperlipidemia.[4,5] Specifically, recent studies have identified an association between the onset of generalized atherosclerotic vascular disease as well as hypertension and the subsequent development of erectile impotence.[6,7] Other causes for erectile dysfunction in the older population include major abdominal vascular surgical procedures and pelvic radiation for the treatment of malignancies of the genitourinary or gastrointestinal tract. Through their effects on large and small vessels, these entities may result in significantly decreased penile arterial inflow.[8,9]

Diabetes mellitus in particular is thought to be responsible for a significant number of cases of erectile failure. The detrimental effects of diabetes on male sexual function appear to be manifestations of generalized damage to both blood vessels and peripheral nerves throughout the body. Peripheral sensory and autonomic neuropathy has been well documented in the diabetic patient population. Evidence also suggests that this disease leads to the development of profound arterial small vessel disease involving the penile arteries and their tributaries. Although controversy exists concerning the primary pathophysiologic mechanism by which diabetes influences erectile function, studies showing the presence of penile vascular disease and arteriogenic impotence in the absence of significant neuropathy indicate that arterial occlusive disease may be more detrimental to male sexual function in the diabetic patient population.[10]

Trauma to the pelvis and/or perineum leading to vascular damage and decreased penile arterial inflow is the most common cause of arteriogenic impotence in men 18 to 35 years of age. Traumatic lesions associated with this form of impotence may be either direct or indirect. Common causes include penetrating and blunt injuries such as gunshot wounds and pelvic fractures during motor vehicle accidents, or blunt perineal injury (bicycle riding).

Veno-occlusive (Venogenic, Venous Leak) Impotence

The venous drainage from the penis can be divided into that of the corpora cavernosa and the corpus spongiosum. The cavernosal venous supply begins in the sinusoidal spaces; travels via venules beneath the tunica albuginea; exits into either the deep dorsal, circumflex, or periurethral veins; and leaves the penis through the cavernous and crural veins that join the internal pudendal vein in the pelvis. The venous supply from the corpus spongiosum begins in the glans, empties into the retrocoronal plexus, and joins the deep dorsal vein, which ultimately exits via the retropubic periprostatic plexus of veins. This system communicates with the cavernosal venous supply through the circumflex veins. The penile skin is drained by the subcutaneous veins that join the superficial dorsal vein and form anastamoses with the saphenous vein.[11]

Physiologically, in addition to a satisfactory arterial inflow, an intact cavernosal veno-occlusive mechanism appears necessary for tumescence of sufficient rigidity for sexual intercourse. The cavernosal veno-occlusive mechanism is thought to function by a mechanism of trabecular smooth muscle relaxation that allows free blood flow from the helicine arteries into the sinusoidal spaces of the corpora. Subsequently, the expansion of the erectile tissue causes compression of the subtunical and emissary veins against the tunica albuginea as this structure is stretched to capacity. Ultimately, the outflow resistance overcomes the inflow hydrostatic pressure and full tumescence and rigidity are achieved.[12]

Several abnormalities of the cavernosal veno-occlusion can result in or contribute substantially to erectile impotence. These abnormalities historically have centered on poor compliance of the corporal sinusoidal system, dysfunction in the relaxation mechanism of the trabecular smooth muscle, or alterations in the structural integrity of the tunica albuginea. Recently, Goldstein et al have demonstrated that there is a diminution of cavernosal smooth muscle and replacement with collagen as the basis for venous leak.[13] In general, these problems share the common link of precipitating penile impotence by restricting the venous outflow resistance of the corpora. These processes (e.g., fibrosis) significantly limit the expansion of the cavernosal smooth muscle and the degree of compression of the subtunical and emissary veins during tumescence.[14-16]

Risk factors for the development of venogenic impotence include diabetes mellitus, hypercholesterolemia, Peyronie's disease, penile trauma (tunical or cavernosal), penile surgery, priapism, and atherosclerotic vascular disease.[17-19] In addition to impairing endothelium-dependent relaxation of the cavernosal tissue, diabetes mellitus has been linked to the nonenzymatic glycosylation of collagen within the corpora cavernosa.[20,21] Hypercholesterolemia has been hypothesized to result in abnormal collagen synthesis and may have a similar effect. Diabetes and atherosclerosis have also been associated with the propagation of cavernosal smooth muscle atrophy, the replacement of trabecular tissue with fibrous scar, and endothelial cell damage. In addition, Peyronie's disease, direct trauma to the penile shaft, surgery that violates the integrity of the tunica albuginea, and priapism are recognized etiologies of venogenic impotence. These penile injuries cause erectile dysfunction via corporal and/or tunical fibrosis, which leads to a disruption in the veno-occlusive capacity of the penis.[22]

NEUROGENIC IMPOTENCE

Neurogenic control of erectile function is driven by cortical, spinal, and peripheral neural pathways. The penis is innervated by both autonomic (parasympathetic and sympathetic) and somatic (sensory and motor) neurons. Autonomic fibers enter the penis via the cavernosal nerves. The somatic innervation is carried by the pudendal nerve and its branches. The penile parasympathetic fibers originate in the sacral spinal cord and join the cavernosal nerves at the level of the pelvic neural plexus. The sympathetic innervation of the penis arises from the thoracolumbar spinal cord and fuses with the parasympathetic neurons to complete the formation of the cavernosal nerves after initially making synapses in the superior hypogastric neural plexus.[23]

Although controversy exists, a normal rigid erection is thought to be evoked by way of the parasympathetic innervation of the corpora cavernosa via cholinergic, VIPergic, and nonadrenergic, noncholinergic (NANC) nerves, whereas stimulation of sympathetic pathways generally results in detumescence. Recent data by Burnett et al[24] using the transgenic mouse deficient in neural nitric oxide synthase (NOS), the enzyme responsible for neural nitric oxide synthesis, have demonstrated an excellent erectile response in these neural NOS-deficient mice upon stimulation of the pelvic nerves. This implies that neurally produced and released nitric oxide may not be as significant in the overall erectile process as previously thought.

Supraspinal pathways in the cerebral cortex have also been shown to influence and modify the normal erectile response to sexual stimulation.[25] In general, there are three main types of erectile response: (1) reflexogenic, whereby somatic afferent stimulation leads directly to parasympathetic efferent impulses and tumescence; (2) psychogenic, in which audiovisual cortical stimuli generate autonomic efferent impulses via the sacral cord to produce an erection; and (3) nocturnal, whereby cortical stimulation of spinal cord pathways during REM sleep facilitates tumescence.

These pathways have been elicited as a result of evaluations of the spinal cord–injured patient.

Neurogenic erectile dysfunction can be caused by injury or disease of the brain, spinal cord, or peripheral nerves serving the penis (autonomic or somatic). Essentially all neurologic lesions that result in erectile failure interfere with the requisite parasympathetic facilitation of corporal smooth muscle relaxation. Cortical disease processes leading to neurogenic impotence include stroke, tumor, epilepsy, Parkinson's disease, and Alzheimer's disease. These processes may result in sexual dysfunction in one of two ways: (1) the loss of libido or (2) overinhibition of spinal erection control pathways. Further, some reports of sexual problems after stroke appear to indicate that penile erection is often possible but that intercourse is problematic because of residual physical limitations in other areas (e.g., extremity sensation and/or motor function).[26]

Spinal cord–level lesions that can result in total penile impotence or erectile dysfunction include spinal cord injury, multiple sclerosis, spina bifida, tabes dorsalis, amyotrophic lateral sclerosis (ALS), syringomyelia, herniated disk, or tumor. The degree of erectile function after a spinal cord traumatic injury depends on the level and magnitude of the injury (i.e., partial versus complete). Many patients with upper motor neuron lesions above the level of the sacral cord retain the ability for reflexogenic erection.[27] Patients with direct lower motor neuron damage to the sacral cord must rely principally on supraspinal psychogenic tumescence mechanisms which may be mediated by intact sympathetic pathways.[28] Similarly, multiple sclerosis, spina bifida, tabes dorsalis, ALS, syringomyelia, spinal cord tumors, and herniated disks affect potency by direct injury to afferent sensory or efferent autonomic neurons.[29,30]

Peripheral neuropathy leading to erectile impotence can be the result of surgical injury or blunt/penetrating trauma to the pelvic plexus, the pudendal nerves, or the cavernosal nerves. Diabetes mellitus, uremia, alcoholism, and vitamin deficiencies can also result in peripheral neurologic dysfunction and impotence; however, the precise pathophysiologic mechanisms have not been clearly elucidated.[31–33]

PSYCHOGENIC IMPOTENCE

Psychogenic impotence can be classified as primary (i.e., no history of normal erections) or secondary (i.e., acquired erectile failure). Primary psychogenic erectile failure is thought to occur in patients who were socialized into a sexually repressive environment (e.g., religious or cultural). Secondary psychogenic impotence can arise from many causes, including performance anxiety, relationship or occupational stress, sexual preference issues, a history of sexual abuse, or fear of sexually transmitted diseases.[34–36] The mechanisms underlying psychogenic erectile dysfunction are poorly understood. Several theories have been advanced and include (1) cortical inhibition of the sacral cord erection center and (2) excessive sympathetic discharge leading to unsuccessful parasympathetic stimulation of cavernosal smooth muscle relaxation.[37,38]

DRUG-INDUCED IMPOTENCE

Many classes of drugs have been implicated in the formation of male sexual dysfunction. Basically, any substance that alters the neural, vascular, or erectile tissue pathways involved in penile tumescence can precipitate pharmacologic impotence. Commonly used medications associated with penile impotence include the antihypertensives, the sedative-hynotics, the neuroleptics, estrogenic/antiandrogenic compounds, and alcohol/illicit drugs.

Antihypertensive medications can be categorized as diuretics, vasodilators, or sympatholytics. These drugs have been found to exert both direct and indirect effects on potency. Diuretics generally have an indirect effect on sexual function.[39] In particular, the thiazide diuretics and spironolactone have been reported to cause impotence possibly linked to diminished libido or hormonal aberrations.[40,41]

Erectile dysfunction is also commonly attributed to the centrally and peripherally acting sympatholytic drugs. Centrally acting agents, including methyldopa, clonidine, and reserpine, have been proven to contribute to penile impotence, decreased libido, and ejaculatory dysfunction. Two possible theories that have been offered to account for the effect of these substances on sexual performance are (1) the inhibition of a proposed hypothalamic erection center (methyldopa/clonidine) and (2) the depletion of central nervous system stores of catecholamine and serotonin (reserpine).[42,43]

The mechanism by which peripherally acting sympatholytics facilitate erectile failure is also unclear. These agents include smooth muscle relaxing agents (e.g., calcium channel blockers, alpha receptor blockers, and ACE inhibitors) and beta receptor blockers. The proposed theory for the influence of these compounds on potency centers on the concept that patients with preexisting vascular occlusive disease (i.e., aortoiliac and pudendal) may require a threshold perfusion pressure to maintain adequate penile inflow. The use of these medications to control moderate/severe hypertension may decrease blood flow to the corporal sinusoids during stimulation and produce inadequate tumescence.[44,45]

The sedative-hypnotic class of drugs may induce abnormal sexual performance mainly by causing a diminished sex drive. This category of medications included the commonly used benzodiazepines diazepam (Valium) and alprazolam (Xanax). Neuroleptic (psychotropic) pharmacologic agents—including the phenothiazines, butyrophenones, tricyclic antidepressants, and monoamine oxidase inhibitors—can also result in disturbances of male sexual function. Although the pathophysiologic pathways involved are poorly understood, possible mechanisms include (1) a sedative effect; (2) an anticholinergic, antidopaminergic, or antihistaminic effect; or (3) the inhibition of catacholamine metabolism.[46]

Other substances that are thought to exert a negative influence on erectile function include H_2 receptor blockers, clofibrate (an antilipemic agent), antiandrogenic drugs (e.g., ketoconazole and cyproterone acetate), and digoxin. Many of these agents affect either androgen metabolism or cellular action and produce changes in libido and/or tumescence. Alcohol and certain illicit drugs (e.g., cannabis, cocaine, and opiate narcotics) have also been linked with impotence.[47,48]

ENDOCRINOLOGIC IMPOTENCE

Several hormonal abnormalities have been found in the impotent patient population. These physiologic derangements may involve many disparate organ systems, such as the pancreas (diabetes mellitus), the thyroid (hypo- and hyperthyroidism), and the hypothalamic–pituitary–gonadal axis (hypo- and hypergonadotropic hypogonadism, hyperprolactinemia). Androgen is responsible for male secondary sex characteristics and may play a role in nocturnal sexual function. Some authors have found an improvement in nocturnal tumescence parameters when hypogonadal men receive replacement testosterone treatment.[49] Male androgen levels are generally recognized to play a secondary role in sexual potency and probably function to enhance erectile quality and libido.[50,51]

Although diabetes mellitus influences erectile function in a complex set of ways (e.g., damage to the penile vasculature, neural networks, and erectile tissue), no specific serum hormone aberrancies except diminished insulin levels have been reported.[52] Hypogonadotropic hypogonadism can be the result of a genetic syndrome (e.g., Kallman's syndrome) or can occur secondary to a pituitary/hypothalamic tumor, surgical injury, aging, or other endocrine disorders (e.g., Cushing's syndrome, thyroid disease). Furthermore, inflammatory processes (e.g., tuberculosis, sarcoidosis), vascular insults (e.g., Sheehan's syndrome), radiation damage, and systemic diseases (e.g., hemochromatosis, amyloidosis) can also destroy the relationship between pituitary and testicular function.[53]

Hypergonadotropic hypogonadism is generally the result of primary testicular failure.[54] This syndrome can be congenital (e.g., Klinefelter's syndrome) or acquired secondary to infection (e.g., mumps, tuberculosis), surgical injury, trauma, testicular tumor, or systemic chemotherapy. Thyroid disease,[55] both hypo- and hyperthyroidism (thyrotoxicosis), is believed to have a negative impact on male erectile performance and sex drive. Although the exact mechanism is unclear, alterations in the free and protein-bound testosterone levels have been identified and implicated as the possible etiology. Hyperprolactinemia resulting from a pituitary tumor, chronic renal failure, or certain medications has been associated with decreased serum testosterone levels and libido. A direct effect of elevated prolactin levels on tumescence has not been clearly established.[56,57]

EVALUATION*

Evaluation for erectile dysfunction scrutinizes the medical variables in the patient and the psychological factors in the man, partner, and couple that coalesce to precipitate and maintain dysfunction. Evaluation can be divided into three tiers, incrementally increasing in invasiveness, expense, and complexity.

Level 1

CLINICAL EVALUATION

Level 1 can be completed in one 3-hour outpatient visit with the mental health professional and urologist working as an interdisciplinary team. The components of the first level include (1) separate clinical interviews of the patient and partner, (2) physical examination and medical history, (3) Doppler examination with calculation of the penile–brachial index, (4) biothesiometry, and (5) hormonal assay. This evaluation occasionally provides sufficient data to delineate the medical and psychological contributions to the dysfunction satisfactorily.

Including the Partner. Erectile dysfunction is not simply a problem for the man whose penis is unreliable. The dysfunction impacts on the man, his partner, and their relationship. Any evaluation that does not include the partner is incomplete. Often the most vital piece of information is a throwaway line from the partner (e.g., "Did he tell you about his drinking problem, not getting that promotion, our daughter's drug problem, his mother's death, my mastectomy, etc."). In addition, meeting the partner allows her to be reassured and to participate in the curative process. A brief partner interview frequently dispels groundless self-recriminations; faulty partner attributions and psychological attitudes that are antithetical to resuming sexual life are also discerned.

Clinicians might encounter some resistance in asking to meet with the partner (e.g., "It's my problem, not hers"; "I don't want to embarrass her"; etc.). These protests generally yield to brief explanations of why it is helpful to interview partners. To go along with such resistance only reinforces the destructive myths that suggest it is simply the man who is "broken."

---

*This section is adapted from Althof SE, Seftel AD: The evaluation and management of erectile dysfunction. *Psychiatr Clin North Am* 1995; 18(1):171–192.

Clinical Psychosocial Interview of the Patient and Partner. The interview focuses on the man's sexual function, the couple's sexual equilibrium, and the social framework in which their lives are embedded. The history of the erectile dysfunction is delineated, and the man is asked to rate the current quality of erections on a 10-point scale (10 equals the most rigid) under a variety of circumstances (e.g., upon awakening, with fantasy, masturbation, foreplay, and intercourse). Unusual and/or disturbing life circumstances coincident to the dysfunction are analyzed.

Other relevant parameters of sexual life are queried, including sexual drive, frequency of lovemaking, orgasmic difficulties, and sexual satisfaction. On occasion it is worthwhile to inquire about gender identity, orientation, and paraphilia because conflicts in these realms may produce erectile dysfunction. It is also important to evaluate the patient's motivation for resuming coitus and/or utilization of a specific treatment option. Obstacles that will negate the potential positive effects of specific treatment alternatives may be detected at this early juncture.

In addition, the magnitude of performance anxiety is assessed, as are the social constructions that augment and disrupt arousal. Dysfunction prompts privately held concerns regarding one's masculinity to surface and become amplified (e.g., "My penis is too small"; "A real man's penis gets hard anywhere, anytime, under any circumstances").

Finally, the quality of the couple's nonsexual relationship is examined, as are conflicts emanating from other sources (e.g., work, finances, partner's health, difficulties with parents or children).

The interview with the partner serves to corroborate the self-report of the patient and to further explicate relevant medical and psychological variables. Her perceptions of the patient and their nonsexual relationship often alters etiologic considerations based solely upon the patient's narrative. In addition, the partner's possible contribution to the genesis and continuity of the dysfunction, her current willingness to resume lovemaking, and her attitude about specific treatment options should be studied.

UROLOGIC EVALUATION

The proper evaluation of the patient with erectile dysfunction includes the history and physical examination, laboratory tests and clinical/radiologic studies. Throughout the investigative process, the physician should be aware of the delicate nature of problems with sexual function and of the importance of patient confidentiality.

The history and physical examination are fundamentally important to the competent evaluation and management of the patient with erectile impotence. The skillfully executed preliminary survey should establish a working diagnosis that identifies and guides the need for appropriate confirmatory laboratory and radiologic tests. In addition, a thorough history and physical examination must define the overall medical condition of the patient and identify pertinent findings that might influence the decision to pursue a medical or surgical course of therapy. Several studies show a good correlation between objective measurements of erectile capacity and patient reports of sexual function in the history and physical portion of the evaluative process. These reports underscore the accuracy and importance of the thorough sexual history in the diagnosis of organic and psychogenic erectile dysfunction.[58,59]

The patient history should include a complete account of the current problem with sexual function. Other important components include the medication summary, a list of drug allergies, a record of current or antecedent medical illnesses and prior surgical procedures, a description of pathologic inherited traits, and documentation of existing or past psychosocial problems. The sexual function history should chronicle the specific nature of the problem. Many patients regard the term *impotence* as a catchall for the broad spectrum of disorders of male sexual function. A detailed inquiry must be made that distinguishes between true erectile dysfunction, the loss of sexual desire, the absence of seminal emission, difficulties achieving orgasm, and premature ejaculation. Once the disorder is outlined, a precise clinical investigation can be begun that may include hormonal studies, a formal evaluation of penile tumescence, a seminal fluid analysis, and psychological counseling.

After a problem of penile erection has been established, the remaining portion of the history should be directed toward ascertaining the patient's potency status, determining the quality of any erections, and identifying an organic or functional etiology for the problem. The potency status describes whether the current erectile capacity is sufficient for intercourse and should identify changes in patient or partner satisfaction with the quality or frequency of sex. The quality of the erection is generally determined by questioning the patient with respect to perceived changes in rigidity, the duration of the erection, the timing of the onset of sexual dysfunction (i.e., sudden versus gradual), and a distinction between tumescence upon awakening from sleep as compared to erections with audiovisual/psychogenic, tactile with partner, or masturbatory stimulation.

The timing of the onset of sexual dysfunction and the comparison of tumescence with differing modes of stimulation can provide important clues in distinguishing organic from functional impotence. The onset of organic impotence is usually slow and insidious, with little difference between erections upon awakening from sleep, with audiovisual/psychogenic stimulation, or upon tactile stimulation. In contrast, functional impotence is often sudden in onset and related to a specific stressful event or a distinct set of chronic psychosocial problems.

The symptoms of arteriogenic erectile impotence ("failure to fill") in the older population appear to reflect a systematic progression of inflow disease, which occurs gradually over a period of years. Initially, patients may experience a delay in the onset of tumescence with stimulation. Subsequently, patients generally develop an inability to obtain an erection of sufficient rigidity for intercourse. Eventually, the complete inability to achieve an erection may ensue. In the younger patient with pelvic or perineal trauma, erectile dysfunction may be an immediate consequence of the injury. The symptoms of impotence secondary to veno-occlusive dysfunction ("failure to maintain") include an inability to achieve optimal rigidity and a poor capacity to sustain an erection adequate for sexual intercourse. Progressively, as in arteriogenic sexual dysfunction, the patient may develop total erectile failure. Moreover, patients with psychogenic erectile failure commonly report normal episodes of tumescence intermittently during a given period of time.

The sexual history should also document the patient's perception of penile rigidity during tumescence. This can be accurately estimated as a percentage of his historical "best erection." Details concerning the duration in which current erections are maintained during intercourse or with other forms of stimulation are also indispensable. These pieces of information can be important indicators of arteriogenic or veno-occlusive impotence. Furthermore, any abnormality of the penis during erection such as curvature that might indicate Peyronie's disease should be noted.

The past medical history should list all medical conditions for which the patient has received treatment. In particular, an inquiry into the presence of conditions related to sexual dysfunction must be made. These conditions include diabetes mellitus, hypertension, metabolic disorders, testicular infections, cryptorchidism, spinal cord injury, coronary artery and peripheral vascular disease, chronic pulmonary problems, changes in bladder/bowel/neurologic function, and tobacco/alcohol/illicit drug use. Furthermore, any history of blunt or penetrating injury to the penis, scrotum, perineum, or pelvis must be recorded. These data may add diagnostic insight or may significantly alter the management of the patient's sexual problem.

The past surgical history should concentrate on treatments that may have led to injuries in the neural, vascular, or erectile tissue structures involved in tumescence. These procedures include previous abdominal/pelvic surgery (e.g., aortoiliac, radical prostatectomy, proctocolectomy, transurethral resection of the prostate), penile surgery, or pelvic/perineal radiation therapy. It is important to note that the temporal relationship of any medical or surgical intervention with the onset of penile impotence should be elicited.

Other essential components of the sexual function history are the medication summary and the list of drug allergies. As stated in the section on pharmacologic impotence, many drugs—including a range of antihypertensives, analgesics, neuroleptics, anticholinergics, and endocrine agents—can affect sexual function. Furthermore, an understanding of the patient's current pharmacologic regimen and any known allergic responses to medications is critical during the perioperative management period after prosthesis placement or penile revascularization surgery. Finally, the family and birth portions of the patient history should document established genetic or congenital disorders such as Klinefelter's syndrome and spina bifida/myelomeningocele that may have long-term urologic sequelae that contribute to penile impotence.

A skillful physical examination is an essential component of the overall investigation of erectile dysfunction. The physical examination can assist in defining the urologic problem and lead to an accurate and precise diagnosis. Prior to beginning the directed genitourinary examination, the practitioner should assess the general medical condition of the patient. In particular, attention should be paid to the cardiovascular and respiratory systems, and any abnormalities of the heart or lungs should be noted. Close scrutiny should also be given to the peripheral vascular examination. The carotid, brachial, femoral, popliteal, dorsalis pedis, and peroneal pulses should be palpated. The carotid arteries should be auscultated for signs of stenosis such as bruits. The abdomen should be palpated to detect signs of an abdominal aortic aneurysm.

A concise neurologic survey should be performed looking for evidence of gross abnormalities in motor strength/coordination, sensation, cranial nerve function, and peripheral reflexes. Particular emphasis should be placed on the sacral nerve distribution using the bulbocavernosus reflex and anal sensation tests to identify deficits in the somatic innervation of the genitalia and perineum. Care should also be taken to record any stigmata of regional or systemic pathology that may directly or indirectly produce changes in sexual function (e.g., sacral skin dimple; spina bifida, lymphadenopathy; occult malignancy, gynecomastia; hypothalamic–pituitary–gonadal axis abnormality, lower-extremity hair loss/skin changes; vascular disease).

A directed genital examination should be performed in any patient with erectile impotence. First, the genitalia are examined by inspection and palpation in the supine and standing positions. Any external lesions of the penis or scrotum as well as the presence of phimosis or paraphimosis should be noted. The presence of hypospadias or epispadias should be recorded because these conditions represent congenital anomalies that may impact treatment options. Palpation of the penis should be performed to detect the presence of Peyronie's plaques.

The examination of the testes and spermatic cord is done in the supine and standing positions. These structures are evaluated by palpation and transillumination. The presence of paired testes should be documented. The size of the testes should be compared to age-matched controls (normal adult testes measure 3 to 4.5 cm in longest dimension). Symmetrically small testes may indicate hypogonadism secondary to testicular failure. A unilaterally small testis may be due to such factors as trauma, infection, torsion, iatrogenic surgical injury, and cryptorchidism. Any deviation from the smooth contour and rubbery consistency of the normal testis that might provide evidence of prior infection or the presence of a mass lesion should be recorded. The cremasteric reflex should be tested and any abnormalities of the spermatic cord, vas deferens, and epididymis should be identified. Finally, any associated hydrocele, spermatocele, varicocele, or hematocele should be reported and investigated with transillumination.

The digital rectal examination is integral to the complete physical examination of the impotent patient. Any abnormalities of the prostate (e.g., enlargement, nodularity, inflammation) or rectum (e.g., mass lesions, blood in stool) should be chronicled. It is important to assess the degree of rectal tone and the bulbocavernosus reflex to obtain evidence of neurologic impairment. The bulbocavernosus reflex is based upon the shared sensory innervation of the glans and the anal sphincter. Afferent somatic fibers travel from these anatomic structures via the pudendal nerve to sacral levels 2 to 4. With an intact spinal reflex arc, gentle compression of the glans should elicit anal sphincter contraction. The absence of this reflex may reflect an underlying sacral nerve injury such as spina bifida occulta. Anal sensation should also be appraised at the time of the rectal examination.

Level 2

DIAGNOSTIC TESTS FOR ERECTILE DYSFUNCTION

Further evaluation is necessary when the etiology is equivocal or enigmatic. The second level of investigation includes nocturnal penile tumescence testing.

The ambulatory nocturnal penile tumescence test (Rigiscan, Dacomed, Minneapolis, MN) has essentially supplanted the stamp test, the snap gauge test, and the visual sexual stimulation test. The nocturnal penile tumescence test (NPT) is based on the theory that normal erections that are independent of supraspinal influences occur regularly during REM sleep. Therefore patients with normal erections during sleep but penile impotence when awake are thought to exhibit psychogenic dysfunction. REM sleep erectile activity is measured with respect to tumescence and rigidity using mercury strain gauges at the base and tip of the penis. Sleep quality is also appraised using EEG and EMG technology.[60,61] The accuracy of nocturnal penile tumescence testing is restricted by a number of factors that limit its sensitivity and specificity. In particular, age, emotional state, sex hormone status, sleep deprivation, and specific medications influence the test results.[62-65] Also, patients with abnormal NPT results suggesting organic impotence have sometimes been reported to have normal ability for intercourse. However, the presence of normal rigid erections with adequate duration during REM sleep in a patient with erectile dysfunction does appear to reflect a psychogenic mechanism.[66] A newer technique, the diurnal penile tumescence test, records the same parameters as in the NPT during daytime napping episodes and appears to correlate well with nocturnal study results. The validity of this test in differentiating psychogenic from organic impotence is still unproven.[67] Visual sexual stimulation, using erotic material to stimulate cortically controlled erection in conjunction with measurements of tumescence and rigidity, has also been reported[68] but is not utilized in our clinic on a routine basis.

Sleep erections are an androgen-dependent phenomenon presumed to reflect the potential of the penis to become rigid unencumbered by psychological conflict, performance anxiety, or interpersonal strife. The subject's sleep is customarily monitored for three consecutive nights either in a sleep laboratory or with portable equipment in the patient's home. NPT data can be evaluated along several dimensions, including (1) number of nightly erection episodes, (2) duration of each episode, (3) increases in penile tumescence at the base and tip, and (4) degree of rigidity at the base and tip. Utilizing these parameters Schiavi reports that the efficiency of NPT (to identify correctly all men with organic impotence and all men free of organic pathology without including false-positives or false-negatives) ranges between 75 and 100%.

Several factors must be considered when interpreting abnormal NPT data. During in-home monitoring, it is important to assess the quality of the subject's sleep, whether the subject properly attached the device to his penis (e.g., only one loop attached, reversal of base and tip leads), and whether the machine is functioning properly. Sleep disorders interfere with nocturnal erection. Obviously, failure to follow standardized technique results in contaminated data. And a machine that is incorrectly calibrated will yield erroneous data. The Rigiscan, a home-monitoring device, does not permit the clinician to perform independent calibrations to ascertain whether or not the machine is providing reliable measurements. Further, NPT appears more responsive to psychological variables than initially thought. Specifically, men who are clinically depressed have abnormal tracings. These return to normal after the depression remits.

There are also significant changes in sleep erections with age. Older men have fewer and shorter periods of nightly erection. Schiavi hypothesized that the "lack of rigid sleep erections in some healthy older men, who report continued ability to have intercourse, may be due to age related changes in central neurobiological process that mediate internally generated sexual arousal." These individuals may compensate by increased reliance on the synergistic effect of direct penile stimulation for the development of reflexogenic erections and maintenance of intercourse capacity. Finally, NPT tracings are generally interpreted in an idiosyncratic manner, with no age-stratified norms. This presents the evaluator with serious concerns regarding the reliability and validity of NPT data interpretation.

Level 3

The diagnostic tests within the third tier should be reserved for those cases where vascular reconstructive surgery is being considered or when the patient wishes to understand further the vasoculopathic entity causing the dysfunction. They include (1) dynamic infusion cavernosometrogram and cavernosogram (DICC), (2) color duplex ultrasonography, (3) angiography.

TESTS FOR VASCULAR IMPOTENCE

Arteriogenic Impotence. Vasculogenic impotence can be caused by defects in arterial inflow or venous outflow resistance. Formal diagnostic testing should be directed by information obtained during the history and physical examination regarding the signs and symptoms of these problems. Current tests to detect arterial perfusion abnormalities are either functional or anatomic and include (1) Doppler penile arterial pressure measurements, (2) duplex/color flow Doppler penile arterial pressure studies, (3) selective penile arteriography, and (4) vasoactive agent injection trials. The Doppler ultrasound and angiographic studies can be performed in either the flaccid or dynamic state (e.g., creation of erection by injection of vasoactive substances or audiovisual stimulation).[69]

The most common initial studies to document arteriogenic impotence are the Doppler penile arterial pressure measurement and the vasoactive agent injection test. The office-based Doppler arterial pressure test utilizes a 10-mHz probe and a penile blood pressure cuff to measure the cavernosal arterial pressure. The penile brachial index (PBI) is then calculated. Reports suggest that a PBI of less than 0.7 probably represents significant cavernosal arterial insufficiency. The PBI is easy to obtain and is noninvasive. However, Doppler penile pressure measurements tend to be nonspecific (difficult to isolate the cavernosal vessels) and to be operator dependent; moreover, if done in the flaccid state, they may not reflect true physiologic conditons.[70–72]

The vasoactive agent injection test is a dynamic study that can be used to attempt to evaluate the function of the penile arteries and erectile tissue. The most commonly used vasoactive agents are papaverine and phentolamine, but newer agents such as PGE_1 are also being investigated.[73] These substances cause direct smooth muscle relaxation of the corporal erectile tissue or endothelium. An abnormal test (poor erection) upon injection of these compounds may indicate arterial inflow insufficiency, veno-occlusive dysfunction, or severe adrenergic tone secondary to anxiety; standing alone, it is of limited usefulness.

Normally, an erection should ensue within 5 to 10 minutes of injection. A normal rigid erection implies a psychogenic or a neurogenic etiology for the patient's sexual dysfunction. An abnormal result in which the erection is either delayed significantly or absent may suggest arterial inflow disease. In cases in which an immediate rigid erection is induced but has short duration, veno-occlusive disease may be present.

The injection test is easy to perform in the physician's office and represents a dynamic test that may approximate the true physiologic environment. However, the injection of vasoactive agents is relatively invasive, is nonspecific, and carries the risks of priapism, systemic hypotension, and localized bleeding. Moreover, heightened sympathetic tone from factors such as pain or test anxiety may suppress normal tumescence and produce a false-positive result. Several reports indicate that the accuracy of the injection test in screening for organic and psychogenic impotence may be enhanced by using concomitant audiovisual or manual stimulation in an attempt to prevent cortical inhibition via sympathetic neural pathways.[74]

In general, the penile Doppler and vasoactive agent injection tests should be interpreted with caution in the initial evaluation of erectile dysfunction. The accuracy of the injection test and the consistency by which it can be performed and interpreted make its use appealing to the general urologist. We routinely employ the Doppler penile-brachial index (PBI) as an office screening tool but limit the office injection for therapeutic, not diagnostic, purposes.

Duplex color flow sonography using pulsed Doppler technology is utilized to increase the accuracy of dynamic penile arterial studies (Fig. 24–1). Pulsed Doppler techniques enhance the specificity of arterial ultrasound by allowing the size of the sampled area to be adjusted and focused on the cavernosal vessels. Duplex and color flow sonography generates data concerning changes in cavernosal artery diameter as well as cavernosal artery peak flow velocity. After the injection of a vasoactive agent, normal values for corporal artery diameter and peak flow velocity have been reported to be more than 0.08 cm and more than 30 cm/sec, respectively. In atherosclerotic disease, patients typically display arterial diameters of less than 0.07 cm and peak velocities of less than 25 cm/sec. We utilize the parameter of flow velocity and avoid diameter in our routine evaluation. Reports indicate that dynamic duplex Doppler analysis correlates better with angiographic findings than with the PBI.[75]

The cavernosal artery systolic occlusion pressure, the maximal arterial pressure deliverable to the corpora cavernosa, can also be measured using duplex Doppler ultrasound and the intracavernous infusion of saline. This test is often performed as part of the dynamic infusion cavernosometry/cavernosography procedure; usually it is not an isolated test. The pressure at which arterial pulsation returns after a maximal elevation of cavernosal pressure by saline infusion is the corporal perfusion pressure. A large gradient between the brachial and perfusion pressures implies arterial inflow disease.

Selective penile arteriography (internal pudendal and penile arteries) provides anatomic information but provides no data concerning erectile physiology (Fig. 24–2). The clinical utility of this study is probably limited to those patients who are appropriate candidates for penile revascularization procedures (e.g., traumatic injuries to the pelvis or perineum in young patients).

Veno-occlusive Impotence. Corporal veno-occlusive dysfunction is diagnosed by the patient history, and the selective utilization of the office-based vasoactive injection test, duplex color flow sonography, or dynamic infusion cavernosometry/cavernosography (DICC; Fig. 24–3). The office injection is fraught with the same limitations as noted earlier. Duplex color flow sonography has been applied to the evaluation of the veno-occlusive mechanism, but controversy exists about its reliability. Cavernosometry appears to be the best discriminator of venogenic impotence. Cavernosometry is based on the theory that the normal erection requires both adequate arterial inflow and, with trabecular smooth muscle relaxation, sufficient venous resistance to maintain tumescence and rigidity. During stimulation or pharmacologic smooth muscle relaxation, there is a significant reduction in the required blood flow to maintain a given intracavernosal pressure.

Generally, the normal "flow-to-maintain" tumescence during dynamic cavernosometry using vasoactive agents is approximately 3 to 5 mL/min.[76] The diagnosis of corporal veno-occlusive dysfunction is made if the flow to maintain a given intracavernous pressure is more than 5 mL/min or if the pressure drop over time from the peak corporal measurement is more than 40 mm Hg/30 sec.[77] Gravity cavernosometry can be performed in an office setting using an infusion of saline by gravity or pump with similar results. Cavernosometry is limited by the ability of the vasoactive agents to overcome sympathetic inhibition of erectile smooth muscle relaxation at physiologically tolerable doses. Recently, Seftel et al and, subsequently, Nehra et al have introduced the concept of redosing during the testing phase to determine complete corporal smooth muscle relaxation, allowing the cavernosometrogram to become standardized utilizing specific test dose conditions.[78,79]

Cavernosography is usually performed after pressure studies indicate a venous leak to document radiographically the anatomic location and degree of veno-occlusive dysfunction. This study can be done after the injection of vasoactive agents, during visual sexual stimulation, or with the passive infusion of saline.[80–82]

Opponents of detailed diagnostic testing to evaluate vasculogenic impotence argue that the current treatment options for most patients are the same irrespective of the underlying etiology (i.e., vacuum erection device, injection therapy, or penile prosthesis), thereby precluding the need for invasive studies. Patients with arteriogenic impotence may, however, respond very differently from individuals with veno-occlusive disease to the same treatment (e.g., injection therapy). Additionally, the modern treatment modalities are each associated with side effects and risks of complications. However, it is our experience that the self-reported history and physical examination may not be truly predictive of the erectile dysfunction, and therefore objective testing is clearly indicated to document the pathophysiology prior to instituting therapy. Our current recommendation therefore is for the urologist to utilize judiciously a series of noninvasive and invasive studies that permit the formulation of a management plan based on rational expectations for the success of each treatment option.

TESTS FOR NEUROGENIC IMPOTENCE

The investigation of the neurogenic component of penile impotence can be either direct or indirect. The neurologic evaluation consists of the physical examination (described earlier) and neurophysiologic testing. It is the aim of neurologic testing to document the extent of the neurologic deficit and identify any possible reversible causes for medical or surgical treatment. After the history and physical examination, specific clinical tests for neurogenic erectile failure are NPT, penile biothesiometry, and neurophysiologic evoked potentials. The physical examination represents a means of identifying gross neurologic defects. General evaluations of sensation and motor function should be obtained, and specific genitourinary tests such as the bulbocavernosus reflex and rectal tone are essential. (See the section on the physical examination.) An abnormal NPT result, in the absence of gross indicators of arteriogenic erectile failure, may indicate a neurologic etiology. In general, detailed evaluations for neurogenic impotence should begin with biothesiometry.

Biothesiometry is an indirect test of the afferent somatic dorsal nerve pathway of the penis. The test utilizes a portable vibrating device with adjustable amplitude to discern differences in the penile vibratory sense. Measurements are taken on key reference points on the index fingers, penile shaft, and glans and are compared to age-specific control ranges.[83,84] Biothesiometry is particularly appealing because it provides a quick-and-easy means of accurately quantifying abnormalities in vibratory sensation that may indicate peripheral neuropathy. A nomogram has been obtained using potent controls. If there is suggestive evidence for sensory loss, then neurophysiologic testing determining dorsal nerve conduction velocity or bulbocavernosus reflex latency testing may identify peripheral and sacral spinal pathology.

The integrity or dysfunction of sensory penile neural pathways can be confirmed with the use of somatosensory evoked potentials. Common pathways tested include (1) the sacral evoked potential and (2) the genitocerebral evoked potential. The sacral evoked potential measures the activity of the sacral spinal reflex arc. This study is performed by recording electrical activity within the bulbocavernosus muscle after stimulation of the penile skin.[85] The genitocerebral evoked potential theoretically investigates the integrity of spinal and supraspinal pathways. In this test, cortical activity, obtained using EEG leads, is recorded during penile stimulation and an attempt is made to extrapolate increased cerebral activity to the presence of intact peripheral, spinal, and cortical neural networks.[86]

New Tests of Erectile Function

SPACE

Currently, efforts to evaluate the structure and function of the erectile tissue remain primitive. Investigative studies in-

Figure 24–1. (A) Normal color Doppler examination of the left cavernosal artery showing color flow in the artery with a pulsed Doppler gate positioned over the artery. Normal pulsed Doppler arterial tracing is shown below with peak systolic velocity of 0.47 m/sec. (See Plate 9.) (B) Normal cavernosal arterial Doppler examination in the flaccid state prior to injection of vasoactive agent. Peak systolic velocity of the artery in this patient is 0.22 m/sec. (C) Normal cavernosal artery Doppler examination 2 minutes after injection of vasoactive agents shows increased flow with elevated peak systolic velocity of 0.45 m/sec.

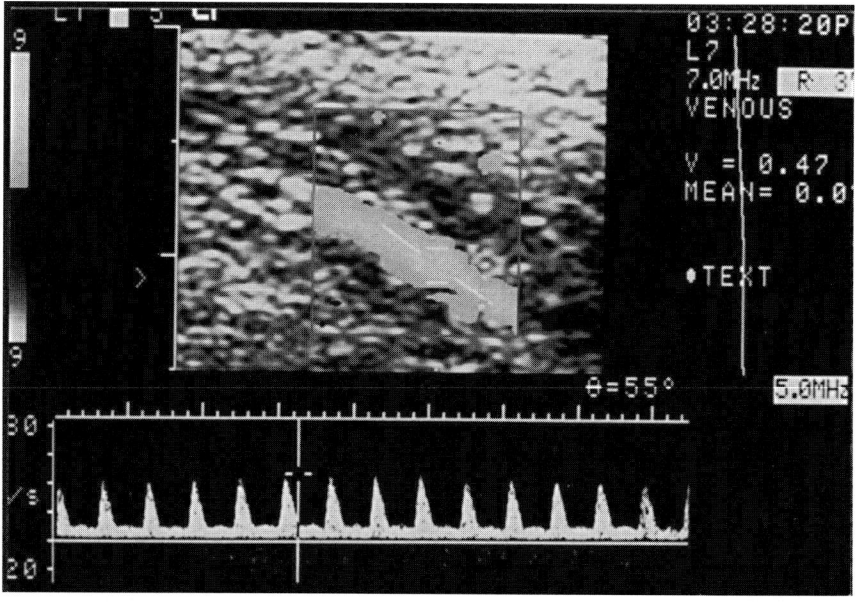

A

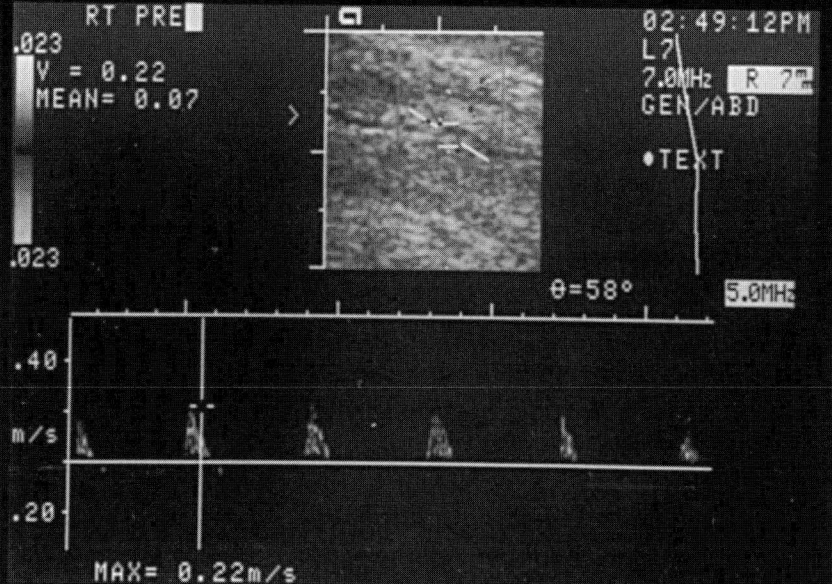

B

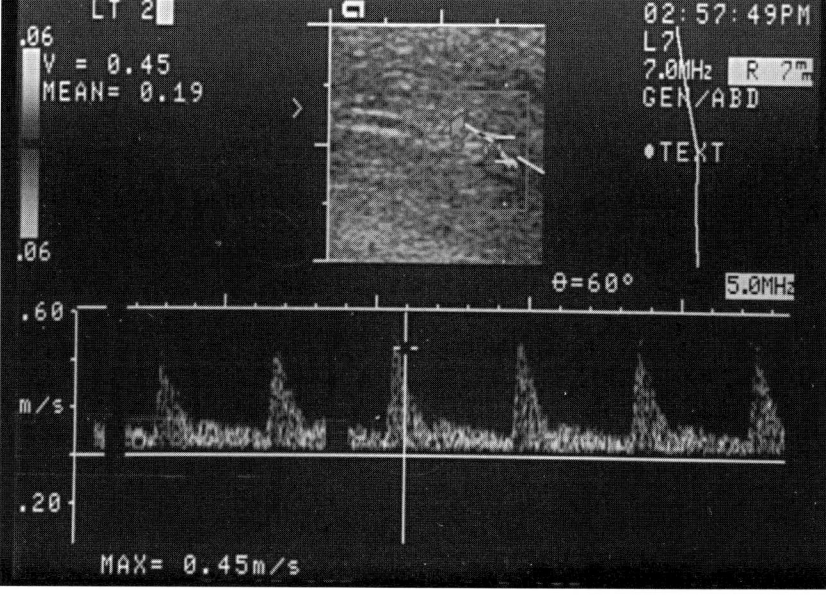

C

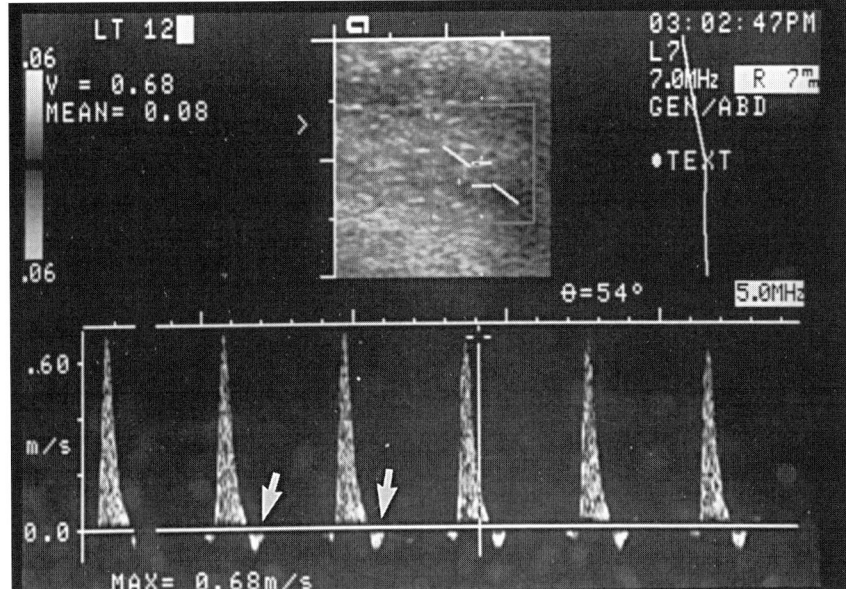
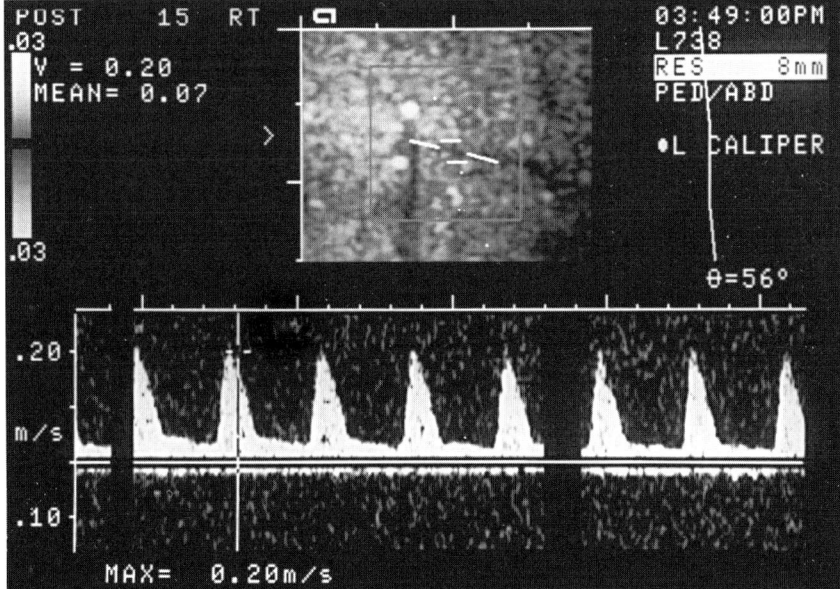

Figure 24–1 Continued. (D) Normal cavernosal artery Doppler examination 12 minutes after injection shows elevated peak systolic velocity to 0.68 m/sec and reversal of diastolic blood flow (arrows). (E) Abnormal Doppler examination of cavernosal artery showing an increase in peak systolic velocity to only 0.20 m/sec consistent with arteriogenic impotence.

clude single potential analysis of cavernosal electrical activity (SPACE) analysis. In general, SPACE analysis has been found to be highly accurate in the diagnosis of cavernous autonomic neuropathy and smooth muscle myopathy. The autonomic cavernous innervation is tested using intracavernosal EMG needles or surface electrodes to analyze the erectile tissue electrical activity.

Using SPACE, specific waveforms indicative of upper and lower motor neuron lesions have been identified.[87–90] Upper motor neuron lesions have been associated with waveforms showing longer duration with occasional whips and bursts. Studies of lower motor neuron lesions have produced characteristic electrical patterns of short duration and variable amplitude. It is important to understand that these tests rely heavily on a detailed knowledge of neural physiology and electrical conduction patterns. Thus this test should only be performed by experienced neurologists or urologists with special training in neurophysiology.

CAVERNOUS BIOPSY

Cavernous tissue biopsy is performed in an attempt to correlate cellular level defects with the clinical diagnosis of erectile failure. Cavernous biopsy using a biopsy gun and subsequent microscopic inspection may produce evidence of smooth muscle changes such as fibrosis, atrophy, and abnormal collagen deposition.[91] These structural changes in cavernous tissue may be responsible for clinical erectile failure.[92] Recent studies have shown evidence that ultrastructural changes of corporal tissue correlate positively with advancing age and are diffuse.[93] Furthermore, recent data using cavernous biopsy demonstrated no significant differ-

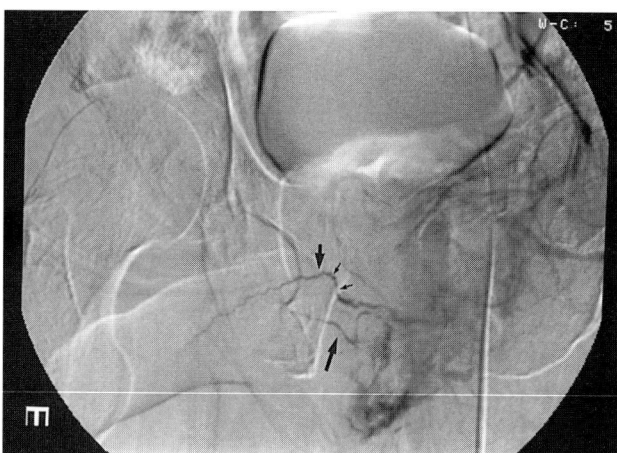

Figure 24–2. Selective penile angiogram showing the dorsal penile artery (short arrow), cavernosal artery (long arrow), and focal stenoses (small arrows) secondary to atherosclerotic disease.

ence in endothelial cell content between impotent and nonimpotent men, giving additional credence to the concept of smooth muscle disease being the focal point of erectile dysfunction.[94]

RADIOISOTOPE MEASUREMENTS OF VENOUS OUTFLOW AND ARTERIAL INFLOW

The use of technetium (Tc-99m)-labeled red blood cells to detect the time in which blood remains within the sinusoidal spaces has been described and represents the forefront of emerging techniques for the diagnosis of corporal venous incompetence. In this test, Tc-99m-labeled autologous red blood cells are used to record the efficiency of the corporal veno-occlusive mechanism. After the injection of vasoactive agents, a gamma camera is used to image the pelvis. A high rate of disappearance of activity has been associated with veno-occlusive disease.[95,96]

A dual isotope technique to evaluate penile arterial inflow has also been developed. During this study, red blood cells are first labeled with Tc-99m in vivo. Xenon-133 in saline is infused into the corpora after stimulating tumescence with vasoactive agents. A gamma camera is then utilized to determine the average peak arterial flow rate. Flow rates below a standard normal value (13.0 mL/min) for potent males are thought to indicate significant penile arterial insufficiency.[97]

NUCLEAR MAGNETIC RESONANCE (NMR, MRI, MAGNETIC RESONANCE IMAGING)

New studies of cavernosal artery perfusion have been introduced. Using nuclear magnetic resonance (NMR) with gadolinium-DTPA as the contrast medium, blood flow within the lacunar spaces of the erectile tissue can be detected and measured. Studies using dynamic NMR in normal penile erections have demonstrated a homogeneous distribution pattern with filling of the entire corporal compartment.[98] In penile arterial inflow disease, an inhomogeneous blood-flow pattern is generally apparent.

PENILE BLOOD GAS

Another new study utilizes the penile blood gas measurement to detect arterial inflow disease. After the injection of vasoactive agents to stimulate erection, the cavernosal blood P_{O_2} is determined over time. Patients with normal arterial perfusion generally show penile blood gas P_{O_2} measurements of more than 97 during tumescence, as reported by

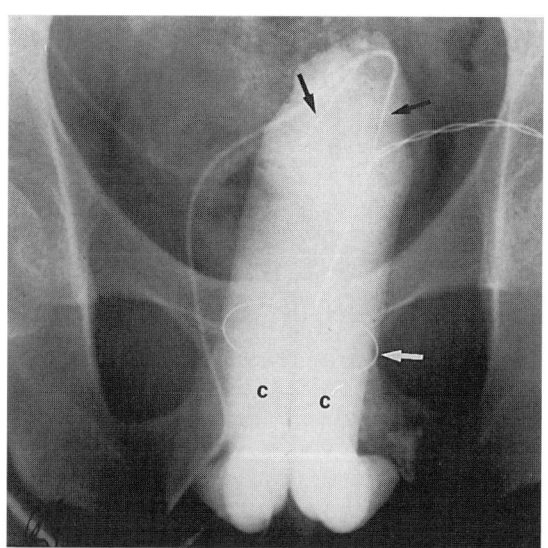
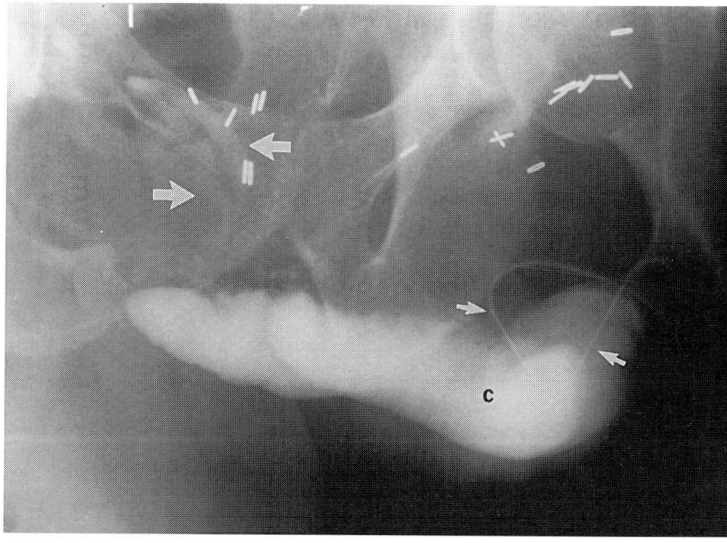

Figure 24–3. (A) Normal cavernosogram showing contrast-enhanced corpus cavernosa (c), infusion cannulae (black arrows), and pressure transducer (white arrow). (B) Venous leak: cavernosogram showing infusion cannulae (small arrows) filling contrast into corpus cavernosum (c) with leak of contrast into pelvic veins (large arrows).

Kim, Vardi et al.[99] Significant decreases in the P_{O_2} measurement may indicate a component of arteriogenic erectile dysfunction.[100] Our own data reveal that the "normal" penile blood gas, 10 minutes after introduction of a pharmacologic erection, is approximately 90 to 95 mm Hg. Arteriogenic impotence is strongly suggested by a P_{O_2} of less than 65 mm Hg, and pure venous leak impotence is heralded by a P_{O_2} of 80 to 85 mm Hg. A clearer understanding of the usefulness of this test will be related to a better understanding of the physiologic aspects of erection and penile oxygenation.

PENILE RIGIDITY

Controversy surrounding the interpretation of many of the diagnostic tests utilized for the evaluation of erectile dysfunction clouds their clinical usefulness. Pitfalls include the subjective assessment of penile rigidity, and the lack of an understanding of penile hemodynamics. In our experience, the assessment of penile rigidity, which indirectly reflects the ability to achieve vaginal penetration, is not uniformly assessable by the physician. Rather, the best discriminator of penile rigidity is the measurement of axial rigidity, by the use of various devices connected to a hand-held force transducer. We believe that based upon the use of penile rigidity, the controversy surrounding the "normal" values for color duplex ultrasound for arteriogenic impotence can be settled. The value that yields an erection with the minimal rigidity for vaginal penetration (we believe to be represented by a 1-kg axial load) appears to be 30 cm/sec. Increasing the flow velocity to 40 cm/sec only appears to improve the rigidity of the erection. Thus the range of 30 to 40 cm/sec appears to represent a continuum of rigidity and should therefore be interpreted as a range of normal values, with 30 cm/sec as the minimum. Arteriogenic impotence would be heralded by a value less than 30 cm/sec.

We have also found that penile rigidity can be useful in understanding the true value of color duplex ultrasound in detecting venous leak impotence. We believe that the established values for venous leak impotence, 3 to 5 cm/sec of end diastolic flow, truly represent venous leak. However, a lack of end-diastolic flow velocity should not preclude the diagnosis of venous leak impotence. Utilizing rigidity and the DICC, we have found a significant incidence of venous leak impotence in patients in the face of no end-diastolic velocity on color duplex ultrasound. The physiology of such an event is speculative. Thus penile rigidity may become an important clinical tool in the evaluation of erectile dysfunction.

CONCLUSION

As our understanding of normal erectile function and the mechanisms leading to impotence improves, the diagnostic testing available to the urologist will certainly become more specific and accurate. The question of whether detailed endocrine evaluations and invasive vascular, neurologic, and erectile tissue testing is necessary and appropriate really depends on whether differentiating the various etiologies of impotence is important to patient management. Certainly, offering the impotent patient an appropriate treatment plan from the full range of modern options requires that urologic specialists be able to make this differentiation based on contemporary knowledge of the pathophysiology of impotence.

REFERENCES

1. Lue T: Physiology of erection and pathophysiology of impotence. In: Walsh PC, Retik AB, Stamey TA, Vaughan ED, eds. *Campbell's Urology, 1*. Philadelphia: WB Saunders, 1992;709–728.
2. Lue T, Takamura T, Umraiya M, et al: Hemodynamics of canine corpora cavernosa during erection. *Urology* 1984;24:347–352.
3. Aboseif S, Lue T: Hemodynamics of penile erection. *Urol Clin North Am* 1988;15:1–7.
4. Goldstein I, Krane R: Diagnosis and therapy of erectile dysfunction. In: Walsh PC, Retik AB, Stamey TA, Vaughan ED, eds. *Campbell's Urology, 3*. Philadelphia: WB Saunders, 1992;3033–3072.
5. Leriche A, Morel A: Syndrome of thrombotic obliteration of aortic bifurcation. *Ann Surg* 1948;127:193–206.
6. Michal V, Ruzbarsky V: Histologic changes in the penile arterial bed with aging and diabetes. In: Waterhouse K, Zorgniotti A, et al, eds. *Vasculogenic Impotence: Proceedings of the First International Conference on Corpus Cavernosum Revascularization*. Springfield, IL: Charles C Thomas, 1980;113–119.
7. Karacan I, Salis P, et al: Erectile dysfunction in hypertensive men: sleep-related erections, penile blood flow and musculovascular events. *J Urol* 1989;142:56–61.
8. Goldstein I, Feldman M, Deckers P, et al: Radiation associated impotence: a clinical study of its mechanism. *JAMA* 1984;251:903–910.
9. Flanigan D, Schuler J, Keifer T, et al: Elimination of iatrogenic impotence and improvement of sexual function after aortoiliac revascularization. *Arch Surg* 1982;117:544–550.
10. Jevitich M, Edson M, Jarman W, et al: Vascular factors in erectile failure among diabetics. *Urology* 1982;19:163–168.
11. Lue T, Tanagho E: Functional anatomy and mechanism of penile erection. In: Tanagho EA, Lue TF, McClure RD, eds. Baltimore: Williams & Wilkins, 1988;39–50.
12. Lue T: Male sexual dysfunction. In: Tanagho EA, McAninch JW, eds. *Smith's General Urology*. Norwalk, CT: Appleton and Lange, 1995;772–792.
13. Nehra A, Moreland R, Saenz de Tejada I, et al: What is venous leak and why is there limited success with venous leak surgery in patients with vasculogenic impotence associated with vascular risk factors? *J Urol* 1995;153:471A. Abstract.
14. Azadzoi K, Goldstein I: Atherosclerosis-induced corporal leakage impotence. *Surg Forum* 1987;38:647–648.
15. Fisher G, Swain M, Cherian K: Increased vascular collagen and elastin synthesis in experimental atherosclerosis in the rabbit. *Atherosclerosis* 1980;35:11–20.
16. Gasior B, Levine F, Howannesian A, Krane R, Goldstein I: Plaque associated corporal veno-occlusive dysfunction in id-

16. iopathic Peyronie's disease: a pharmacocavernosometric and pharmacocavernosographic study. *World J Urol* 1990;8:90–96.
17. Ebbehoj J, Wagner G: Insufficient penile erection due to abnormal drainage of cavernous bodies. *Urology* 1979;13:507–510.
18. Tudoriu T, Bourmer H: The hemodynamics of erection at the level of the penis and its local deterioration. *J Urol* 1983;129:741–745.
19. Lue T, Hricak H, Schmidt R, et al: Functional evaluation of penile veins by cavernosography in papaverine-induced erection. *J Urol* 1986;135:479–482.
20. Jiaan D, Seftel AD, et al: Age-related increase of an advanced glycation end product in penile tissue; potential role in erectile dysfunction. *World J Urol* 1995;13(6):369–375.
21. Hoffman D, Seftel AD, et al: Advanced glycation end-products quench cavernosal nitric oxide. *J Urol* 1995;153(suppl, April):441A. Abstract 849.
22. Penson D, Seftel A, Krane R, Frohrib D, Goldstein I: The hemodynamic pathophysiology of impotence following blunt trauma to the erect penis. *J Urol* 1992;148(4):1171–1180.
23. Benson G, Boileau M: The penis: sexual function and dysfunction. In: Gillenwater JY, Grayhack JT, Howards SS, Duckett JW, eds. *Adult and Pediatric Urology, 2*. St. Louis: Mosby Year Book, 1987;1599–1642.
24. Burnett A, Calvin D, Chamness S, Ricker D, Crone J, Chang T: Characterization of neuronal and endothelial nitric oxide synthase (NOS) isoforms in the penis and urethra of wild type mice and transgenic mice lacking neuronal NOS. *J Urol* 1995;153(suppl April):509A. Abstract 1124.
25. Kedia K, Markland C, Fraley E: Sexual function following high retroperitoneal lymphadenectomy. *J Urol* 1975;114:237–239.
26. Dahlberg C, Jaffe J: *Stroke: a doctor's personal story of his recovery*. New York: Norton, 1977.
27. Bors E, Comarr A: Neurologic disturbances of sexual function with special reference to 529 patients with spinal cord injury. *Urol Surv* 1960;10:191–222.
28. Boller F, Frank E: *Sexual Dysfunction in Neurologic Disorders: Diagnosis, Management, and Rehabilitation*. New York: Raven Press, 1982;33.
29. Cartlidge N: Autonomic function of multiple sclerosis. *Brain* 1972;95:661–664.
30. Van Arsdalen K, Malloy T, Wein A: Erectile physiology, dysfunction and evaluation: II. Etiology and evaluation of erectile dysfunction. *Monogr Urol* 1983;4:165.
31. Ellenberg M: Impotence in diabetics: a neurologic rather than an endocrinologic problem. *Med Aspects Human Sex* 1973;7:12–20.
32. Hansen M, Ertekin C, Larsson L, Pedersen K: A neurophysiological study of patients undergoing radical prostatectomy. *Scand J Urol Nephrol* 1989;23:267–273.
33. Abram H, Hester L, Sheridan W, Epstein G: Sexual functioning in patients with chronic renal failure. *J Nerv Ment Dis* 1975;160:220–226.
34. LoPiccolo J: Diagnosis and treatment of male sexual dysfunction. *J Sex Marital Ther* 1986;11:215–232.
35. Marmor J: Impotence and ejaculatory disorders. In: Kaplan H, Sadock D, Freedman A, *Sexual Experience*. Baltimore: Williams & Wilkins, 1976.
36. Levine S: The psychological evaluation and therapy of psychogenic impotence. In: Seagraves RT, Schoenberg HW, eds. *Diagnosis and Treatment of Erectile Disturbances: A Guide for Clinicians*. New York: Plenum Press, 1985.
37. de Groat W, Steers W: Neuroanatomy and neurophysiology of penile erection. In: Tanagho EA, Lue TF, McClure RD, eds. *Contemporary Management of Impotence and Infertility*. Baltimore: Williams & Wilkins, 1988;3.
38. Benard F, Stief C, Bosch R, et al: Systemic infusion of epinephrine: its effect on erection. In: *Proceedings of the Sixth Biennial International Symposium for Corpus Cavernosum Revascularization and Third Biennial World Meeting on Impotence*. Boston, 1988, p. 16.
39. Bulpitt C, Dollery C: Side effects of hypotensive agents evaluated by a self-administered questionnaire. *Br Med J* 1973;3:485.
40. Hogan M, Wallin J, Baer RM: Antihypertensive therapy and male sexual dysfunction. *Psychosomatics* 1980;21(3):234–237.
41. Papadopoulos C: Cardiovascular drugs and sexuality. *Arch Intern Med* 1980;140(10):1341–1345.
42. Wein A, Van Arsdalen K: Drug-induced male sexual dysfunction. *Urol Clin North Am* 1988;15:23–31.
43. *Medical Letter:* Drugs That Cause Sexual Dysfunction 1983;25:73.
44. Hsieh J, Muller S, Lue T: The influence of blood flow and blood pressure on penile erection. *Int J Impot Res* 1989;1:35–42.
45. Oaks W, Moyer J: Sex and hypertension. *Med Aspects Hum Sex* 1972;61:128.
46. *Medical Letter:* Drugs That Cause Sexual Dysfunction. 1980;22:108.
47. Masters W, Johnson V: *Human Sexual Inadequacy*. Boston: Little, Brown, 1970.
48. Seagraves R, Madsen R, Carter C, et al: Erectile dysfunction associated with pharmacological agents. In: Seagraves RT, Schoenberg HW, eds. *Diagnosis and Treatment of Erectile Disturbances*. New York: Plenum Press, 1985.
49. Cunningham G, Hirshkowitz M, Korenman S, Karacan I: Testosterone replacement therapy and sleep-related erections in hypogonadal men. *J Clin Endocrinol Metab* 1990;70:792–797.
50. Bancroft J, Wu F: Changes in erectile responsiveness during androgen therapy. *Arch Sex Behav* 1983;12:59–66.
51. Benkert O, Witt W, Adam W, Leitz A: Effects of testosterone undecanoate on sexual potency and the hypothalamic–pituitary–gonadal axis of impotent males. *Arch Sex Behav* 1979;8:471–479.
52. Ficher M, Neeb M, Zuckerman M, et al: Study of sexual dysfunction among male diabetics. In: Ficher M, Fishkin RE, Jacobs JA, eds. *Sexual Arousal: New Concepts in Basic Science Diagnosis and Treatment*. Springfield, IL: Charles C Thomas, 1984.
53. Daniels G, Martin J: Neuroendocrine regulation and disease of the anterior pituitary and hypothalamus. In: Braunwald E, Isselbacher KJ, Petersdorf RG, et al, eds. New York: McGraw-Hill, 1987;1694–1718.
54. Nickel J, Morales A, Condra M, et al: Endocrine dysfunction in impotence: incidence, significance, and cost effective screening. *J Urol* 1984;132:40–43.
55. Feingold K, Gavin L, Schambelan M, Sebastian A: The thyroid. In: Andreoli TE, Carpenter CC, Plum F, Smith LH, eds. *Cecil Essentials of Medicine*. Philadelphia: WB Saunders, 1990;456–465.
56. Franks S, Nabarro JD: Prevalence and presentation of hyperprolactinemia in patients with ''functionless'' pituitary tumors. *Lancet* 1977;1:778–780.
57. Miller J, Howards S, McLeod R: Serum prolactin in organic and psychogenic impotence. *J Urol* 1980;123:862–864.
58. Ackerman M, D'Attilio J, Rhamy R, et al: Patient reported sexual symptomatology in predicting functional and insufficient erectile capacity. *Urology* 1991;38(5):437–442.

59. Ackerman M, D'Attilio J, Antoni M, Campbell B: Assessment of erectile dysfunction in diabetic men: the clinical relevance of self-reported sexual functioning. *J Sex Marital Ther* 1991;17(3):191–202.
60. Fisher C, Gross J, Zuch J: Cycle of penile erections synchronous with dreaming (REM) sleep. *Arch Gen Psychiatr* 1965; 12:29–45.
61. Karacan I, Salis P, Williams R: The role of the sleep laboratory in the diagnosis and treatment of impotence. In: Williams, RL, Karacan I, eds. *Sleep Disorder, Diagnosis, Treatment*. New York: John Wiley, 1978.
62. Shvartzman P: The role of nocturnal penile tumescence and rigidity monitoring in the evaluation of impotence. *J Fam Prac* 1994;39(3):279–282.
63. Schiavi R, Schreiner-Engel P, Mandeli J, et al: Healthy aging and male sexual function. *Am J Psychiatr* 1990;147:766–771.
64. Ware J: Evaluation of impotence: monitoring periodic penile erections during sleep. *Psychiatr Clin North Am* 1987; 10:675–686.
65. Thase M, et al: Nocturnal penile tumescence is diminished in depressed men. *Biol Psychiatr* 1988;24:33–46.
66. Seagraves R, Schoenberg H, et al: Evaluation of the etiology of erectile failure. In: Seagraves RT, Schoenberg HW, eds. *Diagnosis and Treatment of Erectile Disturbances*. New York: Plenum Press, 1985.
67. Morales A, Condra M, Heaton J, et al: Diurnal penile tumescence recording in the etiological diagnosis of erectile dysfunction. *J Urol* 1994;152(4):1111–1114.
68. Morales A, Harris C, Condra M, Heaton J: Validation of visual sexual stimulation in the etiological diagnosis of impotence. *Int J. Impot Res* 1990;2(suppl 2).
69. Katlowitz N, Albano G, Morales P, Golimbu M: Potentiation of drug-induced erection with audiovisual sexual stimulation. *Urology* 1993;41(5):431–434.
70. Engel G, Burnham S, Carter M: Penile blood pressure in the evaluation of erectile impotence. *Fertil Steril* 1978;30:687–690.
71. Gewertz B, Zarins C: Vasculogenic impotence. In: Seagraves RT, Schoenberg HW, eds. *Diagnosis and Treatment of Erectile Disturbances: A Guide for Clinicians*. New York: Plenum, 1985;105.
72. Aitchison M, Aitchison J, Carter R: Is the penile brachial index a reproducible and useful measurement. *Br J Urol* 1990;66(2):202–204.
73. Abber J, et al: Diagnostic tests for impotence: comparison of papaverine injection with penile-brachial index and nocturnal penile tumescence monitoring. *J Urol* 1986;135:923–925.
74. Donatucci C, Lue T: The combined intracavernous injection and stimulation test: diagnostic accuracy. *J Urol* 1992; 148(1):61–62.
75. Mueller S, et al: Comparison of selective internal iliac pharmaco-angiography, penile brachial index and duplex sonography with pulsed Doppler analysis for the evaluation of vasculogenic (arteriogenic) impotence. *J Urol* 1990;143(5):928–932.
76. Wespes E, et al: Pharmacocavernosometry-cavernosography in impotence. *Br J Urol* 1986;58:429–433.
77. Padma-Nathan H: Evaluation of the corporal veno-occlusive mechanism: dynamic infusion cavernosometry and cavernosography. *Semin Intervent Radiol* 1989;6:205.
78. Seftel A, Saenz de Tejada I, Frohrib D, et al: Is it possible to achieve maximal smooth muscle relaxation during dynamic cavernosometry and thereby achieve standardization? *J Urol* 1991;145(suppl):343A.
79. Nehra A, Hakim L, et al: A new method of performing duplex Doppler ultrasonography: the effect of re-dosing of vasoactive agents on hemodynamic parameters. *J Urol* 1995; 153(suppl):332A.
80. Wagner G: Erection, physiology and endocrinology. In: Wagner G, Green R, eds. *Impotence: Physiological, Psychological and Surgical Diagnosis and Treatment*. New York: Plenum, 1981;25–36.
81. Lue T, et al: Functional evaluation of penile veins by cavernosography in papaverine-induced erection. *J Urol* 1986; 135:479–482.
82. Wespes E, et al: Cavernosometry-cavernosography: its role in organic impotence. *Eur Urol* 1984;10:229–232.
83. Padma-Nathan H, Goldstein I: Neurologic assessment of the impotent male. In: Montague DK, ed. *Disorders of Male Sexual Functions*. Chicago: Year Book, 1987;86–94.
84. Lavoisier P, Courtois F, et al: Normality criteria for penile sensitivity to pressure, touch and vibration. *Int J Impot Res* 1990;2(suppl 2):89.
85. Krane R, Siroky M: Studies of sacral evoked potentials. *J Urol* 1980;124:872–876.
86. Haldeman S, et al: Pudendal evoked responses. *Arch Neurol* 1982;39:280–283.
87. Stief CG, Djamilian M, Anton P, de Riese W, Allhoff EP, Jonas U: Single potential analysis of cavernous electrical activity in impotent patients: a possible diagnostic method for autonomic cavernous dysfunction and cavernous smooth muscle degeneration. *J Urol* 1991;146(3):771–776.
88. Stief C, Thon W, et al: Single potential analysis of cavernous electrical activity. *Urol Res* 1991;19(5):277–280.
89. Wagner G, et al: Electrical activity of corpus cavernosum during flaccidity and erection of the human penis. *J Urol* 1989;142:723–725.
90. Buvat J, et al: Electromyography of the human penis, including single potential analysis during flaccidity and erection induced by vasoactive agents. *Int J Impot Res* 1990;2(suppl 2):88.
91. Wespes E, et al: Use of biopsy gun for cavernous biopsy. *Eur Urol* 1990;18:81–83.
92. Persson C, et al: Correlation of altered penile ultrastructure with clinical arterial evaluation. *J Urol* 1989;142:1462–1468.
93. Wespes E, Goes PM, Schiffman S, Depierreux M, Vanderhagen JJ, Schulman CC: Computerized analysis of smooth muscle fibers in potent and impotent patients. *J Urol* 1991; 146:1015–1017.
94. Sattar AA, Schulman CC, Wespes E: Objective quantification of cavernous endothelium in potent and impotent men. *J Urol* 1995;153:1136–1138.
95. Grech P, Dave S, et al: Combined papaverine test and radionuclide penile blood flow in impotence: method and preliminary results. *Br J Urol* 1992;69(4):407–417.
96. Kim SC, Kim KB, Oh CH: Diagnostic value of the radioisotope erection penogram for vasculogenic impotence. *J Urol* 1990;144:888–893.
97. Miraldi F, Nelson D, Jones W, Thompson S, Kursh E: A dual-radioisotope technique for the evaluation of penile blood flow during tumescence. *J Nucl Med* 1992;33:41–46.
98. Austoni E, Cazzaniga A, et al: Use of dynamic NMR in the diagnostic evaluation of penile pathology. *Int J Impot Res* 1990;2(suppl 2):161.
99. Kim N, Vardi Y, Nathan HP, et al: Oxygen tension regulates the nitric oxide pathway. *J Clin Invest* 1993;91:437–442.
100. Knipsel HH, Andresen R: Evaluation of vasculogenic impotence by monitoring of cavernous oxygen tension. *J Urol* 1993;149:1276–1279.

25 Neurogenic Bladder

Stephen D. Mark, George D. Webster

Normal voiding relies on coordinated bladder and sphincter function and is a complex neurophysiological event. It is dependent on a variety of integrated neuronal pathways connecting the cerebral cortex, brainstem nuclei in the pons, and sacral spinal cord to the lower urinary tract. Pathologic entities may affect various regions within these pathways, resulting in a neurogenic bladder. Because there is an inexact correlation with the anatomic level of a particular lesion and the urodynamic findings, classification systems have moved away from this anatomic description of the lesion to a more functionally based system. The development of these classification systems has paralleled the increased use of urodynamics, providing an improved understanding of the integration of bladder and sphincter function.

Along with this better understanding of the pathophysiology of neurogenic bladder, therapeutic options have increased markedly. Management should be individualized according to clinical findings along with the patient's intelligence, independence, motivation, dexterity, and capacity for long-term follow-up. With the increased acceptance, safety, and efficacy of clean intermittent catheterization (CIC), more effective pharmacotherapy, and reliability of reconstructive surgery, the length and quality of life in these patients has improved. As a result of these changes the urologist has an increased therapeutic armamentarium; however, because of the unknown long-term effects of some of these management options lifelong care is required.

THE NEUROPHYSIOLOGY OF MICTURITION

The function of the lower urinary tract depends on neuromechanisms that reside in the brain, brain stem, and lumbosacral spinal cord. This neural system exhibits two modes of operation, namely, the storage and elimination of urine. These neural circuits controlling micturition exhibit a switchlike phasic pattern of activity in contrast to the tonic patterns of activity occurring in other autonomic pathways. In addition, the storage and elimination of urine are clearly under voluntary control, unlike other visceral functions. Micturition is dependent upon learned behavior that emerges during maturation of the nervous system and on primitive reflexes that are present from birth. The storage and elimination of urine requires integration and coordination of two systems within the lower urinary tract: (1) a reservoir (the urinary bladder), and (2) the outlet consisting of the bladder neck and the proximal and distal sphincter mechanisms of the urethra. These structures are in turn controlled by three sets of peripheral nerves that are coordinated centrally; two autonomic sets, the sacral parasympathetic (pelvic) nerves and the thoracolumbar sympathetic (hypogastric) nerves; and the sacral "somatic" (pudendal) nerves.

Bradley[1] has described four distinct neuroanatomic loops or circuits and has suggested that the functional integration of these loops provides for coordinated detrusor and sphincter function during storage and elimination of urine.

Loop I. This consists of pathways between the frontal cortex, basal ganglia, thalamic nuclei, cerebellum, and pontomesencephalic reticula formation. These are predominantly inhibitory pathways, and their interruption produces partial or complete loss of volitional control of the micturition reflex, resulting in coordinated unhibited detrusor function. This loop is interrupted in cerebrovascular accidents, brain tumor, head injury, multiple sclerosis, Parkinson's disease, among others.

Loop II. This pathway comprises sensory afferent neurons from the detrusor muscle traveling up the spinal cord in the posterior and lateral columns, "long-routing" to the brain stem micturition center at the level of the pons. Efferent neurons from the center travel down the spinal cord in the reticulospinal tracts, similarly "long-routing" without synapse to the sacral spinal cord. Integrity of this loop is necessary to establish a detrusor reflex of adequate magnitude and duration to accomplish complete bladder emptying. Its partial interruption produces a low-threshold detrusor reflex (a hyperreflexic detrusor) that will also be inadequate and poorly sustained with resultant inefficient emptying. Its complete interruption causes detrusor hyperreflexia after a period of spinal shock during which the patient is unable to generate a voluntary voiding contraction. Clinical situations in which such interruptions occur include spinal cord trauma, multiple sclerosis, and spinal cord tumor.

Loop III. This comprises the detrusor and pudendal motor nuclei and their interneurons within the sacral spinal cord. They provide for coordination between detrusor contraction and striated urethral sphincter relaxation during voiding.

Loop IV. Neurons in this circuit originate in the motor cortex of the frontal lobes and traverse the pyramidal tracts in the lateral columns of the spinal cord, synapsing on the pudendal sphincter nucleus. This circuit provides voluntary control over the striated muscle of the urethral sphincter during bladder storage and voiding.

PERIPHERAL INNERVATION OF THE LOWER URINARY TRACT

The hypogastric pelvic nerves supply the bladder and urethra with sympathetic and parasympathetic efferent innervation, respectively. They also conduct sensory afferent nerves to the spinal cord. The extrinsic component of the striated sphincter receives somatic innervation via the pudendal nerve. The parasympathetic efferent nerves arise from the sacral spinal cord segment S2–3 and S4 and travel in the pelvic nerves to synapse on ganglia in the vesical plexus around the urethrovesical junction and on ganglia within the interstices of the detrusor muscle. These ganglia are the final pathway for integration of motor impulses within the lower urinary tract. Some respond exclusively to parasympathetic innervation and some are exclusively sympathetic; others are either noncholinergic or nonadrenergic (NANC).

The sacral parasympathetic outflow has acetyl choline as its neurotransmitter providing the major excitatory input to the bladder. Thoracolumbar sympathetic pathways elicit a variety of responses in the lower urinary tract, including inhibition of the detrusor muscle, excitation of the bladder base and urethra, and modulation of the cholinergic transmission to the parasympathetic ganglia. They promote the storage of urine and facilitate urinary continence.

Sensory afferent nerves from the bladder conducting proprioceptive (fullness) and enteroceptive (thermal, tactile, and pain) impulses are carried by both the pelvic and hypogastric nerves to the spinal cord, where some will synapse on the pudendal nuclei. Enteroceptive afferents travel in the contralateral spinothalamic tract to the thalamus and ultimately to the sensory cortex. The proprioceptive afferents ascend in the posterior columns to the pontomesencephalic reticula formation and then to the thalamus and sensory cortex.

Interruption of the peripheral nerve supply to the bladder and urethra may result from a variety of lesions. Trauma due to extensive pelvic surgery (such as abdominoperineal resection for carcinoma of the rectum and radical hysterectomy) is a frequent cause. Autonomic neuropathy may result from diabetes, other metabolic lesions, infectious agents, and toxins, including alcohol and heavy metals. Herpes zoster, sacral agenesis, and cauda equina tumors along with injuries may also interrupt the peripheral innervation.

THE NEUROMECHANICS OF THE LOWER URINARY TRACT

The lower urinary tract basically serves two functions: urine storage and urine elimination. Storage requires that the bladder accommodate increasing volumes of urine at low intravesical pressure with appropriate sensation and that there be no inappropriate (uninhibited) bladder contraction until voiding occurs. During bladder filling the outlet remains closed and functionally competent. During bladder elimination a volitional bladder contraction of adequate magnitude and duration must be established together with the co-ordinated relaxation of both the proximal and distal sphincter mechanisms in the absence of anatomic obstruction.

During the storage phase as filling progresses, bladder wall tension increases and volume receptor stimulation occurs with afferent impulses carried by the pelvic and hypogastric nerves rooted to the spinal and bulbar centers. The efferent limb of the storage reflex is predominantly sympathetic and mediated by the hypogastric nerves, resulting in detrusor relaxation and sphincter contraction. In addition, there is a sympathetic inhibitory effect on the parasympathetic ganglion transmission. When the bladder is full and there is maximum afferent stimulation, the voluntary suppression of the detrusor by higher centers is removed when socially appropriate and contraction occurs in response to activation of the parasympathetic motor fibers to the bladder. There is simultaneous inhibition of sympathetic discharge, facilitating detrusor contraction and allowing for relaxation of the smooth musculature at the proximal urethra. Striated muscle sphincter relaxation is mediated by the pudendal nerve synchronously.

Obviously, successful and efficient storage and voiding requires highly coordinated integration of activity at all levels in the central and peripheral nervous system, and the complexity of the system accounts for the susceptibility of the lower urinary tract to neurogenic dysfunction even in the face of subtle neurologic lesions.

CLASSIFICATION OF NEUROGENIC LOWER URINARY TRACT DYSFUNCTION

The purpose of classification systems is to facilitate understanding of the pathophysiology involved and to predict management options and prognosis. Such a system should represent a shorthand mechanism of describing urodynamic findings, give an indication of approximate site and etiology of the offending lesion, and indicate treatment options. A profusion of classification systems is available for lower urinary tract dysfunction based on descriptive, anatomic, and etiologic terminology. More recently, parallel with the increased use of urodynamic evaluation, a descriptive "functional" classification system based on dysfunction of either the bladder or the outlet has been described by Wein.[2] This system has allowed a logical approach to classification and may be expanded to clarify etiology and therapy.

In 1971, Bors and Comar[3] introduced a classification system based on the anatomic location of the lesion from observation of spinal cord–injured patients. This system describes the lesion as upper motor neuron (UMN; suprasacral) or lower motor neuron (LMN; sacral or infrasacral) and comments on the completeness of the lesion and whether the sphincter acts in a coordinated fashion with the bladder. Residual urine estimation is used to determine whether the sphincter and bladder are coordinated (balanced). More than 20% residual in a patient with UMN lesion or 10% in a patient with an LMN lesion is described as unbalanced. The completeness of the lesion is determined by a thorough neurologic examination.

Urodynamic studies have shown there is not an exact relationship between the bladder and sphincter activity and the anatomic location of the neurologic lesion.[4] This system is often difficult to apply to patients with multicentric neurologic disease and is therefore not satisfactory for routine clinical use.

Lapides[5] popularized a widely used, descriptive classification that identifies five categories of neurogenic bladder dysfunction. Two are due to UMN lesions (uninhibited and reflex neurogenic bladder) and the remaining three are due to LMN lesions (autonomous, the sensory paralytic, and the motor paralytic neurogenic bladder). The term *uninhibited bladder* describes a hyperreflexic bladder with a normal or balanced sphincter, whereas the *reflex bladder* describes detrusor hyperreflexia with external sphincter dyssynergia. The *autonomous* neurogenic bladder resulting from a lesion of both sensory and motor limbs of the voiding reflex arc results in an areflexic bladder incapable of contraction or sensation, along with an inactive sphincter mechanism. The *motor paralytic* bladder also results in an areflexic detrusor. In the *sensory paralytic* bladder the primary problem is one of sensory denervation of the bladder, although ultimately bladder overdistention causes myogenic damage and contractile failure.

This classification system is often clinically applicable and easily remembered. Unfortunately, because of incomplete lesions, or an unusual pattern of associated sphincter dysfunction, many patients don't fit neatly into a category.

Urodynamics has become more sophisticated and able to provide objective data for the classification of lower urinary tract dysfunction. Krane[6] among others, has developed a classification in which the detrusor muscle activity is classified according to whether it is functionally normal, hyperreflexic, or areflexic. Hyperreflexia is defined as the presence of involuntary detrusor contractions, most commonly associated with neurologic lesions above the sacral spinal cord. Striated sphincter dyssynergia is most commonly seen after complete suprasacral spinal cord injury, following a period of spinal shock. Smooth sphincter dyssynergia seen in complete lesions above T-6 with an intact sympathetic outflow is characteristically associated with detrusor hyperreflexia

Table 25–1. ICS Classification System

Detrusor:	Normal
	Overactive
	Underactive
Urethra:	Normal
	Overactive
	Underactive
Sensation:	Normal
	Overactive
	Underactive

and striated sphincter dyssynergia. Detrusor areflexia is the inability to generate a voiding contraction and may be secondary to bladder muscle decompensation or to a variety of other conditions that produce inhibition at the level of the brain stem micturition center, the sacral spinal cord, bladder ganglia, or bladder smooth muscle. The International Continence Society (ICS) has proposed an extension and simplification of this urodynamic classification.[7] The storage and voiding phases of micturition are described separately under the headings of urethral and bladder function (Table 25–1).

A more simplistic classification was introduced by Wein,[2] who divided neurogenic lower urinary tract dysfunction into a bladder that failed to store adequately and one that failed to empty adequately (Table 25–2). Storage failure results from bladder abnormalities, outlet abnormalities, or a combination of the two. Emptying failure can likewise result from bladder or outlet abnormalities or from a combination of the two. Failure in either category generally is not absolute but often relative, and this system can be expanded to include etiologic, urodynamic, or therapeutic options. Madersbacher[8] provided a graphic classification system, separating under- and overactive bladder and sphincter function. Each of his four schemas represents a dysfunctional state of the detrusor sphincter system. Again, this system requires urodynamic assessment and cannot be expanded to include every voiding dysfunction. Along with the other functional systems, however, it may be expanded to include therapeutic considerations.

Overall, no classification system for neurogenic bladder is ideal; however, neurourologists should be familiar with only one or two systems. The most complete system involves incorporating a thorough neurologic examination, accurate urodynamic study, and an attempt to categorize each system as described (anatomic, urodynamic, and functional).

Table 25–2. Wein Functional Classification

Failure to store
    Because of bladder
    Because of outlet
Failure to empty
    Because of bladder
    Because of outlet

EVALUATION OF THE PATIENT WITH NEUROGENIC LOWER URINARY TRACT DYSFUNCTION

An orderly approach is recommended to the evaluation of any patient with voiding difficulties.

History

The degree of neurologic impairment will determine the patient's urologic symptomatology. Those with gross deficits may only recognize their inability to remain continent or their inability to void. Others with more subtle neurologic lesions may present with symptoms whose neurogenic etiology is not immediately identifiable that may mimic symptoms of bladder irritation or other obstructive problems. Moreover, other organs with similar innervation to the bladder may cause bowel symptoms, altered perineal sensation, or change in erectile, ejaculatory, or orgasmic function, all of which implicate a neurogenic bladder.

Symptomatology may be valuable in suggesting whether voiding dysfunction represents an abnormality of storage, an abnormality of emptying, or both. Urgency and frequency may be associated with involuntary bladder contractions or reduced bladder compliance. The impending sensation of micturition or urgency may be subdivided into "fear of leakage," where an involuntary bladder contraction (motor urgency) is the likely cause. However, when pain is the prime reason for the urgency, inflammatory disorders are usually responsible. Increased urinary frequency may also result from emptying failure, with a substantial residual urine volume and therefore a decreased functional bladder capacity. Nocturia usually accompanies nonpsychogenic urinary frequency and may be associated on the same basis as increased daytime frequency with either storage or emptying failure.

Neurogenic disease may lead to any of the various forms of urinary incontinence. Stress incontinence may occur as a result of sphincter incompetence caused by sacral cord or peripheral nerve lesions. Urge incontinence is a manifestation of hyperreflexic bladder dysfunction. The patient with intact bladder sensation will recognize the urge to void but may be unable to reach the bathroom in time. In more complete lesions where sensation is lost, unconscious reflex incontinence may occur. Overflow incontinence may result from an areflexic bladder where, upon filling, the intravesical pressure exceeds the urethral closing pressure, causing continuous dribbling of urine. "Total" urinary incontinence occurs when the bladder and urethra are virtually an open conduit. This is rarely seen as a result of neurogenic bladder dysfunction.

Voiding should be initiated voluntarily. Once established, the urinary stream should be continuous and forceful without straining, and the bladder should empty to completion. Each of these factors may be altered in both structural bladder outlet obstruction and neurogenic vesicourethral dysfunction. Pain is a frequent warning symptom of urologic disease. Depending on the level and completeness of the neurologic lesions, such sensations may or may not be perceived by the patient. Hematuria may be the first sign of a serious complication of neurogenic bladder disease and warrants further evaluation.

Overall, the level of independence, intelligence, motivation, and dexterity should be assessed because this will impact significantly on further evaluation and management options.

Neurourologic Examination

The patient with neurogenic bladder dysfunction should undergo a general physical, specific urologic, and thorough neurologic examination.

The neurourologic examination provides evidence of the presence or absence of a neurologic lesion in an attempt to explain a given voiding dysfunction and to determine the patient's ability to accomplish planned urologic management. Mental status is assessed, for it is important to recognize that voiding dysfunction may be secondary to the reduced awareness of sensory input.

Sensory and motor deficits may suggest specific levels of pathology. The abnormalities associated with various neurogenic disorders (e.g., spinal cord injury, Parkinson's disease, multiple sclerosis, and cerebrovascular accident) are usually obvious.

Evaluation of deep tendon reflexes provides an indication of the segmental spinal cord function. LMN lesions are characterized by reduced reflex activity, whereas hyperactivity is seen with UMN lesions. Commonly tested deep tendon reflexes include biceps (C5–6), triceps (C6–7), patella (L2–4), and Achilles (L5, S2). The bulbocavernosus reflex reflects activity of the S2–4 nerve roots. Blaivas et al[9] demonstrated that 98% of normal males and 81% of normal females have an intact bulbocavernosus reflex. The reflex is obtained by penile glans or clitoral stimulation or by stimulation of the bladder mucosa (by pulling on an indwelling Foley catheter), with the efferent pathway leading to perineal contraction. Anal sphincter tone is also an important indicator of intact perineal reflex activity.

In spinal cord lesions it must be remembered that the level of the vertebral lesion usually differs from the spinal cord segmental level. Also, descending degeneration of the spinal cord may occur following injury, leading to a poor correlation between the level of injury and the lower urinary tract function.

The urologic examination should include inspection and palpation of the abdomen, inguinal regions, and external genitalia, including a rectal and pelvic examination. Scars may provide evidence of previous surgery, and cutaneous excoriation of the genitalia may occur secondary to urinary leakage.

Overall, this examination is often rendered difficult in the neurologically impaired patient who is immobile or confined to a wheelchair, making placement of the patient on an examining table time-consuming and difficult. For this reason there is a tendency to examine these patients incompletely.

Laboratory Procedures

URINE ANALYSIS AND URINE CULTURE

Urinalysis is an important part of the patient evaluation because not only may infection worsen the symptoms of storage failure, but neurologically impaired patients may not manifest typical symptoms of urinary infection. Urinary infection is also a major cause of morbidity and mortality in these patients.

In a catheter-free patient the finding of pyuria, microscopic hematuria and bacteriuria, and so on, takes on a significance similar to that in a normal urologic patient and demands further investigation.

In the patient who is managed on CIC or who has a urostomy or continent urinary diversion, or who has had a previous enterocystoplasty, pyuria and microscopic hematuria along with bacteriuria are frequently found. In these patients it seems appropriate to only treat bacteriuria in symptomatic patients suffering from fever, chills, and pyelonephritis. Appropriate antibacterial therapy and further evaluation are also warranted in those patients who have urea-splitting organisms on bacteriologic evaluation.

Because the patient with neurogenic bladder dysfunction is more susceptible to infection and does not always manifest symptoms of infection, urine microscopy and culture should be performed every 3 to 6 months in asymptomatic patients.

BLOOD CHEMISTRIES

Because of the risk of renal impairment, assessment of renal function by serum creatinine is customary. It is important to remember that when using serum creatinine or when calculating glomerular filtration rate (GFR) from the serum creatinine, the muscle wasting that is often seen in spinal cord injury patients will cause renal function to be overestimated.[10] In addition, in patients with enterocystoplasties, reabsorption of urinary electrolytes alters GFR estimation by serum creatinine.[10]

Baseline studies should be obtained in all patients presenting with neurogenic bladder dysfunction and may be repeated as indicated.

RADIOLOGIC STUDIES: UPPER TRACTS

Screening and regular follow-up radiologic evaluation are warranted in all patients with neurogenic lower urinary tract dysfunction because renal deterioration may be asymptomatic.

Vesicoureteral reflux, hydronephrosis, chronic pyelonephritis, and renal calculi are the most common and potentially serious upper tract abnormalities.

Plain Abdominal Film. A plain abdominal film, KUB (kidney, ureters, and bladder) is generally performed as an initial study prior to subsequent evaluation. It may identify opaque urinary calculi.

Excretory Urography. Excretory urography is generally performed as a baseline in all patients with neurogenic bladder. In uncomplicated cases, studies are repeated infrequently (every 3 to 5 years). Although giving excellent anatomic information, the intravenous pyelogram (IVP) provides poor functional information. In a comparison with renal scintigraphy, Lloyd cites the disadvantages of the IVP including adverse reactions to contrast material, the need for bowel preparation and dehydration, and higher radiation exposure.[11] The majority of urologists, however, feel comfortable reading and comparing the time-honored IVP, and this evaluation will remain useful in patients with neuropathic lower urinary tract.

Renal Ultrasound. Renal ultrasound provides anatomic information only and is useful as a frequent noninvasive evaluation of the kidneys, often required in these patients. Ultrasound is a subjective evaluation, and by comparison with the IVP is superior in detecting renal mass lesions but inferior in detecting renal scarring.[12] However, these studies do demonstrate minor changes in upper tract dilatation and can accurately identify renal size and demonstrate both opaque and nonopaque renal calculi. Because there is no radiation exposure, ultrasound is useful for regular follow-up required in these patients, especially in the pediatric population. This study is also useful for indirectly estimating the residual urine volume.

Voiding Cystography. Voiding cystography (VCUG) identifies the morphologic characteristics of the bladder, identifies the presence and grade of vesicoureteral reflux, and hints at the function or status of the sphincter. Because of the requirement for urodynamic studies in the majority of these patients, such information may be obtained during a videourodynamic evaluation; thus the indications for a VCUG alone are controversial.

Nuclear Medicine Evaluation. DMSA (dimercapto succinic acid) scan gives an excellent indication of parenchymal scarring and a differential function.[13] DTPA (diethylene triamine penta-acetic acid) indicates renal function and if combined with diuretics may give information about the presence of obstruction.[14] A delayed film with voiding gives an indirect cystogram, which may be useful to show the presence of reflux.[15] These studies accurately define renal function and scarring and are therefore useful in follow-up to detect subtle changes in upper tract status.

LOWER TRACTS

Endoscopic Procedures. Neurogenic bladder is a disorder of function, and cystoscopy has little to offer in its evaluation. Cystoscopy is indicated, however, for specific abnormalities such as hematuria, recurrent urinary tract infection, and pyuria. Areas suggestive of malignant and premalignant change more common in patients with indwelling catheter or on CIC can be directly observed or biopsied.[16] Autonomic dysreflexia (see later) may be stimulated by cystourethroscopy in patients with complete lesions above T6. Prophylaxis (Nifedipine) may be administered prior to examination.[17] Because of impaired sensation in most patients, general anesthesia is not commonly required. However, spinal or general anesthesia prevents autonomic dysreflexia.

Urodynamic Evaluation. Urodynamic studies measure the physiologic and pathologic factors involved in the storage, transportation, and elimination of urine.[18] These studies are mandatory in the evaluation of the neuropathic lower urinary tract.[19] It is only by accurate identification of the functional abnormalities present that logical therapy may be selected. Various urodynamic studies are available, but, videourodynamics with sphincter EMG gives the most information (Table 25-3). Quantitative data are available from the two discrete phases of micturition—that is, filling/storage and emptying—a concept that fits well into the previously described functional classification of the neurogenic bladder.

Ideally, urodynamic evaluation should answer these important questions:

1. During filling is the bladder hyperreflexic?
2. What is the compliance of the bladder during filling?
3. Are sensation of filling events and the need to void intact?
4. Can the patient generate a voluntary voiding contraction?
5. Is the bladder contraction of significant magnitude and duration to empty completely?
6. Can a voiding contraction be triggered (suprapubic tap)?
7. If voiding is incomplete is it due to detrusor, bladder neck, or external sphincter dysfunction?
8. Is the external sphincter activity coordinated?
9. What is the nature of the motor unit action potential on the EMG recording?
10. What is the latency of impulse transmission in the sacral reflex arc?

Table 25-3. Urodynamic Armamentarium

Uroflowmetry
Cystometry
Pressure flow studies
Videourodynamics
Sphincter EMG
Urethral pressure profilometry
Ambulatory studies

Answers to these questions will not only characterize the bladder dysfunction but also allow prediction of the potential that this dysfunction has for upper tract deterioration.

Certain simple rules aid immeasurably in obtaining the maximum benefit from videourodynamic studies. Not only should correct subtraction of abdominal pressure occur at the beginning of the study, but this should be checked periodically during the study. In addition, during urodynamics one should attempt to reproduce the clinical symptomatology being investigated. These studies are safe, reliable, and reproducible even in the newborn.[20] Blaivas provided an excellent example of the value of urodynamics, finding that 83% of patients had effective treatment when management was based on urodynamic findings but only 27% had effective treatment when management was based on symptoms and signs alone.[21]

Uroflowmetry reflects the activity of both the bladder and outlet, and both the rate and pattern of flow give important information. A normal flow rate, however, does not exclude obstruction. It is important that the flow closely approximates the usual voiding event and that the volumes voided are in excess of 150 mL.

Low flow (≤12 to 15 mL/sec) generally indicates increased bladder outlet resistance, decreased contractility, or both. Intermittent flow may be secondary to abdominal strain or sphincter dyssynergia. Voiding nomograms are useful because flow varies according to sex and age in asymptomatic patients.[22]

The filling cystometrogram and storage phase study is often performed with synchronous monitoring of sphincter activity. The filling medium may be gas, but liquid (water, saline, or contrast) instilled by either urethral or suprapubic catheter is preferable. Sphincter EMG studies permit the monitoring of external striated sphincter activity and may be performed with either needle electrodes, fine wire electrodes, or surface electrodes. During filling cystometry there is a gradual increase in the frequency and amplitude of EMG activity, called recruitment, then at the onset of attempted voiding, activity ceases. The diagnosis of detrusor sphincter dyssynergia may be hinted at by the fluoroscopic appearance of the outlet on videourodynamics during voiding, but it is confirmed with increased sphincter activity on EMG study during voiding. "Pseudo-dyssynergia," described by Barrett and Wein in 1982,[23] may be difficult to differentiate from true dyssynergia and is one example of the difficulties of EMG evaluation.

Involuntary bladder contractions should not occur during filling. The ICS[24] originally restricted abnormal bladder contractions to those above 15 cm of water; however, now they have accepted the presence of any contraction on filling as abnormal, independent of the magnitude.[7] Detrusor hyperreflexia refers to involuntary bladder contractions that are associated with an appropriate neurologic disease. The term detrusor instability should be restricted to involuntary bladder contractions in the absence of neurologic disease.

Compliance (change in volume/change in pressure) is a summation of both the contractile and noncontractile elements within the bladder wall. It is difficult to find stated values for normal compliance on urodynamic evaluation as this will be affected by many factors including the filling rate, and temperature of the filling medium. Abrams stated that a pressure of 3.3 cm H_2O or less at 100 mL/vol would represent normal compliance.[25] McGuire stated that bladder pressure should not exceed 6 cm. of water during normal filling.[19] Reduced compliance should be described as either being in early filling or late filling, as the latter is probably less likely to lead to renal deterioration.

During bladder filling, an increase in sphincter EMG activity is usually seen. Inadequate sphincter competence leads to genuine stress incontinence by definition, with leakage per urethra seen in the absence of a detrusor contraction.[26] This may be visualized directly or seen on fluoroscopy during urodynamic studies. Urethral instability represents a sudden reduction in urethral competence due to sphincter relaxation, usually followed by a detrusor contraction.[27] This may be implicated in the pathophysiology of detrusor instability.

With severe neuropathic sphincter incompetence, it may be difficult to adequately assess bladder function during cystometry as the filling medium leaks around the catheter. Obstruction of the bladder outlet with a Foley catheter balloon impacted at the bladder neck will help resolve this problem.

Ambulatory urodynamic studies (physiologic fill) are becoming increasingly popular and technologic advances are making them more practical. Webb and colleagues were unable to reproduce the poor compliance seen on conventional urodynamics during natural fill ambulatory studies, suggesting it was an artifact of the unphysiologic testing environment.[28]

To evaluate voiding function intra-abdominal pressure, intravesical pressure, uroflow and sphincter EMG are measured simultaneously. The normal adult male voids with a detrusor pressure of 40 to 60 cm of water with a flow rate $\geq$ 15 mL/sec. Voiding pressure is generally lower in females and flow rate is higher.[29] Obstruction is defined by a high pressure, low flow study and simultaneous fluoroscopy may identify the site of the obstruction. Low flow with reduced detrusor pressure represents impaired contractility.[30] With simultaneous recording of sphincter EMG one expects complete silence of sphincter activity during voiding, indicating relaxation. Increase in sphincter activity during the attempt to void generally indicates detrusor sphincter dyssynergia and, a functional obstruction at the level of the external sphincter may be visualized on fluoroscopy.

Further studies of peripheral neurologic integrity may include analyses of motor unit action potential and sacral evoked responses using specialized EMG equipment, and these will not be covered in this chapter. They are reviewed loosely by Galloway and Blaivas.[31]

Urethral pressure profilometry is an attempt to quantify urethral resistance; however, its role in the evaluation of the neuropathic lower urinary tract remains controversial and suspect.[32,33] There is considerable overlap in the values obtained in asymptomatic patients and in those vesicourethral dysfunction of all etiologies.

Common Clinical Findings

The following are frequent clinical findings:

1. *Hyperreflexic detrusor with coordinated urethral sphincter.* This is typical when the lesion is above the pontine micturition center. Depending on the completeness of the neurologic lesion, the patient may or may not have intact bladder sensation. If sensation is intact, the patient will perceive the onset of the uninhibited contraction as urgency and voluntary sphincter contraction will occur until the contraction is lost or until the patient finds a bathroom. In patients who lack bladder sensation, reflex incontinence will occur. Because of the coordinated sphincter relaxation, this condition tends to be less hazardous to the upper tracts.

2. *Hyperreflexic detrusor with dyssynergic external sphincter.* This is typical of complete lesions between the pontine micturition center and the sacral spinal nucleus. Various degrees of dyssynergic activity are seen, presumably dependent on the completeness of the neurologic lesion. The most common is that of crescendo contraction of the external sphincter each time the detrusor contracts. This is a dangerous phenomenon because it causes functional obstruction with detrimental effects on the upper and lower tracts. Patients are generally incontinent with inefficient emptying.

Proximal (smooth muscle) dyssynergia is generally seen in complete lesions above T–6 and is usually associated with external sphincter dyssynergia. Diagnosis is by fluoroscopic evaluation that shows a closed bladder neck during involuntary bladder contractions.

3. *Areflexic detrusor.* Patients with this condition generally have lesions below the sacral spinal cord or are in ''spinal shock'' (see later) and are unable to void because of their inability to generate a micturition contraction. Other potential causes for an acontractile bladder include bladder outlet obstruction, psychogenic inhibition, pharmacologic effects, and myogenic failure.

As in the case of the hyperreflexic detrusor, the sphincter may be variably affected by the neurologic lesion. Where innervation of the sphincter remains intact, the urethra will be functionally competent and continence will be assured, providing the bladder is not allowed to fill to the point of overflow. Reduced compliance may coexist with high detrusor pressures in the absence of a detrusor contraction. If the sphincter mechanism is also denervated, the urethra may be functionally incompetent, resulting in continuous incontinence.

MANAGEMENT OF THE PATIENT WITH NEUROGENIC LOWER URINARY TRACT DYSFUNCTION

There is no single schema for managing patients with neurogenic bladder dysfunction. A variety of general factors will impinge on management selection, such as overall prognosis of the neurologic disease, general neurologic status (e.g., mobility, intelligence, insight, and dexterity), overall medical status, and age. The main objectives in management are preservation of renal function, prevention of urinary infection, and achievement of continence along with complete bladder emptying, preferably without the use of external devices. Table 25–4 is an expansion of the functional classification to incorporate the therapeutic options.

Predicting those patients with neuropathic bladders that place their kidneys at risk is important because prophylactic management in this group has shown prevention of this renal deterioration.[20] In children with myelodysplasia, Bauer noted that 71% of newborns with dyssynergia will develop upper tract deterioration in the first 3 years of life, compared to 17% in the synergic group and 23% of those with completely denervated sphincters.[20] McGuire suggests that reduced bladder compliance causes upper tract deterioration in 63% of cases.[19] Also, a leak point pressure of more than 40 cm H_2O puts patients at risk for upper tract deterioration.[34] Galloway et al[35] used videourodynamic evaluation to determine a hostility score that identifies this high-risk group. It combines the presence or absence of reflux, bladder compliance, detrusor contractility, leak point pressure, and sphincter behavior.

In the past, and largely responsible for the poor prognosis of many patients with neurogenic bladder, an indwelling catheter or supravesical diversion using an ileal conduit was commonly employed. There are few indications for such treatment in the modern medical era.

Therapy to Facilitate Bladder Storage

In some patients storage may be improved and volitional voiding to completion is left intact. In situations where there is significant residual urine, timed bladder emptying either by regular volitional voiding or by CIC must be added.

INTERMITTENT CATHETERIZATION

Voiding by CIC circumvents the problem of bladder emptying and facilitates storage by removing residual urine and allowing an increase in functional bladder capacity. The pioneering work in this field was by Guttman, who, along with Frankel in 1966, reported aseptic intermittent catheterization for managing spinal cord injury patients during spinal shock.[36] However, in rehabilitation centers or at home a clean self-catheterization technique is taught, a concept popularized by Lapides.[37] CIC remains the most effective method of treating the patient whose bladder fails to empty. This technique is safe and effective, and it preserves the independence of patients, allowing them to remain appliance-free. Following cystoplasty CIC is usually required.

A cooperative, dexterous, well-motivated patient or family is a requirement. It is an advantage to have a special nurse who is involved in CIC teach the technique and troubleshoot any subsequent problems. Many patients are initially reluctant to undertake CIC; however, after a thorough explanation most have little difficulty. Neonatal CIC by parents is also well accepted. Graham summarizes the functional aspects required by a patient with neuropathic lower urinary tract disease to perform CIC.[38]

Adult males use a 14 to 16 Fr. catheter and may reuse it after it is washed or microwaved as long as complete bladder emptying is effected.[39] Complications are uncommon; however, they can include urethral false passage or bladder perforation, along with the development of bladder neck ledges with associated obstruction.[40] Bacteriuria is common but symptomatic infection is unusual. There is uncertainty about the long-term effects of bacteriuria and some place patients using CIC on antibiotic chemoprophylaxis.

INHIBITION OF BLADDER CONTRACTILITY

Options include pharmacotherapy, electrical stimulation, denervation procedures, and augmentation cystoplasty. Management options should be used incrementally, moving from initially reversible therapy to the final step of augmentation.

Pharmacologic Therapy. Anticholinergic drugs are used to inhibit bladder contractility, having a direct inhibitory effect on the smooth muscle. Oxybutynin remains the most widely used agent for this purpose. In addition to its anti-

Table 25–4. Expanded Functional Classification

Therapy to Facilitate Bladder Emptying	
Circumventing the problem:	CIC
	Continuous catheterization
	Diversion
Increasing bladder emptying:	External compression
	Reflex voiding "trigger"
	Pharmacologic therapy
	Electrical stimulation
Decreasing Outlet Resistance	
At level of anatomic obstruction:	TURP
	Stricture repair
At level of external sphincter:	Pharmacotherapy
	External sphincterotomy
	Urethral overdilatation
	Stent insertion
At level of bladder neck:	Pharmacotherapy
	Bladder neck incision
Therapy to Facilitate Urine Storage	
Inhibit bladder contractility:	Timed bladder emptying
	Pharmacotherapy
	Bladder overdistention
	Electrical stimulation
	Denervation
	Augmentation cystoplasty
	Detrusor myomectomy
Increasing outlet resistance:	Physiotherapy
	Electrical stimulation
	Pharmacologic therapy
	Cystourethropexy
	Artificial urinary sphincter
Circumventing problem:	CIC

After Wein AJ: Classification of neurogenic voiding dysfunction. *J Urol* 1981; 125:605–609.

cholinergic activity, it has a direct musculotropic effect and some local anesthetic effect on the bladder. It is primarily used orally at a dose of 5 mg b.i.d. to q.i.d. (appropriately lower in children) and appears more effective when given intravesically.[41]

Side effects are commonly noted, including dry mouth, mydriasis, blurred vision, tachycardia, and constipation. These agents are contraindicated in patients with glaucoma and should be used with care in those with bladder outlet obstruction or tachycardia. Other agents include Pro-banthine (adult dose 15 to 30 mg every 4 to 6 hours), flovoxate hydrochloride (adult dose 100 to 200 mg t.i.d.), terbutaline (adult dose 5 mg. t.i.d.) and imipramine hydrochloride (adult dose 25 mg q.i.d.).

Electrical Stimulation (Reflex Inhibition). Electrical stimulation may be used to facilitate bladder storage by inhibiting bladder contractility and increasing outlet resistance. Regular emptying may be facilitated by stimulating detrusor contraction through nerve root stimulation.[42]

By local perineal, anal, or vaginal stimulation, bladder contractility may be reduced by an inhibition of the pudendal to pelvic nerve reflexes. There is, however, disagreement with regard to optimal parameters for electrical stimulation and whether this should be continuous or pulsed. The majority of patients studied have had idiopathic detrusor instability; however, even in those with uninhibited bladder contractions the results appear similar.[43] Functional bladder capacity increases by more than one-third, and more than 30% report a decrease in urinary frequency.[44] Transurethral electrical bladder stimulation has been used in children with myelodysplasia in an attempt to increase functional bladder capacity, again with varying results.[45] The ultimate role for this therapeutic modality is to be determined.

Denervation Procedures. Denervation procedures are reserved for patients with intractable detrusor hyperreflexia unresponsive to other conservative modalities. Selective sacral rhizotomies involve the interruption of either S2, S3, or S4 nerve roots in an attempt to interrupt the motor supply responsible for the involuntary contractions to leave sphincter and sexual function intact. Torrens and Hald[46] have summarized their results showing 81% of patients with neuropathic bladders obtaining successful results. Prior to contemplating such neurosurgical procedures, localization of dominant sacral nerve supplies to the bladder is required.

Both Tanagho and Schmidt[47] and Brindley[48] have used selective dorsal rhizotomy to increase bladder capacity in conjunction with implantation of nerve stimulators to the motor supply of the detrusor. Impotence may occur as a sequela of this; therefore its use in male patients has been restricted. Prevesical denervation using subtrigonal phenyl has become less attractive because of its poor long-term results and potential morbidity.[49]

Bladder Overdistention. Bladder overdistention is performed under epidural anesthesia with specially constructed balloon catheters filled within the bladder until the pressure approximates the systolic blood pressure.[50] This pressure is maintained for four 30-minute periods and results in degeneration of the unmyelinated nerve fibers within the bladder wall. In patients with suprasacral spinal cord lesions the treatment has been used to render the bladder acontractile.[51] This procedure is not without risk, for bladder rupture may result.

Augmentation Cystoplasty. Enterocystoplasty is a major abdominal operative procedure used to enlarge the bladder and disrupt the detrusor hyperreflexic contraction. In patients recalcitrant to other conservative measures, this offers the best method of producing a low-pressure, high-volume bladder.[52] Various bowel segments may be utilized, the ileum and sigmoid being most popular. In neuropathic patients removal of this bowel segment may produce diarrhea.[53]

Detubularization of the bowel is needed to minimize intrinsic bowel contractions. Recently, gastrocystoplasty has been advocated because the stomach has fewer intrinsic contractions, provides an acid milieu free of mucus, and involves a lower incidence of infection. However, this procedure carries the risk of hematuria dysuria syndrome, especially in patients with lower urinary output.[54]

Before contemplating augmentation cystoplasty careful preoperative evaluation is required to determine the presence or absence of reflux and to quantify outlet resistance. Controversy exists as to whether ureteric reimplantation should be performed at the time of augmentation cystoplasty; however, in up to 75% of cases reflux may cease after conversion of the bladder to a low-pressure, high-volume reservoir without reimplantation.[55] Those patients with a suggestion of outlet incompetence either on history or visualized during video urodynamic evaluation or those with a low urethral pressure profilometry (≤ 40 cm H_2O) appear to require a synchronous outlet procedure with cystoplasty. Failure to recognize associated outlet incompetence may lead to persistent incontinence.[56] Several options are available to increase outlet resistance, including bladder neck reconstruction,[57] fascial sling,[58] and implantation of the artificial urinary sphincter.[59] Long-term results with the artificial urinary sphincter are lacking. However, it is clear that CIC can be performed safely through a sphincter cuff.[60] Complications of cystoplasty may be significant, with hyperchloremic metabolic acidosis, mucus production, calculi, and possible long-term increased risk of malignancy.[61]

In wheelchair-bound patients who require cystoplasty, because urethral CIC is required, a continent diversion may be an appropriate alternative to using an abdominal stoma. All operations utilize a detubularized bowel reservoir, antireflux ureteropouch anastomosis, and an efferent valve mechanism. Mitrofanoff[62] created a continence mechanism by tunneling one end of the appendix into the bladder, with the other end brought out to the skin as a catheterizable continent conduit. Recently, Mitchell et al reported that they experienced excellent results with this procedure in these previously difficult patients.[63] Difficulties arise in patients with significant renal impairment and preoperative bowel dysfunction. Lockhart et al recently reported their experience using a gastroileal pouch with good effect in these patients.[64]

INCREASING OUTLET RESISTANCE

As previously discussed, those patients with a history of stress incontinence seen on clinical examination or fluoroscopy, those with low-urethral-pressure profilometry, or those with leak point pressures below 60 cm H_2O should be considered candidates for a procedure to increase outlet resistance. If an outlet procedure is performed alone, careful follow-up is required because a number of patients will have silent upper tract deterioration and require a subsequent cystoplasty.

Pharmacologic Agents. The innervation of the bladder outlet is such that alpha-adrenergic agonists will have a facilitatory effect on the smooth muscle sphincter mechanism. Generally, however, outlet resistance is increased by a variable degree. Because of side effects, these agents have a limited role. Ephedrine, at an adult dose 25 to 50 mg orally q.i.d., showed a good result in 27 of 38 patients with sphincter incompetence.[65] Phenylpropanolamine (50 mg t.i.d) has also been shown to be effective.[66]

Bladder Neck Reconstruction. The Young–Dees principle involves reconstruction of a neourethra from the posterior surface of the bladder wall and trigone. Tanagho recently reported long-term success rates in 60 of 70 patients with his modification.[67] Salle recently described a simplified bladder neck reconstruction that, although effective in the short term, will need longer follow-up.[57]

McGuire popularized sling cystourethropexy as a technique of increasing outlet resistance in patients with a neuropathic sphincter.[58] Success rates of up to 90% have been reported, and the majority of patients are required to perform CIC. Although this procedure is most popular in females, it has also been reported in males, with the sling being positioned beneath the prostatic urethra.[68]

The Brantley Scott artificial urinary sphincter has undergone remarkable development during the past 10 years. Providing stringent implantation criteria are met, its success rate in controlling incontinence is approximately 85%.[69] Results have not been as successful in the pediatric population, and the lower age limit for implantation is still debated. Complications include device malfunction, infection, erosion, or subcuff tissue atrophy with return of incontinence. With surgical care, implantation associated with cystoplasty does not appear to increase the risk of infection, and CIC through the cuff is safe.[70]

Polytef as a periurethral buttressing agent was originally reported in 1973 to increase urethral resistance.[71] It is a thick, sterile paste incorporating particles with a size range of 4 to 100 μm. It has been widely used in the lower urinary tract; however, because of potential migration, caution has been recommended with regard to its use.[72] Highly purified bovine dermal collagen (contigen) cross-linked with glutaraldehyde has been injected into the periurethral bladder neck to increase urethral resistance. Results are similar to those with polytef and show approximately one-third of patients cured, one-third improved, and one-third with no change.[73]

The FDA has recently approved its use. The long-term results of these injectable agents is not yet known.

THERAPY TO FACILITATE BLADDER EMPTYING

Bladder emptying may be facilitated by methods that increase bladder contractility or decrease outlet resistance. These procedures often achieve their end at the expense of continence, in which event they are only appropriate for use in males who can wear an external collecting device. In some cases where external devices do not fit because of inadequate penile length, a semirigid penile prosthesis may be inserted to facilitate placement of such a device.[74]

As previously discussed, intermittent catheterization has revolutionized voiding difficulties because of an inability to volitionally empty to completion. Continuous catheterization is appropriate for short-term bladder drainage, preferably suprapubic. Occasionally in females, long-term suprapubic drainage may be used as a last resort. Lower tract evaluation for malignancy and calculi is recommended because these patients are at increased risk for such complications.[16,75]

Pharmacologic Manipulation. Bethanechol chloride (Urecholine) has acetylcholine-like activity with relatively selective action on the urinary bladder and gut. Although widely used, studies in which it has been used to facilitate voiding have shown disappointing results.[76] In patients with detrusor areflexia, bethanechol will not produce a voiding contraction, although the tone of the detrusor muscle may be increased.

Credé or Valsalva Maneuvers. The increase in abdominal pressure caused by the Valsalva maneuver or by direct extrinsic bladder compression will improve emptying efficiency in patients with low outflow resistance. Such ''voiding'' is unphysiologic and is resisted by a competent outlet mechanism. If adequate emptying does not occur, reduction of outflow resistance may be considered, but at the expense of continence. Vesicoureteral reflux is a relative contraindication to this type of ''voiding'' because increased bladder pressure will be transmitted directly to the upper tracts. In effect, its main use is in a select group of females with detrusor areflexia and in males who have previously undergone a sphincterotomy

Triggering Reflex Bladder Contractions. The areflexic bladder resulting from a sacral or infrasacral lesion does not contract; however, manual stimulation of certain areas within the sacral and lumbar dermatomes may result in a reflex detrusor contraction in patients with hyperreflexic neurogenic bladders. Patients potentially able to induce bladder contractions this way are encouraged to find their own "optimal" trigger points. One must be aware that functional outlet obstruction caused by external sphincter dyssynergia may result in high-pressure obstructed voiding, with potential damage to upper tracts. Balanced lower urinary tract function can be activated in some patients.[77]

Electrical Stimulation. A variety of electrical implants have been tried to augment bladder emptying. Those with promise include either intradural (Brindley)[48] or extradural (Tanagho and Schmidt).[47]

Stimulation of the sacral ventral nerve roots via the sacral anterior root stimulator (SARS) has been extensively reported. This device is neurosurgically implanted intradurally, directly stimulating the ventral nerve roots, which have been shown during implantation to result in bladder contraction.[78] The stimulator is controlled externally by a radiofrequency device to give volitional bladder emptying. The aim is to provide implant-driven voiding with low residuals. Differential nerve stimulation appears to be capable of giving implant-driven erections and defecation.

The candidate for implantation should be intelligent and dexterous, have a stable neurologic lesion, and have an intact S3 efferent nerve with associated detrusor contraction. Direct stimulation of the sacral nerve roots over S2 gives erection in 90% of males and bladder contraction in 60%; stimulation over S3 gives bladder contraction in 90% and anal sphincter contraction in the majority; and stimulation over S4 results in occasional bladder contractions but appears to provide "anti-erectile function."[78] Stimulation is provided by pulses of electrical energy so that detrusor muscle that contracts slowly develops adequate pressure for complete voiding and the urethral striated muscle contracts in short bursts, giving short elevation in an outlet resistance with subsequent dyssynergic voids. Recently, dorsal rhizotomies (S2, S3, S4) have combined with implantation to eliminate this dyssynergia, also removing autonomic dysreflexia and reflex erections. Because of these findings, SARSs are better used in females with suprasacral cord lesions. In males the loss of reflex erections must be addressed prior to implant.

At present, more than 500 implants have been inserted into paraplegic patients and more than 1100 implant years are evaluable. Mechanical problems are rare, with an average of 18.2 implant years per mechanical problem. Sawan has recently reviewed his results of 132 implants.[79] Ninety percent of patients are presently using implant-driven voiding; of these more than 90% are continent. Eleven void with intermittent catheterization and seven have required an artificial urinary sphincter. There has been a significant reduction in the frequency of urinary infections and upper tract deterioration. Patients void four to five times per day, with voiding pressures around 90 cm H_2O with an average residual below 50 mL. Implantation of these devices is currently restricted to special centers.

DECREASING OUTLET RESISTANCE

Pharmacologic Manipulation. Drugs with an alpha-adrenergic blocking activity tend to inhibit and thus relax the proximal sphincter mechanism to reduce outlet resistance. Recently, antiandrogens have become popular to shrink the prostate and are useful in older males to reduce prostatic (anatomic) outlet obstruction.[80] The distal sphincter mechanism may be variably relaxed with such agents as baclofen, dantrolene, or diazepam.[81] These muscle relaxants are nonspecific, and other muscular functions are also affected. Although there are some enthusiastic reports of their use, they rarely improve emptying efficiency dramatically.

Bladder Outlet Surgery. Procedures that have been advocated to reduce outlet resistance include bladder neck incision, transurethral prostatectomy, and external sphincterotomy. To date, external sphincterotomy is the procedure of choice to relieve severe external sphincter dyssynergia in males. Anteromedial (12 o'clock) sphincterotomy is comparatively safe, simple, and very effective.[82] After sphincterotomy balanced voiding with low detrusor pressure can be achieved, but at the cost of incontinence and the necessity of an external collecting device. Sphincterotomy is therefore indicated in males if sphincter dyssynergia cannot be managed otherwise.

Elimination of pudendal nerve activity has been tried previously,[83] but this procedure has been largely abandoned because of the associated loss of reflex erections and incontinence.

More recently, intraurethral stents that hold the external sphincter mechanism open have been advocated. The early results have been encouraging; however, stents may be difficult to remove if malpositioned, and they have been associated with urethral fibrosis and obliteration in the medium term.[84] At present they may have a limited role in those patients who have failed an initial transurethral sphincterotomy.

SPECIFIC NEUROLOGIC PROBLEMS

Diseases Above the Pons

In general, lesions above the pons result in a hyperreflexic bladder with coordinated sphincter relaxation.

CEREBROVASCULAR DISEASE

Urinary retention is common during the initial period after a cerebrovascular accident (CVA). A short period of indwelling Foley catheter drainage is often appropriate. If retention persists, aseptic intermittent catheterization is appropriate until the bladder regains activity. The most common long-term urinary tract dysfunction following a CVA is coordinated detrusor hyperreflexia.[85] Sensation is variably intact. Thus the patient has urgency and urge incontinence if the sphincter mechanism cannot be volitionally controlled. CVAs generally affect elderly patients. There is frequently other lower urinary tract pathology, and urodynamic evaluation should be performed prior to contemplating urologic surgery.

Urinary frequency, urgency, and incontinence resulting from hyperreflexia may be controlled with anticholinergic medications. In patients whose mental status or mobility is severely compromised, a long-term suprapubic catheter remains an alternative.

PARKINSON'S DISEASE

Parkinson's disease is due to dopamine deficiency in the substantia nigra and leads to lower urinary tract dysfunction in 25 to 75% of patients.[86] Both detrusor hyperreflexia and areflexia may result. In addition, the picture is confused by preexisting lower urinary tract anomalies.[87] Medications used in Parkinson's disease may affect the lower urinary tract.

The use of subcutaneous apomorphine prior to urodynamic studies reduces the lower urinary tract symptoms of Parkinson's disease and allows a clearer diagnosis of bladder outlet obstruction resulting from prostatic hypertrophy.[88] Transurethral resection of the prostate is recommended for prostatic obstruction only. If urgency persists postoperatively it may be controlled with anticholinergics.

Diseases Involving the Spinal Cord

SPINAL CORD INJURY

The type of lower urinary tract dysfunction depends upon the level and completeness of the injury. After a significant cord injury, spinal shock results, leading to absent somatic reflex activity and paralysis below this level, along with detrusor areflexia and a functional (competent) bladder neck.[89] Because sphincter tone exists, urinary incontinence does not result unless there is overflow incontinence. Bladder emptying is initially managed with urethral or suprapubic catheterization until the patient is stable; then aseptic CIC is begun. Bladder overdistention in this early phase may result in myogenic failure, so every attempt should be made to empty the bladder regularly. Reflex bladder contractions return usually within 6 to 12 weeks after injury, resulting in involuntary voiding with incomplete emptying between catheterizations. A baseline IVP is customarily obtained during this phase.

In suprasacral spinal injuries, the characteristic lower urinary tract findings are detrusor hyperreflexia, proximal sphincter synergia (lesions below sympathetic outflow), and distal sphincter dyssynergia. Incomplete bladder emptying generally develops. To assess lower urinary tract function, urodynamic evaluation is generally performed once the patient is stable and has reflex contractions. Management depends on the results of these studies, as previously discussed.

Initially, detrusor areflexia with high or normal compliance is seen in patients with sacral spinal cord injury. However, decreased compliance may develop.[90] Autonomic hyperreflexia describes a constellation of mainly cardiovascular symptoms seen in patients with spinal cord injury lesions above T6, the level of sympathetic outflow from the spinal cord. Patients exhibit an exaggerated sympathetic response below the level of this lesion, leading to hypertension, which, rarely, may be fatal because of cerebral hemorrhage. The stimuli for these exaggerated responses commonly arise from the pelvic organs (e.g., urinary infection, cystoscopy, urodynamics). Ideally, any patient susceptible of this should be given prophylaxis prior to such stimuli and oral nifedipine (20 mg) appears adequate.[17] Such prophylaxis, however, does not eliminate the need for careful monitoring during these procedures.

MULTIPLE SCLEROSIS

Multiple sclerosis primarily affects middle-aged women and is characterized by a clinical course of remission and exacerbation. However, the accompanying voiding dysfunction is often progressive. Fifty to 80% of patients complain of voiding symptoms at some time and include urinary retention, urgency, urge incontinence, and voiding inefficiency with incomplete emptying and increased risk of urinary infection.[44] Detrusor hyperreflexia occurs in the majority of patients, and 30 to 65% have associated external sphincter dyssynergia. With this finding, there is the potential for upper tract deterioration.[91]

Because of the variable nature of this disease, aggressive irreversible urologic intervention is not justified. Because of the frequent cerebellar involvement with associated hand dysfunction, CIC programs are often impossible. Specific intervention is dependent on urodynamic findings and the patient's general status.

Diseases of and Below the Sacral Spinal Cord

DISK DISEASE

Because the majority of disk protrusions occur at the L4,5 or L5,S1 level, the urinary retention is seen in only 1 to 18% of patients.[92] Because a laminectomy may not improve bladder function and spinal cord injury is possible, urodynamic studies in patients with lower urinary tract symptoms are recommended prior to this surgery. If required, CIC should be instigated.

RADICAL PELVIC SURGERY

Voiding difficulties may follow AP resection or radical hysterectomy, and in 15 to 20% this may be permanent.[93] In general, detrusor areflexia develops with a nonfunctional bladder neck, and these patients should be begun on CIC. Because there may be a return of bladder function in time, surgery to reduce outlet resistance, such as prostatectomy in males, should be delayed until urodynamics can be performed.

DIABETES MELLITUS

Diabetic peripheral neuropathy may result in bladder dysfunction. Sensory neuropathy causes a lack of awareness of bladder-filling events, and the urge to void is lost. The resulting insidious progressive bladder distention leads to myogenic damage and reduced bladder contractility. A large-capacity, poorly contractile bladder is produced with resultant voiding difficulties, residual urine, and urine infection. Initially, regular timed voiding is utilized because pharmacotherapy to decrease outlet resistance and increase contractility is rarely of value. Because these maneuvers are not always successful, if residual urine is excessive or infection is a problem, CIC is required.

Neurologic Problems of Children

In children, disorders of voiding and continence may be due to structural, functional, or neurogenic etiologies. Functional causes predominate. These often can be differentiated from neurogenic disease on the basis of clinical findings alone. Pediatric neurogenic bladder dysfunction is usually congenital (e.g., myelodysplasia, sacral agenesis) and is rarely acquired (posttraumatic). As in adults, the type of bladder dysfunction that results depends upon the level and completeness of the lesion.

MYELODYSPLASIA

Myelodysplasia, congenital spinal abnormalities, represents the most common etiology of the pediatric neuropathic bladder and occurs once in every 1000 live births. Previously, patients with myelodysplasia were managed expectantly with Credé voiding and vigilant monitoring of the upper tracts. When sinister changes developed, usually manifest as hydronephrosis resulting from obstruction or reflux, management entailed either vesicostomy (young child) or supravesical diversion (older child). The long-term results of the ileal conduit diversion were far from satisfactory because it allowed reflux of infected urine to the upper tracts, thereby promoting renal scarring and atrophy. In addition, a wet urostomy was a distraction from normal physical, sexual, and emotional growth.

Because urodynamic parameters are now quantified to predict the fate of the upper tracts, management has been directed toward preventing this renal deterioration. The factors that predict renal deterioration have been discussed previously.

With this ability to predict upper tract deterioration the timing of evaluation has changed. Newborn assessment generally occurs prior to the child leaving the hospital after delivery and back closure. Evaluation consists of a careful physical examination to determine the clinical neurologic level and degree of completeness, an IVP to determine initial upper tract status and video-urodynamic studies along with sphincter EMG. If evaluation reveals that the lower urinary tract function places the upper tract at risk, prophylactic therapy may be warranted. Contrary to popular belief, CIC in the newborn period is easy for parents to master, even in uncircumcised boys. Management is in accordance with that previously discussed in the text, utilizing regular bladder emptying along with pharmacotherapy to reduce detrusor contractility. Antibiotic chemoprophylaxis is used if reflux is present. Because the neurourologic lesion in myelodysplasia can change with age, sequential urodynamic testing is recommended. Bauer has recently shown that a deterioration in urodynamic findings may be reversed after appropriate neurosurgical evaluation in some patients.[94] Modern management has resulted in urinary diversion becoming rare in this group of patients. Management of persistent incontinence is generally undertaken around age 4 to 6 years, dependent partly on the degree of socialization of the child.

SACRAL AGENESIS

Sacral agenesis—or more correctly, dysgenesis—has been defined as the absence of part or all of two or more lower vertebral bodies. The diagnosis is often delayed until the child fails toilet training and may be indicated on examination by the flattened buttocks along with a short gluteal cleft. When urodynamic findings are undertaken approximately one-third show evidence of suprasacral lesions, one-third have sacral or lower lesions, and one-third have no signs of denervation at all.[95] Management is according to urodynamic findings, as previously discussed.

REFERENCES

1. Bradley WE, Tim GW, Scott FB: Innervation of the detrusor muscle and urethra. *Urol Clin North Am* 1974; 1:3–27.
2. Wein AJ: Classification of neurogenic voiding dysfunction. *J Urol* 1981; 125:605–609.
3. Bors E, Comarr AE: *Neurologic Urology*. Basel: Karger, 1971; 129.
4. Kaplan SA, Chancellor MB, Blaivas JG: Bladder and sphincter behavior in patients with spinal cord lesions. *J Urol* 1991; 146:113–117.
5. Lapides J: Neuromuscular vesical and ureteral dysfunction. In: Campbell MF, Harrison JH, eds. *Urology*, 6th ed. Philadelphia: WB Saunders, 1976; 1343–1370.
6. Krane RJ, Siroky MB: *Clinical Neurourology*. Boston: Little, Brown, 1979; 143.
7. Abrams P, Blaivas J, Stanton S, Andersen J: Standardization of terminology of lower urinary tract function. *Neurourol Urodyn* 1988; 7:403.

8. Madersbacher H: The various types of neurogenic bladder dysfunction: an update of current therapeutic concepts. *Paraplegia* 1990; 28:217–229.
9. Blaivas JG, Zayed AAH, Labib KB: The bulbocavernosus reflex in urology: a prospective study of 229 patients. *J Urol* 1981; 126:197.
10. McDougal WS, Koch MO: Accurate determination of renal function in patients with intestinal urinary diversion. *J Urol* 1986; 135:1175–1178.
11. Lloyd LK: Monitoring the upper tracts in neurogenic bladder dysfunction. *Probl Urol* 1989; 3:72.
12. Rao KG, Heckler RH, Woodlief RM, Ozer MN, Field WR: Real time renal sonography in spinal cord injury patients: prospective comparison with excretory urography. *J Urol* 1986; 135:72.
13. Rushton HG, Majd M, Jantausch B, Wiedermann BL, Belman AB: Renal scarring following reflux and nonreflux pyelonephritis in children: evaluation with DMSA scintigraphy. *J Urol* 1992; 147: 1327–1332.
14. O'Reilly PH, Lupten EW, Tester HJ, Shields RA, Carroll RMP, Chalton EB: The dilated nonobstructed renal pelvis. *Br J Urol* 1981; 53:205–210.
15. Ransley P: Personal communication. 1994.
16. Kaufman JM, Famm B, Jacobs SC, et al: Bladder cancer and squamous metaplasia in spinal cord injury patients. *J Urol* 1977; 118:967.
17. Steinberger RE, Ohl DA, Bennett CJ, McCabe M, Wang SC: Nifedipine pretreatment for autonomic dysreflexia during electroejaculation. *Urology* 1990; 36:228.
18. Webster GD: Urodynamic studies. In: Resnick MI, Older RA, eds. *Diagnosis of Genitourinary Disorders*. New York: Thieme Stratton, 1982; 173–204.
19. McGuire EJ, Woodside JR, Bowdin TA, Weiss RM: Prognostic value of urodynamic testing in myelodysplastic patients. *J Urol* 1981; 126:205.
20. Bauer SB, Hallett M, Khoshbin S, Lebowitz RL, Colodny AH, Retik AB: The predictive value of urodynamic evaluation in the newborn with myelodysplasia. *JAMA* 1984; 152:650.
21. Blaivas JG: Management of bladder dysfunction in multiple sclerosis. *Urology* 1980; 30:12.
22. Haylen BT, Asby D, Sethhurst JR, Frazier MI, West CR: Maximum and average flow rates in normal male and female populations: the Liverpool nomograms. *Br J Urol* 1989; 64:30.
23. Wein AJ, Barrett DM: Etiologic possibilities for increased pelvic floor electromyography activity during bladder filling. *J Urol* 1982; 127:949.
24. Yalla SV, McGuire EJ, Elbadawi A, Blaivas JG: *Neurourology and Urodynamics: Principles and Practice*. New York: Macmillan, 1988.
25. Mundy AR: Clinical physiology of the bladder, urethra and pelvic floor. In: Mundy AR, Stephenson TP, Wein AJ, eds. *Urodynamics: Principles, Practice and Application*. New York: Churchill Livingstone, 1984; 14–25.
26. McGuire EJ: Neuromuscular dysfunction of the lower urinary tract. In: Walsh PC, Gittes RF, Perlmutter AD, Stamey TA, eds. *Campbell's Urology*, 5th ed. Philadelphia: WB Saunders, 1986; 616–638.
27. Sorensen S: Urethral pressure variations in healthy and incontinent women. *Neurourol Urodyn* 1992; 11:549–591.
28. Webb RJ, Stiles RA, Griffiths CJ, Ramsden PD, Neal DE: Ambulatory monitoring of bladder pressure in patients with low compliance as a result of neurogenic bladder dysfunction. *Br J Urol* 1989; 64:150.
29. Robertson AS, Griffiths CJ, Ramsden PD, Neal DE: Bladder function in healthy volunteers: ambulatory monitoring and conventional urodynamic studies. *Br J Urol* 1994; 73:242–249.
30. Resnick NM, Yalla SV: Detrusor hyperactivity with impaired contractile function: an unrecognized but common cause of incontinence in elderly patients. *JAMA* 1987; 257:3076.
31. Galloway NTM, Blaivas JG: Sphincter EMG. In: O'Reilly PH, George NJR, Weiss RM, eds. *Diagnostic Techniques in Urology*. Philadelphia: WB Saunders, 1990; 335–351.
32. Wein AJ, Barrett DM: *Voiding Function and Dysfunction: A Logical and Practical Approach*. Chicago: Year Book, 1988; 14–22.
33. Wein AJ, Barrett DM: *Voiding Function and Dysfunction: A Logical and Practical Approach*. Chicago: Year Book, 1988; 34–39.
34. McGuire EJ, Woodside JR, Borden TA: Upper urinary tract deterioration in patients with myelodysplasia and hypertonia: a follow-up study. *J Urol* 1983; 129:823.
35. Galloway NTM, Mekras J, Helms M, Webster GD: An objective score to predict upper tract deterioration in myelodysplasia. *J Urol* 1991; 145:535–537.
36. Gutman L, Frankel H: The value of intermittent catheterization in the early management of traumatic paraplegia and tetraplegia. *Paraplegia* 1966; 4:63–84.
37. Lapides J, Diokno AC, Silba SJ, Lowe BS: Clean intermittent self-catheterization in the treatment of urinary tract disease. *Trans Am Assoc Genitourin Surg* 1971; 63:92–96.
38. Graham C: Making a catheterization program work in patients with functional limitations. *Probl Urol* 1989; 3:54.
39. Douglas C, Burke B, Kessler OL, Acmonec JF, Bracken RB: Microwave: practical cost effective method for sterilizing urinary catheters at home. *Urology* 1990; 35:219.
40. Percash I, Giroux J: Clean intermittent catheterization in spinal cord injury patients: a follow-up study. *J Urol* 1993; 149:1068–1071.
41. Greenfield SP, Fera M: The use of IV oxybutynin chloride in children with neurogenic bladder. *J Urol* 1991; 146:532–534.
42. Kaplan WE, Richards I: Intravesical transurethral electrotherapy for the neurogenic bladder. *J Urol* 1986; 136:243–246.
43. Ohlsson BL, Fall M, Frankenberg S: Effect of external and direct pudendal nerve maximal electrical stimulation and the treatment of the uninhibited overactive bladder. *Br J Urol* 1989; 64:374.
44. Eriksen BC, Bergmann S, Eik-nes SH: Maximal electrical stimulation of the pelvic floor in female idiopathic detrusor instability and urge incontinence. *Neurourol Urodynam* 1989; 8:219.
45. Decter RM, Snyder P, Laudermilc H: Transurethral electrical bladder stimulation: a follow-up report. Abst American Academy Pediatrics Washington, 1993, No. 87.
46. Torrins M, Hald T: Bladder denervation procedures. *Urol Clin North Am* 1979; 6:283–293.
47. Tanagho EA, Schmidt RA: Electrical stimulation in the clinical management of the neurogenic bladder. *J Urol* 1988; 140:13–31.
48. Brindley GS, Rushton DN: Long term follow-up of patients with sacral anterior root stimulator implants. *Paraplegia* 1990; 28:469–475.
49. Chapple C, Hampson SJ, Turner Warwick R, Worth PT: Subtrigonal phenol infection: How safe and effective is it? *Br J Urol* 1991; 68:483–486.
50. Ramsden PD, Smith JC, Dunn M, Arden GM: Distension therapy for the unstable bladder. Later result including an assessment of repeat dilatations. *Br J Urol* 1976; 48:623–629.
51. Iwatsubo E, Komin S, Yamashita M, et al: Overdistension therapy of the bladder in paraplegic patients using self catheterization: a preliminary study. *Paraplegia* 22:210, 1984.
52. Mundy AR, Stephenson TP: "Clam" ileocystoplasty for the treatment of refractory urge incontinence. *Br J Urol* 1985; 57:641–646.

53. Mark SD, MacDiarmid S, Webster GD: Factors associated with bowel dysfunction following cystoplasty: analysis of 253 patients. *J Urol* 1993; 149(4):108A.
54. Nasrallah PF, Aliabodi MA: Bladder augmentation in patients with neurogenic bladder and vesicoureteral reflux. *J Urol* 1991; 146:563–566.
55. Ralph DJ, Woodhouse CR, Ransley PG: The management of the neuropathic bladder in adolescents with imperforate anus. *J Urol* 1992; 148:366–368.
56. Mark SD, McCrae CU, Arnold EP, Gowland SP: Clam cystoplasty for the overactive bladder: a review of 23 cases. *Aust N Z J Surg* 1994; 64:88–90.
57. Salle JP, Fraga J, Silveira M, Amarante A, Rocito M, Lambertz M, Schmid M: Urethral lengthening with anterior bladder wall flap for urinary incontinence: a new approach. Abst. American Academy Pediatrics 76, Washington, 1993.
58. McGuire EJ, Wang CC, Usitalo H, Savastano J: Modified pubovaginal sling in girls with myelodysplasia. *J Urol* 1986; 135:94.
59. Barrett DM, Parulkar BG: The artificial sphincter (AS800): experience with children and young adults. *Urol Clin North Am* 1989; 16:119.
60. Bosco PJ, Bauer SB, Colodny AH, Mandell J, Retik AB: The long term follow-up of artificial urinary sphincters in children. *J Urol* 1991; 146:396–399.
61. Khoury JM, Webster GD, Timmons SL, Corbel L: Complications of enterocystoplasty. *Urology* 1992; 40:9–14.
62. Mitrofanoff P: Cystométrie continente trans-appendiculaire dans le traitement de vessies neurologiques. *Chir Pédiatr* 1980; 21:297.
63. Somfast JM, Burns MW, Mitchell ME: The Metrofanoff principle in urinary reconstruction. *J Urol* 1993; 150:1875–1878.
64. Lockhart JL, Davies R, Cox C, McAllister E, Helal M, Figueroa TE: The gastroileoileal pouch: an alternative continent urinary reservoir for patients with short bowel acidosis and/or extensive pelvic radiation. *J Urol* 1993; 150:46–50.
65. Diokno A, Taub M: Ephidrene in treatment of urinary incontinence. *Urology* 1975; 5:64.
66. Awad S, Downey J, Kiruluta H: Alpha adrenergic agents in urinary disorders of the proximal urethra: stress incontinence. *Br J Urol* 1978; 50:332.
67. Tanagho EA: Bladder neck reconstruction for total urinary incontinence: 10 years of experience. *J Urol* 1981; 121:321.
68. Herschorn S, Radomski SB: Fascial slings and bladder neck tapering in the treatment of male neurogenic incontinence. *J Urol* 1992; 147:1073–1075.
69. Parulkar BG, Barrett DM, Kramer SA: Experience with AS800 artificial sphincter in pediatric and young adult patients. *Urology* 1993; 42:431–436.
70. Strawbridge LA, Kramer SA, Castillo OA, Barrett DM: Augmentation cystoplasty and the artificial genitourinary sphincter. *J Urol* 1989; 142:297.
71. Berg S: Polytef augmentation urethroplasty. *Arch Surg* 1973; 107:379.
72. Milizia AA, Ryman HM, Myers RP, et al: Migration and granulomatous reaction after periurethral injection of polytef. *JAMA* 1984; 251:3327.
73. Lotenfoe R, O'Kelly JK, Helal M, Lockhart JL: Periurethral polytetrafluoroethylene paste injection in incontinent female subjects: surgical indications and improved surgical technique. *J Urol* 1993; 149:279–282.
74. Van Arsdalen KN, Cline FA, Hackler RH, Brady SM: Penile implants in spinal cord injury patients for maintaining external appliances. *J Urol* 1981; 126:331.
75. Lockie JR, Hall DE, Walzer Y: Incidence of squamous cell carcinoma in patients with long term catheter drainage. *J Urol* 1985; 133:1034.
76. Finkbeiner AE: Is bethanechol chloride clinically effective in promoting bladder emptying? A literature review. *J Urol* 1985; 134:443.
77. Opitz JL: Treatment of voiding dysfunction in spinal cord injured patients: bladder retraining. In: Barrett DM, Wein AJ, eds. *Controversies in Neurourology*. New York: Churchill Livingstone, 1984; 437–451.
78. Brindley GS: Sacral anterior root stimulator implantation: update. International Continence Society, Halifax, 1992.
79. Sawan M, Duval F, Hassouna M, Li JS, Elhilali MM: A transcutaneous implantable bladder controller. *Neurourol Urodyn* 1993; 12:281–284.
80. Gormley GJ, Stoner E, Bruskewitz RC, et al: The effect of Finasteride in men with benign prostatic hyperplasia: the Finasteride study group. *N Engl J Med* 1992; 327:1185–1191.
81. Webster GD: Pharmacologic management of lower urinary tract dysfunction. *Drug Ther* 1983; 15:113–135.
82. Madersbacher H, Scott BF: The 12 o'clock sphincterotomy: technique, indications and results. *Paraplegia* 1976; 14:261–267.
83. Barrett D, Wein AJ: Voiding dysfunction: diagnosis, classification and management. In: Gillenwater JY, Grayhack JT, Howards ST, Duckett JW, eds. *Adult and Pediatric Urology*. Chicago: Year Book, 1987; 863–962.
84. McInerney PD, Vanner TF, Harris SA, Stephenson TP: Permanent urethral stents for detrusor sphincter dyssynergia. *Br J Urol* 1991; 67:291–294.
85. Kahn Z, et al: Predictive correlation of urodynamic dysfunction and brain injury after cerebrovascular accident. *J Urol* 1981; 126:1–86.
86. Marsden C: Parkinson's disease. *Lancet* 1990; 335:948.
87. Sotolongo JR: Voiding dysfunction in Parkinson's disease. *Semin Neurol* 1988; 8:166.
88. Christmas TJ, Chappel CR, Lees AJ, et al: Role of subcutaneous apomorphine in Parkinsonism voiding dysfunction. *Lancet* 1988; 2:1451.
89. Van B, Yalla SV: Vesicourethral dysfunction in spinal cord injury and its management. *Semin Neurol* 1988; 8:150.
90. Thomas DG, Lucus MG: The urinary tract following spinal cord injury. In: Chisholm GD, Fair WR, eds. *Scientific Foundations of Urology*. Chicago: Year Book, 1990; 286–299.
91. Blaivas JG, Kaplan SA: Urologic dysfunction in patients with multiple sclerosis. *Semin Urol* 1988; 8:159.
92. Sandra SD, Fanciullacci F, Politi P, Zonallo A: Urinary disorders in intervertebral disc prolapse. *Neurourol Urodynam* 1987; 6:11.
93. Mundy AR: Pelvic plexus injury. In: Mundy AR, Stephenson TP, Wein AJ, eds. *Urodynamics: Principles, Practices and Applications*. New York: Churchill Livingstone, 1984; 273–277.
94. Lais A, Kasabian NG, Dirow FM, Scott RM, Kelley MD, Bauer SB: The neurosurgical implications of continuous neurourological surveillance of children with myelodysplasia. *J Urol* 1993; 150:1879–1883.
95. Guzman L, Bauer SB, Hellet M, et al: The evaluation and management of children with sacral agenesis. *Urology* 1983; 23:506.

26 Urinary Incontinence

William D. Steers, Burkhardt H. Zorn

Urinary incontinence is the involuntary loss of urine that produces social or hygienic consequences.[1] Incontinence is often perceived as a condition that only affects the elderly or those with neurologic disorders. Yet 15 to 30% of community-dwelling elderly suffer from urinary incontinence, and the prevalence of incontinence is as high as 30 to 58% in healthy middle-aged women.[2] Despite the morbidity of incontinence, less than half of individuals with incontinence seek medical attention.[3] In addition to the psychological impact of urinary incontinence, the financial burden to society exceeds $11 billion annually.[4]

Advances in diagnostic techniques allow identification of the specific etiologies of incontinence. These tests permit therapy to be targeted to the specific type of incontinence that increases the likelihood of a successful outcome. A variety of pharmacologic, behavioral, and surgical treatments have proven effective in treating incontinence. Here we review the diagnostic tools available and discuss their value and application in the evaluation of urinary incontinence.

MECHANISMS OF CONTINENCE

The storage and periodic elimination of urine require an adequate reservoir, comprised of the bladder, and a competent outlet, which includes the bladder neck, urethra, and striated muscles of the pelvic floor.[5] Failure of either of these components can result in urinary incontinence.

The lower urinary tract receives innervation from four sets of nerves: pelvic nerve, hypogastric nerve, sympathetic chain, and pudendal nerve. The pelvic nerve (parasympathetic) arises from the S2 to S4 spinal segments and provides excitatory input to the bladder and inhibitory input to the urethra. Sympathetic input from the T11 to L2 spinal segments conveyed by the hypogastric nerve and sympathetic chain provides excitatory input to the bladder base and urethra. Sympathetic nerves also inhibit the bladder body and modulate excitatory parasympathetic input to the bladder.[6] The net result of these actions is to promote urine storage. Somatic innervation of the pelvic floor muscles is conveyed in the pudendal nerve. This somatic nerve is composed of afferent and efferent axons from the S2 to the S4 sacral spinal cord. The pudendal nerve provides excitatory input to the external urethral sphincter.

Voiding results from the activation of a micturition reflex organized at the level of the pons.[7] Coordinated function of the bladder and its outlet require intact pathways between the pons and sacral spinal cord as well as from the sacral spinal cord to the bladder. A spinobulbospinal micturition reflex is triggered by tension afferents in the bladder wall. These afferents travel in the pelvic nerve and project to the S2 to S4 spinal cord.[7] Detrusor contraction and reflex relaxation of the urethra require efferent input from the sacral spinal cord via the pelvic nerve.

Central inhibitory mechanisms prevent activation of the micturition reflex from inappropriate afferent discharges.[8,9] Alterations in inhibitory mechanisms in neurologic disorders such as multiple sclerosis, Parkinson's disease, or traumatic spinal cord injury can result in bladder contraction at low volumes. Involuntary (uninhibited) contractions associated with a neurologic condition are referred to as detrusor hyperreflexia (DH). Alternatively, uninhibited bladder contractions can also occur from a variety of inflammatory bladder disorders or as a consequence of aging. Uninhibited bladder contractions not associated with a neurologic cause are referred to as detrusor instability (DI).

In addition to excitatory voiding reflexes, a variety of storage reflexes regulate the functions of the bladder neck, urethra, and external urethral sphincter (Fig. 26–1). The intrinsic fibroelastic properties of the bladder neck and proximal urethra act together as a functional proximal sphincter to passively maintain urinary continence.[9] With increased intravesical pressure, neural mechanisms are triggered. Voluntary control of the striated external sphincter via the pudendal nerve serves as a guarding mechanism. The external sphincter mechanism can interrupt micturition or prevent loss of urine during rapid increases in intra-abdominal pressure. Furthermore, afferent discharges resulting from contraction of the striated pelvic floor musculature, including the external urethral sphincter, reflexly inhibit the bladder. These actions of the external sphincter to transiently prevent urine loss have been termed the *guarding reflex*. Extension of smooth muscle from the proximal sphincter serves as a distal intrinsic sphincter mechanism that maintains continence after loss of the proximal sphincter. Continence after radical prostatectomy relies on this distal smooth muscle sphincter mechanism. Thus urinary continence depends on mechanisms that inhibit micturition reflexes and activate storage reflexes.

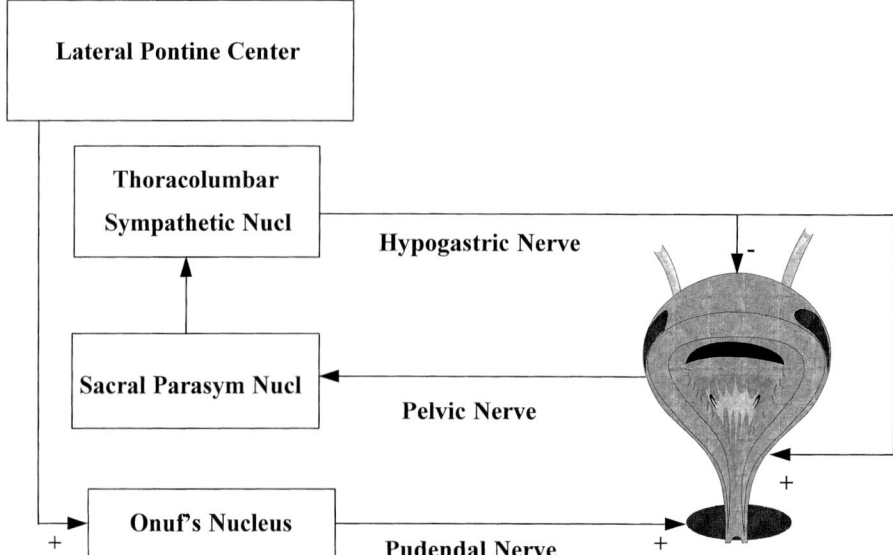

Figure 26–1. Representation of sphincter reflexes: Distention of bladder during filling causes low-level afferent firing. Pelvic nerve afferents trigger (1) hypogastric outflow to bladder, which relaxes (−) the detrusor and contracts (+) the bladder base and urethra, and (2) excitatory pudendal outflow to the external sphincter.

Aside from neurologic etiologies, traumatic or surgical destruction of the urethra may render the bladder outlet incompetent. Inability to transmit intra-abdominal pressure to the outlet because of pelvic floor relaxation may also produce urinary incontinence. In some persons with intact innervation and anatomy, urine is also lost with the inability to get to a toilet because of other physical limitations.

CLASSIFICATIONS OF INCONTINENCE

Urinary incontinence is classified on the basis of symptoms or function. Stress, urge, reflex, total, overflow, and functional incontinence are based on symptoms (Table 26–1).[10] Although other classifications exist, a pure symptom classification is easiest to understand and ascertain from a patient's history.

Stress incontinence results from the inability of the urethra to compensate for increases in abdominal pressure transmitted to the bladder. A rise in intra-abdominal pressure normally occurs with coughing, straining, or laughing. Failure of intra-abdominal pressure transmission to the proximal urethra because of abnormalities in urethral length, mobility, elasticity, or vesicourethral angle produces genuine stress urinary incontinence.[11] Rarely, the inability of the bladder to contract with a normal reflex relaxation of the bladder outlet may produce stress incontinence. This condition is termed *urethral instability*.

Table 26–1. Symptom Classification of Incontinence

Stress
Urge
Reflex
Total
Overflow
Functional

Urge incontinence is characterized by the sudden desire to void followed by the inability to inhibit a micturition reflex. Urgency may also result from inflammation of the bladder due to infection or cancer. Reflex incontinence occurs with the loss of central inhibition from ascending or descending pathways between the brain and sacral spinal cord. An involuntary detrusor contraction often occurs without the sensation of urgency.

At the other extreme, inability of the detrusor to contract or the bladder outlet to relax can cause overflow incontinence. Overflow incontinence develops when bladder pressure exceeds outlet resistance. Likewise, damage to both the proximal and distal intrinsic sphincters may create a maximal urethral closing pressure that is less than resting intravesical pressure. Functional incontinence refers to the inability to access a toilet when voiding is imminent. This condition is common in the elderly and may coexist with other voiding abnormalities.

HISTORY

The history should detail the precise nature of urinary symptoms and accurately quantitate urine loss. Unfortunately, patients are reluctant to admit to incontinence. Diokno found that only 27% of patients with stress incontinence complain to their physicians.[12] Another study found that only 35% of those surveyed informed their health care provider of their incontinence.[13] The Help for Incontinent People (HIP) organization estimates that only one of 12 persons with incontinence seeks treatment.[14]

The reluctance of the patient to admit to urine loss accentuates the need for a more objective measurement of incontinence. A voiding diary is valuable in documenting the frequency, degree, and provocative measures causing incontinence. This diary is also used to assess the efficacy of therapy. A voiding diary should include time and amount of fluid intake; time of void and degree of urge, if present; amount of leakage; and amount voided. Additional information about position or activity at time of leakage is helpful in distinguishing between types of incontinence. Quantitating the number of pads worn and degree of saturation is helpful.

A precipitous loss of urine without warning is consistent with an involuntary detrusor contraction. This history is sufficient to diagnose DI or DH regardless of urodynamic results. A cough or Valsalva maneuver can trigger an involuntary contraction by reducing outlet resistance. This condition is termed *stress hyperreflexia*. Inquiring whether urine leakage is associated with stress or urge is helpful but nondiagnostic in 20% of patients.[15] Therefore urodynamic studies are useful in certain patients.

In addition to the voiding diary, past medical history—including neurologic conditions, prior surgeries, or medical conditions and review of systems—is important. A change in vision, coordination, tremor, paralysis, changes in sensation, or other symptoms associated with specific neurologic conditions may suggest further diagnostic procedures. Neurologic conditions that can affect the bladder or sphincteric function should be queried for specifically. Multiple sclerosis is associated with voiding abnormalities in up to 80% of patients.[16] Diabetes mellitus, myelodysplasia, spinal cord injury, stroke, or Parkinson's disease can all produce incontinence.[17]

Prior surgery, especially gynecologic, urologic, and colorectal procedures, may affect the bladder or its outlet through direct injury to tissues or innervation. Neurologic injuries to peripheral nerves that supply the bladder or sphincter can affect emptying and storage of urine. Pelvic radiation and inflammation contribute to incontinence by decreasing bladder capacity or compliance.

Medications influence the bladder or the function of its outlet. Alpha-adrenergic blockers used to treat hypertension decrease urethral tone. Alpha blockers have been shown to cause stress incontinence. On the other hand, alpha-adrenergic agonists contained in many cold medications may worsen bladder outlet obstruction in men with BPH. Urinary retention can produce overflow incontinence. Cholinergic agonists such as bethanecol can exacerbate involuntary contractions and aggravate urge incontinence. In contrast, anticholinergics, including oxybutynin and Propantheline, can produce retention and result in overflow incontinence. In summary, a voiding diary, medical and surgical history, and review of medications provides insight into the cause of incontinence and aids in formulating a diagnostic plan. The physical examination may confirm previous suspicions with regard to etiology and guide further imaging or urodynamic procedures.

PHYSICAL EXAMINATION

A complete urologic and neurologic examination screens for abnormalities that contribute to incontinence. The neurourologic examination should begin with observation of the patient's gait and demeanor. The abdomen, back, and flanks are examined for masses, hernias, congenital abnormalities, or scars. The neurologic examination should be directed at both sensory and motor systems. Specific lower-extremity reflexes used to assess sacral spinal cord integrity include dorsiflexion of the foot (L4 to S1) plantar flexion of the foot (L5 to S2), and extension of the toes (L4 to S1). The sacral dermatomes are evaluated by assessing perineal sensation, sphincter tone and control, and the bulbocavernosus reflex. Poor tone or inability to contract the anal sphincter voluntarily could signify neurologic damage of the sacral spinal cord or cauda equina. The bulbocavernosus reflex is elicited by squeezing the glans penis or clitoris and detecting contraction of the anal sphincter. The presence of a bulbocavernosus reflex indicates an intact somatic sacral arc consisting of afferents in the dorsal nerve of the penis or clitoris to the sacral spinal cord and efferents in the pudendal nerve. Unfortunately, 30% of neurologically intact women lack this response.[18]

In women with stress urinary incontinence (SUI), provocative maneuvers such as standing, jumping, or squatting may provoke urinary leakage not demonstrated in the supine or lithotomy position. Quantitation of leakage with pads may help with diagnosis or guide treatment. A pad test is performed by ingesting a dye (e.g., pyridium) that is excreted in the urine and changing tampons if a fistula is suspected or incontinence pads every 2 hours for a representative day.[19] The amount and location of staining help to determine the site and degree of urinary leakage. Continuous incontinence in the female with proximal staining of a vaginal tampon suggests a vesicovaginal fistula. Lifelong continuous incontinence mandates an evaluation for an ectopic ureter with an intravenous pyelogram with renal tomograms.

LABORATORY STUDIES

Few laboratory tests are necessary in the initial evaluation of incontinence. A urinalysis is always done. A urine culture may be performed if symptoms and urinalysis suggest infection. If persistent irritative symptoms or involuntary contractions are present in a middle-aged or elderly patient or there is a suspicion of bladder cancer, a urine cytology may be used to screen for carcinoma in situ. Hematuria in the absence of infection should be evaluated with an excretory urogram, urine cytology, and cystoscopy.

URODYNAMIC TECHNIQUES

Urodynamics is an essential tool to determine the etiology of urinary incontinence. Errors as high as 50% in the diagnosis of incontinence based solely on history and examination demonstrate the need for additional testing. Techniques from eyeball urodynamics to multichannel studies with or without fluoroscopy may be used, depending on the patient's history, examination, and previous tests. More complex studies should be employed when simpler tests prove ineffective, incontinence is not demonstrated on clinical examination, urine loss occurs following pelvic surgery, and patients with suspected or known neurologic disorders are evaluated. Multichannel video urodynamics provide the most complete picture of lower urinary tract function in these patients.

Cystometry (CMG) records pressure–volume relationships during filling of the bladder, including bladder sensation, compliance, contractile activity, and capacity (Fig. 26–2). Bladder sensation is noted by recording volumes at the first sensation of bladder filling, at first desire to void, and at strong urgency to void or pain. Compliance reflects the ability of the bladder to accommodate to increased filling. Normally, the pressure remains below 15 mmHg pressure until the bladder has reached its cystometric capacity. A steady rise in detrusor pressure on filling indicates poor compliance that could have deleterious effects on the upper tracts.[20] The overactive detrusor is characterized by detrusor contractions on filling. These contractions may be spontaneous or provoked by any number of stimuli. Maximum cystometric capacity is also demonstrated, but because of unphysiologic filling it may not correspond to actual bladder capacity. A voiding diary is the easiest measure of capacity.

Eyeball or bedside urodynamics is an interactive study between physician and patient. With the patient in the lithotomy position, the bladder is filled through a catheter with the 60-mL syringe attached at a measured height above the pubis. Fifteen centimeters is often chosen. Sensation, compliance, activity, and capacity are determined during filling. The rate of fall or rise of the meniscus in the syringe will demonstrate compliance or involuntary contractions. When the results of this testing do not provide reliable information, more sophisticated urodynamics may be required.

The effect of fill rates has been evaluated and medium fill rates in adults (10 to 100 mL/min) have been found appropriate for most studies.[19] Numerous studies have concluded that a gas or liquid infusant results in the same clinical diagnosis.[21–23] Of note is that with the use of CO_2 gas, filling cystometric parameters sensation, and capacity are reduced by one-third. Modern fiberoptic microtransducer pressure technology allows pressure determinations equivalent to water cystometry while being able to perform cystoscopy synchronously.[24,25] Ambulatory monitoring and telemetry has been compared to conventional testing. Although it may become more widely used in the future, it merely represents an extended cystometrogram with a voiding diary.[26] However, ambulatory cystometry does demonstrate involuntary contractions that would not otherwise be detected on routine urodynamics. Ambulatory urodynamics measures compliance with natural filling of the bladder.

Subtracting the abdominal pressure as measured by rectal pressure from intravesical pressure alleviates posturing and straining artifacts.[27] Unsubtracted cystometric curves reflect both detrusor and abdominal pressure. Simultaneous determination of bladder pressure and intra-abdominal pressure as estimated by the rectal catheter reflects true detrusor pressure. Electronic subtraction of abdominal (rectal) pressure from bladder (vesical) pressure provides the true detrusor pressure.

Electromyography (EMG) can be combined with CMG to evaluate whether the external striated urethral sphincter functions in synchrony with the bladder (Fig. 26–3). Involuntary contraction of the external urethral sphincter during a detrusor contraction is referred to as detrusor sphincter dyssynergia (DSD). An EMG is valuable if a neurologic lesion is suspected. Therefore EMGs are used selectively in

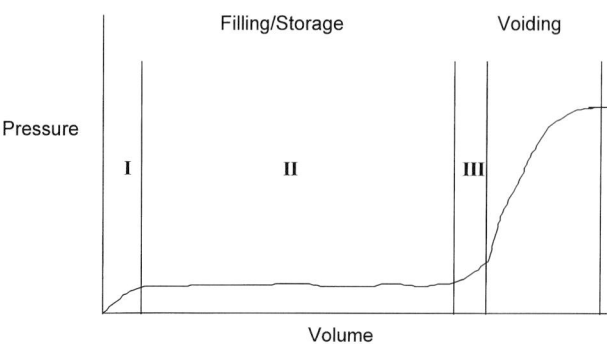

Figure 26–2. Idealized cystometrogram. (**I**). Viscoelastic response to bladder filling (5 to 15 cm H_2O). (**II**). Slight increase in pressure with increased volume (good compliance). (**III**). Bladder stretched to physiologic limit (rarely seen clinically).

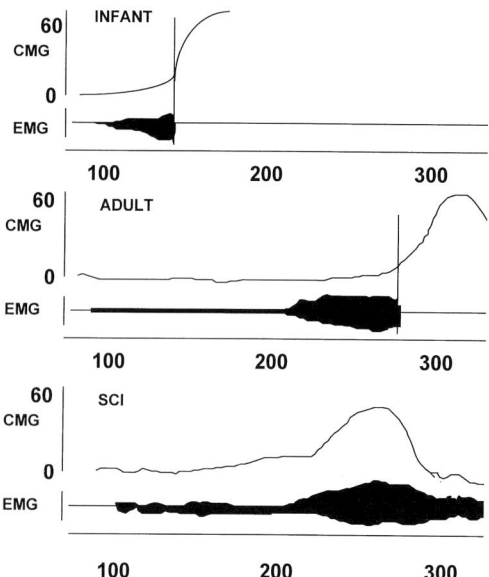

Figure 26–3. Examples of combined cystometry and electromyography. Reflex voiding in infant with coordinated sphincter function. Normal voiding in adult with coordination and ability to inhibit voiding. Reflex voiding in paraplegic with external sphincter dyssynergia.

the evaluation of incontinence. Residual urine, hydronephrosis, or interrupted, low flow rates are suggestive of DSD. Surface or needle electrodes may be employed. In females, placement of needle electrodes in the external sphincter is very difficult because of the minimal amount of striated sphincter present. The advantage of needle electrodes is that they can examine individual motor units rather than the entire perineal floor. Fibrillation potentials and positive sharp waves are indicative of denervation. These findings can only be observed with needle electrodes.[28] Lack of EMG silence at the time of detrusor contraction demonstrates DSD or pseudodyssynergia—voluntary straining. Surface electrodes are easier to use, but most of the signal represents electrical noise. However, global field potentials estimate whether external sphincter relaxation occurs with a bladder contraction.

Uroflow is a simple test that evaluates the volume of urine expelled in relation to time. Uroflow is a common screening test for obstruction in men and is rarely used to evaluate incontinence. The flow rate nomogram described by Siroky corrects for different voided volumes.[29] A minimal voided volume of 150 mL is required to obtain a reliable flow rate. Demographic studies show that flow rates decrease with increasing age.[30] Low flow rates and urge incontinence in the elderly female suggest detrusor hyperactivity with impaired contractility (DHIC). Unfortunately, impaired detrusor contractility and obstruction generate similar curves and absolute values. Thus uroflow is unable to differentiate detrusor hypocontractility from obstruction.[31] A combined pressure–flow study that simultaneously monitors detrusor pressure and flow rate is required to document obstruction. A reduced uroflow with an adequate detrusor contraction defines obstruction. Alternatively, a normal uroflow in the presence of an elevated pressure (more than 100 cm H_2O) indicates obstruction. To perform a combined pressure–flow study a urethral catheter is used to measure detrusor pressure during voiding. Voiding pressures of less than 30 cm H_2O with a flow rate of less than 12 mL/sec indicate detrusor hypocontractility. Voiding pressures of more than 60 cm H_2O with a flow rate less than 12 mL/sec signify bladder outlet obstruction.

Although much is written about urethral pressure profiles, the measurement of this parameter is unnecessary in the evaluation of urinary incontinence.[32] Simple perfusion profilometry, which measures urethral resistance to a constant flow of gas or liquid, is often used. With the bladder filled to capacity, a catheter is slowly withdrawn during urethral pressure measurement. The parameters determined are the maximal urethral closing pressure (MUCP) and functional urethral length (FUL). Although micturitional static urethral pressure profile during voiding may help define the level of obstruction, this test is rarely necessary.[33,34] Leak point pressures provide a better guide to assess the function of the bladder outlet.

The abdominal leak point pressure (ALPP) is a simple test to classify urinary incontinence. McGuire studied women with SUI using fluoroscopy and monitoring detrusor and intra-abdominal pressures. At a bladder volume of 200mL patients increased abdominal pressures by incremental straining. The pressure at which leakage occurred was recorded. The pressure when fluoroscopic or actual leakage occurred defined the ALPP. Patients with an ALPP of less than 60 cm H_2O had type 3 SUI, or intrinsic sphincter deficiency (Fig. 26–4). Type 2 SUI was associated with pressures of more than 90 cm H_2O. Patients with cystoceles also had elevated ALPPs as a result of pressure transmission to the prolapsed bladder. Therefore bladder reduction with a pessary or similar device is necessary to obtain an accurate ALPP. ALPP provides valuable information regarding function of the bladder neck and proximal urethra. This test does not require fluoroscopy to differentiate anatomic incontinence from urethral dysfunction.[35] ALPP can also be estimated by measuring the rectal pressure with straining and observing urine leakage.

Detrusor leak point pressure (DLPP) is very different from ALPP. DLPP represents the pressure in the bladder at which urine exits the urethra. Although urine loss should never occur even at high abdominal pressures, urine can normally exit the urethra at relatively low bladder pressures.

A DLPP of more than 40 cm H_2O is predictive for upper tract deterioration. DLPP is measured by recording detrusor pressure with a No. 7 French urethral catheter. The pressure at which urine exits the urethra without straining represents the DLPP.[36] The DLPP provides prognostic information about future upper tract changes. The ALPP is a provocative dynamic test that mimics circumstances that may cause leakage. In contrast, the DLPP assesses pressures detrimental to renal function.

Ideally, visualizing the lower urinary tract during urodynamics provides the most complete picture of bladder and urethral function. Synchronous multichannel studies combining the previously mentioned techniques of cystometry, uroflow, and EMG with fluoroscopy aid in the evaluation of complex disorders. After obtaining a urinary flow rate, the bladder is catheterized with a triple lumen urinary catheter. A rectal catheter monitors intra-abdominal pressure. Pressures are zeroed at the level of the symphysis pubis. Fifty milliliters of contrast (80% cystografin) is instilled under fluoroscopic monitoring. Radiopaque markers on the urethral and vesical ports aid in catheter placement for determination of detrusor and urethral pressures.

There are multiple advantages of fluoroscopic monitoring of the lower urinary tract during urodynamics. Imaging provides sensitive detection of minimal urinary leakage, detrusor–external sphincter dyssynergia, dysfunction of the internal sphincter, and localization of obstruction.[37] There are a limited number of cystourethrographic radiologic configurations. A closed bladder neck is normal in the resting supine or upright individual undergoing urodynamic filling. Failure to open during micturition may represent smooth muscle dyssynergia or a contracture of the bladder neck. A closed bladder neck can be seen in patients with an areflexic blad-

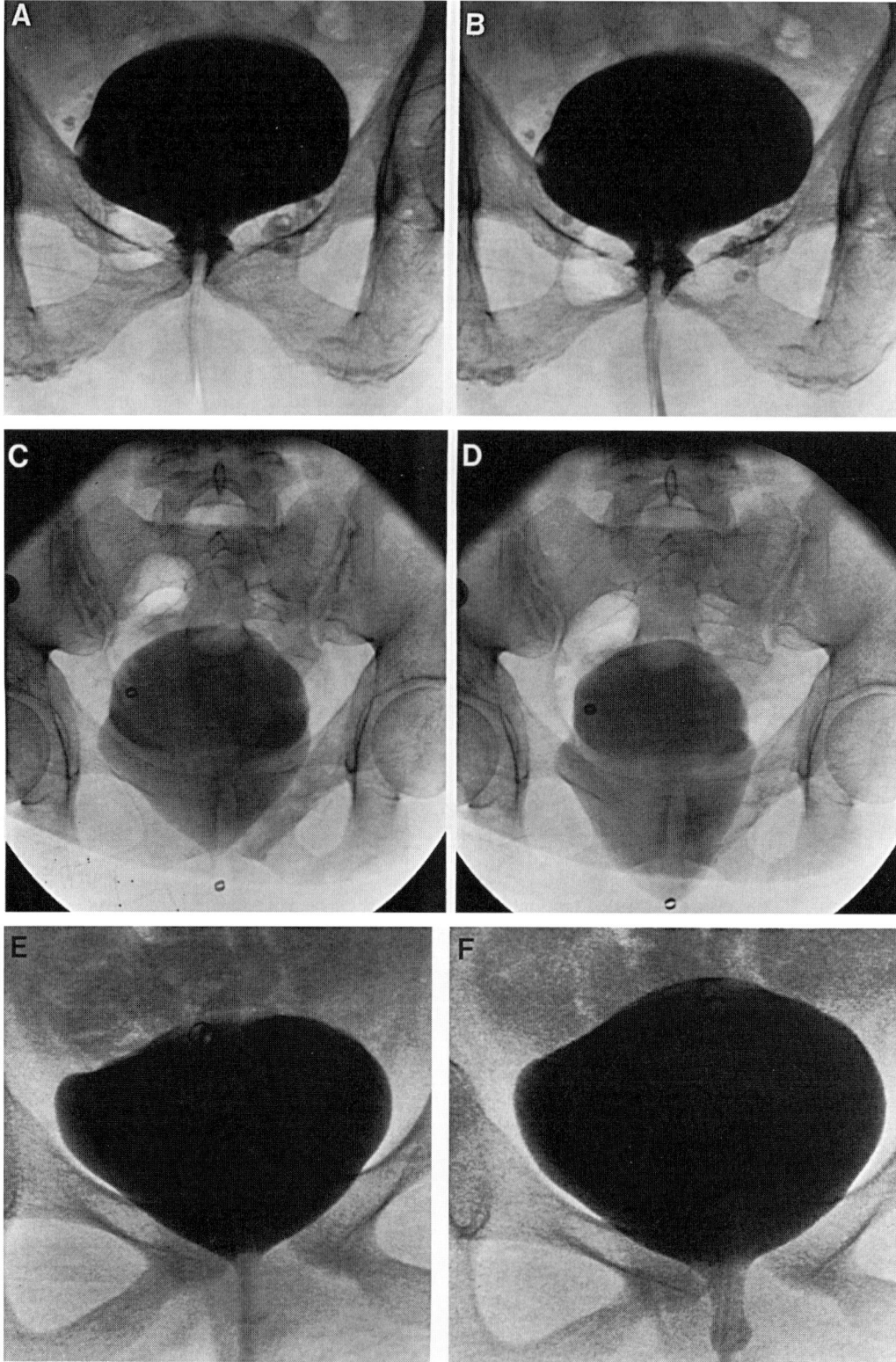

Figure 26–4. Upright cystograms during urodynamic evaluation for urinary incontinence. (**A**) Male with post-TURP incontinence. (**B**) Abdominal leak point pressure (ALPP) of 10 cm H_2O with straining. Diagnosis is type 3 stress urinary incontinence (SUI) or intrinsic sphincter deficiency. (**C**) Female with significant urethral hypermobility and ALPP of 40 cm H_2O with straining. (**D**) Diagnosis is combined type 2 and 3 SUI, successfully treated with pubovaginal fascial sling. (**E**) Female with no urethral hypermobility and ALPP 5 cm H_2O. Diagnosis is type 3 SUI and patient is dry after periurethral collagen injection. (**F**) No hypermobility with straining in upright position.

der. These individuals often strain to void and have a nonfunctioning bladder neck. This closed bladder neck and proximal urethra during voiding may also be seen in patients with benign prostatic hyperplasia (BPH). An open bladder neck is only normal during volitional voiding or with involuntary reflex contractions. If the bladder neck remains open during filling, it is nonfunctional as a result of anatomic or neurologic causes. A closed striated sphincter is normal with urodynamic filling. A closed striated external urethral sphincter during voiding could represent voluntary interruption of urination or inhibition of leakage following an involuntary contraction. It is essential to distinguish the closed external sphincter with a distended proximal urethra that occurs with voluntary contraction from that of external DSD.[38] Appropriate precautions should be taken to avoid excess radiation exposure during fluoroscopy, and the patient must be informed of the risks to instillation of iodinated contrast material. Prophylactic antibiotics are administered during invasive urodynamic studies.

INCONTINENCE IN PATIENTS WITH NEUROLOGIC DISORDERS

Multichannel urodynamic studies provide insight to the pathophysiology of the incontinence and lead to improved management. Patients with voiding disorders associated with stroke, Parkinson's disease, multiple sclerosis (MS), myelodysplasia, spinal cord injury, and other neurologic disorders often warrant multichannel studies (Table 26–2).

Suprapontine lesions such as stroke or other lesions of the brain and lesions caused by Parkinson's disease have variable micturitional profiles. The most consistent urodynamic finding in patients with brain lesions is the loss of voluntary control caused by detrusor hyperreflexia. However, other abnormalities may occur. In a clinical study of 550 patients, Blaivis found that 25% of patients with suprapontine lesions had acontractile bladders. Of the patients with detrusor hyperreflexia, only 50% retained voluntary control of the external sphincter. In those patients with voluntary control, only half were continent.[39,40] Detrusor sphincter dyssynergia does not develop with isolated suprapontine lesions.[39] Patients with suprapontine lesions may have other conditions that contribute to incontinence. For example, Parkinson's disease causes lower urinary tract symptoms, including incontinence. Incontinence in Parkinson's patients results from lack of cortical inhibition and subsequent detrusor hyperreflexia.[41] Although 75% of Parkinson's patients have appropriate external sphincter relaxation, some demonstrate slow or delayed relaxation, termed *sphincter bradykinesia*. In addition, 60% of men with Parkinson's disease were found to have diminished flow rates consistent with bladder outlet obstruction.[41] The inability to empty the bladder completely may exacerbate detrusor hyperreflexia and worsen urge incontinence.

Multiple Sclerosis (MS) is characterized by focal neural demyelinization in the brain and spinal cord. Depending on the site of these plaques, bladder and urethral function can be involved.[42] The posterior and lateral columns of the cervical spinal cord are the most common sites of demyelinization. The lumbar and sacral cords are involved in 40 and 80% of MS patients with bladder dysfunction. The location of these lesions can lead to detrusor hyperreflexia and detrusor sphincter dyssynergia.[43] Indeed, detrusor hyperreflexia has been found in 50 to 90% of patients with MS. DSD occurs in 30 to 66% of MS patients.[43] Incontinence caused by detrusor hyperreflexia can be difficult to manage in MS patients. Patients with neurologic disease are at risk for urologic complications if they (1) are managed with indwelling catheters, (2) have DSD, or (3) demonstrate poor detrusor compliance.[44] MS patients can have any combination of detrusor, urethral, or sensory findings. Detrusor leak point pressures are useful to predict which patients may be at risk of renal deterioration. Therefore urodynamic testing is essential to ascertain the abnormality, implement appropriate therapy, and determine prognosis.

Spinal cord injury produces a spectrum of voiding disorders that are best evaluated with synchronous multichannel studies. Eight thousand to 10,000 new cases of spinal cord injury are seen annually in the United States. The majority are young unmarried males.[45] Most injuries occur at the mid-cervical and the thoracolumbar junction. Although the level

Table 26–2. Neurologic Causes of Incontinence

CONDITION	LEVEL	LESION	CAUSE
Stroke	Suprapontine	Ischemia	Loss of inhibition
Parkinson's disease	Suprapontine	Def Dopa Trans	Loss of inhibition
Multiple sclerosis	Brain/Spine	Focal demyelinization	Loss of inhibition DSD, atonic bladder
Myelodysplasia	Thoracic or lumbar	Denervation	Reflex or atonic bladder, ISD
Spinal cord injury	Variable; rule out second lesion if clinical discrepancies	Loss of ascending/descending tracts	UMN reflex contraction with or without DSD LMN atony with or without ISD

of spinal cord injury or neurologic disorder is predictive for lower urinary tract dysfunction, video urodynamics provides a more accurate diagnosis and prognosis.[46]

Incontinence and upper tract changes are the most common urologic problems encountered in myelodysplastic patients.[47] Myelomeningocele occurs in the lumbosacral cord in 42% of cases, in the thoracolumbar cord in 27%, in the sacral cord in 21%, and in the thoracic and cervical cord in only 10%.[48] Although the vertebral level should determine the type of lower tract dysfunction, it often does not.[49] This disparity has been attributed to associated spinal cord dysplasia, syringomyelia, failure of upward migration of the cord, or tethering.[50] The spectrum of vesicourethral dysfunction is best evaluated by multichannel studies or with the use of fluoroscopy.[37] McGuire found that incontinence in 86% of myelodysplastic children was caused by an open vesical outlet and nonfunctional proximal urethra (type III or intrinsic sphincter deficiency).[36] Fluoroscopy aids in the proper diagnosis and implementation of therapy. In addition, a striking relationship exists between urethral closure pressure and leak point pressure that has prognostic value in prediction of upper tract deterioration. As mentioned previously, patients with a DLPP of greater than 40 cm H_2O risk upper tract deterioration. Therapy should be targeted at increasing bladder compliance.

Incontinent patients should undergo imaging of the nervous system if suspected of having an undiagnosed neurologic disorder. Magnetic resonance imaging (MRI) is valuable in diagnosing spinal cord pathology. Indications for spinal cord imaging include incontinence associated with spinal trauma or surgery or neurologic conditions such as those in MS. Another absolute indication for imaging is the developement of SUI in the male. The acute onset of bladder, bowel, and erectile dysfunction, with or without changes in motor or sensory examination also mandates evaluation of the spinal cord. The new onset of symptoms such as voiding dysfunction in patients with neurologic lesions could indicate the development of spinal cord tethering or syrinx. Stress incontinence in the male without a history of pelvic surgery is due to a neurologic lesion until proven otherwise. This unusual complaint mandates a spinal imaging study. Abnormal physiologic findings direct the spinal level to be imaged. For example, DSD detected by urodynamics implies a suprasacral lesion. An open bladder neck can be found with involvement of sympathetic centers in the thoracolumbar cord. Mass lesions of the spinal canal or spinal cord from neoplasia, trauma, or disk herniation may impinge on the cord or spinal nerves, causing detrusor hyperreflexia. Even though valuable information may be obtained with MRI, the findings must be correlated with urodynamic and clinical findings. A normal MRI does not exclude the possibility of a functional deficit in the central nervous system.

Although the evaluation of patients with neurologic disease is focused on pathology of the spinal cord and brain, workup of female stress incontinence relies on documenting changes in the pelvic anatomy.

FEMALE STRESS URINARY INCONTINENCE

Stress urinary incontinence in the female occurs when abdominal pressure exceeds urethral resistance at times of increased abdominal pressure. Examples of this disturbed relationship include malposition of the bladder neck accentuated by increased abdominal pressure (anatomic incontinence) or intrinsic urethral dysfunction from multiple surgeries, radiation, or trauma.[11] Intact urethropelvic and pubourethral ligaments provide support to the urethra at times of stress. Another important continence mechanism is the coaptation and seal effect of the submucosa and muscular and fibroelastic coat. Transmission of increased abdominal pressure to the bladder neck and urethra augments the closure mechanism during stressful maneuvers. In this fashion, the urethra compensates for increases in intraabdominal pressure.[11] Therapy depends on the exact mechanism of the incontinence and associated defects of the pelvic floor.

Physical examination adds valuable information in planning therapy. The patient should be examined in the lithotomy and upright positions with a full bladder. The level of the bladder neck should be evaluated at rest and with stress, noting any leakage with increases in abdominal pressure. If no leakage occurs, the patient should be repositioned to provoke urine loss. The entire vaginal wall should be inspected for other abnormalities such as cystocele, enterocele, uterine descensus, rectocele, or other vaginal pathology. Treatment should include repair of the pelvic floor at the time of correction of incontinence.

The cotton swab test is a method of evaluating urethral hypermobility. In patients with normal urethral support the cotton swab will remain stationary on straining.[51] However, hypermobility of the urethra can be difficult to establish solely by physical examination. Fluoroscopy or a straining cystogram provides a sensitive measure of urethral position on movement. The Marshall–Marchetti or Bonney test elevates the bladder neck without compressing the urethra as the patient coughs. This test has been thought to be predictive of surgically curable stress incontinence. However, it is nearly impossible to avoid compressing the urethra, thus the usefulness of this test is questioned. After a thorough physical examination there is no consensus on what further tests are absolutely necessary prior to treatment of incontinence. As a guide, the more invasive or morbid the therapy, the more valuable additional testing will be.

Diagnostic imaging may be included in the evaluation of patients with SUI. Clinicians have used x-rays to determine urethral configuration for more than 50 years.[52] In performing a cystourethrogram an 8 or 10 French Robinson catheter is used to measure the postvoid residual. The bladder is then filled with 30% Renografin at low pressure (less than 15 cm H_2O pressure). Bladder sensation, intravesical pressures, and involuntary contractions are noted under fluoroscopic observation with 150 to 200 mL in the bladder. In the upright or nearly vertical position on a tilted fluoroscopic table, relaxing and straining views are performed in the AP and lateral positions. The catheter is then removed, and in the 30% oblique position the function of the bladder neck is recorded as well as the amount of leakage with straining and ability to close the bladder neck after initiating voiding. Bladder configuration, presence of vesicoureteral reflux, and possible urethral abnormalities may also be seen on a voiding cystourethrogram.[53]

Transvaginal endosonography and intraurethral ultrasound have been used recently to evaluate female SUI.[54,55] Although some clinicians are comfortable in formulating therapy with the information obtained with imaging studies and eyeball urodynamics, others prefer information from more sophisticated urodynamic studies.

Cystoscopy is usually performed at the time of corrective surgery. Cystourethrosopy is valuable in patients with a history of multiple surgeries for stress incontinence, radiation, or urethral trauma. The urethra should be inspected for atrophic changes, coaptating ability, fistulas, or diverticula. Vaginoscopy can be undertaken at the same time.

EVALUATION OF INCONTINENCE IN THE MALE

The use of prostate specific antigen (PSA) and transrectal ultrasound techniques has increased the number of patients undergoing radical prostatectomy for prostate cancer. Although the incidence of urinary incontinence after prostatectomy should decrease with refinements in surgical technique, the absolute numbers of incontinent men may increase. A recent sample of Medicare patients was surveyed and 30% reported wearing pads or clamps, 40% dripped urine with full bladders or with coughing, and an additional 23% reported daily wetting of more than a few drops.[56]

Because the proximal sphincter mechanism is destroyed during a prostatectomy, postoperative continence relies on the distal intrinsic sphincter. Although the external striated sphincter can voluntarily interrupt the urinary stream, passive continence is lost without a functioning distal intrinsic sphincter. Tubularization of the bladder neck has been attempted to re-create a continence zone for passive urinary continence. The usefulness of this surgical modification has been debated because the true continence zone appears to be distal to the vesicourethral anastomosis.[57,58] Scar formation at the vesicourethral anastomosis can accentuate urine loss by affecting the dynamics of the bladder neck. Bladder neck contracture can cause obstruction or preclude coaptation of the urethral mucosa. Interruption of the pelvic nerve to the distal bladder and membranous urethra is possible.[59] In addition to anatomic or neural sphincteric damage, bladder dysfunction present before the operation or as a result of surgery may impact on continence and affect treatment.[60]

Sphincteric dysfunction and bladder dysfunction must be evaluated prior to instituting therapy in the postprostatectomy incontinent patient.[61] Of 107 men tested by Leach with CMG and pressure flow studies, only 37% were found to have sphincteric insufficiency, 20% had bladder dysfunction, but 34% had sphincteric insufficiency and high-pressure bladder dysfunction from involuntary contractions or poor compliance.[61] Only 9% of patients had normal urodynamic studies.[62] The difficulty in predicting the cause of incontinence after prostatectomy warrants synchronous multichannel video-urodynamic studies or a combination of CMG, straining cystogram, and ALPP prior to instituting therapy. An ALPP also provides a useful gauge for quantitating results of surgical therapy.

PEDIATRIC INCONTINENCE

The wet child or young adult is frequently seen by the urologist after failure of conservative therapies. Understanding the pathophysiology of nonneurogenic voiding dysfunction and the development of urinary control aids in instituting therapy and reassuring child and parent. The ability to consciously inhibit the infantile voiding reflex is first gained during the day, then at night. Day and night control is achieved by most children between the ages of 2 and 3 (Table 26–3).[63] Continued leakage is termed *primary enuresis* and can occur in the daytime, nighttime, or throughout the day (diurnal). If control is achieved and inability to control urine voluntarily recurs, it is termed *secondary enuresis*. Ten to 20% of 5-year-olds have enuresis, with a 14% spontaneous cure rate. This translates into a 5% rate of incontinence in 10-year-olds, with a 16% annual spontaneous cure rate into adulthood.[64] The prevalence of enuresis in adults is 0.8%.

When children who have not yet acquired the ability to inhibit the voiding reflex or who suffer from painful voiding

Table 26–3. Development of Urinary Control

Infant	Lack of suprapontine control of micturition reflex
Transition phase Ages 2–3	Sensation of fullness, continence attained by volitional contraction of external sphincter
Adult voiding	Awareness of fullness, ability to postpone voiding

disorders (e.g., infection) are put in social situations that require continence, changes to the bladder and bladder outlet can occur. These changes occur secondary to repeated constriction of the external sphincter at the time of bladder contraction—voluntary vesicosphincteric dyssynergia. The high pressures can cause functional and morphologic changes such as ballooning of the proximal urethra, bladder diverticula, vesicoureteral reflux, and upper tract deterioration.[65]

A careful history, physical examination, laboratory studies, and possibly radiologic and urodynamic studies are useful in evaluating incontinence in children.[66] The pattern of wetting is the most important part of the history. In addition, the child or parent should be asked about dysuria, altered stream, urinary tract infection, or constipation. A voiding diary helps to clarify complex voiding patterns. Questioning for symptoms of urgency or tricks used to keep from leaking often shed light on the etiology of the child's condition. The physician should ask if the leakage is constant or intermittent. Questions pertaining to recent stressors may be especially pertinent to those children with secondary enuresis. The physical examination should include evaluation of the abdomen, genitalia, and back to include inspection for signs of spinal dysraphism. For a suspected neurologic cause, a neurourologic examination is performed. A urinalysis is used to screen for proteinuria, infection, glycosuria, or concentrating defects.

Further evaluation depends on associated complaints or physical findings.[67] Pure bedwetters need no further evaluation, and reassurance or treatment should be instituted. Those patients with frequency, urgency, and normal voiding can be managed with smooth muscle relaxants with no further evaluation. Anatomic or neurologic disorders or findings consistent with dysfunctional voiding warrant ultrasonography to assess bladder wall thickness, postvoid residual, and presence of hydronephrosis. Additional imaging depends on ultrasound findings or, as in adults, on whether there is suggestion of neurologic disease. In general, urodynamic studies are rarely required for enuresis or nonneurogenic voiding dysfunction.[67]

EVALUATION OF GERIATRIC INCONTINENCE

Incontinence is not a normal sequela of aging.[68] The principal causes of incontinence in the elderly differ from those in younger adults. An increased incidence of uninhibited bladder contractions occurs in the aged.[69] Detrusor hyperactivity with impaired contractility may mimic SUI in the female and bladder outlet obstruction in men.[69] Although younger people urinate most of their daily ingested fluid before bedtime, the elderly excrete much of their fluid intake at night. Therefore some nocturia is normal with aging. Combined with functional limitations and possibly detrusor instability, nocturia may precipitate enuresis. Pharmaceuticals are a common cause of geriatric incontinence. Sedative, diuretic, anticholinergic, adrenergic drugs, and many other medications have been implicated as a cause of incontinence. A careful medication history eliminates unnecessary testing. The elderly often have more than one condition that contributes to urine loss (Table 26–4). In an attempt to determine bladder changes with aging, Elbadawi has correlated bladder biopsy results with urodynamic findings that may aid in differentiating causes of bladder dysfunction and focus therapy.[70]

Assessment of the severity of symptoms is hindered by inaccurate measuring techniques.[71] Voiding diaries appear to be the most useful and reproducible means of assessing symptoms, but their value in diagnosis or tracking therapy is not defined.[72] Pad-weighing tests have a low sensitivity, especially in the older population.[71,72] The Urilos nappy system, which consists of a pad impregnated with a dry electrode and measures urine volume by changes in capacitance has not shown significant diagnostic value over voiding diaries or pad weighing.[73] A thorough history and physical examination are necessary, but radiologic procedures are rarely indicated.[74] Indications for imaging include recurrent febrile urinary infections, poor bladder compliance, or suspicion of malignancy or fistula.[75]

Multichannel urodynamics is used in the elderly to differentiate multiple conditions that may simultaneously contribute to incontinence. Ouslander compared bedside (eyeball) urodynamics to multichannel studies and found a 75% sensitivity for uninhibited bladder contractions.[75] However, these simplified tests cannot determine if the uninhibited contraction is associated with normal or impaired detrusor function. Detrusor hyperactivity with impaired contractility (DHIC) can mimic any type of incontinence.[76] In men DHIC can mimic prostatism or can contribute to incontinence associated with outlet obstruction. In women leakage can occur secondary to a stress-induced contraction and can be confused with stress incontinence. Although the original description of DHIC was based on multichannel studies, Brandeis demonstrated that most elderly females can be accurately classified by single-channel studies.[76] DuBeau and Resnick concluded that urodynamic studies are indicated

Table 26–4. Mnemonic For Transient Incontinence in Elderly Diappers*

Delirium
Infection
Atrophic urethritis/vaginitis
Pharmaceuticals
Psychological, especially depression
Excessive urine output (cardiac, DM)
Restricted mobility
Stool impaction

*After DuBeau CE, Resnick NM: Evaluation of the causes and severity of geriatric incontinence. *Urol Clin North Am* 1991; 18(2): 243–256.

when empirical therapy puts a patient at risk, previous therapies have failed, complicating co-morbid conditions exist, or corrective surgery is planned.[74]

SUMMARY

Urinary incontinence is a common symptom affecting a large segment of society. The high prevalence of incontinence and the refusal of many individuals to seek medical attention may be attributed in part to the misconception that incontinence is a normal result of aging or childbirth. Effective treatment for urinary incontinence involves an accurate diagnosis aided by understanding the pathophysiology of urinary incontinence. The evaluation of incontinence includes a thorough history and physical examination. Occasionally, imaging and urodynamic testing are required.

REFERENCES

1. Caldwell KP: *Urinary Incontinence*. New York: Grune & Stratton, 1975;7.
2. Herzog AR: Prevalence and incidence of urinary incontinence in a community dwelling population. *NIH Consensus Conference on Urinary Incontinence in Adults: Program and Abstracts*. Bethesda, MD, Oct 3–5 1988;17–21.
3. Burgio KL, Matthews KA, Bernhard TE: Prevalence, incidence and correlates of urinary incontinence in healthy, middle-aged women. *J Urol* 1991;146:1255–1259.
4. Herzog A: Epidemiology and cost of incontinence. *NIH Consensus Conference on Women's Urological Health Research: Program and Abstracts*. Bethesda, MD, March 11–13, 1994; 73.
5. de Groat WC: Anatomy and physiology of the lower urinary tract. *Urol Clin North Am* 1993; 20 (3):383–401.
6. Maggi CA: The dual sensory and efferent function of capsaicin-sensitive sensory nerves in the bladder and urethra. In: *The Autonomic Nervous System: Nervous Control of the Urogenital System, 3*. London: Harwood Academic Publishers, 1993; 383.
7. de Groat WC, Ryall RW: Reflexes to sacral parasympathetic neurons concerned with micturition in the cat. *J Physiol (Lond)* 1969;200:87–105.
8. de Groat WC, Steers WD: Neural control of urinary bladder and sexual organs: experimental studies in animals. In: Bannister R, ed. *Autonomic Failure*. Oxford, England: Oxford University Press, 1987;196–222.
9. Steers WD: Urinary incontinence: advances in neural manipulation. *Surg Rounds* 1988;77:27–34.
10. Raz S: Evaluation of the incontinent patient. In: Krane RJ, Siroky MB eds. *Clinical Neurology*. Boston: Little, Brown, 1979;123–134.
11. Staskin DR, Zimmern PE, Hadley HR, Raz S: The pathophysiology of stress incontinence. *Urol Clin North Am* 1985; 12:271–278.
12. Diokno AC, Brock BM, Brown MB: Prevalence of urinary and other urological symptoms in the noninstitutionalized elderly. *J Urol* 1986;136:1022–1026.
13. Nygaard I, Delancey JOL, Arnsdorf L, et al: Exercise and incontinence. *Obstet Gynecol* 1990;75:63–67.
14. Jeter KF: *Incontinence in the American Home: Facts Not Myth*. Union, SC HIP, 1985.
15. Stanton S, Tanagho E: *Surgery of Female Incontinence*. New York: Springer-Verlag, 1986;23–54.
16. Goldstein I, Siroky MB, Sax DS, Krane RJ: Neurourologic abnormalities in multiple sclerosis. *J Urol* 1982;128:541–546.
17. Chancellor MB, Blaivis JG: Diagnostic evaluation of incontinence in patients with neurological disorders. *Comp Ther* 1991;17(2):37–43.
18. Blaivas JG, Zayed AAH, Labib KB: The bulbocavernosus reflex in urology: a prospective study of 299 patients. *J Urol* 1981;126:197–199.
19. Blaivas JG: Techniques of evaluation. In: Yalla SV, McGuire EJ, Elbadawi A, et al, eds. *Neurourology and Urodynamics: Principles and Practice*. New York, Macmillan, 1988;155–198.
20. McGuire EJ, Woodside JR, Borden TA: The prognostic significance of urodynamic testing in myelodysplastic patients. *J Urol* 1981;125:205–209.
21. Cass AS, Ward BD, Markland C: Comparison of slow and rapid fill cystometry using liquid and air. *J Urol* 1970; 104:104–107.
22. Gleason DM, Bottacini MR, Reilly RJ: Comparison of cystometrograms and urethral profiles with gas and water media. *Urology* 1977;9:155–159.
23. Jorgenson L, Lose G, Anderson JT: Cystometry : H_2O and CO_2 as filling medium? A literature survey of the influence of the filling medium on the qualitative and quantitative cystometric parameters. *Neurourol Urodynam* 1988;7: 343–349.
24. Belville WD, Swierzewski SJ, Wedemeyer G, Faerber G, McGuire EJ: Synchronous cystoscopy and cystometry in the management of neurogenic bladder dysfunction. *J Urol* 1993; 150:431–433.
25. Belville WD, Swierzewski SJ, Wedemeyer G, McGuire EJ: Fiberoptic microtransducer pressure technology: urodynamic implications. *Neurourol Urodynam* 1993; 12:171–178.
26. van Waalwijk van Doorn ESC, Remmers A, Janknegt RA: Extramural ambulatory urodynamic monitoring during natural filling and normal daily activities: evaluation of 100 patients. *J Urol* 1991;146:124–131.
27. Webster GD, Older RA: The value of subtracted bladder pressure measurement in routine urodynamic studies. *Urology* 1980;16:656–659.
28. Siroky MB: Electromyography of the Perineal Striated Muscles. In: Krane RJ, Siroky MB, eds. *Clinical Neurourology*, 2nd ed. Boston: Little, Brown, 1991;245–254.
29. Siroky MB, Olsson CA, Krane RJ: The flow rate nomogram II: clinical correlation. *J Urol* 1980;123:208–210.
30. Balslev JJ, Jensen KM-E, Bille-Brahe NE, et al: Uroflowmetry in asymptomatic elderly males. *Br J Urol* 1986;58:390–394.
31. Chancellor MB, Blaivis JG, Kaplan SA, Axelrod S: Bladder outlet obstruction versus impaired detrusor contractility: the role of uroflow. *J Urol* 1991;145:810–812.
32. Blaivas JG, Awad SA, Bissada N, et al: Urodynamic procedures: recommendations of the urodynamic society—procedures that should be available for routine urologic practice. *Neurourol Urodynam* 1982;1:51–55.
33. Yalla SV, Sharma GVRK, Barsamin EM: Micturitional static urethral pressure profile: a method of recording urethral pressure profile during voiding and the implications. *J Urol* 1980; 124:649–656.
34. Yalla SV, Waters WB, Snyder H, Varady S, Blute R: Urodynamic localization of isolated bladder neck obstruction in men: studies with micturitional vesicourethral static pressure profile. *J Urol* 1981; 125:677–684.
35. Fitzpatrick CC, McGuire EJ, Wan J, et al: Abdominal leak point pressure as index of urethral sphincter function. *Inter-*

national Urogynecology Journal: 1993 Annual Scientific Meeting Abstracts. p. 387. Abstract 1.
36. McGuire EJ, Fitzpatrick CC, Wan J, et al: Clinical assessment of urethral sphincter function. *J Urol* 1993;150:1452–1454.
37. McGuire EJ, Woodside JR: Diagnostic advantages of fluoroscopic monitoring during urodynamic evaluation. *J Urol* 1981;125:830–834.
38. Blaivas JG, Sinha HP, Zayed AAH, Labib KB: Detrusor–external sphincter dyssynergia. *J Urol* 1981;125:542–544.
39. Blaivas JG: The neurophysiology of micturition: a clinical study of 550 patients. *J Urol* 1982;127:958–962.
40. Kahn Z, Hertinu J, Yang WC, Melman A, Lieter E: Predictive correlation of urodynamic dysfunction in brain injury and cerebrovascular accident. *J Urol* 1981;126:86–89.
41. Pavlakis AJ, Siroky MB, Goldstein I, Krane RJ: Neurourologic findings in Parkinson's disease. *J Urol* 1983;129:80–83.
42. McDonald WI: Pathophysiology in multiple sclerosis. *Brain* 1974;97:179–196.
43. Blaivas JG, Bhimani G, Labib KB: Vesicourethral dysfunction in multiple sclerosis. *J Urol* 1979;122:342–347.
44. Blaivas JG, Barbalin GA: Detrusor–external sphincter dyssynergia in men with multiple sclerosis: an ominous urologic condition. *J Urol* 1984;131:14–17.
45. Woolsey RM, Young RR: Disorders of the spinal cord. *Neurol Clin* 1991;9:551.
46. Kaplan SA, Chancellor MB, Blaivas JG: Bladder and sphincter behavior in patients with spinal cord lesions. *J Urol* 1991;146:113–117.
47. Smith ED: *Spina bifida and total care of spinal myelomeningocele.* Springfield, IL, Charles C Thomas, 1965.
48. Kaplan GW: Myelomeningocele and related disorders. *JCE Urol* 1978;15.
49. Barson AJ: Spina bifida: the significance of the level and extent of defect to the morphogenesis. *Dev Med Child Neurol* 1970;12:129–137.
50. Rudy DC, Woodside JR: The incontinent myelodysplastic patient. *Urol Clin North Am* 1991;18:2:295–308.
51. Bruskewitz R: Female incontinence: signs and symptoms. In: Raz S, ed. *Female Urology*. Philadelphia: WB Saunders, 1983;45–50.
52. Shapiro RA, Raz S: Clinical applications of the radiologic evaluation of female incontinence. In: Raz S, ed. *Female Urology*. Philadelphia: WB Saunders, 1983;123–136.
53. Zimmern PE: The role of voiding cystourethrography in the evaluation of the female lower urinary tract. *Probl Urol* 1991;5(1):24–41.
54. Johnson JD, Lamensdorf H, Hollander IN, Thurman AE: Use of transvaginal endosonography in the evaluation of women with stress urinary incontinence. *J Urol* 1992;147:421–425.
55. Klein H, Kirshner-Hermanns R, Lagunilla J, Gunther RW: Assessment of incontinence with intraurethral US: preliminary results. *Radiology* 1993;187:140–143.
56. Fowler FJ, et al: Patient-reported complications and follow-up treatment after radical prostatectomy: the national Medicare experience: 1988–1990. *Urology* 1993;42:622–629.
57. Presti JC Jr, Schmidt RA, Narayan PA, et al: Pathophysiology of urinary incontinence after radical prostatectomy. *J Urol* 1990;143:975–979.
58. Myers RP: Male urethral sphincteric anatomy and radical prostatectomy. *Urol Clin North Am* 1991;18:2:211–227.
59. O'Donnell PD, Finan BF: Continence following nerve-sparing radical prostatectomy. *J Urol* 1989;142:1227–1230.
60. Foote J, Yun S, Leach GE: Post-prostatectomy incontinence: pathophysiology, evaluation, and management. *Urol Clin North Am* 1991;18:2:229–241.
61. Leach GE, Yip CM, Donovan BJ: Post-prostatectomy incontinence: the influence of bladder dysfunction. *J Urol* 1987;138:574–579.
62. Leach GE, Yun SK: Post-prostatectomy incontinence. Part 1: the urodynamic findings in 107 men. *Neurourol Urodynam* 1992;11:91–97.
63. Klimberg I: The development of voiding control. *American Urological Association Update Series*, 1988, Lesson 21.
64. Forsythe WI, Redmond A: Enuresis and spontaneous cure rate: study of 1129 enuretics. *Arch Dis Child* 1974;49:259–263.
65. Kondo A, Kobayashi M, Otani T, et al: Children with unstable bladder: clinical and urodynamic observation. *J Urol* 1983;129:88–93.
66. Himsl KK, Hurwitz RS: Pediatric urinary incontinence. *Urol Clin North Am* 1991; 18(2):288–293.
67. Resnick NM: Voiding dysfunction in the elderly. In: Yalla SV, McGuire EJ, Elbadawi A, eds. *Neurourology and Urodynamics*. New York: Macmillan, 1988;303.
68. Brocklehurst JC, Dillane JB: Studies of the female bladder in old age: cystometrograms in non-incontinent women. *Geront Clin* 1966;8:285–290.
69. Resnick NM, Yalla SV: Detrusor hyperactivity with impaired contractile function: an unrecognized but common cause of incontinence in elderly patients. *JAMA* 1987;257:3076–3080.
70. Elbadawi A, Yalla SV, Resnick NM: Structural basis of geriatric voiding dysfunction. I: Methods of a prospective ultrastructural/urodynamic study and an overview of the findings. *J Urol* 1993;150:1650–1656.
71. Wyman JF, Choi SC, Harkins SW, et al: The urinary diary in evaluation of incontinent women: a test–retest analysis. *Obstet Gynecol* 1988;71:812–816.
72. Kromann-Anderson B, Jakobsen H, Anderson JT: Pad weighing tests: a literature survey on test accuracy and reproducibility. *Neurourol Urodyn* 1989;8:237–242.
73. Eadie AS, Glen ES, Rowen D: The Urilos Recording Nappy System. *Br J Urol* 1983;55:301–305.
74. DuBeau CE, Resnick NM: Evaluation of the causes and severity of geriatric incontinence. *Urol Clin North Am* 1991; 18(2):243–256.
75. Ouslander J, Leach G, Abelson S: Simple versus multichannel cystometry in the evaluation of bladder function in an incontinent geriatric population. *J Urol* 1988;140:1482–1487.
76. Brandeis GH, Baumann MM, Yalla SV: Detrusor hyperactivity with impaired contractility: the great mimic. *J Urol* 1990;143:223A. Abstract.

27 Diagnosis of Adrenal Disorders

Robert A. Older, Alexander D. Zwart, Helmy M. Siragy

The scope of clinical problems related to adrenal disease has changed over the last decade, mostly because of the incidentally discovered adrenal mass on abdominal or chest imaging for reasons other than adrenal imaging. It has proved difficult to reach a consensus on what to do with these "incidentalomas," both regarding biochemical and additional imaging workup and regarding indications for surgery.

This chapter approaches adrenal problems from two perspectives. The first addresses imaging studies and biochemical tests that are useful and/or indicated in suspected adrenal problems. The second addresses the issues that are raised when adrenal masses are discovered with an imaging study done for nonadrenal reasons.

Diagnostic imaging studies and biochemical studies are important in the management of adrenal disorders because a variety of adrenal disorders require surgical intervention, whereas others can be observed.

A general rule for suspected adrenal disorders, from an endocrinologic standpoint, is to image after the biochemical workup is completed. This allows the clinician to decide which imaging study to obtain and can save patients from unnecessary surgery. Conversely, in case of an incidentaloma, biochemical testing next to the history and physical examination will help the clinician decide whether more or other imaging studies are needed and whether surgery or observation is indicated.

IMAGING MODALITIES

Imaging of the adrenal glands continues to evolve with the major changes currently occurring in better characterization of lesions. Computed tomography (CT) continues to be the cornerstone of adrenal imaging, with improvements in CT scanners helping to improve detection of lesions. In addition, progress with magnetic resonance imaging (MRI) and nuclear medicine studies has provided alternate methods of detection and new methods of characterizing lesions. These have improved both sensitivity and specificity of adrenal lesion detection. Table 27–1 lists imaging studies used in adrenal disease.

Generally Available Techniques

ABDOMINAL RADIOGRAPHY

Although very limited in the information it can provide, the supine abdominal radiograph may be worthwhile as an initial screening examination in selected cases. Although further studies will always be necessary, the abdominal radiograph can provide useful information when adrenal lesions are large or calcified.[1–3] Calcification is common in adrenal carcinoma, being present in approximately one-third of cases.[1] Punctate calcification is present in 30 to 50% of neuroblastomas, and calcification is found in pheochromocytoma, adrenal cysts, adrenal hemorrhage, tuberculosis, and rarely a benign adenoma.[2,4–9]

ULTRASOUND

Although able to demonstrate both normal and abnormal adrenal glands,[10] ultrasound has not developed as a routine procedure for adrenal evaluation, largely because of the availability and greater accuracy of CT. Although consistent visualization of the normal and abnormal adrenal has been shown,[10] much of this work has been done by a limited number of individuals and its accuracy is probably related to operator skill, experience, and interest.

Although ultrasound has not developed as a routine study for evaluation of suspected adrenal pathology in the adult, it is the primary study in the evaluation of suspected adrenal masses in the pediatric population, with CT and MRI used as secondary studies.[11] Ultrasound has been recommended as the procedure of choice in suspected neonatal hemorrhage,[12] which can present as a solid adrenal mass because of its early detection while still echogenic. Acute hemorrhage becomes echogenic immediately, with liquefaction beginning approximately 24 hours after hemorrhage and a

Table 27–1. Imaging Studies for Adrenal Disease

Currently used and generally available:
  Computed tomography
  MRI
  Ultrasound
  Adrenal venous sampling
  Abdominal radiograph [primarily children]
Currently used, but with limited availability:
  Scintigraphic scanning
    NP-59 [131-I-6B-iodomethyl-19-norcholesterol]
    MIBG [131-I-metaiodobenzylguanidine]

530   Diagnosis of Genitourinary Disease

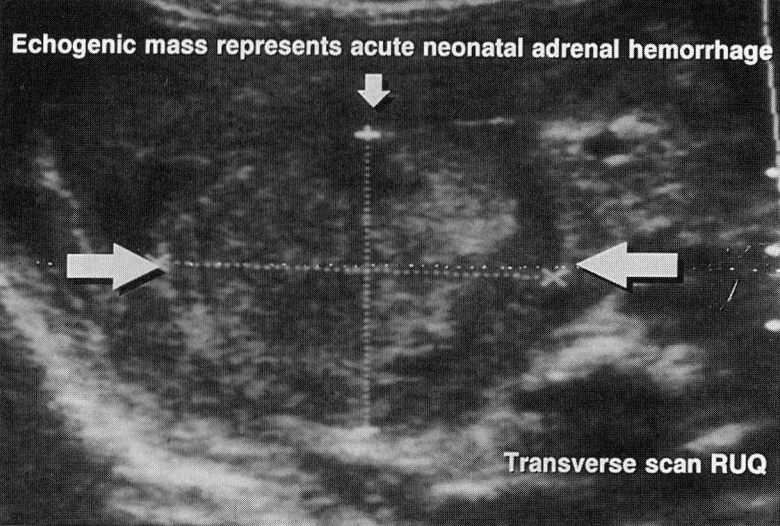

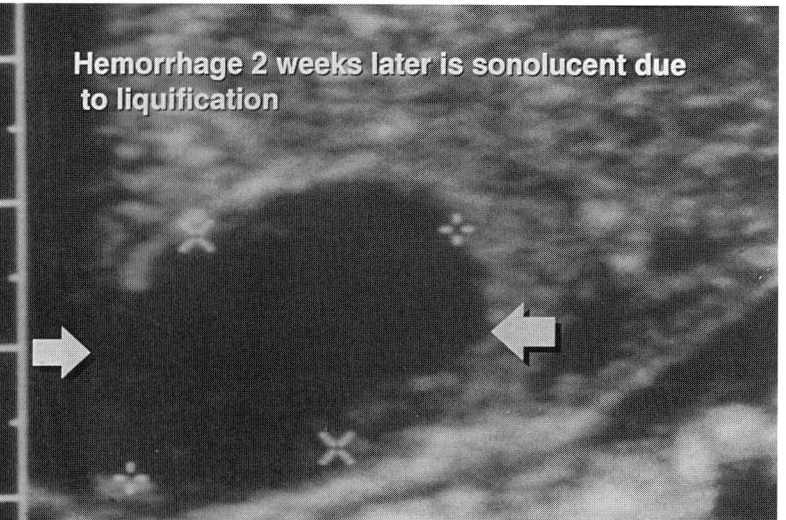

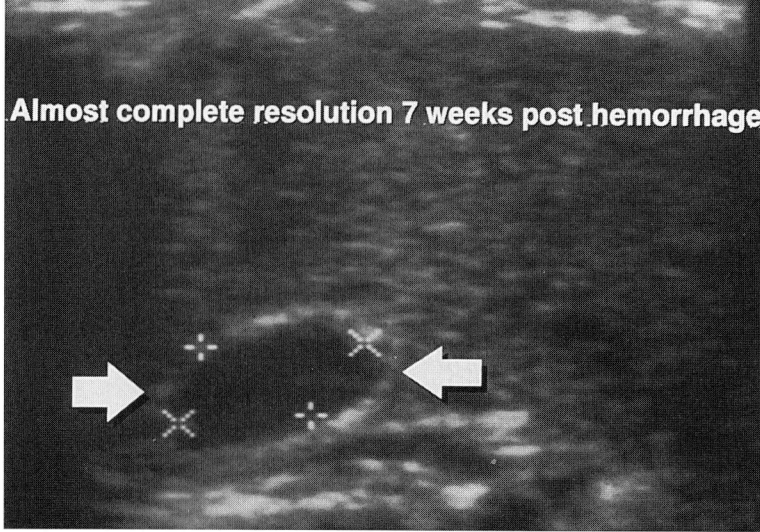

Figure 27–1. Evolution of neonatal adrenal hemorrhage. (**A**) Large echogenic mass representing acute adrenal hemorrhage. (**B**) Two-week follow-up shows sonolucent mass due to liquification. (**C**) Almost complete resolution of the mass at 7 weeks.

gradual decrease in echogenicity leading to a sonolucent appearance at about 96 hours (Fig. 27–1).[12–14]

Ultrasound may play an important role in the diagnosis of adrenal cysts. Although uncommon, these lesions are well evaluated by ultrasound.[15,16] In areas where CT is not readily available or where financial restraints limit the number of CT machines and there is a long wait, ultrasound may assume greater importance, as has been suggested by Yamakita.[17]

COMPUTED TOMOGRAPHY

CT is the mainstay of adrenal diagnosis. The normal adrenal glands are visible on essentially all CT scans done with current-generation equipment, especially if 5-mm images are obtained. The medial limb of the right adrenal gland is generally easier to see than the lateral limb and presents as a linear density immediately posterior to the inferior vena cava. The lateral limb is smaller and has a more horizontal appearance (Fig. 27–2). An inverted V or Y appearance can be seen on the right, but this appearance is most common with the left adrenal. Less commonly, the left adrenal has a triangular appearance. The thickness of the limbs of either adrenal is generally in the 5- to 7-mm range. A width greater than 1 cm is considered abnormal. The limbs of the left gland are generally thicker than those of the right.[18] The length of the limbs is variable and ranges from 2 to 4 cm.[18]

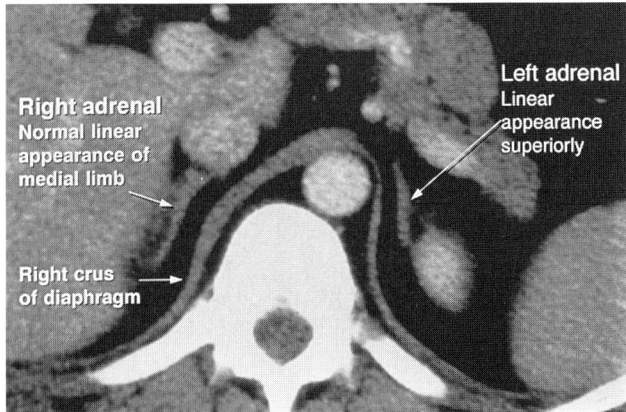
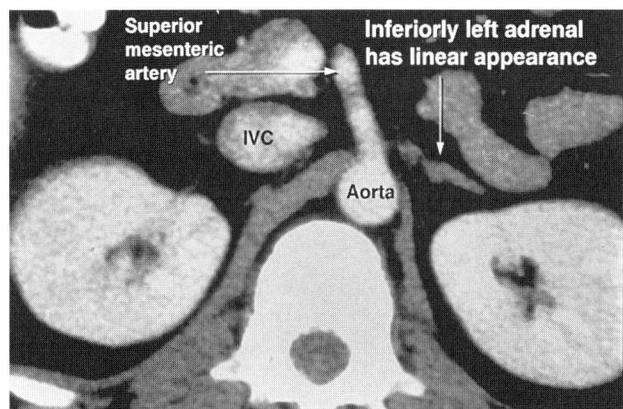
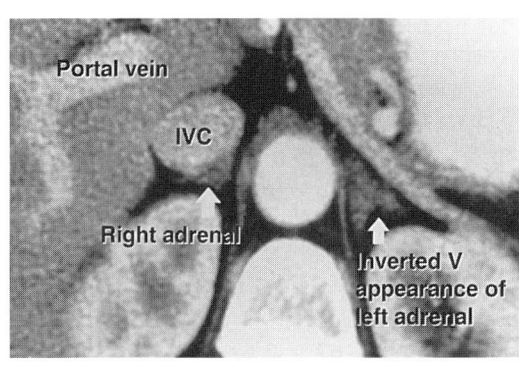
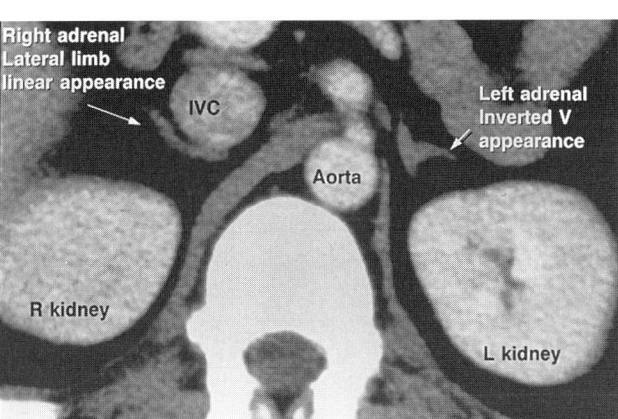
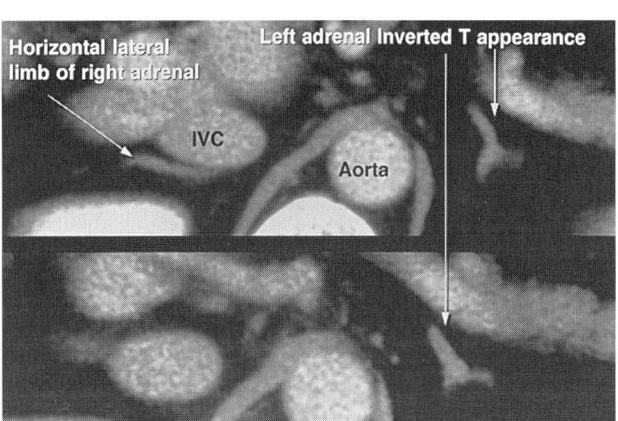

Figure 27–2. Variations in the appearance of normal adrenal glands. (**A, B**) Case 1. (**C, D**) Case 2. (**E**) Case 3. (**F**) Case 4.

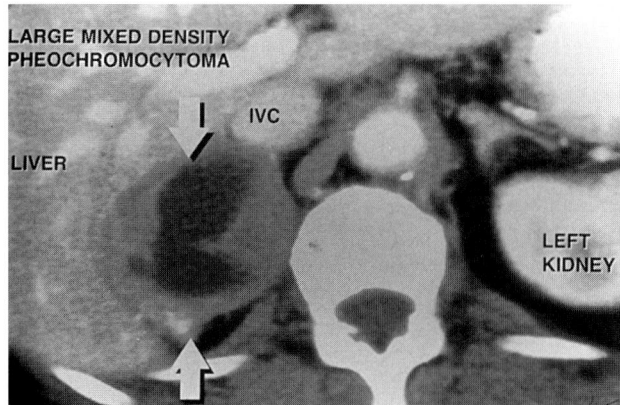

Figure 27–3. Computed tomography of a large right adrenal pheochromocytoma.

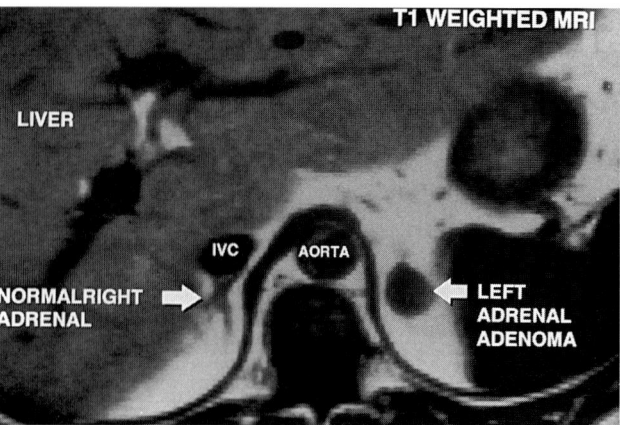

Figure 27–5. Adrenal MRI (T1) shows a normal right gland and a small adenoma on the left.

CT is excellent for detecting lesions of the adrenal. Both large (Fig. 27–3) and small (Fig. 27–4) lesions can be demonstrated, but with lesions of less than 1 cm, such as those in primary aldosteronism, the sensitivity does decrease. CT is primarily a method of detection and is not as good for characterizing lesions.

MAGNETIC RESONANCE IMAGING

MRI has added greatly to the evaluation of adrenal lesions. Normal glands can be demonstrated in the majority of patients (Fig. 27–5).[19] Although it can be used to detect the initial lesion, its primary use is in characterization of lesions. Initially, this was done using heavily weighted T1 or T2 sequences[20] where metastases, carcinomas, and pheochromocytomas were shown to have higher signal intensities on T2-weighted images than did adenomas.[21,22] Further studies using both visual and quantitative analysis of the T2 intensity of adenomas and nonadenomas compared to the intensity of liver confirmed initial impressions that nonadenomas show higher signal intensity than adenomas.[23] T1-weighted images had less success in lesion separation.[24] Dynamic enhanced MR scans with analysis of signal increase following contrast and evaluation of the speed with which the contrast enhancement and washout occurred compared favorably with CT of the same patients but still showed an 8% equivocal rate and 4% false-positive or false-negative.[25] Although these techniques could separate many types of lesions, they were not totally successful with significant areas of overlap.[20]

The most recent MRI techniques have concentrated on the large amount of cytoplasmic lipid generally contained in adenomas and usually not found in metastases, pheochromocytomas, or carcinomas. These techniques, termed *chemical shift imaging*, take advantage of the fat content of benign adenomas to separate these from other lesions. The fat content produces a decrease in signal intensity when opposed-phase images are used.[26] Multiple studies using chemical shift imaging have shown excellent results in separating benign adenomas from nonadenomas,[26–30] but further studies are necessary to confirm the reliability of chemical shift imaging before it is accepted as an alternative to biopsy. There is variability in the fat content in malignant lesions as well as adenomas, a potential problem for this technique. Further data will be necessary to determine if there is significant "overlap" of benign and malignant lesions with this technique.[20] Chemical shift imaging, however, does appear to have considerable promise for differentiating these lesions without biopsy.[28]

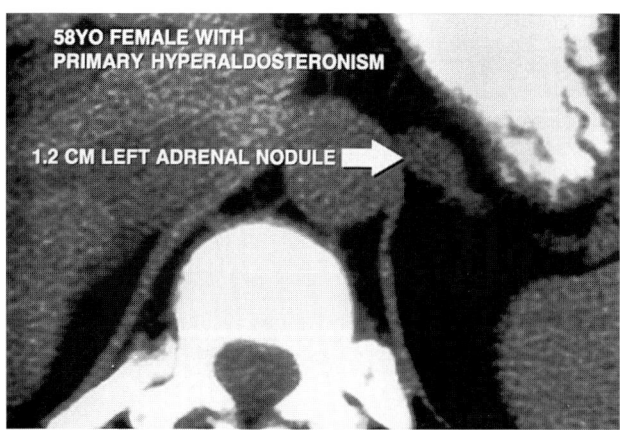

Figure 27–4. Small nodule on CT in a patient with primary hyperaldosteronism.

ADRENAL VENOUS SAMPLING

Adrenal venous sampling consists of selective catheterization of the adrenal veins to obtain blood samples for analysis of aldosterone and/or cortisol levels. A venogram is often obtained to confirm the position of the catheter, but the venogram is not the prime diagnostic tool, and care must be taken not to overinject contrast in an attempt to obtain a venogram because this can produce complications. Venous sampling requires considerable expertise and experience if it is to be successful. This technique is most useful in patients with primary aldosteronism and will be further discussed in that section.

Techniques with Limited Availability

ADRENAL SCINTIGRAPHY

The availability of adrenal scintigraphy is limited because NP-59, which it requires is not FDA approved in the United States, and although 131-I-metaiodobenzylguanidine (MIBG) is approved, it must be specially ordered.

Radiopharmaceuticals used to detect and localize adrenal cortical abnormalities are radiolabeled analogs of cholesterol. These include NP-59, 75Se-B-selenomethylnorcholesterol, and the original agent 131-I-19-iodocholesterol. These radiopharmaceuticals are carried in the circulation bound to low-density lipoproteins and then are absorbed by specific receptors on adrenocortical cells, after which they are internalized and esterified to form a pool of cholesterol ester substrate. Unlike native cholesterol, the radiocholesterol analogs are not further metabolized to adrenocortical hormone precursors.[31,32] Uptake of NP-59 is increased by adrenocorticotrophic hormone and decreased by the uses of dexamethasone. The uptake of NP-59 can also be reduced by very high serum cholesterol levels.[31] Although readily available in much of the world, NP-59 is still not commercially available in the United States. It is available as an investigational new drug from the University of Michigan.[31] The routine dose of NP-59 is 1.0 mCi NP-59 per 1.73 m^2 to a maximal dose of 2 mCi. The imaging intervals and the use of baseline versus dexamethasone suppression studies are determined by the clinical problem being evaluated.[32]

In cases of primary aldosteronism the role of imaging is to separate an aldosterone-secreting adenoma from bilateral hyperplasia. Because these adenomas are small and hyperplasia may not significantly alter the size or shape of the adrenals, pharmacologic manipulation is used to enhance the sensitivity of NP-59 scanning. Dexamethasone suppression allows detection of small adenomas by reducing the uptake in the normal surrounding adrenal cortex. Four milligrams dexamethasone is given orally for 7 days prior to administration of NP-59 and continued during the usual 5 to 7 days of imaging. Dexamethasone suppression causes biochemical suppression of cortisol and its metabolites, and thus helps to distinguish normal from abnormal. The normal adrenal cortex is not seen before the fifth day after NP-59 administration, whereas an adenoma can be seen as a unilateral focus of activity prior to the fifth day (Fig. 27–6). Bilateral adrenal visualization prior to the fifth day would indicate bilateral adrenal hyperplasia.[32] If adrenal visualization only occurs on or after the fifth day, the study is not diagnostic. Dexamethasone suppression has improved the accuracy of NP-59 scanning in primary aldosteronism to approximately 90%, a number comparable to thin-section CT scanning.[32]

NP-59 scintigraphy is also used in Cushing's syndrome (CS), although the very high accuracy of CT makes it less necessary. Scanning is performed without suppression, and unilateral increased uptake is indicative of an adenoma. The contralateral gland is suppressed by the increased blood cortisol levels. Carcinoma producing CS presents as bilateral nonvisualization because the carcinoma takes up too little tracer to be seen and the contralateral gland is suppressed.[32] An area where scintigraphy may play a greater role is CS resulting from ACTH-independent bilateral cortical nodular hyperplasia (CNH). CT is less accurate in this setting and may only detect the largest lesion on one side, leading to an erroneous diagnosis of a unilateral adenoma. The NP-59 scan shows uptake in both glands and can determine the bilateral nature of the process.[32] Experience with this test, however, is neither extensive nor widespread.

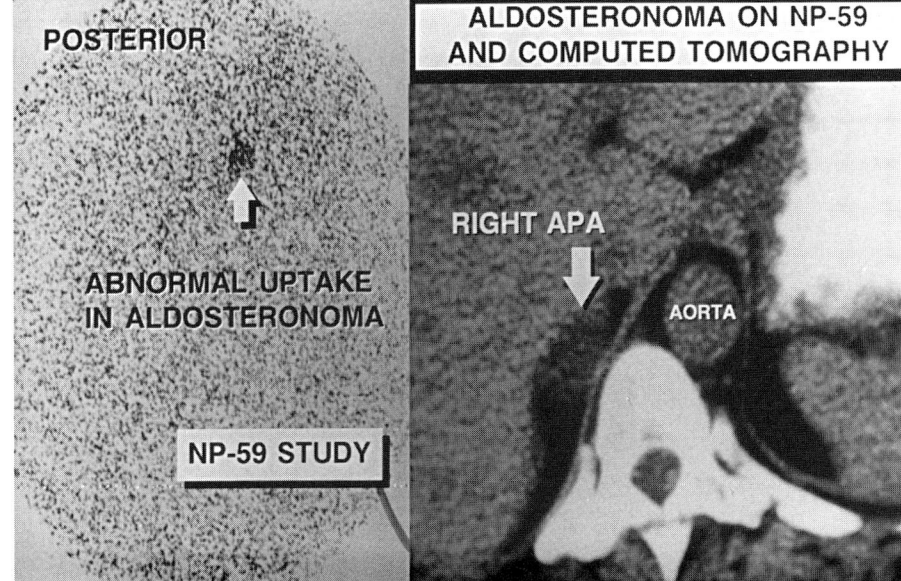

Figure 27–6. Aldosteronoma demonstrated with NP-59 study and computed tomography.

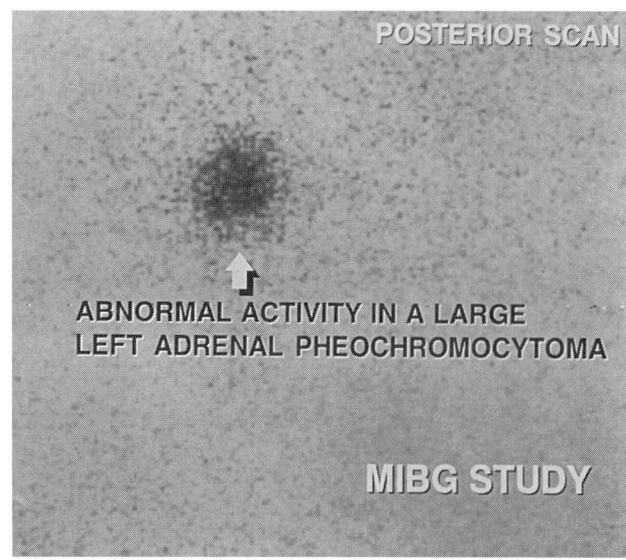 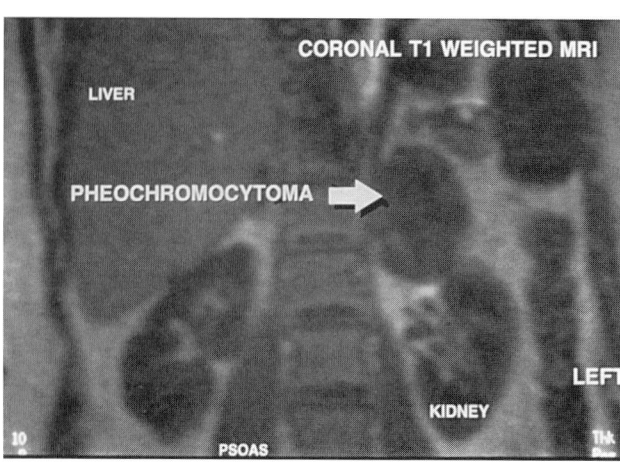

Figure 27–7. (A) MIBG study demonstrating obvious uptake in a left adrenal pheochromocytoma, confirming the etiology of the mass detected with MRI (B).

NP-59 scanning can also be used in the evaluation of the incidentally discovered nodule. NP-59 accumulation in an adrenal mass has been shown to be an indicator of function as well as an indicator of benign lesion. Masses with decreased or absent uptake require further evaluation. Adrenal scintigraphy may help reduce the need for invasive procedures such as biopsy.[32]

MIBG is an analog of guanethidine. It localizes in the adrenergic nerve terminals of the chromaffin storage granules in which norepinephrine is normally stored. I-131-labeled MIBG can visualize the adrenal medulla or overactive sympathetic tissues in other areas of the body (Fig. 27–7).[33] To perform the study the patient receives an intravenous dose of 0.5 to 1.0 mCi of 131-I-MIBG and is then scanned 48 and 72 hours later. The normal adrenals are not visualized with 131-I-MIBG but can be seen if 123-I-MIBG is used. If available on a regular basis, 123-I-MIBG is superior for most types of imaging. Cost and logistics, however, limit its availability.[32]

Activity is normally demonstrated in the salivary glands, myocardium, spleen, and liver.[34] MIBG scans are limited by cost, availability, and radiation dose, which includes approximately 50 rad to the adrenals, 4 rad to the bladder, and 0.1 rad to the whole body.[33]

MIBG scanning takes advantage of the total-body screening ability of the scintigraphic approach. Simultaneous scintigraphy with other radiopharmaceuticals to demonstrate specific organs such as liver or kidney has also proven useful, especially in extra-adrenal lesions.

EVALUATION OF SPECIFIC DISORDERS

Imaging in the evaluation of adrenal disorders involves both functioning and nonfunctioning lesions. Functioning lesions can present as Cushing's syndrome (CS), can present as primary aldosteronism (PA), or can have the manifestations associated with a pheochromocytoma. Nonfunctioning lesions usually represent nonfunctioning adenomas, but they must be differentiated from metastatic lesions and adrenal cancer. The latter problem is quite common because of the incidental detection of adrenal masses with CT and more recently with MRI.

Cushing's Syndrome

DEFINITION

In the 1950s Cushing's syndrome (CS) was defined as a syndrome resulting from chronic excess of cortisol.[35] The clinical features of CS are outlined in Table 27–2.[36] The symptomatology depends on the cause of hypercortisolism. Patients with pituitary Cushing's disease usually present with a classic Cushingoid clinical picture, whereas patients with lung cancer and ectopic overproduction of corticotropin (ACTH) can present acutely with wasting and hypokalemic alkalosis.[37,38] The full clinical syndrome is mostly seen in long-standing disease. However, when the diagnosis is made, subtle symptomatology can usually be traced back many years before the patient presents to the physician.

CLASSIFICATION

CS can be classified as ACTH dependent or ACTH independent. The ACTH-dependent CS is mainly due to ACTH-secreting pituitary tumor and less frequently due to ectopic oversecretion of ACTH. *Cushing's disease* is a term reserved for demonstrated pituitary-dependent ACTH overproduction that causes CS.[36] A rare cause of ACTH-dependent CS is ectopic oversecretion of corticotropin-releasing

Table 27–2. Clinical Features of Cushing's Syndrome

CLINICAL FEATURE	REPORTED INCIDENCE (%)
Centripetal obesity	79-97
Weakness/proximal myopathy	29-90
Hypertension	74-87
Skin changes	
Thin skin/bruising	23-84
Acne, greasy skin	26-80
Hirsutism	64-81
Plethora	50-94
Abdominal striae	51-71
Infection (e.g., tinea vesicolor)	30
Pigmentation	4-16
Psychiatric changes	31-86
Oligo/amenorrhea	55-80
Impotence	55-80
Osteoporosis	
Backache	
Vertebral collapse	> 40-50
Pathologic fracture	
Thirst/polyuria	25-44
Glucose intolerance	39-90
Ankel edema	28-60
Renal calculi	15-19
Exophthalmos	0-33
Headache	0-47
Abdominal pain	0-21

Adapted from Howlett TA, Rees LH, Beeser GM: Cushing's Syndrome. *Clin Endocrinol Metab* 1985; (14)4:911–945.

hormone. The ACTH-independent CS, which is much less common than ACTH-dependent CS, is caused by adrenal adenoma, adrenal carcinoma, and micronodular adrenal disease.[36–39] Iatrogenic administration of exogenous glucocorticoids is, however, the most common cause of clinical CS.

Adrenal lesions producing CS may be bilateral adrenal hyperplasia, adenoma, or carcinoma. Bilateral adrenal hyperplasia results from excessive ACTH secretion. In such cases the hyperplasia, and the CS, is reversible after removal of the source of excessive ACTH secretion.[36] Micronodular hyperplasia is an uncommon cause of CS, and usually it cannot clearly be demonstrated whether the adrenal lesion is ACTH dependent or not.[40,41] The pigmented form of micronodular hyperplasia is even more uncommon and usually is ACTH independent. Nodular hyperplasia is also referred to as macronodular hyperplasia, depending on the size of the nodules. Massive macronodular hyperplasia is usually autonomous.[42] The pathogenesis of these nodular adrenal lesions is not well understood, and the biochemical features are inconsistent.[40] Fortunately, these are uncommon presentations of CS.

Adrenal carcinomas producing CS are rare but frequently have a rapidly progressive course.[43] They tend to hypersecrete different adrenocortical hormones and to be larger (>3.5 cm) at diagnosis. Metastatic disease is frequent.

In summary, the lesion producing CS are:

Bilateral adrenal hyperplasia—ACTH dependent in 70 to 90%
  Most due to an ACTH-secreting pituitary adenoma Cushing's disease
  Ectopic ACTH-producing tumors—oat cell carcinoma; bronchial carcinoid, thymomas, medullary thyroid cancer, pheochromocytoma
Adrenal adenoma—ACTH independent
Adrenal carcinoma—ACTH independent
Macronodular hyperplasia—ACTH dependent and independent
Massive macronodular hyperplasia—rare
Primary pigmented nodular adrenal disease—rare
Ectopic CRH—rare

DIAGNOSIS

The first hurdle to jump in suspected CS is to exclude exogenous administration of glucocorticoids, including injections for pain syndromes or inflammatory conditions, which many patients do not remember well. The next step is to establish definite endogenous overproduction of cortisol.[36]

A useful screening test is a 24-hour urinary free cortisol (UFC) excretion. If normal, CS is virtually excluded, and if very high it can be diagnostic of CS. Interfering substances in the assay and incorrect collections are well-recognized problems. It is recommended to obtain total urinary creatinine for correlation. Another useful screening test is the overnight low-dose dexamethasone test (1 mg at 11 P.M.).[44] CS is unlikely if the following morning at 8 the plasma cortisol is less than 5 mg/dL. Borderline results in both tests can be seen in obesity, stress such as hospitalization, depression, and alcoholism. The latter two disorders can lead to suggestive Cushingoid features. The clinical suspicion of these disorders (pseudo-CS) is important to avoid diagnostic errors.

To establish the diagnosis of CS definitely, a two-day low-dose dexamethasone suppression test (0.5 mg q 6 hr, while collecting urine for two consecutive 24-hour determinations of UFC should be performed.[44] If UFC suppresses to less than 20 mg/24 hour, the diagnosis of CS can be rejected. Alternatively, normal subjects suppress 17-OH-corticosteroids to less than 4 mg/24 hour with this 2-day test.[44]

ADDITIONAL TESTING

Recent developments have allowed more reliable measurements of plasma ACTH concentrations. This can be a very helpful tool to differentiate between an adrenal cause of CS and ACTH dependency. Undetectable plasma ACTH is virtually diagnostic of primary adrenal disease.[39,44] Occasionally, ACTH structure is altered (e.g., in some ectopic ACTH syndromes) and not picked up by certain assays.[45]

The following tests are used in differentiating pituitary from ectopic ACTH production. They rely on the concept that in pituitary-dependent disease the pituitary gland is responsive to high concentrations of glucocorticoids,[35] whereas ectopic ACTH production usually follows a more autonomous course.[40] The high-dose dexamethasone suppression test (2 mg dexamethasone q 6 hour for 48 hours while collecting two consecutive 24-hour urine collections) can differentiate Cushing's disease from adrenal tumors or ectopic ACTH production. It was recently demonstrated that combined use of suppression of UFC by more than 90% and of 17-hydroxycorticosteroids by more than 64% was associated with 100% specificity for pituitary disease in a large group of patients, whereas sensitivity for the combined test was 83%.[46]

Metyrapone inhibits 11-beta-hydroxylase, thus reducing circulating cortisol. This stimulates ACTH secretion in normal subjects and in pituitary-dependent CS but not in patients with adrenal tumors. The increase in ACTH manifests itself as an increase in urinary 17-OH-corticosteroids and/or plasma 11-deoxycortisol. It can be done as an overnight test and as a full 24-hour test.

IMAGING

It should be kept in mind that in normal subjects incidental adrenal lesions can be found in 1 to 10%[47] and that incidental pituitary lesions can be found in 4 to 20% of patients getting a head CT scan for nonpituitary reasons.[48] Moreover, pituitary imaging does not demonstrate a tumor in 33 to 50% of patients with proven Cushing's disease.[44,49] This stresses the importance of sequential biochemical testing in patients with suspected CS. It will guide the physician to what imaging study to obtain, and it will limit false-positive imaging results.

Imaging is generally used to determine the site of a functioning adenoma, or less likely, carcinoma. Radiology, however, can also aid in the evaluation of patients with CS and excess ACTH production. This can be due to a pituitary tumor or an ectopic source. Petrosal sinus sampling is an accurate way of making this differentiation. Comparison of ACTH levels in the inferior petrosal sinuses with peripheral levels allows differentiation between ectopic and pituitary ACTH production.[50] Thin-section chest CT can help identify pulmonary sources of ectopic ACTH production.

If laboratory tests indicate that a functioning adrenal tumor is most likely, the role of imaging is to identify which adrenal gland contains the lesion. Because most cases of adenoma producing Cushing's are relatively large lesions, with an average of 5 cm, these are readily apparent on CT, giving CT a high sensitivity for detection. Carcinomas tend to be even larger and are easily detected. CT is therefore the primary imaging modality for adrenal causes of Cushing's syndrome.

Of all the forms of Cushing's syndrome, macronodular hyperplasia is often the most difficult to diagnose correctly, especially if ACTH independent. When characterized by a dominant nodule it can be confused with a unilateral adenoma on CT. This type of hyperplasia may not show typical responses on endocrine tests, further compounding the problem. Hyperplasia of the contralateral gland and remaining portions of the ipsilateral gland indicates an ACTH-dependent hyperplasia as opposed to an autonomous adenoma in which the contralateral gland would be small, as would be the uninvolved parts of the ipsilateral gland.[42]

Massive macronodular hyperplasia and primary pigmented nodular adrenal disease are two rare forms of Cushing's syndrome that have characteristic CT appearances (Fig. 27–8).[42,51] The former shows massively enlarged glands with multiple nodules and is relatively easily diagnosed. Primary pigmented nodular adrenal disease has been described as having a "string of beads" appearance,[42] but demonstration of the fine nodularity of this disease requires thin-section images, and some studies have suggested a normal appearance for primary pigmented nodular adrenal disease. The fine nodularity in one or both glands with intervening hypoplastic tissue[52] may be difficult to demonstrate, and this disease can therefore present as "knobby," a unilateral nodule, or normal.[51]

Other than for cortical nodular hyperplasia, radiolabeled cholesterol (NP-59) is of limited use in the diagnosis of Cushing's syndrome because of the high accuracy of CT, which is nearly 100% for adenoma or carcinoma.[32] Radiocholesterol (NP-59) shows bilateral adrenal uptake in hyperplasia, unilateral concordant activity in functioning adenoma, and no activity in carcinoma because of lack of uptake in the carcinoma and suppression of the contralateral gland.[53]

NP-59 can be quite helpful if adrenal deposits are left behind at surgery, especially in malignant disease. Increased activity in these functioning deposits can be detected with NP-59, whereas detection with other imaging techniques may be more difficult.[54] NP-59 has been helpful in massive macronodular hyperplasia and primary pigmented nodular adrenal disease, two rare forms of Cushing's syndrome. Iodocholesterol scans showed bilateral uptake in five out of six patients with these entities. Identification of the bilaterality of this process is important because the therapy is bilateral adrenalectomy.[51] MRI currently has little role in Cushing's syndrome, largely because of the accuracy of CT. MRI cannot separate functioning from nonfunctioning adenomas, and although adenomas can be separated to some degree from carcinomas on the basis of T2 characteristics, there is still a moderate-sized indeterminate group (21%).[55]

Imaging Summary.

CT: primary study will detect almost all adenomas and carcinomas NP-59: Recurrent or residual disease

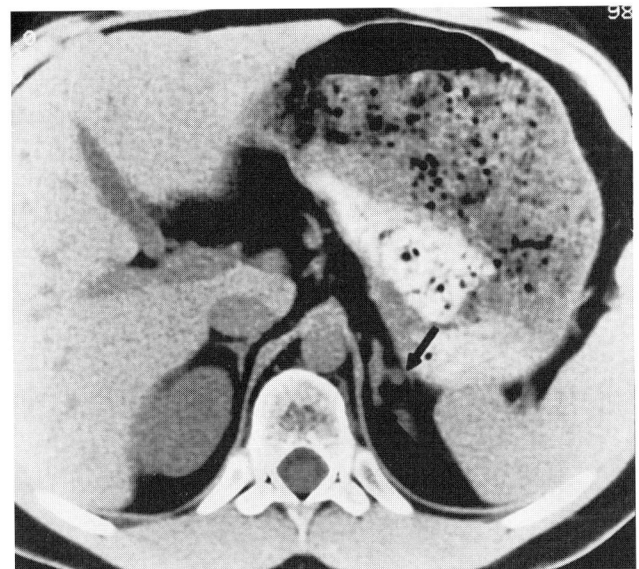
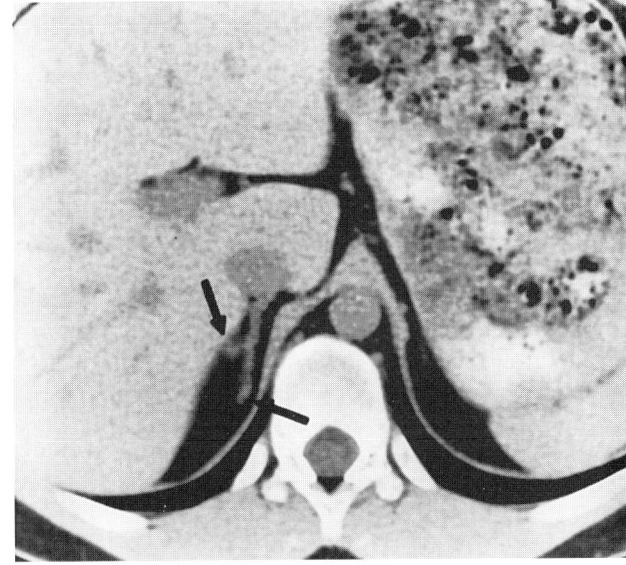
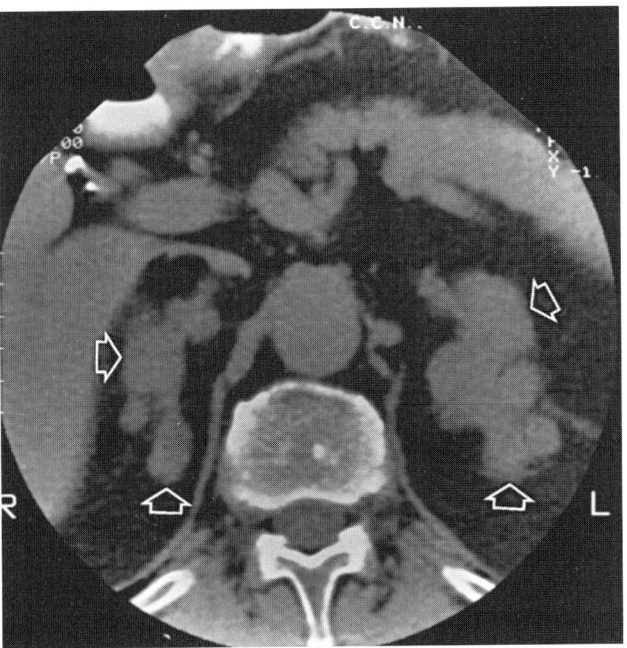

Figure 27–8. (**A**) CT of primary pigmented nodular hyperplasia. (Courtesy of Dr. John Doppman. Reproduced from The dilemma of bilateral adrenocortical nodularity in Conn's and Cushing's syndromes. *Radiol Clin North Am* September 1993. With permission from WB Saunders.) (**B**) CT of massive macronodular hyperplasia. Bilateral large nodules (open arrows) deform the adrenal. (Courtesy of Dr. John Doppman. Reproduced from The dilemma of bilateral adrenocortical nodularity in Conn's and Cushing's syndromes. *Radiol Clin North Am*, September 1993. With permission from WB Saunders.)

ACTH-independent cortical nodular hyperplasia, bilateral uptake differentiates from adenoma

Petrosal sinus sampling:
  Differentiation of pituitary or ectopic source of ACTH

TREATMENT

Surgical resection of the lesion-producing CS is most likely to be curative. Bilateral adrenalectomy has been long replaced by transsphenoidal adenectomy for pituitary Cushing's disease.[40] Adrenalectomy is the treatment of choice for adrenal adenoma or carcinoma-causing CS. Radiotherapy, including gamma knife treatment, is considered when sellar surgery is contraindicated, or for recurrent Cushing's disease. Long-term complications of radiation therapy may include hypothalamic–pituitary hypofunction.[56] Although CS can be treated medically by a variety of medications that inhibit cortisol production (ketoconazol, metyrapone, aminogluthemide) or work as an "adrenolytic" agent (mitotane), none of these are curative. However, they can be useful to control clinical CS in inoperable patients.

Primary Hyperaldosteronism

DEFINITION

Aldosterone plays an important role in the regulation of arterial blood pressure and body fluid and electrolyte homeostasis. The primary action of aldosterone is to stimulate distal tubular sodium reabsorption and potassium excretion in the kidney. Primary aldosteronism is a syndrome of hypertension and spontaneous hypokalemia associated with elevated plasma aldosterone concentrations and low plasma renin activity.[57] In primary aldosteronism plasma renin activity (PRA) is suppressed secondary to the autonomous elevation of plasma aldosterone. The prevalence of primary aldosteronism in the hypertensive population probably is less than 1%.[58,59] This is a potentially curable disease.[58] The prevalence of primary aldosteronism in hypertensive, spontaneous hypokalemic patients may be as much as 50%. It may occur predominantly in females. Peak age at diagnosis is between the third and fifth decades.[59] Clinical findings, next to hypertension, are primarily due to the hypokalemic state, which is absent in 10 to 20% of patients.[59,60] Symptoms include muscular weakness, parasthesias, polyuria, polydipsia, periodic paralysis, and tetany.[59]

CLASSIFICATION

Primary aldosteronism can be classified based on anatomic and biochemical findings. About 60% of patients with primary aldosteronism have an aldosterone-producing adenoma (APA); 40% have bilateral adrenal hyperplasia.[59] Aldosterone-producing adenoma is generally unilateral and can be cured surgically. Adenomas typically have higher aldosterone plasma concentrations and are typically smaller than 2 cm.[59] In normal subjects an increase in angiotensin II, as in the upright position or with dehydration, leads to increase in plasma aldosterone concentration (PAC). In patients with APA the PAC tends not to change or paradoxically decrease on upright posture.[57]

Bilateral adrenal hyperplasia occurs more frequently in older patients and can present in various forms. Idiopathic hyperaldosteronism (IHA) is due to diffuse hyperplasia and is the most frequent form. Plasma aldosterone concentration usually increases in the upright position, indicating renin responsiveness, and 18-OH-corticosterone increases less than with APA. Macronodular hyperplasia biochemically mimics APA but is rare.[57]

Glucocorticoid suppressible hyperaldosteronism is a familial disorder.[58] Patients are diagnosed at a young age and there are no gross adrenal abnormalities, pathologically characterized by bilateral micronodular hyperplasia. Patients typically respond to replacement glucocorticoid therapy.

Adrenal carcinoma is a very rare cause of primary aldosteronism; PAC can be markedly elevated. Usually tumors are large (> 30 g).[61]

DIAGNOSIS

Patients with unprovoked hypokalaemia should be evaluated for PA. All medication that can interfere with the renin-angiotensin system should be discontinued. First, primary aldosteronism needs to be demonstrated biochemically. A useful screening test is 24-hour urinary potassium excretion. If this value is over 30 mEq/day, it is very suggestive for mineralocorticoid overactivity in patients with low serum potassium and normal sodium intake.[62] Sodium restriction can decrease renal potassium wasting.[58] Another screening test is the concomitant measurement of PAC and PRA. The higher the PAC/PRA ratio, the higher the suspicion for primary aldosteronism (e.g., >40).[62] It is important to measure both, because many patients with essential hypertension have low PRA. These values change with position and sodium intake.[58] Because both renin and aldosterone secretion are controlled in part by the level of sodium intake, 24-hour urinary sodium excretion should be measured just before sampling for renin and aldosterone.

The diagnosis of primary aldosteronism is confirmed by increased urinary excretion of aldosterone in the setting of normal sodium intake and suppressed PRA[59,63] or by non-suppressibility of PAC by saline infusion demonstrated by PA of more than 10 ng/dL.[59]

Secondary hyperaldosteronism can be ruled out if plasma renin activity is not suppressed, as seen in cirrhosis, hypoalbuminemia, congestive heart failure, malignant hypertension, renal artery stenosis, renin-producing tumors, and Bartter's syndrome. Laxatives and diuretics can cause hypokalemia. Cushing's syndrome, certain types of congenital adrenal hyperplasia, licorice, and chewing tobacco can cause hypokalemia and hypertension.[58,63]

ADDITIONAL TESTING

The next step is to distinguish between APA and IHA, because the treatment of choice is surgical in APA, whereas medical treatment is indicated for IHA.[59] During the diagnostic workup, alpha methyldopa and alpha-blockers are preferred as antihypertensive agents because they do not interfere with the diagnostic workup. Potassium supplements should be given to correct the hypokalemia. Serum potassium should be greater than 3.5 mEq/L. Plasma aldosterone concentration and urinary aldosterone excretion tend to be more markedly increased in APA. 18-OH-corticosterone is usually more than 100 μg/dL in APA.[57] After overnight supine position measurements of PAC at 8 A.M. and after 4 hours of upright posture will show an increase in PAC in most patients with IHA, presumably because it is under partial angiotensin control. Patients with APA usually do not respond to the upright posture and can even show a paradoxical decrease in PAC.[59] It is of great importance in all these studies that patients are in sodium balance with a diet containing more than 100 mEq Na for several days.

IMAGING

In many institutions adrenal CT scanning is the first study done after a biochemical diagnosis of primary aldosteronism. Because aldosterone-producing adenomas tend to be small, a high-resolution technique should be employed. Patients with IHA can have normal-appearing adrenal glands or hyperplastic nodules. Bilateral APA is rare, but incidentally discovered adrenal masses are common, and these may

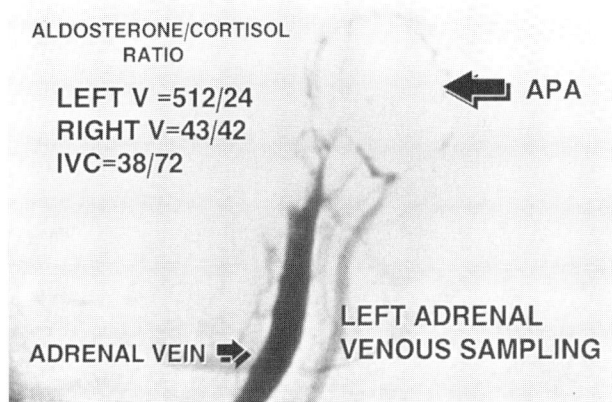

Figure 27–9. CT of aldosteronoma (**A**), confirmed with adrenal venous sampling (**B**). The depiction of the mass with venous injecton is incidental and not necessary for diagnosis.

cause confusion.[62] Thus the finding of an adrenal mass on CT is not necessarily diagnostic of APA. Diagnostic accuracy has varied from 73 to 90%.[62,64–66] If combined use of results of endocrine studies and CT findings are not satisfactory to manage the individual patient,[67] other diagnostic modalities are available. Bilateral adrenal vein sampling is invasive and technically difficult but is viewed as the gold standard. Iodocholesterol scintigraphy occasionally has false-negative results in IHA.[59,62] Both studies employ signs of lateralization.

Although CT is generally accepted as the primary imaging modality for primary aldosteronism, there is considerable controversy about the implications of the CT findings and how these relate to the patient's endocrine studies. The CT findings can be divided into three main categories: unilateral nodule, bilateral nodules, and normal or hyperplastic glands.

A unilateral mass detected with CT is reliable evidence of an aldosteronoma as the cause of the clinical syndrome,[66] but only if endocrine studies also indicate this diagnosis (Fig. 27–9). If both endocrine studies and CT are in agreement, a diagnosis can be made, but if they differ other studies such as NP-59 scanning or adrenal venous sampling are necessary.[42,67]

Bilateral nodules at CT cause the greatest diagnostic dilemma. These most likely represent IHA (Fig. 27–10), but the rare bilateral aldosterone-producing adenomas (APA) are also a possibility, as is an aldosteronoma in association with an incidental nonfunctioning nodule.[42] Diagnosis is dependent on correlation of endocrine and clinical data. If endocrine studies are in favor of hyperplasia, a trial of medical therapy is justified. However, if clinical studies are equivocal, then the possibility of a unilateral or, less likely, bilateral adenoma must be excluded with further studies such as adrenal venous sampling.

The reliability of CT is decreased when bilateral nodules are detected. Most missed adenomas occurred in this group of patients.[68] Adrenal venous sampling in these patients will provide a more accurate diagnosis but does require an invasive study.[42,68] If technically successful, venous sampling has an accuracy of approximately 95% not only for localizing the side of an aldosteronoma, but also in separating unilateral from bilateral disease.[50] Aldosterone/cortisol ratios are measured for the right and left adrenal veins as well as the inferior vena cava. A ratio of greater than 1.5 between the aldosterone/cortisol ratio in an adrenal vein compared with the aldosterone/cortisol ratio in the inferior vena cava is indicative of an aldosteronoma in that gland.[50] Ratios greater than 1.5 from both adrenal veins as compared with the inferior vena cava indicate hyperplasia.[50] ACTH stimulation with adrenal vein sampling increases diagnostic accuracy. An aldosterone/cortisol level on the "normal" side that remains below the peripheral vein ratio is strong evidence against hyperplasia, which would produce a bilateral response to ACTH.[42]

With normal-appearing or diffusely enlarged glands there must be correlation with endocrine studies to diagnose IHA. Without this correlation a small unilateral adenoma could be overlooked; therefore either adrenal venous sampling[42] or

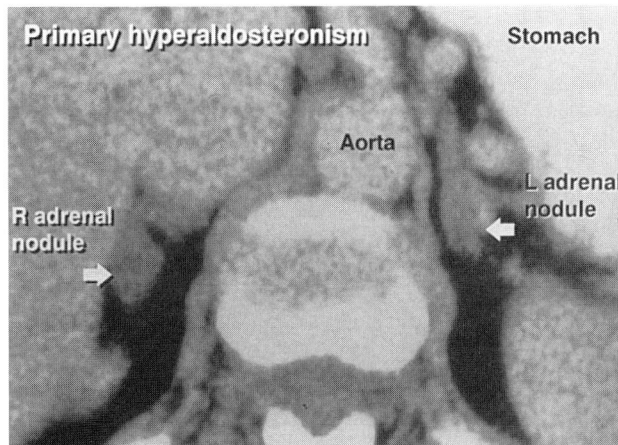

Figure 27–10. CT of bilateral adrenal nodules in a patient with primary aldosteronism.

NP-59 studies are needed. A negative CT does not have the same reliability as a positive study and does not exclude adenoma.[66]

The NP-59 isotope scan has shown variable sensitivity and specificity for detection of aldosteronomas (Fig. 27–11).[34,65,69] It does take several days to perform and is not generally available because it is not FDA approved. If NP-59 is available it would be the next logical test if the combination of CT and clinical studies does not give a definitive diagnosis.

Ultrasound has no significant use in the diagnosis of primary aldosteronism. Yamakita used ultrasound in studying 13 patients with aldosterone-producing adenoma and detected fewer than 50% of the adenomas. This was improved with a second study but was still inferior to CT.[17]

Imaging Summary.

Computed tomography—primary study
Adrenal venous sampling—needed if CT and clinical data do not agree or are equivocal (and if the patient is a good surgical candidate)

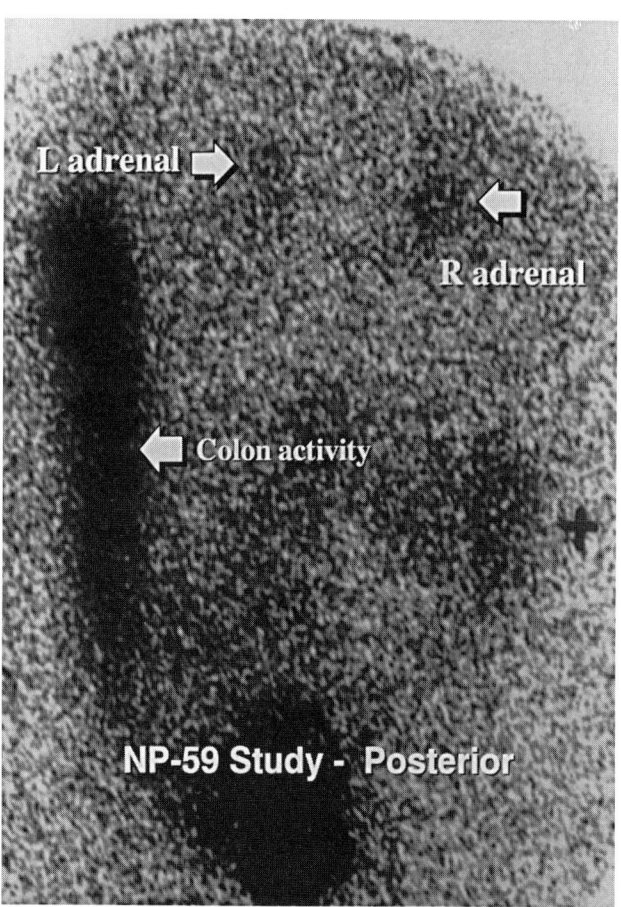

Figure 27–11. Incorrect NP-59 diagnosis. Increased activity bilaterally was interpreted as hyperplasia, but subsequent tests and surgery proved a diagnosis of right-sided aldosteronoma.

NP-59—alternate to adrenal venous sampling as a secondary procedure, if available.

TREATMENT

Only surgery can offer cure for patients with APA. If a 100% cure is not achieved, hypokalemia and hypertension are easier to control medically.[59] In poor surgical candidates and in patients with IHA, medical treatment is indicated.

Spironolactone, an aldosterone receptor blocker, is used in doses from 100 to 400 mg/day. Hypokalemia responds more promptly than hypertension, and hypertension may be resistant to spironolactone in IHA.[57,62] In male patients high doses of spironolactone can have serious side effects because it blocks androgen synthesis and action. Patients unable to tolerate this medication may also be treated with potassium-sparing diuretics such as amiloride or triamterene.[57,62] Also, angiotensin-converting enzyme inhibitors can present an alternative.[59]

Pheochromocytoma

DEFINITION

The clinical diagnosis of pheochromocytoma is made when a catecholamine-producing tumor is demonstrated. A catecholamine-producing tumor can be found anywhere in the paraganglion system, composed of chromaffin cells originating from the neural crest.[70,71] The majority of clinical pheochromocytomas arise from the adrenal medulla, with only 10% being extra-adrenal (usually called functioning paragangliomas) in the adult population[70] and less than 10% being bilateral. The majority of extra-adrenal pheochromocytomas are intra-abdominal.[72] Malignancy is often difficult to demonstrate pathologically. The reported incidence for adrenal pheochromocytomas ranges from 3 to 14%.[70] In familial pheochromocytomas and in children the incidence of bilateral adrenal and extra-adrenal disease is generally higher.[71,73] Pheochromocytomas can occur as sporadic disease (90%) and as familial syndromes (10%). They can also be part of several distinct clinical syndromes, such as von Hippel–Lindau, multiple endocrine neoplasia II, neurofibromatosis, tuberous sclerosis, and Sturge–Weber syndrome, all of which frequently are familial diseases.[74] Atypical presentations were noted by Kotzerke who recommended aggressive screening for pheochromocytomas in Multiple Endocrine Neoplasia families. These lesions, which can be a major cause of death in these families, can often be detected by age 30 with an extensive workup. Kotzerke found MIBG to be the most sensitive screening study for this group of patients.[75] A recently discovered familial form of pheochromocytoma is called familial extra-adrenal pheochromocytoma.[76]

Although an uncommon cause of hypertension (<1%) pheochromocytomas are potentially fatal. However, they can be cured surgically, which makes diagnosis crucial. The diagnosis is usually best established with clinical and laboratory data, leaving imaging to determine the location of the lesion.[33]

The most common symptoms in pheochromocytomas are severe or accelerated hypertension, lability of blood pressure, and paroxysms (''spells'') of palpitations, diaphoresis, and headache.[70] In a normotensive patient and in the absence of these paroxysms, more than 99.9% of pheochromocytomas are clinically excluded.[77] Other associated symptoms include pallor, anxiety, visual disturbances, weakness, fatigue, nausea, vomiting, and chest or abdominal pain.[77] Hypertension or spells during abdominal examination, after trauma, or after glucagon or metoclopromide administration should alert the physician to the possibility of an underlying pheochromocytoma.[70]

DIAGNOSIS

The biochemical diagnosis of pheochromocytoma is based on excessive 24-hour urinary excretion of free catecholamines (norepinephrine and epinephrine) and its metabolites (normetanephrines, metanephrines, and vanillylmandelic acid (VMA).[70] Sensitivity and specificity reports vary for the individual tests and are dependent on the assay. Traditional spectrophotometric and fluorometric methods are replaced by sensitive and specific chromatographic methods.[77,78] Medications (which can also lower catecholamine excretion), exercise, or situations accompanied by stress, such as hospitalization, can elevate urinary excretion of catecholamines and metabolites.[70]

Specificity rises with increase in urinary free catecholamine excretion,[70] with values of more than 150 to 200% usually having good specificity. Sensitivity and specificity for urinary free catecholamines range from 92 to 95% and 92 to 96%, respectively.[70,77] For normetanephrines and metanephrines, corresponding values are 91 to 95% and 95% respectively.[77] For VMA, depending on the upper limit of the normal range, 71 to 100% is found for sensitivity, with specificity approaching 100% for results in tests with a high upper limit of normal. Extra-adrenal pheochromocytomas do not convert norepinephrine to epinephrine, so that in extra-adrenal lesions the urine norepinephrine level is high, whereas in adrenal lesions the urine epinephrine is elevated.[79]

It is advisable to communicate with the laboratory where the assay is performed about possible interfering substances and medications that alter catecholamine excretion or metabolism. Some advocate the use of combined testing of urinary excretion of free catecholamines, and normetanephrines and metanephrines,[77] based on the fact that some tumors may excrete predominantly catecholamines or their metabolites. Timed specimens may be useful in patients with ''spells'' and normal 24-hour urinary excretion.[70]

Other tests in the diagnosis of pheochromocytoma have been used. Plasma measurements of catecholamines are labile and not as sensitive as urinary testing. Clonidine can suppress plasma catecholamine concentration in normal subjects but not in patients with pheochromocytoma.[77,80] It may be useful in selected patients (e.g., when urine studies are borderline abnormal).[81]

IMAGING

The three imaging studies currently used for the detection of pheochromocytoma are CT, MRI, and MIBG scans. Preference often depends on local expertise and availability as well as on the patient population. Referral centers likely to see difficult, recurrent, or multifocal lesions may prefer a ''total body'' type of study such as an MIBG scan, if available. Essentially all institutions have CT available, and most have MRI. Only a few have MIBG available. Experience with each study must also be considered. Most radiologists have experience with CT but fewer are experienced with body MRI.

Pheochromocytomas are usually at least moderate in size. CT, with a sensitivity of 90 to 95%, is the prime screening study.[64,82] Both adrenal and extra-adrenal lesions can be detected with CT, but accuracy for intra-adrenal lesions such as the typical sporadic pheochromocytoma is greater (Fig. 27–12). In nonoperated patients with clear biochemical evidence of pheochromocytoma, CT is the best initial study and will detect most lesions.[83]

MIBG scanning depends on the active transport of the radionuclide into viable tumor cells and is the most specific test for pheochromocytoma, with a sensitivity of approximately 80%.[84] MIBG screens the entire body and is particularly useful for extra-adrenal disease, postoperative situations,[33] and metastatic diseases (Fig. 27–13), where CT is less effective; it is also useful in distinguishing metastatic from locally recurrent disease.[32] Because MIBG is very specific for pheochromocytoma it can be useful when endocrine studies are not conclusive. For these situations[33] and for children in whom extra-adrenal lesions are increased, MIBG can be used as a primary study.[85] Following whole-body scintigraphic screening, more detailed CT or MRI can be performed for any suspicious areas.

MRI can be used both for detection and for characterization of lesions. The high signal intensity on a T2-weighted image (Fig. 12B, 27–14) allows detection of a pheochromocytoma and suggests its etiology. MRI does have a decreased spatial resolution as compared to CT, but the hyperintensity of pheochromocytoma on T2 images can counterbalance the decreased spatial resolution of MRI and allow easier detection of metastatic, recurrent, and extra-adrenal lesions such as those in the bladder or pericardium,[55,64] which may be missed on CT.[86] The very high signal intensity on T2 helps distinguish pheochromocytoma from an adrenal adenoma[64] and can be particularly helpful

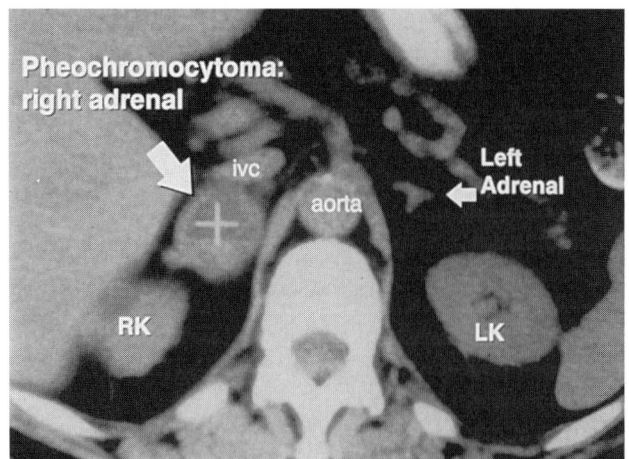
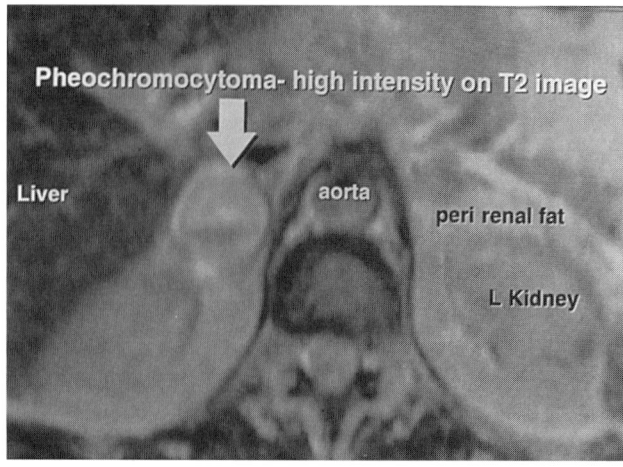

Figure 27–12. CT (**A**) and MRI (**B**) demonstration of pheochromocytoma.

if chemical tests are not conclusive for pheochromocytoma.[55] MRI, however, is not specific with overlap between the appearance of pheochromocytoma and other lesions.[87]

Imaging Summary.

Pheochromocytoma—diagnosis
    Adults—no familial disease
        Computed tomography
        MIBG if CT negative
        MRI
    Adults—familial, recurrent, residual
        MIBG for screening
        CT/MRI—further anatomic detail
    Children
        MIBG for screening
        CT/MRI

TREATMENT

Although patients can be treated medically, surgery is the only available definitive therapy. Medical therapy is used to prepare patients for surgery and has been shown to decrease surgical morbidity.[70] Usually phenoxybenzamine, an alpha-blocker, is started at 20 mg/day in divided doses. Dosing is then increased every several days until patient is normotensive. The maximal dose is usually 80 to 160 mg/day. Complete alpha-blockade may take several weeks and is clinically evident by the presence of normotension and the absence of orthostatic hypotension. Liberal fluid and salt intake will help normalize weight and orthostasis. If tachycardia develops, a beta-blocker can be started only after sufficient alpha-blockade has been achieved.[70,71]

During anesthesia and hypertensive crisis, nitroprusside, phentolamine, and beta-blockers (for life-threatening arrhythmias) have proven to be very useful drugs.[70,71]

Clinically Silent Adrenal Masses

Probably the most common adrenal lesion is the incidentally detected adrenal mass. Patients studied with high-resolution imaging techniques for reasons other than suspected adrenal disease reportedly are diagnosed as having clinically silent

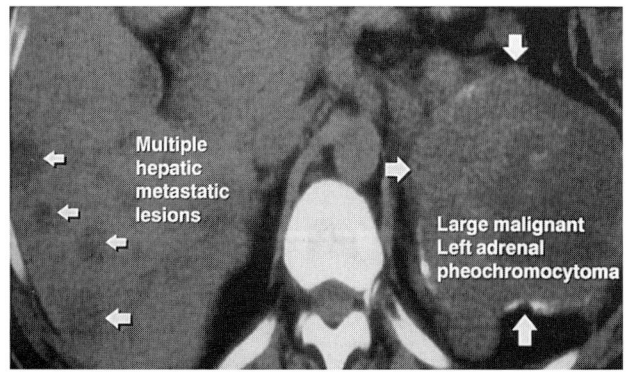
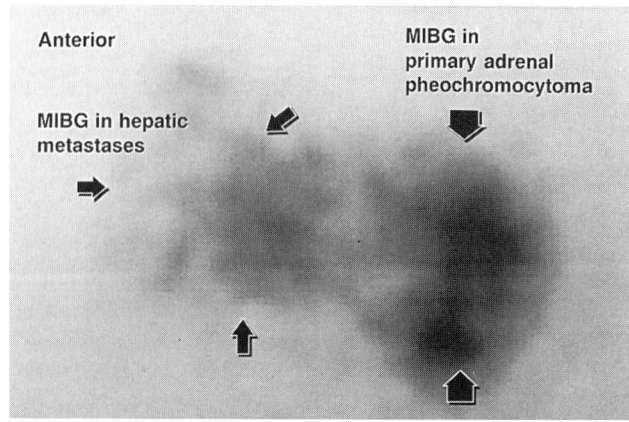

Figure 27–13. CT (**A**) and MIBG (**B**) showing both primary pheochromocytoma and metastatic lesions in the liver.

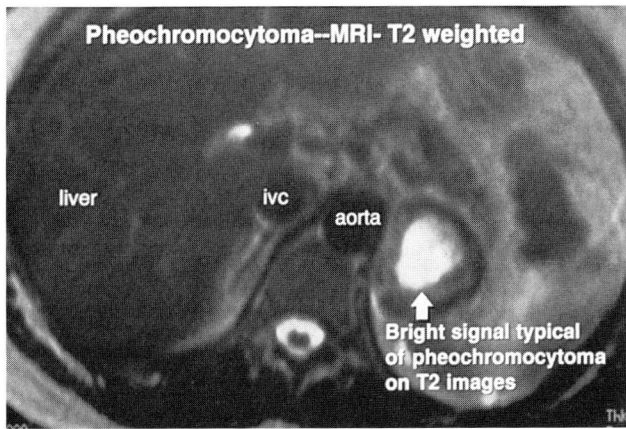

Figure 27–14. (A) MRI of left-sided pheochromocytoma.

adrenal masses in 1 to 10% of cases.[47] Other data indicate that with improved imaging techniques, at least a .6 to 2% of patients undergoing imaging studies for nonadrenal reasons will be incidentally found to have an adrenal mass.[55,88] Autopsy series have documented adrenal masses in 2 to 9% of patients without a history of adrenal disease. Causes of those incidentally discovered adrenal masses are listed in Table 27–3[47]

The evaluation and treatment of those "incidentalomas" remain controversial. By far the most common lesion will be a nonfunctioning benign adenoma. In determining further evaluation or therapy it is necessary to separate these adrenal lesions according to whether the patient does or does not

Table 27–3. Incidentally discovered adrenal masses

Adrenal cortex
  Adenoma
  Nodullar hyperplasia
  Carcinoma
Adrenal medulla
  Pheochromocytoma
  Ganglioneuroma
  Ganglioneuroblastoma
Other adrenal masses
  Myelolipoma
  Neurofibroma
  Hamartoma
  Teratoma
  Xanthomatosis
  Amyloidosis
  Cyst
  Hematoma
  Granulomatosis
Metastases
  Breast carcinoma
  Lung cancer
  Lymphoma
  Leukemia
  Other

Reprinted from Gross MD, Shapiro B: Clinically silent adrenal masses. *Clin Endocrinol Metab* 1993; 77 (4):885-888.

have a primary malignancy. The vast majority of adrenal metastases occurs in the presence of obvious primary disease. Some lung and breast cancers can present, however, with adrenal metastases.[47]

Occasionally, some benign lesions can be diagnosed by CT characteristics alone, such as simple cysts, myelolipomas, and adrenal hemorrhage.[88]

The estimated prevalence of conditions associated with hypersecretion in 100,000 patients with incidentalomas is as follows: pheochromocytoma, 6500; aldosterone-producing adenoma (APA), 7000; glucocorticoid-producing adenoma, 35; and adrenal cancer,[68,88] These estimates are based on certain assumptions but can be of help in clinical decision making. The absence of any type of spell or hypertension makes a pheochromocytoma unlikely. It is generally recommended, however, that all patients with an incidentaloma be screened for a pheochromocytoma, because it is relatively frequent and potentially lethal,[47,88,89] and treatment can be curative. The absence of spontaneous hypokalemia and/or hypertension makes primary aldosteronism unlikely.[88] Because APA can be a relatively frequent finding in patients with incidentaloma, initial screening has been recommended.[47] In the absence of obesity and hypertension Cushing's syndrome is not likely present. Screening in the absence of clinical features of CS is generally not recommended.[47,88]

Feminization and virilization should alert the physician for functioning adrenal tumors or for functioning adrenal carcinoma in the setting of virilization without clinical hypercortisolism.[90] Urinary ketosteroid excretion and serum DHEAS concentration are often high in patients with adrenal cancer.

Bilateral adrenal enlargement can also be a result of chronic pituitary overstimulation, as in Cushing's disease and in congenital adrenal hyperplasia.[91]

DIAGNOSIS: NONONCOLOGY POPULATION

Fine Needle Aspiration Biopsy. In the nononcologic population fine needle aspiration biopsy (FNA) is generally considered not useful because it lacks specificity. It has difficulty differentiating between benign and malignant adrenal lesions.[47,92] Biopsy is most specific for metastatic carcinoma[47] and thus is most useful in the patient with lung or breast cancer and no other known metastatic disease. Before even considering a FNA, a pheochromocytoma has to be ruled out biochemically in every patient because of the possibility of a lethal hypertensive crisis.[47] In cystic lesions, FNA can be helpful. Clear fluid is uniformly associated with benign lesions, whereas bloody fluid can be indicative of either benign or malignant disease.[92,93]

Size and Density as Clinical Factors. In using size of the incidentally discovered adrenal mass to assess the indication for surgery, most authors agree that tumors larger than 5 or 6 cm should be removed,[92,94] unless the mass is clearly cystic

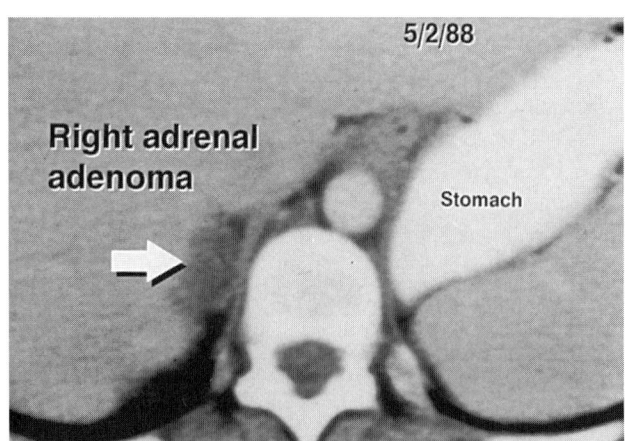 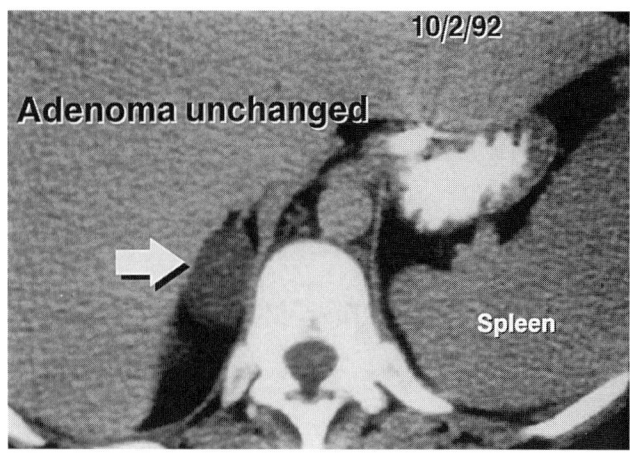

Figure 27–15. (A, B) Typical low-density adrenal adenoma detected incidentally with CT and unchanged over 4 years.

and a cyst puncture shows clear fluid. Lesions less than 3 cm can be observed by serial imaging (e.g., every 3 to 6 months for 1 to 2 years).[95] This leaves a gray zone for masses between 3 and 5 cm where recommendations vary,[47] although statistically most lesions will be benign.[36,96] Within this group younger patients are of more concern.

These lesions will usually be detected with CT and there are CT criteria in addition to size and shape that can increase confidence for a benign lesion. An attenuation coefficient of less than 10 HU on an unenhanced scan has been shown to have a greater than 95% likelihood of being benign (Fig. 27–15).[97] Often an attenuation in this range can be obtained even on an enhanced scan and strongly suggests a benign lesion. This additional information can limit or even eliminate the need for follow-up in this group of patients with no known primary malignancy. Berland has suggested no further follow-up in benign-appearing lesions because of the very low incidence of malignancy and the low cost/benefit ratio of further evaluating these lesions.[98]

Scintigraphy. Iodocholesterol scintigraphy is cumbersome and not widely available, but it is a potentially useful adjunct in the differentiation between benign, functioning (with positive uptake) and malignant, nonfunctioning (with no uptake) lesions.[72] This is especially helpful in the tumors of 3 to 5 or 6 cm in size.

Specific Nonfunctioning Adrenal Lesions.

Adrenal Cyst. Adrenal cysts are uncommon lesions[16,99,100] that unless large enough to produce symptoms, are usually incidentally detected during a radiologic examination. These may be congenital, secondary to neonatal adrenal hemorrhage, acquired as a consequence of infarction, or the consequence of an infection or parasitic infestation such as amoebiasis. Four types of adrenal cyst have been classified: (1) parasitic cysts (7%), (2) epithelial cysts (9%), (3) endothelial cysts (45%), and (4) pseudocysts (39%), which occur secondary to hemorrhage in children and adults.[15] Unless the cyst is associated with an infection or parasitic disease, it usually has no clinical significance other than the mechanical problem posed by renal displacement or distortion. Depending upon the clinical presentation, adrenal cysts may be managed expectantly, by surgical intervention, or by percutaneous aspiration.

Diagnosis of an adrenal cyst depends on the type of cyst. A simple adrenal cyst shows an anechoic appearance with ultrasound, as well as smooth walls and increased through transmission. With CT a simple cyst will be homogeneous, sharply marginated, and of water density.[100] A simple cyst, of insufficient size to cause mechanical problems, can be followed with ultrasound. Large lesions may require percutaneous aspiration[16] or surgery.

Adrenal pseudocysts, which are the second most common type of adrenal cyst, often have a complex appearance on CT or MRI, making differentiation from carcinoma difficult (Fig. 27–16).[100,101] Thick walls, solid-appearing tissue, and even neovascularity on angiography can present a picture indistinguishable from malignancy. These lesions are often the result of previous adrenal hemorrhage.[15,100,101]

Myelolipoma. Although many incidental adrenal lesions detected with CT or ultrasound represent diagnostic dilemmas, myelolipomas generally have sufficiently characteristic features to make a specific diagnosis. The presence of fat within the lesions is usually detected with CT by the negative attenuation numbers, which can range from −30 to −150 (Fig. 27–17).[99] These lesions show an increase in attenuation following contrast enhancement, and although in most cases the fatty nature of the lesion is still apparent on contrast-enhanced scans, the enhancement can occasionally mask the negative attenuation values of the fat. Precontrast scans are therefore needed to avoid errors.[99] Most incidental lesions are detected on enhanced scans being obtained for other reasons. With suspicion that a lesion could be a myelolipoma, a follow-up unenhanced scan would be a simple way to confirm this benign diagnosis. If studied with ultrasound myelolipomas are almost always hyperechoic because of their

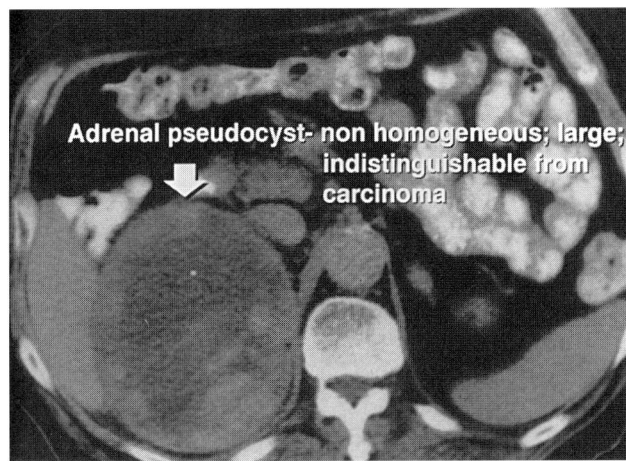

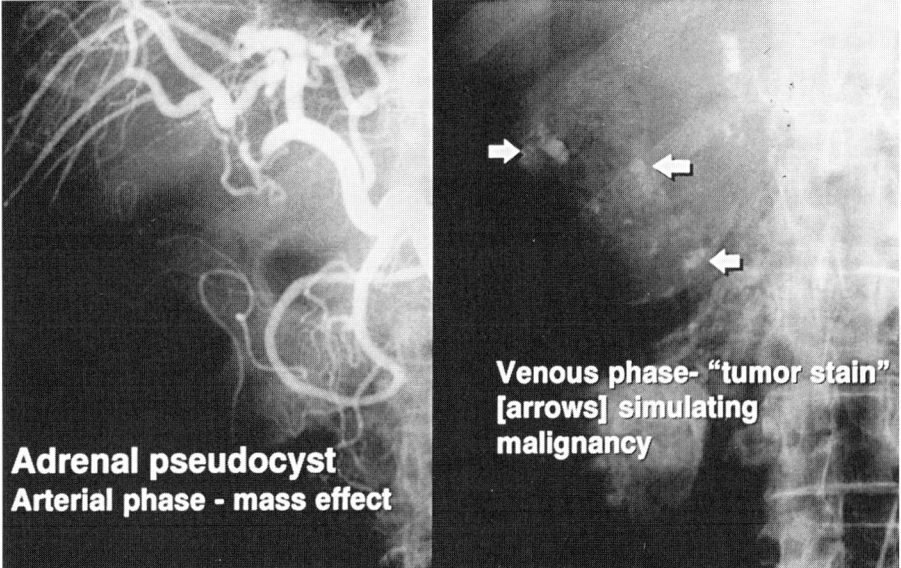

Figure 27–16. Adrenal pseudocyst. (**A**) CT and (**B**) angiography. Neither study clearly differentiates this lesion from adrenal carcinoma.

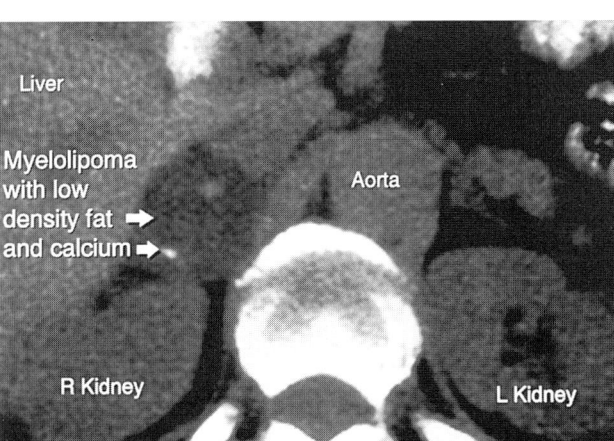

Figure 27–17. CT of a myelolipoma of the right adrenal gland.

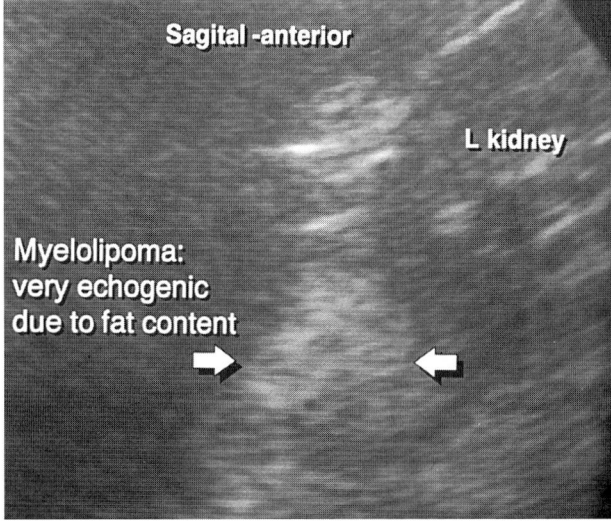

Figure 27–18. Ultrasound of adrenal myelolipoma seen as an echogenic mass.

high fat content (Fig. 27–18).[99] Ultrasound could therefore be useful in clarifying a questionable lesion on CT because this could be done the same day without the need to return for an unenhanced scan. When there is predominantly myeloid tissue the lesions may be hypoechoic and therefore nonspecific.[99]

PATIENTS WITH KNOWN MALIGNANCY

In a patient with a known primary malignancy, evaluation of an adrenal mass is a more complex issue. The adrenal glands are routinely specifically included on chest CT scans because of the high incidence of detecting adrenal metastases in otherwise operable patients.[102,103] Several series evaluating adrenal lesions in patients who were otherwise operable candidates have shown that approximately 50% are benign and 50% are metastatic lesions.[104–108] Any adrenal lesion in this population therefore may represent a metastatic lesion, but the incidence of benign disease is high enough to warrant further studies to resolve this point.

Katz[107] recommended CT-guided FNA on all adrenal masses if there was no other evidence of systemic disease and no clinical evidence of adrenal hyperfunction. She found 13 metastases and 10 adenomas in patients with various primary malignancies. Most metastatic lesions were in patients with lung cancer. Adenomas, however, were also found in lung cancer, breast cancer, and melanoma, all of which have a propensity to metastasize to the adrenals. Biopsy was needed not only to detect metastatic lesions, but to avoid misdiagnosis of a benign adenoma as metastatic.[107] The need for a definitive diagnosis even in this high-risk group was also emphasized by Oliver, who found only 8 of 25 adrenal masses to be metastases in patients with non–small cell carcinoma of the lung. Seventeen of these lesions proved to be adenomas.[105]

In patients with a malignancy likely to metastasize to the adrenals such as breast (54%) or lung (36%) and in whom such a metastasis would change the therapeutic approach, needle biopsy has been used extensively. This is related to the nonspecific appearance of adrenal tumors on CT and the difficulty in separating benign from malignant disease.[105] At present percutaneous biopsy, with an accuracy of greater than 90%,[108–110] is the gold standard short of surgery, and other imaging studies must be compared against this. CT-guided needle biopsy has been shown to be highly accurate not only in confirming metastatic disease, but also in excluding it (Fig. 27–19).[108–110]

The diagnostic options short of biopsy include computed tomography, MRI, and NP-59 scanning. Because most adrenal masses will be detected with CT, it is reasonable to consider this first. The attenuation coefficients of adrenal lesions have been studied in a primarily oncologic population, and an attenuation coefficient of less than 0 HU was found to be 100% accurate for a benign adenoma.[97] This is

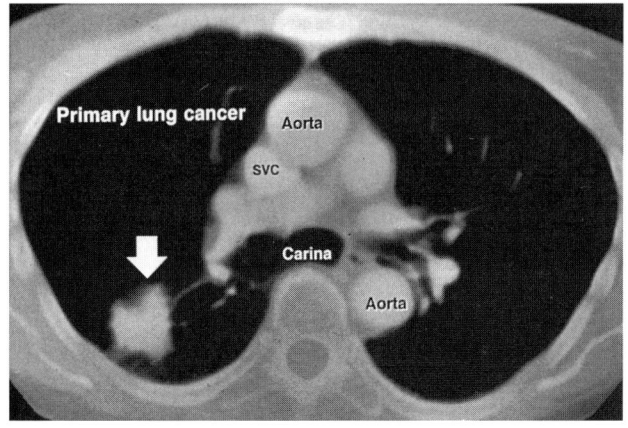

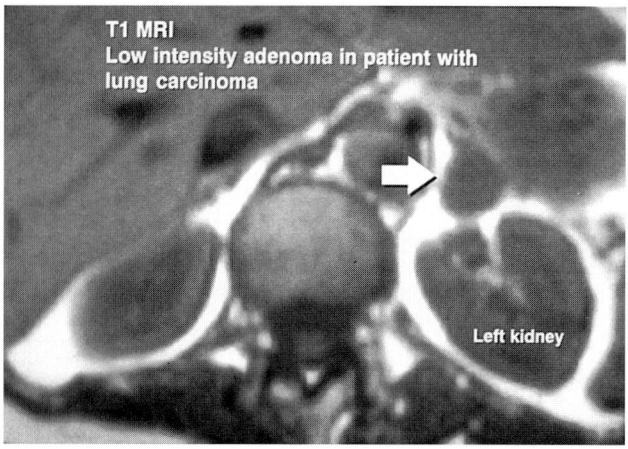

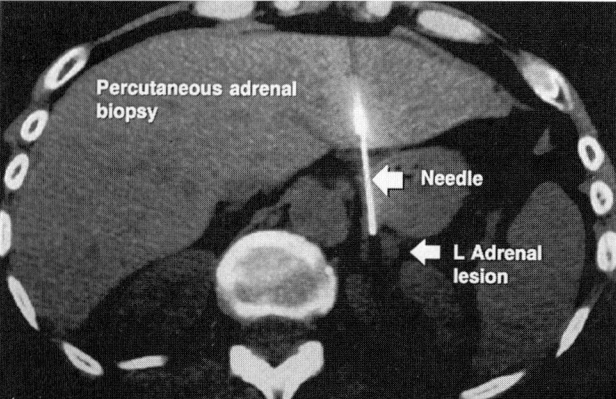

Figure 27–19. (**A**) CT showing primary lung cancer. (**B**) Adrenal MRI most consistent with left adrenal adenoma. (**C**) CT-guided biopsy of adrenal mass.

due to the high cellular fat content of a benign adenoma. Lesions less than 10 HU were also highly likely to be adenoma, but the accuracy dropped to 96%. These data have been substantiated by Korobkin who used a threshold value of +18 Hounsfield units (HU) in separating adenoma from nonadenoma.[111] Dynamic enhanced CT was shown to be accurate in detecting malignant lesions, but many benign lesions were considered indeterminate or malignant.[98]

Multiple studies have been done to evaluate the potential use of MRI in differentiating adrenal lesions. Initial studies showed a tendency for adenomas to have a lower signal intensity compared to the liver on T2 images than did metastases, other malignant lesions, or pheochromocytomas. Considerable overlap was present, however,[112] limiting usefulness in the oncologic population.

Glazer,[23] using a 0.35-T unit, compared the visual and quantitatively measured intensity of adenomas and nonadenomas to liver intensity on T2 images. Nonadenomas were visually more intense in 16 of 19 cases and had an adrenal/liver ratio of .83 more in 19 of 20 cases. Reinig was also able to accurately separate benign adenomas from metastases and other malignant lesions by virtue of the high T2 signal intensity of the latter (Fig. 27–20).[22] Others have found the adrenal mass/fat signal ratio the most useful in separating adenomas from nonadenomas. Lesions with a ratio above 0.8 were malignant and those with a ratio below 0.6 were benign. However, 31% of cases fell between these levels and were indeterminate.[113]

Results using T1-weighted images have been less successful, with approximately one-third of cases falling into an equivocal category.[24] Baker was unable to differentiate adenomas from nonadenomas using a T1 signal intensity ratio,[114] and in contrast to prior studies did not find the adrenal mass liver ratio on T2-weighted images helpful in differentiation of adenomas from other lesions. He did, however, use a 1.5-T unit in contrast to other studies.[23,114]

Krestin compared CT and MR in evaluating adrenal lesions in patients with known primary malignancy and was able to show a greater accuracy with less indeterminate cases when pre- and postcontrast dynamic MR scans were used. Using MR without enhancement gave results similar to those of CT.[25]

The most promising MRI technique is "chemical shift," based on the relatively consistent difference in lipid content between benign and malignant adrenal lesions.[26] Lesions containing a high fat and water content will "cancel out" and have a lower intensity. Tsushima[27] used chemical shift imaging and determined a signal intensity (SI) index = (SI on in phase-SI on out of phase)/(SI on in phase × 100). A positive index occurred if a lesion contained significant fat because this would produce a decreased intensity on the out-of-phase images. All adenomas had an SI of greater than 5%, whereas metastatic lesions and pheochromocytomas were all less than 5%, with no overlapping cases. No significant difference was present between functioning and nonfunctioning adenomas.[27]

Mitchell[26] also used chemical shift imaging to successfully separate benign from malignant lesions. A total of 26 out of 27 benign cortical masses showed a loss of signal intensity on the chemical shift, and no such decrease was demonstrated in 12 metastatic lesions. Relative signal intensity loss on opposed phase imaging was the most accurate technique.[26] Three presentations at the 1994 Roentgen Ray Society Meeting support the value of this technique and indicate a potential for an accuracy high enough to eliminate the need for biopsy in many cases.[28–30]

NP-59, although not as widely used, has shown success in further evaluation of nonfunctioning adrenal lesions. Francis studied 28 lesions; all 14 lesions in which there was definite uptake of NP-59 proved to be adenomas. Those with no uptake were either metastatic lesions (9) or cysts (2). Three cases were indeterminate.[115]

The evaluation of nonfunctioning adrenal masses in the oncology population is still evolving, but it does appear that MR, CT and NP-59 can help characterize lesions and increase the probability of benign versus malignant disease. McNicholas has proposed a combined imaging algorithm which uses noncontrast CT attenuation values as the initial step with chemical-shift MR for indeterminate lesions.[116] Data regarding these techniques are still limited, making it

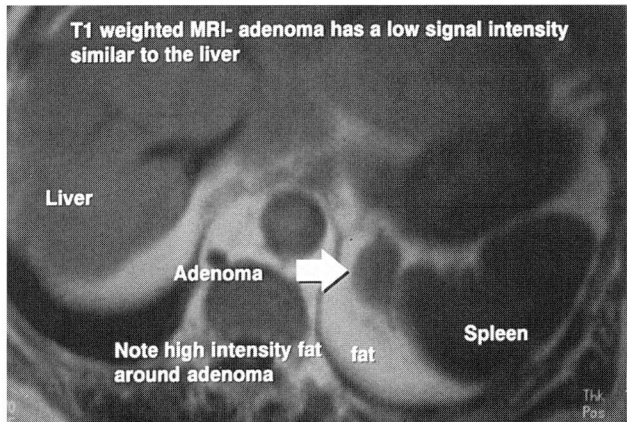
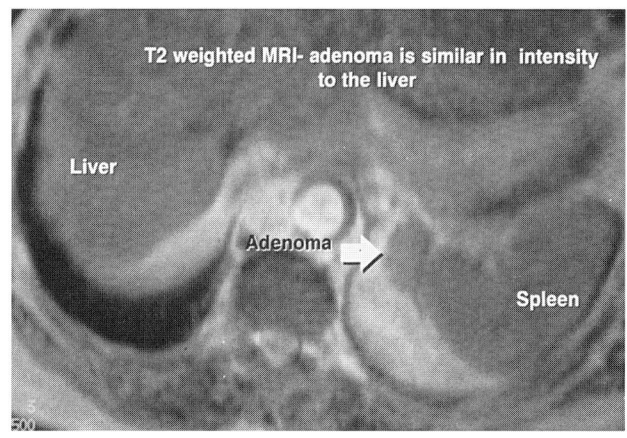

Figure 27–20. MRI of an adrenal adenoma with (**A**) T1 and (**B**) T2 weighting.

difficult to draw definite general conclusions, but in specific cases where biopsy might be more difficult or dangerous they offer an alternate method of diagnosis.

REFERENCES

1. Meyers MA: Disease of the adrenal glands. Springfield, IL: Charles C Thomas, 1963.
2. Starer F: The radiology of suprarenal masses. *Br J Hosp Med* 1970 (August):207.
3. Sutton D: The radiological diagnosis of adrenal tumors. *Br J Radiol* 1975;48:237.
4. Abeshouse GA, Goldstein RB, Abeshouse BS: Adrenal cysts: review of the literature and report of three cases. *J Urol* 1959; 51:711.
5. Glenn JF: Neonatal adrenal hemorrhage. *J Urol* 1962;87:634.
6. Grainger RG, Lloyd GAS, Williams JL: Egg-shell calcifications: a sign of phaeochromocytoma. *Clin Radiol* 1967; 18:282.
7. Kincaid OW, Hodgson JR, Dockerty MB: Neuroblastoma: a roentgenologic and pathological study. *AJR* 1957;78: 420–436.
8. McDonald P, Hiller HG: Angiography in abdominal tumors in childhood with particular reference to neuroblastoma and Wilms' tumor. *Clin Radiol* 1968;19:1.
9. Paster SB, Rosen RT: Calcification in benign adrenal adenomas. *J Urol* 1974;3:646.
10. Yeh H: Adrenal gland and non-renal retroperitoneum. *Urol Radiol* 1987;9:127–140.
11. Gooding GAW: Adrenal, pancreatic and scrotal ultrasound in endocrine disease. *Radiol Clin North Am* 1993;31:1069–1083.
12. Wu C: Sonographic spectrum of neonatal adrenal hemorrhage: report of a case simulating solid tumor. *J Clin Ultrasound* 1989; 17:45–49.
13. Lillehei KO, Chandler WF, Knake JE: Real time ultrasound characteristics of the acute intracerebral hemorrhage as studied in the canine model. *Neurosurgery* 1984;14:48–51.
14. Coelho JCU, Sigel B, Ryva JC, et al: B-mode sonography of blood clots. *J Clin Ultrasound* 1982;10:323–327.
15. Barki Y, Eilig I, Moses M, Golcman L: Sonographic diagnosis of a large hemorrhagic adrenal cyst in an adult. *J Clin Ultrasound* 1987;15:194–197.
16. Tung GA, Pfister RC, Papanicolaou N, Yoder IC: Adrenal cysts: imaging and percutaneous aspiration. *Radiology* 1989; 173:107–110.
17. Yamakita N, Yasuda K, Miura K: Ultrasonography in the diagnosis of aldosterone-producing adenoma: is it useful? *Inter Med* 1992;31:589–582.
18. Montagne JP, Kressel HY, Korobkin M, Moss AA: Computed tomography of the normal adrenal glands. *AJR* 1978; 130: 963–967.
19. Chang A, Glazer HS, Lee JKT, et al: Adrenal gland: MR imaging. *Radiology* 1987;163:123–128.
20. Reinig JW: MR imaging differentiation of adrenal masses: has the time finally come? *Radiology* 1992;185:339–340.
21. Geatti O, Shapiro B: Adrenal cortical adenoma causing Cushings's syndrome: correct localization by functional scintigraphy despite nonlocalizing morphological imaging studies. *Clin Nucl Med* 1990;15:168–171.
22. Reinig JW, Doppman JL, Dwyer AJ, et al: Adrenal masses differentiated by MR. *Radiology* 1986;158:81–84.
23. Glazer GM, Woolsey EJ, Borrello J, et al: Adrenal tissue characterization using MR imaging. *Radiology* 1986;158:73–79.
24. Chezmar JL, Robbins SM, Nelson RC, et al: Adrenal masses: characterization with T1-weighted MR imaging. *Radiology* 1988;166:357–359.
25. Krestin GP, Friedman G, Fishbach R, et al: Evaluation of adrenal masses in oncologic patients: dynamic contrast-enhanced MR vs CT. *Comput Assist Tomogr* 1991;15(1):104–110.
26. Mitchell DG, Crovello BS, Matteucci T, et al: Benign adrenocortical masses: diagnosis with chemical shift MR imaging. *Radiology* 1992;185:345–351.
27. Tsushima Y, Ishizaka H, Matsumoto M: Adrenal masses: differentiation with chemical shift, fast low-angle shot MR imaging. *Radiology* 1993;186:705–709.
28. Bilbey J, Chan N, Wilkins GE, et al: Characterization of adrenal masses with chemical shift MR imaging. Presented at American Roentgen Ray Society, April 25, 1994, New Orleans, LA.
29. Mayo-Smith W, Lee MJ, Boland GW, et al: Evaluation of adrenal masses with chemical shift imaging. Presented at American Roentgen Ray Society, April 25, 1994, New Orleans, LA.
30. Korobkin M: Differentiation of adrenal adenomas from nonadenomas using chemical shift and gadolinium enhanced MR imaging. Presented at American Roentgen Ray Society, April 25, 1994, New Orleans, LA.
31. Sandler MP, Delbeke D: Radionuclides in endocrine imaging. *Radiol Clin North Am* 1993;31:909–921.
32. Gross MD, Shapiro B: Scintigraphic studies in adrenal hypertension. *Semin Nucl Med* 1989;19:122–143.
33. Velchik VG, Alavi A, Kressel HY, et al: Localization of pheochromocytoma: MIBG, CT, and MRI correlation. *J Nucl Med* 1989;30:328–336.
34. Lamki M, Haynie TP: Role of adrenal imaging in surgical management. *J Surg Oncolo* 1990;43:139–147.
35. Liddle GW: Tests of pituitary–adrenal suppressibility in the diagnosis of Cushing's syndrome. *J Clin Endocrinol Metab* 1969;20(12):1539–1561.
36. Siragy HM: Cushing's syndrome. In: Carey RM, ed. *Adrenal Disorders*. New York: Thieme, 1989.
37. Bagshawe KD: Hypokalemia, carcinoma and Cushing's syndrome. *Lancet* 1960;2:284.
38. Schteingart DE: Ectopic secretion of peptides of the proopiomelanocortin family. *Endocrinol Metab Clin North Am* 1991;20(3):453–471.
39. Loriaux DL: The treatment of Cushing's syndrome and adrenal cancer. *Endocrinol Metab Clin North Am* 1991; 20(4):767–771.
40. Schteingart DE: Cushing's syndrome. *Endocrinol Metab Clin North Am* 1989;18(2):311–338.
41. Anon DC, Dindling JW, Fitzgerald PA, et al: Pituitary ACTM dependency of nodular adrenal hyperplasia in Cushing's syndrome. *Am J Med* 1981;71:302–305.
42. Doppman JL: The dilemma of bilateral adrenocortical nodularity in Conn's and Cushing's syndromes. *Radiol Clin North Am* 1993;31:1039–1050.
43. Hutter AM, Kayhoc DE: Adrenal cortical carcinoma: clinical features of 138 patients. *Am J Med* 1966;41:572–580.
44. Kaye TB, Crapo L: The Cushing syndrome: an update on diagnostic tests. *Ann Intern Med* 1990;112(6):434–444.
45. Odell WD: Bronchial and thymic carcinoids and the ectopic ACTM syndrome. *Am Thorac Surg* 1990;60:5–6.
46. Flack MR, Oldfield EH, Cutler GB, et al: Urine free cortisol in the high-dose dexamethasone suppression test for the differential diagnosis of the Cushing syndrome. *Ann Intern Med* 1992;116(3):211–217.
47. Gross MD, Shapiro B: Clinical review 50: clinically silent adrenal masses. *J Clin Endocrinol Metab* 1993;77(4):885–888.

48. Motlich ME, Russell EJ: The pituitary "incidentiloma." *Ann Int Med* 1990;112:925–931.
49. Ludecke DK: Transnasal microsurgery of Cushing's disease 1990: overview including personal experience with 256 patients. *Pathol Res Pract* 1991;187(5):608–612.
50. Miller DM: Endocrine angiography and venous sampling. *Radiol Clin North Am* 1993;31:1051–1067.
51. Zeiger MA, Nieman LK, Cutler GP, et al: Primary bilateral adrenocortical causes of Cushing's syndrome. *Surgery* 1991;110:1106–1115.
52. Doppman JL, Travis WD, Nieman L, et al. Cushing syndrome due to primary pigmented nodular adrenocortical disease: findings at CT and MR imaging. *Radiology* 1989;172:415–420.
53. Shamma FN, Abrahams JJ: Imaging in endocrine disorders. *Repro Med* 1992;37:39–45.
54. Harris RD, Herwig KR: Unusual cause for recurrent Cushing syndrome and its diagnosis by computed tomography and NP-59 radiocholesterol scanning. *Urology* 1990;36(3):277–279.
55. Bretan PN Jr., Lorig R: Adrenal imaging: computed tomographic scanning and magnetic resonance imaging. *Urol Clin North Am* 1989;16(3):505–513.
56. Constine LS, Woolf PD, Cann D, et al: Hypothalamic–pituitary dysfunction after radiation for brain tumors. *N Engl J Med* 1993;328:87–94.
57. Siragy HM, Carey RM: Management of primary aldosteronism. *Drug Ther* 1986, 89–101.
58. Noth RH, Biglieri EG: Primary hyperaldosteronism. *Med Clin North Am* 1988;72(5): 1117–1130.
59. Melby JC: Clinical review. 1: Endocrine hypertension. *J Clin Endocrinol Metab* 1989;69(4):697–703.
60. Conn JW, Rovner DR, Cohen EL, Nesbit RM: Normokalemic primary aldosteronism: its masquerade as "essential hypertension." *JAMA* 1966;195(1):111–116.
61. Neville AM, Symington T. Pathology of primary aldosteronism. *Cancer* 1966;12:1854.
62. Young WF Jr, Hogan MJ, Klee GG, et al: Primary aldosteronism: diagnosis and treatment. *Mayo Clin Proc* 1990;65(1):96–110.
63. Case records of the Massachusetts General Hospital, Case 24–1192. *N Engl J Med* 1992;326(24):1617–1623.
64. Dunnick NR. Adrenal imaging: current status. *AJR* 1990;154:927–936.
65. Ikeda DM, Francis IR, Glazer GM, et al: The detection of adrenal tumors and hyperplasia in patients with primary aldosteronism: comparison of scintigraphy, CT, and MR imaging. *AJR* 1989;153:301–306.
66. Dunnick NR, Leight GS, Roubidoux MA, et al: CT in the diagnosis of primary aldosteronism: sensitivity in 29 patients. *AJR* 1993;160:321–324.
67. Radin RD, Manoogian C, Nadler JL: Diagnosis of primary hyperaldosteronism: importance of correlating CT findings with endocrinologic studies. *AJR* 1992;158:553–557.
68. Doppman JL, Gill JR Jr, Miller DL, et al: Distinction between hyperaldosteronism due to bilateral hyperplasia and unilateral aldosteronoma: reliability of CT. *Radiology* 1992;184:677–682.
69. Kazerooni EA, Sisson JC, Shapiro B, et al: Diagnostic accuracy and pitfalls of (Iodine-131) 6-Beta-Iodomethyl-19 Norcholesterol (NP59) imaging. *J Nucl Med* 1990;31:526–534.
70. Sheps SG, Jiang NS, Klee GG, et al: Recent developments in the diagnosis and treatment of pheochromocytoma. *Mayo Clin Proc* 1990;65(1):88–95.
71. Whalen RK, Althausen AF, Daniels GH: Extra-adrenal pheochromocytoma. *J Urol* 1992;147:1–10.
72. Francis IR, Gross MD, Shapiro B, et al: Integrated imaging of adrenal disease. *Radiology* 1992;184(1):1–13.
73. Fonkalsrud EW: Pheochromocytoma in childhood. *Prog Pediatr Surg* 1991;26:103–111.
74. Kalff V, Shapiro B, Lloyd R, et al: The spectrum of pheochromocytoma in hypertensive patients with neurofibromatosis. *Arch Intern Med* 1982;142(12):2092–2098.
75. Kotzerke J, Stibane C, Dralle H, et al: Screening for pheochromocytoma in the MEN 2 syndrome. *Henry Ford Hosp Med J* 1989;37:129–131.
76. Greene JP, Guay AP: New perspectives in pheochromocytoma. *Urol Clin North Am* 1989;16:487–503.
77. Stein PP, Black HR: A simplified approach to pheochromocytoma: a review of the literature and report of one institution's experience. *Medicine* 1991;70(1):46–66.
78. Rosano TG, Swift TA, Hayes LW: Advances in catecholamine and metabolite measurements for diagnosis of pheochromocytoma. *Clin Chem* 1991;37(10, pt 2):1854–1867.
79. Shimizu H, Ueda Y, Makino K, et al: Multiple endocrine neoplasia type 2A. *Intern Med* 1992;31:798–802.
80. Bravo EL, Tarazi RC, Fouad FM, et al: Clonidine-suppression test. *N Engl J Med* 1981;305(11):623–626.
81. Sjoberg RJ, Simcic KJ, Kidd GS: The clonidine suppression test for pheochromocytoma. *Arch Intern Med* 1992;152:1193–1197.
82. Radin RD, Ralls PW, Boswell DW, et al: Pheochromocytoma: detection by unenhanced CT. *AJR* 1986;146:741–744.
83. Maurea S, Cuocolo A, Reynolds JC, et al: Iodine-131-metaiodobenzylguanidine scintigraphy in preoperative and postoperative evaluation of paragangliomas: comparison with CT and MRI. *Nucl Med* 1993;34:173–179.
84. Schwarz RJ, Schmidt N: Efficient management of adrenal tumors. *Am Surg* 1991;161:576–579.
85. Khafagi FA, Shapiro B, Fisher M, et al: Phaeochromocytoma and functioning paraganglioma in childhood and adolescence: role of iodine 131 metaiodobenzylguanidine. *Eur J Nucl Med* 1991;18:191–198.
86. Beland SS, Vesely DL, Watson CA, et al: Localization of adrenal and extraadrenal pheochromocytomas by magnetic resonance imaging. *South Med J* 1989;82:1410–1413.
87. Lee MJ: Characterization of adrenal pheochromocytoma: diagnostic specificity of MR imaging. Presented at American Roentgen Ray Society, April 25, 1994, New Orleans, LA.
88. Ross NS, Aron DC: Hormonal evaluation of the patient with an incidentally discovered adrenal mass. *N Engl J Med* 1990;323(20):1401–1405.
89. Edwards GA, Smythe GA, Graham PE, et al: The impact of recent advances in diagnostic technology on the clinical presentation of phaeochromocytoma *Med J Aust* 1992;156:153–157.
90. Bertagna C, Orth DN: Clinical and laboratory findings and results of therapy in 58 patients with adrenocortical tumors admitted to a single medical center (1951 to 1978). *Am J Med* 1981;71:855–875.
91. Mokshagundam S, Surks MI: Congenital adrenal hyperplasia diagnosed in a man during workup for bilateral adrenal masses. *Arch Intern Med* 1993;153:1389–1391.
92. Copeland PM: The incidentally discovered adrenal mass. *Ann Surg* 1983;199(1):116–122.
93. Copeland PM: The incidentally discovered adrenal mass. *Ann Intern Med* 1983;98:940–945.
94. Khafagi FA, Gross MD, Shapiro B et al: Clinical significance of the large adrenal mass. *Br J Surg* 1991;78:828–833.
95. Older RA, Moore AV Jr, Glenn JF, et al: Diagnosis of adrenal disorders. *Radiol Clin North Am* 1984;22:433–455.
96. Bernardino ME: Management of the asymptomatic patient with a unilateral adrenal mass. *Radiology* 1988;166:121–123.

97. Lee MJ, Hahn PJ, Papanicolaou N, et al: Benign and malignant adrenal masses: CT distinction with attenuation coefficients, size and observer analysis. *Radiology* 1991;179:415–418.
98. Berland LL, Koslin DB, Kenney PJ, et al: Differentiation between small benign and malignant adrenal masses with dynamic incremented CT. *AJR* 1988;151:95–101.
99. Musante F, Derchi LE, Zappasodi F, et al: Myelolipoma of the adrenal gland: sonographic and CT features. *AJR* 1988; 151:961–964.
100. Johnson CD, Baker ME, Dunnick NR: CT demonstration of an adrenal pseudocyst. *J Compu Assis Tomogr* 1985;9:817–819.
101. Aisen AM, Ohl DA, Chenevert DL, et al: MR of an adrenal pseudocyst. *Magn Reson Imaging* 1992;10:997–1000.
102. Whittlesey D: Prospective computed tomographic scanning in the staging of bronchogenic carcinoma. *J Thorac Cardiovasc Surg* 1988;95:876–882.
103. Nielsen ME Jr, Heaston DK, Dunnick NR, et al: Preoperative CT evaluation of adrenal glands in non–small cell bronchogenic carcinoma. *AJR* 1982;139:317–320.
104. Ettinghausen SE, Burt ME: Prospective evaluation of unilateral adrenal masses in patients with operable non-small-cell lung cancer. *J Clin Oncol* 1991;9:1462–1466.
105. Oliver TW Jr., Bernardino ME, Miller JI, et al: Isolated adrenal masses in non-small-cell bronchogenic carcinoma. *Radiology* 1984;153:217–218.
106. Pagani JJ: Non–small cell lung carcinoma adrenal metastases: computed tomography and percutaneous needle biopsy in their diagnosis. *Cancer* 1984;53:1058–1060.
107. Katz RL, Shirkoda A: Diagnostic approach to incidental adrenal nodules in the cancer patient: results of a clinical, radiologic and fine-needle aspiration study. *Cancer* 1985; 55:1995–2005.
108. Bernardino ME, Walther MM, Phillips VM, et al: CT guided adrenal biopsy: accuracy, safety and indications. *AJR* 1985; 144:67–69.
109. Berkman WA, Bernardino ME, Sewell CW, et al: The computed tomography–guided adrenal biopsy: an alternative to surgery in adrenal mass diagnosis. *Cancer* 1984;53:1098–2103.
110. Heaston DK, Handel DB, Ashton PR, et al: Narrow gauge needle aspiration of solid adrenal masses. *AJR* 1981; 138:1143–1148.
111. Korobkin M, Brodeur FJ, Yutzy GG, et al: Differentiation of adrenal adenomas from nonadenomas using CT attentuation values. *AJR* 1996 (in press)
112. Falke THM, te Strake L, Shaff MI, et al: MR imaging of the adrenals: correlation with computed tomography. *J Comput Assist Tomogr* 1986;10:242–253.
113. Chang A, Glazer HS, Lee JKT, et al: Adrenal gland: MR imaging. *Radiology* 1987;163:123–128.
114. Baker ME, Blinder R, Spritzer C, et al: MR evaluation of adrenal masses at 1.5 T. *AJR* 1989;153:307–312.
115. Francis IR, Smid A, Gross MD, et al: Adrenal masses in oncologic patients: functional and morphologic evaluation. *Radiology* 1988;166:353–356.
116. McNicholas MMJ, Lee MJ, Mayo-Smith, et al: An imaging algorithm for the differential diagnosis of adrenal adenomas and metastases. *AJR* 1995;165:1453–1459.

28 Renal Transplantation

Bashir R. Sankari, Andrew C. Novick

The success rate of renal transplantation has improved dramatically during the last decade.[1] Newer immunosuppressive agents and improved surgical techniques and postoperative care have contributed to this success rate. Renal transplantation has become the preferred treatment for suitable patients with end-stage renal disease. The participation of urologists in renal transplantation varies with different programs.[2] This involvement includes the various aspects of renal transplantation, from donor and recipient evaluation, surgical procedures, and postoperative immunosuppression and management. The urologists should continue to have an active role in kidney transplantation because they are the surgeons and physicians best suited to understand and manage renal transplant patients.[3] This chapter is intended to give a thorough review of the various problems encountered in renal transplantation and to give the reader a working plan in diagnosing and managing the different disease entities encountered in kidney transplantation.

ACUTE TUBULAR NECROSIS

Acute tubular necrosis (ATN) may occur immediately after kidney transplantation or may follow an initial short period of allograft function. ATN is related to both donor and recipient factors. It is more common in cadaveric kidneys from older donors who have sustained some warm ischemia time or prolonged hypotensive periods requiring increased vasopressors.[4] Prolonged preservation time will subject the kidney to an increased ATN rate. The use of University of Wisconsin intracellular cold flushing and storage solution has resulted in prolongation of cold ischemia preservation time of transplant kidneys.[5] Hypovolemia and low systolic blood pressure in the recipient at the time of engraftment will aggravate the ATN rate. ATN of renal allograft results in oliguria or frank anuria. Use of calcium channel blockers, albumin, osmotic, and loop diuretics may decrease the severity of oliguria.[6] If diuresis does not occur, the patient returns to dialysis with the expectation of recovery of renal function usually within 3 weeks, although the process can take longer. The diagnosis of ATN in renal allograft is by exclusion of other factors. Traditional signs of ATN, such as tubular casts, urine osmolality of 300 mOsm or less, or urine concentration over 60 mEq/L, are not reliable in patients whose native kidneys also elaborate urine.[7] The renal ultrasound is noncontributory. The nuclear renal scan shows a well-perfused kidney with variable uptake of radionuclide, depending on the severity of ATN, with no excretion. As long as the kidney is viable and no signs of rejection occur, one can wait. During this period efforts are made to avoid severe volume depletion. Immunosuppressive therapy is continued. Suggestions exist in the literature that induction with cyclosporine in cadaveric kidney transplant results in an increased ATN rate because of its nephrotoxicity.[8] Many transplant centers have modified their immunosuppressive protocol to include the prophylactic use of an antilymphocyte preparation and to introduce cyclosporine at a later date, when renal allograft diuresis is acceptable.[9] Serial renograms are beneficial in determining the viability of oliguric kidneys in ATN and in predicting recovery or deterioration.[10] At any suggestion of rejection or if the oliguria lasts longer than anticipated, renal allograft biopsy is done to document the process and appropriate therapy is instituted. Current evidence suggests that kidney allografts undergoing an initial period of ATN perform as well over the long term as those that function immediately.[11] ATN of renal allografts results in an increased cost from additional hospitalization, dialysis, and use of antilymphocyte preparation.[12]

RENAL ALLOGRAFT REJECTION

Despite improvement in tissue typing and immunosuppression, renal allograft rejection remains the limiting factor in the success of renal transplantation. Rejection is currently the principal cause of renal allograft failure.[13] The autoimmune response to foreign antigens is complex and not completely understood.[14] Allografts can be damaged by both cellular and humoral mechanisms. Prevention of renal allograft rejection depends on avoiding cytotoxic antibodies against donor antigens and manipulation of the host immune system by various immunosuppressive agents. Renal allograft rejection results in a significant rise of serum creatinine and may be the only sign of an ongoing rejection. Serum creatinine is considered increased if it is 20% more than the baseline.[15] Additional signs depend on the timing of rejection and may include fever, allograft tenderness, and decreased urine output.

Hyperacute Rejection

Hyperacute rejection occurs rapidly, often within minutes of establishing blood flow. The reaction is due to the presence in the recipient of preformed antibodies against antigens of the donor. These antibodies are usually the result of previous blood transfusions in which leukocytes are the source of the sensitizing antigens. Additional causes include pregnancy and a previous allograft.[16] One of the most dramatic examples occurs when kidneys from blood group A or B donors are transplanted into blood group O recipients, who normally process preformed isohemagglutinins against A and B antigens.[17] These grafts are rejected so quickly that they never become vascularized. The diagnosis of hyperacute rejection is clinical and is usually made on the operative field. The donor organ becomes mottled, cyanotic, and swollen, and transplant function ceases. Histologically, the reaction is characterized by heavy platelet deposition, endothelial damage of both large and small vessels, leukocyte clumping in glomerular capillaries, prominent polymorphonuclear leukocyte infiltration, platelet thrombi, and relatively scant lymphocyte infiltration.[18] This rejection process is irreversible, so prevention is essential. Theoretically, hyperacute rejection ought to be preventable by preoperative cross-matching. Current cross-match protocols that include highly sensitive techniques, such as cytotoxicity with antihuman immunoglobulin antibodies and flow cytometry cross-match, have markedly reduced the incidence of hyperacute rejection in kidney transplantation.[19]

Accelerated Rejection

Accelerated rejection occurs between days 1 and 5 posttransplant, too early to be primary acute rejection. It is characterized by an acute decline in renal function following a brief period of allograft function, often associated with local or systemic evidence of inflammation such as fever and allograft tenderness. Hyperacute rejection is probably due to low levels of undetected humoral sensitization to human leukocyte antigen (HLA) or vascular endothelial cell.[20] Cellular immune response is also active in this reaction. Deterioration of renal blood flow on the renal scan is noted. Diagnosis depends on histologic findings on renal allograft biopsy. Vascular lesions with lymphocytic penetration of the endothelium are prominent, with fibrinoid necrosis, interstitial hemorrhage, thrombotic lesions, tubulitis, and focal interstitial infiltrates, usually with small lymphocytes, macrophages, and plasma cells. In severe cases polymorphonuclear leukocytes (polys) are noted in the glomeruli and capillaries (Fig. 28–1). Treatment should be aggressive and prompt. Intravenous methylprednisolone bolus is usually not effective,[21] and primary therapy should include monoclonal antilymphocyte antibodies (OKT$_3$).[22] In severe cases with polys, plasmapheresis should be considered.[23] The outcome of renal allograft following accelerated rejection is usually poor, with severely impaired function and failure within a year.[24]

Acute Rejection

Acute allograft rejection continues to be a common cause of allograft loss in transplantation.[1] It usually occurs 7 days or more after transplantation. The onset is heralded by a rise in serum creatinine, with a variable degree of decreased urine output. Additional signs occur uncommonly, depending on the severity of rejection, and include fever, leukocytosis, hypertension, allograft swelling, and tenderness. In the majority of cases, the diagnosis of renal allograft rejection is

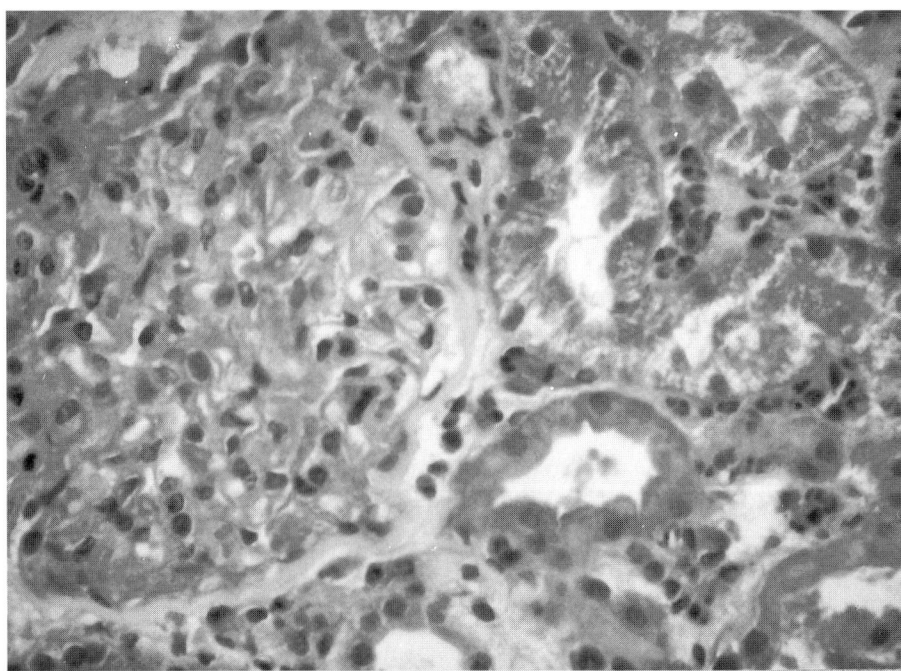

Figure 28–1. Accelerated renal allograft rejection. H&E (hematoxylin and eosin) stain of kidney biopsy revealing vasculitis with inflammatory cells mainly polymorphonuclear around the capillary endothelium and glomerulus (× 250). Patient received a retransplant kidney sharing a common HLA-DR mismatch with his previously failed transplant kidney. Kidney function deteriorated 4 days after surgery. Patient was treated with OKT$_3$ and plasmapheresis, with recovery of kidney function. (Courtesy of Dr. Ho Huang Chang, Department of Pathology, Charleston Area Medical Center, Charleston, WV.)

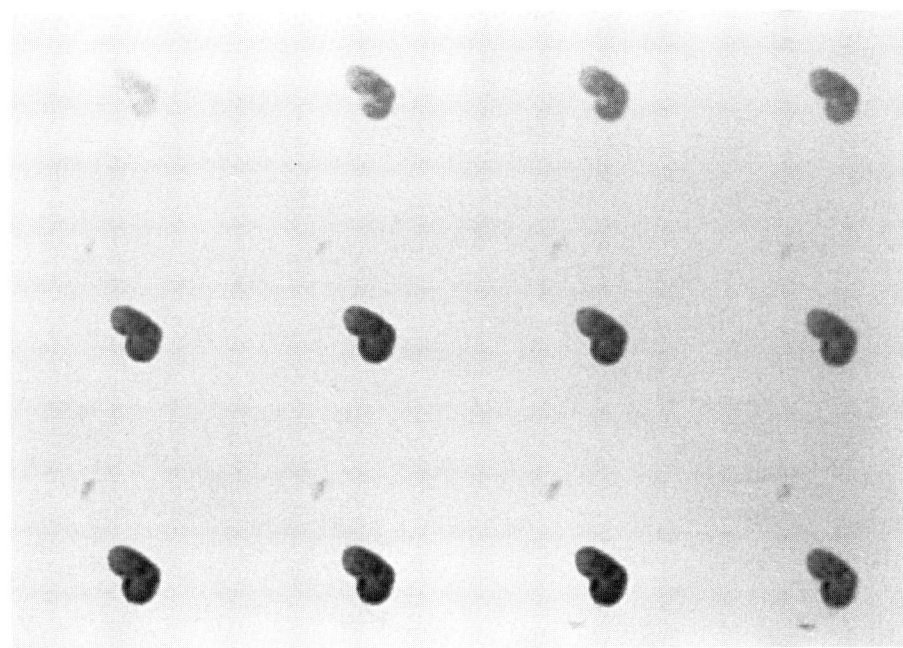

Figure 28–2. Renal allograft rejection. Renal scan with MAG-3 (technetium-99m mercaptoacetyltriglycine) taken at an interval of 2 mins/frame shows decreased uptake and excretion of radionuclide. Compare this with the normal renal scan in Figure 28–3.

evident based on clinical and laboratory findings. Renal allograft sonography may show an edematous renal parenchyma but is noncontributory in most of the cases. However, renal ultrasound is important to rule out other causes of renal allograft dysfunction such as urinary obstruction and perirenal fluid collection.[25] Renal scan will show deterioration of kidney function with variable degree of decreased blood flow proportional with the severity of the rejection (Figs. 28–2, 28–3). Poor uptake of the radionuclide by the renal tubules is also noted with blunting of the excretion curve. In severe cases of acute rejection little or no flow to the renal allograft exists and will warrant establishing the presence of a viable kidney by a renal angiogram. In doubtful cases the diagnosis of rejection is best established by a renal allograft biopsy. The allograft biopsy will also provide information on the likelihood of response to antirejection therapy.[21] The hallmark of acute rejection on histology is a widespread lymphocytic infiltration of the renal cortical tubules (tubulitis) and interstitium (Fig. 28–4). Other cellular elements include monocytes, lymphoblasts, plasma cells, and occasional eosinophils. The presence of excessive tissue eosinophilia correlates with the presence of a severe acute rejection episode.[26] Vascular changes are present occasionally with swelling of the endothelium of the peritubular capillaries,

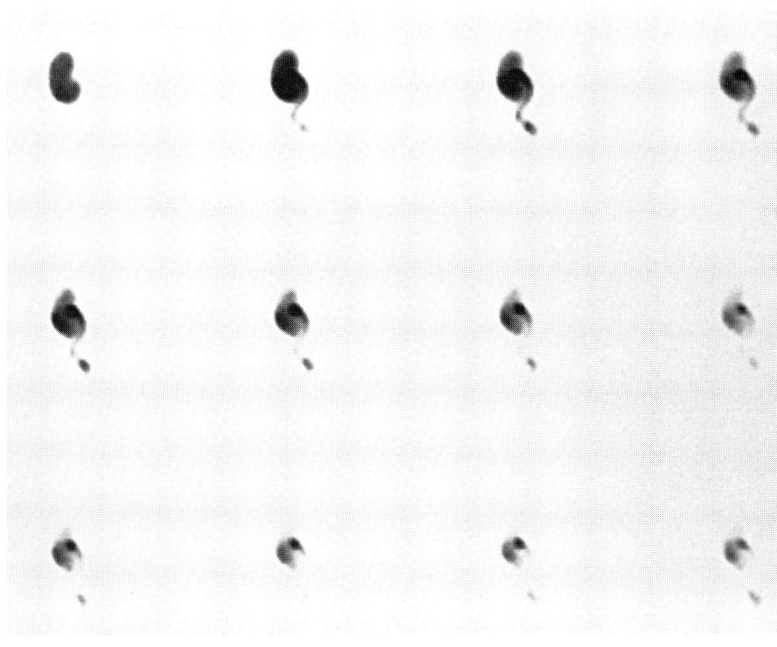

Figure 28–3. Normal renal allograft. Renal scan with MAG-3 (2 mins/frame) shows prompt uptake and excretion of radionuclide by the transplant kidney.

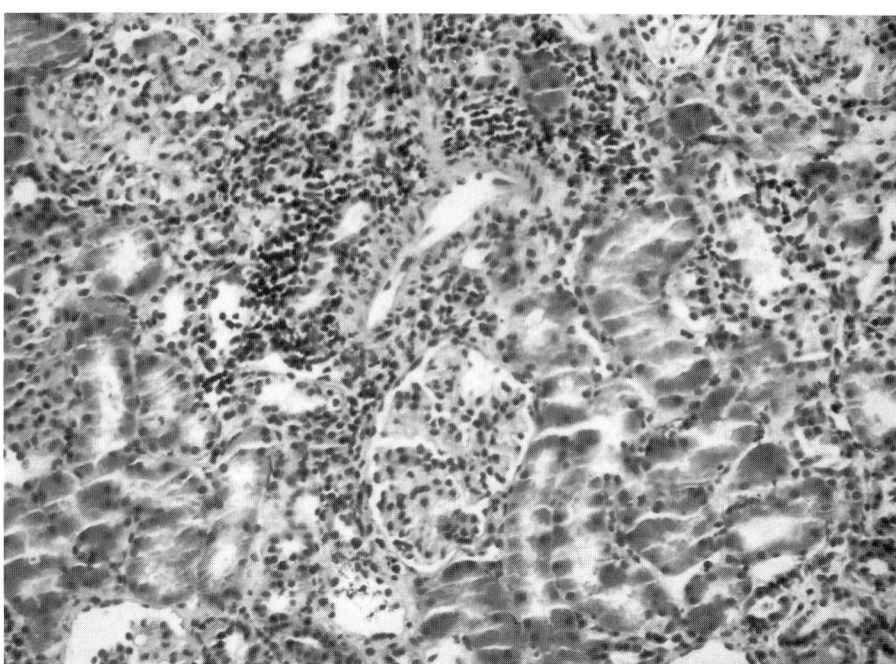

Figure 28–4. Acute cellular rejection. H&E stain of renal allograft biopsy showing lymphocytic infiltrates in the proximal renal tubules (tubulitis) and interstitium (× 250). (Courtesy of Dr. Ho Huang Chang, Department of Pathology, Charleston Area Medical Center, Charleston, WV.)

glomeruli, and arterioles. In severe cases foci of fibrinoid necrosis are present in the wall of small arteries and arterioles, and fibrin thrombi with platelet aggregation in the small venules and in the glomerular and peritubular capillaries, the precursor of diffuse cortical necrosis and intravascular or glomerular thrombosis. The response to treatment depends on the timing and severity of the rejection episodes. The treatment of acute rejection is most often effective within the first 3 months after transplant. For uncomplicated first rejection, successful therapy is possible even beyond 1 year. The type of cellular rejection that responds best to therapy is characterized by infiltration with large lymphoblastoid cells. Cellular rejection becomes more refractory as the lymphoid cells become smaller and plasma cells become more prevalent.[15] Treatment of acute rejection consists of boluses of intravenous methylprednisolone (IVMP). The most common schedule is to use 500 mg IVMP daily for 3 days. Response should occur within 48 hours but can be as prolonged as 5 days. If response does not occur in a timely fashion, treatment with an antilymphocyte preparation should be initiated.[27] In cases of severe acute rejection with vascular involvement treatment with IVMP is usually not effective and therapy with an antilymphocyte preparation should be initiated from the beginning. In cases with substantial cortical necrosis, diffuse glomerular thrombosis, and widespread interstitial hemorrhage, aggressive treatment with immunosuppressants should be withheld, because treatment of these conditions is futile and creates an unacceptable benefit-to-risk ratio.

Chronic Rejection

Chronic rejection occurs over many months to years and is the usual cause of progressive late failure of long-surviving renal allografts. The major clinical manifestation is a gradual rise in serum creatinine with proteinuria, hypertension, and progressive anemia. The most dominant histologic picture in chronic rejection is proliferation of the intima and narrowing of the arteries. This picture of arteriosclerosis is often associated with nephrosclerosis and interstitial fibrosis (Fig. 28–5). Presumably, these changes are due to chronic immunologic inflammation mediated by antibodies directed against vascular endothelium, with formation of platelets and fibrin aggregates.[28] The cellular elements of immunologic response are also present to a variable intensity.[29] Some have suggested that chronic rejection involves antibody-dependent cell-mediated cytotoxicity, an effector mechanism that combines humoral and cellular components of the immune system.[30] Nonimmunologic causes may contribute to graft loss in chronic rejection caused by the reduced renal mass and result in glomerular capillary hypertension with hyperperfusion and hyperfiltration.[31] The outcome of chronic rejection is a relentless deterioration of renal function as a result of failure to respond to therapy. Because chronic rejection is the largest cause of renal allograft failure over a prolonged period of time, it constitutes an important immunobiological process that needs to be better understood if the survival of renal allograft is to be prolonged. Current literature suggests that appropriate immunosuppression with adequate cyclosporine dosages can delay the occurrence of chronic rejection and prolong the survival of renal allografts.[32,33]

SURGICAL COMPLICATIONS

Surgical problems following renal transplantation are related to either vascular or urologic complications. Improvements

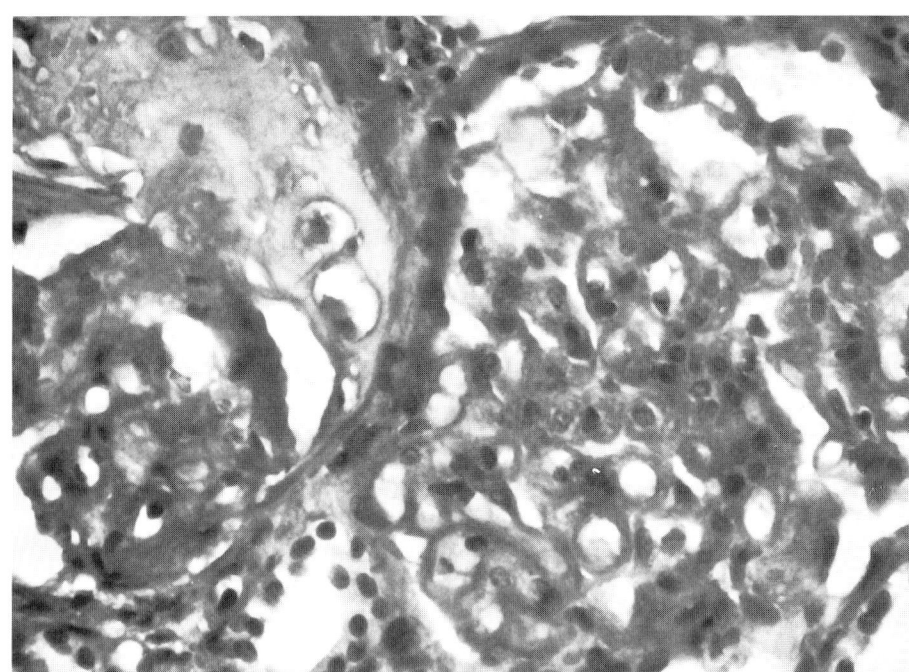

Figure 28–5. Final outcome of chronic rejection on renal allograft. Biopsy showing glomerulopathy with thickening of glomerular basement membrane. Partial obliteration and sclerosis of glomerulus on the left side is also evident. PAS (periodic acid–Schiff) stain (× 250) (Courtesy of Dr. Ho Huang Chang, Department of Pathology, Charleston Area Medical Center, Charleston, WV.)

in surgical techniques and attention to both the donor operation and preparation of the recipient bed have led to a remarkable decrease in the surgical complication rate. Though infrequent, vascular complications are associated with a high morbidity and mortality and require immediate attention. Early vascular complications include hemorrhage, rupture of the renal allograft, renal artery thrombosis, and renal vein thrombosis. Late vascular complications of clinical importance include renal artery stenosis. Urologic complications may present early or late in the transplant period and consist of either urinary leak or obstruction.

Hemorrhage

Acute postoperative hemorrhage can result from dehiscence of a vascular suture line. Additional causes include inadequate preparation of the graft bed, undetected or poorly ligated branch of the hypogastric artery, inappropriately ligated epigastric vessels, an unrecognized vessel in the renal pelvis, abnormal coagulation mechanisms of the recipients, and spontaneous graft rupture. The incidence of postoperative hemorrhage is increased when hemodialysis is required in the immediate postoperative period. The diagnosis of postoperative hemorrhage is usually evident on clinical grounds. The patient complains of excruciating pain around the kidney and in the back and flank. Hypovolemic shock can develop rapidly. Perinephric hematoma formation can cause functional allograft impairment by compression of the renal parenchyma, renal vessels, or ureter. Emergency exploration is usually necessary. If vascular repair or reconstruction cannot be accomplished within a reasonable time, allograft nephrectomy will be indicated. Evacuation of the hematoma is important to prevent bacterial infection.[34]

Late hemorrhage, arising months or years after transplantation, is rare but can occur as a result of rupture of a pseudoaneurysm at the anastomotic site. Hemorrhage as a result of percutaneous needle allograft biopsy has also been reported.[35] The use of smaller-gauge automated needle biopsy under real-time ultrasound guidance should decrease this complication rate.[36] Rupture of a mycotic aneurysm is another disastrous event that is fortunately rare.[37] It is usually the result of a deep-wound infection with secondary involvement of the vascular suture line. Transplant nephrectomy with ligation of the iliac artery and drainage of the area is the most expeditious and effective procedure.[38] Salvage of the ipsilateral limb is possible with an extra-anatomic revascularization procedure through either a femoral–femoral or axillo–femoral bypass graft.

Renal Allograft Rupture

Spontaneous rupture of the renal allograft is becoming rare in the era of more effective immunotherapy. It is usually the result of rapid parenchymal swelling with acute rejection early in the transplant period.[39] Rupture at the site of a previous open renal biopsy has also been reported.[40] Immediate exploration is indicated. Renal salvage should be attempted by approximating the fracture edges with mattress sutures placed over Teflon pledgets or by prolonged pressure exerted over the kidney. Nephrectomy becomes necessary when these maneuvers fail.

Renal Artery Thrombosis

Thrombosis of the renal artery is a rare complication following renal transplantation. Renal artery stenosis may occur as a result of faulty surgical techniques, postoperative hypotension, trauma to the intima of the donor artery during retrieval or perfusion, atherosclerosis of the recipient iliac artery, and redundancy of the renal artery with subsequent kink.[41] Cyclosporine toxicity has been implicated in some cases of renal artery thrombosis on the basis of a hypercoagulable state.[42] Thrombosis of the renal artery should be suspected when a period of anuria followed an acceptable diuresis. Renal flow scan will show no uptake of the isotope by the kidney (Fig. 28–6). Renal angiogram is diagnostic (Fig. 28–7). In most cases, by the time the diagnosis is obtained, the kidney is beyond salvage. The transplanted kidney lacks collateral circulation and its ischemia tolerance time is less than an hour.[43] Transplant nephrectomy is the treatment of choice.

Renal Vein Thrombosis

Renal vein thrombosis following renal transplantation is also a rare complication.[41] It may result from faulty surgical technique in performing the vascular anastomosis, ipsilateral femoroiliac thrombosis with propagation into the renal vein,[44] or external compression of the iliac or renal vein by a perirenal fluid collection. Anatomic compression of the left common iliac vein between the sacral promontory and the right common iliac artery or aorta has been described as predisposing to renal vein thrombosis following transplantation in the left iliac fossa.[45] Additional causes in pediatric recipients include extrinsic compression in the iliac fossa[46] and kidneys from donors less than 5 years old.[47] An increased incidence of venous thromboembolism has also been noted in the cyclosporine era.[48] Renal vein thrombosis results in acute renal failure with oliguria, enlargement of the renal allograft, and ipsilateral lower-extremity edema. Renal flow scan shows delayed uptake with no or very little excretion of the isotope (Fig. 28–8). Venous Doppler studies reveal thrombosis of the ipsilateral femoral and iliac venous system. Venography is diagnostic and is useful in delineating the extent of the thrombus (Fig. 28–9). Graft survival depends on the timing of venous thrombosis following transplantation. Renal allograft survival has generally been poor, with renal vein thrombosis occurring within a month of transplantation. Early diagnosis and prompt thrombectomy may occasionally result in some graft salvage,[49] but more commonly, prolonged venous stasis will lead to a nonviable graft when surgical intervention is undertaken and nephrectomy becomes the most effective option.[50] Contrary to the arterial system, collateral venous circulation does occur in transplanted kidneys and becomes well established 1 month after transplantation.[51] Renal vein thrombosis occurring at that time can be treated with thrombolytic and anticoagulation therapy with good results toward graft salvage.

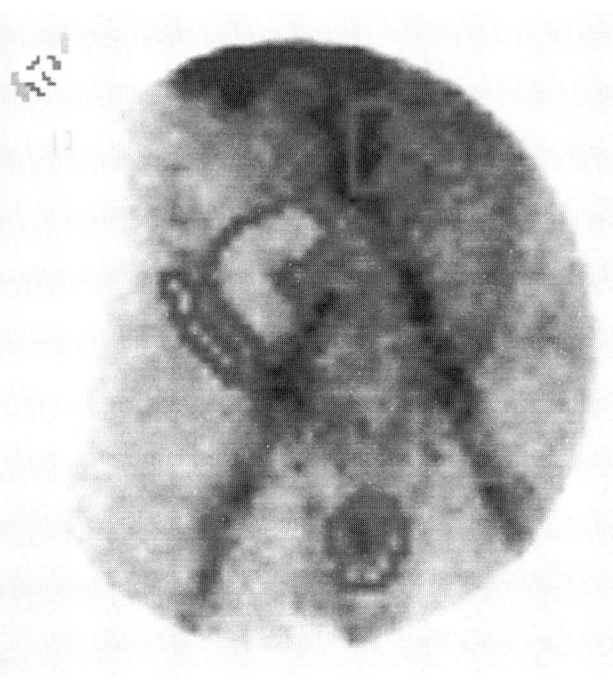

Figure 28–6. Renal artery thrombosis. Renal flow scan with MAG-3 showing no perfusion to the renal allograft (cold spot in the kidney area within the cursor).

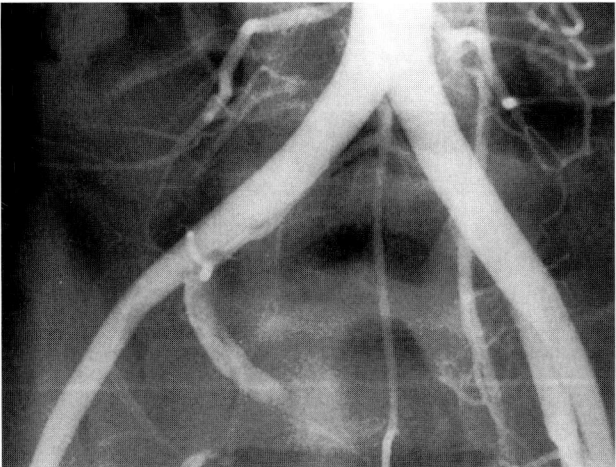

Figure 28–7. Renal artery thrombosis. Angiogram showing total occlusion of the transplant renal artery, anastomosed end to end to the right hypogastric artery.

Renal Artery Stenosis

Hypertension is a common problem after renal transplantation. It occurs in approximately 50 to 60% of long-term recipients with functioning grafts.[52,53] The etiology of hypertension after transplantation is complex (Table 28–1) and includes many variables such as acute and chronic rejection, steroids therapy, cyclosporine therapy, diseased native kidneys, recurrence of original disease, preexisting essential hypertension, and/or transplant renal artery stenosis.[54] Of these, transplant renal artery stenosis (RAS) represents a potentially curable cause of posttransplant hypertension, the treatment of which might also help preserve kidney function. The incidence of posttransplant RAS is reported to be between

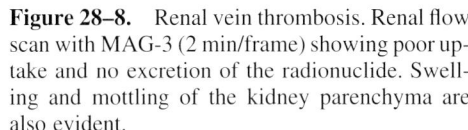

Figure 28–8. Renal vein thrombosis. Renal flow scan with MAG-3 (2 min/frame) showing poor uptake and no excretion of the radionuclide. Swelling and mottling of the kidney parenchyma are also evident.

1 and 12% in different series, largely depending on the definition of the degree of significant stenosis and the indication for angiography.[55–59] The location of the stenosis in relation to the suture line could be proximal because of recipient atherosclerotic disease, anastomotic, or distal in the donor renal artery.[60] Anastomotic stenosis is generally regarded as technical due to faulty surgical techniques.[61] The etiology of distal stenosis is less clear but is considered to be related to immunologic causes.[62,63] Additional causes of posttransplant RAS include damage to the donor arterial intima during perfusion, improper apposition of the donor and recipient vessels with torsion, and excessive length of the renal artery leading to angulation.[41] Posttransplant RAS should be suspected when the recipient has severe hypertension poorly responsive to medical therapy with unexplained deterioration in renal function. A bruit over the renal allograft is not a good clinical indication of RAS because it can be present in 25% of normotensive renal transplant patients and can merely indicate a good blood flow to the renal allograft.[64] The importance of peripheral renin or selective renal vein renin values in the diagnosis of posttransplant RAS is debatable.[65–68] However, a deterioration of renal function as a result of treatment with angiotensin-converting enzyme inhibitors (captopril test) is highly suspicious of posttransplant

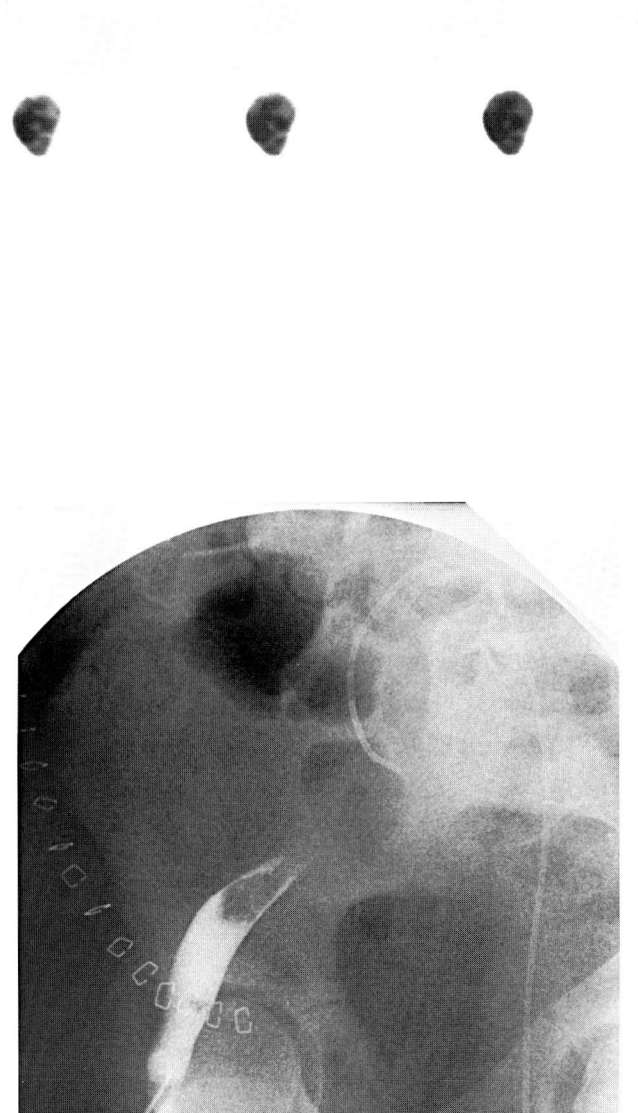

Figure 28–9. Renal vein thrombosis. Venogram showing thrombus in the external iliac vein with occlusion of the renal transplant venous drainage.

Table 28–1. Causes of Posttransplant Hypertension

Chronic rejection
Acute rejection
Steroids
Cyclosporine
Recurrent disease
Native kidney disease
Essential hypertension
Renal artery stenosis

RAS.[68-70] The diagnosis of RAS requires invasive angiography (Fig. 28-10). The use of intra-arterial digital subtraction angiography allows excellent visualization of the arterial anatomy with the use of less radiocontrast material and is currently the procedure of choice for the diagnosis of posttransplant RAS.[71] A systolic pressure gradient across the stenosis of 60 mm Hg or more correlates highly with a hemodynamically significant lesion.[59] Intervention is indicated when medical therapy fails and renal allograft biopsy shows absence of chronic rejection or intrarenal disease. The treatment of choice of posttransplant RAS is percutaneous balloon angioplasty (Fig. 28-11), which should be attempted as a primary treatment modality.[57,59] For those lesions that fail angioplasty surgical intervention is indicated. A variety of reconstructive procedures have been described that are technically very complex operations. An intraperitoneal approach with the use of a saphenous vein bypass graft from the common or external iliac arteries and segmental resection with reanastomosis have resulted in a better success rate with decreased mortality and morbidity and are the preferred methods of treatment.[55,58,59]

Urinary Extravasation

Urinary extravasation after renal transplantation occurs in 1 to 8% of cases and is associated with an increased morbidity

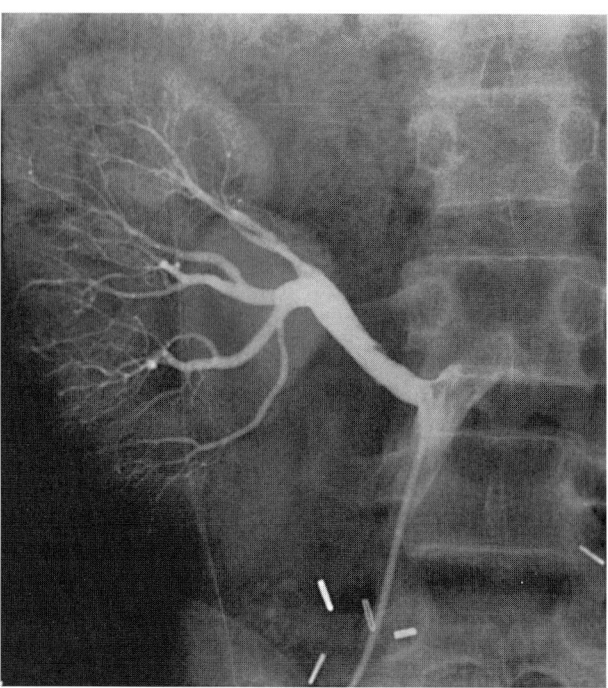

Figure 28-11. Results of percutaneous balloon angioplasty of the renal artery stenosis lesion of Figure 28-10.

and mortality.[72] Prompt diagnosis and management are necessary. The anterior bladder suture line and the ureterovesical junction anastomosis are the two most common sites for urinary extravasation.[73] Additional sites can occur at any point along the urinary collecting system of the transplanted kidney, either because of a calyceal cutaneous fistula or because of ureteral necrosis. Preexisting recipient bladder condition may contribute to urinary leak related to increased bladder pressure such as the presence of bladder outlet obstruction, posterior urethral valves, and neurogenic bladder.[74] Urine leak at the anterior cystotomy line has decreased tremendously by adopting the modified anterior extravesical ureteroneocystotomy technique as opposed to the more traditional transvesical Leadbetter–Politano technique.[75] Urinary leak is generally the result of vascular insufficiency resulting from inadequate preservation of ureteral blood supply during donor nephrectomy. Unlike the native ureter, which is nourished by several vessels, the ureter of the transplanted kidney receives its blood supply exclusively from the renal vessel branches that course the hilar and upper periureteral tissues. With interruption and/or thrombosis of these small branches, the distal portion of the ureter may necrose. Therefore to ensure preservation of ureteral blood supply, a large periureteral fatty tissue should be removed en bloc with the kidney and ureter, and dissection in the perihilar area should be avoided. The shortest practical length of ureter should be used and any twisting should be avoided.[76] Ureteral infarction occurs more commonly in allografts with multiple renal arteries, particularly those with a smaller lower pole artery. Kidneys from living related do-

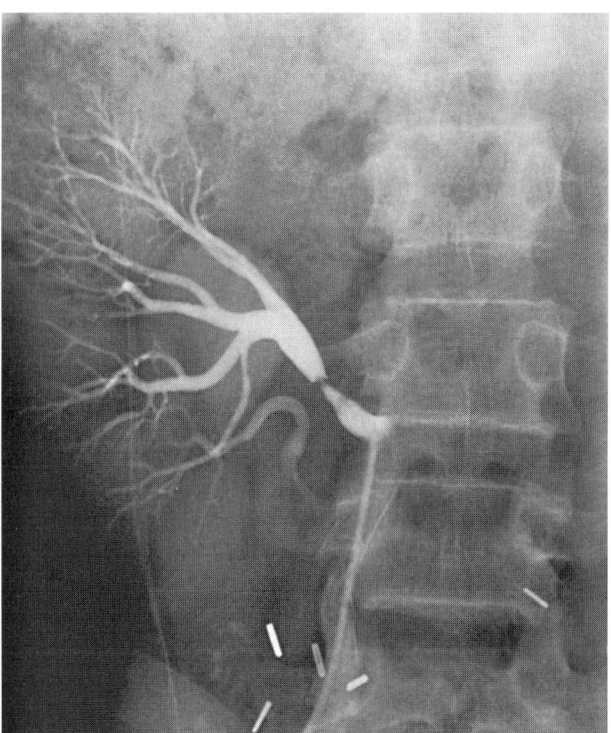

Figure 28-10. Renal artery stenosis. Angiogram shows two renal arteries to the transplant kidney with a high-grade stenosis of the main upper renal artery distal to the end-to-side anastomosis with the common iliac artery.

nors are at increased risk because of the limited exposure. Segmental infarction of renal parenchyma may also result in urinary extravasation caused by the development of a calyceal cutaneous fistula, especially if the involved vessel supplies more than 10% of the renal parenchyma.[77] Urinary extravasation usually occurs early in the postoperative period. Diagnosis is heralded by a decrease in urinary output, unexplained fever, and wound drainage. Additional signs include progressive allograft tenderness and edema of the scrotum, labia, or ipsilateral thigh. The diagnosis is usually established by a cystogram (Fig. 28–12) and/or an intravenous pyelogram in patients with normal kidney function. Percutaneous antegrade pyelogram may be needed to establish the site of extravasation in those patients with poor renal function and to rule out ureteral necrosis (Fig. 28–13). Ultrasound and/or computerized axial tomography (CT) scan will show a fluid collection around the kidney (Fig. 28–14). Urinary extravasation occurring within a few days of transplantation is best treated by immediate exploration. Ureteral reimplantation in the bladder is the procedure of choice if enough viable transplant ureter exists. Cases with total ureteral necrosis or inadequate ureteral length can be salvaged by a ureteropyelostomy (native ureter to transplant renal pelvis).[78] The ipsilateral native kidney does not need to be uniformly removed when the ureter is used. Additional useful techniques include a direct pyelovesical anastomosis with a

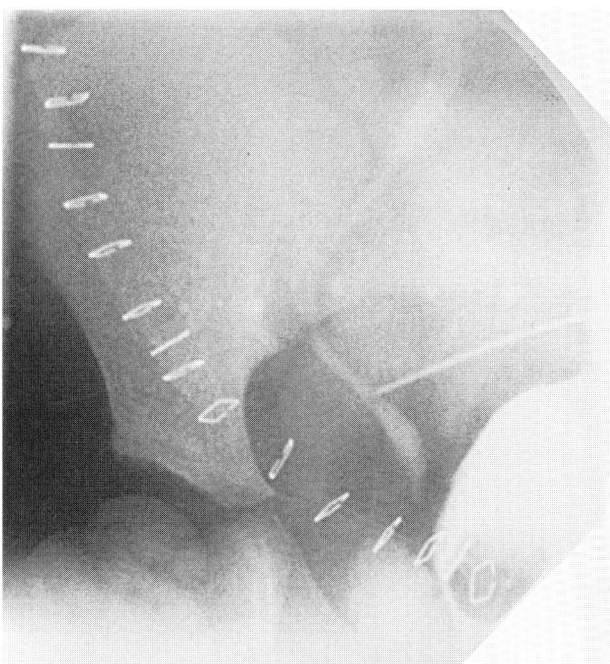

Figure 28–13. Antegrade nephrostogram of the case in Figure 28–12 showing intact transplant ureter with the urinary extravasation located at the level of ureterovesical junction.

psoas hitch or Boari flap.[79] Urinary diversion either with an indwelling ureteral stent or with a nephrostomy tube is a useful adjunct to urinary reconstruction. Small leak at the site of ureteroneocystotomy can be treated occasionally with prolonged Foley catheter drainage.[80] Additional cases of ureteral extravasation have been treated nonoperatively with percutaneous nephrostomy tube[81] and/or combined nephrostomy ureteral stenting.[82] In these cases the accompanying urinoma need not be drained unless it is infected.[83] Open repair is indicated when these maneuvers fail. The percutaneous nephrostomy tube will still serve a purpose to optimize the patient's condition and control sepsis before urinary tract reconstruction. In addition, it will protect the urologic repair postoperatively. Management of calyceal cutaneous fistula is complicated by the frequently associated urinary infection, perinephric abscess, and sepsis. Salvage of such kidneys is unusual. Nephrostomy and adequate sump drainage have been notably unsuccessful. Occasional grafts have been salvaged by surgical excision of the infarcted segment and closure of the defect, with a muscle or omental flap providing bulk for suture closure.[84]

Urinary Obstruction

Ureteral obstruction can occur acutely in the early postoperative period from edema at the site of anastomosis, hematoma in the bladder submucosal tunnel, ureteral torsion, or slough of the distal ureteral tip. This early event is usually a total obstruction that results in diminishing urine output or

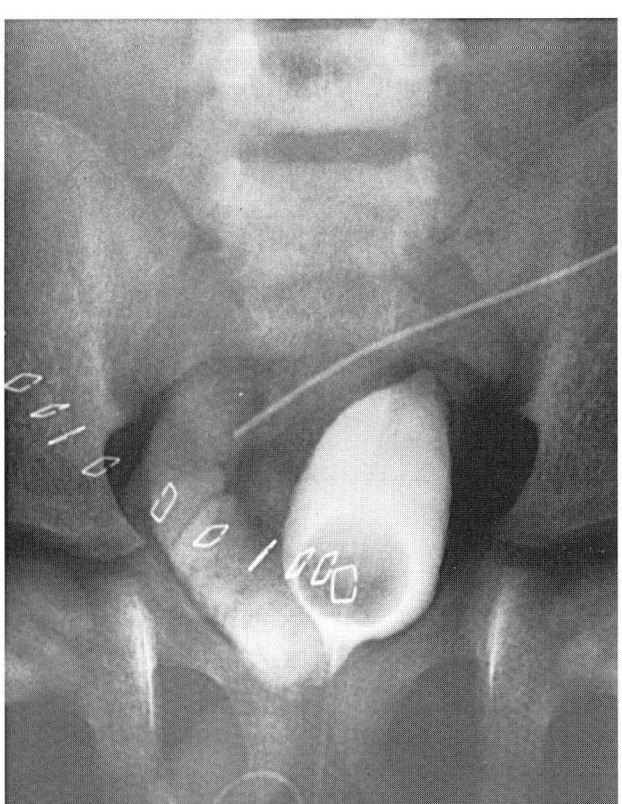

Figure 28–12. Cystogram showing urinary extravasation. The peritoneal dialysis catheter is also shown.

560 Diagnosis of Genitourinary Disease

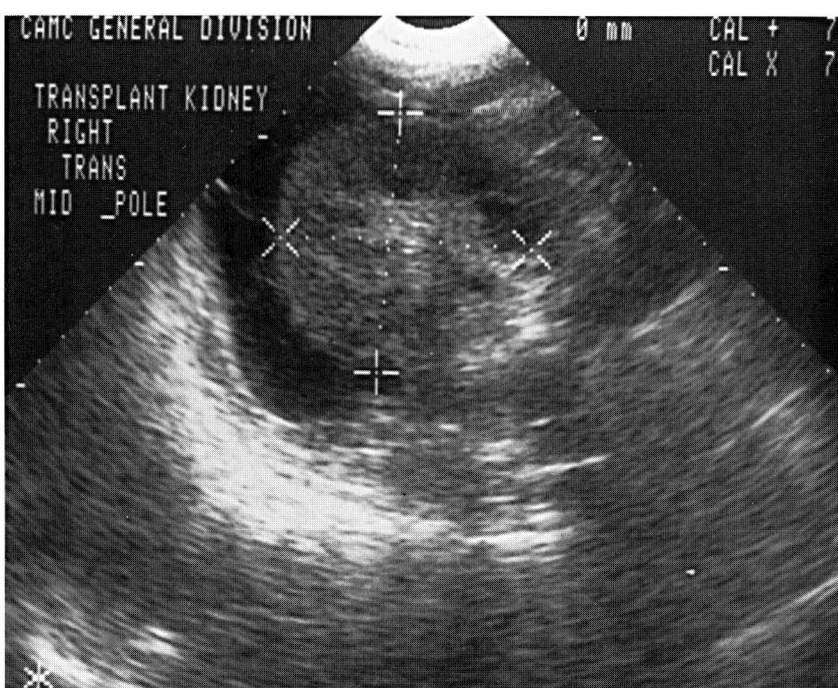

Figure 28–14. Urinary extravasation. Ultrasound of transplant kidney showing urinoma collection around the renal allograft. The renal allograft is marked with cursors.

even anuria. Reoperation is indicated to salvage the renal allograft. More commonly, ureteral obstruction is a late complication, occurring in 1 to 10% of kidney recipients.[85] The site of obstruction can be anywhere along the course of the ureter, but most commonly at the ureterovesical junction (Fig. 28–15). Causes of obstruction include local host immunologic responses, ischemia, fibrosis, and scarring of surrounding tissues. Additional causes include acute angulation of the ureter (Fig. 28–16), extrinsic compression from spermatic cord,[86] or lymphocele collection. Clinically, ureteral obstruction is manifested by renal allograft dysfunction. Fluctuation or decrease in urine output may occur but is not consistent because in most cases the ureteral obstruction is partial. Ultrasound is the diagnostic method of choice in patients showing significant hydronephrosis (Fig. 28–17). Kidney function may be impaired enough to preclude intravenous pyelography and diuretic renal scan. An element of hydronephrosis of the renal allograft may exist as a result of vesicoureteral reflux or may be present without physiologic significance. A voiding cystogram and a diuretic renal scan will be helpful under these circumstances to assess the significance of obstruction. Percutaneous antegrade pyelography is indicated to assess the site of obstruction (Figs. 28–15, 28–16). This can be done safely under ultrasound or CT guidance. The positioned catheter may be left indwelling for percutaneous nephrostomy drainage to allow recovery of kidney function prior to any intervention. Many cases of ureteral obstruction can be managed nonoperatively with balloon dilatation and stenting.[83] This is most successful when the obstruction involves a very short segment. Surgical intervention is indicated when percutaneous techniques fail.

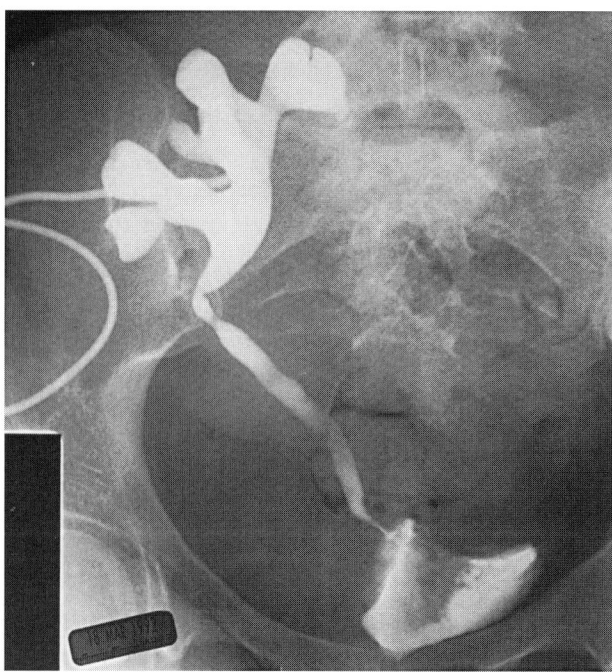

Figure 28–15. Antegrade pyelogram showing urinary obstruction at the level of the ureterovesical junction of transplant kidney.

Distal obstruction at the vesicoureteral junction can sometimes be repaired by a ureteroneocystomy. In most cases this is not feasible because of severe scarring and poor lower ureteral blood supply. Reconstruction is best accomplished by ureteroureterostomy or ureteropyelostomy.[78] If the native ureter is unavailable, repair can be successfully done with a direct anastomosis of renal pelvis or proximal ureter to the bladder with the help of a psoas hitch or Boari flap. A tapered piece of bowel is another helpful alternative for ureteral replacement.[87]

Lymphocele

Lymphocele formation is a well-known complication of renal transplantation. It is caused by lymphatic leakage from the allograft bed or the allograft itself. The incidence has ranged from 1 to 22%, depending on the definition of lymphocele, length of follow-up, and frequency of radiologic investigation.[88,89] Contributing factors implicated in the development of lymphoceles include extensive perivascular dissection of native vessels, hilar lymphatics of the renal allograft, acute rejection episodes, high-dose steroids, and anticoagulants. Retransplantation has also been implicated in the development of lymphoceles.[90] Care in ligation of perirenal lymphatics during donor nephrectomy, graft preparation, and dissection of the recipient iliac fossa is essential in the prevention of lymphocele formation posttransplantation. The majority of lymphoceles are asymptomatic and require no treatment.[89] Intervention is indicated when lymphoceles become symptomatic. The most common initial sign and symptoms are urinary frequency, suprapubic pres-

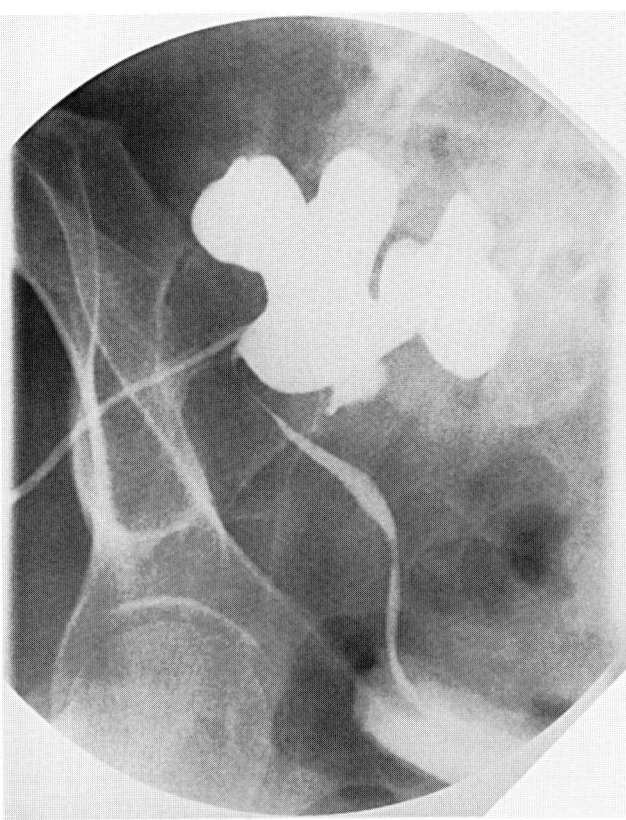

Figure 28–16. Antegrade pyelogram showing obstruction of the upper ureter of transplant kidney caused by acute angulation of the ureter with the kidney lying transversely.

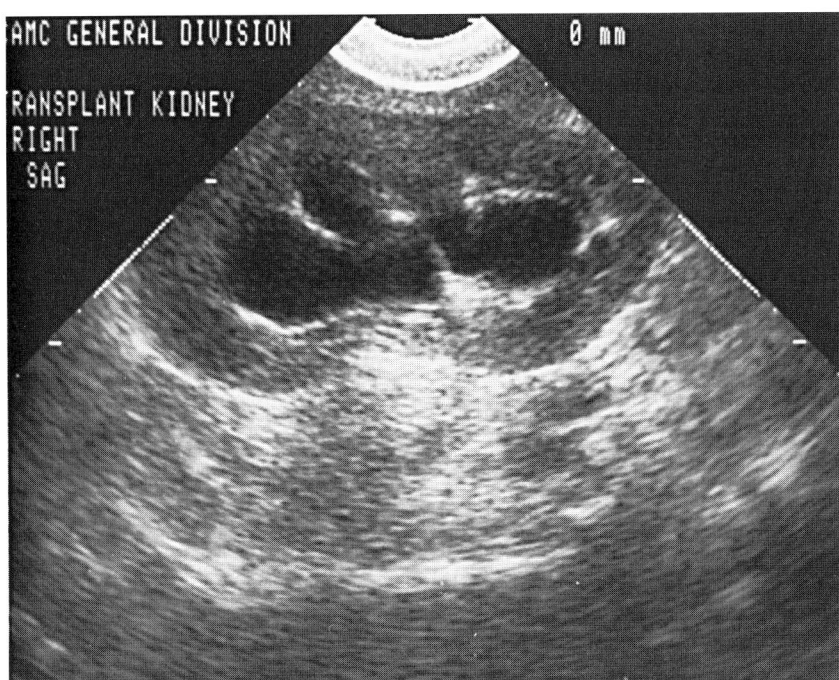

Figure 28–17. Ultrasound showing significant hydronephrosis of transplant kidney resulting from ureteral obstruction.

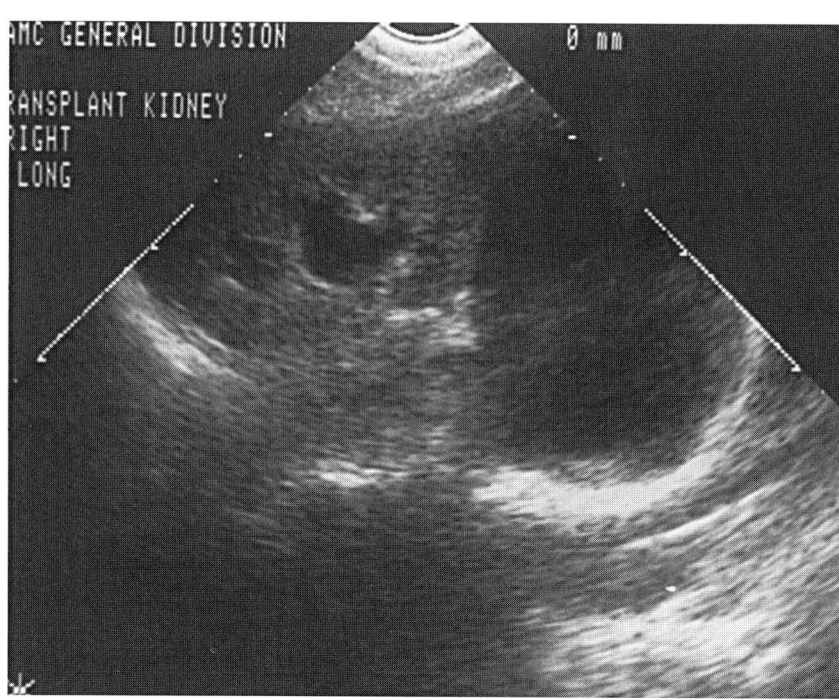

Figure 28–18. Posttransplant lymphocele shown on ultrasound medial to the kidney with associated hydronephrosis of the renal allograft.

sure, palpable mass adjacent to the renal allograft, and edema of the ipsilateral thigh and genitalia. Renal dysfunction with increase in serum creatinine is usually present. Ultrasonography (Fig. 28–18) and CT scanning (Fig. 28–19) are the two most helpful diagnostic studies for establishing the presence, location, and extent of perinephric fluid collection. Hydronephrosis may be associated with lymphocele formation because of extrinsic compression of the ureter (see Fig. 28–18). Urinoma should be considered in the differential diagnosis. Needle aspiration and determination of creatinine and urea content of the fluid collection will establish the diagnosis. Lymphocele fluid will have the same creatinine and urea concentration as the plasma. Different treatment modalities exist for symptomatic lymphoceles (Table 28–2). Simple needle aspiration usually results in recurrence and subjects the patient to increased risk of infection of the lymphocele cavity.[91] Needle aspiration of posttransplant lymphocele has a limited value as a treatment modality and

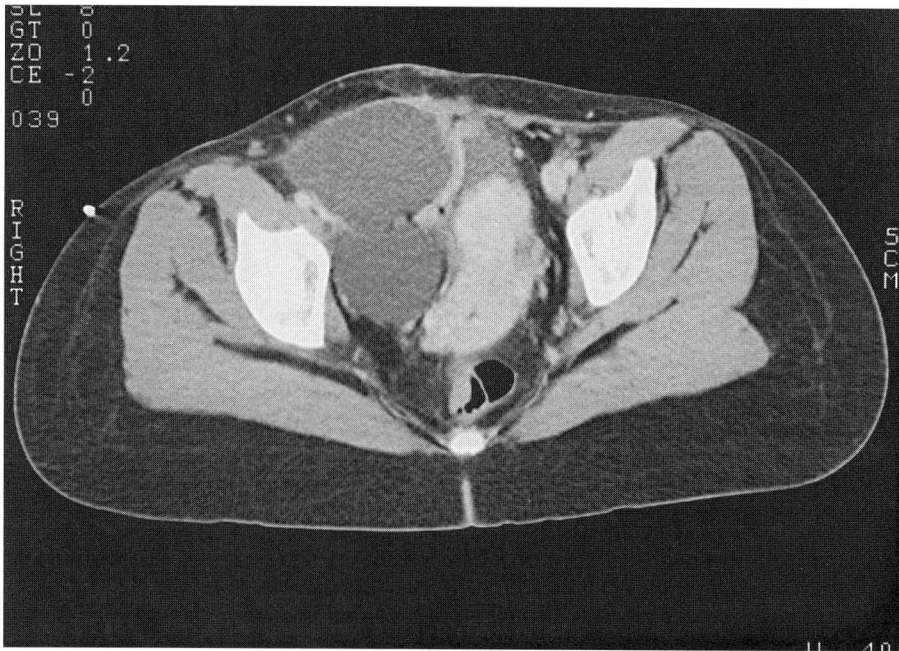

Figure 28–19. CT scan showing a large multilocular pelvic lymphocele with deviation of the bladder medially.

Table 28–2. Treatment Modalities of Symptomatic Lymphoceles

External marsupialization
Needle aspiration
Betadine irrigation
Sclerotherapy
Intraperitoneal drainage: operative, laparoscopy

should be used only for diagnostic purposes. Aspiration combined with betadine irrigation[92] or sclerotherapy[93] has resulted in a well-documented success rate. Catheter drainage with antibiotic irrigation is recommended for infected lymphoceles.[89] External marsupialization of the lymphocele cavity through the transplant incision is effective but is time-consuming and requires prolonged hospitalization with packing of the wound until healing with granulation tissue occurs.[94] Its use should be limited to cases with infected lymphoceles and lymphatic fistulas. Intraperitoneal drainage of lymphoceles is the most effective and physiologic way of lymphocele drainage and is currently the preferred method of treatment.[95] This is usually achieved through an intraperitoneal approach with marsupialization of the lymphocele cavity in the peritoneum. The same procedure can now be achieved through a laparoscopic approach with minimum morbidity.[96,97] Infection of the lymphocele cavity represents a contraindication to intraperitoneal drainage.

Hydrocele

The incidence of ipsilateral hydrocele formation after renal transplantation has been reported to be as high as 68% in cases in which the spermatic cord has been transected at transplantation.[98] This practice has since been abandoned. Transection of the spermatic cord results in interference with lymphatic drainage of the testicle and leads to accumulation of hydrocele fluid. In addition, the testicle is rendered ischemic because of interruption of the main blood supply, making its viability totally dependent on collateral circulation. Hydrocelectomy in these patients is fraught with the possibility of serious complications, including testicular loss and abscess formation.[98] Aspiration of hydrocele with tetracycline sclerotherapy is an alternative noninvasive and effective treatment for hydroceles following renal transplantation.[99] Fortunately, the majority of hydroceles after renal transplantation are asymptomatic and only a few require treatment. Symptoms are usually related to discomfort, pain, interference with sexual activity, and/or embarrassment related to size. The diagnosis is usually evident on physical examination and by transillumination. Ultrasound may be used to document the size and pattern of the hydrocele and to assess the testicle; it can also be used as an adjunct to aspiration and sclerotherapy.

RENAL ALLOGRAFT DYSFUNCTION

Renal allograft dysfunction after renal transplantation is multifactorial, depending on the time frame from the transplant operation. Knowledge of the various pathologic conditions will help expedite the diagnostic studies and optimize therapy. Based on the previous discussion, renal allograft dysfunction can be divided into three distinct categories:

1. *Very early dysfunction*—occurring less than 1 week posttransplant.
2. *Early dysfunction*—occurring between 1 week and 3 months posttransplant.
3. *Late dysfunction*—occurring more than 3 months posttransplant.

The differential diagnosis of very early renal allograft dysfunction and a suggested algorithm for its work-up are summarized in Table 28–3 and Figure 28–20.

The differential diagnosis of early renal allograft dysfunction and a suggested algorithm for its work-up are summarized in Table 28–4 and Figure 28–21.

The differential diagnosis of late renal allograft dysfunction and a suggested algorithm for its work-up are summarized in Table 28–5 and Figure 28–22.

Acknowledgment. The authors would like to thank Barbara Eldridge for her excellent secretarial support.

Table 28–3. Differential Diagnosis of Very Early Renal Allograft Dysfunction

Surgical catastrophe: renal artery occlusion, renal vein thrombosis
Urinary obstruction: mechanical urethral catheter, transplant ureter
Urinary extravasation
Accelerated vascular rejection
Acute tubular necrosis

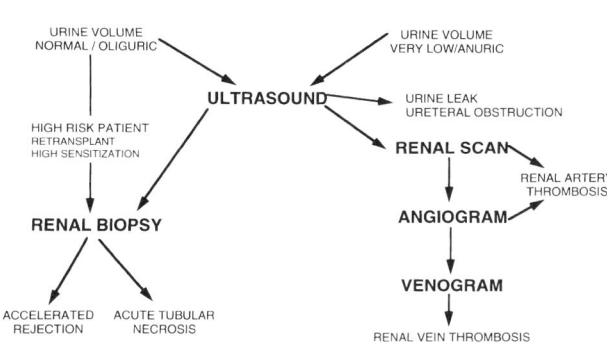

Figure 28–20. Algorithm for the workup of very early renal allograft dysfunction.

Table 28–4. Differential Diagnosis of Early Renal Allograft Dysfunction

Acute cellular rejection
Cyclosporine toxicity
Urinary obstruction
Urinary extravasation
Lymphocele

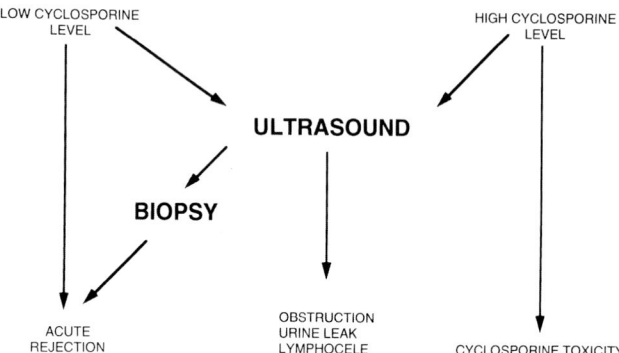

Figure 28–21. Algorithm for the workup of early renal allograft dysfunction.

Table 28–5. Differential Diagnosis of Late Renal Allograft Dysfunction

Late acute cellular rejection
Chronic rejection
Cyclosporine toxicity
Recurrent or de novo renal disease
Urinary obstruction
Renal artery stenosis

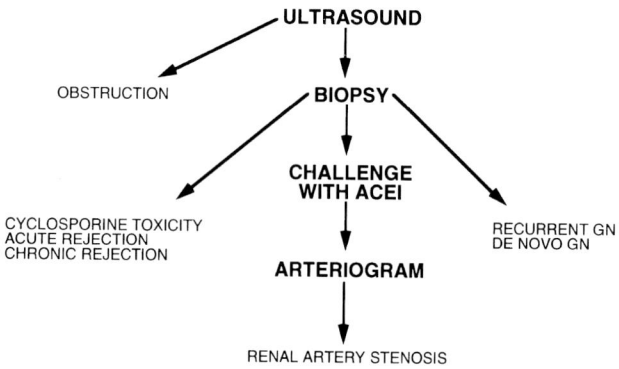

Figure 28–22. Algorithm for the workup of late renal allograft dysfunction.

REFERENCES

1. Ceska J, Terazaki P: The UNOS scientific renal transplant registry 1991. In: Terazaki PI, ed. *Clinical Transplants 1991.* Los Angeles: UCLA Tissue Typing Laboratory, 1991; 1–11.
2. Novick AC, Flechner S: The integration of clinical transplantation into urology residency training. *J Urol* 1988; 139:568–569.
3. Peters PC: The future of urology. *J Urol* 1989; 142:929–930.
4. Finn WF: Prevention of ischemic injury in renal transplantation. *Kidney Int* 1990; 37:171–182.
5. Belzer FO, Southard JH: Principles of solid organ preservation by cold storage. *Transplantation* 1988; 45:673–676.
6. Byrick RJ, Rose DK: Pathophysiology and prevention of acute renal failure: the role of the anesthetist. *Can J Anaesth* 1990; 37:457–467.
7. Finn WF: Diagnosis and management of acute tubular necrosis. *Med Clin North Am* 1990; 74:873–891.
8. Myers BD: Cyclosporine nephrotoxicity. *Kidney Int* 1986; 30:964–974.
9. Novick AC: The role of antilymphocyte globulin in cadaver renal transplantation. *Transplant Proc* 1986; 18:22–27.
10. Diethelm AG, Duvosky EV, Whelchel JD, Hartley MW, Tauxe WN: Diagnosis of impaired renal function after kidney transplantation using renal scintigraphy, renal plasma flow and urinary excretion of hippurate. *Ann Surg* 1980; 191:604–616.
11. Fischer J, Kirste G, Keller H, Wilms H: Does ATN influence renal transplant function negatively. *Transplant Proc* 1988; 20:908–909.
12. Rosenthal JT, Danovitch GM, Wilkinson A, Ettenger RB: The high cost of delayed graft function in cadaveric renal transplantation. *Transplantation* 1991; 51:1115–1117.
13. Perez RV, Matas AJ, Gillingham KJ, et al: Lessons learned and future hopes: three thousand renal transplants at the University of Minnesota. In: Terazaki PI, ed. *Clinical Transplants 1990.* Los Angeles: UCLA Tissue Typing Laboratory, 1990; 217–231.
14. Krensdy AM, Weiss A, Crabtree G, Davis MM, Parham P: T-lymphocyte antigen interactions in transplant rejection. *N Engl J Med* 1990; 322:510–517.
15. Braun WE: Treatment of allograft rejection. In: Glassock RJ, ed. *Current Therapy in Nephrology and Hypertension-2.* Philadelphia: Decker, 1987; 345–354.
16. Sanfilippo F, Vaghn WK, Bollinger RR, Spees EK: Comparative effects of pregnancy, transfusion, and prior graft rejection on sensitization and renal transplant results. *Transplantation* 1982; 34:360–366.
17. Hume DM, Merrill JP, Miller BF, Thorn JW: Experiences with renal homotransplantation in humans: report of nine cases. *J Clin Invest* 1955; 26:327–382.
18. Williams GM, Hume D, Hudson R, Morris P, Kano K, Milgrom F: Hyperacute renal homograft rejection in man. *N Engl J Med* 1968; 279:611–618.
19. Gebel HM, Lebeck LK: Crossmatch procedures used in organ transplantation. *Clin Lab Med* 1991; 11:603–620.
20. Barger BO, Shroyer TW, Hudson SL, et al: Early graft loss in cyclosporine A treated cadaveric renal allograft recipients receiving retransplants against previous mismatched HLA-A, -B, -DR donor antigens. *Transplant Proc* 1988; 20 (suppl 1): 170–172.
21. Finkelstein FO, Siegel NJ, Bast LC, Forrest JN, Kashgarian M: Kidney transplant biopsies in the diagnosis and treatment of acute rejection reactions. *Kidney Int* 1976; 10:171–178.
22. Ettenger RB, Marik J, Rosenthal JT, et al: OKT$_3$ for rejection

reversal in pediatric renal transplantation. *Clin Transpl* 1988; 2:180–184.
23. Fassbinder W, Ernst W, Stuttle HJ, Scheuermann E, Fursch A, Schoeppe W: Reversal of acute vascular rejection by plasma exchange. *Int J Artif Organs* 1983; 6 (suppl 1) :57–60.
24. Lindholm A, Lundgren G, Fehraman I, et al: Acute rejection episodes in cyclosporine treated cadaveric kidney recipients. *Clin Transpl* 1988;2:194–200.
25. Matas AJ, Simmons RL, Kjellstrand CM, Najarian JS: Pseudorejection: factors mimicking rejection in renal allograft recipients. *Ann Surg* 1977;186:51–59.
26. Kormendi F, Amend WJC: The importance of oesinophil cells in kidney allograft rejections. *Transplantation* 1988;45:537–539.
27. Thistlethwaite JR, Gaber AO, Hagg BW, et al: OKT_3 treatment of steroid resistant renal allograft rejection. *Transplantation* 1987;43:176–184.
28. Porter K: The effect of antibodies on human renal allografts. *Transplant Proc* 1976, 8:189–197.
29. Busch GJ, Schamberg JF, Moretz RC, Strom TB, Tilney NL, Carpenter CB: Four patterns of human renal allograft rejection: a cytologic and in vitro analysis of the infiltrate in 24 irreversibly rejected kidneys. *Transplant Proc* 1977;9:37–42.
30. Thomas J, Thomas F, Kaplan AM, Lee HM: Antibody dependent cellular cytotoxicity and chronic renal allograft rejection. *Transplantation* 1976;22:94–100.
31. Barrientos A, Portoles J, Herrero JA, et al: Glomerular hyperfiltration as a nonimmunologic mechanism of progression of chronic renal rejection. *Transplantation* 1994;57:753–755.
32. Almond PS, Matas A, Cullingham K, et al: Risk factors for chronic rejection in renal allograft recipients. *Transplantation* 1993;55:752–757.
33. Knight RJ, Kerman RH, Welsh M, et al: Chronic rejection in primary renal allograft recipients under cyclosporine–prednisone immunosuppressive therapy. *Transplantation* 1991; 51:355–359.
34. Goldman MH, Tilney NL, Vineyard GC, Laks H, Kahan MG, Wilson RE: A twenty year survey of arterial complications of renal transplantation. *Surg Gynecol Obstet* 1975; 141: 758–760.
35. Waltzer WC, Miller F, Arnold A, Jao S, Anaise D, Rapaport FT: Value of percutaneous core needle biopsy in the differential diagnosis of renal transplant dysfunction. *J Urol* 1987; 137:1117–1121.
36. Erturke E, Rubens DJ, Panner BJ, Cerilli JG: Automated core biopsy of renal allografts using ultrasonic guidance. *Transplantation* 1991;51:1311–1312.
37. Kyriakides GK, Simmons RL, Najarian JS: Mycotic aneurysms in transplant patients. *Arch Surg* 1976; 111:472–476.
38. Gorey TF, Bulkley GB, Spees EK, Sterioff S: Iliac artery ligation: the relative paucity of ischemic sequelae in renal transplant patients. *Ann Surg* 1979;190:753–757.
39. Goldman M, DePauw L, Kinnaert, et al: Renal allograft rupture: possible causes and results of surgical conservative management. *Transplantation* 1981;32:153–155.
40. Salaman JR, Calne RY, Pena J, Sells RA, White HJO, Yoffa D: Surgical aspects of clinical renal transplantation. *Br J Surg* 1969;56:413–417.
41. Palleschi J, Novick AC, Braun WE, Magnusson MO: Vascular complications of renal transplantation. *Urology* 1980;16:61–67.
42. Rigotti J, Flechner SM, VanBuren CT, Payne WT, Kahan BD:Increased incidence of renal allograft thrombosis under cyclosporine immunosuppression. *Int Surg* 1986;71:38–41.
43. Novick AC: Renal hypothermia: in vivo and ex-vivo. *Urol Clin North Am* 1983;10:637–644.
44. Rao KV, Smith EJ, Alexander WJ, Fidler JP, Pemmaraju SR, Pollack VE: Thromboembolic disease in renal allograft recipients. *Arch Surg* 1976;111:1086–1092.
45. Sorensen BL, Hald T, Nissen HM: Silent iliac compression syndrome as a cause of renal vein thrombosis after transplantation. *Scand J Urol Nephrol* 1972; 6 (suppl 15):75–77.
46. Borowicz MR, Hanevold CD, Cfer JB, et al: Extrinsic compression in the iliac fossa can cause renal vein occlusion in pediatric kidney recipients but graft loss can be prevented. *Transplant Proc* 1994;26:119–120.
47. Harmon WE, Stablein D, Alexander SR, Tejani A: Graft thrombosis in pediatric renal transplant recipients: a report of the American Pediatric Renal Transplant Cooperative Study. *Transplantation* 1991;51:406–412.
48. Vanrenterghem Y, Roel SL, Lerut T, Gruwez J, Michielsen P: Thromboembolic complications and haemostatic changes in cyclosporine treated cadaveric kidney allograft recipients. *Lancet* 1985;1:999–1002.
49. Delbeke D, Sacks GA, Sandler MP: Diagnosis of allograft renal vein thrombosis. *Clin Nucl Med* 1989;14:415–420.
50. Nerstrom B, Ladefoged J, Lund FL: Vascular complications in 155 consecutive kidney transplantations. *Scand J Urol Nephrol* 1972;6 (suppl 15):65–74.
51. Schwarz GR, Banowski LH, Peter ET, Blakeley WR, Klingler EL: Inferior vena cava interruption in renal transplant recipients. *Am Surg* 1974;40:178–180.
52. Pollini J, Guttman RD, Beaudouin JG, Morehouse DD, Klassen J, Knaack J: Late hypertension following renal allotransplantations. *Clin Nephrol* 1979;11:202–212.
53. Hamilton DV, Carmichael DJS, Evans DB, Caline RY: Hypertension in renal transplant recipients on cyclosporine A and azathioprine. *Transplant Proc* 1982;12:597–600.
54. Waltzer WC, Turner S, Frohnert P, Rapaport FT: Etiology and pathogenesis of hypertension following renal transplantation. *Nephron* 1986;42:102–109.
55. Dickerman RM, Peters PC, Hull AR, Curry TS, Atkins C, Fry WJ: Surgical correction of post-transplant renovascular hypertension. *Ann Surg* 1980;192:639–644.
56. Benoit G, Hiesse C, Icard P, et al: Treatment of renal artery stenosis after transplantation. *Transplant Proc* 1987;19:3600–3601.
57. Greenstein SM, Verstandig A, Mclean G, et al: Percutaneous transluminal angioplasty: the procedure of choice in the hypertensive renal allograft recipient with renal artery stenosis. *Transplantation* 1987;43:29–32.
58. Lacombe M: Renal artery stenosis after renal transplant. *Ann Vasc Surg* 1988;2:155–160.
59. Roberts JP, Ascher NL, Fryd DS, et al: Transplant renal artery stenosis. *Transplantation* 1989;48:580–583.
60. Lacombe M: Arterial stenosis complicating renal allotransplantation in man: a study of 38 cases. *Ann Surg* 1975; 181:283–288.
61. Chandrasoma P, Aberle AM: Anastomotic line renal artery stenosis after transplantation. *J Urol* 1986;135:1159–1162.
62. Smith RB, Cosimi AB, Lordon R, Thompson AL, Ehrlich RM: Diagnosis and management of arterial stenosis causing hypertension after renal transplantation. *J Urol* 1976;115:639–642.
63. Schacht RA, Martin DG, Singam RK, Wheeler CS, Lansing AM: Renal artery stenosis after renal transplantation. *Am J Surg* 1976;131:653–657.
64. Ricotta JJ, Schaff HV, Williams GM, Rolley RT, Whelton PK, Harrington DM: Renal artery stenosis following transplantation: etiology, diagnosis, and prevention. *Surgery* 1978;84: 595–602.
65. Hsu AC, Balfe JW, Olley PM, Kidd BSL, Arbus GS, Churchill BM: Allograft renal artery stenosis: increased peripheral renin

activity as an early indication of uncontrolled hypertension. *Clin Nephrol* 1978;10:232–238.
66. Luke RG, Curtis JJ, Jones P, Whelchel JD, Diethelm AG: Mechanism of post transplant hypertension. *Am J Kidney Dis* 1985;5:A79–A84.
67. Bennett WM, McDonald WJ, Lawson RK, Porter GA: Post transplant hypertension: studies of cortical blood flow and the renal pressor system. *Kidney Int* 1974;6:99–108.
68. Curtis JJ, Luke RG, Whelchel JD, Diethelm AG, Jones P, Dustan H: Inhibition of angiotensin-converting enzyme in renal transplant recipients with hypertension. *N Engl J Med* 1983; 308:377–381.
69. Ogborn MR, Crocker JFS: Captopril and transplant renal artery stenosis. *Nephron* 1988;48:333–334.
70. Dubovsky EV, Curtis JJ, Luke RC, et al: Captopril as a predictor of curable hypertension in renal transplant recipients. *Contrib Nephrol* 1987;56:117–123.
71. Roeren T, Hauenstein K, Kinkel E, Kirste G: Intraarterial digital subtraction angiography of renal transplants. *Urol Radiol* 1986;8:77–80.
72. Barry JM, Hatch DA: Parallel incision, unstented extravesical ureteroneocystotomy: follow-up of 203 kidney transplants. *J Urol* 1985;134:249–251.
73. Schiff M, McGuire EJ, Weiss RM, Lytton B: Management of urinary fistulas after renal transplantation. *J Urol* 1976; 115:251–256.
74. Groenewegen AAM, Sukhai RN, Nauta J, Scholtmeyer RJ, Nijman RJM: Results of renal transplantation in boys treated for posterior urethral valves. *J Urol* 1993;149:1517–1520.
75. Konnak JW, Herwig KR, Finkbeiner A, Turcotte JG, Freier DT: Extravesical ureteroneocystotomy in 170 renal transplant patients. *J Urol* 1975;113:299–301.
76. Salvatiera O, Olcott C, Amend WJ, Cochrum KC, Feduska NJ: Urological complications of renal transplantation can be prevented or controlled. *J Urol* 1977;117:421–424.
77. Goldman MH, Burleson RL, Tilney NL, Vineyard GC, Wilson RE: Calyceal cutaneous fistulae in renal transplant patients. *Ann Surg* 1976;184:679–81.
78. Anderson MJ, Middleton RG: Secondary pyloureterostomy with an intact ureter. *J Urol* 1982;128:247–248.
79. Kennelly MJ, Konnack JW, Herwig KR: Vesicopyeloplasty in renal transplant patients: a 20 years follow-up. *J Urol* 1993; 150:1118–1120.
80. Zaontz MR, Hatch DA, Firlit CF: Urological complications in pediatric renal transplantation: management and prevention. *J Urol* 1988;140:1123–1128.
81. Goldstein I, Cho S, Olsson CA: Nephrostomy drainage for renal transplant complications. *J Urol* 1981;126:159–163.
82. Sankari BR, Wyner LM, Chiang ML, Sparks DA, Reifsteck JE, Morrison DR: A customized nephroureteral stent for the nonoperative treatment of urine leak in pediatric renal transplantation. *Transplant Proc* 1994;26:37–38.
83. Streem SB, Novick AC, Steinmuller DR, Musselman PW: Percutaneous techniques for the management of urological renal transplant complications. *J Urol* 1986;135:456–459.
84. Fox M, Tottenham RC: Urinary fistula from segmental infarction in a transplanted kidney: recovery following surgical repair. *Br J Urol* 1972;44:336–338.
85. Lodghlin KR, Tilney NL, Richie JP: Urologic complications in 718 renal transplant patients. *Surgery* 1984;95:297–302.
86. Karmi SA, Dagher FJ, Ramos E, Young JD: Spermatic cord: cause of ureteral obstruction in renal allotransplant recipients. *Urology* 1978;11:380–383.
87. Fontana I, Arcuri V, Verrina E, et al: Tapered bowel segment for ureteral replacement in renal transplantation. *Transplant Proc* 1994;26:117–118.
88. Braun WE, Banowski LH, Straffon RA, et al: Lymphoceles associated with renal transplantation: report of 15 cases and review of the literature. *Am J Med* 1974;57:714–729.
89. Khauli RB, Stoff JS, Lovewell T, Ghavamian R, Baker S: Post transplant lymphoceles: a critical look into the risk factors, pathophysiology and management. *J Urol* 1993; 150:22–26.
90. Stephanian E, Matas AJ, Gores P, Sutherland DER, Najarian JS: Retransplantation as a risk factor for lymphocele formation. *Transplantation* 1992;53:676–678.
91. Lindstedt E, Lindholm T, Gustavsson J: Lymphocele: an important post transplantation complication. *Scand J Urol Nephrol* 1976;10:94–96.
92. Teruel JL, Martin Escobar E, Quereda C, Mayayo T, Ortuno J: A simple and safe method for management of lymphocele after renal transplantation. *J Urol* 1983;130:1058–1059.
93. Williams G, Howard N: Management of lymphatic leakage after renal transplantation. *Transplantation* 1981;31:134.
94. Zincke H, Woods JE, Anguilo JJ, et al: Experience with lymphoceles after renal transplantation. *Surgery* 1975;77:444–450.
95. Kay R, Fuchs E, Barry JM: Management of postoperative pelvic lymphoceles. *Urology* 1980;15:345–347.
96. Clayman RV, Samuel SKS, Jendrisak MD, Hanto DW: Laparoscopic drainage of the post transplant lymphocele. *Transplantation* 1991;51:725–727.
97. Khauli RB, Mosenthal AC, Caushaj PF: Treatment of lymphocele and lymphatic fistula following renal transplantation by laparoscopic peritoneal window. *J Urol* 1992; 147:1353–1355.
98. Penn I, Mackie G, Halgrimson CG, Starzl TE: Testicular complications following renal transplantation. *Ann Surg* 1972; 176:697–699.
99. Sankari BR, Boullier JA, Garvin PJ, Parra RO: Sclerotherapy with tetracycline for hydroceles in renal transplant patients. *J Urol* 1992;148:1188–1189.

29 Genitourinary Manifestations of HIV Infection

Carole A. Sable, Brian Wispelwey

HUMAN IMMUNODEFICIENCY VIRUS (HIV)

In the late 1970s a rare malignancy (Kaposi's sarcoma) and an unusual infection (*Pneumocystis carinii* pneumonia) were reported in young homosexual men.[1] These reports represented the initial cases of a new acquired human immunodeficiency symdrome. Several explanations for this syndrome surfaced, but when other groups of people (intravenous drug users and hemophiliacs) developed a similar illness, it became clear that the etiology was a common transmissible agent. The virus responsible for this syndrome, human immunodeficiency virus, was initally isolated from patients in 1983 and can now be detected in more than 99% of persons with AIDS.

Life Cycle

HIV is a member of the lentivirus subfamily of human retroviruses and contains three genes that encode viral structural proteins (gag, pol, and env) as well as at least seven other genes responsible for a variety of regulatory functions (including *tat*, *rev*, and *nef*). HIV initially attaches to the CD4 receptor on target cells such as T helper lymphocytes, macrophages, microglial cells, and dendritic cells via its gp 120. The CD4 receptor may not be the only receptor for HIV, but it is the most efficient means by which HIV enters target cells. Once the virus enters the cell, it uncoats and the viral reverse transcriptase produces double-stranded DNA from viral RNA. The DNA integrates into the host genome and subsequently exists as proviral DNA. HIV infection can remain clinically latent and largely localized in lymphoid tissue for a period of years. Eventually, increased viral replication occurs and the infection spreads by the release of infectious virions or cell fusion with uninfected cells. There are many strains of HIV and an individual may be infected with several strains simultaneously. Each strain possesses slightly different characteristics of cell tropism, viral resistance, and virulence.[2] A second, related virus, HIV-2, has been identified primarily in West Africa but also in Europe, South America, and the United States.

The primary feature of HIV infection is that it attacks the host defense mechanisms that are specifically designed to protect the host from infection. Immunologic abnormalities can be detected in patients with HIV infection early in the course of their disease even before there is a decline in the number of T helper lymphocytes. The exact mechanisms by which HIV infection produces cell death have been increasingly clarified and remain an area of intensive investigation.

Epidemiology

The estimated number of HIV-infected people in the United States is 1 to 1.5 million. The first 100,000 cases of AIDS in the United States were diagnosed over 8 years, but only 2 years had elapsed when the second 100,000 cases had occurred. The number of reported AIDS cases in the United States as of September 1992 was 242,146 and in 1995 was approaching 400,000. Initially, the epidemic affected large metropolitan areas, but recently, increasing numbers of cases in small cities and rural areas have been seen. In the United States, homosexual men accounted for the largest percentage of AIDS cases in the early years of the epidemic, followed by intravenous drug users. More recently, heterosexual transmission has become the major mode of HIV transmission in this country. The incidence of HIV infection and AIDS in women has increased dramatically. In 1992 AIDS was the leading cause of death in U.S. men aged 25 to 44 and was the fourth leading cause of death in women in the same age group.[3,4]

Worldwide the problem is even more dramatic and supports the view that this is a pandemic out of control. By 1992 an estimated 14 million people in the world were infected with HIV. The World Health Organization estimates that the number will reach 30 to 40 million by the end of the century. Others estimate that closer to 110 million people will be infected. As of 1993, an estimated 2.5 million people had AIDS; at least 80% were from the developing world. Sub-Saharan Africa has been the most severely affected, but Southeast Asia and India have been suffering from an exponential increase in cases. It is suggested that Southeast Asia will have the largest number of HIV-infected individuals by the year 2000.[5] Dealing with AIDS in the developing world is complicated by cultural differences and lack of resources. There is no indication that the current trends will reverse in the near future.

TRANSMISSION

Epidemiologic and virologic studies have identified the primary modes of HIV transmission to be parenteral exposure to blood, sexual contact, and perinatal transmission.[6] Heterosexual transmission is the primary mode of transmission worldwide and is responsible for 75% of the estimated 10 million persons infected. No type of sexual contact is completely safe, but various sexual practices are associated with different levels of risk of HIV transmission. Receptive anal intercourse carries the highest risk for heterosexual as well as homosexual partners.

Heterosexual transmission occurs in both directions, but is much less efficient from women to men than from men to women. In the United States the majority of women who have acquired the disease heterosexually have had sex with an injection drug user. Overall, sexual transmission is estimated to be 0.1 to 0.2% per sexual contact. Several factors may increase heterosexual transmission, including advanced stage of HIV infection, early HIV infection (before the development of antibodies), viral strain, genital ulcer disease, other sexually transmitted diseases, lack of circumcision, traumatic sex, and cervical ectopy.

Injection drug use is responsible for 25% of AIDS cases and occurs primarily in developed countries. The prevalence of HIV infection in injection drug users varies dramatically, from a low of less than 5% in Australia to at least 30% in Italy and Spain. Other drug use is also associated with an increased risk of HIV infection, usually through enhancement of other risk behaviors.

Perinatal transmission can occur either in utero or at birth and results in HIV infection in approximately 30% of births to HIV-infected mothers. The exact time of greatest risk for transmission has not been determined. Infants may have immunologic abnormalities at birth associated with the presence of HIV and develop rapidly progressive disease and death. Alternatively, infants may have no detectable abnormality at birth and develop disease later. Several studies have demonstrated that the firstborn twin has a higher incidence of being HIV infected in discordant pairs, and cesarean section is not protective. Transmission can also occur through breast milk and is highest in women who have primary HIV infection or seroconvert during pregnancy or in the postpartum period (29% risk versus a 14% risk for those women already known to be HIV infected). Recent data (unpublished) demonstrated a decrease in the rate of HIV transmission to infants of seropositive mothers from 23 to 8% when AZT was administered to the mothers during pregnancy. No adverse effects on the infants were seen.

Transmission also occurs through infected blood or blood products and accounts for 5% of all AIDS cases. The number of cases has been steadily declining since antibody testing became widely available in 1985. The high proportion of hemophiliacs with HIV infection is related to transfusions of large quantities of blood products prior to 1985. Although markedly decreased, the risk from transfusion is not zero; transmission can occur in the window period before conventional antibody tests become positive. Seroconversion typically occurs within 6 months of becoming infected. In 1990, the risk of HIV infection in the United States was approximately one in 225,000 donations. Transmission can also occur via transplantation of infected organs and tissues.

More than 40 health care workers have developed HIV infection because of a percutaneous injury from a needle stick or similar parenteral injury with blood from an HIV-positive patient. The estimated risk from a single needle stick is 0.3%. Transmission of HIV from health care worker to patient is very rare. The most publicized case involved a dentist in Florida who transmitted to patients, probably because of poor infection control practices.[7] A number of other HIV-infected health care workers have been studied and have not transmitted infection to patients when appropriate precautions were taken.

Despite careful investigation a small number of persons remains with an undefined means of HIV exposure. In most cases the reason is that the information is incomplete. Recent studies have revealed an isolated number of persons who became infected after living with an HIV-infected person. These cases include a child who was HIV-negative at birth (tested because he was born to an HIV-positive mother) and later seroconverted after living in the same household with another HIV-positive infant.[8] There was no definite blood or body fluid exposure, though the newly infected child did have a weeping skin rash and the source child had frequent nosebleeds and bloody diarrhea. The viral strains of the two children were nearly identical and different from either child's mother. In another case there was transmission between two hemophiliac brothers in whom there would have been opportunity for contamination with infected blood.[9] Other reports have occurred very rarely and are associated with variable degrees of certainty.[10] It is important to remember that there have been several studies of household contacts without any documented transmission by casual contact, so the risk, although real, is very small.[11–13]

NATURAL HISTORY OF HIV INFECTION

HIV infection results in a continued, progressive decline in immune function. The median time to development of AIDS is 10 years, though the time varies considerably and depends on host and viral factors and on interventions such as treatment and prophylaxis.[14,15] The classification of disease related to HIV infection has evolved since its discovery. The most recent classification system is from the CDC in January 1993. The newest definition of AIDS includes all prior AIDS-defining illnesses (see Table 29–1) as well as a CD4 count of less than 200/mm^3 and three new diseases—pulmonary tuberculosis, recurrent bacterial pneumonia, and cervical cancer. This system relies heavily on CD4 counts.

Table 29–1. Nephrotoxic Agents Used in HIV-Positive Patients and Proposed Mechanisms of Nephrotoxicity

Agents

Acyclovir	IL-2
Aminoglycosides	Pentamidine
Amphotericin	Radiocontrast dye
AZT	Rifampin
Dapsone	Sulfadiazine
Foscarnet	Trimethoprim (TMP)/sulfa (SMX)

Proposed Mechanisms of Nephrotoxicity

Amphotericin: renal insufficiency, distal renal tubular antigen, and hypokalemia

Dapsone: Unknown but produces proteinuria and papillary necrosis

Interferon, interleukin, suramin: may lead to proteinuria

Pentamidine: mild reversible azotemia, increased with underlying renal disease and concurrent nephrotoxic agents

Rifampin: tubulointerstitial nephritis and acute renal failure

TMP/SMX: sulfa causes acute interstitial nephritis, TMP causes an increase of about 30% in serum creatinine concentration (TMP competes with creatinine for tubular secretion)

A general caution is that the CD4 count is prone to several sources of error: There can be diurnal variation in CD4 count of up to 100 cells (less with lower counts), wide variation from one laboratory to another, changes with delays in processing or improper handling, and altered values with different total white blood cell counts. The CD4 percentage is less susceptible to these variations, and some consider it a better predictor of immune status.

ACUTE SEROCONVERSION ILLNESS

The acute seroconversion is generally asymptomatic, but up to 50% experience an acute mononucleosis-like syndrome 2 to 6 weeks after exposure to HIV. The most common symptoms include fever, lymphadenopathy, pharyngitis, transient rash, and myalgias or arthralgias. A small percentage of patients develop oral thrush, pneumocystis pneumonia, encephalopathy, or various forms of neuropathy. Symptoms usually resolve in 2 weeks but can persist for as long as 2 months. During seroconversion there is marked lymphopenia with reductions of both CD4 and CD8 lymphocytes. A significant number of atypical lymphocytes may be seen. This is followed by a period of lymphocytosis with an increase and eventual return to normal of CD8 cells. The CD4 cells also increase but do not return to baseline. A more accelerated course of HIV is seen in patients who have prolonged symptoms with seroconversion and in those whose CD4 counts remain suppressed after initial symptoms. Seroconversion is also associated with high levels of viremia and detectable levels of p24 antigen, followed by an antibody response within 3 weeks. An acute HIV seroconversion can be diagnosed in the correct clinical situation by positive p24 antigen and negative antibody tests to HIV.

CD4 ABOVE 500: EARLY ILLNESS

When patients have CD4 counts greater than 500 they are generally asymptomatic, although lymphadenopathy may be present. Possible symptoms include determatologic disorders such as seborrheic dermatitis, psoriasis, or a pruritic papular dermatitis (eosinophilic folliculitis). Oral lesions also occur and include oral hairy leukoplakia and aphthous ulcers. The likelihood of developing AIDS within 24 months is less than 5% in these patients.

Despite the apparent clinical stability during this period, there is a continuous decline in CD4 count and an increase in viral burden, though the total quantity of virus remains low (1 in 1000 to 1 in 10,000 cells infected). As stated earlier, several mechanisms have been elucidated to explain the progressive decline in CD4 cells besides direct viral infection.

CD4 COUNTS 200–500: MIDSTAGE DISEASE

Most patients remain asymptomatic in the midstage of the disease, although the symptoms that occurred earlier may persist or worsen. Other features develop, including diarrhea, intermittent fever, weight loss, and recurrent herpesvirus infections. Oral or vaginal yeast infections may occur intermittently or continuously. Bacterial infections are common, and the pathogens are typically those seen in community-acquired infections. Antiretroviral therapy is typically started during this time and is associated with an initial increase in CD4 counts. Patients in this stage of illness who are not treated have a 20 to 30% possibility of developing AIDS within the next 24 months.

CD4 BELOW 200: LATE DISEASE

Once patients reach the late stage they are at risk for the number of opportunistic infections and malignancies associated with AIDS. Prophylaxis against *Pneumocystis carinii* pneumonia (PCP) is initiated in patients with CD4 counts of less than 200. The frequency and severity of constitutional symptoms also increase, and the possibility of developing a new AIDS-related illness or dying is 50 to 70% in the following 24 months.

Despite interventions, the likelihood of developing a new AIDS-related condition or dying is very high for the group of patients with CD4 counts of less than 50. Accompanying this profound immunosuppression is an increased prevalence of certain diseases, including disseminated mycobacterium avium complex (MAC), cytomegalovirus retinitis, cryptococcal meningitis, disseminated histoplasmosis, and lymphoma. Multiple diseases may occur at the same time, and for many relapse is common if treatment is discontinued.

Neurologic symptoms are more pronounced, and many patients develop AIDS-related dementia or progressive multifocal leukoencephalopathy (PML), a lethal complication caused by a papovavirus. The routine use of prophylaxis for PCP has reduced the incidence of PCP, but other diseases—including MAC, candidal esophagitis, wasting syndrome, and CMV retinitis—have become more common.

DISEASE PROGRESSION

The course of HIV infection is varied, and although the median time for patients to develop AIDS is 10 to 20 years, some patients experience a markedly different course.[16] Studies of persons with known or estimated dates of seroconversion have demonstrated that transfusion recipients have the most rapid progression to AIDS, with a median time of 7 to 8 years. A number of both clinical and laboratory parameters have also been associated with more rapid disease progression. These were determined in a cohort study of homosexual men in San Francisco. Predictive factors included oral thrush, oral hairy leukoplakia, recurrent varicella zoster, and constitutional symptoms. Laboratory predictors include low CD4 count, rapidly falling CD4 percentage, elevated beta-2 microglobulin, elevated neopterin, +HIV p24 antigenemia, and syncytia-inducing strains of HIV. It is important to note that these natural history studies were conducted on patients who were not receiving antiretroviral therapy or PCP prophylaxis.

Testing

The laboratory methods available for the diagnosis of HIV include serology, antigen detection, cell culture, and gene amplication. The most commonly used method of determining infection with HIV is serology.[17]

The initial screening test is an enzyme-linked immunoadsorbent assay (ELISA), which has a sensitivity of greater than 99.7% and a specificity of at least 98.5%. If the prevalence of HIV is low there will be a number of false-positives even though the test is very sensitive. Because of this, a repeatedly positive ELISA must be confirmed by a second test such as radioimmunoprecipitation or Western blot (WB).

The WB not only determines the presence of anti-HIV antibodies, but also allows determination of the specific antigens to which the antibodies are directed. A positive WB is generally considered positive bands from two of the three major antigen groups (gag, pol, env), although the exact definition is controversial. The CDC requires two of the following bands for a positive result: p24, gp41, or gp160/120. A negative WB contains no bands for HIV, and an indeterminate is any other result.

The p24 antigen test measures the amount of free viral protein in the plasma or tissue culture supernatant. P24 is most prevalent at the time of seroconversion and in advanced HIV infection but has low sensitivity in asymptomatic patients.

Viral culture techniques are also available but are much more labor intensive and require a long time to produce positive results.

The newest technique is PCR (polymerase chain reaction), which can amplify target DNA present in very small amounts (as little as one copy of HIV in 100,000 cells) so that the virus can be detected. The one caution is that the extreme sensitivity of PCR means that even minimal inadvertent contamination can result in false-positive results.

It is important to remember that there is a window period in HIV infection that represents the time between infection with the virus and the production of a specific antibody response that can be detected by standard serologic methods. A patient is infectious during this process and so can transmit HIV, although the routine tests for HIV are negative. During the window period it is possible to detect HIV directly for viral components. Methods include detection of p24 antigen and PCR for HIV-1 DNA or RNA. Early reports of prolonged latency in HIV infection do not appear to be correct; seroconversion generally occurs within 6 months of infection with HIV.

GENITOURINARY DISEASES AND HIV INFECTION

The first description of renal diseases in HIV was by Gardenswartz in 1984.[18] Early reports of diseases related to HIV mentioned only rare involvement of the genitourinary system. Since 1990 it has become obvious that genitourinary disease is an important component of the illness of HIV. Renal manifestations of HIV infection occur commonly, and 38 to 68% exhibit azotemia, proteinuria, hematuria, or pyuria at some time during their illness.[19] The diseases that occur are diverse and include intrinsic renal disease secondary to HIV, intrarenal infection, and acute renal failure secondary to a number of causes.[18,20] Most of the diseases are associated with radiologic abnormalities, and in one study of 60 patients, 46 (77%) had abnormalities on renal ultrasound; 12 out of 18 patients (67%) had abnormalities on CT.[21] In addition, a review of retroperitoneal and pelvic CT of 86 patients with HIV demonstrated the following abnormalities: enlarged kidneys in 34 (40%), hilar LN in 30 (35%), renal calcifications in 7 (8%), adnexal mass in 5 (6%), hydronephrosis in 4 (5%), pyelonephritis in 3 (3%), abscess in 3 (3%), and solid masses in 3 (3%).[22] It is important to note that the patients reviewed had imaging studies done for clinical indications and that the information is not meant to be indicative of incidence of disease.

We will focus on the abnormalities that are unique to HIV and those diseases whose manifestations are different in the setting of HIV infection.

Intrinsic Renal Disease

HIV NEPHROPATHY

HIV nephropathy occurs in approximately 10% of HIV-positive patients. It was initially described by Rao in 1984 and is characterized by focal and segmental glomerulosclerosis (FSGS).[23] Although initally postulated, it is not the same disease as heroin nephropathy. Clinically, patients develop mild hypertension and proteinuria that may be in the nephrotic range. Progressive renal failure develops over a period as short as a few months.[22,24]

The kidneys are enlarged and are swollen on gross appearance. Histologically, the disease is manifested by mesangial hypocellularity, sparse interstitial infiltrate, tubular degenerative changes, and tubular ectasia with protein casts throughout the cortex and medulla.[25] Bowman space dilatation, edema, and inflammation are also present. Glomerular capillaries are collapsed and obliterated with hyaline deposits.[21,26]

HIV nephropathy can develop at any time in the course of HIV disease but is more common in blacks and in men. Treatment is for the renal failure that eventually develops and includes either hemodialysis or peritoneal dialysis. Early reports of HIV nephropathy described a wasting syndrome and rapid death despite treatment with hemodialysis.[23] More recent information supports dialysis as an effective therapy for this disease; survival depends more on the stage of HIV infection than on the presence of HIV nephropathy.

IMAGING

Ultrasound reveals enlarged kidneys with increased cortical echogenicity (Fig. 29–1).[20,26,27] There is no correlation between the degree of echogenicity and the extent of renal disease. On CT there is global enlargement of the kidneys without hydronephrosis or cortical scarring, and increased attenuation in the medulla. After the administration of contrast, a striated nephrogram can be seen, resulting from the presence of dilated tubules filled with protein.[27,28] On MRI the kidneys are enlarged and demonstrate nonspecific loss of the normal corticomedullary differentiation on T1-weighted images.

The findings of HIV nephropathy on ultrasound are nonspecific. Increased echogenicity can be seen in a number of diseases associated with HIV infection, including glomerular lesions such as focal segmental glomerulosclerosis, mesangial hypercellularity, diffuse proliferative glomerulonephritis (GN), and membranous GN; acute tubular necrosis; focal interstitial nephritis; nephrocalcinosis; and tubular atrophy. An abnormal ultrasound, although not diagnostic in this population, does raise the concern of intrinsic renal disease.

OTHER GLOMERULAR LESIONS

HIV nephropathy is not the only glomerular abnormality seen in patients with HIV infection.[29] Immune complex mediated glomerulopathies have been reported, and, rarely, other antigens such as hepatitis B (surface and e antigens), CMV, and EBV have been identified in renal tissue. Diffuse or focal mesangial hypercellularity with deposits of IgM and C3 have been identified as isolated renal manifestations. Minimal change disease and hemolytic uremic syndrome have also been identified in patients with HIV infection.

Infections

Recurrent infections of the genitourinary tract may occur in as many as 50% of HIV-positive patients and can take the form of cystitis, pyelonephritis, lobar nephronia, or renal

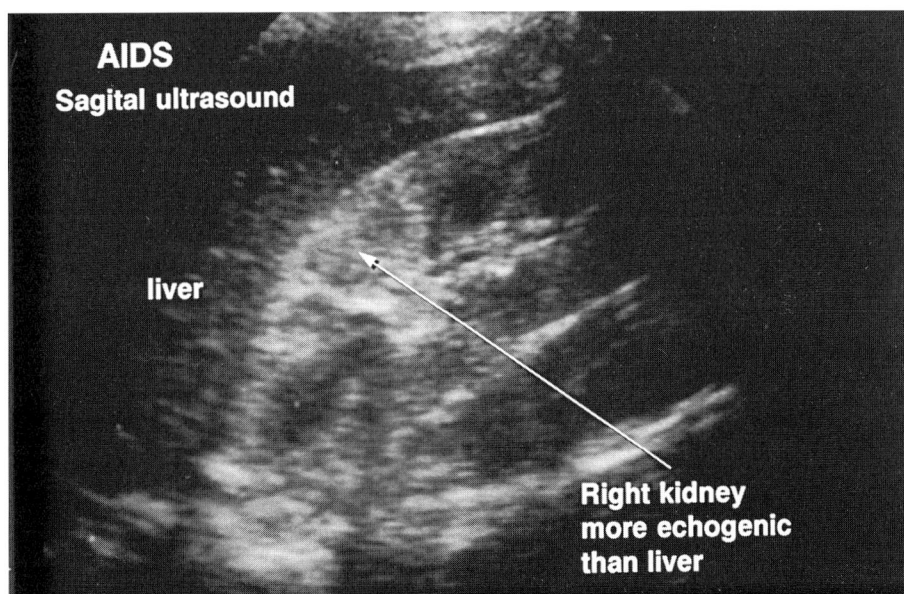

Figure 29–1. Sagittal ultrasound of a kidney with AIDS nephropathy. Parenchyma has increased echogenicity.

abscess.[30] Intravenous drug users are also at risk for the development of septic emboli.

Urinary tract infections may be secondary to atypical pathogens such as species of *Candida, Salmonella,* and *Acinetobacter* as well as typical urinary organisms.[19] Prostatitis may result from infection with a variety of pathogens, including *Staphylococcus aureus, Mycobacterium tuberculosis, Cryptococcus neoformans, Histoplasma capsulatum, H. parainfluenzae,* and salmonella as well as routine enterobacteriaceae. If present, prostatic abscesses require surgical drainage in addition to antimicrobial therapy. This may be accomplished transurethrally or by open perineal drainage. The optimal method for diagnosis of prostatic abscess is CT.

Epididymo-orchitis also occurs and can be caused by a number of pathogens, including *Candida albicans, Toxoplasma gondii, Histoplasma capsulatum,* cytomegalovirus (CMV), and salmonella.[31-33] Infections caused by salmonella can be fatal and must be treated aggressively. As with salmonella sepsis, patients frequently relapse if not placed on prophylactic antibiotics after treatment of the acute infection.

Another common abnormality is chronic dysuria with negative routine cultures. Under these circumstances, atypical pathogens, including acid-fast bacilli and viruses, must be considered as possible etiologies. The viral pathogens that have been implicated include CMV, human papilloma virus (HPV), and herpes simplex virus (HSV).[30,34,35] Medications may also cause dysuria by damaging the epithelial cells lining the urethra. In HIV-positive patients routinely taking a number of drugs, it may be difficult to determine the causative agent.

IMAGING

The CT appearance of cystitis is that of bladder wall thickening. In acute pyelonephritis the kidneys are swollen, with patchy nephrograms that may have either areas of increased or decreased echogenicity. A renal abscess is seen as a focal, low-attenuation lesion that may have a rim of enhancement. Thickening of Gerota's fascia may be the manifestation of perirenal inflammatory changes.[22] None of these abnormalities is specific for, or indicative of, HIV infection. All can be seen with any bacterial infection of the kidney.

ATYPICAL PATHOGENS

Pneumocystis carinii is one of the most common infections in patients with HIV and typically occurs when the CD4 count is less than 200. Pulmonary symptoms, including dry cough and progressive dyspnea and exertion, are the most common presenting manifestations. Extrapulmonary pneumocystosis is unusual but can occur in the setting of inhaled pentamidine used for PCP prophylaxis. Many sites of disease have been reported, including the choroid, liver, lymph nodes, bone marrow, spleen, and kidneys.

Typical radiographic findings of renal involvement include punctate calcifications confined to the cortex. Calcifications in PCP, unlike other diseases, are not necessarily indicative of healed, inactive disease.[36-38] It is important to perform nonenhanced CT scans because IV contrast may obscure the presence of calcifications. Of note, nephrocalcinosis is not diagnostic for *Pneumocystis carinii* and can be seen with a variety of diseases, including hypercalcemia and hypercalciuria, *Mycobacterium avium* complex (MAC), CMV, and histoplasmosis.[39,40] Diagnosis is made by biopsy of the involved tissue with special stains, including methenamine silver and toluidine blue. Pulmonary disease may also be present and provide an additional site for diagnosis.

Disseminated *Mycobacterium avium* complex (MAC) occurs in as many as 55% of AIDS patients with advanced disease (CD4 counts of less than 100). Disease can involve the bone marrow, lungs, liver, gastrointestinal tract, lymph nodes, spleen, and kidneys. There is typically diffuse adenopathy involving the para-aortic, renal hilar, and mesenteric nodes. Presenting symptoms vary, depending on the organ systems involved, but commonly patients report a systemic illness with fever, night sweats, weight loss, and abdominal pain.

When the kidneys are involved in MAC infections, partial nephrocalcinosis of the cortex and medulla is seen. One characteristic finding on CT is decreased attenuation within the lymph nodes corresponding to areas of necrosis. Mesenteric nodal abscesses may occur as a result of confluent nodal masses. Although a number of diseases can produce bulky lymphadenopathy in AIDS patients, these two features would be unusual.[41]

Extrapulmonary *Mycobacterium tuberculosis* (TB) represents approximately 50% of the tuberculosis seen in HIV infection and is common at any stage of HIV disease. Tuberculosis occurs more commonly in patients who have other risks for the disease, including using intravenous drugs, living under crowded conditions, and being black or Hispanic. Patients with renal TB present with urinary symptoms of dysuria and hematuria, and "sterile" pyuria and microscopic hematuria are evident in most patients. Renal involvement can be seen as single or multiple hypoechoic lesions on renal ultrasound.[42] Abnormalities will be seen on intravenous pyelogram in more than 90% of patients and include evidence of pyelonephritis in early disease (calyceal blunting and reflex of contrast). Later changes are more diagnostic and include ureteral strictures, corkscrewing, beading, focal calcification, hydronephrosis, and parenchymal cavitation. The abnormalities may be bilateral, even though in most patients symptomatic disease is unilateral.

A diagnosis of mycobacterial disease can be made by fine needle aspiration of the involved organ or tissue. Mycobacteria may involve several organ systems simultaneously, and a renal or lymph node biopsy may not be needed to confirm the diagnosis. In patients with MAC, systemic symptoms are typically present and blood cultures are often positive. However, multiple diseases may be present simultaneously in

AIDS patients, and a failure to respond to therapy should prompt further diagnostic evaluation, including biopsy.

Candida produces multiple small masses that are usually low attenuation on CT and hypoechoic on ultrasound. It may also result in the formation of fungus balls and obstruction of the ureter or renal pelvis. Other fungi such as histoplasmosis and aspergillus may also involve the kidneys in HIV-positive patients. Histoplasma can produce multiple non-shading echogenic areas on ultrasound that vary widely in size.[43]

Cryptosporidia has been reported to cause an enterovesicular fistula in a patient with AIDS.[44] Cryptosporidia is an enteric protozoan that causes self-limited diarrhea in immunocompetent patients. It is transmitted by the fecal–oral route from pets, farm animals, and other people. In immunocompromised patients the disease manifests as chronic, watery diarrhea for which there is no proven effective therapy. In the case reported, the fistula was demonstrated only by CT. All other studies, including barium enema, cystoscopy, flexible sigmoidoscopy, and colonoscopy, were negative.

Findings consistent with the diagnosis of a fistula on imaging studies include intravesical air, focal bladder wall thickening, thickening of the adjacent bowel wall, paravesical mass, adherence of bowel to bladder, and presence of orally or rectally injected contrast in the bladder. There are a number of causes of fistulas, including diverticulitis, Crohn's disease, colon cancer, pelvic tumors, radiation therapy, trauma, appendiceal abscesses, ulcerative colitis, TB, syphilis, and schistosomiasis.

Cytomegalovirus (CMV) causes both direct and indirect effects on the kidneys. CMV is a disease of significant immunosuppression in HIV infection and is typically not seen until CD4 counts are less than 100. (GI disease can occur with higher CD4 counts of around 200.) The most common manifestation of CMV in AIDS is retinitis, followed by GI disease with esophagitis and colitis. CMV can also be isolated from the urine of patients with advanced HIV disease. Symptomatic cystitis also occurs and may be accompanied by hematuria and pyuria.[34]

SEXUALLY TRANSMITTED DISEASES

Because HIV is a sexually transmitted disease (STD), it is common for other STDs to occur simultaneously with HIV.[45] The majority have characteristics similar to the general population and are discussed elsewhere. Two diseases deserve mention, pelvic inflammatory disease and genital warts.

Pelvic inflammatory disease (PID) can be more severe in HIV-infected women. They require hospitalization more frequently and have a higher incidence of complications, including tubo-ovarian abscess. Because of this, caution must be exercised in dealing with this population.[46]

Genital warts, caused by human papilloma viruses (most commonly types 6 and 11), can cause large exophytic masses in homosexual men. If the lesions are intraurethral they may result in urinary obstruction. Exophytic lesions can also occur in the rectum and produce obstruction of the GI tract. The oncogenic types of HPV (16 and 18) are related to an increased risk of carcinoma in situ of the cervix and invasive cervical carcinoma. Women with HIV have been found to have more advanced cervical neoplasia at diagnosis and to be more likely to have recurrent disease, perianal involvement, and disease more commonly associated with evidence of HPV infection. HIV-infected homosexual men with significant immunosuppression are at increased risk for developing HPV-related anal neoplasia.[47]

Malignancy

LYMPHOMA

Lymphoma in patients with AIDS is typically non-Hodgkins lymphoma and is characteristically B cell in origin. It is an aggressive disease and is widely disseminated at the time of diagnosis.[48,49] Lymphoma may be the initial manifestation of AIDS, and the diagnosis of an aggressive, disseminated B cell lymphoma should raise the question of HIV infection. Among patients with AIDS-related lymphoma, 6 to 12% have renal involvement, which usually manifests as bilateral, discrete parenchymal masses rather than as a diffuse increase in size such as that seen in lymphoma in patients without AIDS.[50–52] There may also be invasion of the kidneys or obstruction of the collecting system or ureters by lymphadenopathy.[53] Involvement is typically multifocal, so CT is the diagnostic modality of choice.[54]

KAPOSI'S SARCOMA

Kaposi's sarcoma (KS) occurs in 25% of patients with HIV and is commonly multicentric.[48] The most common sites include skin, lymph nodes, lungs, GI tract, liver, and spleen.[55] Renal involvement occurs less frequently. The disease is usually microscopic and consists of irregular dilatation of the vascular space coated with swollen endothelial cells. KS is frequently found on autopsy and is not evident on imaging studies.[22] Lesions are seen on the skin of the penis in approximately 20% of patients with KS and may result in urinary retention if they involve the glands. Conservative treatment of penile lesions is recommended and may involve excisional biopsy, local radiation, or laser therapy. Systemic treatment is generally reserved for widely disseminated or visceral disease.

If KS involves the retroperitoneal lymph nodes, bulky lymph nodes will be seen on CT and obstructive uropathy may develop. By the time KS involves the retroperitoneum, there is typically evidence of disease elsewhere.[48] Other unusual sites of involvement in the GU tract include the prostate, testes, seminal vesicles, and bladder.[20] The presence of large, bulky adenopathy is nonspecific and can be seen with MAC or lymphoma as well as with KS.

OTHER MALIGNANCIES

Testicular tumors, including both germ cell and lymphoma, have been reported to occur more commonly in patients with HIV infection. An increase in germ cell tumors has not been demonstrated in every study. Lymphoma is a common problem in patients with AIDS, so it is not surprising that testicular lymphoma is more common in this group than in the general population. Renal cell carcinoma has also been reported.[20]

ACUTE RENAL FAILURE

One of the most common causes of acute renal failure in patients with HIV infection is acute tubular necrosis (ATN) secondary to toxic or hemodynamic abnormalities, including sepsis, shock, or drugs (Table 29–2). Acute interstitial nephritis also occurs.[19,24,30]

ATN can result from hypovolemia associated with vomiting or diarrhea, hypotension secondary to shock, or drug toxicity. Although the possible initiating events may be more numerous in HIV-infected individuals, the diagnosis and treatment are the same as for those not infected with HIV.

SUMMARY

The genitourinary manifestations of HIV infection are diverse and occur relatively commonly (in approximately 10% of patients). The diseases typically reflect the stage of immunosuppression. Early in HIV infection, when the patient's immune system is relatively intact, infections are the same as those that occur in the general population. In addition, HIV may directly affect the kidney at any stage of HIV infection and may result in HIV nephropathy. As the patient's immunosuppression progresses and AIDS develops, opportunistic infections and malignancies become more common. Some of the diseases are unique to HIV infection; others exhibit unique clinical features in patients with HIV infection.

An understanding of the diagnostic possibilities allows us to develop a logical approach to an HIV-positive patient with genitourinary disease.

REFERENCES

1. CDC: Pneumocystis pneumonia—Los Angeles, *MMWR* 1981; 30:250–252.
2. Levy JA: HIV pathogenesis and long-term survival. *AIDS* 1993;7:1401–1410.
3. CDC: Update: mortality attributable to HIV infection among persons aged 25–44 years—United States, 1991 and 1992. *MMWR* 1993;42:869–872.
4. CDC: Update: AIDS—United States, 1992. *MMWR* 1993; 42:547–556.
5. Mann J, Tarantola DJM, Netter TW: The HIV pandemic: status and trends. In: Mann J, Tarantola DJM, Netter TW, eds. A *Global Report: AIDS in the World*. Cambridge: Harvard University Press, 1992;11–132.
6. CDC: The HIV/AIDS epidemic: the first 10 years. *MMWR* 1991;40:357–368.
7. CDC: Possible transmission of HIV to a patient during an invasive dental procedure. *MMWR* 1990;39:489–493.
8. Fitzgibbon JE, Gaur S, Frenkel LD, et al: Transmission from one child to another of HIV type I with a zidovudine-resistance mutation. *N Engl J Med* 1993;329:834–841.
9. Morbidity Mortality Weekly Report: HIV infection in two brothers receiving intravenous therapy for hemophilia. *MMWR* 1992;41:228–231.
10. Wahn V, Kramer HH, Vort T, Bruster HT, et al: Horizontal transmission of HIV infection between two siblings. *Lancet* 1986;2:694.
11. Rogers MF, White CR, Sanders R, et al: Lack of transmission of HIV from infected children to their household contacts. *Pediatrics* 1990;85:210–214.
12. Fischl MA, Dickinson GM, Scott AB, et al: Evaluation of heterosexual partners' children, and household contacts of adults with AIDS. *JAMA* 1987;257:640–644.
13. Friedland GH, Saltzman BR, Rogers MF, et al: Lack of transmission of HTLVIII/LAV infection to household contacts of patients with AIDS or AIDS-related complex with oral candidiasis. *N Engl J Med* 1986;314:344–349.
14. Lifson AR, et al: Progression and clinical outcome of infection due to HIV. *Infect Dis Clin* 1992;14:966–972.
15. Pantaleo G, Grazrosi C, Fauci AS: The immunopathogenesis of human immunodeficiency virus infection. *N Engl J Med* 1993;328:327–335.
16. Ward JW, Bush TJ, Perkins HA, et al: The natural history of transfusion-associated infection with HIV: factors influencing the rate of progression to disease. *N Engl J Med* 1989;321:947–952.
17. Sloand EM, Pitt E, Chiarello RJ, Nemo GJ: HIV testing: state-of-the-art. *JAMA* 1991;266:2861–2866.
18. Gardenswartz MH, Lerner CW, Seligson GR, et al: Renal disease in patients with AIDS: a clinicopathologic study. *Clin Nephrol* 1984;21:197–204.
19. Glassock RJ, Cohen AH, Donovitch G, Parsa KP: HIV infection and the kidney. *Ann Intern Med* 1990;112:35–49.
20. Miles BJ, Melser M, Farah R, et al: The urologic manifestation of AIDS. *J Urol* 1989;142:771–773.

Table 29–2. Renal Disease and HIV Infection

Infectious organisms	Glomerulonephritis
Viral: HIV, CMV	Membranous
Mycobacteria: *M. tuberculosis, M. avium* complex	Membranoproliferative Mesangial proliferative
Bacteria (including salmonella):	**Acute renal failure**
Fungi: *Candida* sp.	Acute tubular necrosis: sepsis, toxins, hypovolemia
Cryptococcus neoformans	
Histoplasma capsulatum	
Aspergillus sp.	Acute interstitial nephritis
Pneumocystis carinii	Vascular: infarction, vasculitis, hemolytic–uremic syndrome
Malignancy	
Non–Hodgkin's lymphoma	
Hodgkin's disease	
Kaposi's sarcoma	
Hypernephroma	

21. Miller FH, Parikh S, Gore RM, et al: Renal manifestation of AIDS. *Radiographics* 1993;13:587–596.
22. Kuhlman JE, Browne D, Shermak M, et al: Retroperitoneal and pelvic CT of patients with AIDS: 1 & 2 involvement of the genitourinary tract. *Radiographics* 1991;11:473–483.
23. Rao TKS, Filippone EJ, Nicastri AD, et al: Associated focal and segmental glomerulosclerosis in AIDS. *N Engl J Med* 1984;310:669–673.
24. Rao TKS, Friedman EA, Nicastri AD, et al: The types of renal disease in AIDS. *N Engl J Med* 1987;316:1062–1068.
25. Pardo V, Aldana M, Colton RM, et al: Glomerular lesions in AIDS. *Ann Intern Med* 1984;101:429–434.
26. Hamper VM, Goldblum LE, Hutchins GM, et al: Renal involvement in AIDS: sonographic–pathologic correlation. *AJR* 1988;150:1321–1325.
27. Schaffer RM, Schwartz AE, Becker JA, et al: Renal ultrasound in AIDS. *Radiology* 1984;153:511–513.
28. Kuhlman JE: Renal and urinary tract complications. In: Kuhlman JE, ed. CT of the immunocompromised host. *Contemporary Issues in CT*. New York: Churchill Livingstone 1990; 89–114.
29. Van der Reyden HJ, Schipper MEI, Danner SA, Arisz L, et al: Glomerular lesions and opportunistic infections of the kidney in AIDS: an autopsy study of 47 cases.
30. Vaziri ND, Barbari A, Licorush K, et al: Spectrum of renal abnormalities in AIDS. *J Natl Med Assoc* 1985;77:369–375.
31. Haskell L, Fusco MJ, Ares L, Sublay B: Case report: disseminated toxoplasmosis presenting as symptomatic orchitis and nephrotic syndrome. *Am J Med Sci* 1989;298:185–190.
32. Nistal M, Santana A, Paniagua R, Palacios J: Testicular toxoplasma in two members with AIDS. *Arch Pathol Lab Med* 1986;110:744–746.
33. Chabon AB, Stenger RJ, Grabstald H: Histopathology of testis in AIDS. *Urology* 1987;29:658–663.
34. Benson MC, Kaplan MS, O'Toole K, Romagnoli M: A report of CMV cystitis and a review of other genitourinary manifestations of AIDS. *J Urol* 1988;40:153–154.
35. Lucas SB, Parr DC, Wright E, et al: AIDS presenting as CMV cystitis. *Br J Urol* 1989; 64:2129–2130.
36. Radin DR, Baker EL, Klatt EC, et al: Visceral and nodal calcifications in patients with AIDS-related *Pneumocystis carinii* infection. *AJR* 1990;154:27–31.
37. Bargman JM, Wagner C, Cameron R: Renal cortical nephrocalcinosis: a manifestation of extrapulmonary *Pneumocystis carinii* infection in AIDS. *Am J Kidney Dis* 1991;17:712–715.
38. Sponge AR, Wilson ST, Gopinath N, et al: Extrapulmonary *Pneumocystis carinii* in a patient with AIDS: sonographic findings. *AJR* 1990;155:76–78.
39. Manz F, Jaschke W, van Kaick A, et al: Nephrocalcinosis in radiographs, CT, ultrasound and histology. *Pediatri Radiol* 1980;9:19–26.
40. Bray HJ, Lail VJ, Cooperberg PL, et al: Tiny, echogenic foci in the liver and kidney in patients with AIDS: not always due to disseminated *Pneumocystis carinii*. *AJR* 1992;158:181–182.
41. Falkoff GE, Rigsby CM, Rosenfield AT: Partial combined cortical and medullary nephrocalcinosis: ultrasound and CT patterns in AIDS-associated MAI infection. *Radiology* 1987;162:343–344.
42. Pitchenik AE, Feitel D: Tuberculosis and non-tuberculosis mycobacterial disease. *Med Clin North Am* 1992;76:121–152.
43. Kay CJ: Renal diseases in patients with AIDS: sonographic findings. *AJR* 1992;159:551–554.
44. Meyers SA, Kuhlman JE, Fishman EK: Enterovesical fistula in a patient with cryptospordia and AIDS. CT demonstration. *Clin Imaging* 1990;14:143–145.
45. Wasserhert JN: Epidemiological synergy: interrelationships between HIV and other STDs. *Sex Transm Dis* 1992;19:61–77.
46. Hoegsberg B, Abulafia O, Sedlis A, et al: Sexually transmitted diseases and HIV infection among women with pelvic inflammatory disease. *Am J Obstet Gynecol* 1990;163:1135–1139.
47. Vermund SH, Kelley KF, Klein BS, et al: High risk of human papillomavirus infection and cervical squamous intraepithelial lesions among women with symptomatic HIV infection. *Am J Obstet Gynecol* 1991;165:392–400.
48. Nyberg DA, Federle MP: AIDS-related Kaposi sarcoma and lymphomas. *Semin Roentgenol* 1987;22:54–65.
49. Levine AM: AIDS-associated lymphoma. *Med Clin North Am* 1992;76:253–268.
50. Townsend RR: CT of AIDS-related lymphoma. *AJR* 1991;156:969–974.
51. Cohan RH, Dunnich NR, Leden RA, Baker ME: Computed tomography of renal lymphoma. *J Comput Assist Tomogr* 1990;14:933–938.
52. Nyberg DA, Jeffrey RB, Federle MP, et al: AIDS-related lymphomas: evaluation by abdominal CT. *Radiology* 1986;159:59–63.
53. Spector DA, Katz RS, Fuller H, et al: Acute non-dilating obstructive renal failure in a patient with AIDS. *Am J Nephrol* 1989;9:129–132.
54. Townsend RR, Laing FC, Jeffrey RB, Bottles K: Abdominal lymphoma in AIDS: evaluation with ultrasound. *Radiology* 1989;171:719–724.
55. Krown SE, Myskowski PL, Paredes J: Kaposi's sarcoma. *Med Clin North Am* 1992;76:239–252.

Index

(Page numbers followed by *t* indicate tables.)

Abdominal examination, 8–9
Abdominal leak point pressure, 521
Abdominal masses, 8
Abdominal radiography, 35–44
  of adrenal gland, 527
  in bladder outlet obstruction, 329
  calcification, 38–41
  in excretory urography, 57–58, 61
  gas collections, 41–44
  in neurogenic bladder, 505
  normal, 35
  postcompression, 61
  reviewing, 35
  in soft tissue abnormalities, 35–38
Abscess
  prostate, *see* Prostate, abscess
  renal, *see* Renal abscess
"Absent kidney sign", 156
Absorptive hypercalciuria, 304
Accelerated renal allograft rejection, 552
Accessory gland fungal infection, 296
Acquired renal cystic disease, 88
Acute bacterial prostatitis, 263, 448
Acute bacterial pyelonephritis, 267–275
  in children, 268
  physical examination, 267–268
  radionuclide scan of, 268
  urinalysis in, 268
Acute lobar nephronia, pediatric, 247
Acute renal allograft rejection, 552–554
Acute renal failure
  AIDS-related, 574
  causes of, 146
  radionuclide imaging of, 145–149
Acute tubular necrosis, 146
  AIDS-related, 574
  as renal transplant complication, 551
    radionuclide imaging of, 152
    ultrasound in, 97
Adenocarcinoma
  of bladder, 400–403
  of collecting system, 173
  of prostate, 454
  renal, *see* Renal cell carcinoma
Adenoma
  magnetic resonance imaging of, 185
  renal, 185, 382
  of renal collecting system, 171–172
Adenomatoid tumor, 474
ADPKD, *see* Autosomal dominant polycystic kidney disease
Adrenal gland, 529–548
  abdominal radiography of, 527
  adrenal venous sampling, 532–533

Cushing's syndrome, 534–537
cysts, 544
hemorrhage, neonatal, 252–253
imaging modalities, 529t–534
  computed tomography, 174–175, 531–532
  magnetic resonance imaging, 252–253, 532
  scintigraphy, 533–534
  ultrasound, 81–82, 529–531
masses of
  clinically silent, 542–548
  computed tomography in, 174
  diagnosis, 543–546
  evaluation with known malignancy, 546–548
  incidentally discovered, 543t
pheochromocytoma, *see* Pheochromocytoma
primary hyperaldosteronism, 537–540
trauma to, 174, 425
Adrenal venous sampling, 532–533
Adult polycystic renal disease, *see* Autosomal dominant polycystic kidney disease
Advanced urodynamics, 27
Adverse reactions to contrast media, 50–53
Agenesis
  renal, 231
  sacral, 513
AIDS-related disorders, 570–574
  see also HIV infection
  computed tomography in, 165–166, 171, 572
  genitourinary tuberculosis, 285, 290, 572
  infections, 571–572
  mycobacterial infections, *see* Mycobacterial infections, AIDS-related
  renal, 574t
    intrinsic renal disease, 571
    ultrasound of renal involvement, 93
Allergic reactions to contrast media, 50–51
Ambulatory urodynamics, 27–28
Angiography, *see* Renal angiography
Angiomyolipoma, 384–385
  in children, 421–423
  imaging in, 384–385
    computed tomography, 172, 385
    magnetic resonance imaging, 185, 385
    ultrasound, 90
  of renal collecting system, 172
Aniridia, 412
Antegrade descending-voiding urethrography, 69–71
Antegrade pyelography, 215–216
  in urinary stone disease, 313
  in urothelial tumors, 378
Antegrade pyeloureterography, 215–216, *see also* Antegrade pyelography
Antibody coating, 276

Antihypertensives, erectile dysfunction from, 487
Antituberculosis drugs, 290–293
Arteriogenic impotence, 485–486
  diagnostic tests for, 114–115, 492
  symptoms of, 489–490
  ultrasound in, 114–115
Arteriography
  penile, 492
  renal, 344, 413
Arteriovenous fistula
  following renal transplantation, 98
  renal angiography in, 225
  ultrasound in, 98
ATN, *See* Acute tubular necrosis
Augmentation cystoplasty, 509–510
Autosomal dominant polycystic kidney disease
  computed tomography in, 167
  magnetic resonance imaging in, 184
  pediatric, 249
  ultrasound in, 87
Autosomal recessive polycystic kidney disease, 249
  disease types, 249t
  ultrasound in, 87–88

Bacteria, in urinalysis, 14
Bacterial cystitis, 257–259
Bacteriuria, 257
  causes, 258
  in pregnancy, 280
  urine culture for, 14–16, 257–258
Beckwith-Wiedeman syndrome, 412
Bell clapper deformity, 111
Benign neoplasms
  see also specific neoplasms
  of bladder, 395–396
  of collecting system, 190
  computed tomography in, 171–172
  renal, 382–387
    ultrasound in, 90–91
  of testes, 476
  of urethra, 407
Benign prostatic hypertrophy, 335–337, 450–454
  clinical findings, 450–451
  definition, 450
  diagnosis, 450–451
  etiology, 450
  hesitancy in, 323
  imaging in, 118–119, 451
    magnetic resonance imaging, 451
    transrectal ultrasound, 118–119, 451
  physical examination, 327
  treatment, 337, 452–454
  urographic alterations from, 329t

577

Bifid scrotum, 466
Biothesiometry, 493
Birth history, 2
Bladder
　anatomy, 438
　cancer, see Bladder cancer
　computed tomography of, 175–177
　cystography, see Cystography
　focal disease of, 194
　foreign bodies in, 207
　hernia of, 175
　infectious lesions, 100–101
　inflammatory lesions
　　computed tomography in, 176
　　magnetic resonance imaging in, 193
　　ultrasound evaluation of, 100–101
　　and urinary tract infections, 260–262
　injuries to, 438, 439–440, 442
　magnetic resonance imaging of, 193–196
　pain from, 3–4
　physical examination of, 9
　rupture
　　computed tomography in, 175–176
　　pelvic fractures causing, 439–440
　tuberculosis in, 290
　tumors, see Bladder tumors
　ultrasound evaluation of, see Ultrasound, of bladder
Bladder cancer, 396–403
　etiology and pathogenesis, 396–397
　magnetic resonance imaging in, 195–196
　metastatic disease, 196
　schistosomiasis associated with, 300
　transitional cell carcinoma, see Transitional cell carcinoma, bladder
Bladder capacity, 23
　reduced, 5
Bladder compliance, 23–24
Bladder contractility
　inhibition of, 508–510
　triggering, 510–511
Bladder function, cystometry measuring, 22–25
Bladder neck
　obstruction of, 337–338
　reconstruction in neurogenic bladder, 510
Bladder neck dyssynergia, 338
Bladder outlet
　decreasing resistance in neurogenic bladder, 511
　increasing resistance in neurogenic bladder, 510
　obstruction, see Bladder outlet obstruction
　surgery in neurogenic bladder, 511
　urethral pressure studies of, 28–30
Bladder outlet obstruction, 323–340
　and acute renal failure, 146
　etiologies, 324t, 335–339
　hematuria in, 326
　irritative symptoms, 324–325
　laboratory studies, 328
　obstructive symptoms, 323–324
　physical examination, 327–328
　prostatism and, 325t, 327t
　radiography in, 329–330
　residual urine volume in, 328
　symptoms, 323–327
　symptom scores, 326–327

　treatment, 339–340
　urinary incontinence in, 325
　urinary retention in, 326
　urodynamic studies of, 330–335
　urologic pain in, 325–326
　in women, 337
Bladder overdistention, 509
Bladder tumors, 395–407
　benign, 395–396
　cancer, see Bladder cancer
　computed tomography in, 176–177, 404–406
　cystography in, 404
　cystoscopy in, 404
　cytology in, 404
　excretory urography, 404
　flow cytometry of, 404
　magnetic resonance imaging in, 194–197, 406
　radionuclide bone scans in, 406
　ultrasound evaluation of, 100, 404
Bladder wall, 193
Blood chemistries, in neurogenic bladder, 505
Blood in urine, see Hematuria
Blood urea nitrogen, 17
Blunt trauma
　renal, 425–426
　scrotal, 479
Bone metastases
　radionuclide bone scans monitoring, 156
　renal angiography in, 224
Bone scans, 154–156
　in bladder tumors, 406–407
Bony pelvis
　anatomy, 438
　physical examination of, 9
Bowel preparation, in urography, 54
BPH, see Benign prostatic hypertrophy
Brachytherapy, 460
Breath-hold imaging, in MRI, 180–181
Broth dilution method, in urine culture, 16–17
Brush biopsy, 377
BUN, 17

Calcification
　abdominal radiographs in, 38–41
　of bladder tumors, 176
　renal, see Renal calcification
　scrotoliths, 108
Calcium stones, 304–306
Candida albicans infection, 293–294
　AIDS-related, 573
Candidiasis, 293–294
　magnetic resonance imaging in, 190
Carcinoma
　adenocarcinoma, see Adenocarcinoma
　embryonal cell, 104, 475
　penile, 116
　renal cell, see Renal cell carcinoma
　small cell, 401–402
　squamous cell, see Squamous cell carcinoma
　transitional cell, see Transitional cell carcinoma
　urethral, 198
　yolk sac, 475
Cardiac abnormalities, from contrast media, 51
Casts, in urinalysis, 14
Cavernosography, 492–493

Cavernous biopsy, 495–496
CDU, see Color Doppler ultrasound
Cerebrovascular accident, and neurogenic bladder, 511–512
Chemotherapy in Wilm's tumor, 416, 418–419
Children
　development of urinary control, 525t
　medullary cystic disease in, 250–253
　neurogenic bladder in, 513
　obstruction and reflux in, 232–250
　pyelonephritis in, 247
　　acute bacterial, 268
　radionuclide imaging of, 136–145
　renal agenesis and ectopia in, 231–232
　renal tumors in, 411–423
　spinal dysraphism in, 32–33
　undescended testes in, 479–481
　urinary incontinence in, 525–526
　urinary tract abnormalities in, 231t
　urinary tract infection in, 245–247, 259
　uroradiology of, 231–254
　Wilm's tumor in, see Wilm's tumor
Chills, 3
Choriocarcinoma of scrotum, 475
　ultrasound in, 105
Chronic atrophic pyelonephritis, 278, see also Reflux nephropathy
Chronic bacterial prostatitis, 263–265, 448–449
Chronic bacterial pyelonephritis, 275–278
Chronic epididymitis, 468
Chronic renal allograft rejection, 554
Chronic renal disease, 149–152
Chyluria, 7
CMG, 22
CMN, see Congenital mesoblastic nephroma
CMV, AIDS-related, 166, 573
　computed tomography in, 166
CO_2 cystometry, 22
Collecting system
　chronic bacterial pyelonephritis affecting, 277
　computed tomography of, 172
　duplication anomalies of, 237–239
　excretory urography of, 60
　filling defect, see Filling defect
　magnetic resonance imaging of, 190–191
　stones in, 172, 190–191
　transitional cell carcinoma of, 172–173, 190
Colle's perineal fascia, 438–439
Color Doppler ultrasound, 79
　in arteriogenic impotence, 492
　of kidneys, 80–81
　　transplant complications, 97–98
　of scrotum, 466
　　blunt trauma, 479
　　inflammation, 110–111
　of testes
　　inflammation, 110–111
　　tumors, 107
　in urinary obstruction, 83
Complete blood count, 328
Complex renal cysts, 349–359
　angiography in, 359
　class 3, 352–355
　class 5, 355
　classes 1 and 2, 349–352
　classification of, 349

Complex renal cysts *(Continued)*
    computed tomography in, 166–167, 349–357
    magnetic resonance imaging in, 357–359
    pitfalls in diagnosis, 355–357
    spiral CT of, 359
    ultrasound in, 349–352, 355–357
Computed tomography, 161–177
    of adrenal gland, 174–175, 531–532
    in AIDS-related disorders, 165–166, 171, 572
    anatomy in, 161
    in angiomyolipoma, 172, 385
    in bladder tumors, 176–177, 404–406
    in extrarenal lesions, 173–174
    in genitourinary tuberculosis, 290
    in oncocytoma, 171–172, 382
    in primary hyperaldosteronism, 538–540
    of prostate, 447–448
        in cancer staging, 458–459
    renal
        abscess, 274
        acute bacterial pyelonephritis, 269
        autosomal dominant polycystic kidney disease, 87
        complex cysts, 166–167, 349–357
        congenital anomalies, 162
        metastases, 171, 387–388
        renal cell carcinoma, 168–170, 186–187, 363–368
        simple cysts, 86, 345–346t
        Wilm's tumor, 413
        xanthogranulomatous pyelonephritis, 164–165, 279
    in schistosomiasis, 299
    single photon emission, 156
    technique, 161–162
    in upper tract obstruction and dilatation, 318–319
    in urinary stone disease, 172, 312t
    urography and, 46
    in urothelial tumors, 172–173, 376–377
Condyloma acuminata in urethra, 407
Coned kidney radiograph, with abdominal compression, 60–61
Congenital anomalies
    agenesis
        renal, 231
        sacral, 513
    computed tomography in, 162
    of kidney, *see* Kidney, congenital anomalies
    and neurogenic bladder, 513
    of scrotum, 466–467
    urethral, 197
Congenital mesoblastic nephroma, 419–421
Constant infusion technique, 134
Continuous incontinence, 6
Contrast media
    see also specific types
    in cystography, 66–68
    in magnetic resonance imaging, 199–200
    in urography, 46–54
        adverse reactions, 50–53
        allergic reaction, 46
        dosage, 53–54
        method of injection, 57
        molecular structure, 46–48
        physiology, 46–48
        uroradiographic quality, 48–49

Contrast nephropathy, 177
Cortical renal abscess, 273
Crede maneuvers, 510
Cryoablation of prostate, 120
Cryptorchidism, 479–481
    see also Undescended testes
    ultrasound in, 112
Cryptosporidia, AIDS-related, 573
Crystals, in urinalysis, 14
Cushing's syndrome, 534–537
Cyclosporin, in renal transplant, 152
    toxicity from, 97
Cystadenoma of epididymis, 474
Cystic disease of kidneys, 248t
    autosomal dominant polycystic kidney disease, *see* Autosomal dominant polycystic kidney disease
    classification of, 247
    complex cysts, *see* Complex renal cysts
    computed tomography in, 166–167
    hemodialysis causing
        magnetic resonance imaging in, 184
        pediatric, 250
    indeterminate lesions, 220–224, 346–347
    magnetic resonance imaging in, 182–185
    malformations, associated with, 250t
    pediatric, 247–250, 250
    simple cysts, *see* Simple renal cysts
    ultrasound in, 86–88, 249
Cystine stones, 306
Cystitis
    bacterial, 257–259
    cystica, 260–261
    emphysematous, 42–43, 259–260
    eosinophilic, 262
    glandularis, 261–262
    hemorrhagic, 166, 193–194
    interstitial, 262
    ultrasound in, 100–101
Cystitis cystica, 260–261
Cystitis glandularis, 261–262
Cystography, 66–68
    bladder
        foreign bodies in, 207
        injuries to, 442
        tumors of, 404
    contrast media in, 66–68
    radionuclide, 134–135, 244–245
    retrograde, 66–68, 206
    in schistosomiasis, 298
    urethral, 207
    in urinary tract infections, 259
Cystometrogram, 22
Cystometry, 22–25
    in bladder outlet obstruction, 330–331
    involuntary contractions during, 24
    misinterpretation of, 24–25
    in urinary incontinence, 520
Cystoscopes, 205–206
Cystoscopy, 205–218
    in bladder tumors, 404
    in cystitis cystica, 261
    in emphysematous cystitis, 260
    in interstitial cystitis, 262
    in malakoplakia, 262
    in urinary tract infections, 259
    in urothelial tumors, 378

Cyst puncture, 344–345t
Cytology
    in bladder tumors, 404
    in urothelial tumors, 377
Cytomegalovirus, AIDS-related, 166, 573
    computed tomography in, 166

Daytime urinary frequency, 5
Denervation procedures, in neurogenic bladder, 509
Deny-Drash syndrome, 412
Dermatologic disorders, 7
Detrusor leak point pressure, 521
Detrusor pressure, 22–23
Detrusor-sphincter dyssynergia, 338–339
    sphincter electromyography in, 30
Diabetes
    and emphysematous cystitis, 259–260
    irritative voiding symptoms from, 5
Diabetes mellitus
    arteriogenic impotence due to, 485
    and neurogenic bladder, 513
Diffuse renal disease, 93–94
Digital fluororadiography, 64, 65–66
Digital luminescent radiography, 64–65
Digital radiography, 64–66
Digital rectal examination, 10
    in bladder outlet obstruction, 327–328
    in erectile dysfunction, 491
    in prostate cancer, 119, 454–455
Dip-slide culture, 16
Disc dilution method, in urine culture, 17
Disc disease, 512
Discoloration of urine, 7
Diuretic renal scintigraphy, 235
Diuretic renography
    of hydronephrosis, 135
    of upper obstruction and dilatation, 319–320
    urography and, 45
DMSA scan, 505
DNA ploidy, 398–399
Doppler penile arterial pressure measurement, 492
Doppler ultrasound
    color, *see* Color Doppler ultrasound
    of kidneys
        pulse Doppler ultrasound, 80–81
        in transplant rejection, 97
    pulsed, 80–81
    in venogenic impotence, 115
Double balloon technique, in retrograde urethrography, 73
Drug allergy history, 1
Drug-induced impotence, 487–488
Duplication anomalies, 237–239
    ultrasound in, 238–239
Dysuria, AIDS-related, 572

Ectopic kidney, 231
Effective renal plasma flow
    iodine-131 and iodine-123 in, 131
    nonimaging measurement of, 134
Electrical stimulation, 509, 511
Electromyography
    in bladder outlet obstruction, 334–335
    sphincter, *see* Sphincter electromyography

Electromyography *(Continued)*
 in urinary incontinence, 520–521
Emboli, renal, 188–189
Embolization, preoperative, 220
Embryonal cell carcinoma, 104, 475
Emphysematous cystitis, 42–43, 259–260
Emphysematous pyelonephritis, 42, 270–272
 computed tomography in, 164
 treatment, 271–272
Endocrinologic impotence, 488
Endoscopy, 205–218
 in bladder outlet obstruction, 329
 of lower tract, 205–208
 in neurogenic bladder, 506
 percutaneous nephroscopy, *see* Percutaneous nephroscopy
 ureteropyeloscopy, *see* Ureteropyeloscopy
 of urinary diversion, 218
Endourology, *see* Endoscopy
Enuresis, 5
Eosinophilic cystitis, 262
Epidermoid cysts, of testes, 476
 ultrasound in, 107
Epididymitis, 467–468
Epididymo-orchitis
 AIDS-related, 572
 pediatric radionuclide imaging in, 144, 145
 ultrasound in, 110
Epinephrine in renal angiography, 224
Erectile dysfunction, 6, 485–497
 clinical evaluation, 488–489
 diagnostic tests, 491
 drug-induced impotence, 487–488
 endocrinologic impotence, 488
 evaluation, 488–497
 neurogenic impotence, 486–487, 493
 physical examination, 489–491
 psychogenic impotence, 487
 urologic evaluation, 489–491
 vasculogenic impotence, *see* Vasculogenic impotence
Erectile function tests, 493–497
 cavernous biopsy, 495–496
 nuclear magnetic resonance imaging, 496
 penile blood gas measurement, 496–497
 penile rigidity assessment, 497
 radionuclide imaging, 496
 single potential analysis of cavernosal electrical activity, 493–495
Erythrocytes, 14
Evoked responses, in sphincter EMG, 32
Excretory urography, 45–64
 in acute bacterial pyelonephritis, 268
 in bladder tumors, 404
 complications of, 46
 contrast media in, 46–54
 in cystitis cystica, 261
 in cystitis glandularis, 262
 indications for, 46
 intravenous urogram, *see* Intravenous urography
 in neurogenic bladder, 505
 patient preparation in, 54–57
 performance of, 57–61
 in renal cell carcinoma, 363
 technical factors, 62
 in tuberculosis, 288–290
 in urinary tract infections, 259
 in urothelial tumors, 376
Excretory voiding urethrography, 69–70
External genitalia
 dermatologic disorders of, 7
 female, 10
 male, 9–10
 physical examination of, 9–10
 symptoms in, 3–7
Extratesticular abnormalities, 474
 ultrasound in, 107–110

Family history, 2
Fast low-angle shot technique, in MRI, 180
Fecaluria, 7
Fever, 3
Fibromas, renal, 385
Filariasis, 300–301
Filling defect
 cystoscopy in, 207
 differential diagnosis, 312t
 intravenous pyelography in, 312t
 magnetic resonance imaging in, 190–191
Fistulae
 AIDS-related, 573
 arteriovenous, 98, 225
 gastrointesitnal-genitourinary, 152
FLASH technique, in MRI, 180
Flow cytometry, 404
Fluid collections, following renal transplant, 96
Fluid cystometry, 22
Fluid restriction, in urography, 54–57
Fluoroscopy
 in urinary incontinence, 521–522
 videourodynamics and, 28
Focal bacterial nephritis
 acute, 165
 computed tomography in, 165
 ultrasound in, 91
Focal pyelonephritis, 389–390
Foreign bodies of bladder and urethra, 207
Frequency-selective fat suppression, in MRI, 180
Fungal infection, 285, 293–296
 Candida albicans, 293–294, 573
 interventional radiography, 296
 pharmacology, 295–296
 radiology in, 294–295
 treatment of, 294, 295–296
 ultrasound in, 93

Gallium scanning
 of renal abscess, 274
Gas collections, 41t–44
Gastrointesitnal-genitourinary fistula, 152
Genital warts, 573
Geriatric incontinence, 526–527
Germ cell tumors of testes, 103–104
GFR, *see* Glomerular filtration rate
Glomerular filtration rate, 17
 nonimaging measurement of, 134
 technetium-99m use in measuring, 131
Glomerulocystic disease, pediatric, 249–250
Glomerulonephritis, 93–94
Gonadal stromal tumors, 105–106
Gonadoblastoma, 106
Gram staining, 258

Granulomatous prostatitis, 265–266
Grawitz tumor, *see* Renal cell carcinoma
Gross hematuria, 7
Gynecomastia, 8

Hemangiomas of scrotum, 467
Hematocele, 473–474
Hematoma
 computed tomography in, 162, 173
 following renal transplant, 96
 retroperitoneal, 173
Hematospermia, 8
Hematuria, 7
 in bladder outlet obstruction, 326
 cystoscopy in, 207
 renal angiography in, 225–227
 ureteroscopy for, 212
 urinalysis in, 14
Hemihypertrophy, 412
Hemodialysis, renal cysts and
 magnetic resonance imaging in, 184
 pediatric, 250
Hemorrhage
 adrenal, pediatric, 252–253
 renal
  magnetic resonance imaging in, 189
  as transplant complication, 555
Hemorrhagic cyst, 167
Hemorrhagic cystitis
 in AIDS patients, 166
 computed tomography in, 166
 magnetic resonance imaging in, 193–194
Hesitancy, 323
Heterozygous cystinuria, 305
HIV infection, 567–574
 see also AIDS-related disorders
 acute seroconversion illness, 569
 CD4 counts, 569–570
 epidemiology, 567–570
 genitourinary diseases and, 571–574
 life cycle, 567
 malignancies associated with, 573–574
 natural history of, 568–569
 nephrotoxic agents used in, 569t
 progression of, 569–570
 sexually transmitted diseases and, 573
 testing, 570
 transmission, 568
HIV nephropathy, 571
 computed tomography in, 165
Hormonal therapy, 481
Horseshoe kidney, 231–232
 computed tomography in, 162
 radionuclide imaging of, 132
 uroradiology of, 231–232
Hydrocele, 471
 as renal transplant complication, 563
 ultrasound in, 107–108
Hydronephrosis
 diuretic renography in, 135
 following renal transplant, 96–97
 pediatric
  radionuclide imaging in, 132–142
  uroradiology in, 232–235
 ultrasound, conditions simulating on, 317t
Hydronephrosis of pregnancy, 83–84
Hyperacute renal allograft rejection, 552

Hypernephroma, *see* Renal cell carcinoma
Hyperoxaluria, 305
Hypertension
 in chronic renal disease, 149–152
 renal artery stenosis and, 149, 150
 from upper urinary tract disorders, 3
Hypertrophy
 benign prostatic, *see* Benign prostatic hypertrophy
 of bladder wall, 193
 hemihypertrophy, 412
Hyperuricosuria, 305
Hypocitraturia, 305
Hypomagnesuria, 305

Immunocompromised individuals
 AIDS, *see* AIDS-related disorders
 HIV infection, *see* HIV infection
 infection in, 285
  AIDS-related, 285, 290, 571–572
  fungal, 294
Impotence
 erectile dysfunction, *see* Erectile dysfunction
 ultrasound in, 113–115
Incontinence, *see* Urinary incontinence
Indeterminate renal masses, 346–347
 angiography in, 220–224
Infantile polycystic disease, *see* Autosomal recessive polycystic kidney disease
Infection
 fungal, *see* Fungal infection
 HIV infection, *see* HIV infection
 mycobacterial, *see* Mycobacterial infection
 parasitic, *see* Parasitic infection
 renal, *see* Renal infection
 urinary tract, *see* Urinary tract infection
Infectious stones, 306
Inferior vena cava, 220
Infertility
 erectile dysfunction, *see* Erectile dysfunction
 impotence, male, 113–115
 seminal vesicles and, 121
 varicocele and, 108–109
Intermittency, 5
 in bladder outlet obstruction, 324
Intermittent catheterization, 508
Interstitial cystitis, 262
Interstitial seed radiation, 460
Interventional radiology
 in fungal infection, 296
 in genitourinary tuberculosis, 293
 in schistosomiasis, 299
Intrarenal reflux, 245
Intravenous pyelography
 see also Intravenous urography
 in bladder outlet obstruction, 329
 filling defect, differential diagnosis of, 312*t*
 in simple renal cysts, 344
 in Wilm's tumor, 412–413
Intravenous urography, 231
 see also Intravenous pyelography
 in renal abscess, 273
 in renal sinus cysts, 87
 in upper tract obstruction and dilatation, 317–318
 in urinary stone disease, 309–311
Intrinsic renal disease, AIDS-related, 571

Inverted papilloma of bladder, 395
Iodine-123, 131
Iodine-131, 131
Ionic contrast
 molecular structure and physiology of, 47–48
 nonionic contrast versus, 49
 uroradiographic quality of, 48–49
IRR, 245
Irritative voiding symptoms, 4–5
Ischemia
 renal, 188–189
 testis, 111
IVP, *see* Intravenous pyelography
IVU, *see* Intravenous urography

Juvenile nephronophthisis, 250
 see also Medullary cystic disease
Juxtaglomerular cell tumors, 171
Juxtarenal processes, 192

Kaposi's sarcoma, 573
 computed tomography in, 171
Kidney, 82
 AIDS-related disorders, *see* AIDS-related disorders, renal
 computed tomography, *see* Computed tomography, renal
 congenital anomalies
  agenesis, 231
  computed tomography in, 162
  magnetic resonance imaging in, 181–182
  radionuclide imaging in, 136–142
 Doppler ultrasound of, 80–81
  transplant rejection, 97
 failure of, *see* Renal failure
 infection, *see* Renal infection
 magnetic resonance imaging of, *see* Magnetic resonance imaging, of kidneys
 masses of, *see* Renal masses
 neoplasms, *see* Renal neoplasms
 obstruction of
  magnetic resonance imaging in, 188
  as renal transplant complication, 96–97, 559–561
 parenchyma, *see* Renal parenchyma
 physical examination of, 8–9
 radionuclide imaging of, *see* Radionuclide imaging, renal imaging
 stone disease in, 41, 84–85
 symptoms in, 3
 trauma, 425–432, *see also* Renal injuries
 ultrasound of, *see* Ultrasound, renal

Labia, pain in, 4
Laboratory examination, 13–18
Lactic dehydrogenase isoenzyme, 276–277
Laparoscopy, 460
Latency, nerve conduction studies in, 31–32
LDH isoenzyme, 276–277
Leak point pressure, 29–30
Leiomyomas, renal, 385
Leukemia
 renal, 89
 testicular, 476
Leukocytes, 14, 258
Leukoplakia, renal, 92

Leydig cell tumors, 475
 ultrasound in, 105–106
Libido, loss of, 6
Lipomas, renal, 385
Lipomatosis, pelvic, 194
Lower urinary tract
 bladder, *see* Bladder
 endoscopy of, 205–208
 function of, 21
 infection of, 257–260
 innervation of, 502
 neuromechanics of, 502
 penis, *see* Penis
 symptoms in, 3–7
 trauma to, 438–443
 urethra, *see* Urethra
Low semen volume, 8
LPP, 29–30
Lymphocele
 as renal transplant complication, 96, 561–563
 treatment modalities in, 563*t*
Lymphoma
 HIV infection associated with, 573
 renal, *see* Renal lymphoma
 of testes, 475–476

MAG3, 131–132
Magnetic resonance imaging, 179–200
 of adrenal gland, 532
  neonatal hemorrhage, 252–253
 in angiomyolipoma, 185, 385
 of bladder, 193–196
  tumors, 194–197, 406
 breath-hold imaging, 180–181
 of collecting system, 190–191
 contrast agents in, 199–200
 frequency-selective fat suppression, 180
 future of, 199–200
 of juxtarenal processes, 192
 of kidneys, 181–192
  abscess, 274
  acute bacterial pyelonephritis, 269–270
  complex cysts, 357–359
  renal cell carcinoma, 185–187, 369–372
  simple cysts, 346*t*
  Wilm's tumor, 187, 413
  xanthogranulomatous pyelonephritis, 190, 279
 physics of, 179–180
 principles of, 179–181
 of prostate, 448
  benign prostatic hypertrophy, 451
  cancer staging, 459
  radionuclide bone scans compared, 156
  rapid acquisition with relaxation enhancement, 181
 of retroperitoneum, 192–193
 saturation pulses, 181
 of scrotum, 466
 specialized coils, 199
 techniques of, 180, 199
 of ureter, 192–193
Malacoplakia, 262
 ultrasound in, 92
Malignant melanoma, of bladder, 402

Malignant non-germ cell tumors, of scrotum, 105
Malignant tumors
  see also specific types of malignancies
  bladder cancer, see Bladder cancer
  carcinoma, see Carcinoma
  of collecting system, 190
  HIV infection associated with, 573–574
  metastases, see Metastases
  prostate cancer, see Prostate cancer
  scrotum, 104–107
Masses
  see also specific types of masses
  abdominal, 8
  of adrenal gland, see Adrenal gland, masses of
  extrinsic lesions, 99
  indeterminate renal, 220–224, 346–347
  renal, see Renal masses
  scrotal, see Scrotum, mass lesions
  of spermatic cord, 10
  ultrasound in, 99
  ureteral, differential diagnosis of, 99
Medical history, 1
  in erectile dysfunction, 490
Medication summary, 1
  in erectile dysfunction, 490
Medullary cystic disease
  see also Juvenile nephronophthisis
  pediatric, 250–253
  ultrasound in, 88
Medullary sponge kidney, 184
Megaureter, 235–237
Mesenchymal neoplasms, of bladder, 396, 403
Mesothelioma, paratesticular, 474
Metastases
  to adrenal glands, 546–548
  to bladder, 196
  of bladder carcinoma, 177, 196
  bone
    radionuclide bone scans monitoring, 156
    renal angiography in, 224
  of prostate cancer, 154–156
  renal, 387–389
    angiography in, 224
    computed tomography in, 171, 387–388
    magnetic resonance imaging in, 188
  to renal collecting system, 190
  to testes, 476
Methylglucamine cation, 48–49
Microscopic hematuria, 7
Micturitional urethral pressure profile, 335
Micturition cycle, 21
  neurophysiology of, 501–502
Mixed germ cell tumors of scrotum, 105
MRI, see Magnetic resonance imaging
Multicystic dysplastic kidney
  computed tomography in, 167
  pediatric, 250–251
  ultrasound in, 88
Multilocular cystic nephroma
  computed tomography in, 171
  magnetic resonance imaging in, 184–185
  ultrasound in, 91
Multilocular masses, 167
Multiple sclerosis, 512, 523
Mumps orchitis, 469
Mycobacterial infections, 285
  AIDS-related, 572–573
    computed tomography in, 166
    tuberculosis, 285, 290, 572
  tuberculosis, genitourinary, see Tuberculosis, genitourinary
Myelodysplasia, 513, 524
Myelolipoma, of adrenal gland, 544–546

National Wilm's Tumor Studies, 416–417
Nausea, 3
Needle-aspiration biopsy, see Percutaneous needle aspiration
Neoplasms
  benign, see Benign neoplasms
  extratesticular, 109–110
  malignant, see Malignant tumors
  renal, see Renal neoplasms
  of testes, 474–478
Nephrectomy, 293
Nephrocalcinosis, 85
Nephrogenic adenoma, of bladder, 396
Nephronia
  acute lobar, pediatric, 247
  computed tomography in, 165
Nephrotomography
  in excretory urography, 63–64
  of simple renal cysts, 344t
Nerve conduction studies, 31–32
Neuroblastoma
  in adrenal medulla, 175
  pediatric, 143–144
Neuroendocrine tumors, 152
Neurofibromatosis, 194
Neurogenic bladder, 501–513
  in children, 513
  classification of, 502–503
  clinical findings, 507
  decreasing outlet resistance, 511
  expanded functional classification, 508t
  facilitation of bladder emptying, 510–511
  facilitation of bladder storage, 508–510
  ICS classification system, 503t
  increasing outlet resistance, 510
  innervation, 502
  laboratory procedures, 505–507
  management of, 507–511
  neurophysiology of micturition, 501–502
  neurourological examination, 504–505
  patient evaluation, 504–507
  patient history, 504
  specific problems, 511–513
  ultrasound evaluation of, 101
  Wein functional classification, 503t
Neurogenic impotence, 486–487
  diagnostic tests, 493
Neurogenic obstruction, 338–339
Neurologic disorders, urinary incontinence and, 523–524
Neuropathic bladder, 5
  videourodynamics for, 28
Neurourological examination, of bladder, 504–505
Nocturnal penile tumescence test, 491
Nocturnal urinary frequency, 5
Nonbacterial prostatitis, 265, 449
Non-germ cell neoplasms, 475

Nonionic contrast
  dosage of, 53–54
  ionic contrast versus, 49
  molecular structure and physiology of, 48
Nonseminomatous germ cell tumors, 475, 478
  ultrasound in, 104–105
Nonurachal adenocarcinoma, 401
Nuclear magnetic resonance imaging, 496

Oblique-view radiographs, 61
Obstruction
  of renal artery and vein, 146
  urinary, see Urinary tract obstruction
Obstructive voiding
  causes of, 5–6
  symptoms of, 5
  urodynamic studies in, 33
Oncocytoma, 382–384
  computed tomography in, 171–172, 382
  ultrasound in, 90, 382
Orchitis, 469
Orgasm, absence of, 7
Overflow incontinence, 6

Pain, as symptom, 2–7
  in bladder outlet obstruction, 325–326
  differential diagnosis, 2, 3
Papillomas, of bladder, 194
Parapelvic cysts, 184
Parasitic infection, 285, 296–301
  filariasis, 300–301
  rare forms of, 301
  schistosomiasis, 297–300
Parkinson's disease, 512
Patient history, 1–8
  in blunt renal trauma, 425
  in neurogenic bladder, 504
  in penetrating renal trauma, 426
  in urinary incontinence, 518–519
Patient preparation, in urography, 54–57
Patient selection, in urography, 45–46
Pediatrics, see Children
Pelvic inflammatory disease, 573
Pelvic lipomatosis, 194
Pelvis
  fractures, urologic injury from, 439–440
  surgery, and neurogenic bladder, 512–513
Penetrating renal trauma, 426–427t
Penile arteriography, 492
Penile blood gas measurement, 496–497
Penis
  anatomy of, 112–113
  pain in, 4
  physical examination of, 9
  physiology of, 113
  ultrasound of, 112–116
Penoscrotal transposition, 466–467
Percutaneous needle aspiration
  in adrenal masses, 543
  in genitourinary tuberculosis, 293
  in renal abscess, 274–275
  in renal cell carcinoma, 375–376
Percutaneous nephroscopy, 213–218
  anatomy, 213–214
  antegrade pyeloureterography, 215–216, see also Antegrade pyelography
  complications, 217–218

Percutaneous nephroscopy *(Continued)*
  indications, 217
  instrumentation, 214–215
  technique, 216–217
Percutaneous transcatheter embolization, 225–227
Percutaneous transluminal angioplasty, 228
Peyronie's disease, ultrasound in, 115–116
Pharmacologic therapy
  in fungal infection, 295–296
  in genitourinary tuberculosis, 290–293
  in neurogenic bladder, 508–509, 510
  in schistosomiasis, 299
Pheochromocytoma, 540–542
  bladder, 194, 402–403
  diagnosis, 541
  imaging in, 541–542
    computed tomography, 175
    magnetic resonance imaging, 194
    radionuclide imaging, 152
  treatment, 542
Physical examination, 1–10
  abdominal examination, 8–9
  in acute bacterial pyelonephritis, 267–268
  in benign prostatic hypertrophy, 327
  in bladder outlet obstruction, 327–328
  in blunt renal trauma, 425
  in erectile dysfunction, 489–491
  of external genitalia, 9–10
  general principles, 8
  in penetrating renal trauma, 426
  of scrotum, 9, 465–466
  in urinary incontinence, 519
  in urinary stone disease, 307
Plate dilution method, in urine culture, 17
Pneumaturia, 7–8
Pneumocystis carinii infection of kidneys, 572
  computed tomography in, 166
Polyps of urethra, 407
Polyuria, 5
POM, *see* Primary obstructive megaureter
Poor force of urinary stream, 324
Posterior urethral valves, 239–243
Postvoid radiographs, 61
Pregnancy
  bacteriuria in, 280
  hydronephrosis in, 83–84
  pyelonephritis in, 280–281
Premedication of contrast media, 51
Preoperative embolization, 220
Preoperative evaluation, renal angiography in, 220
Pressure-flow studies
  in bladder outlet obstruction, 332–334
  computer-assisted analysis of, 333–334
Primary hyperaldosteronism, 537–540
Primary nonobstructive nonrefluxing megaureter, pediatric, 236–237
Primary obstructive megaureter, pediatric, 235–236
Primary refluxing megaureter, pediatric, 236
Prone radiographs, 61
Prostadynia, 449
Prostate, 445–461
  abscess, 449–450
    from fungal infections, 296
    ultrasound in, 120–121

anatomy, 116–117, 445
benign prostatic hypertrophy, *see* Benign prostatic hypertrophy
computed tomography of, 447–448
inflammation of, 448–450
  prostatitis, *see* Prostatitis
  ultrasound in, 120–121
magnetic resonance imaging of, *see* Magnetic resonance imaging, of prostate
pain from, 4
physical examination of, 10, 445–446
ultrasound of, 116–121
  transrectal, *see* Transrectal ultrasound
Prostate cancer, 454–461
  adenocarcinoma, 454
  computed tomography staging, 458–459
  digital rectal examination in
    in screening, 454–455
    in staging, 455
    transrectal ultrasound and, 119
  expectant management of, 461
  grading, 455
  laparoscopic staging, 460
  magnetic resonance imaging in staging, 459
  metastases of, 154–156
  outlet obstruction from, 339
  prostate specific antigen, *see* Prostate specific antigen
  radionuclide bone scans of, 154–156
  screening, 454–455
  staging, 455–460
  transrectal ultrasound in, 456–457
    and biopsy, 119–120, 458
    in screening, 455
    in staging, 457–458
  treatment, 460–461
Prostate specific antigen, 17–18, 119, 454–455
  in bladder outlet obstruction, 328
  as marker, 17–18
  monitoring treatment response with, 18
  in staging of cancer, 18, 456
  and ultrasound, 119
Prostatic acid phosphatase, 456
Prostatic intraurethral stents, 453–454
Prostatism
  AUA Symptom Index, 327*t*
  benign prostatic hypertrophy, *see* Benign prostatic hypertrophy
  and bladder outlet obstruction symptoms, 325*t*, 335–337
Prostatitis, 262–266, 448–450
Prostatodynia, 265
Prune-belly syndrome, 243–244
Pseudoaneurysms, in renal transplant, 98
Pseudohematuria, 7
Psychogenic impotence, 487
Psychosocial interview in erectile dysfunction, 489
Pulsed Doppler ultrasound, 80–81
Purified protein derivative testing, 286–287
Pyelonephritis, 267
  acute bacterial, 267–275
  chronic bacterial, 275–278
  computed tomography in, 164
  emphysematous, *see* Emphysematous pyelonephritis
  focal, 389–390

  magnetic resonance imaging in, 189
  pediatric, 247, 268
  in pregnancy, 280–281
  radionuclide imaging in, 142
  ultrasound in, 91
  xanthogranulomatous, *see* Xanthogranulomatous pyelonephritis
Pyonephrosis, 91–92
Pyuria, 7
  in urinary tract infections, 258

Radiation therapy
  for prostate cancer, 460
  for Wilm's tumor, 416, 418–419
Radical prostatectomy, 460–461
Radiography
  see also specific imaging methods
  abdominal, *see* Abdominal radiography
  of chronic bacterial pyelonephritis, 277
  cystography, *see* Cystography
  digital, 64–66
  of emphysematous pyelonephritis, 271–272
  of genitourinary tuberculosis, 287
  in renal abscess, 272–273
  seminal vesiculography, 73–74, 266–267
  urethrography, *see* Urethrography
  of urinary tract, *see* Excretory urography
Radiology
  in fungal infection, 294–295
  in schistosomiasis, 297–299
Radionuclide bone scans, 154–156
  in bladder tumors, 406–407
Radionuclide cystography, 134–135
  of vesicoureteral reflux, 244–245
Radionuclide imaging, 131–157
  cystograms, *see* Radionuclide cystography
  diuretic renogram, *see* Diuretic renography
  in erectile function testing, 496
  imaging procedures, 132–136
  instrumentation, 132
  in neurogenic bladder, 505
  pediatric, 136–145
  renal imaging, 132–133, 145–149
    abscess, 274
    acute bacterial pyelonephritis, 268
    clinical applications, 145–157
    congenital anomalies, 136–142
    function quantitation, 133–134
    masses, 361
    pediatric trauma, 143
    simple cysts, 344
    transplantation evaluation, 152–154
  of upper tract obstruction and dilatation, 319–320
Radiopharmaceuticals, 131–132
Rapid acquisition spin echo, in MRI, 181
Rapid acquisition with relaxation enhancement, in MRI, 181
RAS, *see* Renal artery stenosis
RAT, *see* Renal artery thrombosis
RCC, *see* Renal cell carcinoma
Referred pain, 2
Reflex inhibition, in neurogenic bladder, 509
Reflux
  pediatric, 232–250
  vesicoureteral, *see* Vesicoureteral reflux

Reflux nephropathy, 278
  see also Chronic atrophic pyelonephritis
  magnetic resonance imaging in, 189
  ultrasound in, 92
Rejection of renal transplant, see Renal allograft rejection
Renal abscess, 272–275
  computed tomography in, 165
  magnetic resonance imaging in, 189–190
  predisposing factors, 272
  ultrasound in, 91
Renal adenocarcinoma, see Renal cell carcinoma
Renal agenesis, 231
Renal allograft dysfunction, 563–564
  differential diagnosis of, 563t, 564t
Renal allograft rejection, 551–554
  magnetic resonance imaging in, 192
  ultrasound in, 97
Renal angiography, 220–229
  in abscess, 273–274
  in acute bacterial pyelonephritis, 270
  in complex cysts, 359
  in hematuria, 225–227
  in indeterminate masses, 220–224
  in preoperative evaluation, 220
  in renal cell carcinoma, 375
  of renal donors, 228–299
  in renovascular hypertension, 228
  in transplantation, 228
  in trauma, 227
  in xanthogranulomatous pyelonephritis, 280
Renal arteriography
  in simple renal cysts, 344
  in Wilm's tumor, 413
Renal artery
  obstruction of, 146
  pediatric trauma to, 143
  radionuclide imaging of, 143
  stenosis, see Renal artery stenosis
  thrombosis, see Renal artery thrombosis
Renal artery stenosis
  angiography in, 228
  nuclear screening tests for, 149–150
  percutaneous transluminal angioplasty for, 228
  as renal transplant complication, 556–558
    detection of, 152
    radionuclide imaging in, 154
    ultrasound in, 98
Renal artery thrombosis
  computed tomography in, 163
  as renal transplant complication, 555–556
  ultrasound in, 98
Renal calcification
  abdominal radiographs in, 38–41
  computed tomography in, 167
  in indeterminate renal masses, 346–347
Renal cell carcinoma, 361–376
  and adenomas, 382
  in children, 423
  differential diagnosis of, 389–390
  examination, 362
  focal pyelonephritis compared, 389–390
  imaging in, 363–368
    computed tomography, 168–170, 186–187, 363–368

excretory urography, 363
magnetic resonance imaging, 185–187, 369–372
renal angiography, 220, 224, 375
ultrasound, 88–89, 363
laboratory studies, 362
percutaneous needle aspiration of, 375–376
presentation, 361–362
renal infarct compared, 389–390
staging of, 186–170, 368–369, 370t
Renal clear cell carcinoma, see Renal cell carcinoma
Renal colic, 3
Renal collecting system, see Collecting system
Renal collecting tubular ectasia, 184
Renal cysts, see Cystic disease of kidneys
Renal donors, 228–229
Renal dysplasia
  classification of, 248
  radionuclide imaging in, 132
Renal emboli, 188–189
Renal failure
  acute, see Acute renal failure
  chronic, 149–152
  radionuclide imaging in, 149–152
  ultrasound in, 93
  urography in, 46
Renal function, 17
  magnetic resonance imaging of, 191–192
  nonimaging quantitation, 134
  radionuclide imaging of, 133–134
Renal hypercalciuria, 304–305
Renal infarct, 389–390
Renal infection
  acute renal failure and, 146–149
  computed tomography in, 164–165
  magnetic resonance imaging in, 189–190
  pyelonephritis, see Pyelonephritis
  radionuclide imaging in, 142, 146–149
  tuberculosis, 92, 288
  ultrasound in, 91–93
Renal injuries, 425–432
  angiography in, 227
  blunt trauma, 425–426
  classification of injuries, 427t
  indications for surgery, 428
  magnetic resonance imaging in, 191
  nonoperative management, indications for, 428–430
  penetrating trauma, 426–427t
  radiographic staging of, 427–428
  radionuclide imaging in, 143
  surgery, 428, 430–432
Renal leukemia, 89
Renal lymphoma
  computed tomography in, 170–171
  magnetic resonance imaging in, 187–188
  ultrasound in, 89
Renal masses
  see also specific masses
  angiography in, 220–229
  calcification in, 41, 346–347
  cysts, see Cystic disease of kidneys
  differential diagnosis of, 389–390
  imaging techniques, 361
    computed tomography, 167–172

radionuclide imaging, 149
ultrasound, 88–91
indeterminate lesions, 220–224, 346–347
neoplasms, see Renal neoplasms
Renal neoplasms
  see also specific types of neoplasms
  benign neoplasms, 382–387
    ultrasound in, 90–91
  in children, 411–423
  computed tomography in, 167
  cystic, 167
  cysts and malignancy, 343
  metastases, see Metastases, renal
  radionuclide imaging in, 143–144
  renal angiography in, 220
  ultrasound in, 88–91
Renal parenchyma
  magnetic resonance imaging in, 182–190
  radiographs in excretory urography, 58–60
Renal sinus cysts, 87
Renal stone disease
  abdominal radiographs in, 41
  ultrasound in, 84–85
Renal toxicity
  as contrast media reaction, 51–53
  of iodinated contrast media, 46
Renal transplantation, 551–564
  acute tubular necrosis following, see Acute tubular necrosis, as renal transplant complication
  angiography following, 228
  cyclosporin in, 152
  dysfunction following, 563–564
  magnetic resonance imaging in, 192
  postimplant hypertension, 557t
  radionuclide evaluation of, 133, 152–154
  rejection of, see Renal allograft rejection
  rupture as complication, 555
  surgical complications, 554–563
  ultrasound in, 96–98
Renal tuberculosis, 288
  ultrasound in, 92
Renal tubular acidosis, 305–306
Renal vein
  obstruction, 146
  stenosis, as renal transplant complication, 98
  thrombosis, see Renal vein thrombosis
  venogram of, 220
Renal vein thrombosis
  computed tomography in, 163
  pediatric, 251–252
  as renal transplant complication, 556
    ultrasound in, 98
  ultrasound in, 98, 252
Reninomas, 171
Renography
  diuretic renography, see Diuretic renography
  of renovascular hypertension, 149–150
Renovascular disease
  see also Renal artery and Renal vein
  computed tomography in, 163
Renovascular hypertension
  angiography in, 228
  renogram of, 149–150
Residual urine volume, 26
Resorptive hypercalciuria, 305
Retrograde cystography, 66–68, 206

Retrograde pyelography
 in upper tract obstruction and dilatation, 320
 in urinary stone disease, 312–313
Retrograde ureteropyeloscopy, 209
Retrograde urethrography, 206
 in bladder outlet obstruction, 329–330
 normal anatomy, 73
 in urethral trauma, 441
Retroperitoneal lymphadenopathy, 193
Retroperitoneum
 computed tomography in, 173–174
 fibrosis
  computed tomography in, 173–174
  magnetic resonance imaging in, 192–193
 hematoma of, 173
 magnetic resonance imaging of, 192–193
 sarcoma of, 174
Rhabdomyosarcoma, paratesticular, 474

Sacral agenesis, 513
Sarcoidosis, 305–306
Saturation pulses, in MRI, 181
Schistosomiasis, 297–300
Scintigraphy
 of adrenal gland, 533–534
  masses of, 544
 diuretic renal, 235
 nuclear, 466
Scintillation camera, 132
Screening tests
 prostate specific antigen as, 17–18
 for renal masses, 168
Scrotal ectopia, 467
Scrotal hypoplasia, 466
Scrotoliths, 108
Scrotum, 465–481
 anatomy, 465
 color Doppler imaging, see Color Doppler ultrasound, of scrotum
 congenital abnormalities of, 466–467
 differential diagnosis of pain, 4
 hemangiomas of, 467
 inflammatory processes, 467–469
  ultrasound in, 110–111
 magnetic resonance imaging of, 466
 mass lesions, 8, 471–474
  malignant tumors, 104–107
  ultrasound in, 103–107
 nuclear scintigraphy of, 466
 pediatric, 144–145
 physical examination of, 9, 465–466
 radionuclide imaging of, 135–136
  pediatric, 144–145
 trauma, 478–479
  ultrasound, 111–112
 ultrasound of, 101–112, 466
  blunt trauma, 479
  color Doppler imaging, see Color Doppler ultrasound, of scrotum
  extratesticular abnormalities, 107–110
  inflammation, 110–111
  malignant tumors, 104–107
  mass lesions, 103–107
  normal anatomy, 101–102
  trauma, 111–112
  vascular supply, 103

Secondary nonobstructive nonrefluxing megaureter, pediatric, 237
Secondary refluxing megaureter, pediatric, 236
Sedative-hypnotic drugs, erectile dysfunction from, 487–488
Seminal emission, absence of, 6–7
Seminal vesicles
 anatomy, 117–118
 bacterial infection of, 266–267
 ultrasound of, 116–121
Seminal vesiculitis, 266–267
Seminal vesiculography, 73–74, 266–267
Seminoma, 475, 478
 staging of, 478t
 ultrasound in, 104
Seminomatous germ cell neoplasms, 475
Sertoli cell tumors, 475
 ultrasound in, 106
Serum acid phosphatase, 18
Serum creatinine, 17
Sexual dysfunction, male, 6–7
 erectile dysfunction, see Erectile dysfunction
 infertility, see Infertility
Sexual history, 1–2
 in erectile dysfunction, 490
Sexually transmitted diseases, 573
Signs, urologic, 7–8
Simple renal cysts, 343–346
 computed tomography in, 86, 345–346t
 pediatric, 251
 radiography in, 343–346
 surgical exploration of, 345
 ultrasound in, 86–87, 345t
Single photon emission computed tomography, 156
Single potential analysis of cavernosal electrical activity, 493–495
Small cell carcinoma, of bladder, 401–402
Snapshot gradient echo, in MRI, 181
Sodium cation, 48–49
Soft tissue abnormalities, 35–38
Somatosensory evoked potentials, 493
SPACE, 493–495
SPECT, 156
Spermatic cord
 in erectile dysfunction, 490–491
 masses of, 10
 pain from, 4
 physical examination of, 9, 10, 490–491
 torsion of, 469–471
Spermatocele, 473
Sphincter electromyography, 30–32
 in bladder outlet obstruction, 334–335
 evoked responses in, 32
 kinesiologic studies in, 30
 nerve conduction studies in, 31–32
 in neurogenic bladder, 506–507
 neurophysiologic recordings in, 31
Spinal cord disorders
 disc disease and, 512
 and neurogenic bladder, 512, 523–524
 urodynamic studies in, 33
Spinal dysraphism, 32–33
Squamous cell carcinoma
 of bladder, 399–400
 computed tomography in, 173

renal, 90
 of renal collecting system, 173
 ultrasound in, 90
Streak plate culture, 16
Stress urethral pressure profile, 29
Stress urinary incontinence, 6
 female, 524–525
 magnetic resonance imaging in, 198
 physical examination, 524
 urethral pressure profilometry for, 29
 urodynamic studies in, 33
 videourodynamics for, 28
Struvite stones, 306
SUI, see Stress urinary incontinence
Surgical history, 1
 in erectile dysfunction, 490
SV, 73–74, 266–267
Sympatholytic drugs, in erectile dysfunction, 487
Symptoms, urologic, 2–7

Tamm-Horsfall protein, 277
Tc-99m DTPA, 131
Tc-99m glucoheptonate, 131
Tc-99m mercaptoacetyltriglycine, 131
Technetium-99m, 131
 in erectile function testing, 496
Teratocarcinoma, of scrotum, 104
Teratoma, of scrotum, 475
 ultrasound in, 104
Testes
 color Doppler ultrasound of, 107, 110–111
 cryptorchidism, see Cryptorchidism
 cysts, 106–107
 mass lesions, 474–478
  imaging in, 103–107, 476
  staging of, 476–477, 478t
  ultrasound in, 103–107
 physical examination of, 9–10
 in erectile dysfunction, 490–491
 torsion, 471
  ischemia from, 111
  pediatric radionuclide imaging in, 144–145
 ultrasound of
  cryptorchidism, 112
  inflammation, 110–111
  ischemia, 111
  mass lesions, 103–107
  rupture, 111–112
  trauma, 111–112
 undescended, 479–481
Testicular microlithiasis, 107
Tomography
 computed, see Computed tomography
 in excretory urography, 63–64
 nephrotomography, 63–64
 in urinary stone disease, 308–309
Torsion
 spermatic cord of, 469–471
 testes, see Testes, torsion
Total incontinence, 6
Transitional cell carcinoma
 bladder, 397–399
  computed tomography in, 176
  ultrasound in, 100

Transitional cell carcinoma *(Continued)*
  DNA ploidy in, 398–399
  prognostic markers, 398–399
  renal, 90
  of renal collecting system
    computed tomography in, 172–173
    magnetic resonance imaging in, 190
  ultrasound in, 90, 100
Transitional cell papilloma, 395
Transrectal ultrasound
  in benign prostatic hypertrophy, 451
  of prostate, 446–447
  in prostate cancer, *see* Prostate cancer, transrectal ultrasound in
Transurethral resection of prostate, 453
Transurethral ultrasound, 404
Trauma
  arteriogenic impotence due to, 485
  to bladder, 438, 439–440, 442
  computed tomography in, 162–163
  to kidney, 425–432, *see also* Renal injuries
  to lower urinary tract, 438–443
  to pediatric renal artery, 143
  to penis, 116
  to scrotum, 111–112, 478–479
  to testes, 111–112
  ultrasound in, 111–112, 116
  to upper urinary tract, 425–436
  to ureter, 432–436
TRUS, *see* Transrectal ultrasound
Tuberculosis, genitourinary, 285–293
  AIDS-related, 285, 290, 572
  in bladder, 290
  computed tomography in, 290
  diagnosis, 285–287
  interventional radiology, 293
  pharmacology, 290–293
  renal, 92, 288
  surgery, 293
  ultrasound in, 92, 290
  ureteral, 288–290
  urography in, 288–290
Tuberous sclerosis, 421
Tubular ectasia
  renal collecting, 184
  of testes, 107
Tumors, *see* Neoplasms

Ultrasound, 79–121
  of adrenal gland, 81–82, 529–531
    neonatal hemorrhage, 252
  of bladder, 100–101
    bladder outlet obstruction, 330
    tumors, 100, 404
  color Doppler, *see* Color Doppler ultrasound
  Doppler, *see* Doppler ultrasound
  in duplication anomalies, 238–239
  in genitourinary tuberculosis, 290
  instrumentation, 79–80
  normal anatomy, 80
  of penis, 112–116
  in posterior urethral valves, 239
  of prostate, 116–121, 446–447
    benign prostatic hypertrophy, 118–119, 451
  in prune-belly syndrome, 244

  renal, 82, 84–98
    abscess, 274
    acute bacterial pyelonephritis, 268, 269
    benign neoplasms, 90–91
    cystic disease, 86–88, 249
    diffuse renal disease, 93–94
    infections, 91–93
    masses of, 88–90
    in neurogenic bladder, 505
    renal cell carcinoma, 88–89, 363
    simple cysts, 86–87, 345t
    transplantation evaluation, 96–98
    vascular disease, 94–96
    Wilm's tumor, 412
  of scrotum, *see* Scrotum, ultrasound of
  of seminal vesicles, 116–121
  techniques, 79–80
  of ureter, 98–100
    primary obstructive megaureter, 236
  in ureteropelvic junction obstruction, 235
  in urinary stone disease, 311–312
  in urinary tract obstruction, *see* Urinary tract obstruction, ultrasound in
  urography and, 45–46
  in urothelial tumors, 376
Undescended testes, 479–481
  see also Cryptorchidism
Upper urinary tract
  infection of, 259, 267–281
  kidney, *see* Kidney
  obstruction and dilatation of, 315–322
  symptoms in, 2–3
  trauma to, 425–436
  ureter, *see* Ureter
Upright radiographs, 61
Urachal adenocarcinoma, 400–401
Ureter
  injuries to, 432–436
  magnetic resonance imaging of, 192–193
  obstruction of
    acute renal failure and, 146
    radionuclide imaging in, 136–142, 146
  perforations of, 213
  stones in, 99, 212
  stricture of, 212–213
  symptoms in, 3
  tuberculosis in, 288–290
  ultrasound evaluation of, 98–100
  ureteroscopy of, *see* Ureteroscopy
Ureterocele
  pediatric, 239
  ultrasound evaluation of, 100
Ureteroileal anastomosis, strictures of, 218
Ureteropelvic junction obstruction
  pediatric, 235
  ultrasound in, 83, 235
Ureteropyeloscopy, 208–213
  see also Ureteroscopy
  retrograde, 209
Ureteroscopy, 212–213
  see also Ureteropyeloscopy
  of urothelial tumors, 377–382
Ureterovesicle junction obstruction, pediatric, 235–237

Urethra
  benign tumors of, 407
  carcinoma of, 198
  congenital anomalies of, 197
  cystography of, 207
  discharge from, 8
  diverticula, 407
    magnetic resonance imaging in, 197–198
  female
    cancer in, 198, 407–408
    magnetic resonance imaging of, 196–197, 198
    urethral caruncle, 408
  foreign bodies in, 207
  magnetic resonance imaging of, 196–198
  male
    anatomy, 438
    cancer in, 198, 407
    magnetic resonance imaging of, 197, 198
    trauma to, 441
    ultrasound of, 116, 117
  obstruction of, 239–243
  pain from, 4
  posterior urethral valves, 239–243
  trauma to, 438
    magnetic resonance imaging in, 198
    pelvic fractures causing, 439
    retrograde urethrogram of, 441
    treatment, 442–443
  tumors of, 198, 407–408
Urethral caruncle, 408
Urethral pressure profile, 28–29
  in urinary incontinence, 521
Urethral pressure profilometry, 29
Urethral pressure studies, 28–30
  leak point pressure, 29–30
  urethral pressure profile, 28–29, 521
Urethral stricture disease, 339
  cystography in, 207
Urethrography, 68–73
  excretory voiding, 69–70
  retrograde, *see* Retrograde urethrography
  voiding cystourethrography, *see* Voiding cystourethrography
Urge incontinence, 6
Urgency, 5, 324
Uric acid stones, 306
Urinalysis, 13–14
  in acute bacterial pyelonephritis, 268
  in bladder outlet obstruction, 328
  in blunt trauma to kidneys, 425–426
  collection technique, 13
  dipstick analysis, 13–14
  gross inspection of urine in, 13
  in neurogenic bladder, 505
  in penetrating renal trauma, 426–427
  specific gravity of urine, 13
Urinary beta-2 microglobulin, 277
Urinary bladder, *see* Bladder
Urinary diversion, endoscopy of, 218
Urinary extravasation, 558–559
Urinary frequency, 324
  clinical events influencing, 325t
  daytime, 5
  nocturnal, 5

Urinary incontinence, 6, 517–527
  in bladder outlet obstruction, 325
  in children, 525–526
  classifications of, 518
  geriatric incontinence, 526–527
  laboratory studies, 519
  in males, 525
  mechanisms of continence, 517–518
  neurologic disorders and, 523t–524
  patient history, 518–519
  physical examination, 519
  stress, see Stress urinary incontinence
  symptom classification, 518t
  transient incontinence in elderly persons, 526t
  urodynamic techniques, 519–523
Urinary retention, 326
Urinary sedimentation examination, 14
Urinary stone disease, 303–313
  abdominal radiographs in, 41
  antegrade pyelography in, 313
  calcium stones, 304–306
  clinical presentation, 306–308
  computed tomography in, 172, 312t
  cystine stones, 306
  epidemiology, 306–307
  epitaxy theory of, 303
  inhibitors theory of, 303–304
  intravenous urography, 309–311
  laboratory examination, 307–308
  magnetic resonance imaging in, 190–191
  matrix theory of, 303
  pathophysiology of, 304–306
  physical examination, 307
  plain films, 308–309
  precipitation-crystallization theory of, 303
  radiologic evaluation, 308–313
  renal, 41, 84–85
  in renal collecting system, 172, 190–191
  retrograde pyelography in, 312–313
  signs and symptoms, 307
  struvite stones, 306
  theories of formation, 303–304
  tomography, 308–309
  ultrasound in, 84–85, 99, 311–312
  ureteral, 99, 212
  ureteroscopy for, 212
  uric acid stones, 306
Urinary tract dilatation, upper, 315–322
Urinary tract infection, 257–281
  AIDS-related, 572
  cystoscopy in, 207
  incidence, 258–259
  inflammatory bladder lesions and, 260–262
  of lower urinary tract, 257–260
  pediatric, 245–247, 259
  prostatitis, 262–266
  radionuclide imaging in, 142
  seminal vesiculitis, 266–267
  upper, 259, 267–281
  uroradiology in, 246–247
  vesicoureteral reflux and, 245
Urinary tract obstruction
  of bladder outlet, see Bladder outlet obstruction

  of kidneys
    magnetic resonance imaging in, 188
    as renal transplant complication, 96–97, 559–561
    pediatric, 232–250
    ultrasound in, 82–85
      bladder outlet obstruction, 330
      following renal transplant, 96–97
      upper urinary tract, 315–317
      ureteropelvic junction obstruction, 83, 235
    upper, 315–322
      conditions not detected by ultrasound, 317t
  of ureter
    acute renal failure and, 146
    radionuclide imaging in, 136–142, 146
  ureteropelvic junction obstruction
    pediatric, 235
    ultrasound in, 83, 235
  urethral, 239–243
Urine
  cultures, see Urine culture
  discoloration of, 7
  urinalysis, see Urinalysis
Urine culture, 14–17
  in bacteriuria, 14–16, 257–258
  in bladder outlet obstruction, 328
  in genitourinary tuberculosis, 286
  Gram staining in, 258
  in neurogenic bladder, 505
  susceptibility tests in, 16–17
  in urosepsis, 258
Urinoma
  computed tomography in, 173
  following renal transplant, 96
Urodynamic studies, 21–33
  in bladder outlet obstruction, 330t–335
  cystometry, see Cystometry
  history of, 21
  lower urinary tract function in, 21
  in neurogenic bladder, 506t–507
  patient preparation in, 22
  role of, 22
  sphincter electromyography, see Sphincter electromyography
  in urinary incontinence, 519–523
  uroflowmetry, see Uroflowmetry
  usage of, 32–33
  videourodynamics, see Videourodynamics
  voiding studies, 26–28
Uroflowmetry, 25–26
  in bladder outlet obstruction, 331–332
  in neurogenic bladder, 506–507
  in urinary incontinence, 521
Urogenic diaphragm, 438
Urography, see Excretory urography
Urologic history, 1–8
  in erectile dysfunction, 489–491
Urosepsis, 258
Urothelial tumors, 376–382
  antegrade pyelography in, 378
  brush biopsy of, 378
  computed tomography in, 172–173, 376–377
  cystoscopy in, 378
  cytology in, 378
  excretory urography in, 376

  signs and symptoms, 376
  staging, 382
  ultrasound in, 376
  ureteroscopy in, 378–382

Valsalve maneuvers, 510
Varicocele, 471–473
  ultrasound in, 108–109
Vascular disorders
  impotence from, see Vasculogenic impotence
  renal
    as transplant complication, 97–98
    ultrasound in, 94–96
  ultrasound in, 94–96, 97–98
  varicocele, 108–109
Vasculogenic impotence, 485–486
  diagnostic tests for, 492–493
  ultrasound in, 114–115
Vas deferens, 74
Vasoactive agent injection test, 492
Venogenic impotence, 486
  see also Veno-occlusive impotence
  ultrasound in, 115
Venogram
  of inferior vena cava, 220
  renal masses, detecting, 224
  of vas deferens, 74
Veno-occlusive impotence, 486
  see also Venogenic impotence
  diagnostic tests for, 492–493
Venous leak impotence, 486
  see also Venogenic impotence
Vesicoureteral reflux
  computed tomography in, 165
  pediatric, 165
  radionuclide imaging in, 142
  voiding cystourethrography in, 244–245
Videourodynamics, 28
  in bladder outlet obstruction, 334
  in neurogenic bladder, 506–507
Villous adenoma of bladder, 396
Virilism, 8
Visual laser ablation of prostate, 453
Voiding cystourethrography, 70–71, 231
  in bladder outlet obstruction, 330
  in neurogenic bladder, 505
  in pediatric urinary tract infections, 259
  in posterior urethral valves, 241
  in prune-belly syndrome, 244
  in vesicoureteral reflux, 244–245
Voiding studies, 26–28
Vomiting, from upper urinary tract disorders, 3
Von Hipple-Lindau disease
  magnetic resonance imaging in, 184
  renal angiography in, 224
Von Recklinghausen disease, 194
Vulva, pain associated with, 4

Wilm's tumor, 411–419
  adult, 419
  associated anomalies, 411–412
  bilateral, 417
  chemotherapy for, 416
    complications of, 418–419
    preoperative, 418

Wilm's tumor *(Continued)*
  congenital mesoblastic nephroma and, 420
  imaging studies, 412–413
    magnetic resonance imaging, 187, 413
  incidence, 411
  laboratory tests, 413
  National Wilm's Tumor Studies, 415t, 416–417
  neonatal, 419
  nephrogenic rests in, 415
  pathogenesis, 411
  pathology, 413
  presentation, 411
  radiation therapy for, 416
    complications of, 418–419
  small stage I, 417
  staging, 415
  subtypes of, 414–415
  surgical management, 415–416
  survival in, 416t
  treatment scheme, 417t

Xanthogranulomatous pyelonephritis, 278–280
  computed tomography in, 164–165, 279
  magnetic resonance imaging in, 190, 279
  treatment, 280
  ultrasound in, 92, 279

Yolk sac carcinoma, 475

RC
874
.D47

```
RC            Diagnosis of
874              genitourinary
.D47             disease.
1997

                                    43771
$169.95
```

SOUTH UNIVERSITY
709 MALL BLVD.
SAVANNAH, GA 31406

BAKER & TAYLOR